ROCKWOOD AND WILKINS'

Fractures in Children

TENTH EDITION

ROCKWOOD AND WILKINS'
Fractures in Children

TENTH EDITION

EDITORS

Peter M. Waters, MD, MMSc
Hendrick Family Endowed Professor
Department of Orthopaedic Surgery
Atrium Health
OrthoCarolina
Charlotte, North Carolina

David L. Skaggs, MD, MMM
Professor
Department of Orthopaedic Surgery
Cedars-Sinai Medical Center
Los Angeles, California

John M. Flynn, MD
Professor and Chair of Pediatric Orthopedic
  Surgery
Department of Surgery
Division of Orthopedic Surgery
University of Pennsylvania, Children's
  Hospital of Philadelphia
Philadelphia, Pennsylvania

ASSOCIATE EDITORS

Lindsay Andras, MD
Assistant Professor of Orthopaedic Surgery
Keck School of Medicine of USC
Children's Orthopaedic Center
Children's Hospital Los Angeles
Los Angeles, California

Donald S. Bae, MD
Department of Orthopaedic Surgery
Boston Children's Hospital
Professor of Orthopaedic Surgery
Harvard Medical School
Boston, Massachusetts

Keith D. Baldwin, MD, MSPT, MPH
Associate Professor
Division of Orthopedic Surgery
Department of Surgery
University of Pennsylvania, Children's
  Hospital of Philadelphia
Philadelphia, Pennsylvania

Jonathan G. Schoenecker, MD, PhD
Professor
Department of Orthopaedics
Vanderbilt University
Nashville, Tennessee

Philadelphia • Baltimore • New York • London
Buenos Aires • Hong Kong • Sydney • Tokyo

Acquisitions Editor: Tulie McKay
Development Editors: Stacey Sebring
Editorial Coordinators: Sean Hanrahan and Janet Jayne
Marketing Manager: Kirsten Watrud
Production Project Manager: Kirstin Johnson
Manager, Graphic Arts & Design: Stephen Druding
Illustrator: Bernie Kida
Manufacturing Coordinator: Lisa Bowling
Prepress Vendor: Aptara, Inc.

10th edition

Copyright © 2025 Wolters Kluwer.

9 8 7 6 5 4 3 2 1

Printed in Mexico

978-19752-1173-8

Library of Congress Cataloging-in-Publication data available upon request

I want to acknowledge my wife Mary and children Erin, Colleen, John, and Kelly for patience and understanding while I dedicated many hours to this project. They understand that Dad has homework too. Also, I would like to recognize the injured children, medical students, residents, and fellows who count on this textbook to be the trusted source of information for fracture care; their needs are the inspiration that drive us to create an excellent final product.

Jack Flynn

Time passes, a lot changes, and yet much remains the same. All of us are lucky and blessed in our professional lives; and for me, even more so, in my personal life. It just keeps getting better. Indebted.

Peter M. Waters

I want to most of all thank my wife Val for always being there for me. Thanks to my children Kira, Jamie, and Clay for being good friends and giving me great life and career advice. Please welcome my daughter Kira the ortho resident to our club. And thanks to my nurse Elaine who has improved our patients' care for the last 15 years along with Trauma Chief/partner/son Ken Illingworth.

David L. Skaggs

Joshua M. Abzug, MD
Professor, Orthopaedics
University of Maryland
Baltimore, Maryland

Alexandre Arkader, MD
Associate Professor of Orthopedic Surgery
Pediatric Orthopedics and Orthopedic Oncology
Perelman School of Medicine at University of
    Pennsylvania
The Children's Hospital of Philadelphia
Philadelphia, Pennsylvania

Haleh Badkoobehi, MD, MPH
Pediatric Orthopaedic Surgeon
Residency Program Director, Orthopaedic Surgery
Harbor-UCLA
Torrance, California

Donald S. Bae, MD
Professor of Orthopaedic Surgery
Department of Orthopaedic Surgery
Boston Children's Hospital/Harvard Medical School
Boston, Massachusetts

Courtney E. Baker, MD
Orthopedic Surgeon, Orthopedics
Vanderbilt University Medical Center
Nashville, Tennessee

Keith D. Baldwin, MD, MSPT, MPH
Associate Professor
Division of Orthopedic Surgery
Department of Surgery
University of Pennsylvania, Children's Hospital
    of Philadelphia
Philadelphia, Pennsylvania

Andrea S. Bauer, MD
Associate Professor, Orthopaedic Surgery
Boston Children's Hospital
Boston, Massachusetts

Douglas Brockmeyer, MD
Pediatric Neurosurgeon
Department of Neurosurgery
University of Utah
Salt Lake City, Utah

James E. Cassat, MD, PhD
Associate Professor
Pediatrics; Pathology, Microbiology, and Immunology;
    and Biomedical Engineering
Vanderbilt University Medical Center
Nashville, Tennessee

Jaime R. Denning, MD, MS
Associate Professor, Orthopaedic Surgery
Cincinnati Children's Hospital Medical Center
Cincinnati, Ohio

Eric W. Edmonds, MD
Professor, Orthopaedic Surgery
University of California San Diego and Rady Children's
    Hospital San Diego
San Diego, California

Mark A. Erickson, MD, MMM
Professor, Orthopedic Surgery
University of Colorado School of Medicine
Denver, Colorado

John M. Flynn, MD
Professor and Chair of Pediatric Orthopedic Surgery
Department of Surgery
Division of Orthopedic Surgery
University of Pennsylvania, Children's Hospital
    of Philadelphia
Philadelphia, Pennsylvania

Andrew D. Franklin, MD, MBA
Associate Professor of Anesthesiology
Department of Anesthesiology
Vanderbilt University Medical Center
Nashville, Tennessee

Sumeet Garg, MD
Associate Professor of Orthopedics
Children's Hospital Colorado
University of Colorado
Aurora, Colorado

Benton E. Heyworth, MD
Attending, Orthopedic Surgery
Department of Orthopedic Surgery
Boston Children's Hospital
Boston, Massachusetts

Christine Ann Ho, MD, FAAOS, FAAP, FAOA
Texas Scottish Rite Hospital for Children
Division Director, Department of Pediatric Orthopaedics
Children's Health Dallas
Professor, Department of Orthopaedics
University of Texas Southwestern Medical School
Dallas, Texas

Oduche Igboechi, MD, MPH, MBA
Assistant Professor, Orthopaedic Surgery
University of Maryland School of Medicine
Baltimore, Maryland

Kenneth D. Illingworth, MD
Director of Pediatric Orthopaedic Trauma
Pediatric Spine/Orthopaedics
Assistant Professor of Orthopaedics
Pediatrics and Neurosurgery
Cedars-Sinai Medical Center
Los Angeles, California

Rajiv Iyer, MD
Assistant Professor, Neurosurgery
University of Utah
Salt Lake City, Utah

Robert M. Kay, MD
Chief, Division of Orthopaedic Surgery
Director, Jackie and Gene Autry Orthopedic Center
Director, Neuromuscular Program
Associates Chair in Orthopedics
Children's Hospital Los Angeles
Los Angeles, California

Mininder S. Kocher, MD, MPH
Professor of Orthopaedic Surgery
Boston Children's Hospital/Harvard Medical School
Boston, Massachusetts

Ryan J. Koehler, MD, MS
Assistant Professor
Pediatric Orthopaedics
Children's Mercy Hospital
Kansas City, Missouri

Dennis E. Kramer, MD
Assistant Professor, Orthopaedic Surgery
Harvard Medical School
Boston, Massachusetts

Nathaniel Lempert, MD
Assistant Professor, Orthopaedics & Rehabilitation
Vanderbilt University Medical Center
Nashville, Tennessee

Ying Li, MD
Frederick J. Fischer MD Professor of Orthopaedic Surgery
Chief, Section of Pediatric Orthopaedic Surgery
ACU Medical Director, C&W Pediatric Multispecialty Surgery
Fellowship Program Director, Pediatric Orthopaedic Surgery/
    C.S. Mott Children's Hospital
Michigan Medicine
Ann Arbor, Michigan

Kevin J. Little, MD
Director, Pediatric Hand and Upper Extremity Surgery
Division of Pediatric Orthopaedics
Cincinnati Children's Hospital Medical Center
University of Cincinnati College of Medicine
Cincinnati, Ohio

Karim Masrouha, MD
Assistant Professor
Director
New York Ponseti Clubfoot Center
Division of Pediatric Orthopedic Surgery
Division of Orthopedic Oncology
Department of Orthopedic Surgery; NYU Langone Health,
    NYU Langone Orthopedic Hospital
New York, New York

Amy L. McIntosh, MD
Professor, Orthopedic Surgery
Scottish Rite Hospital for Children
Dallas, Texas

Stephanie N. Moore-Lotridge, PhD
Assistant Professor, Orthopaedic Surgery
Vanderbilt University Medical Center
Nashville, Tennessee

Jon Niconchuk, MD
Assistant Professor of Pediatric Anesthesiology
Department of Anesthesiology
Vanderbilt University Medical Center
Nashville, Tennessee

Kenneth J. Noonan, MD
Professor, Pediatric Orthopedics
University of Wisconsin—Madison
Madison, Wisconsin

Jonas K. Owen, MD
Assistant Professor, Orthopedic Surgery
Department of Orthopedic Surgery
Children's Hospital Los Angeles
Los Angeles, California

Chinmay Paranjape, MD, MHSc
Pediatric Orthopaedic Surgery Fellow, Orthopaedic
    Surgery
Rady Children's Hospital
San Diego, California

Vince W. Prusick, MD
Pediatric Orthopaedic Surgeon, Orthopaedic Surgery
Shriners Medical Center Lexington/University of Kentucky
Lexington, Kentucky

Julia S. Sanders, MD
Assistant Professor
Department of Orthopedic Surgery
University of Colorado School of Medicine
Aurora, Colorado

Wudbhav N. Sankar, MD
Professor of Orthopaedic Surgery
Division of Orthopaedic Surgery
Children's Hospital of Philadelphia
Philadelphia, Pennsylvania

Jeffrey R. Sawyer, MD
Professor of Orthopaedic Surgery
Pediatric Orthopaedic Surgery and Spinal Deformity
Campbell Clinic, Memphis, Tennesse

Brian P. Scannell, MD
Residency Program Director
Department of Orthopaedic Surgery
Carolinas Medical Center, Atrium Health
Charlotte, North Carolina

Jonathan G. Schoenecker, MD, PhD
Professor
Department of Orthopaedics
Vanderbilt University
Nashville, Tennessee

Apurva S. Shah, MD, MBA
Assistant Professor of Orthopaedic Surgery
Director of Clinical Research
Director of the Brachial Plexus Injury Program
The Children's Hospital of Philadelphia
Perelman School of Medicine at the University of Pennsylvania
Philadelphia, Pennsylvania

Benjamin W. Sheffer, MD
Assistant Professor, Orthopaedic Surgery
University of Tennessee HSC—Campbell Clinic Orthopaedics
Memphis, Tennessee

Benjamin J. Shore, MD, MPH, FRCSC
Associate Professor, Orthopedic Surgery
Department of Orthopaedic Surgery
Boston Children's Hospital
Boston, Massachusetts

Sarah E. Sibbel, MD
Orthopedic Surgeon
Department of Orthopedics
Children's Hospital Colorado
University of Colorado School of Medicine
Aurora, Colorado

David L. Skaggs, MD, MMM
Professor
Department of Orthopaedic Surgery
Cedars-Sinai Medical Center
Los Angeles, California

Milan V. Stevanovic, MD, PhD
Professor of Orthopaedic Surgery (Clinical Scholar)
Department of Orthopaedic Surgery
Keck School of Medicine of University of Southern California
Los Angeles, California

Vishwas Talwalkar, MD, FAAOS, FAAP
Professor, Orthopaedic Surgery and Pediatrics
Shriners Hospital for Children Medical Center/
    University of Kentucky
Lexington, Kentucky

Vidyadhar Upasani, MD
Professor of Orthopedic Surgery, Orthopedic Surgery
University of California San Diego
San Diego, California

Eric J. Wall, MD
Director, Sports Medicine
Department of Orthopaedics
Cincinnati Children's Hospital Medical Center
Cincinnati, Ohio

Lindley Wall, MD, MSc
Professor, Orthopedic Surgery
Washington University School of Medicine
Saint Louis, Missouri

Peter M. Waters, MD, MMSc
Hendrick Family Endowed Professor
Department of Orthopaedic Surgery
Atrium Health
OrthoCarolina
Charlotte, North Carolina

Brendan A. Williams, MD
Assistant Professor of Orthopaedic Surgery
Department of Orthopaedic Surgery
Children's Hospital of Philadelphia
Philadelphia, Pennsylvania

Benjamin R. Wilson, MD
Assistant Professor
Department of Orthopaedic Surgery and Sports Medicine
University of Kentucky
Lexington, Kentucky

The quantity of information available to pediatric musculoskeletal caregivers, surgeons, and researchers continues to accelerate in the 21st century. Learners and practitioners at all stages of their careers need expertise to guide them in decision making and technical performance. Even in the world of short operative videos and small size knowledge content, we believe detailed, filtered evidence by subject matter experts with clear direction on the present state-of-the-art care for injured children is important and impactful.

Our goal is that the 10th edition of *Rockwood and Wilkins' Fractures in Children* enhances your care delivery for your patients. In each chapter, subject matter experts offer their overviews and analyses of existing clinical research and provide the very best evidence-based recommendations possible. The "author's preferred method" at the end of each chapter serves as a concise and practical algorithm for treating children with fractures and dislocations.

There is in-depth content as well as callouts, including checklists for preoperative planning and key surgical steps,

tables of potential pitfalls and preventative measures, and short lists of key annotated references. We have retained the author's preferred treatment section, which has been popular since its introduction several editions ago.

This edition is a transition volume. The senior editors (PW, DS, JF) have been honored to work together on editions 7 through now 10. We started our Rockwood and Wilkins journey as Associate Editors with Drs. Beaty and Kasser; and now have the good fortune to be joined by Associate Editors Drs. Lindsay Andras, Don Bae, Keith Baldwin, and Jon Schonecker. Your learning is in good hands going forward. We all collaborated in our relentless desire to help you improve your patient care for injured children. We know and appreciate how well you do your jobs, how hard you work, and how much you care.

Peter M. Waters, MD, MMSc
David L. Skaggs, MD, MMM
John M. (Jack) Flynn, MD

CONTENTS

SURGICAL PROCEDURE VIDEOS

FUNDAMENTALS OF PEDIATRIC FRACTURE CARE

1

Epidemiology of Fractures in Children

Ryan J. Koehler and Benjamin J. Shore

INTRODUCTION

An understanding of the epidemiology of pediatric trauma is a prerequisite to developing an evidence-based approach to prevention and treatment. Epidemiology is defined as the study of the distribution and determinants of health and disease. Various epidemiologic methods including surveillance and descriptive studies can be used to investigate the distribution of frequency, pattern, and burden of disease whereas analytical methods can be used to study the determinants of disease.

Injuries in children and adolescents present a significant public health challenge globally, affecting pediatric patients, families, and health care providers alike. Accidental injuries are the leading cause of death among children in the United States. However, fatalities represent just a fraction of the impact unintentional injuries have on children. In 2019 alone, there were more than 5.6 million nonfatal unintentional injuries reported in children, with estimated medical costs exceeding $3.1 billion for nonfatal unintentional falls in the United States (Centers for Disease Control Web-based Injury Statistics Query and Reporting System; www.cdc.gov/injury/wisqars/index.html).

Considering the far-reaching consequences of pediatric musculoskeletal injuries on public health, comprehending the epidemiology of pediatric fractures becomes crucial for maximizing efforts toward prevention and optimal treatment. Pediatric trauma often leads to temporary activity limitation and hospitalization, and in rarer cases, permanent disability.[2,44] Further, being the leading cause of death and disability in children, presents a significant challenge to child health. However, it also provides a crucial opportunity for making a positive societal impact. Therefore, the primary objective should be to minimize the burden of accidental fractures, especially those resulting in mortality and long-term consequences. Moreover, in situations where prevention is not entirely feasible, optimizing care becomes paramount to minimize potential long-term complications and alleviate the social and economic burdens faced by families.

ETIOLOGY OF FRACTURES IN CHILDREN

THREE BROAD CAUSES

Broadly, fractures have three main causes: accidental trauma, nonaccidental trauma (child abuse), and pathologic conditions. Accidental trauma forms the largest etiologic group and can occur in a variety of settings, some often overlapping others. Nonaccidental trauma and fractures resulting from pathologic conditions are discussed in later chapters of this book.

SPORTS-RELATED ACTIVITIES

The last two decades have seen an increase in youth participation in organized athletic participation, especially among younger children. Wood et al. studied the annual incidence of sports-related fractures in children aged 10 to 19 years presenting to hospitals in Edinburgh. The overall incidence was 5.63 per 1,000 population per year, with males accounting for 87% of fractures. Soccer, rugby, and skiing were responsible for nearly two-thirds of the fractures among the 30 sporting activities that adolescents participated in. Upper-extremity fractures were by far the most common injury accounting for 84% of all fractures with most being low-energy injuries and few requiring operative intervention.[70] A retrospective study over a 16-year time period from an emergency department at a level 1 trauma center in the Netherlands examined risk factors for upper-extremity injury in sports-related activities. Most injuries occurred while playing soccer and upper-extremity injuries were most common. Risk factors for injury were young age and playing individual sports, no-contact sports, or no-ball sports. Women were at risk in speed skating, in-line skating, and basketball, whereas men mostly were injured during skiing and snowboarding.[105]

In the United States, football- and basketball-related injuries are common complaints presenting to pediatric emergency departments, with fractures occurring more frequently in football.[25] In a 5-year survey of the National Electronic Injury Surveillance System (NEISS)-All Injury Program, injury rates ranged from 6.1 to 11 per 1,000 participants per year as age increased, with fractures and dislocations accounting for nearly 30% of all injuries receiving emergency room evaluation.[64]

Accidental Recreational Activities and Devices

In addition to increasing participation in sports, new activities and devices[65] have emerged that expose children to increased fracture risk. Traditional activities such as skateboarding, roller skating, alpine sports, and bicycling have taken on a new look in the era of extreme sports where such activities now involve high speeds and stunts. Many of these activities have safety equipment available but that does not assure compliance. Organizations such as Pediatric Orthopaedic Society of North America (POSNA), American Academy of Pediatrics (AAP), and the American Academy of Orthopaedic Surgeons (AAOS) have issued position statements regarding the proper use and supervision of such devices, but it remains within the duty of the physician to educate and reinforce to patients and families to promote safety around these activities.[57]

Playground Equipment

Play is an essential element of a child's life. It enhances physical development and fosters social interaction. Unfortunately, unsupervised or careless use of some play equipment can endanger life and limb.[48] When Mott et al.[66] studied the incidence and pattern of injuries to children using public playgrounds, they found that approximately 1% of children using playgrounds sustained injuries. Swings, climbers, and slides are the pieces of playground equipment associated with 88% of the playground injuries.[60]

In a study of injuries resulting from playground equipment, Waltzman et al.[101] found that most injuries occurred in boys (56%) with a peak incidence in the summer months. Fractures accounted for 61% of these injuries, 90% of which involved the upper extremity and were sustained in falls from playground equipment such as monkey bars and climbing frames. Younger children (<4 years old) were more likely to sustain fractures than older children. Lillis and Jaffe[54] made similar observations in a study in which upper-extremity injuries, especially fractures, accounted for most of hospitalizations resulting from injuries on playground equipment. Older children sustained more injuries on climbing apparatus, whereas younger children sustained more injuries on slides. Loder[56] used the NEISS dataset to explore the demographics of playground equipment injuries in children. Monkey bars were the most common cause of fractures. In another study looking specifically at injuries from monkey bars, the peak age group was the 5- to 12-year-old group, with supracondylar humeral fractures being the most common fracture sustained.[61] The correlation of the hardness of the playground surface with the risk of injury has been confirmed in numerous studies.[47,56] Changing playground surfaces from concrete to more impact-absorbing surfaces such as bark reduced the incidence and severity of head injury but increased the tendency for long-bone fractures (40%), bruises, and sprains. Public playgrounds appear to have a higher risk for injuries than private playgrounds because they usually have harder surfaces and higher pieces of equipment,[74] although playground injury was most likely to occur at school compared to home, public, and other locations.[75]

To potentially improve playground safety, close supervision of children and prioritizing age-appropriate and well-maintained equipment are essential measures. In addition, utilizing impact-absorbing surfaces and carefully considering playground safety standards could help reduce the risk of head injuries. However, it is important to balance impact absorption with the potential for other types of injuries. Public playgrounds may have a higher risk of injuries compared to private ones due to factors such as harder surfaces and taller equipment. Implementing these measures speculatively could contribute to a safer playground environment, reducing the occurrence of serious injuries during playtime.

Bicycle Injuries

Bicycle injuries are a significant cause of mortality and morbidity for children.[77] Bicycle mishaps are the most common causes of serious head injury in children.[103] Boys in the 5- to 14-year age group are at greatest risk for bicycle injury (80%). Puranik et al.[77] studied the profile of pediatric bicycle injuries in a sample of 211 children who were treated for bicycle-related injury at their trauma center over a 4-year period. They found that bicycle injuries accounted for 18% of all pediatric trauma patients. Bicycle/motor vehicle collisions caused 86% of injuries. Sixty-seven percent had head injuries and 29% sustained fractures. More than half of the incidents occurred on the weekend. Sixteen percent were injured by ejection from a bicycle after losing control, hitting a pothole, or colliding with a fixed object or another bicycle. Fractures mainly involved the lower extremity, upper extremity, skull, ribs, and pelvis in decreasing order of incidence. Over the last decade, youth participation in mountain biking has seen an increase and with that so has the number of injuries related to mountain biking increased with many caused by unpredictable terrain and falls as one rides downhill.[3,4] As public awareness of both the severity and preventability of bicycle-related injuries grows, the goal of safer bicycling practices and lower injury rates can be achieved.[77]

Skateboarding

Skateboarding and in-line skating have experienced a renewed surge in popularity over the past three decades. Since the late 1990s, there has been an increase in the number of skateboard injuries.[45] Because the nature of skateboarding encompasses both high-speed and extreme maneuvers, high-energy fractures and other injuries can occur, as highlighted by several published reports.[28,72] Studies have shown that skateboarding-related injuries are more severe and have more serious consequences than roller skating or in-line skating injuries.[72] In a study of skateboarding injuries, Fountain et al.[28] found that fractures of the upper or lower extremity accounted for 50% of all skateboarding injuries. Interestingly, more than one-third of those injured sustained injuries within the first week of skateboarding. Most injuries occurred in preadolescent boys (75%) from 10 to 16 years of age; 65% sustained injuries on public roads, footpaths, and parking lots. In a study over a 5-year period of time using data from the National Trauma Data Bank, skateboarding injuries were associated with a higher incidence of closed-head injuries and long-bone fractures with children under age 10 more likely to sustain a femur fracture.[58] Several authors[28] have recommended safety guidelines and precautions such as use of helmets, knee and elbow pads, and wrist guards, but such regulations seldom are enforced.

Trampolines

Trampolines are a significant cause of morbidity in children. Several studies have noted a dramatic increase in the number of pediatric trampoline injuries starting in the 1990s, deeming this mechanism as a "national epidemic."[29,92] Using the NEISS data, Smith[92] estimated that there are roughly 40,000 pediatric trampoline injuries per year. Younger children had a higher incidence of upper-extremity fractures and other injuries. Furnival et al.,[29] in a retrospective study over a 7-year period, found that the annual number of pediatric trampoline injuries tripled between 1990 and 1997. In contrast to other recreational activities in which boys constitute the population at risk, patients with pediatric trampoline injuries were predominantly girls, with a median age of 7 years. Nearly a third of the injuries resulted from falling off the trampoline. Fractures of the upper and lower extremities occurred in 45% and were more frequently associated with falls off the trampoline. In a later study, Sandler et al.[81] reported injuries requiring surgery in over 60% of patients with 20% requiring operative fixation for upper-extremity fractures. These researchers, along with others,[29] concluded that use of warning labels, public education, and even direct adult supervision were inadequate in preventing these injuries and have called for a total ban on the recreational, school, and competitive use of trampolines by children.[23,29,81,92,93]

Motor Vehicle Accidents

This category includes injuries sustained by occupants of a motor vehicle accident (MVA) and victims of vehicle–pedestrian accidents.

The injury patterns of children involved in MVAs differ from those of adults. In all types of MVAs for all ages, children constitute a little over 10% of the total number of patients injured.[49,83] Only about 18% of all the persons injured as motor vehicle occupants are children. Whereas about 29% of vehicle-versus-pedestrian accidents involve children. Of the total number of children involved in MVAs, 56.4% were vehicle–pedestrian accidents and 19.6% were vehicle–bicycle accidents.[26]

The fracture rate and type of fractures observed in children involved in MVAs differ from that of adults. When considering the total number of vehicle–pedestrian accidents, about 22% of the children sustained fractures, compared to 40% of adults sustaining fractures from MVAs. This has been attributed to the fact that children are more likely to "bounce" when hit.[26] In addition, children are twice as likely as adults to sustain a femoral fracture when struck by an automobile; in adults, tibial and knee injuries are more common in the same type of accident. This seems to be related to where the car's bumper strikes the victim.[11,12] MVAs also produce a high proportion of rare pediatric injuries such as spinal and pelvic fractures.[11]

All-Terrain Vehicles

Recreational all-terrain vehicles (ATVs) have emerged as a new cause of serious pediatric injury. Despite product training and safety education campaigns, ATV accidents continue to cause significant morbidity and mortality in children and adolescents.[31,34,41,43,82,85] In contrast to other etiologies of injury, children who sustained ATV-related fractures had more severe injuries and a higher percentage of significant head trauma, with 1% of these injuries resulting in in-hospital death. These statistics point to the failure of voluntary safety efforts to date and argue for much stronger regulatory control.

In a review of 96 children who sustained injuries in ATV-related accidents during a 30-month period, Kellum et al.[41] noted age-related patterns of injury. Younger children (≤12 years) were more likely to sustain an isolated fracture and were more likely to sustain a lower-extremity fracture, specifically a femoral fracture, than older children. Older children were more

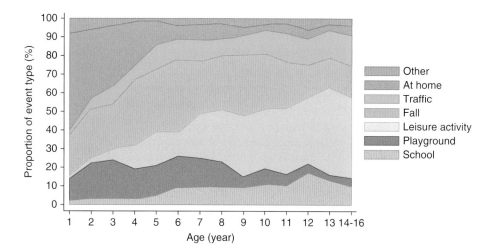

Figure 1-1. Accident types correlated to age. There is a predominance of fractures due to accidents at home throughout the first 4 years of life, whereas leisure activities become the leading cause during school age and adolescence. (Redrawn from Joeris A, et al. An epidemiological evaluation of pediatric long bone fractures: a retrospective cohort study of 2716 patients from two Swiss tertiary pediatric hospitals. *BMC Pediatr.* 2014;14:314. © Joeris et al.; licensee BioMed Central. 2014.)

likely to sustain a pelvic fracture. In a recent review of the Kids' Inpatient Database, Sawyer et al.[82] found that despite the known risks associated with ATV use in children, their use and injury rate continue to increase. The injury rate for children from ATV accidents has increased 240% since 1997, whereas the spinal injury rate has increased 476% over the same time frame. The authors found that injuries to the spinal column occurred in 7.4% of patients with the most common level of fracture being thoracic (39%), followed by lumbar (29%) and cervical (16%). Pelvic fractures were the most common associated fractures, accounting for 44% of all musculoskeletal injuries, followed by forearm/wrist fractures (15%) and femoral fractures (9%). Despite educational and legislative efforts, children account for a disproportionate percentage of morbidity and mortality from ATV-related accidents. The sport of motocross has also been shown to have a high rate of musculoskeletal injuries requiring hospitalization in children.[50]

The etiologic aspects of children's fractures are summarized in Figure 1-1.

Gunshot and Firearm Injuries

Gunshot or missile wounds arise from objects projected into space by an explosive device. Gunshot wounds have become increasingly common in children in the United States. Firearms are second only to motor vehicles as the leading cause of death in youths. In considering the prevalence of firearms in the United States, it has been estimated that there are about 200 million privately owned guns in the United States and that approximately 40% of U.S. households contain firearms of some type.[27]

Two epidemiologic reports from pediatric trauma centers, orthopaedic injuries related to firearms, demonstrated varying rates of complications and need for operative intervention (35% and 54%) in gunshot wound–related injuries and complications.[69,73] Perkins et al.[73] found that in 46 patients with 50 injuries, gunshot-related fractures had an increased incidence of permanent neurologic deficits, infection (11%), and fracture nonunion rates (9%).

The two most common complications associated with firearm-related injuries are growth arrest and infection. Other complications included delayed union and malunion. The treatment of fractures associated with gunshot wounds in children is never simple. Bone defects, associated peripheral nerve injuries, and involvement of the joint can negatively influence outcomes.[6]

Firearm-related injury and safety have received much attention nationally and internationally in the wake of the events over the last decade. Reducing the number of these injuries presents a complex problem that requires modifying behavioral or environmental risk factors. Strategies to reduce firearm-related injuries and deaths among the youth include firearm safety education, reducing the number of guns in the environment through restrictive legislation, gun buy-back programs, gun taxes, physician counseling, and modifying the design of guns to make them more childproof and prevent unauthorized and unintended use.

In summary, children through increased exposure to recreational sports and activities are at increased risk for fractures and injuries. It is essential to understand common patterns of injury found in these activities. Understanding these risks can help providers educate patients and families to the inherent risk of recreational devices such as bicycles, trampolines, and ATVs. In addition, understanding how high-risk devices and activities contribute to the overall burden of pediatric trauma can help with advocacy for safety interventions to prevent pediatric injuries.

INCIDENCE OF FRACTURES IN CHILDREN

"CLASSIFICATION BIAS": DIFFICULTIES DEFINING DISEASE

Gathering comprehensive epidemiologic data on pediatric fractures presents challenges due to the lack of consistent definitions and classifications. However, efforts have been made to develop standardized systems for classifying pediatric fractures, aiding in future studies and enhancing comparability. An international study group has developed and performed early validation of

Figure 1-2. The AO PCCF for fracture classification with bone, segment, and subsegment nomenclature. (From Slongo TF, Audigé L; AO Pediatric Classification Group. Fracture and dislocation classification compendium for children: the AO Pediatric Comprehensive Classification of Long Bone Fractures (PCCF). *J Orthop Trauma.* 2007;21(10 Suppl): S135–S160.)

a standardized classification system of pediatric fractures.[88–91] The authors of an agreement study found that with appropriate training, the AO Pediatric Comprehensive Classification of Long Bone Fractures (PCCF) system could be used by experienced surgeons as a reliable classification system for pediatric fractures for future prospective studies (Fig. 1-2).[88,89] In addition, follow-up studies have provided useful epidemiologic reporting of pediatric long-bone fractures using the AO PCCF.[36–38] Despite validation and use for epidemiologic studies this classification system has not gained widespread acceptance in clinical practice but could be a useful tool for improving communication and understanding of common pediatric fracture patterns.

GLOBAL INCIDENCE OF PEDIATRIC FRACTURES

The incidence of pediatric fractures varies due to geographical, environmental, sex, and age differences. Understanding these variations provides valuable insights into fracture patterns and aids in developing preventive strategies. Early studies on the incidence of fractures in children formed a knowledge base about fracture healing in children. Landin's 1983 report on 8,682 fractures remains a landmark study on the incidence of fractures in children.[49] He reviewed the data on all fractures in children that occurred in Malmö, Sweden, over 30 years and examined the factors affecting the incidence of children's fractures. By studying two populations, 30 years apart, he determined that fracture patterns were changing and suggested reasons for such changes. His initial goal was to establish data for preventive programs, so he focused on fractures that produced clean, concise, concrete data. An update from Malmö, Sweden, over the years 2005 to 2006 noted that previously reported declines in overall fracture rate remained unchanged and may have been related to a change in the region's demographics. There was, however, a decrease in rate among girls. The pediatric fracture rate during the period 2005 to 2006 was 1,832 per 10,000 person-years

(2,359 in boys and 1,276 in girls), with an age-adjusted boy-to-girl ratio of 1.8 (1.6%–2.1%).[51] Recent follow-up to this study has shown that the fracture rate in this population has remained stable in boys and girls over the past 35 years.[9]

Rennie et al. conducted a similar review of pediatric fractures in Edinburgh, Scotland and found the overall incidence was 20.2 per 1,000 children annually.[79] This incidence was similar to 201/10,000 among children and adolescents reported in northern Sweden between 1993 and 2007 with a 13% increase during the years between 1998 and 2007. The authors also reported the accumulated risk of sustaining a fracture before the age of 17 being 34%.[32] In Landin's series from Malmö, Sweden, the chance of a child sustaining a fracture during childhood (birth to age 16) was 42% for boys and 27% for girls.[49] When considered on an annual basis, 2.1% of all the children (2.6% for boys; 1.7% for girls) sustained at least one fracture each year. These figures were for all fracture types and included those treated on an inpatient basis and an outpatient basis. The overall chance of fracture per year was 1.6% for both girls and boys in a study from England of both outpatients and inpatients by Worlock and Stower.[106] The chance of a child sustaining a fracture severe enough to require inpatient treatment during the first 16 years of life is 6.8%.[15] Thus, on an annual basis, 0.43% of the children in an average community will be admitted for a fracture-related problem during the year. The overall incidence and lifetime risk of children's fractures are summarized in Table 1-1.

Early reports of children's fractures grouped the areas fractured together, and fractures were reported only as to the long bone involved (e.g., radius, humerus, femur). More recent reports have split fractures into the more specific areas of the long bone involved (e.g., the distal radius or the distal humerus). In children, fractures in the upper extremity are much more common than those in the lower extremity.[107] Overall, the radius is the most fractured long bone, followed by the humerus. In the lower extremity, the tibia is more commonly fractured than the femur (Table 1-2).[38]

The individual reports agree that the most common area fractured in children is the distal radius. The next most common area involves the hand (phalanges and metacarpals), clavicle, and distal humerus.[68,78,79]

Physeal Fractures

The incidence of physeal injuries overall varied from 14.8% to as high as 30% in the literature across various series.[40,79,97] The rate of premature physeal closure varies by fracture type and

TABLE 1-1. Overall Frequency of Fractures

Percentage of children sustaining at least one fracture from 0 to 16 years of age:

  Boys, 42–60%

  Girls, 27–40%

Percentage of children sustaining a fracture in 1 year: 1.6–2.1%

Annual rate of fracture in childhood: 12–36 per 1,000 persons

TABLE 1-2. Incidence of Fractures in Long Bones	
Bone	%
Radius/ulna	59
Humerus	21
Tibia/fibula	15
Femur	5

From Joeris A, et al. An epidemiological evaluation of pediatric long bone fractures: a retrospective cohort study of 2716 patients from two Swiss tertiary pediatric hospitals. *BMC Pediatr.* 2014;14:314 © Joeris et al; licensee BioMed Central. 2014.

Figure 1-3. Incidence of fractures by age. Boys (*blue*) peak at 13 years whereas girls (*red*) peak earlier, at 12 years, and then decline. (Reprinted from Rennie L, et al. The epidemiology of fractures in children. *Injury.* 2007;38(8):913–922. Copyright © 2007 Elsevier Ltd. With permission.)

location. Distal radius physeal fractures are the most common physeal fracture with premature physeal closure occurring in 18%.[42] Lower extremity fractures are more commonly impacted by postfracture premature physeal arrest. In the distal tibia, premature physeal closure occurred in 13% of all cases and was highest in Salter–Harris IV fractures. Distal femur physeal fractures have a complication rate as high as 40% with the most common complication being complete physeal arrest in 30% of cases.[1]

Open Fractures

The overall reported incidence of open fractures in children has changed over time ranging from 1.5% to 2.6% in older series[4,106] to 0.7% to 1% in recent reports.[38,79] Regional trauma centers often see patients exposed to more severe trauma, so there may be a higher incidence of open fractures in these patients. The incidence of open fractures was 9% in a report of patients admitted to an urban trauma center.[11] In this large series, the most common location for open fracture is the lower leg (tibia/fibula) followed by the forearm (radius/ulna).

In summary, the study of pediatric fracture epidemiology presents challenges due to inconsistent definitions and classifications. However, advancements in standardized classification systems, such as the PCCF, have improved comparability and classification reliability. Landmark studies have provided insights into the incidence and patterns of pediatric fractures, emphasizing their significant likelihood during childhood. Specific fracture areas, such as the distal radius, upper extremity, and lower leg, are more commonly affected. Complications, such as premature physeal closure and open fractures, have been studied, guiding effective management strategies. Nevertheless, there are still knowledge gaps to address, and further research is required to overcome the heterogeneity of risk factors, practice patterns, and data collection infrastructure in pediatric trauma.

PATIENT FACTORS THAT INFLUENCE FRACTURE INCIDENCE AND FRACTURE PATTERNS

Age

Fracture incidence in children demonstrates an age-related increase, with various factors influencing age-specific fracture patterns and locations. These factors encompass age-dependent

activities and changes in intrinsic bone properties, contributing to the observed variations in fracture occurrence throughout childhood and adolescence. Starting with birth and extending to age 12, all the major series that segregated patients by age have demonstrated a linear increase in the annual incidence of fractures with age (Fig. 1-3). The peak age for fracture occurrence is age 11 to 12 in girls and age 13 to 14 in boys.[22,31,39,78,79]

Although there is a high incidence of injuries in children aged 1 to 2 years, the incidence of fractures is low with most fractures being related to accidental or nonaccidental trauma from others.[19,46] The anatomic areas most often fractured seem to be the same in the major series, but these rates change with age. Rennie et al.[79] demonstrated in their 2000 study from Edinburgh that the incidence of fractures increased and fracture patterns changed as children aged. Fracture incidence curves for each of the most common fractures separated by sex were shown on six basic incidence curves similar to Landin's initial work (Fig. 1-4).[49] When Landin compared these variability patterns with the common etiologies, he found some correlation. For example, late-peak fractures (distal forearm, phalanges, proximal humerus) were closely correlated with sports and equipment etiologies. Bimodal pattern fractures (clavicle, femur, radioulnar, diaphyses) showed an early increase from lower-energy trauma, then a late peak in incidence caused by injury from high- or moderate-energy trauma likely caused by MVAs, recreational activities, and contact sports in the adolescent population. Early-peak fractures (supracondylar humeral fractures are a classic example) were mainly caused by falls from high levels.

Age is a significant determinant of fracture incidence and patterns in children. The linear increase in annual fracture incidence with age, as demonstrated in various studies, highlights the importance of considering age-specific activities and bone characteristics when understanding fracture epidemiology. Fracture rates and locations shift with age, correlating with specific etiologies such as sports-related injuries, high-energy trauma, and falls from high levels.

Sex

Here is a sex-based difference in the incidence of injuries, location of injuries, and etiology of injuries across all age groups. For

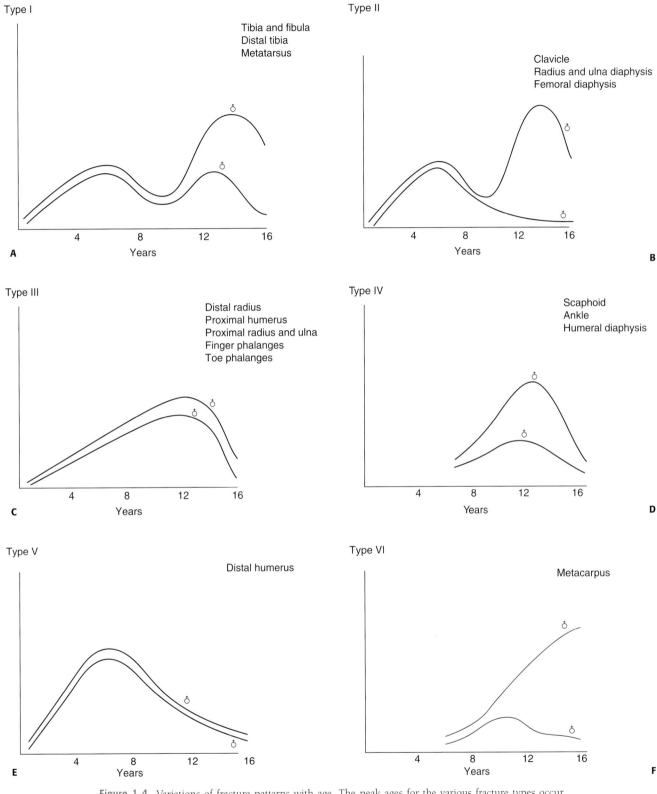

Figure 1-4. Variations of fracture patterns with age. The peak ages for the various fracture types occur in one of six patterns. (Reprinted from Rennie L, et al. The epidemiology of fractures in children. *Injury.* 2007;38(8):913–922. Copyright © 2007 Elsevier Ltd. With permission.)

all age groups, the overall ratio across a number of series of boys to girls who sustain a single fracture is about 1.5:1.[22,32,33,39,79]

In some areas, there is little difference in the incidence of fractures between boys and girls. For example, during the first 2 years of life, the overall incidence of injuries and fractures is nearly equal. During these first 2 years, the injury rates for foreign-body ingestion, poisons, and burns have no significant gender differences. With activities in which there is a male difference in participation, such as with sports equipment and bicycles, there is a marked increase in the incidence of injuries in boys.[14] The injury incidence may not be caused by the rate of exposure alone; behavior may be a major factor.[98] For example, one study found that the incidence of auto/pedestrian childhood injuries peaks in both sexes at ages 5 to 8.[80] When the total number of street crossings per day was studied, both sexes did so equally. Despite this equal exposure, boys had a higher number of injuries. Thus, the difference in the rate between the sexes begins to develop a male predominance when behaviors change. In Sweden, the greatest difference in rate of fractures was observed at age 15 where the fracture ratio was 4.3:1 male to female.[9]

Socioeconomic and Cultural Differences

The incidence of pediatric fracture varies in different geographic settings, socioeconomic climates, and differing ethnicities. Two studies from the United Kingdom looked at the relationship of affluence to the incidence of fractures in children and had differing conclusions. Lyons et al.[59] found no difference in the fracture rates of children in affluent population groups compared to those of children in nonaffluent families. On the other hand, Stark et al.[94] in Scotland found that the fracture rates in children from nonaffluent social groups were significantly higher than those in affluent families. There are also contradictory results in the literature with regard to fracture risk associated with living in urban versus rural settings.[24,33] In the United States, the increased rate of pediatric femur fractures was influenced by adverse socioeconomic and sociodemographic fractures.[35] Wren et al.[107] in a large prospective cohort studied the association of race and ethnicity as a risk factor for fracture in children and adolescents. They found that fracture rates were higher, regardless of sex, for White children compared with all other racial and ethnic groups. Thus, fracture incidence varies based on geographic settings, socioeconomic climates, and ethnicities. Studies report contradicting results regarding the relationship between affluence and fracture rates, as well as urban versus rural living settings. Adverse socioeconomic factors can influence fracture rates, and racial and ethnic disparities exist in fracture rates among children.

Clinical Factors

There are a number of clinical factors associated with fractures in children such as obesity and low bone mineral density (BMD).[13,71,84] Obesity in children and adolescents represents a complex interaction of host and environmental factors, making it the most prevalent nutritional problem for children in the United States. In a retrospective chart review, Taylor et al.[96]

noted that overweight children had a higher reported incidence of fractures and musculoskeletal complaints. Although Leonard et al.[53] found increased BMD in obese adolescents, the lack of physical activity often seen in obesity may in fact lead to reduced muscle mass, strength, and coordination resulting in impaired proprioception, balance, and increased risk of falling and fracture. In a recent study, Valerio et al.[99] confirmed a greater prevalence of overweight/obesity in children and adolescents with a recent fracture when compared to age- and sex-matched fracture-free children and found that obesity rate was increased in girls with upper limb fractures and girls and boys with lower limb fractures. Obese patients are also more likely to have a greater fracture displacement and potential for surgical complications when compared with normal-weight patients even with low-energy mechanisms.[13,71,84]

Low BMD and decreased bone mass in children is a complex problem that can result from a variety of causes including dietary nutritional deficiency, lack of adequate weight-bearing activity, and ineffective metabolic processing. In the adult population, low BMD is linked to increased fracture risk; however, in children, the relationship is less clear with a meta-analysis showing some association between fracture risk and low BMD.[18] In 2006, Clark examined in a prospective fashion the association between bone mass and fracture risk in childhood. Over 6,000 children at 9.9 years of age were followed up for 2 years and the study showed an 89% increased risk of fracture per standard deviation (SD) decrease in size-adjusted BMD.[16] In a follow-up study of this same cohort, the risk of fracture following slight or moderate to severe trauma was inversely related to bone size relative to body size perhaps reflecting the determinants of volumetric BMD such as cortical thickness on skeletal fragility.[17]

In summary, patient factors, such as age, sex, socioeconomic and cultural differences, and clinical factors, significantly impact fracture incidence and patterns in children. Considering these variables is crucial for a comprehensive understanding of pediatric fracture epidemiology and the development of effective preventive strategies.

THE IMPACT OF ENVIRONMENTAL FACTORS ON FRACTURES IN CHILDREN

Seasonal and Climatic Differences

Fractures are more common during the summer when children are out of school and exposed to more vigorous physical activities. An analysis of seasonal variation in many studies shows an increase in fractures in the warmer months of the year.[14,15,32,49,78,79,87,102,106]

Children in colder climates, with ice and snow, are exposed to risks different from those of children living in warmer climates. The exposure time to outdoor activities may be greater for children who live in dry and warm weather climates.[86] The most consistent climatic factor appears to be the number of hours of sunshine. Masterson et al.,[62] in a study from Ireland, found a strong positive correlation between fracture admissions and months with greater sunshine. Overall, the average number of fractures in the summer was 2.5 times that in the winter. On

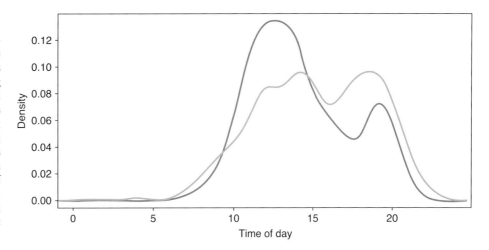

Figure 1-5. Distribution of fractures during time of day by summertime (*green*) and wintertime (*blue*). Density estimates are computed using kernel-smoothing method with normal kernel function and suitable bandwidth. The x-axis represents the hours in 5-hour intervals throughout the day (i.e., *0*, midnight; *5*, 5 AM; *10*, 10 AM; *15*, 3 PM; and *20*, 8 PM), and the y-axis represents the probability density that a fracture would occur at any given time of day. (Redrawn from Randsborg PH, et al. Fractures in children: epidemiology and activity-specific fracture rates. *J Bone Joint Surg Am.* 2013;95:e42.)

days with more sunshine hours than average, the average fracture admission rate was 2.31 per day; on days with fewer sunshine hours than average, the admission rate was 1.07 per day.

Time of Day

The time of day in which children are most active seems to correlate with the peak time for fracture occurrence. Seasonal variation and geographic location seem to play a role as to what time during the day injury occurs (Fig. 1-5).[62] In a Swedish study, the incidence peaked between 2 PM and 3 PM,[78] whereas in a study out of Texas by Shank et al.,[104] the hourly incidence of fractures formed a well-defined bell curve peaking at about 6 PM.

Home Environment

Fractures sustained in the home environment are defined as those that occur in the house and surrounding vicinity. These generally occur in a supervised environment and are mainly caused by falls from furniture, stairs, fences, and trees as well as from injuries sustained from recreational equipment (trampolines and home jungle gyms). Falls can vary in severity from a simple fall while running, to a fall of great magnitude, such as from a third-story window. In falling from heights, adults often land on their lower extremities, accounting for the high number of lower-extremity fractures, especially the calcaneus. Children tend to fall head first, using the upper extremities to break the fall. This accounts for the larger number of skull and radial fractures in children. Femoral fractures also are common in children falling from great heights. In contrast to adults, spinal fractures are rare in children who fall from great heights. In one study, children falling three stories or less all survived. Falls from the fifth or sixth floor resulted in a 50% mortality rate.[8,63]

Interestingly, a Swedish study showed that an increased incidence of fractures in a home environment did not necessarily correlate with the physical attributes or poor safety precautions of the house.[8] Rather, it appears that a disruption of the family structure and presence of social handicaps (alcoholism, welfare recipients, etc.) are important risk factors for pediatric fracture.

School Environment

The supervised environments at school are generally safe, and the overall annual rate of injury (total percentage of children injured in a single year) in the school environment ranges from 2.8% to 16.5%.[104] Most injuries occur because of use of playground or recreational equipment or participation in athletic activity. True rates may be higher because of inaccurate reporting, especially of mild injuries. The annual fracture rate of school injuries is thought to be low. Of all injuries sustained by children at school in a year, only 5% to 10% involved fractures.[55] In Worlock and Stower's series of children's fractures from England,[106] only 20% occurred at school. Most injuries (53%) occurring in school are related to athletics and sporting events,[106] and injuries are highest in the middle school children, with one study citing a 20% fracture rate in school-aged children of those injured during physical education class.[52]

In summary, pediatric trauma should be viewed as a seasonal disease with environmental risk factors that directly contribute to exposure and incidence. Understanding these seasonal and environmental factors can be useful for risk mitigation and resource allocation, especially during the predictably busy warmer months.

EVOLVING EPIDEMIOLOGY OF FRACTURES IN CHILDREN

COVID-19 PANDEMIC

The COVID-19 pandemic and societal lockdowns have created new challenges for treating pediatric orthopaedic trauma. During the pandemic, the overall volume of pediatric fractures decreased by 2.5-fold due to lack of exposure to high-risk activities such as playground equipment and the discontinuation of sports programs.[10] As countries have eased restrictions, there has been a corresponding rise in pediatric trauma volume. It will take time to determine the full effects of the global pandemic to determine what impact the pandemic as well as prolonged periods of sedentary activity may have on the overall incidence of pediatric orthopaedic injuries.

PREVENTIVE PROGRAMS

While studying the epidemiology of fractures, it is important to focus on the etiology of fractures and the settings in which they occur. Fractures do not occur in a vacuum, and well-researched studies that analyze the physical and social environment in which they occur are extremely valuable. Efforts can be made toward creating a safer environment for play and recreation. It is hoped that by targeting these areas, programs can be designed to decrease the risk factors.

NATIONAL CAMPAIGNS

Several national organizations have developed safety programs. The foremost is the AAP, that has committees on injury and poison prevention and sports medicine and fitness that has produced guidelines for athletics,[21] playgrounds, trampolines,[23] ATVs,[5] and skateboards.[20] The AAOS has also produced a program designed to decrease the incidence of playground injuries. These programs offer background data and guidelines for various activities, but their effectiveness has not been fully studied. In addition, the AAOS, the Orthopaedic Trauma Association (OTA), and POSNA have issued updated position statements regarding the safe use of ATVs, trampolines, skateboards, and in-line skating.

EXPANDED OPPORTUNITIES TO EXAMINE THE EPIDEMIOLOGY OF PEDIATRIC TRAUMA

Several sources of administrative, national, and regional data have recently become available, providing significantly improved investigation into various areas within pediatric trauma. The Healthcare Cost and Utilization Project (HCUP) is a family of databases including the State Inpatient Databases (SID), the Nationwide Inpatient Sample (NIS), and the Kids' Inpatient Database (KID). Although administrative data may lack clinical detail for certain purposes, these datasets provide a comprehensive overview of health care utilization in the United States and are available without purchase (http://www.ahrq.gov/research/data/hcup/index.html).[95] The KID database has been increasingly used to examine the incidence of pediatric trauma as well as practice patterns in pediatric trauma. Data for KID are collected and published every 3 years. In 2011 study, using the 2006 HCUP KID dataset, Gao[30] reported on lower-extremity fractures requiring hospitalization and found that there were about 11,500 admission records for children aged 0 to 20 years with lower-extremity fractures. Urban hospitalizations accounted for 93% of cases and 66% of admissions were to teaching hospitals in Gao's study. There was an increased mortality risk among patients cared for in nonteaching hospitals and hospitals located in a rural region. In an additional study using this dataset, Nakaniida et al.[67] found femur and humerus fractures as the most common injuries requiring hospitalization, with pelvic and vertebral fractures largely due to MVAs representing the most costly injuries.

Trauma registries are another source for injury data that document clinical and demographic information regarding acute care delivered to hospitalized patients with injuries at trauma centers. These databases are designed to provide information that can be used to study the effectiveness and quality of trauma care, collect information on rare injuries,[76,100] and identify areas for quality improvement. Although the amount of information available through regional and national databases allowed is immense, the creation and maintenance of these registries require a significant amount of time and financial resources. Several limitations of these databases include the focus on adult over pediatric injuries and the data that do not always reflect population-based samples. The American College of Surgeons National Trauma Data Bank serves as the largest database, producing annual reports on pediatric injury from trauma centers in the United States and Canada (www.facs.org/quality-programs/trauma/quality/national-trauma-data-bank/). In the future, databases such as these may provide the infrastructure needed to study pediatric musculoskeletal trauma care.

ACKNOWLEDGMENTS

With appreciation to Kaye Wilkins, Brian Brighton, and Michael Vitale for their work on previous editions of this chapter.

Annotated References

Reference	Annotation
Bergman E, Lempesis V, Nilsson JÅ, et al. Time trends in pediatric fractures in a Swedish city from 1950 to 2016. *Acta Orthop.* 2020; 91(5):589–604.	Epidemiologic studies on pediatric fractures have been ongoing in the Swedish city of Malmö since 1950. This most recent report describes the fracture epidemiology including etiology, comparing this to historical data and describes changes in age- and sex-adjusted pediatric fracture incidences to identify time trends independent of changing population demographics.
Clark EM, Ness AR, Bishop NJ, Tobias JH. Association between bone mass and fractures in children: a prospective cohort study. *J Bone Miner Res.* 2006;21(9):1489–1495.	The largest prospective study on bone mass in nearly 6,000 children demonstrated low bone density as a risk factor for fractures in children.

Annotated References

Reference	Annotation
Garay M, Hess J, Armstrong D, Hennrikus W. Pediatric ATV injuries in a statewide sample: 2004 to 2014. *Pediatrics.* 2017;140 (2):e20170945.	Data over an 11-year period from a statewide trauma database was reviewed to report the incidence of ATV-related injuries, mortality rates, as well as associated fracture patterns.
Hedstrom EM, Waernbaum I. Incidence of fractures among children and adolescents in rural and urban communities: analysis based on 9,965 fracture events. *Inj Epidemiol.* 2014;1(1):14.	In a study of nearly 10,000 fracture events in children, known risk factors of age and sex were predictive of fracture incidence. The authors also found a lower rate of fractures in rural and less densely populated municipalities.
Joeris A, Lutz N, Wicki B, et al. An epidemiological evaluation of pediatric long bone fractures: a retrospective cohort study of 2716 patients from two Swiss tertiary pediatric hospitals. *BMC Pediatr.* 2014;14:314.	Using the AO PCCF, the morphologic patterns of over 2,700 upper- and lower-extremity fractures are presented along with age, sex, and injury data.
Monteilh C, Patel P, Gaffney J. Musculoskeletal injuries associated with hoverboard use in children. *Clin Pediatr (Phila).* 2017;56(10):909–911.	Hoverboards, which are self-balancing, elevated motorized scooters, have recently been introduced as recreational devices to children and adolescents. This early report describes the increase in fractures especially of the upper extremity with falls associated with this device.
Naranje SM, Gilbert SR, Stewart MG, et al. Gunshot-associated fractures in children and adolescents treated at two level 1 pediatric trauma centers. *J Pediatr Orthop.* 2016;36(1):1–5.	A recent retrospective review from two trauma centers reports on 49 patients with 58 gunshot-associated fractures in the pediatric population. While nearly two-thirds of patient's fractures were successfully managed nonoperatively, more than one-third required surgery to manage their fracture or associated complications.
Wren TAL, Shepherd JA, Kalkwarf HJ, et al. Racial disparity in fracture risk between white and nonwhite children in the United States. *J Pediatr.* 2012;161(6):1035–1040.	A longitudinal study of nearly 1,500 children with data collected on diet, activity, ethnicity, and body composition including DXA measures reported on risk factors for fracture. Skeletal age 10–14 years and White race along with increased sports participation were some predictors of fracture risk in this population.

REFERENCES

1. Adams AJ, Mahmoud MAH, Wells L, et al. Physeal fractures of the distal femur: does a lower threshold for surgery lead to better outcomes? *J Pediatr Orthop B.* 2020;29(1):40–46.
2. Aitken ME, Jaffe KM, DiScala C, Rivara FP. Functional outcome in children with multiple trauma without significant head injury. *Arch Phys Med Rehabil.* 1999;80(8):889–895.
3. Aitken SA, Biant LC, Court-Brown CM. Recreational mountain biking injuries. *Emerg Med J.* 2011;28(4):274–279.
4. Aleman KB, Meyers MC. Mountain biking injuries in children and adolescents. *Sports Med.* 2010;40(1):77–90.
5. All-terrain vehicle injury prevention: two-, three-, and four-wheeled unlicensed motor vehicles. *Pediatrics.* 2000;105(6):1352–1354.
6. Arslan H, Subasi M, Kesemenli C, et al. Problem fractures associated with gunshot wounds in children. *Injury.* 2002;33(9):743–749.
7. Audigé L, Slongo T, Lutz N, et al. The AO pediatric comprehensive classification of long bone fractures (PCCF). *Acta Orthop.* 2017;88(2):133–139.
8. Barlow B, Niemirska M, Gandhi RP, Leblanc W. Ten years of experience with falls from a height in children. *J Pediatr Surg.* 1983;18(4):509–511.
9. Bergman E, Lempesis V, Nilsson JÅ, et al. Time trends in pediatric fractures in a Swedish city from 1950 to 2016. *Acta Orthop.* 2020;91(5):589–604.
10. Bram JT, Johnson MA, Magee LC, et al. Where have all the fractures gone? The epidemiology of pediatric fractures during the COVID-19 pandemic. *J Pediatr Orthop.* 2020;40(8):373–379.
11. Buckley SL, Gotschall C, Robertson W Jr, et al. The relationships of skeletal injuries with trauma score, injury severity score, length of hospital stay, hospital charges, and mortality in children admitted to a regional pediatric trauma center. *J Pediatr Orthop.* 1994;14(4):449–453.
12. Centers for Disease Control and Prevention (CDC). Nonfatal motor-vehicle-related backover injuries among children—United States, 2001–2003. *MMWR Morb Mortal Wkly Rep.* 2005;54(6):144–146.
13. Chang CH, Kao HK, Lee WC, Yang WE. Influence of obesity on surgical outcomes in type III paediatric supracondylar humeral fractures. *Injury.* 2015;46(11):2181–2184.
14. Cheng JC, Ng BK, Ying SY, Lam PK. A 10-year study of the changes in the pattern and treatment of 6,493 fractures. *J Pediatr Orthop.* 1999;19(3):344–350.
15. Cheng JC, Shen WY. Limb fracture pattern in different pediatric age groups: a study of 3,350 children. *J Orthop Trauma.* 1993;7(1):15–22.
16. Clark EM, Ness AR, Bishop NJ, Tobias JH. Association between bone mass and fractures in children: a prospective cohort study. *J Bone Miner Res.* 2006;21(9):1489–1495.
17. Clark EM, Ness AR, Tobias JH. Bone fragility contributes to the risk of fracture in children, even after moderate and severe trauma. *J Bone Miner Res.* 2008;23(2):173–179.
18. Clark EM, Tobias JH, Ness AR. Association between bone density and fractures in children: a systematic review and meta-analysis. *Pediatrics.* 2006;117(2):e291–e297.
19. Clarke NMP, Shelton FRM, Taylor CC, et al. The incidence of fractures in children under the age of 24 months–in relation to non-accidental injury. *Injury.* 2012;43(6):762–765.
20. Committee on Injury and Poison Prevention, American Academy of Pediatrics. Skateboard and scooter injuries. *Pediatrics.* 2002;109(3):542–543.
21. Committee on Sports Medicine and Committee in School Health; Washington RL, Bernhardt DT, Gomez J, et al. Organized sports for children and preadolescents. *Pediatrics.* 2001;107(6):1459–1462.
22. Cooper C, Dennison EM, Leufkens HGM, et al. Epidemiology of childhood fractures in Britain: a study using the general practice research database. *J Bone Miner Res.* 2004;19(12):1976–1981.
23. Council on Sports Medicine and Fitness, American Academy of Pediatrics; Briskin S, LaBotz M. Trampoline safety in childhood and adolescence. *Pediatrics.* 2012;130(4):774–779.
24. Danseco ER, Miller TR, Spicer RS. Incidence and costs of 1987–1994 childhood injuries: demographic breakdowns. *Pediatrics.* 2000;105(2):E27.
25. de Putter CE, van Beeck EF, Looman CWN, et al. Trends in wrist fractures in children and adolescents, 1997–2009. *J Hand Surg Am.* 2011;36(11):1810–1815.e12.
26. Derlet RW, Silva J Jr, Holcroft J. Pedestrian accidents: adult and pediatric injuries. *J Emerg Med.* 1989;7(1):5–8.
27. Dowd MD, Sege RD; Council on Injury, Violence, and Poison Prevention Executive Committee, American Academy of Pediatrics. Firearm-related injuries affecting the pediatric population. *Pediatrics.* 2012;130(5):e1416–e1423.
28. Fountain JL, Meyers MC. Skateboarding injuries. *Sports Med.* 1996;22(6):360–366.
29. Furnival RA, Street KA, Schunk JE. Too many pediatric trampoline injuries. *Pediatrics.* 1999;103(5):e57.
30. Gao Y. Children hospitalized with lower extremity fractures in the United States in 2006: a population-based approach. *Iowa Orthop J.* 2011;31:173–180.
31. Garay M, Hess J, Armstrong D, Hennrikus W. Pediatric ATV injuries in a statewide sample: 2004 to 2014. *Pediatrics.* 2017;140(2):e20170945.
32. Hedstrom EM, Svensson O, Bergström U, Michno P. Epidemiology of fractures in children and adolescents. *Acta Orthop.* 2010;81(1):148–153.
33. Hedstrom EM, Waernbaum I. Incidence of fractures among children and adolescents in rural and urban communities: analysis based on 9,965 fracture events. *Inj Epidemiol.* 2014;1(1):14.
34. Helmkamp JC, Furbee PM, Coben JH, Tadros A. All-terrain vehicle-related hospitalizations in the United States, 2000–2004. *Am J Prev Med.* 2008;34(1):39–45.
35. Hinton RY, Lincoln A, Crockett MM, et al. Fractures of the femoral shaft in children. Incidence, mechanisms, and sociodemographic risk factors. *J Bone Joint Surg Am.* 1999;81(4):500–509.

36. Joeris A, Lutz N, Blumenthal A, et al. The AO pediatric comprehensive classification of long bone fractures (PCCF). *Acta Orthop.* 2017;88(2):123–128.
37. Joeris A, Lutz N, Blumenthal A, et al. The AO pediatric comprehensive classification of long bone fractures (PCCF). *Acta Orthop.* 2017;88(2):129–132.
38. Joeris A, Lutz N, Wicki B, et al. An epidemiological evaluation of pediatric long bone fractures: a retrospective cohort study of 2,716 patients from two Swiss tertiary pediatric hospitals. *BMC Pediatr.* 2014;14:314.
39. Jones IE, Williams SM, Dow N, Goulding A. How many children remain fracture-free during growth? a longitudinal study of children and adolescents participating in the Dunedin Multidisciplinary Health and Development Study. *Osteoporos Int.* 2002;13(12):990–995.
40. Kawamoto K, Kim WC, Tsuchida Y, et al. Incidence of physeal injuries in Japanese children. *J Pediatr Orthop B.* 2006;15(2):126–130.
41. Kellum E, Creek A, Dawkins R, et al. Age-related patterns of injury in children involved in all-terrain vehicle accidents. *J Pediatr Orthop.* 2008;28(8):854–858.
42. Khan H, Green G, Arnander M, et al. What are the risk factors and presenting features of premature physeal arrest of the distal radius? A systematic review. *Eur J Orthop Surg Traumatol.* 2021;31(5):893–900.
43. Kirkpatrick R, Puffinbarger W, Sullivan JA. All-terrain vehicle injuries in children. *J Pediatr Orthop.* 2007;27(7):725–728.
44. Kopjar B, Wickizer TM. Fractures among children: incidence and impact on daily activities. *Inj Prev.* 1998;4(3):194–197.
45. Kyle SB, Nance ML, Rutherford GW Jr, Winston FK. Skateboard-associated injuries: participation-based estimates and injury characteristics. *J Trauma.* 2002;53(4):686–690.
46. Laffoy M. Childhood accidents at home. *Ir Med J.* 1997;90(1):26–27.
47. Laforest S, Robitaille Y, Lesage D, Dorval D. Surface characteristics, equipment height, and the occurrence and severity of playground injuries. *Inj Prev.* 2001;7(1):35–40.
48. Lam KY, Kumar GS, Mahadev A. Severity of playground-related fractures: more than just playground factors? *J Pediatr Orthop.* 2013;33(3):221–226.
49. Landin LA. Fracture patterns in children. Analysis of 8,682 fractures with special reference to incidence, etiology and secular changes in a Swedish urban population 1950–1979. *Acta Orthop Scand Suppl.* 1983;202:1–109.
50. Larson AN, Stans AA, Shaughnessy WJ, et al. Motocross morbidity: economic cost and injury distribution in children. *J Pediatr Orthop.* 2009;29(8):847–850.
51. Lempesis V, Rosengren BE, Nilsson JÅ, et al. Time trends in pediatric fracture incidence in Sweden during the period 1950–2006. *Acta Orthop.* 2017;88(4):440–445.
52. Lenaway DD, Ambler AG, Beaudoin DE. The epidemiology of school-related injuries: new perspectives. *Am J Prev Med.* 1992;8(3):193–198.
53. Leonard MB, Shults J, Wilson BA, et al. Obesity during childhood and adolescence augments bone mass and bone dimensions. *Am J Clin Nutr.* 2004;80(2):514–523.
54. Lillis KA, Jaffe DM. Playground injuries in children. *Pediatr Emerg Care.* 1997;13(2):149–153.
55. Linakis JG, Amanullah S, Mello MJ. Emergency department visits for injury in school-aged children in the United States: a comparison of nonfatal injuries occurring within and outside of the school environment. *Acad Emerg Med.* 2006;13(5):567–570.
56. Loder RT. The demographics of playground equipment injuries in children. *J Pediatr Surg.* 2008;43(4):691–699.
57. Lovejoy S, Weiss JM, Epps HR, et al. Preventable childhood injuries. *J Pediatr Orthop.* 2012;32(7):741–747.
58. Lustenberger T, Talving P, Barmparas G, et al. Skateboard-related injuries: not to be taken lightly. A National Trauma Databank Analysis. *J Trauma.* 2010;69(4):924–927.
59. Lyons RA, Delahunty AM, Heaven M, et al. Incidence of childhood fractures in affluent and deprived areas: population based study. *BMJ.* 2000;320(7228):149.
60. Mack MG, Hudson S, Thompson D. A descriptive analysis of children's playground injuries in the United States 1990–4. *Inj Prev.* 1997;3(2):100–103.
61. Mahadev A, Soon MYH, Lam KS. Monkey bars are for monkeys: a study on playground related extremity fractures in Singapore. *Singapore Med J.* 2004;45(1):9–13.
62. Masterson E, Borton D, O'Brien T. Victims of our climate. *Injury.* 1993;24(4):247–248.
63. Meller JL, Shermeta DW. Falls in urban children: a problem revisited. *Am J Dis Child.* 1987;141(12):1271–1275.
64. Monroe KW, Thrash C, Sorrentino A, King WD. Most common sports-related injuries in a pediatric emergency department. *Clin Pediatr (Phila).* 2011;50(1):17–20.
65. Monteilh C, Patel P, Gaffney J. Musculoskeletal injuries associated with hoverboard use in children. *Clin Pediatr (Phila).* 2017;56(10):909–911.
66. Mott A, Evans R, Rolfe K, et al. Patterns of injuries to children on public playgrounds. *Arch Dis Child.* 1994;71(4):328–330.
67. Nakaniida A, Sakuraba K, Hurwitz EL. Pediatric orthopaedic injuries requiring hospitalization: epidemiology and economics. *J Orthop Trauma.* 2014;28(3):167–172.
68. Naranje SM, Erali RA, Warner WC Jr, et al. Epidemiology of pediatric fractures presenting to emergency departments in the United States. *J Pediatr Orthop.* 2016;36(4):e45–e48.
69. Naranje SM, Gilbert SR, Stewart MG, et al. Gunshot-associated fractures in children and adolescents treated at two Level 1 pediatric trauma centers. *J Pediatr Orthop.* 2016;36(1):1–5.
70. Nelson NG, Alhajj M, Yard E, et al. Physical education class injuries treated in emergency departments in the US in 1997–2007. *Pediatrics.* 2009;124(3):918–925.
71. Nhan DT, Leet AI, Lee RJ. Associations of childhood overweight and obesity with upper-extremity fracture characteristics. *Medicine (Baltimore).* 2021;100(18):e25302.
72. Osberg JS, Schneps SE, Di Scala C, Li G. Skateboarding: more dangerous than roller skating or in-line skating. *Arch Pediatr Adolesc Med.* 1998;152(10):985–991.
73. Perkins C, Scannell B, Brighton B, et al. Orthopaedic firearm injuries in children and adolescents: an eight-year experience at a major urban trauma center. *Injury.* 2016;47(1):173–177.
74. Petridou E, Sibert J, Dedoukou X, et al. Injuries in public and private playgrounds: the relative contribution of structural, equipment and human factors. *Acta Paediatr.* 2002;91(6):691–697.
75. Phelan KJ, Khoury J, Kalkwarf HJ, Lanphear BP. Trends and patterns of playground injuries in United States children and adolescents. *Ambul Pediatr.* 2001;1(4):227–233.
76. Prentice HA, Paxton EW, Hunt JJ, et al. Pediatric hip fractures in California: results from a community-based hip fracture registry. *Perm J.* 2017;21:16–81.
77. Puranik S, Long J, Coffman S. Profile of pediatric bicycle injuries. *South Med J.* 1998;91(11):1033–1037.
78. Randsborg PH, Gulbrandsen P, Saltytė Benth J, et al. Fractures in children: epidemiology and activity-specific fracture rates. *J Bone Joint Surg Am.* 2013;95(7):e42.
79. Rennie L, Court-Brown CM, Mok JYQ, Beattie TF. The epidemiology of fractures in children. *Injury.* 2007;38(8):913–922.
80. Routledge DA, Repetto-Wright R, Howarth CI. The exposure of young children to accident risk as pedestrians. *Inj Prev.* 1996;2(2):150–161.
81. Sandler G, Nguyen L, Lam L, et al. Trampoline trauma in children: is it preventable? *Pediatr Emerg Care.* 2011;27(11):1052–1056.
82. Sawyer JR, Bernard MS, Schroeder RJ, et al. Trends in all-terrain vehicle-related spinal injuries in children and adolescents. *J Pediatr Orthop.* 2011;31(6):623–627.
83. Schalamon J, Sarkola T, Nietosvaara Y. Injuries in children associated with the use of nonmotorized scooters. *J Pediatr Surg.* 2003;38(11):1612–1615.
84. Seeley MA, Gagnier JJ, Srinivasan RC, et al. Obesity and its effects on pediatric supracondylar humeral fractures. *J Bone Joint Surg Am.* 2014;96(3):e18.
85. Shults BA, West BA, Rudd RA, Helmkamp JC. All-terrain vehicle-related nonfatal injuries among young riders in the United States, 2001–2010. *Pediatrics.* 2013;132(2):282–289.
86. Sinikumpu JJ, Pokka T, Hyvönen H, et al. Supracondylar humerus fractures in children: the effect of weather conditions on their risk. *Eur J Orthop Surg Traumatol.* 2017;27(2):243–250.
87. Sinikumpu JJ, Pokka T, Sirniö K, et al. Population-based research on the relationship between summer weather and paediatric forearm shaft fractures. *Injury.* 2013;44(11):1569–1573.
88. Slongo TF, Audigé L; AO Pediatric Classification Group. Fracture and dislocation classification compendium for children: the AO pediatric comprehensive classification of long bone fractures (PCCF). *J Orthop Trauma.* 2007;21(10 Suppl):S135–S160.
89. Slongo T, Audigé L, Clavert JM, et al. The AO comprehensive classification of pediatric long-bone fractures: a web-based multicenter agreement study. *J Pediatr Orthop.* 2007;27(2):171–180.
90. Slongo T, Audigé L, Lutz N, et al. Documentation of fracture severity with the AO classification of pediatric long-bone fractures. *Acta Orthop.* 2007;78(2):247–253.
91. Slongo T, Audigé L, Schlickewei W, et al. Development and validation of the AO pediatric comprehensive classification of long bone fractures by the Pediatric Expert Group of the AO Foundation in collaboration with AO Clinical Investigation and Documentation and the International Association for Pediatric Traumatology. *J Pediatr Orthop.* 2006;26(1):43–49.
92. Smith GA. Injuries to children in the United States related to trampolines, 1990–1995: a national epidemic. *Pediatrics.* 1998;101(3 Pt 1):406–412.
93. Smith GA, Shields BJ. Trampoline-related injuries to children. *Arch Pediatr Adolesc Med.* 1998;152(7):694–699.
94. Stark AD, Bennet GC, Stone DH, Chishti P. Association between childhood fractures and poverty: population based study. *BMJ.* 2002;324(7335):457.
95. Steiner C, Elixhauser A, Schnaier J. The healthcare cost and utilization project: an overview. *Eff Clin Pract.* 2002;5(3):143–151.
96. Taylor ED, Theim KR, Mirch MC, et al. Orthopedic complications of overweight in children and adolescents. *Pediatrics.* 2006;117(6):2167–2174.
97. Tiderius CJ, Landin L, Düppe H. Decreasing incidence of fractures in children: an epidemiological analysis of 1,673 fractures in Malmo, Sweden, 1993–1994. *Acta Orthop Scand.* 1999;70(6):622–626.
98. Valerio G, Gallè F, Mancusi C, et al. Pattern of fractures across pediatric age groups: analysis of individual and lifestyle factors. *BMC Public Health.* 2010;10:656.
99. Valerio G, Gallè F, Mancusi C, et al. Prevalence of overweight in children with bone fractures: a case control study. *BMC Pediatr.* 2012;12:166.
100. von Heyden J, Hauschild O, Strohm PC, et al. Paediatric acetabular fractures. Data from the German Pelvic Trauma Registry Initiative. *Acta Orthop Belg.* 2012;78(5):611–618.
101. Waltzman ML, Shannon M, Bowen AP, Bailey MC. Monkeybar injuries: complications of play. *Pediatrics.* 1999;103(5):e58.
102. Wareham K, Johansen A, Stone MD, et al. Seasonal variation in the incidence of wrist and forearm fractures, and its consequences. *Injury.* 2003;34(3):219–222.
103. Weiss BD. Bicycle-related head injuries. *Clin Sports Med.* 1994;13(1):99–112.
104. Westfelt JAN. Environmental factors in childhood accidents: a prospective study in Göteborg, Sweden. *Acta Paediatr Scand Suppl.* 1982;291:1–75.
105. Wood AM, Robertson GA, Rennie L, et al. The epidemiology of sports-related fractures in adolescents. *Injury.* 2010;41(8):834–838.
106. Worlock P, Stower M. Fracture patterns in Nottingham children. *J Pediatr Orthop.* 1986;6(6):656–660.
107. Wren TAL, Shepherd JA, Kalkwarf HJ, et al. Racial disparity in fracture risk between white and nonwhite children in the United States. *J Pediatr.* 2012;161(6):1035–1040.

2

Fracture Repair in Children

Courtney E. Baker and Jonathan G. Schoenecker

INTRODUCTION

Roughly 20% of children will sustain a fracture at some point, and the incidence of these injuries is on the rise.[30,47,64] Pediatric fractures are not only a significant orthopaedic issue but also a matter of broader societal health concern. The bones of a child are encased in thicker periosteum,[89] heal more rapidly,[16,45] and have a substantially greater potential for remodeling compared to adults. These physiologic differences necessitate distinct approaches in the treatment of fractures in children.

Fracture healing in children is influenced by a combination of biologic and biomechanical factors, underscoring the importance of understanding the complexities of bone healing.[16,45,67,89] Pediatric bones, distinguished by their unique healing characteristics and the presence of growth plates, typically exhibit fracture patterns that are less comminuted than those in adults and thus necessitate tailored treatment approaches. The growth plate, or physis, is often the most susceptible part of a child's bone to injury, potentially leading to either temporary or permanent growth arrest.[64] Despite this susceptibility, children possess an extraordinary capacity for fracture remodeling, enabling the correction of even initially misaligned fractures. For instance, deformities in the distal radius can remodel at a rate of approximately one degree per month, particularly when aligned with the wrist's natural flexion–extension motion. The role of the periosteum and physes introduces additional complexity into the management of pediatric fractures. Consequently, the choice of treatment, ranging from casting to the use of surgical implants, has a significant impact on the healing process.[16,40,50,65]

This overview focuses on the distinctive aspects of pediatric fracture healing, emphasizing a healing model that integrates biomechanics with vascularity, and underscores the periosteum's critical role.[16,45] As a key provider of pluripotent cells and vascularity for fracture repair, the periosteum is central to our comprehensive approach to diagnosing and managing pediatric fractures, particularly those involving the physis. A thorough grasp of these biologic and biomechanical factors is vital for effective pediatric fracture care.

ANATOMIC CONSIDERATIONS OF THE IMMATURE SKELETON

Long bones in children are distinguished by three key regions: the epiphyses, which are the bulbous ends covered in articular cartilage, taper into the funnel-shaped metaphyses, and the diaphysis sits centrally between these metaphyses (Fig. 2-1).[45] The epiphyseal and metaphyseal regions are separated by the physis, a cartilaginous structure critical for bone's longitudinal growth. Larger long bones like the clavicle, humerus, radius, ulna, femur, tibia, and fibula feature physes at both ends, whereas smaller tubular bones such as metacarpals, metatarsals, and phalanges typically have an

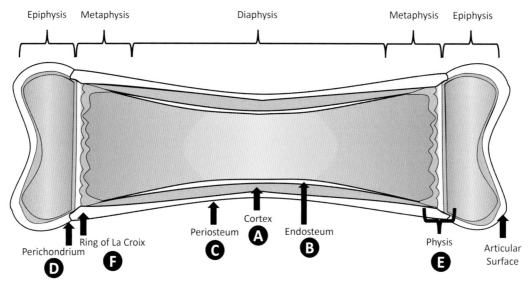

Figure 2-1. Bone can be divided into three regions: the epiphysis, metaphysis, and diaphysis. The diaphysis makes up the shaft of long bone. The epiphysis is situated at either end of long bones and forms the articular surface. Between the diaphysis and the epiphysis is the metaphysis, an area of bone that begins to fan out and widen. Cortical bone (*A*), referred to as the cortex, is a thick external shell of compact bone that contains Haversian canals for blood vessel passage. Two fibrovascular layers surround the cortex. The innermost layer is the endosteum (*B*), which separates the cortical bone from the medullary space. The medullary space contains trabecular, spongy bone that is less dense and hematopoietically active. The periosteum (*C*) surrounds the external side of the cortex except at the articular surface of the epiphysis. The periosteum is a highly vascularized reservoir of stem cells known as pericytes. The periosteum is contiguous with the perichondrium (*D*), another thick fibrovascular tissue. The perichondrium circumferentially surrounds the cartilage of the developing bone at the physis and articular surface in children. The physis (*E*) is a bone-forming machine of multiple layers spanning from the zone of ossification to the epiphyseal plate. Within the physis is a cartilaginous, avascular area that separates the metaphyseal and epiphyseal vascularity as no blood vessels cross this structure. Adjacent to the germinal cells of the physis is the epiphyseal plate which mechanically supports the physis and prevents epiphyseal blood vessels from touching the physeal germinal cells. The ring of La Croix (*F*) is an area near the physis containing perivascular stem cells that proliferate and migrate into the physis to promote longitudinal bone growth. (Copyright © 2024 J. Schoenecker.)

active physis at only one end. The proportional growth contribution of proximal and distal physes varies across these bones, as illustrated for upper and lower extremities in (Fig. 2-2).[17,78,88]

EPIPHYSIS

The epiphysis of a long bone, situated between the bone's end and the growth plate or physis, is primarily cartilaginous at birth, known as chondroepiphysis, except in certain bones like the distal femur and occasionally the proximal tibia. A secondary ossification center, forming at specific stages, enlarges and gradually replaces the cartilaginous areas with bone by the time of skeletal maturity. Accurately diagnosing and treating fractures around children's joints requires a thorough understanding of each epiphysis's unique development, including the timing of ossification center formation and its fusion to the metaphysis at the end of growth (Figs. 2-3 and 2-4). As these centers mature, there's an increase in the bone end's rigidity, altering the fracture patterns with age. Notably, some chondroepiphyses, like the proximal ends of metacarpals 2 to 5, do not develop secondary ossification centers and ossify directly through vascular invasion at the time of physeal closure.[17,78,88]

The external surface of the epiphysis is composed of articular cartilage or perichondrium, to which muscle fibers, tendons, and ligaments anchor. The perichondrium contributes to the centrifugal enlargement of the epiphysis and seamlessly transitions into the periosteum. This continuity bolsters the structural integrity of the epiphyseal/metaphyseal junction, notably at the zone of Ranvier (Fig. 2-5).[5,15,22,94] Beneath the articular cartilage, hyaline cartilage facilitates the growth of the epiphysis. Upon reaching skeletal maturity, a distinct tidemark forms, demarcating the transition from articular to calcified epiphyseal hyaline cartilage.

PHYSIS

At the core of longitudinal bone growth in children is the physis, or growth plate, a highly organized and dynamic structure integral to bone elongation (see Fig. 2-5). The physis comprises chondrocytes in various stages of proliferation, differentiation, and complex extracellular matrix formation, all of which contribute to ongoing bone growth. The matrix is primarily made up of type II collagen fibers, supplemented with aggrecans and noncollagenous proteins such as cartilage oligomeric protein

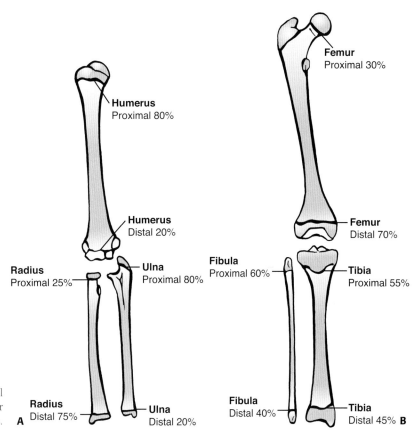

Figure 2-2. Approximate percentage of longitudinal growth provided by the proximal and distal physes for each long bone in the upper (**A**) and lower (**B**) extremities.

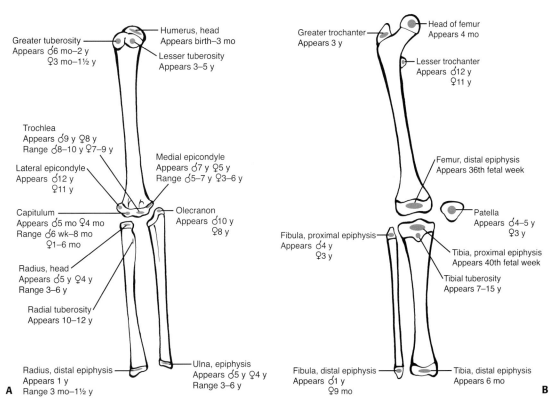

Figure 2-3. Typical age (and range) of development of the secondary ossification centers of the epiphyses in the upper (**A**) and lower (**B**) extremities.

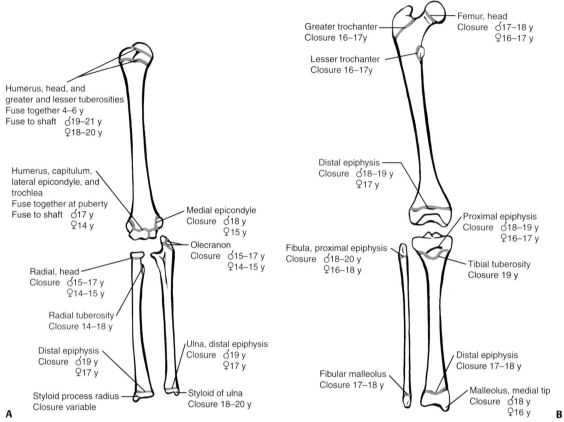

Humerus, head, and
greater and lesser tuberosities
Fuse together 4–6 y
Fuse to shaft   ♂19–21 y
            ♀18–20 y

Humerus, capitulum,
lateral epicondyle, and
trochlea
Fuse together at puberty
Fuse to shaft   ♂17 y
            ♀14 y

Radial, head
Closure   ♂15–17 y
        ♀14–15 y

Radial tuberosity
Closure 14–18 y

Distal epiphysis
Closure   ♂19 y
        ♀17 y

Styloid process radius
Closure variable

Medial epicondyle
Closure   ♂18 y
        ♀15 y

Olecranon
Closure   ♂15–17 y
        ♀14–15 y

Ulna, distal epiphysis
Closure   ♂19 y
        ♀17 y

Styloid of ulna
Closure 18–20 y

A

Greater trochanter
Closure 16–17y

Lesser trochanter
Closure 16–17y

Femur, head
Closure   ♂17–18 y
        ♀16–17 y

Distal epiphysis
Closure   ♂18–19 y
        ♀17 y

Fibula, proximal epiphysis
Closure   ♂18–20 y
        ♀16–18 y

Proximal epiphysis
Closure   ♂18–19 y
        ♀16–17 y

Tibial tuberosity
Closure 19 y

Fibular malleolus
Closure 17–18 y

Distal epiphysis
Closure 17–18 y

Malleolus, medial tip
Closure   ♂18 y
        ♀16 y

B

Figure 2-4. Typical age (and range) of closure of physes the upper (**A**) and lower (**B**) extremities.

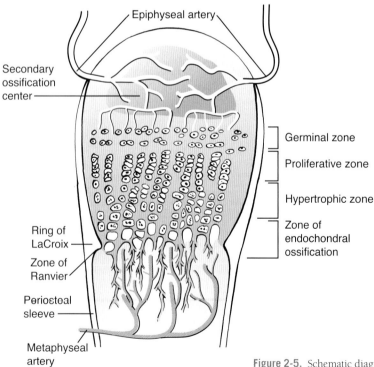

Epiphyseal artery

Secondary
ossification
center

Germinal zone

Proliferative zone

Hypertrophic zone

Zone of
endochondral
ossification

Ring of
LaCroix

Zone of
Ranvier

Periosteal
sleeve

Metaphyseal
artery

Figure 2-5. Schematic diagram of the organization of the physis. Four zones are illustrated: the germinal, proliferative, hypertrophic, and provisional calcification (or endochondral ossification) layers. Note also the groove of Ranvier and the perichondral ring of LaCroix.

and matrilin-3. Notably, the synthesis of type X collagen within the hypertrophic zone signifies chondrocyte maturation, distinguishing this part of the growth plate.[4,6,7,17,62,88]

Zones of the Physis

The growth plate is segmented into distinct morphologic zones, each with a specific role in bone development (see Fig. 2-5):

- **Germinal bone:** The reserve area with undifferentiated chondrocytes, characterized by horizontally oriented collagen fibers, indicative of a less active role in immediate growth.
- **Proliferative zone:** Active cellular division occurs here, with vertically aligned collagen fibers reflecting growth and the columnar arrangement of chondrocytes.
- **Hypertrophic zone:** This zone sees cellular enlargement and matrix production, crucial for the cartilage-to-bone transition.
- **Provisional calcification zone:** The final stage before the metaphysis, where calcification peaks in preparation for ossification.
- **Zone of ossification:** Located in the metaphysis, this vascularized zone is where chondrocytes either undergo apoptosis or transdifferentiate into osteoblasts, forming the primary spongiosum.

Each zone has a unique response to mechanical stress, with the proliferative and hypertrophic zones being particularly susceptible to greater strains under compression.

The physis also includes two specialized peripheral areas:

- **Zone of Ranvier:** A triangular microscopic structure housing fibroblasts, chondroblasts, and osteoblasts, responsible for the physis' peripheral growth.
- **Perichondral ring of LaCroix:** A fibrous structure connecting the metaphyseal periosteum to the cartilaginous epiphysis, essential for stabilizing the epiphysis to the metaphysis.

These structures are crucial for the mechanical integrity and peripheral growth of the physis.

Vascularity of the Physis

The chondrocytic portion of the physis is avascular but surrounded by a vital vascular network necessary for nutrient diffusion and repair mechanisms (Fig. 2-6).[45] The epiphyseal and

Figure 2-6. Vascular anatomy of developing bone. Bone is a highly vascular organ. Nutrient arteries (*A*) are large-caliber blood vessels that penetrate the diaphysis and metaphysis of developing bone. Alternatively, epiphyseal arteries (*B*) must enter at the epiphysis, where they centripetally provide blood pumped from the heart to bone. Once inside the bone (*C*), this external blood supply is combined with blood produced from the medullary cavity and is recycled to the rest of bone in a centrifugal fashion. Transcortical vessels (*D*) facilitate centrifugal perfusion. These vessels (both arterial and venous) traverse the endosteum and cortex to connect the bone marrow to the periosteum (*E*) and are an important facilitator of bone perfusion and venous drainage. At the ends of long bone, the physis separates the blood supply of the epiphysis from the metaphysis. Abutting the metaphyseal side of the physis are metaphyseal vessels (*F*) that end at the growth plate as large capillary loops with slow flow. The ingress of these blood vessels into the physis enables the production of primary spongiosum, creating the zone of ossification. Subchondral bone of the epiphysis (*G*) is supplied solely by epiphyseal arteries which additionally provide nutrients and oxygen to the germinal cells of the physis via diffusion across the epiphyseal plate. Therefore, a disruption in the epiphyseal vasculature can also affect the germinal cells of the physis. (Copyright © 2024 J. Schoenecker.)

metaphyseal blood vessels, along with circumferential perichondrial vasculature, play a significant role in growth plate nutrition. This diverse vascular supply is key in maintaining the physis and in revascularization after injury. The epiphyseal vascularity mainly nourishes the chondrocytic portion of the physis through diffusion, while the metaphyseal vascularity forms the primary spongiosum in the zone of ossification.[38,52,59,99,100] Understanding these vascular dynamics is critical when considering growth plate injuries, as injuries to the metaphyseal vascularity don't typically lead to physeal arrest, whereas epiphyseal vascularity injuries can jeopardize long-term physeal integrity (see Fig. 2-5).[31,38,59,99,100]

There are also distinct types of epiphyseal blood supply, classified as type A (e.g., proximal humeral and femoral epiphyses) and type B (e.g., proximal and distal tibia, distal radius).[31,59,99,100] These types differ in their susceptibility to vascular compromise, with type A epiphyses particularly at risk of extensive ischemic damage to the physis.[31,59,99,100]

Cell Signaling

Chondrocyte development, from mesenchymal stem cells into osteochondroprogenitor cells, is significantly influenced by the Wnt/β-catenin signaling pathway. This pathway plays a pivotal role in determining whether these cells differentiate into osteoblasts or chondrocytes. The hedgehog (Hh) signaling pathway, especially Indian Hh (IHH), is integral in regulating chondrocyte fate in the growth plate, functioning within a feedback loop with parathyroid hormone–like hormone (PTHrP) and bone morphogenic proteins (BMPs) to finely tune chondrocyte differentiation.[4,12,19,62]

METAPHYSIS

The metaphysis, the flared section at each end of the diaphysis, features thinner cortical thickness and a higher volume of trabecular bone within the secondary spongiosa. Endochondral modeling centrally and peripherally forms the primary spongiosa, which is then remodeled into the more mature secondary spongiosa by osteoclasts and osteoblasts. This region experiences considerable bone turnover compared to other bone areas. Its cortex, thinner and more porous than the diaphysis, contains cortical fenestrations with fibrovascular soft tissue elements linking the metaphyseal marrow spaces to the subperiosteal region. The metaphysis develops extensive secondary and tertiary haversian systems only in late stages of skeletal maturation. These anatomic changes correlate with varying fracture patterns over time, explaining why buckle (or torus) fractures are more common than complete metaphyseal or epiphyseal/physeal fractures in this region.[58,75,101]

The periosteum, loosely attached to the diaphysis, firmly anchors to the metaphysis due to the fibrous tissue continuity through metaphyseal fenestrations. It attaches densely to the peripheral physis and merges into the zone of Ranvier and the epiphyseal perichondrium (see Fig. 2-5). The zone of Ranvier, between bone and cartilage formation, contributes to growth plate remodeling over time.[22,94] The fenestrated metaphyseal cortex extends to the physis as the osseous ring of LaCroix (see Fig. 2-5), with no significant direct muscle attachments to the

metaphyseal bone except for the medial distal femoral attachment of the adductor muscles.

DIAPHYSIS

The diaphysis, comprising the bulk of each long bone, evolves from bone remodeled from the metaphysis. It is characterized by mature, lamellar bone, and the developing diaphyseal bone is highly vascular. In cross-section, the central area is less dense than in older children, adolescents, and adults. Growth leads to increased complexity in the haversian (osteonal) systems and formation of more extracellular matrix, reducing cross-sectional porosity and enhancing hardness. Some bones, like the tibia, may experience decreased vascularity as they mature, affecting healing rates and nonunion risks.[80,81] Bone vascularity is crucial not only for nutrient delivery but also because pericyte cells around blood vessels contribute to new osteoblast formation.[13]

PERIOSTEUM

A child's periosteum is thicker and more easily elevated than in adults, possessing greater osteogenic potential.[89] In young children, even complete diaphyseal removal, if the periosteum is left intact, can lead to bone regrowth.[5,15] The periosteum's thickness and strength influence fracture displacement, ease of closed reduction, and new bone formation capacity. It is typically torn on the tension side and intact on the compression side during injuries. The intact periosteal hinge or sleeve can limit fracture fragment displacement and assist in reduction. The periosteum enables tissue continuity across fractures, allowing subperiosteal new bone to quickly bridge the fracture gap, leading to early healing and stability.[5,15]

The periosteum consists of two tissue layers: an outer fibroblast layer providing fibrous attachment to connective tissues, and an inner cambium layer housing cells supporting bone formation and repair. The periosteum serves as the origin for muscle fibers along the metaphysis and diaphysis, coordinating growth between bone and muscle units. Exceptions include muscle fiber attachments near the linea aspera and the medial distal femoral metaphysis. Radiographs in these areas are often misinterpreted as showing pathologic responses, although they reflect normal skeletal development variations.[53] The periosteum in growing children also plays a crucial role in remodeling, forming new bone over the concave side of a deformity and resorbing bone on the convex side, ultimately resulting in a straight diaphysis.[53,96]

APOPHYSIS

An apophysis is composed of fibrocartilage, growing mainly in response to tensile forces and usually attached to muscular structures. Secondary ossification centers can form in the apophysis during growth. Due to their distinct histologic composition, these structures fail differently than other bone parts, with excessive tensile stress possibly causing avulsion, especially during late closure stages. Such injuries can produce substantial new bone, potentially mistaken for tumors, particularly around the pelvis. Healing of a displaced fragment to an underlying nondisplaced secondary center creates symptomatic reactive overgrowth, as seen in Osgood–Schlatter lesions in the tibial tuberosity apophysis.[70]

UNIFYING THEORY OF FRACTURE REPAIR

GENERAL PRINCIPLES

The most primary concerns following a fracture are the prevention of hemorrhage and infection. Both are early, life-threatening complications. From a practical perspective, if someone does not survive the hemorrhage or early infection after fracture, whether the fracture is able to heal over the subsequent weeks is of no consequence. Fortunately, life-threatening hemorrhage and infection are rare in modern society thanks to millennia of evolutionary pressure and modern resuscitation practices. Such topics are discussed in greater detail in other resources.[16,71,83,102]

Once overall survival following a fracture is ensured, the body sets upon the major work of healing the bone. There are two osseous problems after a fracture: mechanical dysfunction and hypoxia. To address the mechanical aspect, orthopaedic surgeons use a variety of techniques and implants to foster an environment most conducive to the body's innate bone healing biology. Orthopaedic surgeons do this by controlling strain—the measure of deformation a structure undergoes relative to its original length—through a variety of well-molded casts and implants. Through years of clinical practice and pattern recognition, orthopaedic surgeons are well adept at controlling strain, however, interestingly, it is never objectively measured at the time of surgery.[82,101]

The presence of hypoxia, a less apparent yet potentially more critical consequence of a fracture, must also be addressed. Bone, a highly vascularized tissue, experiences not only a disruption of its structural integrity but also a severance of its blood supply upon fracturing, resulting in an extensive area of oxygen-deprived tissue. In the healing process, reestablishing vascular union across a fracture site is just as crucial as achieving bony continuity and invariably precedes bone formation.[13,37,59]

It is essential to understand that the balance between strain and vascularity at the fracture site dictates the pathway of healing—whether it be primary or secondary bone healing, as depicted in (Fig. 2-7).[2,16] An environment that maintains adequate vascularity and minimal strain is conducive to primary fracture repair. Conversely, secondary fracture repair occurs under conditions of compromised vascularity and/or moderate strain levels. Recognizing the central roles of strain and vascularity is not only required to understand the fracture healing process but also enables the clinician to effectively leverage these factors in the repair process.

THE TWO TYPES OF FRACTURE REPAIR

Bone formation occurs through two distinct processes: intramembranous and endochondral ossification. Intramembranous ossification involves the direct transformation of pericytes into osteoblasts, which then deposit bone matrix directly into pre-existing connective tissue. This process is characteristic of primary bone healing and contributes to the peripheral ossification seen in secondary bone healing. In contrast, endochondral ossification occurs in areas of strain or hypoxia and involves the creation of a cartilage scaffold that is subsequently replaced by bone through a process initiated by intramembranous ossification.[1,16,67]

Primary Fracture Repair

In microenvironments with low strain and sufficient vascularity, bone heals through primary fracture repair. Primary bone healing occurs through intramembranous ossification, a process requiring intact blood supply at the fracture site, as depicted in (Fig. 2-8). The surrounding healthy periosteum and endosteum ensure adequate oxygen levels. Rigid fixation applied under compression minimizes mechanical strain and facilitates an optimal environment for pericytes to differentiate into osteoblasts. These osteoblasts, in close association with endothelial cells, secrete essential ossification materials (hydroxyapatite, collagen type I, and BMP) and vascular endothelial growth factor (VEGF), which sustains revascularization and mimics natural bone remodeling.[16,17,66]

Secondary Fracture Repair

Secondary fracture repair occurs in microenvironments with moderate strain and/or insufficient vascularity. Secondary bone healing is a more complex process that incorporates both endochondral ossification at the core and intramembranous ossification at the periphery of the fracture, as illustrated in (Fig. 2-9). Fractures with displacement disrupt normal blood circulation patterns, causing hypoxia and inflammation, leading to bone necrosis. The severity of necrosis correlates with the initial fracture displacement's impact on blood flow and the bone's inherent vascular network. Pericytes migrate to the fracture site and adapt to the low-oxygen environment by differentiating into "spring" chondrocytes. These cells manage strain by synthesizing collagen types II and IX and additional matrix proteins, forming a soft tissue callus. The degree of callus formation is proportional to the motion—or strain—at the fracture site. Greater motion leads to greater strain, and larger stimulus for

Figure 2-7. Strain and vascularity. The type of bone healing that occurs is dependent on the mechanics and biology of the fracture. In areas with low strain and sufficient vascularity, primary bone healing is possible. In areas with either medium strain or insufficient vascularity, secondary bone healing can occur. However, if the strain is too high or vascularity too low, then the fracture will not heal.

Strain (Motion at Fracture Site)

Vascularity	Low	Medium	High
Sufficient	Primary	Secondary	Nonunion
Insufficient	Secondary	Nonunion	Nonunion

Type of Bone Healing

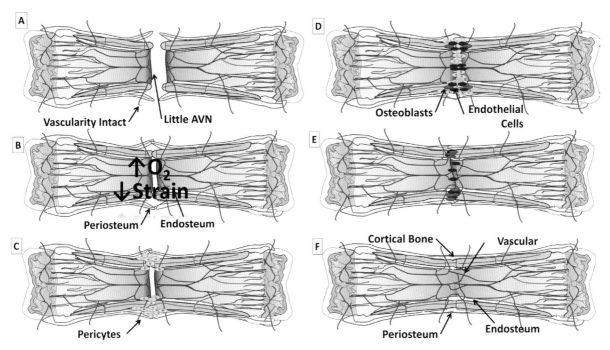

Figure 2-8. Intramembranous ossification. In fractures with intact vascularity (**A**), little avascular necrosis, low strain (**B**), and sufficient oxygenation with healthy periosteum and endosteum, intramembranous ossification is possible. **C:** In intramembranous ossification healing, pericytes that are capable of differentiating into osteoblasts invade the fracture site. **B, D:** They are followed by endothelial cells and the pericytes transition into osteoblasts as in the normal process of remodeling. The osteoblasts (**E**) gradually achieve bony union that includes (**F**) union of cortical bone, intramedullary vascularity, periosteum, and endosteum. (Copyright © 2024 J. Schoenecker.)

spring chondrocyte development, ultimately a larger callus to stabilize and bridge the fracture ends.[7,16,69]

Once the fracture is bridged with callus and strain reduced, "spring" chondrocytes evolve into hypertrophic chondrocytes, especially in regions farthest from the fracture where the strain is lowest. These cells release VEGF, orchestrating the orderly migration of endothelial cells, pericytes, and osteoblasts into the formerly avascular callus, culminating in hard callus formation. Concurrently, intramembranous ossification occurs on the well-vascularized periosteum of the unaffected peripheral cortical bone, contributing to the hard callus and stability.[9,16,89]

Upon the transformation of the soft tissue callus to a hard callus, the fracture site consists of stable, vascularized bone. The body then embarks on remodeling, harnessing its osteogenic and angiogenic capacities to sculpt the bone into a structurally sound and mechanically efficient form. Mechanical stresses guide this process, causing the intramedullary vasculature to expand and the cortical diameter to decrease. Adhering to Wolff's law, the dynamic balance between osteoclast-mediated bone resorption and osteoblast-led bone formation allows the bone to regain its original shape and structural integrity.[15,36]

CELLULAR COORDINATION DURING FRACTURE REPAIR

Fracture healing is a highly coordinated process, characterized by teams of cells that work to address the mechanical challenges (strain) and vascular discontinuity (hypoxia) following a fracture

(see Fig. 2-7). Depending on the microenvironment of the fracture, these teams of cells "fix" fractures using either intramembranous (primary fracture repair) or a combination of intramembranous and endochondral ossification (secondary fracture repair).[66]

To understand the differences between these processes, one must distinguish the major cell types involved: pericytes, prehypertrophic (or "spring") chondrocytes, hypertrophic chondrocytes, endothelial cells, osteoblasts, and osteoclasts. The pericyte acts as the "stem cell," responsible for generating most of the new tissue required to bridge a fracture. Normally part of the blood vessel boundary within bone, pericytes become activated and proliferate when a vessel is damaged due to fracture.[3,69] The activation of pericytes leads to their differentiation into osteoblasts or chondrocytes, influenced by the local microenvironment. The periosteum and endosteum vasculature serve as the primary sources of pericytes for fracture healing.[5,89]

Chondrocytes, which are derived from pericytes, are well suited for the hypoxic environment at a fracture site and are key players in endochondral ossification and callus formation. "Spring" chondrocytes are so named because they work to resolve high strain near the fracture by producing a biomechanical matrix that stabilizes the fracture site. These cells, which also exist in healthy articular cartilage, proliferate in response to strain and synthesize organized extracellular matrix proteins, primarily type II collagen.[6,16,36]

When "spring" chondrocytes have effectively reduced interfragmentary strain, they evolve into hypertrophic chondrocytes.[16]

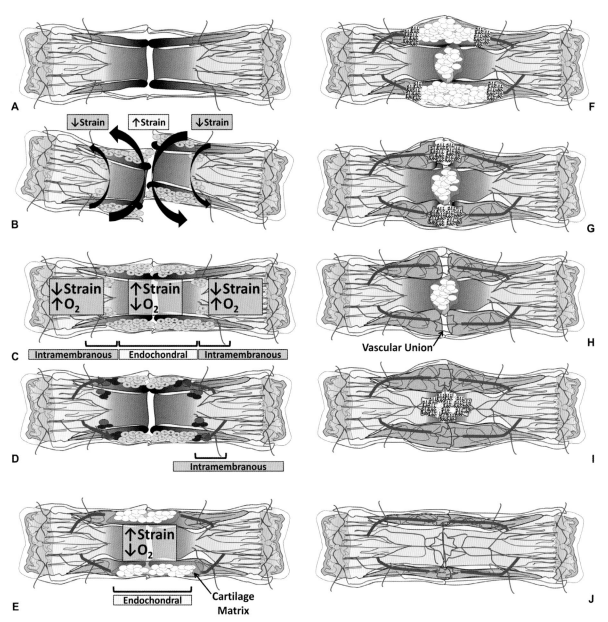

Figure 2-9. Endochondral ossification. **A:** After most fractures, the vascular supply to the fracture site is disrupted, leading to hypoxia and avascular necrosis of bone. **B:** In response to the injury, pericytes enter the fracture site, to resolve the strain and motion at the fracture and begin the reparative process. Depending on the conditions of strain and oxygen supply within the fractured bone, either intramembranous (**C**) or endochondral ossification will proceed. **D:** Osteoblasts accompanied by endothelial cells supplied by the centrifugal blood supply begin the process of intramembranous ossification at the edges of the fracture. **E:** At the middle of the fracture site, "spring" chondrocytes survive in the hypoxic environment, proliferate based on strain and motion, and resolve strain by depositing extracellular matrix proteins. **F:** When strain has been sufficiently resolved, these chondrocytes undergo hypertrophy and become the bone bomb. **G:** Hypertrophic chondrocytes promote vascular invasion and osteogenesis by depositing BMP, VEGF, and hydroxyapatite. **H:** Vascular union always precedes bony union in a fracture site as the endothelial cells are necessary for ossification. **I:** With bony union of the fracture callus, the fracture is stabilized, and the remaining chondrocytes become hypertrophic. **J:** The fracture is now healed and remodeling proceeds as in a healthy bone to make it more structurally efficient. (Copyright © 2024 J. Schoenecker.)

These cells are crucial for the next phase as they accumulate cytokines, growth factors, and other elements necessary for subsequent bone growth. Literature suggests that these hypertrophic chondrocytes release alkaline phosphatase-coated microvesicles, which are filled with nanohydroxyapatite to seed new bone formation. Along with type X collagen, these structures are precursors to calcified cartilage, critical for subsequent ossification. In addition, the microvesicles carry VEGF and BMP-2, which promote angiogenesis and osteogenesis.[7,49]

Endothelial cells facilitate the transition from a chondroid soft tissue callus to a hard tissue callus. They depend on "spring" chondrocytes to resolve strain before entering the callus and are attracted by the hypertrophic chondrocyte-produced VEGF. Osteoblasts, following endothelial cells, migrate into the callus and lay down collagen type I, hydroxyapatite, and BMP, advancing revascularization. These osteoblasts continue ossification, eventually encapsulating themselves with hydroxyapatite to become osteocytes. The summation of this process is an immature, structurally inefficient "hard callus" which provides both vascular and bony union across the fracture gap and is histologically identified as woven bone.[9,16,27]

With the reestablishment of blood vessels, macrophages arrive, fusing into osteoclasts to break down the large hydroxyapatite crystals created by osteoblasts. Osteoclasts remodel the woven bone into structurally efficient lamellar bone, ensuring an organized blood supply sufficient to sustain osteocytes.[13,14]

THE ESSENTIAL ROLE OF VASCULARITY IN FRACTURE REPAIR

Vascularity is fundamental to intramembranous and endochondral ossification and therefore pivotal for bone repair. Surgeons appreciate how vascular bone is when attempting to fix an acute fracture; however, it is commonly viewed as collateral injury and of secondary importance to the osseous injury. It is common to hear the phrase "respect the soft tissues" in orthopaedic trauma, referencing the AO principles. However, this phrase falls well short in describing the specific function and absolute necessity of vascularity to successful fracture healing. Studies have shown restoring vascular continuity is required prior to osseous union. Without vascular union, there can be no fracture healing. Therefore, understanding the patterns and phases of revascularization is key to treating fractures. Outside of the operating room, the best surgical outcomes are achieved when addressing systemic factors that negatively affect vascularity and thus hinder bone healing: smoking and diabetes, among others.[16,26,56,61]

Historical perspectives on revascularization in fracture healing have varied over time. Kolodny,[61] in 1923, proposed the "centripetal model," suggesting that revascularization postfracture was driven primarily by the periosteum. In contrast, Trueta, through mid-20th–century research, presented the "centrifugal model," emphasizing the dominance of the intramedullary blood supply.[99,100] These seemingly opposing models were harmonized by Rhinelander in the 1960s and 1970s, who determined that fracture morphology dictated revascularization.[87] Nondisplaced fractures supported Trueta's findings with rapid reformation of intramedullary vessels. In displaced fractures,

a periosteal vascular response occurred first, as Kolodny had described, followed by the reestablishment of intramedullary blood supply. This demonstrated that both models are correct within their respective fracture types.[16]

Contemporary understanding of fracture repair begins with recognizing the anatomical and vascular complexity of bone. The primary builders of bone, osteoblasts, rely on a rich vascular network to provide the necessary oxygen and nutrients. The intricate vascular system of bone is composed of a mix of metaphyseal/epiphyseal, diaphyseal, endosteal, and periosteal arteries, forming a sinusoidal network that sustains both cortical and cancellous bone structures.[105] Central to this system are the nutrient arteries, penetrating the bone in a centripetal fashion, then branching extensively, and eventually linking the central and peripheral aspects of the bone.[16,86]

THE CRUCIAL ROLE OF PERIOSTEUM IN FRACTURE REPAIR

Periosteum is a multilayered tissue enveloping the bone, aptly named from the Greek words for "around" (peri) and "bone" (osteon). It consists of a robust outer fibrous layer harboring blood vessels, and an inner cambium layer rich with progenitor cells. Periosteum's role in bone formation was a point of scientific curiosity and debate for centuries. From Leeuwenhoek's initial microscopic explorations to Duhamel du Monceau's 18th-century comparisons with tree growth, scientists have long identified periosteum's significant contributions to bone development. Subsequent work using lineage-tracing models concretely established periosteal cells as central to bone fracture healing as well.[79,89]

Periosteum is not only an anatomical structure but an active participant in fracture healing, particularly in children. The two primary ways periosteum contributes to fracture healing physiology are by[1] providing most of the pluripotent cells for healing and[2] serving as a dominant source of vascularity.

The periosteum serves as a reservoir of pericytes—stem cells capable of differentiating into various cell types for healing, including chondrocytes and osteoblasts. Pericytes play an adaptive role in fracture healing by responding to the local injury microenvironment. In areas of high strain or low oxygen, they differentiate into chondrocytes, promoting endochondral ossification. In contrast, with minimal strain and adequate oxygen, these cells become osteoblasts, contributing to intramembranous ossification. Periosteum's ability to support both intramembranous and endochondral ossification through its pericyte reserves as dictated by the fracture pattern demonstrates its essential and dynamic role in fracture repair.[16,45,60]

Periosteum responds robustly to fractures, facilitating a vascular shunt that channels blood flow to the affected area. Revascularization patterns vary based on fracture type as discussed previously. In displaced fractures, the periosteum is the initial source of vascular regeneration and thereby an essential structure in most fractures. At the fracture edges, preserved vascularity and low mechanical strain within the periosteum promote intramembranous ossification as opposed to the hypoxia-driven endochondral ossification that occurs in the fracture center.[11,16,29,45,105]

CLINICAL APPLICATION OF A PERIOSTEUM-CENTRIC FRACTURE THEORY

Periosteum is undeniably a crucial element of normal bone physiology. Pediatric orthopaedists can utilize it in various ways to benefit children. Although its presence (and functional absence) is not directly visible, clinical examinations and radiographic assessments can infer its status to assist in the reduction and fixation of pediatric fractures. Understanding the biology of the periosteum in fracture repair is fundamental for the treatment of pediatric fractures.

Addressing pediatric fractures necessitates an approach that aligns with the unique properties of a child's periosteum. Typically, fractures in children result from falls that exert a compressive force across a long bone. Rarely is this force perfectly axial, leading instead to one side of the bone being compressed while the opposite side experiences tension. Should the injury involve a significant rotational component, shear forces may prevail, potentially transforming a transverse fracture into a spiral one.[20,27]

The periosteum and bone exhibit different levels of tolerance to compressive and tensile forces, a concept known as biomechanical anisotropy. Fractures often begin at points of maximum tensile stress, where the periosteum and bone are most susceptible. Typically, the periosteum fails first, followed by the cortical bone. Certain fracture types, like toddler's fractures or occult supracondylar humerus fractures, might primarily involve the periosteum. A robust enough force will cause the fracture to extend from the tensile to the compressive side, culminating in a complete fracture. Greenstick fractures occur when the energy from the injury dissipates before affecting the compression side of the bone.[18,42]

In cases of complete fractures, the periosteum on the compression side typically remains intact due to its higher resilience to compressive forces. As the fracture displaces, the periosteum delaminates from the cortex.

In summary, the periosteum around a fracture typically disrupts at the site of greatest tensile force and stays intact but separates in relation to the displacement of the distal fragment on the compression side of the fracture.[60,85]

FOUR ESSENTIAL TASKS FOR MANAGING PEDIATRIC FRACTURES

A principle-based strategy for managing pediatric fractures involves four essential tasks:

1. Identify where the periosteum is torn.
2. Evaluate adjacent soft tissue injury.
3. Employ intact periosteum for fracture reduction.
4. Replace torn periosteum.

Task 1: Identify Where the Periosteum is Torn

The periosteum is characteristically torn at the site of the highest tensile stress and remains intact on the side subjected to compression. Identifying where the periosteum has been torn can often be deduced from clinical signs and radiographic indicators. The forces that tear the periosteum are the same which will impart greatest damage on surrounding periosteum. Therefore, hematoma, swelling, skin discoloration, or an open wound are all clinically observable hallmarks of the location of greatest tension. In cases where the path of fracture displacement poses a threat to neurovascular structures, symptoms such as nerve palsy or a loss of blood flow can also help identify the periosteum's rupture site. For instance, a Gartland type 3B supracondylar humerus fracture generally involves a tear in the anterior and medial periosteum due to a posterior and medial tensile force, with the distal fragment moving posteriorly and laterally. The resultant bruising is typically located anteriorly and medially, correlating with the location of the proximal metaphyseal spike. These injuries may coincide with median nerve palsy or a compromised brachial artery due to their proximity to the trajectory of the displaced fracture.

Radiographs can also help identify the torn periosteum. Prior to any manipulation or management, the distal fracture fragment generally shifts away from the maximal tensile force. A simple way to remember this is in simple transverse fractures is "the fracture apex points toward the side of maximum tension" and the location where the periosteum is likely torn. In addition, fracture features such as comminution and Thurston-Holland fragments and comminution arise from compressive forces and are therefore found opposite the tensile side where the periosteum is disrupted.

In extreme cases, the periosteum can be circumferentially torn, which might occur in traumatic, near-amputation events or because of overly vigorous attempts at fracture reduction. However, these instances are the exception rather than the rule. More commonly, the clinical and radiographic evidence provides a reliable map to pinpoint the anatomical location of the periosteal tear and, by extension, the sections where the periosteum remains intact.

Task 2: Determine the Soft Tissue Collateral Damage

The previously discussed concept highlights that the soft tissues most at risk for damage from displacement of a fracture are located adjacent to the periosteal rupture. Once the bone/periosteum structure fails, any remaining energy of injury is transferred to the surrounding soft tissues. Soft tissues are most vulnerable to tension and so the structures on the tension side of the injury are most at risk. Secondarily, the fracture displacement with distal fragment shifting away from the tension side causes the soft tissues to be draped over the jagged, exposed bony fracture edge. This threatens laceration of any soft tissue structures on the tension side, up to and including the skin.

Using the Gartland Type 3B supracondylar humerus fracture as an illustrative case, the tension side of the injury is anteromedial because the distal fragment is seen displaced posterolateral. The anteromedial/tension side with its torn periosteum and exposed fracture ends poses a threat to adjacent structures—brachial artery and median nerve—and might even lead to an open fracture through the skin. This explains why brachial artery and median nerve injuries are common in significantly displaced Gartland Type 3B supracondylar humerus fractures. A retrospective analysis of 128 cases of supracondylar humerus fractures that had concomitant neurovascular injury found a significant association between the presence of anteromedial bruising and median nerve injuries, as well as between antero-lateral bruising and radial nerve injuries.[91] Every patient who suffered a vascular injury also exhibited anterior or anterome-dial bruising.

Such findings underscore the utility of bruising patterns and radiographic evaluations in identifying neurovascular injuries. The study indicated that bruises alone pinpointed 60.2% of neuro-vascular injuries, while radiographic assessments alone identified 64.1%. However, when both clinical and radiographic findings were combined, they correctly identified 82.0% of neurovascular injuries.[91] Therefore, identifying the site of the torn periosteum with the aid of clinical signs and radiographic evidence is crucial. It enables a high-yield examination to determine status of those critical soft tissue structures most at risk following a fracture.

Task 3: Use the Intact Periosteal Hinge to Reduce the Fracture

The bedrock fracture treatment in pediatric orthopaedics is reduc-tion and casting. Despite being practiced for thousands of years, manual reduction of fractures can still be a challenge. Leveraging the strong biomechanical properties of the periosteum in children makes all reductions easier. This robust periosteum can endure the forces of reduction and assist in maintaining the fracture align-ment postreduction. This approach contrasts sharply with adult fractures, where the periosteum is often circumferentially com-promised, inadequate for reduction support, or the fracture is too comminuted to stay aligned.

In pediatric cases, the periosteum is usually intact on the compression side. The usual displacement of the distal frag-ment is away from the tension side and toward the compression side. Consequently, the reduction maneuver involves moving the distal fragment toward the tension side, relying on the intact periosteum on the compression side to maintain alignment once achieved. Since the periosteum is not elastic and does not stretch beyond its original size, achieving proper length in a completely displaced fracture may require initially increas-ing the fracture displacement toward the compression side—accentuating the injury—to extend the intact periosteum, then hinging the distal fragment back into place.

Understanding these principles is relatively straightforward in the context of direct transverse fractures, such as a simple distal forearm fracture without a rotational component. How-ever, the concept becomes more complex in fractures with rota-tion, like a midshaft forearm fracture resulting from a pronation movement. In both-bone fractures at the same level but with torsion, the reduction process requires derotation to engage the intact periosteum and ensure stabilization.

From these scenarios, the critical takeaway is identifying and leveraging the intact periosteum in pediatric fracture reduction.

Task 4: Replace the Torn Periosteum to Stabilize the Fracture

Understanding that the periosteum plays a role not only in reducing but also securing a fracture is crucial. A torn perios-teum renders any reduction incompletely stable. Predictably,

the fracture is prone to redisplace through the tension side. Therefore, following a reduction, one most "replace the torn periosteum," ensuring the fracture remains in the optimal posi-tion until it achieves inherent stability.

In most pediatric fractures, a well-molded cast suffices to replicate the structural function of torn periosteum. However, significant injuries necessitate more robust internal stabilization using implants such as wires, plates and screws, or intramed-ullary devices. While the biology behind these choices will be covered later, the specific applications for each type of fracture are elaborated upon in their respective chapters.

From a biologic standpoint, given the periosteum is the source of all regenerative materials for fracture healing, it is no surprise that the earliest signs of healing occur at the site of the intact periosteum. Callus formation, the earliest radiographic sign of fracture healing, will be observed on the compressive side of the fracture. Early callus formation can provide valuable confirmation of fracture repair progress and construct stability in cases fixed with relative stability.

FRACTURE FIXATION IN PEDIATRIC ORTHOPAEDICS

In pediatric orthopaedic practice, when fractures cannot be sta-bilized by casting alone, alternative fixation methods become necessary. For fractures where the periosteum is partially intact and strong, minimally invasive techniques like percutaneous pinning or wiring may suffice to hold the fragments in place during healing. However, more significant hardware, such as plates and screws or intramedullary devices, may be required in certain situations. It's important to understand that while these devices offer biomechanical advantages, they can also impact the biologic environment essential for fracture healing. Sur-geons aim to balance strain and vascularity with the fixation method chosen to foster optimal conditions for bone union, highlighting the importance of selecting implants based on a comprehensive understanding of their interaction with the healing process.

PLATING STRATEGIES

For fractures where primary bone healing is the objective, sur-geons might opt for plating methods that ensure absolute stabil-ity. This approach is suitable when there is good blood supply at the fracture ends, and plates and screws are used to compress the fracture, minimizing strain. By reducing the conditions that typically induce endochondral ossification—strain and lack of blood supply—these fractures heal through direct bone forma-tion without needing a cartilage callus. Techniques such as pre-bending plates to increase compression on the opposite cortex are used to encourage primary healing and faster union.[63]

In some cases, achieving absolute stability might be unfea-sible or even detrimental. Striving for such stability might lead to nonunion where (a) proper alignment cannot be achieved, (b) significant portions of the fracture are avascular due to injury, or (c) plating disrupts blood flow excessively. These situations call for a healing approach that can navigate increased strain and vascular challenges, areas where endochondral ossification excels. In these instances, the approach shifts toward providing relative stability.[16,49,93]

Direct measurements of strain and vascularity at the fracture site are not currently possible, but surgeons estimate these based on the fracture's characteristics and the condition of surrounding tissues. It's recognized that fractures with extensive comminution, significant soft tissue damage, or located in areas with poor blood supply necessitate constructs that allow for some movement. Plates can still be an option if used in a manner that permits micromotion at the fracture site, enhancing callus development—a concept known as "biologic plating."[14,16,85]

Achieving the right level of stability with plating is a careful balancing act. While some degree of movement stimulates callus growth, too much can lead to a nonunion. On the other hand, too much rigidity can impede the natural healing process. Maintaining the integrity of the vascularized soft tissues and periosteum at the fracture site is crucial, given their vital role in healing. The design of modern implants, such as limited-contact plates, reflects the importance of preserving the periosteum, allowing bone to contact the implant only around the screw holes.[18,90]

INTRAMEDULLARY NAILING STRATEGIES

Intramedullary nailing is a predominant treatment for many diaphyseal fractures, embodying key healing principles. These nails act as load-sharing devices, fostering relative stability and the micromotion that supports chondrocyte activity and subsequent endochondral ossification. Importantly, this technique spares the periosteum's integrity around the fracture, vital for successful healing.[16]

The reaming process, a prerequisite for intramedullary nailing, does impact the bone's internal blood supply. Although reaming temporarily interrupts the endosteal vascular network, the resulting ischemia is short lived, largely mitigated by an enhanced blood flow from the periosteum. Opting for a larger diameter nail may improve stability postreaming but risks further cortical damage, potentially delaying the recovery of the medullary blood flow. This highlights the critical balance in nail selection—ensuring sufficient stability while minimizing vascular disruption.[85,87]

PHYSEAL FRACTURES

In most fracture scenarios, vascularity and stability are the twin pillars for ensuring a good outcome. However, in cases of periphyseal fracture, vascularity maintains a primacy above that of stability. Depending on the location and the condition of the blood supply, a fracture can either heal efficiently due to the proximity of bone regrowth machinery, or it may lead to significant complications if the fracture disrupts the delicate physeal biology. Therefore, how a periphyseal fracture affects the physis becomes a pivotal consideration for both treatment and outcome predictions. Typically, fractures that are primarily metaphyseal in nature, do not cross the physis, and spare the epiphyseal circulation tend to heal more favorably. This is because the germinal layer of the physis and the blood supply to the epiphysis are preserved, allowing for resumption of normal physeal development postinjury, which generously accommodates for most postfracture healing abnormality. Conversely, fractures that impair the blood flow to the epiphysis can severely and permanently hinder subsequent physeal function. An exception to this is seen with Salter–Harris I or II fractures that are severely displaced, potentially compromising epiphyseal arteries at a distance from the epiphysis.[61,64]

SALTER–HARRIS CLASSIFICATION

The Salter–Harris classification (Fig. 2-10), widely recognized in the field, catalogs five types of physeal injuries. The first four types draw from earlier works by Poland (types I, II, and III)

I   II   III   IV   V

Figure 2-10. Salter–Harris classification of physeal fractures. In Salter–Harris type I fractures, the fracture line is entirely within the physis, referred to by Poland as type I. In Salter–Harris type II fractures, the fracture line extends from the physis into the metaphysis; described by Poland as type II and Aitken as type I. In Salter–Harris type III fractures, the fracture enters the epiphysis from the physis and almost always exits the articular surface. Poland described this injury as type III and Aitken as type II. In Salter–Harris type IV, the fracture extends across the physis from the articular surface and epiphysis, to exit in the margin of the metaphysis. Aitken described this as a type III injury in his classification. Salter–Harris type V fractures were described by Salter and Harris as a crush injury to the physis with initially normal radiographs with late identification of premature physeal closure.

Metaphysis

Endochondral ossification

Hypertrophic

Physis

Proliferative zone

Germinal zone

Epiphysis

Figure 2-11. Scheme of theoretic fracture plane of Salter–Harris type I fractures. Because the hypertrophic zone is the weakest zone structurally, separation should occur at this level. Experimental and clinical studies have confirmed that the fracture plane is more complex than this concept and frequently involves other physeal zones as well.

and Aitken (whose type III became Salter–Harris type IV). Salter and Harris introduced a fifth type, proposing it to be a compression injury that initially appears normal on radiographs but can result in late physeal closure.

Salter–Harris Type I

Salter–Harris type I fractures traverse the physis without any extension into the adjacent metaphysis or epiphysis (Fig. 2-11). Consequently, radiographs may appear normal apart from possible soft tissue swelling, underscoring the importance of a thorough clinical assessment. The Olmstead County Survey found these fractures most common in the phalanges, metacarpals, distal tibia, and ulna. For infants, separations often occur in the upper and lower ends of the humerus and the upper end of the femur. If clinical suspicion is high for a type I injury, additional imaging modalities like ultrasound, MRI, or intraoperative arthrography may be used for diagnosis.[27,66,69]

The fracture line in type I injuries typically lies within the hypertrophic zone of the physis, which offers the least resistance to traumatic forces. This theoretically spares the resting and proliferative zones, thereby reducing the risk of growth disturbances provided there's no vascular damage to these areas. However, this traditional view has been challenged by evidence of uneven loading and physis irregularities, indicating that any physis zone could be vulnerable in such injuries.

Since the articular surface and the critical germinal and proliferative layers of the physis are usually not displaced in type I injuries, and the epiphyseal blood supply remains undisturbed, the focus of treatment is on careful repositioning of the epiphysis atop the metaphysis and providing necessary stabilization for the healing fragments.

Salter–Harris Type II

Salter–Harris type II fractures are characterized by both physeal and metaphyseal involvement, where the fracture line begins at one edge of the growth plate, crosses part of it, and exits through the metaphysis, forming the Thurston-Holland fragment (Fig. 2-12). Despite the damage, since the fracture spares the germinal zone and the epiphyseal blood supply unless it's highly displaced, the risk of growth disturbances is minimal. Treatment mirrors type I, aiming to preserve the articular surface integrity through appropriate alignment and stabilization.[24,33]

Salter–Harris Type III

These fractures start within the epiphysis and cut through the articular surface before traversing the growth plate peripherally (Fig. 2-13). They leave an epiphyseal fragment that is completely isolated from the rest of the bone, attached to the metaphysis. With type III fractures, the risk of subsequent growth disturbance is significantly increased from injury to the vascular supply of the resting zone in the physis. The fracture will heal but likely with a physeal bar in the area with compromised epiphyseal blood supply. These fractures commonly require surgical stabilization for restoration of the articular surface, and stabilization to prevent growth complications is key (Fig. 2-14).[100]

Salter–Harris Type IV

Type IV fractures are essentially vertical shear injuries that disrupt the articular surface and span all layers of the growth plate, posing a significant risk to the epiphyseal blood supply (Fig. 2-15). Again, physeal bars are common as a result of death to the resting and proliferative physeal zones. These fractures are often seen in areas like the medial malleolus and necessitate anatomic reduction along with stabilization in the operating room.[57]

Salter–Harris Type V

Type V fractures, initially proposed by Salter and Harris, represent compression injuries that may not be evident on initial radiographs but can lead to early physeal closure. While some

Figure 2-12. Fracture plane of Salter–Harris type II fractures. The fracture extends from the physis into the periphery of the metaphysis.

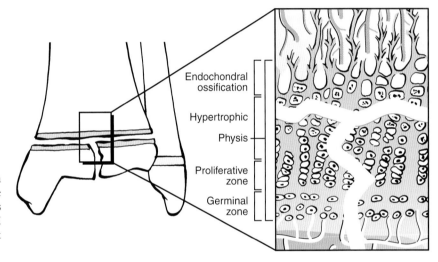

Figure 2-13. Scheme of fracture plane in Salter–Harris type III fractures. The fracture plane extends from the physis into the epiphysis and articular surface. "Extra-articular" type III fractures in which the articular surface is intact have been reported but are quite rare.

Figure 2-14. A: Salter–Harris type III fracture of the distal femur. **B:** Fixation with cannulated screws.

Figure 2-15. Scheme of the Salter–Harris type IV fracture. **A:** The fracture line extends across the physis from the epiphysis and articular surface into the peripheral metaphysis. **B:** Displacement of the fragments can lead to horizontal apposition (and cross-union) of the epiphyseal and metaphyseal bones.

debate exists regarding the nature of these injuries, examples like the closure of the tibial tubercle suggest that such injuries do indeed occur. They might stem from vascular rather than compression trauma, and advanced imaging techniques like MRI may reveal physeal damage not visible on x-rays. Regardless of the exact mechanism, these injuries are considered valid and clinically significant.[43,72]

PETERSON CLASSIFICATION OF PHYSEAL FRACTURES

Acknowledging limitations within the Salter–Harris system, Peterson and colleagues developed a revised classification (Fig. 2-16). It incorporates Salter–Harris types I to IV (renumbered as Peterson types II–V) and introduces two additional types, which are commonly encountered in practice and worth noting.

Peterson's type I involves a transverse metaphyseal fracture that extends longitudinally to the physis, with variations depending on the degree of comminution and fracture pattern (Fig. 2-17).

Peterson's type VI refers to partial loss of the growth plate, often occurring with traumatic injuries such as those from lawn mowers or abrasive road incidents. These injuries may also involve soft tissue damage, neurovascular compromise, and articular surface impairment, making them particularly complex and severe.

ACUTE TREATMENT OF PHYSEAL INJURIES

Evaluation

A variety of imaging techniques are available for assessing physeal injuries, each offering unique insights. The standard initial approach typically involves plain radiographs, which are highly effective for evaluating most physeal injuries. When a physeal injury is suspected, it is crucial to obtain targeted views specifically centered over the suspected physis to minimize parallax and enhance detail. Oblique views can also be instrumental, especially for identifying minimally displaced injuries.

While plain radiographs often provide sufficient detail for assessing and treating most physeal injuries, there are instances where more intricate anatomical details are necessary. In such cases, computed tomography (CT) scans can be invaluable (Fig. 2-18). CT scans, particularly those utilizing reconstructed images, offer excellent visualization of bony structures. They are particularly useful for examining complex or highly comminuted fractures and assessing the articular congruency in cases of minimal displacement.

Magnetic resonance imaging (MRI) scans excel in revealing soft tissue lesions and bone bruises that may be invisible with standard radiographic techniques.[23,28,41,54,55,84,97] MRI has also

I	II	III	IV	V	VI
Metaphysis → Physis	Metaphysis and physis	Physis	Epiphysis and physis	Metaphysis and physis and epiphysis	Physis missing
	Poland II Aitken I Salter–Harris II	Poland I Salter–Harris I	Poland III and IV Aitken II Salter–Harris III	Aitken III Salter–Harris IV	

Figure 2-16. Peterson classification of physeal fractures. Type I is a fracture of the metaphysis extending to the physis. Peterson type VI is epiphyseal (and usually articular surface) loss. Lawn mower injuries are a frequent mechanism for type VI injuries.

proved effective in detecting entrapped periosteum in incomplete closed reductions of Salter–Harris type II fractures. In addition, arthrography,[3,32,46,68,104] MRI, and ultrasound[21,34,35,51,92] can be used to evaluate the congruency of articular surfaces. Arthrography and MRI are especially helpful in young patients with small or nonexistent secondary ossification centers in the epiphyses.

In certain scenarios, particularly for diagnosing epiphyseal separation in infants, ultrasonography emerges as a useful tool.

Its noninvasive nature and the absence of radiation exposure make it an attractive option for this purpose.[21,32,34,35,51]

Treatment

The management of physeal fractures, like all fractures in children, follows a systematic approach. This includes a comprehensive assessment and stabilization of the child, particularly

Figure 2-17. Peterson type I injury of the distal radius. These injuries typically have a benign course with respect to subsequent growth disturbance.

Figure 2-18. CT scans with or without reconstructed images can be helpful in the assessment of physeal fractures. Coronal (**A**) and sagittal (**B**) reconstructions of a triplane fracture of the distal tibia.

if they are polytraumatized, alongside a thorough evaluation of the neurovascular and soft tissue status of the affected limb. The approach to reduction and the decision on what is considered an "acceptable" reduction depend partly on the specific fracture pattern and the potential for remodeling of the fracture site.

Intra-articular fractures, notably Salter–Harris types III and IV, necessitate anatomic reduction. This precision is crucial to restore the integrity of the articular surface and to avert the risk of epiphyseal–metaphyseal cross-union. On the other hand, Salter–Harris type I and II fractures, especially those resulting from low-energy trauma, generally pose minimal risk of growth disturbances, with the exception of those occurring in the distal femur and proximal tibia. These fractures exhibit excellent potential for remodeling in most cases. Nonetheless, care must be taken during surgical intervention to avoid causing additional physeal damage through excessive force or overly invasive reduction techniques.

When performing closed reductions of physeal fractures, the principle of "90% traction, 10% translation" should be adhered to. This approach is designed to minimize iatrogenic injury to the growth plate, which can occur if the physis is subjected to abrasive contact against the sharp edges of the metaphysis.

Repetitive stress physeal injuries are a unique entity to the developing skeleton. Continuous physical activities in children can lead to stress-related physeal injuries, resembling stress fractures. These are commonly observed in the distal radius or ulna of competitive gymnasts, the proximal tibia in sports like soccer, and the proximal humerus in baseball pitchers. Management involves rest, careful resumption of activities, and ongoing observation for potential physeal growth disturbances.

GROWTH DISTURBANCE AFTER PHYSEAL INJURY

Growth disturbance stands as a singular complication predominantly associated with physeal injuries. Often, this disturbance manifests as a form of tethering, known as physeal bar or arrest. However, it's important to note that growth disturbances can sometimes occur without an apparent tether or bar (Fig. 2-19). In some cases, there may even be an acceleration of growth. In addition, growth disturbances can arise even in the absence of an overt injury to the physis.[77]

Physeal growth disturbance, though relatively rare, is a significant complication of physeal fractures. Its potential ramifications include angular deformities, limb-length discrepancies, epiphyseal distortion, or a combination of these issues. The development and severity of these abnormalities depend on several factors: the specific physis involved, the location of the

A, B   **C**

Figure 2-19. Growth deceleration in the absence of a true physeal arrest. This patient sustained concurrent ipsilateral femoral shaft and Salter–Harris type IV distal femoral epiphyseal fractures. **A:** Anteroposterior radiograph of the healed femur. Both fractures were treated with internal fixation. **B:** The patient developed valgus deformity of the distal femur because of asymmetric growth of the distal femoral physis. Note that the distance between the screws on either side of the physis has increased asymmetrically, confirming asymmetric growth rather than cessation of growth laterally. **C:** The angular deformity was treated with medial distal femoral epiphyseal stapling.

disturbance within the physis, the duration for which the disturbance has been present, and the patient's stage of skeletal maturity.[8–10,44,48]

The manifestation of physeal growth disturbance can vary. It might appear as a radiographic abnormality on serial radiographs in a patient known to be at risk post fracture or infection. Clinically, it can present with established limb deformity, such as angular deformity or shortening, or it may be incidentally discovered on radiographs taken for other reasons. The classic radiographic features include the loss of the normal physeal contour and a well-defined radiolucency between the epiphyseal and metaphyseal bones. Frank physeal arrests are typically characterized by sclerosis in the arrest region, and if asymmetric growth has occurred, there may be a tapering growth arrest line, angular deformity, epiphyseal distortion, or limb shortening. Physeal growth disturbance without a complete arrest usually presents as a thinner or thicker physeal area with an indistinct metaphyseal border, indicating altered endochondral ossification.

When a growth arrest is suspected in a skeletally immature child, further diagnostic evaluation is often necessary. CT scans with sagittal and coronal reconstructions can clearly reveal areas of bone bridging the physis (Fig. 2-20). MRI is another sensitive method for assessing physeal architecture, capable of providing detailed images of the physis and the area of growth disturbance (Fig. 2-21). It can also assess the organization of the remaining

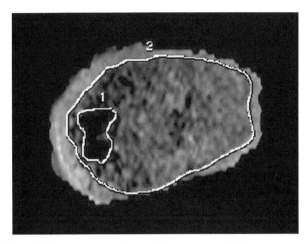

Figure 2-21. Reconstructed MRIs allow estimation of the percentage of surface area of the physis affected by a growth arrest. This workstation reconstruction delineates the perimeter of normal physis (border 2) and that of the physeal arrest (border 1). Surface area affected can be calculated from these reconstructions.

physis, indicating its relative "health," which is particularly useful in cases of infection, irradiation, or tumor in determining the feasibility of arrest resection.

In addition to advanced imaging, conventional radiographic evaluation remains valuable. Radiographs of the entire affected

Figure 2-20. Harris growth arrest line tapering to the physis at the level of the growth arrest can serve as an excellent radiograph confirmation of the presence of the true growth arrest. Although most commonly noted on plain radiographs, these arrest lines can be seen on CT scans and MRIs as well. **A:** Anteroposterior radiograph of the distal tibia after Salter–Harris type IV fracture demonstrates a Harris growth arrest line (*arrows*) tapering to the medial distal tibial physis, where a partial physeal arrest has formed. **B:** Harris growth arrest line (*arrows*) as noted on CT. CT scans with coronal (**C**) and sagittal (**D**) reconstructions corrected for bone distortion provide excellent images of the location and size of the arrest.

limb are important for documenting the extent of any angular deformity and for assessing existing limb-length inequality using a scanogram. Estimating the predicted growth remaining in the unaffected contralateral physis, based on the child's skeletal age and appropriate growth tables, is also a critical component of the overall assessment.

Many bones show transversely oriented, dense trabecular linear bone patterns within the metaphysis, known as Harris or Park growth slowdown or arrest lines. These lines emerge following events that temporarily slow growth or increase mineralization, such as illnesses, bisphosphonate drug treatments, infection, or growth plate trauma. After normal growth resumes, these lines, left behind in the metaphysis, gradually remodel and eventually disappear (see Fig. 2-21). In systemic issues affecting bone growth, these lines appear symmetrically throughout the skeleton, being thickest in the rapidly growing bones' metaphyses. They are crucial for analyzing the impact of fractures on growth, as they can corroborate femoral overgrowth postdiaphyseal fracture or medial eccentric overgrowth post–proximal tibia metaphyseal fracture. A line converging toward a physis indicates localized growth damage that could result in an osseous bridge, risking angular deformity (see Fig. 2-8).

Growth Disturbance Without Arrest

Growth deceleration, distinct from a total cessation of growth, is characterized radiographically by changes in the appearance of the physis, typically showing a relative widening with indistinct metaphyseal boundaries. Clinically, this may be accompanied by deformities, particularly if the disturbance is significant and longstanding. Differentiating between growth deceleration without complete arrest and true physeal arrest is crucial, as the management strategies and outcomes for these two conditions differ significantly.

Unlike physeal arrests, these cases do not display a sclerotic area of arrest on plain radiographs. Any growth arrest line present may appear asymmetric but will not taper directly to the physis, indicating growth asymmetry rather than a complete halt. In addition, the resulting deformity may not always progress relentlessly and can sometimes show improvement over time.

On the other hand, growth acceleration is most commonly seen after proximal tibial fractures and femur fractures in young patients (Fig. 2-22). This acceleration typically resolves spontaneously.

Management of Growth Disturbance

In situations where the radiographic abnormality is stable, regular and meticulous observation may be sufficient. However, it is crucial to monitor the condition closely, as any progressive deformity will necessitate intervention.

If angular deformity is present or progressing, several treatment options are available. These include hemiepiphysiodesis or physeal tethering using staples, screws, or tension plates and corrective osteotomy, with or without completion of the epiphysiodesis.[25,39,73,74,76,95,98,103] When there's no clear physeal arrest, hemiepiphysiodesis or tethering on the convex side of the affected physis can gradually correct the deformity. Upon

Figure 2-22. A: AP radiograph of the tibia of a 4-year-old shows a proximal metaphyseal fracture with minimal displacement in the fibula intact. **B:** Two years later, note the significant valgus deformity.

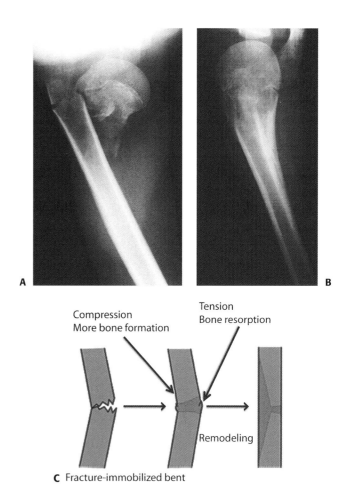

Figure 2-23. Remodeling of a fracture. Initial (**A**) and follow-up (**B**) radiographs of a proximal humeral fracture, illustrating an impressive degree of remodeling. **C:** How bone deposition and resorption result in straightening of the deformity over time. Efficient remodeling requires an open growth plate, and as such is a unique feature of childhood injury.

correction, further options include completing the epiphysiodesis (potentially alongside contralateral epiphysiodesis to avoid significant limb-length disparity) and removing the tethering device, followed by careful observation for any recurrence or overcorrection of the deformity. Despite various techniques and implants available for physeal tethering, there is currently no conclusive evidence favoring one method.

Corrective osteotomy is another viable approach for managing established angular deformity due to growth disturbance. The surgeon must determine whether to perform epiphysiodesis on the affected physis, possibly along with contralateral epiphysiodesis, to prevent recurrence.

The development of a bony bridge across a segment of the physis can lead to partial physeal arrest. Partial physeal arrests can cause angular deformity, joint distortion, limb-length inequality, or a combination thereof. The specific outcome depends on the location of the arrest, the remaining growth rate and extent in the involved physis, and the overall health of the residual affected physis.

BONE REMODELING AFTER A FRACTURE

In children, the ongoing process of bone growth can correct malunited fractures, reducing the need for anatomic reduction compared to adults.[22,65,94] This remodeling occurs in response to body weight, muscle action, joint reaction forces, and intrinsic mechanisms like the periosteum's influence. The likelihood of spontaneous and complete correction is higher in younger children, when fractures are near the physis, and when the angulation aligns with the joint's normal plane of motion (see Fig. 2-23). This is particularly noticeable in hinge joints like the knee, ankle, elbow, or wrist, where corrections in the normal motion plane happen relatively swiftly. For example, the distal radius can correct deformities at a rate of one degree per month. However, spontaneous correction is less likely for angular deformities in planes outside of normal motion, such as cubitus varus deformity following a supracondylar humerus fracture. Similarly, rotational deformities generally do not correct spontaneously.

Annotated References

Reference	Annotation
Baker CE, Moore-Lotridge SN, Hysong AA, et al. Bone fracture acute phase response: a unifying theory of fracture repair: clinical and scientific implications. *Clin Rev Bone Miner Metab.* 2018;16(4):142–158.	The proposed model for bone fracture repair addresses five key challenges—bleeding, infection, hypoxia, strain, and weight bearing—by integrating advances in molecular biology and clinical practices into a comprehensive framework. Centered around the acute phase response (APR), it outlines a sequential approach to "survival" and "repair," emphasizing the need for balanced interventions to prevent complications and ensure effective healing. This framework serves both as a guide for clinicians in optimizing fracture management and as a basis for future research into the complex process of bone regeneration.
Hajdu KS, Baker CE, Moore-Lotridge SN, Schoenecker JG. Sequestration and involucrum: understanding bone necrosis and revascularization in pediatric orthopedics. *Orthop Clin North Am.* 2024;55(2):233–246.	While focused on the pathophysiology of sequestration and involucrum, this article provides the most up-to-date description of vascular anatomy of developing bone and repair.
Mangialardi G, Cordaro A, Madeddu P. The bone marrow pericyte: an orchestrator of vascular niche. *Regen Med.* 2016;11(8):883–895.	The understanding of pericytes has transformed from seeing them merely as sources of trophic support and vascular stability to recognizing their multipotent nature, especially as key stem cells in bone biology. This review focuses on the perivascular population in bone marrow, examining their relationships with other niche components, their linkage to bone marrow stromal stem cells, and how they differ from perivascular populations in the vessel/wall niche. The discussion ends by exploring the regenerative capabilities of these cells in bone biology and the obstacles to their use in cell therapy.
Marsell R, Einhorn TA. The biology of fracture healing. *Injury.* 2011;42(6):551–555.	Fracture healing is a complex biologic process that involves specific regenerative patterns and changes in gene expression, with both anatomical and biochemical pathways thoroughly investigated. Indirect healing is more common and involves an initial acute inflammatory response, followed by the formation of a cartilaginous callus that undergoes revascularization, calcification, and remodeling to restore normal bone structure. Direct healing, requiring anatomical reduction and stable conditions, regenerates lamellar bone and Haversian systems without remodeling but is less common due to the stringent conditions it necessitates.

Annotated References	
Reference	**Annotation**
Roberts SJ, van Gastel N, Carmeliet G, Luyten FP. Uncovering the periosteum for skeletal regeneration: the stem cell that lies beneath. *Bone*. 2015;70:10–18.	The periosteum, recognized for its cartilage- and bone-forming capabilities, is a crucial source of skeletal progenitor cells, playing a significant role in bone development, growth, and fracture healing. Advances in research tools and techniques have enhanced our understanding of periosteal cells' specific roles and regulatory mechanisms. This article reviews periosteal cell biology, including its cellular composition, molecular regulation, and the potential of periosteum-derived cells in bone tissue engineering and regenerative medicine, highlighting its significance in a special issue on stem cells and bone.

REFERENCES

1. Abram LJ, Thompson GH. Deformity after premature closure of the distal radial physis following a torus fracture with a physeal compression injury. Report of a case. *J Bone Joint Surg Am*. 1987;69(9):1450–1453.
2. Aitken AP. The end results of the fractured distal tibial epiphysis. *J Bone Joint Surg Am*. 1936;18:685–691.
3. Akbarnia BA, Silberstein MJ, Rende RJ, et al. Arthrography in the diagnosis of fractures of the distal end of the humerus in infants. *J Bone Joint Surg Am*. 1986;68(4):599–602.
4. Akiyama H, Kim JE, Nakashima K, et al. Osteo-chondroprogenitor cells are derived from Sox9 expressing precursors. *Proc Natl Acad Sci U S A*. 2005;102(41):14665–14670.
5. Allen MR, Hock JM, Burr DB. Periosteum: biology, regulation, and response to osteoporosis therapies. *Bone*. 2004;35(5):1003–1012.
6. Amini S, Mortazavi F, Sun J, et al. Stress relaxation of swine growth plate in semi-confined compression: depth dependent tissue deformational behavior versus extracellular matrix composition and collagen fiber organization. *Biomech Model Mechanobiol*. 2013;12(1):67–78.
7. Amini S, Veilleux D, Villemure I. Tissue and cellular morphological changes in growth plate explants under compression. *J Biomech*. 2010;43(13):2582–2588.
8. Anderson M, Green WT. Lengths of the femur and the tibia; norms derived from orthoroentgenograms of children from 5 years of age until epiphysial closure. *Am J Dis Child (1911)*. 1948;75(3):279–290.
9. Anderson M, Green WT, Messner MB. Growth and predictions of growth in the lower extremities. *J Bone Joint Surg Am*. 1963;45-A:1–14.
10. Anderson M, Messner MB, Green WT. Distribution of lengths of the normal femur and tibia in children from one to eighteen years of age. *J Bone Joint Surg Am*. 1964;46:1197–1202.
11. Antabak A, Papes D, Haluzan D, et al. Reducing damage to the periosteal capillary network caused by internal fixation plating: an experimental study. *Injury*. 2015;46(Suppl 6):S18–S20.
12. Arikawa T, Omura K, Morita I. Regulation of bone morphogenetic protein-2 expression by endogenous prostaglandin E2 in human mesenchymal stem cells. *J Cell Physiol*. 2004;200(3):400–406.
13. Armulik A, Genové G, Betsholtz C. Pericytes: developmental, physiological, and pathological perspectives, problems, and promises. *Dev Cell*. 2011;21(2):193–215.
14. Augat P, Simon U, Liedert A, Claes L. Mechanics and mechano-biology of fracture healing in normal and osteoporotic bone. *Osteoporos Int*. 2005;16(suppl 2):S36–S43.
15. Augustin G, Antabak A, Davila S. The periosteum. Part 1: anatomy, histology and molecular biology. *Injury*. 2007;38(10):1115–1130.
16. Baker CE, Moore-Lotridge SN, Hysong AA, et al. Bone fracture acute phase response: a unifying theory of fracture repair: clinical and scientific implications. *Clin Rev Bone Miner Metab*. 2018;16(4):142–158.
17. Ballock RT, O'Keefe RJ. Physiology and pathophysiology of the growth plate. *Birth Defects Res C Embryo Today*. 2003;69(2):123–143.
18. Barthelemi S, Robinet J, Garnotel R, et al. Mechanical forces-induced human osteoblasts differentiation involves MMP-2/MMP-13/MT1-MMP proteolytic cascade. *J Cell Biochem*. 2012;113(3):760–772.
19. Bitgood MJ, McMahon AP. Hedgehog and Bmp genes are coexpressed at many diverse sites of cell-cell interaction in the mouse embryo. *Dev Biol*. 1995;172(1):126–138.
20. Bleuel J, Zaucke F, Brüggemann GP, Niehoff A. Effects of cyclic tensile strain on chondrocyte metabolism: a systematic review. *PLoS One*. 2015;10(3):e0119816.
21. Broker FH, Burbach T. Ultrasonic diagnosis of separation of the proximal humeral epiphysis in the newborn. *J Bone Joint Surg Am*. 1990;72(2):187–191.
22. Burkus JK, Ogden JA. Development of the distal femoral epiphysis: a microscopic morphological investigation of the zone of Ranvier. *J Pediatr Orthop*. 1984;4(6):661–668.
23. Carey J, Spence L, Blickman H, Eustace S. MRI of pediatric growth plate injury: correlation with plain film radiographs and clinical outcome. *Skeletal Radiol*. 1998;27(5):250–255.
24. Cass JR, Peterson HA. Salter-Harris Type-IV injuries of the distal tibial epiphyseal growth plate, with emphasis on those involving the medial malleolus. *J Bone Joint Surg Am*. 1983;65(8):1059–1070.
25. Castaneda P, Urquhart B, Sullivan E, Haynes RJ. Hemiepiphysiodesis for the correction of angular deformity about the knee. *J Pediatr Orthop*. 2008;28(2):188–191.
26. Castillo RC, Bosse MJ, MacKenzie EJ, Patterson BM; LEAP Study Group. Impact of smoking on fracture healing and risk of complications in limb-threatening open tibia fractures. *J Orthop Trauma*. 2005;19(3):151–157.
27. Claes LE, Heigele CA. Magnitudes of local stress and strain along bony surfaces predict the course and type of fracture healing. *J Biomech*. 1999;32(3):255–266.
28. Close BJ, Strouse PJ. MR of physeal fractures of the adolescent knee. *Pediatr Radiol*. 2000;30(11):756–762.
29. Colnot C, Zhang X, Knothe Tate ML. Current insights on the regenerative potential of the periosteum: molecular, cellular, and endogenous engineering approaches. *J Orthop Res*. 2012;30(12):1869–1878.
30. Cooper C, Dennison EM, Leufkens HGM, et al. Epidemiology of childhood fractures in Britain: a study using the general practice research database. *J Bone Miner Res*. 2004;19(12):1976–1981.
31. Dale GG, Harris WR. Prognosis of epiphysial separation: an experimental study. *J Bone Joint Surg Br*. 1958;40-B(1):116–122.
32. Davidson RS, Markowitz RI, Dormans J, Drummond DS. Ultrasonographic evaluation of the elbow in infants and young children after suspected trauma. *J Bone Joint Surg Am*. 1994;76(12):1804–1813.
33. Deckers MM, van Bezooijen RL, van der Horst G, et al. Bone morphogenetic proteins stimulate angiogenesis through osteoblast-derived vascular endothelial growth factor A. *Endocrinology*. 2002;143(4):1545–1553.
34. Dias JJ, Lamont AC, Jones JM. Ultrasonic diagnosis of neonatal separation of the distal humeral epiphysis. *J Bone Joint Surg Br*. 1988;70(5):825–828.
35. Diaz MJ, Hedlund GL. Sonographic diagnosis of traumatic separation of the proximal femoral epiphysis in the neonate. *Pediatr Radiol*. 1991;21(3):238–240.
36. Dy P, Wang W, Bhattaram P, et al. Sox9 directs hypertrophic maturation and blocks osteoblast differentiation of growth plate chondrocytes. *Dev Cell*. 2012;22(3):597–609.
37. Einhorn TA. The cell and molecular biology of fracture healing. *Clin Orthop Relat Res*. 1998;(355 Suppl):S7–S21.
38. Farnum CE, Lenox M, Zipfel W, et al. In vivo delivery of fluoresceinated dextrans to the murine growth plate: imaging of three vascular routes by multiphoton microscopy. *Anat Rec A Discov Mol Cell Evol Biol*. 2006;288(1):91–103.
39. Fraser RK, Dickens DR, Cole WG. Medial physeal stapling for primary and secondary genu valgum in late childhood and adolescence. *J Bone Joint Surg Br*. 1995;77(5):733–735.
40. Friberg KS. Remodelling after distal forearm fractures in children. I. The effect of residual angulation on the spatial orientation of the epiphyseal plates. *Acta Orthop Scand*. 1979;50(5):537–546.
41. Gabel GT, Peterson HA, Berquist TH. Premature partial physeal arrest. Diagnosis by magnetic resonance imaging in two cases. *Clin Orthop Relat Res*. 1991;(272):242–247.
42. Gaston MS, Simpson AHRW. Inhibition of fracture healing. *J Bone Joint Surg Br*. 2007;89(12):1553–1560.
43. Gerber HP, Vu TH, Ryan AM, et al. VEGF couples hypertrophic cartilage remodeling, ossification and angiogenesis during endochondral bone formation. *Nat Med*. 1999;5(6):623–628.
44. Green WT, Anderson M. Skeletal age and the control of bone growth. *Instr Course Lect*. 1960;17:199–217.
45. Hajdu KS, Baker CE, Moore-Lotridge SN, Schoenecker G. Sequestration and involucrum: understanding bone necrosis and revascularization in pediatric orthopedics. *Orthop Clin North Am*. 2023. https://doi.org/10.1016/j.ocl.2023.09.005
46. Hansen PE, Barnes DA, Tullos HS. Arthrographic diagnosis of an injury pattern in the distal humerus of an infant. *J Pediatr Orthop*. 1982;2(5):569–572.
47. Hedstrom EM, Svensson O, Bergström U, Michno P. Epidemiology of fractures in children and adolescents. *Acta Orthop*. 2010;81(1):148–153.
48. Hensinger R. Linear growth of long bones of the lower extremity from infancy to adolescence. In: Hensinger R, ed. *Standards in Pediatric Orthopaedics: Table, Charts, and Graphs Illustrating Growth*. Raven Press Books; 1986:232–233.
49. Hirao M, Tamai N, Tsumaki N, Yoshikawa H, Myoui A. Oxygen tension regulates chondrocyte differentiation and function during endochondral ossification. *J Biol Chem*. 2006;281(41):31079–31092.
50. Houshian S, Holst AK, Larsen MS, Torfing T. Remodeling of Salter-Harris type II epiphyseal plate injury of the distal radius. *J Pediatr Orthop*. 2004;24(5):472–476.

51. Howard CB, Shinwell E, Nyska M,Meller I. Ultrasound diagnosis of neonatal fracture separation of the upper humeral epiphysis. *J Bone Joint Surg Br.* 1992; 74(3):471–472.

52. Hunter LY, Hensinger RN. Premature monomelic growth arrest following fracture of the femoral shaft. A case report. *J Bone Joint Surg Am.* 1978;60(6):850–852.

53. Jacobsen FS. Periosteum: its relation to pediatric fractures. *J Pediatr Orthop B.* 1997;6(2):84–90.

54. Jain R, Bielski RJ. Fracture of lower femoral epiphysis in an infant at birth: a rare obstetrical injury. *J Perinatol.* 2001;21(8):550–552.

55. Jaramillo D, Kammen BF, Shapiro F. Cartilaginous path of physeal fracture-separations: evaluation with MR imaging–an experimental study with histologic correlation in rabbits. *Radiology.* 2000;215(2):504–511.

56. Jiao H, Xiao E, Graves DT. Diabetes and its effect on bone and fracture healing. *Curr Osteoporos Rep.* 2015;13(5):327–335.

57. Kasser JR. Physeal bar resections after growth arrest about the knee. *Clin Orthop Relat Res.* 1990;(255):68–74.

58. Keaveny TM, Hayes WC. A 20-year perspective on the mechanical properties of trabecular bone. *J Biomech Eng.* 1993;115(4B):534–542.

59. Kim HK, Stephenson N, Garces A, et al. Effects of disruption of epiphyseal vasculature on the proximal femoral growth plate. *J Bone Joint Surg Am.* 2009;91(5):1149–1158.

60. Knothe Tate ML, Ritzman TF, Schneider E, Knothe UR. Testing of a new one-stage bone-transport surgical procedure exploiting the periosteum for the repair of long-bone defects. *J Bone Joint Surg Am.* 2007;89(2):307–316.

61. Kolodny A. Periosteal blood supply and healing fractures. *J Bone Joint Surg Am.* 1923;5:698–711.

62. Kronenberg HM. Developmental regulation of the growth plate. *Nature.* 2003; 423(6937):332–336.

63. Kubiak EN, Fulkerson E, Strauss E, Egol KA. The evolution of locked plates. *J Bone Joint Surg Am.* 2006;88(Suppl 4):189–200.

64. Landin LA. Fracture patterns in children. Analysis of 8,682 fractures with special reference to incidence, etiology and secular changes in a Swedish urban population 1950–1979. *Acta Orthop Scand Suppl.* 1983;202:1–109.

65. Larsen E, Vittas D, Torp-Pedersen S. Remodeling of angulated distal forearm fractures in children. *Clin Orthop Relat Res.* 1988;(237):190–195.

66. Mangialardi G, Cordaro A, Madeddu P. The bone marrow pericyte: an orchestrator of vascular niche. *Regen Med.* 2016;11(8):883–895.

67. Marsell R, Einhorn TA. The biology of fracture healing. *Injury.* 2011;42(6):551–555.

68. Marzo JM, d'Amato C, Strong M, Gillespie R. Usefulness and accuracy of arthrography in management of lateral humeral condyle fractures in children. *J Pediatr Orthop.* 1990;10(3):317–321.

69. Matthews BG, Grcevic D, Wang L, et al. Analysis of αSMA-labeled progenitor cell commitment identifies notch signaling as an important pathway in fracture healing. *J Bone Miner Res.* 2014;29(5):1283–1294.

70. Mayba II. Avulsion fracture of the tibial tubercle apophysis with avulsion of patellar ligament. *J Pediatr Orthop.* 1982;2(3):303–305.

71. McKibbin B. The biology of fracture healing in long bones. *J Bone Joint Surg Br.* 1978;60-B(2):150–162.

72. Mendez AA, Bartal E, Grillot MB, Lin JJ. Compression (Salter-Harris Type V) physeal fracture: an experimental model in the rat. *J Pediatr Orthop.* 1992;12(1):29–37.

73. Metaizeau JP, Wong-Chung J, Bertrand H, Pasquier P. Percutaneous epiphysiodesis using transphyseal screws (PETS). *J Pediatr Orthop.* 1998;18(3):363–369.

74. Mielke CH, Stevens PM. Hemiepiphyseal stapling for knee deformities in children younger than 10 years: a preliminary report. *J Pediatr Orthop.* 1996;16(4):423–429.

75. Moen CT, Pelker RR. Biomechanical and histological correlations in growth plate failure. *J Pediatr Orthop.* 1984;4(2):180–184.

76. Nouth F, Kuo LA. Percutaneous epiphysiodesis using transphyseal screws (PETS): prospective case study and review. *J Pediatr Orthop.* 2004;24(6):721–725.

77. Ogden JA. Growth slowdown and arrest lines. *J Pediatr Orthop.* 1984;4(4):409–415.

78. Ogden JA. Skeletal growth mechanism injury patterns. *J Pediatr Orthop.* 1982; 2(4):371–377.

79. Ozaki A, Tsunoda M, Kinoshita S, Saura R. Role of fracture hematoma and periosteum during fracture healing in rats: interaction of fracture hematoma and the periosteum in the initial step of the healing process. *J Orthop Sci.* 2000;5(1):64–70.

80. Pearson OM, Lieberman DE. The aging of Wolff's "law": ontogeny and responses to mechanical loading in cortical bone. *Am J Phys Anthropol.* 2004;(Suppl 39):63–99.

81. Peinado Cortés LM, Vanegas Acosta JC, Garzón Alvarado DA. A mechanobiological model of epiphysis structures formation. *J Theor Biol.* 2011;287:13–25.

82. Perren SM. Physical and biological aspects of fracture healing with special reference to internal fixation. *Clin Orthop Relat Res.* 1979;(138):175–196.

83. Peters W, Irving J, Letts M. Long-term effects of neonatal bone and joint infection on adjacent growth plates. *J Pediatr Orthop.* 1992;12(6):806–810.

84. Petit P, Panuel M, Faure F, et al. Acute fracture of the distal tibial physis: role of gradient-echo MR imaging versus plain film examination. *AJR Am J Roentgenol.* 1996;166(5):1203–1206.

85. Pfeifer R, Sellei R, Pape HC. The biology of intramedullary reaming. *Injury.* 2010;41(Suppl 2):S4–S8.

86. Rhinelander FW. The normal microcirculation of diaphyseal cortex and its response to fracture. *J Bone Joint Surg Am.* 1968;50(4):784–800.

87. Rhinelander FW. Tibial blood supply in relation to fracture healing. *Clin Orthop Relat Res.* 1974;(105):34–81.

88. Rivas R, Shapiro F. Structural stages in the development of the long bones and epiphyses: a study in the New Zealand white rabbit. *J Bone Joint Surg Am.* 2002;84-A(1):85–100.

89. Roberts SJ, van Gastel N, Carmeliet G, Luyten FP. Uncovering the periosteum for skeletal regeneration: the stem cell that lies beneath. *Bone.* 2015;70:10–18.

90. Schmal H, Strohm PC, Jaeger M, Südkamp NP. Flexible fixation and fracture healing: do locked plating 'internal fixators' resemble external fixators? *J Orthop Trauma.* 2011;25(Suppl 1):S15–S20.

91. Schultz JD, Rees AB, Wollenman LC, et al. bruise location in supracondylar humerus fractures predicts specific neurovascular injuries. *J Pediatr Orthop.* 2022;42(3): e250–e256.

92. Sferopoulos NK. Fracture separation of the medial clavicular epiphysis: ultrasonography findings. *Arch Orthop Trauma Surg.* 2003;123(7):367–369.

93. Shao J, Zhang Y, Yang T, et al. HIF-1α disturbs osteoblasts and osteoclasts coupling in bone remodeling by up-regulating OPG expression. *In Vitro Cell Dev Biol Anim.* 2015;51(8):808–814.

94. Shapiro F, Holtrop ME, Glimcher MJ. Organization and cellular biology of the perichondrial ossification groove of Ranvier: a morphological study in rabbits. *J Bone Joint Surg Am.* 1977;59(6):703–723.

95. Shin SJ, Cho TJ, Park MS, et al. Angular deformity correction by asymmetrical physeal suppression in growing children: stapling versus percutaneous transphyseal screw. *J Pediatr Orthop.* 2010;30(6):588–593.

96. Siffert RS, Katz JF. Growth recovery zones. *J Pediatr Orthop.* 1983;3(2):196–201.

97. Smith BG, Rand F, Jaramillo D, Shapiro F. Early MR imaging of lower-extremity physeal fracture-separations: a preliminary report. *J Pediatr Orthop.* 1994;14(4):526–533.

98. Stevens PM, Pease F. Hemiepiphysiodesis for posttraumatic tibial valgus. *J Pediatr Orthop.* 2006;26(3):385–392.

99. Trueta J, Little K. The vascular contribution to osteogenesis. II. Studies with the electron microscope. *J Bone Joint Surg Br.* 1960;42-B:367–376.

100. Trueta J, Morgan JD. The vascular contribution to osteogenesis. I. Studies by the injection method. *J Bone Joint Surg Br.* 1960;42-B:97–109.

101. Tschegg EK, Celarek A, Fischerauer SF, et al. Fracture properties of growth plate cartilage compared to cortical and trabecular bone in ovine femora. *J Mech Behav Biomed Mater.* 2012;14:119–129.

102. Wattenbarger JM, Gruber HE, Phieffer LS. Physeal fractures, part I: histologic features of bone, cartilage, and bar formation in a small animal model. *J Pediatr Orthop.* 2002;22(6):703–709.

103. Wiemann JM IV, Tryon C, Szalay EA. Physeal stapling versus 8-plate hemiepiphysiodesis for guided correction of angular deformity about the knee. *J Pediatr Orthop.* 2009;29(5):481–485.

104. Yates C, Sullivan JA. Arthrographic diagnosis of elbow injuries in children. *J Pediatr Orthop.* 1987;7(1):54–60.

105. Yuasa M, Mignemi NA, Barnett JV, et al. The temporal and spatial development of vascularity in a healing displaced fracture. *Bone.* 2014;67:208–221.

3

Pharmacology of Pediatric Fracture Care

Stephanie N. Moore-Lotridge, James E. Cassat, Jon Niconchuk, Andrew D. Franklin, and Nathaniel Lempert

ANALGESICS

PRINCIPLES OF ACUTE PAIN RELIEF

In 1986, the World Health Organization (WHO) formulated the "ladder" strategy for stepwise escalation of analgesic therapy, and this concept remains applicable for the management of acute pain following pediatric fracture.[29] This approach states that if a pharmacologic agent is needed to manage pain, it is most appropriate to start with simple analgesics (acetaminophen, ibuprofen) and progress to opioids if significant pain persists. Physicians should consider the patient's age, weight, comorbidities, and allergies/intolerances when selecting the appropriate analgesics for pediatric patients. This section will review recent evidence regarding best practices for the pharmacologic management of acute pain in pediatric fracture care (Table 3-1).

Enteral administration of analgesics is common in the context of acute injury. Analgesics may be provided by medical providers in the emergency department or caregivers following an injury. The most common analgesics include acetaminophen, nonsteroidal anti-inflammatory drugs (NSAIDs), and opioids. Over the past 15 years, multiple clinical trials have been conducted to determine the most efficacious analgesic regimens for pediatric fracture care.[3,4] Notably, a randomized trial conducted in 2014 compared the use of oral ibuprofen to oral morphine in pediatric fracture patients and concluded that despite no differences in analgesic efficacy between the two groups, a significantly greater number of adverse events, including nausea and vomiting, were seen in the morphine cohort. The authors thus suggested the use of ibuprofen for outpatient pain management of uncomplicated fractures.[31]

Given the frequent use of ibuprofen for pediatric fracture care, numerous retrospective and prospective clinical trials have studied the impact of NSAID use on bone healing. When assessed in adult patients, NSAID use is weakly associated with increased rates of delayed union or nonunion,[39] but these results have not been replicated in pediatric studies. A prospective randomized clinical trial from the University of Missouri of 102 pediatric patients found that the administration of NSAIDs, specifically ibuprofen, did not impair clinical or radiologic healing parameters of long bone fractures.[34] Likewise, a retrospective study of 808 pediatric patients found that exposure to ibuprofen did not alter the healing of extremity fractures. Finally, a recent systematic review confirmed that NSAID use in pediatric patients provides adequate analgesia without increasing the risk of nonunion in long bone fractures.[16]

In cases of more severe displaced fractures requiring reduction and/or operative fixation, multimodal pharmacologic approaches aimed at providing both anxiolysis and analgesia should be utilized in pediatric patients (see Table 3-1). Anxiety and emotional distress in children with acute fractures may be mitigated by pharmacologic and nonpharmacologic interventions. In patients requiring fracture reduction in the emergency department, analgesics are often administered concomitantly with agents used for conscious sedation. Nitrous oxide, benzodiazepines, opioids, ketamine, and propofol are commonly utilized to achieve analgesia and/or sedation.[7] In addition to pharmacologic therapy, distraction techniques may reduce anxiety and emotional distress.

TABLE 3-1. Common Pediatric Analgesics

Drug	Dosage	Maximum Dose	Oral Liquid Available?	Common Concentrations
Acetaminophen (Tylenol)	10 mg/kg PO/IV every 6 hours	4,000 mg/day or 60 mg/kg/day	Yes	160 mg/5 mL, 500 mg/5 mL
Ibuprofen (Motrin)	10 mg/kg PO every 6 hours	2,400 mg/day or 40 mg/kg/day	Yes	100 mg/5 mL
Ketorolac (Toradol)	0.5 mg/kg IV every 6 hours	30 mg/dose, 90 mg/day	No	
Cyclobenzaprine (Flexeril)	2.5–10 mg every 8 hours	10 mg/dose	No	
Tizanidine (Zanaflex)	2–4 mg per dose; 0.3 mg/kg/day (in 3–4 divided doses)	24 mg/day	Yes	1 mg/mL (prepared by pharmacy)
Diazepam (Valium)	0.1–0.2 mg/kg/dose 2–4 times per day	10 mg/dose	Yes	1 mg/mL
Oxycodone (Roxicodone)	0.1–0.2 mg/kg every 4–6 hours PRN	5–10 mg/dose	Yes	5 mg/5 mL (i.e., 1 mg/mL)
Gabapentin (Neurontin)	5 mg/kg	300 mg every 8 hours (may increase to 900 mg every 8 hours); 3,600 mg/day	Yes	250 mg/5 mL

Children may be provided a toy, book, or an electronic device to divert focus and provide distraction during the procedure. Recent studies have highlighted how virtual reality (VR) platforms and music can be utilized in children receiving treatment in the emergency department to provide sufficient distraction to result in anxiolysis and reduced pain perception.[2,6,13] Physicians can also engage the child in conversation or encourage breathing exercises to activate the parasympathetic nervous symptom and help with relaxation. Finally, physicians should consider involving the parents/caretaker, nurses, or ancillary staff in the process to help reduce anxiety. Certified child life specialists (CCLSs) are formally trained professionals with proficiency in helping children during stressful events. While variable between institutions, CCLSs can be used during multiple stages of pediatric fracture management, including pre- and postoperative periods, cast application and removal, and physical therapy.

Highly potent opioid analgesics have historically been utilized as monotherapy to effectively mitigate fracture-related pain. However, recent studies report that children undergoing closed reduction and percutaneous pinning (CRPP) for displaced supracondylar humerus fracture (SCHF) receive adequate analgesia with nonopioid agents with fewer side effects compared to opioid therapy.[38] Given that NSAIDs and acetaminophen are relatively safe and well tolerated, these analgesics represent an effective first-line therapy for providing prompt analgesia following injury. Another benefit of nonopioid analgesic therapy is increased ability to reliably detect signs of compartment syndrome, which is particularly important in pediatric patients with high-energy fractures.[1]

OPIOID STEWARDSHIP

Opioids are often indicated to mitigate pain in pediatric patients undergoing orthopaedic care, and opioid stewardship strategies help limit overprescribing, overuse, misuse, diversion, dependence, and withdrawal.

Nelson et al. reported that following CRPP for SCHF, pediatric patients' requirement for opioid analgesia was minimal after 3 postoperative days.[32] This study recommended that a prescription for seven opioid doses after discharge is sufficient for analgesic coverage in most pediatric SCHF patients. In further support of limiting opioid prescriptions and standardization of postoperative pain medication management for SCHF, Nationwide Children's Hospital implemented educational modules for patients, families, and orthopaedic providers that resulted in a decline in opioid prescribing and use. As part of this work, 45.5% of surgical SCHF patients were discharged without an opioid prescription, with no increase in postdischarge requests for additional analgesics.[41] Future studies are warranted to assess the need for opioid use at all and optimal prescribing limits when indicated.

Prior studies have clearly demonstrated that children can manifest withdrawal symptoms from the abrupt cessation of opioids after as little as 5 to 7 days. Withdrawal symptoms, often missed or misinterpreted in pediatric inpatients, can include anxiety, agitation, insomnia, and tremors.[40] Patients who have been in intensive care units for prolonged periods are at high risk of withdrawal due to the use of opioids for both pain and sedation. Current guidelines suggest that children who have had opioids for 14 days or more should be weaned with a gradually tapering dose. Children who have been exposed for 7 to 14 days should be monitored for withdrawal symptoms and considered for opioid tapering if symptoms appear. Abrupt discontinuation of opioids is generally well tolerated by children who have received opioids for less than 2 days.[17]

ANTIBIOTICS

Antibiotics may be prescribed to prevent or treat infections that can occur in the setting of fractures. This is especially important for open fractures (fractures that penetrate the skin), those associated with significant soft tissue damage, and fractures that are grossly contaminated. While accounting for less than 10% of all pediatric fractures, open fractures are considered surgical emergencies and carry a significant risk for infection and associated morbidity.[24] A recent retrospective study by Kuhn et al. reviewed 303 open long bone fractures and found that 24 (~8%) patients developed a deep infection following injury. These patients were found to have higher severity injuries and a longer time between injury and hospital presentation. Importantly, this study found that for every minute of delayed presentation, the odds of a deep infection increased by 1%.[25]

ANTIBIOTIC CHOICE

A consistent aspect of pediatric fracture management across institutions is the immediate administration of antibiotics and tetanus prophylaxis in cases of open fractures. While it is well established that antibiotics should be started urgently, the suggested class of antibiotics and duration of administration has varied between studies.[18] Following an extensive literature review, the Surgical Infection Society (SIS) published a recommendation that prompt administration of first-generation cephalosporins (Table 3-2) be the first-line antibiotic administered for pediatric open fractures.[9,21] For those patients with severe beta-lactam allergy, clindamycin or vancomycin are recommended. These guidelines were also endorsed by the Infectious Diseases Society of America, the American Society of Health-System Pharmacists, and the Society for Healthcare Epidemiology of America. Paralleling the SIS recommendations, the Eastern Association for the Surgery of Trauma (EAST) recommends coverage of gram-positive bacteria with systemic antibiotics such as first-generation cephalosporins in open fractures.[22] Importantly, although antibiotics are clearly indicated for severe open fractures (e.g., Gustilo type III), some experts recommend that type I and type II open fractures be grouped

TABLE 3-2. Cephalosporins

Drug Name	Route
First-Generation Cephalosporins	
Cefazolin	IV
Cephalothin	
Cephapirin	
Cefadroxil	Oral
Cephalexin	
Cephradine	IV or oral
Second-Generation Cephalosporins	
Cefmetazole	IV
Cefotetan	
Cefoxitin	
Cefprozil	Oral
Cefuroxime	IV or oral

within a risk stratification that includes clean orthopaedic procedures, in which antibiotic prophylaxis is not clearly indicated.[9]

ANTIBIOTIC DURATION

Many intravenous cephalosporins have short half-lives and may need to be given more frequently in patients with normal renal function. Cefazolin and ceftriaxone have a longer half-life and therefore do not need to be dosed as often.[10] Randomized controlled trials examining short-term (1 day) or long-term (3–5 days) antibiotic administration in open fractures found equal infection rates when first- or second-generation cephalosporins were administered.[11] From these findings, a short course of antibiotics is suggested for open pediatric fractures, particularly severe type III open fractures.

PERIOPERATIVE ANTIBIOTICS

Across many fracture types, standard of practice at many institutions is to provide perioperative antibiotics to reduce surgical site or pin track infection. Typically, this will involve the administration of a first- or second-generation cephalosporin 30 to 60 minutes prior to surgery (see Table 3-2).[12] A 2004 Cochrane Review analyzing eight trials concluded that antibiotics are effective in reducing the incidence of wound infection following open limb fracture.[20] This is particularly true in operative cases where any foreign material is implanted (i.e., K-wires, pins, screws, etc.).

Recent retrospective studies as well as position statements by the Peri-Operative Prophylaxis in Neonatal and Paediatric Age (POP-NeoPed) Study Group have challenged this long-held practice, suggesting that perioperative antibiotics are not always necessary.[35] This includes bloodless fracture reductions that are managed in the OR and SCHFs managed with a CRPP.[8] Retrospective review of 845 pediatric patients with SCHFs treated with CRPP found that infections were a rare complication and that infection rates were not significantly different between patients receiving or not receiving perioperative antibiotics. With increased attention around antibiotic stewardship, the authors suggest that it is important to eliminate unnecessary antibiotic use while continuing to maintain a low rate of surgical site infection.[8] However, for the care of open fractures, if an open surgical approach is required, the POP-NeoPed Study Group still suggests administering a first-generation cephalosporin 30 minutes prior to surgery.[35] This recommendation is likewise suggested for higher severity injuries where amputations may be required.

ANTICOAGULANTS IN PEDIATRIC TRAUMA CARE

Given that traumatic injuries and large surgical procedures can predispose adult patients to venous thromboembolisms (VTEs), such as deep vein thromboses and pulmonary embolisms, much consideration has been given to the use of anticoagulants in children and adolescents under these clinical conditions. Compared to the adult population, the rate of VTE following a lower extremity orthopaedic trauma in a pediatric patient is extremely low (0.058%).[30] In patients that did experience a VTE, retrospective studies have identified that these patients many times are adolescents (>15 years of age) with polytraumatic injuries.[30] Furthermore, pediatric patients at increased risk for a VTE following injury include those with a prior history of VTE, reduced mobility longer than 48 hours, known genetic conditions such as thrombophilia, or acquired conditions such as cardiovascular disease or malignancy.[15,23] From this foundation, many institutions have developed clinical practice guidelines for prophylactic treatment of VTE, where pediatric patients at low risk receive no prophylaxis with early ambulation recommended, while patients with a moderate or high VTE risk can receive mechanical and/or pharmacology prophylaxis in addition to early ambulation. Commonly, low–molecular-weight heparin (Enoxaparin) is safe and efficacious for pharmacologic prophylaxis of VTE in patients under 18 years of age. In very young children (<2 months of age), recommended prophylactic dosing is 0.75 mg/kg dose subcutaneously every 12 hours, which is increased in children over 2 months of age through adolescence to 0.5 mg/kg subcutaneously every 12 hours.[27,28,33,37]

There is scant research to support mechanical prophylaxis in the pediatric population although many institutional protocols recommend intraoperative use of pneumatic compression devices in adolescent patients expected to undergo procedures lasting more than 60 minutes.[23] In many instances, appropriate sizes may not be available for smaller patients (i.e., <40 kg). Proper hydration and early mobilization are important considerations in the surgical and postsurgical populations.

In summary, prior to initiating prophylactic anticoagulation, a careful assessment of the risk/benefit profile for the patient should be considered. In most pediatric cases, even in adolescents, routine pharmacologic prophylaxis does not appear to be indicated. While significant variability exists between institution protocols, mechanical prophylaxis consisting of early mobilization and sequential compression devices (SCDs) are recommended by most institutional protocols despite limited scientific support.

VITAMIN D SUPPLEMENTS

Vitamin D, a fat-soluble hormone synthesized and metabolized by all mammals, is a critical component for calcium homeostasis and has a significant impact on bone quality and mineralization. Vitamin D is first synthesized as a provitamin, 7-dehydrocholesterol, in the skin where subsequent exposure to sunlight converts 7-dehydrocholesterol to vitamin D (cholecalciferol). Vitamin D can also be obtained from dietary supplementation where it is absorbed from the small intestine and circulated in the blood. While the primary function of vitamin D is the regulation of calcium homeostasis, it is now well understood that vitamin D also plays an important role in bone mineralization.

Recent clinical reports have demonstrated that vitamin D deficiency is common in the pediatric population. This has been observed with increasing frequency since the 1980s.[14] Given that vitamin D is associated with bone formation and mineralization, studies have suggested that vitamin D be supplemented in children. The American Academy of Pediatrics recently recommended a vitamin D dietary allowance of 400 IU or 10 µg daily from the time of infancy through adolescence.[4] Beyond the time of adolescence and skeletal development, the recommendations for optimal vitamin D levels are less precise, resulting in reports recommending daily vitamin D intake be anywhere from 200 to 4,000 IU/day. The use of vitamin D supplements was further supported by recent case-control study suggesting that vitamin D supplementation—but not serum 25-hydroxyvitamin D level or milk intake—was associated with reduced fracture risk among healthy young children.[5] Given that the therapeutic side effects and adverse consequences of vitamin D supplementation are rare, many physicians support vitamin D supplementation in both healthy children and following a fracture to support bone health. In patients who are found to be deficient (i.e., <30 ng/mL), it has been shown that daily dosing of 1,000 to 5,000 IU/day of D3 orally is safe and effective in patients older than 12 months. Alternative dosing strategies include 50,000 IU/wk orally for 3 months.

CALCIUM

Calcium is a key nutrient for adequate skeletal mineralization with recommended intakes best achieved through a healthy diet. Pathologic calcium insufficiency is less common than vitamin D deficiency. Calcium supplementation in childhood was recently investigated by a meta-analysis showing only a small effect on bone mineral density unlikely to alter fracture risk.[36] Routine calcium supplementation is not recommended for healthy children and adolescents, but increased dietary intake to meet daily requirements is encouraged.[19] Higher daily supplementation may be required in children with malabsorption or medications that impair calcium retention or absorption such as diuretics or glucocorticoid therapy.

BISPHOSPHONATES

Bisphosphonates have been used by clinicians for more than 40 years to improve bone quality in cases of osteoporosis. Bisphosphonate therapy is typically reserved for children with a history of low-trauma fractures, such as osteogenesis imperfecta (OI), and those patients with reduced potential for recovery due to permanent or persistent osteoporosis risk factors.[26] When administered to children with moderate to severe OI, bisphosphonates have been found to increase bone mineral density and reduce fracture risk. While short-term use of bisphosphonates is considered safe and well tolerated in pediatric patients,[26] their use in healthy children to promote bone formation following fractures is not clinically warranted.

Annotated References

Reference	Annotation
Ali S, Manaloor R, Johnson DW, et al; Pediatric Emergency Research Canada. An observational cohort study comparing ibuprofen and oxycodone in children with fractures. *PLoS ONE.* 2021;16(9):e0257021.	This prospective study compared the effectiveness and safety of prescribing ibuprofen and oxycodone for at-home management of children's fracture pain. The study found that ibuprofen and oxycodone had similar analgesic effectiveness, but oxycodone was associated with more adverse events and negatively impacted function. Level of Evidence: II
Bernaerts S, Bonroy B, Daems J, et al. Virtual reality for distraction and relaxation in a pediatric hospital setting: an interventional study with a mixed-methods design. *Front Digit Health.* 2022;4:866119.	This study investigated the feasibility, acceptability, tolerability, and preliminary effectiveness of a VR application prototype called Relaxation-VR for pain and anxiety management in pediatric patients aged 4–16 years. The study found that VR use for distraction and relaxation is acceptable, feasible, and tolerable for pediatric patients, as well as clinicians, and can reduce anxiety, pain, and stress, and increase happiness in a hospital setting. Level of Evidence: II
Bloomer AK, Coe KM, Brandt AM, et al. Hold the antibiotics: are preoperative antibiotics unnecessary in the treatment of pediatric supracondylar humerus fractures? *J Pediatr Orthop.* 2022;42(5): e474–e479.	This retrospective study evaluated the use of preoperative antibiotics for children undergoing CRPP for SCHFs. The study found that the use of antibiotics did not significantly decrease the rate of surgical site infections compared to not using antibiotics, suggesting that absence of antibiotics was not clinically inferior in this population. Level of Evidence: IV; case series
Chang Y, Bhandari M, Zhu KL, et al. Antibiotic prophylaxis in the management of open fractures: a systematic survey of current practice and recommendations. *JBJS Rev.* 2019;7(2):e1.	This article discusses the results of a systematic survey conducted to assess current practices and recommendations regarding antibiotic prophylaxis for patients with open fractures of the extremities. Current practice and recommendations strongly support early systemic antibiotic prophylaxis for patients with open fractures of the extremities. The survey likewise identified variations in antibiotic regimens, doses, and durations of administration, and highlights the need for well-designed randomized controlled trials to establish optimal practice in the future. Level of Evidence: V
Hauser CJ, Adams CA Jr, Eachempati SR; Council of the Surgical Infection Society. Surgical Infection Society guideline: prophylactic antibiotic use in open fractures: an evidence-based guideline. *Surg Infect (Larchmt).* 2006;7(4):379–405.	This systematic review of clinical trials on the use of prophylactic antibiotics for open fractures suggests that a short course of first-generation cephalosporins, used in combination with prompt orthopaedic fracture wound management, significantly lowers the risk of infection. However, there was insufficient evidence to support other common management practices such as prolonged courses of antibiotics or the use of local antibiotic therapies. Large, randomized, blinded trials are needed to prove or disprove the value of these traditional approaches. Level of Evidence: III
Kelly D, Sheffer B, Elrod R, et al. Infections after open fractures in pediatric patients: a review of 288 open fractures. *J Surg Orthop* Adv. 2022;31(2):73–75.	This retrospective study of 288 open fractures in children at a Level 1 children's trauma center reported an overall infection rate of 8.3% and identified obesity as a significant risk factor for infection. Although methicillin-resistant staphylococcus aureus was responsible for only one infection in this study, the authors suggest continued monitoring for antibiotic-resistant organisms in open fracture patients. Level of Evidence: III
Laine J, Kadado A, James C, Novotny IS. The role of bisphosphonates in pediatric orthopaedics: what do we know after 50 years? Current concept review. *J Pediatr Orthop Soc North Am.* 2019;1(1).	Bisphosphonates have been used for 50 years in pediatric patients with conditions such as osteoporosis and bone fragility. However, there are currently no established guidelines on treatment regimen or duration. While bisphosphonates have shown promise in pediatric secondary osteoporosis, more studies are needed to inform clinical management, and clinical studies of bisphosphonate use in avascular necrosis have not been as promising as animal models. Level of Evidence: III
Naveen P, Gina B, Kangrui L, et al. Oral administration of morphine versus ibuprofen to manage postfracture pain in children: a randomized trial. *CMAJ.* 2014;186(18):1358.	This study compared the efficacy of orally administered morphine and ibuprofen in managing pain related to uncomplicated fractures in children. The results showed that there was no significant difference in pain reduction between the two groups, but morphine was associated with more adverse effects than ibuprofen. Level of Evidence: I

Annotated References

Reference	Annotation
Nuelle JAV, Coe KM, Oliver HA, et al. Effect of NSAID use on bone healing in pediatric fractures: a preliminary, prospective, randomized, blinded study. *J Pediatr Orthop.* 2020;40(8).	This study investigated whether NSAIDs used in the acute phase of bone healing in children with fractures result in delayed union or nonunion. The results showed that ibuprofen is an effective medication for fracture pain in children and its use does not impair clinical or radiographic long bone fracture healing in skeletally immature patients. Level of Evidence: I; therapeutic
Wheatley BM, Nappo KE, Christensen DL, et al. Effect of NSAIDs on bone healing rates: a meta-analysis. *J Am Acad Orthop Surg.* 2019;27(7).	This meta-analysis aimed to determine whether the use of NSAIDs leads to delayed union or nonunion. The authors found that across literature, NSAID exposure increased the risk of delayed union or nonunion in adult patients, but not in pediatric patients. Level of Evidence: II

REFERENCES

1. Abzug JM, Herman MJ. Management of supracondylar humerus fractures in children: current concepts. *J Am Acad Orthop Surg.* 2012;20(2):69–77.
2. Addab S, Hamdy R, Thorstad K, et al. Use of virtual reality in managing paediatric procedural pain and anxiety: an integrative literature review. *J Clin Nurs.* 2022;31(21–22):3032–3059.
3. Ali S, Gourlay K, Yukseloglu A, et al. Quantifying the intensity of adverse events with ibuprofen and oxycodone: an observational cohort study. *BMJ Paediatr Open.* 2022;6(1):e001428.
4. Ali S, Manaloor R, Johnson DW, et al; Pediatric Emergency Research Canada. An observational cohort study comparing ibuprofen and oxycodone in children with fractures. *PLoS One.* 2021;16(9):e0257021.
5. Anderson LN, Heong SW, Chen Y, et al; TARGet Kids Collaboration. Vitamin D and fracture risk in early childhood: a case-control study. *Am J Epidemiol.* 2017;185(12):1255–1262.
6. Bernaerts S, Bonroy B, Daems J, et al. Virtual reality for distraction and relaxation in a pediatric hospital setting: an interventional study with a mixed-methods design. *Front Digit Health.* 2022;4:866119.
7. Bin K, Rony L, Henric N, Moukoko D. Pediatric fracture reduction in the emergency department. *Orthop Traumatol Surg Res.* 2022;108(1S):103155.
8. Bloomer AK, Coe KM, Brandt AM, et al. Hold the antibiotics: are preoperative antibiotics unnecessary in the treatment of pediatric supracondylar humerus fractures? *J Pediatr Orthop.* 2022;42(5):e474–e479.
9. Bratzler DW, Dellinger EP, Olsen KM, et al; American Society of Health-System Pharmacists (ASHP), Infectious Diseases Society of America (IDSA), Surgical Infection Society (SIS), Society for Healthcare Epidemiology of America (SHEA). Clinical practice guidelines for antimicrobial prophylaxis in surgery. *Surg Infect (Larchmt).* 2013;14(1):73–156.
10. Bui T, Preuss CV. Cephalosporins. [Updated 2023 March 24]. In: *StatPearls* [Internet]. StatPearls Publishing; 2023. https://www.ncbi.nlm.nih.gov/books/NBK551517/.
11. Chan JKK, Aquilina AL, Lewis SR, et al. Timing of antibiotic administration, wound debridement, and the stages of reconstructive surgery for open long bone fractures of the upper and lower limbs. *Cochrane Database Syst Rev.* 2022;4(4):CD013555.
12. Chang Y, Bhandari M, Zhu KL, et al. Antibiotic prophylaxis in the management of open fractures: a systematic survey of current practice and recommendations. *JBJS Rev.* 2019;7(2):e1.
13. Chiu CC, Lin YT, Wang Y, et al. Immersive virtual reality to distract from pain in children treated with L-asparaginase by intramuscular injection. *Cureus.* 2023;15(1):e34317.
14. Contreras JJ, Hiestand B, O'Neill JC, et al. Vitamin D deficiency in children with fractures. *Pediatr Emerg Care.* 2014;30(11):777–781.
15. Cunningham AJ, Dewey E, Lin S, et al. Pediatric trauma venous thromboembolism prediction algorithm outperforms current anticoagulation prophylaxis guidelines: a pilot study. *Pediatr Surg Int.* 2020;36(3):373–381.
16. DePeter KC, Blumberg SM, Dienstag Becker S, Meltzer JA. Does the use of ibuprofen in children with extremity fractures increase their risk for bone healing complications? *J Emerg Med.* 2017;52(4):426–432.
17. Galinkin J, Koh JL; Committee on Drugs, Section on Anesthesiology and Pain Medicine, American Academy of Pediatrics. Recognition and management of iatrogenically induced opioid dependence and withdrawal in children. *Pediatrics.* 2014;133(1):152–155.
18. Godfrey J, Pace JL. Type I open fractures benefit from immediate antibiotic administration but not necessarily immediate surgery. *J Pediatr Orthop.* 2016;36:S6–S10.
19. Golden NH, Abrams SA; Committee on Nutrition. Optimizing bone health in children and adolescents. *Pediatrics.* 2014;134(4):e1229–e1243.
20. Gosselin RA, Roberts I, Gillespie WJ. Antibiotics for preventing infection in open limb fractures. *Cochrane Database Syst Rev.* 2004;2004(1):CD00376.
21. Hauser CJ, Adams CA Jr, Eachempati SR; Council of the Surgical Infection Society. Surgical Infection Society guideline: prophylactic antibiotic use in open fractures: an evidence-based guideline. *Surg Infect (Larchmt).* 2006;7(4):379–405.
22. Hoff WS, Bonadies JA, Cachecho R, Dorlac WC. East Practice Management Guidelines Work Group: update to practice management guidelines for prophylactic antibiotic use in open fractures. *J Trauma.* 2011;70(3):751–754.
23. Jinks S, Arana A. Venous thromboembolism in paediatrics. *BJA Educ.* 2019;19(9):305–312.
24. Kelly D, Sheffer B, Elrod R, et al. Infections after open fractures in pediatric patients: a review of 288 open fractures. *J Surg Orthop Adv.* 2022;31(2):73–75.
25. Kuhn AW, Troyer SC, Martus JE. Pediatric open long-bone fracture and subsequent deep infection risk: the importance of early hospital care. *Children (Basel).* 2022;9(8):1243.
26. Laine J, Kadado A, James C, Novotny IS. The role of bisphosphonates in pediatric orthopaedics: what do we know after 50 years? Current concept review. *J Pediatr Orthop Soc North Am.* 2019;1(1).
27. Massicotte P, Adams M, Marzinotto V, et al. Low-molecular-weight heparin in pediatric patients with thrombotic disease: a dose finding study. *J Pediatr.* 1996;128(3):313–318.
28. Massicotte P, Julian JA, Marzinotto V, et al. Dose-finding and pharmacokinetic profiles of prophylactic doses of a low molecular weight heparin (reviparin-sodium) in pediatric patients. *Thromb Res.* 2003;109(2–3):93–99.
29. McGrath PA. Development of the world health organization guidelines on cancer pain relief and palliative care in children. *J Pain Symptom Manage.* 1996;12(2):87–92.
30. Murphy RF, Naqvi M, Miller PE, et al. Pediatric orthopaedic lower extremity trauma and venous thromboembolism. *J Child Orthop.* 2015;9(5):381–384.
31. Naveen P, Gina B, Kangrui L, et al. Oral administration of morphine versus ibuprofen to manage postfracture pain in children: a randomized trial. *CMAJ.* 2014;186(18):1358.
32. Nelson SE, Adams AJ, Buczek MJ, et al. Postoperative pain and opioid use in children with supracondylar humeral fractures: balancing analgesia and opioid stewardship. *J Bone Joint Surg Am.* 2019;101(2):119–126.
33. Nohe N, Flemmer A, Rümler R, et al. The low molecular weight heparin dalteparin for prophylaxis and therapy of thrombosis in childhood: a report on 48 cases. *Eur J Pediatr.* 1999;158(Suppl 3):S134–S139.
34. Nuelle JAV, Coe KM, Oliver HA, et al. Effect of NSAID use on bone healing in pediatric fractures: a preliminary, prospective, randomized, blinded study. *J Pediatr Orthop.* 2020;40(8):e683–e689.
35. Opri F, Bianchini S, Nicoletti L, et al; on behalf of the Peri-Operative Prophylaxis in Neonatal ind Paediatric Age Pop-NeoPed Study Group. Surgical antimicrobial prophylaxis in patients of neonatal and pediatric age undergoing orthopedic and hand surgery: a RAND/UCLA appropriateness method consensus study. *Antibiotics (Basel).* 2022;11(3):289.
36. Parry J, Sullivan E, Scott AC. Vitamin D sufficiency screening in preoperative pediatric orthopaedic patients. *J Pediatr Orthop.* 2011;31(3):331–333.
37. Revel-Vilk S, Chan AKC. Anticoagulation therapy in children. *Semin Thromb Hemost.* 2003;29(4):425–432.
38. Swanson CE, Chang K, Schleyer E, et al. Postoperative pain control after supracondylar humerus fracture fixation. *J Pediatr Orthop.* 2012;32(5):452–455.
39. Wheatley BM, Nappo KE, Christensen DL, et al. Effect of NSAIDs on bone healing rates: a meta-analysis. *J Am Acad Orthop Surg.* 2019;27(7):e330–e336.
40. Whelan KT, Heckmann MK, Lincoln PA, Hamilton SM. Pediatric withdrawal identification and management. *J Pediatr Intens Care.* 2015;4(2):73–78.
41. Winslow L, Holstine J, Samora JB. Reducing the use of opioids for pediatric patients with supracondylar humerus fractures. *Jt Comm J Qual Patient Saf.* 2020;46(10):581–587.

4

Cast and Splint Immobilization

Vince W. Prusick and Vishwas Talwalkar

INTRODUCTION

The past several decades have seen amazing enhancements in the management of adult orthopaedic trauma; one of the most significant is the ability to operatively reduce fractures and to stabilize them safely with internal implants. These methods have resulted in less reliance on fracture manipulation and stabilization with external devices such as traction, splint, and cast immobilization. Gone are the days of extended skeletal traction and spica cast application for adult femur fractures; tibia shaft fractures in adults are rarely treated with time-honored methods of reduction in the emergency ward, long-leg cast application, followed by months of patellar tendon bearing a short-leg cast application. Although still used with some frequency in adult trauma, upper extremity cast and splint application is often considered temporary until definitive internal fixation.

Parallel to changes in fracture management, medicine has seen similar changes in medical education as well as who delivers certain health care. For instance, as a result of specialization, many adult orthopaedists manage fewer traumas, rarely place casts, and even more rarely will they educate residents in the safe and effective use of these methods. As reimbursement for health care changes, orthopaedic surgeons are called to do those things that only they can do: operate. Many other aspects of patients' care are assumed by advanced practitioners such as nurse practitioners or physician assistants (NPs or PAs) or other allied health specialists. In many emergency rooms and in most outpatient clinics, the patient who requires definitive cast immobilization will usually have these applied by cast technicians or nurses. As a result, large fracture clinics where orthopaedic residents learn from senior residents or faculty to manage fractures with casting are replaced by cast technicians while residents learn who needs operations and how.

To a lesser degree and similar to adults, decades of advances in imaging and development of appropriate operative methods and implants have also benefited pediatric patients with orthopaedic trauma. Despite wide changes in adult trauma, cast and splint methodology is still used with great frequency in the management of pediatric trauma. In children, requisite attention to perfect reduction and extensive immobilization is not needed because of the rapidity of fracture healing and the remodeling potential seen in children. Over 90% of adult forearm fractures are treated with surgery; in children, 90% of forearm fractures are treated with reduction and cast immobilization.

The purpose of this chapter is to review in detail the methods and pitfalls of nonoperative treatment that are common to all areas of pediatric trauma. In addition, we will review unique characteristics of children that are also of importance in all fracture locations and trauma. It is desired that this chapter and its figures will serve as a primer of nonoperative pediatric orthopaedic trauma management.

PAIN MANAGEMENT AND SEDATION FOR FRACTURE MANAGEMENT

In normally sensate children, reduction and immobilization of fractures is always associated with pain and anxiety. Advances in fracture management have been accompanied by improvements in methods to diminish anxiety, provide muscle relaxation, and to decrease pain during these noxious events. The most optimal location to perform these procedures is within the operating room (OR) where complete pain control, relaxation, and amnesia are provided by the anesthesia team.[51] This setting is ideal as it allows the orthopaedist to focus completely on the fracture without worrying about the safety of the child, without the distractions of a suffering child, and without parents looming in the background. Unfortunately, this resource is not often available for our patients in a timely manner and the costs associated with general anesthesia and possible admission far outweigh the costs of fractures that are treated equally well in the emergency department (ED).[30] In addition, the risks of general anesthesia are currently being evaluated and it is suspected that multiple long anesthetics may have some effect on child development. Yet one should consider reduction and cast application in the OR for children with autistic spectrum disorders (ASDs); children with medical comorbidities that preclude safe sedation in the ED; and in cases of fractures which could be very difficult to reduce (significant displacement and swelling) and will likely need operative stabilization anyway.

Procedural sedation methods include different routes of drug delivery (intranasal, intravenous [IV], or inhalational) and can utilize differing combinations of agents. Although not an exhaustive list, a contemporary listing of systemic drugs used for these injuries include combinations of etomidate, ketamine, narcotics, midazolam, propofol, and nitrous oxide.[1,8,47,51,68] Some centers do not monitor these children who are sedated for procedures with nitrous oxide and oxygen.[8] Yet most centers recommend at least pulse oximetry and noninvasive blood pressure monitoring for all conscious sedation including nitrous oxide and oxygen.[61]

Ketamine appears to be a very popular agent for use in the ED with good sedative, amnestic, and analgesic effects; and reported doses include 0.75 to 2.0 mg/kg delivered IV or 2 to 4 mg/kg delivered Intramuscular (IM). Its advantages include wide use and experience as a solitary agent, and that it can be administered IV or IM.[18] Side effects include nystagmus, lacrimation, salivation, vocalization, respiratory depression, and dissociative reactions that can occur at higher doses (2.5 mg/kg IV). Ketamine at lower doses may have decreased side effects but may require some redosing.[38] Some studies have augmented ketamine with small boluses of propofol (with its good antiemetic and anxiolytic properties); ketamine is helpful in mitigating the occasional hypotensive effects seen with propofol.[1,60]

Another popular agent for sedation is 50:50 nitrous oxide and oxygen (anxiolytic and analgesic), which is appealing because children don't need to be NPO and it is fast-acting, reversible, and doesn't require special staff to administer it. Nitrous oxide can be supplemented with hematoma block after a steady state of sedation has been achieved. Procedural sedation in combination with local block does have the advantage of not needing as much systemic sedation.

Some have suggested that regional anesthesia such as hematoma block could be the first line of pain management for upper extremity fractures as it is quicker and is well tolerated.[5,67] Conversion to sedation with ketamine of midazolam may be needed in a small proportion.[5] Regional Bier blocks have also been used in children with forearm and wrist fractures with good efficacy and have been shown to be safe, efficient, cost-effective, and do not require patients to be fasting. When using a dose of 3.33 mg/kg of lidocaine, there are very few complications except for tourniquet pain. Techniques for ultrasound-guided hematoma blocks have also been described.[63] Despite the efficacy of regional blocks, recent research has suggested local hematoma block may not be as widely used today as many EDs are using ketamine or midazolam.[17]

GENERAL

Because of the growth and remodeling potential of pediatric bones, acceptable alignment rather than exact anatomic reduction is sufficient for many fractures, allowing the majority of pediatric fractures to be managed in a cast. Similarly, joint stiffness is not typically a long-term problem in children treated in a cast.[7] The goals of pediatric cast treatment are to protect and provide stability to the broken bone, maintain alignment, and protect from further injury until sufficient healing has occurred. In general, the alignment maintained in the cast should allow the child to eventually remodel to anatomic "normal" by the cessation of growth. The younger the child, the more malalignment may be acceptable. Likewise, deformity closer to the growth plate and in the plane of motion will typically remodel more than those elsewhere.

The duration of cast treatment is both age and site specific. Very young children, infants, and newborns will generally heal fractures more quickly than adolescents. In general, fractures of the hands and feet require 4 weeks of immobilization; elbow fractures 3 to 6 weeks; and tibial shaft fractures may take 12 to 16 weeks, whereas most other fractures require 6 weeks. Before discontinuing cast immobilization, fracture healing should be documented on radiographs and the child should be nontender at the fracture site.

In general, casts are utilized to *maintain* alignment. If a fracture is nondisplaced or has an acceptable alignment, the cast's purpose is to keep the child comfortable and maintain that alignment until the bone has healed. If a fracture has an unacceptable alignment, it should be reduced to an acceptable alignment and the cast placed to maintain that alignment. Fractures that should be treated operatively include injuries in which adequate alignment or length cannot be easily obtained or maintained, displaced intra-articular fractures, and many fractures involving the physis. Postoperatively, the limb may be protected with a splint or a cast if necessary. Problems may arise when a cast is used to *obtain* acceptable alignment.

Pressure sores and soft tissue injuries have been documented when casts are used in this manner and should be done so with caution.[42,53]

To minimize motion at the fracture site, casts are placed to span the joint proximal, distal, or both. In general, the more proximal a fracture, the more likely joints at each end of the bone will be spanned. Increasing the length of the cast increases the resistance to rotation.[40] To maintain correct alignment, limbs may be casted in different positions to counteract specific displacing forces on the proximal or distal fragment of a given fracture. For example, in a subtrochanteric femur fracture, the proximal fragment is pulled into flexion, abduction, and external rotation by attached muscles, so the distal fragment must be positioned with this in mind. The distal fragment must be brought into a position of flexion to match the flexed proximal femur from pull of the psoas muscle.

CAST COMPLICATIONS

Although casting is often viewed as "conservative" treatment, the treating physician and family should recognize that this does not imply that this treatment is without complications. Although the true incidence of cast complications is unknown, a litigation history of a large multispecialty multilocation pediatric group showed that casts were the number one cause of litigation. Over 25% of children treated in a hip spica cast have been shown to have skin complications.[22] Over a 5-year period at one institution, 168 unplanned visits to the emergency room were because of cast issues. Twenty-nine percent of these visits were for a wet cast, 23% for a tight cast, and 13% for a loose cast.[59] Over a 10-year period, Physicians Insurers Association of America (PIAA) reported 1,023 claims on problems of immobilization and traction for which 16% of all claims had an associated issue including failure of consent. This implies that many physicians and patients may expect cast immobilization to be without risk. Thus, it is important to inform patients and their caregivers of the risks associated with cast treatment. For instance, a child with a tibia fracture can be told to expect pain in the pretibial area but they should also be aware that pain in other locations (such as over the point of the heel) is not fracture related and may imply an impending heel sore. When the expectations of cast immobilization are explained and risks of treatment are given, it is beneficial that these risks be written and delivered to the patient and their family.[37]

The Wet and Soiled Cast

Wet casts that are not made with fiberglass and waterproof liners (and thus can dry quickly) should be changed. Failure to do so may result in skin irritation, breakdown, and possible infection. Light moisture or spotting may be dried with a hair dryer on cool or low heat, with instructions to check the temperature of the dryer with their hand to ensure that it is not too warm. A frankly wet cast or cast padding that cannot be dried as described above usually requires inspection of the skin and cast change (Fig. 4-1). Although most limbs in these casts will only demonstrate skin maceration,[22] serious

Figure 4-1. Examples of dermatitis related to wet casts. **A:** A soiled hip spica cast. **B:** Upper extremity cast that was wet. (Property of UW Pediatric Orthopaedics.)

life-threatening complications such as toxic shock syndrome and necrotizing fasciitis have been reported.[20,54] Hip spica casts are often applied in the OR and their removal and exchange at times require a general anesthetic. Parents should be well instructed on positioning to avoid soiling, frequent diaper changes, and inspecting the children for skin irritation. Anesthetic risks must be weighed with the perceived soft tissue and skin risk.

Thermal Injury

Plaster and fiberglass, the two most common casting materials, harden through exothermic chemical reactions. Plaster has a much higher setting temperature than fiberglass and therefore a higher risk for thermal injury when a cast is placed. Two factors strongly associated with thermal injuries are dip water temperature and the thickness of cast material.[34,43,69] Several studies have shown that risk of thermal injury is significant if the dip water temperature is too hot (>50 °C) or if the casts are too thick (>24 ply).[27,35] Each plaster manufacturer has recommended dip water temperatures that should not be exceeded. Using warmer temperatures to "speed up" the setting time beyond that recommended should be avoided. Casts in excess of 24 ply are rarely encountered; however, increased amounts of casting material are often placed in the concavities of extremities (antecubital fossa and dorsum of the ankle) because of material overlap.[35] Incorporating splints on the convexity, thus decreasing overlap in the concavity, can minimize this. Similarly, clinicians placing plaster splints of 10 to 15 ply on an extremity may breech safe thicknesses when the splint is too long and the edges are folded over, thus creating a focal area of 20 to 30 ply, a thickness at which temperatures do become a risk.[35] Studies have shown that temperatures high enough to cause significant thermal injuries can also be reached when the clinician places a curing cast on a pillow.[27,35] The practice of reinforcing a curing plaster cast with fiberglass may place the limb at significant risk because the fiberglass overlap prevents heat from effectively dissipating. The plaster must be allowed to cure before setting the casted limb on a support or applying fiberglass reinforcement. Failure to wait may place the insulated portion of the limb at significant risk.[35] Case reports demonstrating this potential complication do exist.[9] Those patients undergoing regional or general anesthesia may be at increased risk as they will not report burning pain that is associated with thermal injury.

Areas of Focal Pressure: Impending Pressure Sores

A key to preventing loss of fracture reduction is in the application of a well-molded cast. Cast padding should be applied between three and five layers thick over the limb being casted.[52,62] Bony prominences (heel, malleoli, patella, ASIS, and olecranon) and cast edges should be additionally padded to prevent irritation yet allow a cast to be molded to fit snugly without undue pressure. The use of foam padding in such areas may help decrease the incidence of pressure sores.[26]

Families and patients should be instructed to refrain from placing anything between a cast and the patients' skin, food, toys, writing utensils, money, and other items have been found down casts, and we have seen them erode through patients' skin.[11,66] Any patient with a suspected foreign body down their cast should have the cast removed and skin inspected (Fig. 4-2).

Figure 4-2. Examples of foreign bodies found under splints/casts. **A:** A bracelet that was not removed prior to immobilization. **B:** A plastic knife that was found down a lower extremity cast. **C:** A coin found down a long-arm cast. **D:** A toy tank found under a cast. (Property of UW Pediatric Orthopaedics.)

A loose cast (either too much padding from poor application or decreased swelling) may result in skin sores as a result of shear forces repeatedly applied to the limb or a loss of reduction.[36] Distal fingers or toes are often noted to "migrate" proximally (disappearing toes/fingers sign) when this occurs and should alert the parent and the clinician that there is a problem.[71] In a lower extremity cast, which migrates distally, the dorsum of the foot and ankle receives pressure from the anterior ankle crease of the cast, while the heel is pulled up and rests along the posterior calf portion of the cast. Prolonged positioning in such a manner may result in pressure sores.

Detecting Cast Complications

That "there are no hypochondriacs in casts" is an important aphorism to remember and every effort should be taken to resolve the source of complaint in an immobilized patient. A complication of casting should be considered whenever an immobilized patient has an unexplained increase in pain, irritability, or unexplained fevers.[20]

Some cast complications such as soiling and wetness can be detected on physical examination, whereas others may be more difficult to diagnose. A foul-smelling cast may be a sign of wound infection and the cast should be removed or windowed to inspect the source of the smell. Pressure sores may be diagnosed if the patient can localize an area of discomfort away from the fracture or operative site. Complaints of pain in high-risk areas such as the heel, dorsum of the foot, popliteal fossa, patella, and olecranon, must alert the clinician of an impending problem. However, with pediatric patients, localization may not be possible. One must correlate history and the clinical examination findings, such as the "disappearing toes sign," with radiographs. These images can be used to critically evaluate not only the alignment of the fractured bone but also the outline and contour of the cast padding and material, especially in the antecubital, the popliteal fossa, and over the dorsum of the foot. If there is a suspicion of a problem, the cast should be windowed or removed and the area inspected.

Certain pediatric patients may be at a higher risk for cast complications. These include the very young, developmentally delayed, or patients under anesthesia or sedation who may have difficulty responding to noxious stimuli such as heat or pressure during the cast application. Discerning problems in this group may be quite difficult and cast sores can occur despite appropriate and careful application.

Similarly, patients with impaired sensation are at increased risk for injuries related to excessive heat and pressure. In this group are those with spinal cord injuries,[64] myelomeningocele,[49] Charcot–Marie–Tooth disease, and systemic disorders such as diabetes mellitus.[31] Patients with CP are at increased risk for complications due to communication difficulties and poor nutrition, in addition to their spasticity.[45]

TREATING CAST COMPLICATIONS

Dermatitis

The majority of dermatitis under casts has to do with maceration of the skin and continued contact with wetness including fluids such as urine or feces. Often, removal of the cast, cleansing of the skin, and allowing the skin to "dry out" is all that is required. Some recommend applying over-the-counter skin moisturizers.[22] If fungal infection is suspected, half-strength nystatin cream and 1% hydrocortisone cream may be applied, followed by miconazole powder dusting twice daily.[22] If unstable, the fracture may be managed by a newly applied dry split cast or splint, allowing time for the skin to recover. In rare cases, internal or external fixation may be chosen to manage the fracture and to allow treatment of the skin issues. Often, the skin will improve dramatically after a few days and a new cast may be applied. If significant concern for cellulitis exists, such as induration or fevers, laboratory tests should be ordered and empiric oral antibiotics prescribed.

Pressure Sores

Pressure sores are the result of a focal area of pressure, which exceeds perfusion pressure. Although there may be initial pain associated with this pressure, this can be difficult to separate from the pain of the fracture or surgery. Any pain away from the injured area should be suspected to have a problem with focal pressure. The heel is the most common site. These sores may vary from areas of erythema, to black eschars, to full-thickness soft tissue loss and exposed bone (Fig. 4-3). In the benign cases, removal of the cast over the heel and either cessation or careful reapplication is all that is necessary. Typically, black eschars imply partial- to full-thickness injuries. If they are intact, nonfluctuant, nondraining, and mobile from the underlying bone, they may be treated as a biologic dressing with weekly wound checks. If any concern exists, a wound team and/or plastic surgery consult should be sought earlier rather than later. Often, dressing changes using topical enzymatic ointments and antibiotic ointments can be used to treat these wounds (Fig. 4-4). Whenever exposed bone is present, osteomyelitis is a concern requiring aggressive intervention and possible IV antibiotic therapy. In these severe cases, vacuum-assisted closure (VAC) therapy, skin grafting, or flap coverage may be necessary.[44]

Joint Stiffness and Muscle Contractures

Determination of cast immobilization duration is often multifactorial; however, the clinician must recognize that unwanted physiologic changes may occur. Although these changes are less pronounced in children than adults, excessive length of immobilization may lead to problems such as stiffness,[24] muscle atrophy, cartilage degradation, ligament weakening, and osteoporosis.[7,13,14,32,65] This must be weighed against the bony healing gained in prolonged immobilizations. Alternatives such as Pavlik harness bracing for infants with femur fractures,[55] patellar tendon bearing casts versus long-leg casts for tibial fractures, short-arm casts for distal forearm fractures, and other functional braces may minimize some of the risks of cast immobilization or at least decrease the duration of cast treatment.

The ankle, elbow, and fingers are often locations prone to stiffness. The duration of immobilization should be minimized if at all possible.

Figure 4-3. Examples of heel pressure sores. Mild erythema and superficial skin damage (**A**), intact eschar (**B**), and partial/full-thickness injury with exposed bone and fascia (**C**). (Property of UW Pediatric Orthopaedics.)

Compartment Syndrome

Most limbs with fresh fractures are more comfortable after immobilization. Therefore, increasing pain or neurovascular change should be fully evaluated to detect the above complications and possibly compartment syndrome. Fractures and surgery can result in progressive soft tissue swelling that might not have been present at the time of cast application and may lead to compartment syndrome. Other systemic conditions may also raise the risk for this devastating complication in an otherwise straightforward clinical picture. In this scenario,[59]

Figure 4-4. A: Picture of heel ulcer at clinical follow-up after operative debridement. **B:** After roughly 2 months of topical enzymatic and antibiotic treatment with dressing changes. (Property of UW Pediatric Orthopaedics.)

the first intervention should be relieving the circumferential pressure by splitting the cast and all underlying padding, as leaving the padding intact has been shown to not fully relieve compartment pressure. Should splitting the cast fail to alleviate symptoms, cast removal should be considered. Fractures of the tibia,[25,29] forearm,[29] and elbow have increased risk of compartment syndrome. High-energy fractures resulting from motor vehicle accidents, crush injuries, or two-level injuries such as a floating elbow should raise the treating physician's awareness to the possibility of an impending compartment syndrome. Any child unable to detect pain normally (a nerve injury or regional anesthesia) must be followed closely for the development of compartment syndrome and treated appropriately.

Children do not usually exhibit the classical four Ps (pallor, paresthesias, pulseless, pain with passive stretch) associated with compartment syndrome until myonecrosis may be starting. Instead, the "three As" of increased agitation, anxiety, and analgesic requirements have been documented as the earliest signs of compartment syndrome in children. Any child exhibiting these symptoms that are not relieved with cast splitting should have the cast removed and limb inspected with a high suspicion of compartment syndrome. One should be ready to take the child to the OR for formal compartment evaluation and decompression if needed.

Fractures with associated neurovascular injuries are at significant risk of developing a compartment syndrome and require frequent neurovascular checks. These limbs may be stabilized with a splint as opposed to circumferential cast application, which could worsen the risk of compartment syndrome. These limbs are most often treated with operative stabilization using internal or external fixation and/or splint immobilization. This allows continued neurovascular assessment, palpation of compartments, and inspection of the limb. For instance, the child with a floating elbow fracture and associated nerve palsy (at high risk for compartment syndrome) is usually best treated with internal fixation of the fractures, and either a splint, bivalved cast that is easily opened, or cast with thick foam to allow for swelling, with the volar forearm exposed to assess the compartments as well as the pulses.

Disuse Osteopenia and Pathologic Fractures Adjacent to Cast

Patients with paralytic conditions or cerebral palsy patients and those taking anticonvulsants may experience further disuse osteopenia with immobilization.[64] These patients are at significantly higher risk of pathologic fracture while casted or upon cast removal.[2,45] Strategies to prevent this includes minimizing immobilization (<4 weeks), weight-bearing casts, and the use of less rigid immobilization such as Soft Cast (3M Health Care Ltd., Loughborough, England) and splints and braces.

Delayed Diagnosis of Wound Infections

Many children are placed in postsurgical casts. The vast majority does well without incident. However, casts over wounds or pins may cause a delay in the diagnosis of a wound infection (Fig. 4-5). For instance, an estimated 1% to 4% of all pediatric supracondylar humerus fractures treated with pinning the

Figure 4-5. After getting a postoperative cast wet, dermatitis and possible cellulitis were found at the incision following a gastrocnemius recession. (Property of UW Pediatric Orthopaedics.)

elbow will develop a postoperative pin-tract inflammation or infection.[4,24] Therefore, unexplained fever beyond the perioperative period, increase in pain at pin sites, foul smell, or discharge from a cast should be evaluated by a member of the orthopaedic team. The wound should be examined either with cast windowing or cast removal. Laboratory tests including CBC, ESR, and CRP may be advisable. In cases of early pin-site infection where the fracture is not yet healed, oral antibiotics may control the infection long enough to allow more fracture healing prior to pin removal. Infections of pins used for certain fractures may have a high chance of joint penetration (lateral condyle, supracondylar humerus, distal femoral physeal, and proximal humerus) and thus superficial pin-tract infection could lead to a septic joint. This is much more serious than simple pin-site infections and most often must be treated with surgical irrigation and debridement, and pin removal should be considered despite the status of fracture healing.

TYPES OF CASTING MATERIALS

Before placing a cast, the limb must be inspected. Any dirt, operative skin prep, or jewelry should be removed before the cast is applied. Often, appropriate size stockinette or liner is applied against the skin, under the cast and cast padding. Although not essential, these liners minimize skin irritation and allow nice well-padded and polished edges to the cast to be applied. They also minimize the tendency of some children to "pick out" their cast padding. These liners are made of cotton, water-friendly synthetic materials such as polyester, sliver-impregnated cotton (to minimize bacterial growth), or Gore-Tex (W.L. Gore & Associates, Inc.; Newark, DE). Some in the care of children who require spica cast application favor water-impermeable liners such as Gore-Tex. In addition to being more convenient for patients, these newer materials minimize skin irritation.

Cast Padding

Different materials are used to pad the extremity between the cast material and the patient's skin. A thin layer (3–5 layers) of padding is applied to the portion of the extremity that is not prone to pressure sores and it is applied without wrinkles.[52,62] Additional layers may be placed over bony prominences to minimize pressure in these areas. Cotton is the cheapest and is historically most commonly used. But casts with cotton padding cannot be made waterproof as the cotton padding retains water. Newer synthetic materials have variable water resistance and, when paired with fiberglass, can allow patients to bathe and swim. However, these materials are considerably more expensive than their cotton counterparts. In addition, some synthetic padding is less resistant to a cast saw. If one applies Gore-Tex padding, the blue DE FLEX safety strip can be placed along the path that the cast saw will take to remove the cast.

Cast edges are often a source of skin irritation and abrasion. This is especially true for fiberglass casts. When making a cast, applying the stockinette and cast padding at least 1 cm beyond the edge of the fiberglass, and folding the stockinette and padding back over the first layer of fiberglass, will make a cast with well-padded edges. Closed-cell adhesive foam may also be applied to the edges of a cast and to pad bony prominences. It is important to recognize that some foam padding will accumulate moisture and will not be effectively wicked away from the liner and skin. Should difficulty be found in folding back the underlying stockinette or liner, the cast edges may be petaled with tape or moleskin adhesive. This involves placing a 1- to 2-inch piece of tape on the inside of the liner and folding the taped liner over the opening of cast. Most commonly, petaling is performed on hip spica casts but may be performed on any cast.

Plaster of Paris

Plaster-impregnated cloth is a time-tested form of immobilization. It was first described in 1852 and has been the gold standard for cast immobilization for many years. This material is generally less expensive than fiberglass. Some surgeons find plaster easier and better to mold, and some surgeons find fiberglass superior for molding. Inconveniences associated with plaster include its poor resistance to water and its lower strength-to-weight ratio resulting in heavier (thicker) casts.

Plaster of Paris combines with water in a reaction that results in gypsum. In the process of setting up, the conversion to gypsum is an exothermic reaction with thermal energy as a by-product. In general, the amount of heat produced is variable between each of the manufactured plasters. However, within each product line, faster-setting plasters can be expected to

produce more heat. As the speed of the reaction, amount of reactants, or temperature of the system (dip water and/or ambient temperature) increase, the amount of heat given off can cause significant thermal injury.[27,35] The low strength-to-weight ratio may also increase risk of thermal injury as those unfamiliar with the amount (ply) of plaster to use may inadvertently use too much, resulting in a burn.

Fiberglass

Fiberglass casting tape has a long history of safe and effective use. These materials have the benefit of being significantly lighter in weight, stronger, and more durable. In addition, these materials can be combined with waterproof liners to allow patients to bathe and swim in their casts. They are also more radiolucent, allowing better imaging within the cast.

Risk of thermal injury is much lower and is a major advantage over plaster.[35] However, because of the increased stiffness, some feel these casts are more difficult to mold, whereas others prefer fiberglass as the strength of the molded portion is greater.

When fiberglass is applied correctly with the stretch–relax technique, it has been shown to generate significantly lower pressure than plaster cast and it better accommodated simulated swelling without the need to sacrifice the structural integrity of the cast.[19]

Although fiberglass is more expensive than plaster, in a randomized prospective study of military personnel and their dependents, the overall cost of casting a fracture is similar, as the plaster casts needed to be replaced more frequently. In addition, fiberglass short-leg casts were significantly more comfortable and had fewer effects on activities of daily living than plaster short-leg casts.[41]

Overall, fiberglass is steadily replacing plaster in most pediatric centers for fracture care and spicas. Compared to plaster, fiberglass provides superior strength, durability, and imaging, as well as lighter weight, excellent molding, and ability to be used as a "water-friendly" cast.

Other Casting Materials

In addition to the standard rigid casting materials of plaster and fiberglass, a less rigid class of synthetic casting material is available. Although less rigid than standard casting materials, this Soft Cast (3M Health Care Ltd., Loughborough, United Kingdom) has several potential advantages. Experimental studies have shown that this material is more accommodating to increases in pressure than the other casting materials.[21] As this material is less rigid, it may be an ideal material to immobilize patients with severe osteopenia. Finally, this material can be removed without using a cast saw, which eliminates the risk of cast saw injury.[10]

Combination of Materials

Some combine plaster and fiberglass casting materials. One may reinforce a thin well-molded plaster cast by overwrapping it with fiberglass to increase its durability and minimize its weight. With this technique, one must ensure that the plaster has set before overwrapping with the fiberglass. Failure to do so may result in a thermal injury.[35] Shortcomings of this technique include the fact that the two layers of material may obscure fine radiographic detail. Finally, great care must be taken when removing such casts as it may be difficult to "feel" the depth of the cast saw blade and blade temperatures may be more elevated than usual. To avoid the increased risks of burns, it may be advantageous to use plastic protection strips under the cast when using a standard vibrating cast saw for cast removal. Because of the many shortcomings and dangers of a plaster cast overwrapped by fiberglass, we do not recommend routine use and prefer proper technique with fiberglass casting.

GENERAL CAST APPLICATION PRINCIPLES

While pain control and sedation are often required, techniques are needed for calming and distracting a child during cast application. Speaking with a soft voice and sitting and placing oneself at a level at or below that of the child are all useful techniques to present a less intimidating stature. Initial examination techniques should be soft and distant from the site of concern, progressing slowly to the area of concern.

Talking to the child and their parents helps identify the best approach for an individual child, and use of child life specialists proves extremely helpful in implementing the preferred approach.[15,58] For infants and toddlers, soft music, toys (especially those with lights or moving parts), and some interactive applications on handheld devices help with distraction and relaxation.[48] When using a cast saw for cutting the cast or cast removal, ear protection helps decrease anxiety.[12] For children with cognitive disorders, behavioral disorders, or ASD, discussion of possible approaches with the parents reaps rewards as they have the best sense of what will be calming, as well as stimulatory, for their child.

Plaster of Paris depends on excellent handling techniques to maximize the benefits of mold ability and fit and also to maximize strength. Some like the plaster to be wet to mold better; others would like a drier roll to ease application (less slippery) and speed the curing process. It is optimal to keep the plaster roll in contact to the limb to avoid wrapping the material too tight (Fig. 4-6). The plaster should be unrolled with overlaps of one-half to one-third the width of the roll and tucks are taken to avoid the tendency of pulling and stretching the material (thus increasing tightness) to get a good distribution and fit of the plaster around the difficult concave areas of the ankle, knee, elbow, and thumb. The optimal cast technique requires frequent rubbing and incorporation of the plaster rolls as the cast is being applied (i.e., initial molding) and will improve the fit but will also flatten the tucks and incorporate the mineral portion of the plaster into the fiber mesh for optimal strength. Plaster splints should be dipped and vigorously molded together before applying to the convexity of the limb (back of elbow or ankle) or where additional strength is needed (anterior knee [long-leg cast] or posterior thigh [spica cast]).

Once the plaster cast is applied and the initial molding has been accomplished, the cast is supported by broad surfaces such as the palm of a hand; the thorax of the surgeon is an excellent

Figure 4-6. Plaster roll is not lifted off of the cast but kept in contact during application as it is "rolled" up the extremity with an overlap of 30% to 50%. (Property of UW Pediatric Orthopaedics.)

broad surface to hold the plantar foot in neutral flexion and extension (Fig. 4-7A). Statically holding a cast with the tips of fingers as it dries will leave indentations that can lead to pressure sores. If fingers are needed for molding, pressure should be applied and then withdrawn as the plaster reaches the final curing at which point, terminal molding of the cast can be done. Terminal molding is that point at which the plaster is fairly firm, somewhat pliable and warm; yet can be gently deformed without cracking the plaster of Paris. This is the appropriate time to do the final mold and hold of fracture fragments. As the cast goes through the final curing process, it can be supported on pillows, provided the cast is not too hot (the pillow prevents heat loss and will increase the temperature at the skin surface). A leg cast should be supported under the calf and allowing the heel to hang free (Fig. 4-7B) and thus prevent a gradual deformation of the heel into a point of internal skin pressure.

Fiberglass material is applied and molded in a slightly different manner and requires some specific techniques in comparison to plaster of Paris. Fiberglass material should be removed from its package and dipped in water just prior to application as it will cure and harden in the air. Fiberglass is often tacky in nature and therefore increased tension is needed to unroll the fiberglass and can inadvertently result in a cast that is circumferentially too tight. To avoid this, fiberglass should be applied

Figure 4-7. A: The foot is supported on the surgeon's thorax, and this holds the foot at 90 degrees while the rest of the cast is molded. **B:** While the cooled cast is supported on the pillow, the heel is allowed to hang free and thus be at less risk for deformation and a heel sore. The cast is univalved with a cast saw that is supported by the surgeon's index finger. (Property of UW Pediatric Orthopaedics.)

in a stretch relaxation manner; the fiberglass roll is lifted off of the limb (in contradistinction to plaster which stays in contact); unrolled first then wrapped around the limb (Fig. 4-8). Particular caution should be observed when wrapping a wide roll into a concavity (anterior elbow or ankle) as just the right amount of tension will allow the fiberglass to lay flat without compressing across the joint too tightly. Small relaxing cuts in the fiberglass may be needed, as fiberglass does not tuck as easily as plaster of Paris. Fiberglass is not as exothermic as plaster of Paris and risk of burns is lower when used without underlying plaster. The other principles of holding the cast as the fiberglass cures are the same as with plaster of Paris.

CAST SPLITTING

Casts are cut and split to decrease the pressure the limb experiences after trauma or surgery. In general, the more trauma (either from the trauma or the surgery performed) a limb experiences, the more swelling that will ensue. Thus, minimally displaced fractures can often be managed without splitting a cast, while those requiring a closed or open reduction may initially need to be managed in a split cast or one padded with thick foam. Although splitting may be done prophylactically or as symptoms develop, the experienced clinician will often choose the former to avoid having to split the cast at a later time when the child is in pain, crying, anxious, and usually in the middle of the night. When splitting a cast, one must ensure that the plaster or fiberglass has set, that is hardened and cool, and that the blade temperature remains cool throughout the splitting process. Attempting to split a plaster cast before it is warm and hard (curing) or less than 10 minutes after application is more difficult and prone to result in inadvertent skin touches.

The effect of cast splitting depends on the material used, how it was applied, and whether the associated padding is split.

Figure 4-8. The fiberglass is applied with stretch relaxation method. The fiberglass is unrolled first then placed over the body. (Property of UW Pediatric Orthopaedics.)

Figure 4-9. **A, B:** Foam padding is placed on skin, followed by cast padding, then fiberglass casting material. This allows for welling and provides strength but does not hold fracture reduction. Ideally, stockinette at the ends of the cast would make for better edges. (Property of Children's Hospital of Los Angeles.)

Plaster cast cutting and spreading (univalve) can be expected to decrease 40% to 60% of the pressure and release of padding may increase this by 10% to 20%.[28,50] Fiberglass casts applied without stretch relaxation are known to be two times tighter than those applied with plaster and in these cases, bivalving the fiberglass cast would be needed to see similar decreases in pressure. Casts that are applied with the stretch relaxation method are among the least constrictive of fiberglass casts and therefore univalving may be sufficient as long as the cast can be spread and held open with commercially available plastic cast wedges.

Although splitting casts is the traditional means of relieving cast tightness and allowing for swelling, use of thick foam is gaining acceptance at many centers (Fig. 4-9). Half-inch sterile foam can be used on most postoperative casts when concern for swelling is present. The foam is placed directly on skin to ensure circumferential pressure is not caused by cast padding. Stockinette and cast padding are then applied, followed by fiberglass. This type of cast is not used to hold a closed reduction with cast molding but works well for fractures made stable with internal fixation.

Instead of splitting the cast, the editor (D.L.S.) recommends foam placed under fiberglass if the cast may need to accommodate swelling.

CAST REMOVAL

Casts are removed using an oscillating cast saw designed to cut the hard cast material and not soft material such as padding or skin. In one report, the incidence of cast saw burns occurring with the removal of casting material was found to be 0.72% (Fig. 4-10).[3] Studies have shown that increased cast thickness, decreased padding, and dull blade use result in higher blade temperatures.[39] The technician who removes the cast must be well trained in the use of the saws. One common pitfall is to slide the oscillating saw along the cast, thus increasing the

chance of a cut or burn. Proper technique dictates that the blade be used by alternating firm pressure with relaxation into the material and then withdrawn before replacing it at a different location.[62] Furthermore, the technician should intermittently feel the blade and pause during the removal process when necessary to allow the blade to cool.

Various safety shields are available that, at the time of cast removal, may be slid between the skin and the padding to prevent saw injury. In general, cast saw burns should be exceedingly rare if protective plastic strips are used at the time of cast removal, and the cast saw is used only over these strips. Often, the safety shield cannot be slid up the entirety of the cast, so extreme care must be taken in these areas where the skin is not protected. Alternatively, safety strips may be incorporated into the cast at the time of cast application (Fig. 4-11). Finally, new advances in differing types of saws may improve the safety of cast removal.

CAST WEDGING

In a fresh fracture (usually <2 weeks old and prior to significant callus formation) in which initial reduction was obtained and subsequently is found to have an unacceptable loss of reduction, cast wedging of a well-fitting cast may be attempted. Many techniques for cast wedging have been described; however, the most recent description by Bebbington[6] appears to be easy to apply for simple angular deformities. The radiograph of the malaligned limb is used to trace the long axis of the bone onto a sheet of paper, which is then cut along this line. The cut edge of the paper is traced onto the cast, matching the position of the apex of the paper with the apex of the deformity. The cast is then cut, nearly circumferentially at this level, leaving a bridge of intact plaster or fiberglass only at the apex. Corks or cast wedges are applied opposite this bridge until the line transferred on the cast is straight.

Figure 4-10. Examples of cast saw burns. Initial injury photo (**A**) and after healing (**B**). **C:** A separate injury.

Figure 4-11. **A:** A cutaway picture showing the DE FLEX (W.L. Gore & Associates; Newark, Delaware) strip under the fiberglass casting tape. **B:** This strip will protect the skin from cast saw that may cut or burn through synthetic cast padding. (Property of UW Pediatric Orthopaedics.)

If this fails, the cast may need to be removed and the fracture either remanipulated or treated in some other fashion. Great care should be taken when performing cast wedging, especially in the tibia and in fractures where the patient may be already partially healed. The patient and family should be warned that the procedure will be uncomfortable at the time of wedging. The clinician needs to ensure that no excessive focal pressure is exerted at the bridge, causing a pressure ulcer or nerve compression. There are techniques described for closing wedge cast modification, but the authors have no experience with this technique. If any concern exists for excessive pressure or unsafe positioning following wedging, a new cast should be applied or a different treatment course taken.

CASTING OVER SURGICAL WOUNDS AND IMPLANTS

Often, casts are applied over surgical wounds. While the majority of these heal uneventfully, special attention should be given to casts applied over traumatic or surgical wounds. When applying a stockinette over a surgical wound, care should be taken to ensure the dressing is not bunched up under the liner. It is vitally important that wounds should not be dressed with circumferential cotton gauze as they may become constrictive with dried blood over time and act as a tourniquet. We prefer to use sterile cast padding, which is able to stretch with swelling and we limit placement of the gauze to directly over the wound itself. Applying nonstick dressings directly to the wound aids in decreasing the anxiety of wound inspection during the cast removal process. Should unexplained pain, fevers, foul odors, drainage, or worsening pain occur, wounds should be inspected; without these, however, routine inspection is often not necessary.

Bending the exposed ends of pins under a cast prevents excessive migration and allows for easy removal; however, migration of the bent end of the pin can occur. Sterile felt or antibiotic dressing may be placed at the pin site to help provide mechanical protection of soft tissue from migrating pins. Be aware that pin caps may become displaced and cause pressure sores. Cast padding should be placed over the pins to prevent them from sticking to the casting material as it hardens.

Although the technique of pins and plaster has largely disappeared from adult orthopaedics, it can be used occasionally in pediatric orthopaedics. In this technique, a fracture is reduced using pins that are placed percutaneously and incorporated into a cast to act essentially as an external fixator. The pin sites should be managed as any other exposed pin with an antibiotic dressing and/or sterile felt at the pin/skin interface. This technique allows the pins to be removed when callus formation is observed without removing the entire cast.

To inspect any area of concern under a cast, the cast can be removed, split, or windowed. The process of windowing involves localizing the area of concern and removing the overlying cast in this area without disrupting the alignment of the underlying bone. One may consider removing this window as a circular or oval piece to avoid creating any stress risers in the cast that may alter its structural integrity. However, attempting to cut "curves" with an oscillating saw places torque on the blade, increasing blade temperature. These factors should be remembered when windowing a cast. Once the cast and padding materials are removed, the wound can be inspected. Once satisfied, equal depth of padding should be replaced over the wound and the window replaced. It may be taped in place if serial examinations are required, or it may be overwrapped with casting tape. Failure to replace the window can lead to swelling through the window aperture.

MEDICAL COMORBIDITIES THAT AFFECT CAST CARE

Even with application of a "perfect" cast, numerous medical issues may complicate tolerance of casting or lead to complications.[33] Children with myelomeningocele are susceptible to a number of casting complications. Pressure sores commonly occur in insensate children who do not experience or exhibit discomfort when irritation arises under the cast. Caution should be taken to avoid areas of increased pressure or overmolding when casting. In addition, the many fractures in children with myelomeningocele result from casting used for immobilization following elective surgery.[49] Iatrogenic fracture risk can be minimized by utilizing casting for as short a time frame as possible and/or use of a soft fiberglass casting material or a soft, bulky dressing that creates less of a stress riser on the bone.[49] Children with cerebral palsy are also at increased risk for pressure sores due to poor nutrition and an inability to articulate pain. The contractures that likely contributed to the fracture may make casting or splinting difficult.[56] Similar

approaches may be considered in children with malnutrition, renal osteodystrophy, or other bone fragility disorders. An additional consideration in cases of malnutrition and diminished bone health includes increased duration of fracture healing that may require longer periods of protection to prevent refracture.[23]

Children with obesity present their own complications. Although there are no studies documenting the outcomes of casting in obese children, studies on surgical treatment have demonstrated complications of refracture, wound infection, and failure of surgical fixation,[46,70] issues that likely have nonoperative correlates. Loss of alignment when adequate molding cannot occur because of increased soft tissues can occur. When casting an obese child, inclusion of an extra joint above and/or below the fracture may be required to maintain cast position. Furthermore, additional assistants may be necessary for appropriate limb positioning and holding. Diligent monitoring of alignment allows intervention with recasting, wedging, or transition to surgical intervention. Obese patients are more likely to undergo surgical treatment, as opposed to closed reduction, although it is unclear whether this is related to fracture severity or concerns regarding fracture stabilization.[57]

Alterations in casting materials or approaches may also be necessary in children with behavioral issues. Children with ASD present additional complexity during cast application (see discussion on distraction techniques), but even prior to cast application, considering their behavior guides decision making regarding the most appropriate immobilization. Children with violent tendencies pose even more risk once a cast is applied, not only to others but also to themselves. Administration of behavioral medications may improve tolerance of casting.[16] Soft splinting or cast bracing may be preferable, accepting some risk of malunion over likely secondary injury. Discussion and shared decision making with the parents result in the best management for an individual child and their family.

Children with dermatologic conditions require other considerations when deciding on best methods of immobilization. Children with atopic dermatitis may react to synthetic padding, so cotton may be more preferable. Splinting allows for better skin management, but when casting is required, minimizing duration or performing frequent cast changes allows for monitoring of skin conditions or early transition to splinting. Soft casting material contains diisocyanate which has been suspected, but not proven, as a skin irritant in isolated cases; avoiding such material in children with significant skin sensitivity or disorders seems prudent. Windowing the cast over an area of skin breakdown or infection allows for monitoring of the area. Varicella presents an even more complex issue as widespread skin breakdown occurs, predisposing to superinfection and development of bacterial pyomyositis. Casting helps prevent skin breakdown by covering itchy lesions, but monitoring lesions is not possible. Again, splinting may be preferable to allow for monitoring if it does not compromise maintenance of fracture reduction; otherwise, windowing or frequent cast changes may allow for skin monitoring. There should be a low threshold for removal of the cast if the child complains of pain to assess for not only compartment syndrome or infection but also necrotizing fasciitis.[20]

SUGAR-TONG SPLINT IMMOBILIZATION

Sugar-tong splints provide effective temporary support to the wrist and forearm until definitive reduction and casting or internal fixation, while allowing for swelling. Sugar-tong splints can be used for definitive treatment, provided the splint is comfortable and is retightened after 5 to 10 days to accommodate the decrease in swelling. At that point, reapplication of an elastic bandage or overwrapping with fiberglass is appropriate.

Before treating, the contralateral uninjured limb may be used as a template to measure and prepare an appropriate slab of casting material that should be wide enough to fully support the volar and dorsal surfaces of the arm (without radial and ulnar overlap) and long enough to span the arm from the volar

MP flexion crease in the hand, around the elbow (flexed at 90 degrees), and dorsally to the metacarpal heads (Fig. 4-12A). It is important that plaster splints are no more than 10 layers thick and of appropriate length so that edges do not have to be folded over (increasing thickness and the heat from curing). The slab is further customized to cut out material around the thumb base and tuck cuts are made at the elbow to prevent bunching of the material during the application.

The injured arm is reduced and positioned as described above, it is wrapped with three to four layers of cotton padding from the hand and around the elbow (similar thickness as that used for long-arm casting). The slab is dipped in cool water, excess water is removed, and the material is vigorously rubbed together so that the layers incorporate for strength. The ends of the slab have two to three layers of padding applied that will fold back and make the edges soft (Fig. 4-12B). The splint is applied and held with one roll of cotton and then an elastic bandage is tightly applied until the material is hardened (Fig. 4-12C). After hardening, the tight elastic bandage is removed and replaced with a new self-adherent elastic bandage applied without significant tension (Fig. 4-12D). This method ensures an optimal fit without having the splint be too tight.

A. B

D

C

Figure 4-12. A: The plaster roll for the sugar-tong splint is measured and is chosen to be wider than the arm without allowing for overlapping once the plaster slab is dipped and applied. **B:** After being dipped and applied, the slab is held on by one layer of cotton while tucks are cut in the plaster at the elbow to allow for overlap and minimal bunching. **C:** An elastic bandage is wrapped tightly to assist with terminal molding of the splint. **D:** The elastic bandage has been removed and replaced with a self-adherent elastic tape that has been loosely applied. (Property of UW Pediatric Orthopaedics.)

In the method described above, the arm is circumferentially wrapped with cotton and then a slab of plaster with padded ends is applied over it. This method is advantageous in ensuring a smooth interface of cotton without bunching under the plaster slab. If the clinician fears a lot of circumferential cotton padding could worsen swelling, an alternative method exists. In this instance, a long strip of padding is made by layering three to five layers of cotton and then the plaster slab is laid on top of it. The cotton is long and wide enough to ensure that there are no rough edges. The padded slab is then applied and wrapped as described above.

LONG-ARM 90-DEGREE CAST IMMOBILIZATION

Fracture reduction and long-arm cast application are best done in a setting where the child is adequately sedated and where enough qualified personnel can apply the cast under fluoroscopic guidance, although this may not be possible in many locations. Fracture reduction technique may consist of longitudinal traction, manipulation recreating the deformity, or reducing the fracture and placing the intact periosteum on tension. Three-point molding can be used in completely displaced fractures at the same level in the forearm; hand rotation is the final position to account for, based on angulation. In both-bone forearm fractures in which the fractures are at differing levels, apex volar greenstick angulation is reduced with pronation and apex dorsal angulation is reduced with supination (Fig. 4-13). It may be helpful to remember the (literal) "rule of thumb": rotating the thumb toward the apex of the deformity aids in reduction. Thus, an apex volar greenstick is reduced with pronation and an apex dorsal with supination. Optimal hand and wrist rotations can be ensured with fluoroscopy prior to cast application.

Finger traps and an IV pole or an assistant are necessary for successful casting. In this instance, longitudinal traction is used with the assistance of finger traps. Prior to securing the fingers, the appropriate length of stockinette should be placed on the

Figure 4-13. The deformity is accentuated with hyperflexion followed by reduction to allow the displaced ends to become opposed. (Property of UW Pediatric Orthopaedics.)

arm (Fig. 4-14A). A thin layer of cotton padding is applied circumferentially around the hand and arm. Individual strips of cotton are placed and torn with tension to fit intimately on the posterior elbow, thus avoiding too much anterior padding (Fig. 4-14B). Cotton is rolled high in the axilla to ensure enough padding for the proximal trimline. After padding is applied to the entire arm, fiberglass is applied from distal to proximal (Fig. 4-14C). One technically challenging area is the first web space. Multiple techniques exist for passing the fiber glass around this area, including cutting across approximately three-fourths of the roll, twisting the roll, or folding the roll to the appropriate size. Regardless of technique, the key is ensuring there is adequate padding on the thumb and index finger metacarpal head to avoid irritation. The fiberglass is then rolled up the arm to the level of the elbow to focus on one joint at a time. This allows you to mold the wrist or forearm as needed before extending it proximally above the elbow. As the fiberglass begins to harden, terminal molding of the arm is performed under fluoroscopy by flattening over the apex of the deformity, molding the ulnar border with the flat of the hand, and finally with some interosseus molding that will make the cast flatter and less cylindrical in cross-section (Fig. 4-14D). This method of applying the cast in two stages has the potential downside of edges of the short-arm cast digging into soft tissue proximally, so this must be avoided. The humerus portion is molded terminally by flattening the posterior humerus and molding along the supracondylar ridges (Fig. 4-14E). At this point, the stockinette edges can be folded back and a final layer of fiberglass can be applied to capture these edges (Fig. 4-14F). Final fluoroscopic or radiographic images are obtained while the child is still sedated, and if alignment is good, the forearm cast is univalved or bivalved and spread depending on preference (Fig. 4-14G). In general, the cast should be univalved and spread on the side of the arm that is opposite the direction of initial displacement; a fracture with a propensity for dorsal displacement should be split volarly and a fracture with a propensity for volar displacement should be split and spread along the dorsal surface.

SHORT-ARM CAST IMMOBILIZATION

As there are now good quality, randomized prospective studies showing that distal third both-bone fractures are treated equally well in short- or long-arm casts, short-arm cast immobilization is appropriate for most distal radius and ulnar fractures. The technique of application is similar to that presented above; however, it is important that the distal cast be oval in cross-section and the cast index (ratio of the AP cast width to lateral cast depth) to be near 0.7.

LONG ARM–THUMB SPICA EXTENSION CAST IMMOBILIZATION

In some instances, the fracture loses reduction when flexed to 90 degrees and the arm must be casted in extension. Including a thumb spica extension in this cast will fully control forearm

Figure 4-14. A: Stockinette is applied to the hand and arm along with a thin layer of cotton padding. **B:** To pad the convexity of the elbow without excessively padding the concavity, cotton strips are placed and torn over the elbow to prevent cotton from bunching up in the antecubital fossa. **C:** Fiberglass is partially cut to allow passage around the thumb to avoid skin irritation. **D:** Interosseus mold is applied to the forearm. **E:** Supracondylar mold is applied to prevent cast from sliding on the arm. **F:** Stockinette edges are folded back and a final layer of fiberglass is applied to complete the cast. **G:** Cast has been univalved and a spacer applied to keep edges distracted.

rotation while additionally maintaining the fracture out to length, which is obtained during the casting under traction. To prevent pressure sores over the thumb, extra padding is placed over the radial aspect of the anatomic snuffbox and thumb (Fig. 4-15A). The thumb spica portion of fiberglass is placed carefully out to the tip of the thumb while holding the thumb in neutral abduction and opposition (Fig. 4-15B). The fiberglass is applied with 50% overlap and using the stretch relaxation technique, fluoroscopy is again utilized while terminal molding of the short-arm portion is performed in slight pronation and with broad pressure over the apex of the deformity (Fig. 4-15C). The upper arm portion is next applied once the forearm portion is

hardened and with the reduction confirmed under fluoroscopic imaging. As the upper fiberglass hardens, a supracondylar mold is applied with the arm in gentle traction as the butt of the surgeon's hand and thenar eminence terminally mold the fiberglass (Fig. 4-15D); this mold in concert with the thumb spica mold should help to maintain rotation and length of the reduction. Final trimming and finishing the edges with the previously placed stockinette is done in the hand and the palmar trimline is cut back to allow MP finger flexion (Fig. 4-15E). Finally, the dorsum of the cast can be univalved with a cast saw to allow for swelling; with fiberglass, the cut edges of the cast need to be held open with commercially available spacers or other such

Figure 4-15. A: The thumb spica cotton padding is applied. A moderate amount of padding is applied at the dorsal radial aspect of the thumb base. **B:** Fiberglass is applied with the stretch relaxation method. **C:** Initial molding of the fiberglass is performed over the apex of the deformity. **D:** Supracondylar mold is applied above the elbow; this will prevent the cast from slipping down. **E:** The hand portion is trimmed back to allow finger MP flexion and the spica portion of the cast is out to the tip of the thumb, which is neutrally placed. (Property of UW Pediatric Orthopaedics.)

material to keep the cast from springing closed; this is in contra-distinction to plaster, which can remain open once a terminally molded cast is spread.

THUMB SPICA CAST IMMOBILIZATION

Usual incorporation of the thumb is needed for the extension cast described above as well as carpal injuries. Some surgeons include the thumb in all short-arm casts too. Regardless, it's important to ensure the thumb is well padded and casted in

a neutral position thumb abduction and opposition with well-padded distal trimline.

Shoulder Immobilization

Immobilization about the shoulder and the clavicle is somewhat limited when compared with other areas of the skeleton. Because of anatomic constraints about the shoulder, it is often very challenging to gain a reduction of a bone (proximal humerus, clavicle); and it is not practical to expect the fracture fragment to be firmly held in a reduced position. One historical exception may be the use of the shoulder spica cast for displaced proximal humerus fractures. Practically speaking, this cast was challenging to apply and for the patient to wear; pediatric orthopaedic trauma surgeons today would use internal fixation to maintain fracture reduction.

Despite the difficulty encountered when attempting reduction and firmly maintaining reduction with closed means, immobilization about the shoulder is used to provide comfort to the injured child. For clavicle fractures, a figure-of-eight collar or a shoulder sling can support the shoulder. Although the figure-of-eight collar was designed to retract the shoulder posteriorly and thus potentially reduce a shortened clavicle; practically the effect is minimal and the force needed to hold the shoulder back is often a challenge to the patient. Most patients find a personal preference between figure-of-eight collar and shoulder sling that is acceptable given equal clinical results between the two.

A proximal humerus fracture (whether treated nonoperatively or operatively) may be protected with immobilization with a sugar-tong splint. This splint is applied in stages. A slab of fiberglass or plaster is cut to a length that spans the proximal medial humerus (not too high in the axilla) and extends over the elbow and up the lateral aspect of the humerus up over the shoulder (Fig. 4-16). After dipping in water, the slab is placed on appropriate padding and then applied to the arm. We find it helpful to wrap sugar-tong splints very tightly with an elastic bandage as this improves the mold and fit. The elastic bandage is removed when the splint material is hard and is replaced loosely with a new one. The common pitfalls with this type of immobilization include the medial splint edge in the axilla that is too thick or too high. In addition, when the lateral splint edge is too low and ends close to a fracture level, it does not immobilize and actually increases the lever arm forces at the fracture. This is due to the fact that the adjacent

Figure 4-16. The plaster of a sugar-tong upper arm splint is folded over the shoulder and above the fractured proximal humerus fracture. (Property of UW Pediatric Orthopaedics.)

joints that are immobilized, and that could normally move and decrease the length of the lever arm, cannot function as such.

Hanging arm casts can be used in proximal humerus surgical neck fractures and humeral shaft fractures. These long-arm casts are applied with the concept that gravity will act upon the humerus fracture and can be effective in gradually improving alignment in children with fractures that are minimally angulated or bayonet opposed. The children will have to sleep in an upright position for several weeks until the fracture is healed enough to be converted to splint immobilization. These casts are simple long-arm casts that do not require intimate molding; the weight of the cast will provide gradual distraction that aligns the fracture. Common pitfalls include a patient who cannot sleep upright and placing the neck collar attachment on the forearm too close to the elbow, which could increase anterior angulation; or placing the attachment too close to the wrist, which could lead to posterior angulation.

SHORT-LEG CAST APPLICATION

Short-leg casts are applied with goals of fully immobilizing the lower leg and keeping the ankle at 90 degrees while avoiding complications such as pressure sores. After applying stockinette, the limb is wrapped with cotton padding and the ankle is held at 90 degrees. A potential pitfall is that as the casting material is placed, the ankle drifts into equinus; then as ankle flexion is restored to 90 degrees, casting material bunches up at the anterior ankle, which can cause soft tissue damage over time as well as neurovascular constriction. Care must be taken to ensure the position is held constant to avoid this. The ankle can be held at 90 degrees by the surgeon's torso and the fiberglass is carefully molded around the malleoli and the pretibial crest. The cast should be hard and well cured before cutting; bivalving a wet cast will weaken it and the foot can drift into equinus. The cooled cast can be supported on a pillow with the heel hanging free. Once hardened, the cast can be univalved and spread anteriorly, if needed, to accommodate swelling; if significant swelling is expected, the cast can be bivalved and spread with release of the cotton padding. Using fiberglass for short-leg casts generally results in a lighter and stronger cast, but if fiberglass is improperly applied too tightly, it can cause compartment syndrome.

LONG-LEG CAST APPLICATION

Long-leg cast application incorporates all of the techniques above; once the short-leg portion has hardened, the upper thigh is wrapped with padding and the knee (held in the chosen degree of flexion) and thigh are overwrapped with cast material. Care is needed to make sure the posterior trimline of the short-leg cast is not too high and which could be compressing in the popliteal fossa. The anterior knee portion can be reinforced with a splint and thus further decreasing the cast load in the popliteal fossa. Finally, a medial and lateral supracondylar mold (similar to that in long-arm cast) can be used to support the weight of the cast and prevent distal migration. Plaster long-leg casts can be heavy, as such, we will use an all fiberglass cast or consider a composite cast whereby the short-leg portion is molded with plaster of Paris and then when hardened, the proximal portion is placed with fiberglass.

SHORT-LEG SPLINT APPLICATION

Posterior short-leg splints are commonly used to immobilize the foot and ankle prior to definitive operative or nonoperative treatment and additionally to support the limb in the immediate postoperative period. These splints can accommodate significant swelling following trauma or surgery. Supplemental stirrup application may be needed in larger patients whose foot position cannot be controlled with a single posterior slab. In these cases, similar application methods and principles are used as seen in the upper extremity sugar-tong splint application.

Fundamental application includes holding the foot and ankle in 90 degrees of flexion while the limb is wrapped with four to six layers of cotton padding from the toes to the knee. A posterior slab of plaster is selected and should be wide enough to provide a medial and lateral trimline of an inch. It should be 10 layers thick and measured similarly to that seen in short-leg cast application described above. If needed, a U-stirrup of plaster five layers thick is measured and is usually 1 to 2 inches narrower than the posterior plaster slab; this allows overlap of the two pieces of plaster without completely covering the anterior foot, ankle, and leg. Both the stirrup and the posterior slab are dipped in water and the proximal and distal trimlines are padded with three to four more layers of cast padding. The slab is applied posteriorly; any redundant material at the level of the heel can be cut away before the U-stirrup is applied with some overlap of the stirrup and the slab. The plaster is held in place with one layer of cast padding. An elastic bandage is applied tightly until the plaster is hard, and then removed to prevent constriction. This last layer of cast padding allows for easy removal of the final layer of loosely applied elastic bandage or self-adherent elastic tape.

Variances to this method are similar to sugar-tong splint application described above. For instance, some practitioners prefer to layer the wet plaster splint with 5 thicknesses of padding and apply the padded splint directly to the limb. This has advantages in minimizing circumferential wrapping of the limb with cotton; yet, great care is needed to prevent inadvertent bunching or slipping of the padding.

SPICA CAST APPLICATION

Spica casts can be applied from infants to adolescents and the location of application can vary according to age and clinical problem. For instance, infants and most children with painful injuries will require sedation and application in the supine position on a spica table. In contrast, a single-leg spica cast can be used as an adjunct to internal fixation for femur fracture in large children or adolescents. These latter casts can be applied in a supine or even a standing position with a compliant and comfortable patient. Because of the size of the casts, most spica casts are constructed with synthetic cast material.

Spica cast application in children is performed on a well-padded spica table that should be firmly attached to the OR bed or cart; one person should be responsible for managing the torso and making sure the child does not fall off the table; one to two assistants will support the legs while the anesthesia team manages the head and airway—this leaves the last of a four- or five-person team to apply the cast.

Before placing the child on the spica table, a waterproof pantaloon or stockinette is applied to the torso and legs in some centers. Place a 2- to 4-inch thick towel or other pad on the stomach and under the liner or stockinette that will be removed when the cast is dry, to have room for food and respiration. Note that if the patient starts to desaturate during spica cast application, pulling out the abdomen padding frequently resolves this. The child is lifted onto the table and 3 to 6 thicknesses of padding are applied, with more at bony prominences such as over the patella and heels. It is also wise to completely cover the perineum with padding and high over the thorax; it is extremely hard to add padding once the cast material is applied (Fig. 4-17A). After padding is appropriately applied, the thorax is wrapped with fiberglass cast material (see Fig. 4-8) and extended down over the uninjured thigh; care is needed to cover the "intern's triangle"; this is the posterior area of the cast at the junction of the thigh, buttock, and thorax. Once the uninjured leg portion is hardened, the injured leg is casted from proximal to distal. We recommend casting from the thorax, over the hip, to the distal thigh, and then extending over the knee and onto the distal leg as soon as the hip and thigh portion is firm; once the knee and leg portion is hardened, then extend it down to include the foot and ankle. Care must be taken not to apply a short-leg cast first, and use it to apply traction across the femur as this is associated with soft tissue problems and compartment syndrome. In general, we include the foot in neuromuscular patients who are prone to develop an equinus contracture and whose distal tibia is osteoporotic and prone to fracture at the level of the distal trimline. The risk of including the foot in a spica cast is soft tissue problems over the dorsal ankle. Once the final cast is hardened, the perineal region is trimmed out and patient is removed from the spica table. The abdominal pad is removed and in some children, a hole can be cut for further room (Fig. 4-17B,C). Next, appropriate radiographs are obtained and the trimlines are padded from rolling back the under padding and lining and incorporated with trim fiberglass. The decision to apply a bar from leg to leg is made based on the structural integrity of the cast. Usually, this is not needed in small children and infants. Should a bar be needed, then it is wise to wait until the cast is fully cured and the chance of a pressure sore is decreased. Non–toilet-trained infants and children need to have an absorbent pad (small diaper, ABD pad, or sanitary napkin) placed in the perineal region and then a diaper is placed over this (Fig. 4-17D). Simply placing a diaper over the cast will not absorb the waste material, as the diaper will not be in contact before it tracks under the cast.

For length-stable diaphyseal femoral shaft fractures, many centers are now moving toward a single-leg spica cast, which does not include the contralateral thigh and positions the hip

Figure 4-17. A: This 5-year-old child with a femur fracture is supported with four assistants as cotton padding is applied to the patient's body, which is covered with a waterproof liner over a stack of towels placed as a spacer for his belly. **B, C:** The abdominal pillow is removed after trimming away the perineal region. **D:** When finished, the spica edges are well padded and incorporated into the cast. A small diaper is placed into the perineal region and then another diaper will be placed over this to hold it in place. (Property of UW Pediatric Orthopaedics.)

and knee in less flexion and gives the child the opportunity to ambulate with a walker or crutches.

CONCLUSION

In this chapter, we highlight the pearls and pitfalls of cast and splint application in children with pediatric orthopaedic trauma. This orthopaedic subspecialty is one of the few in which an injury is more likely treated with these methods than surgical treatment. A dearth of prospective studies means that much art and personal preferences remain in cast and splint application. As time moves along and there are more innovative methods to treat fractures with surgery, the role of casting will not be supplanted. There will always be a need for a technically well-done cast that helps speed recovery in pediatric trauma. In our minds, the many complications result from inappropriate use of the cast or splint to *obtain* correction; in contrast, the cast or splint should be used to *maintain* reduction achieved either open or closed. Tight casts and bandages are also commonly associated with compartment syndrome. Problems such as tight casts, wet casts leading to infection, foreign objects in casts, and pressure ulcers are not uncommon. It is important to educate parents that small children may not adequately communicate problems occurring under a cast. It is good for us all to remember that in the words of Chad Price, MD, "there are no hypochondriacs in a cast."

ACKNOWLEDGMENTS

The authors thank Blaise A. Nemeth, Matthew A. Halanski, and Kenneth J. Noonan for the chapter in the last edition on which this revision was based.

REFERENCES

1. Aarons CE, Fernandez MD, Willsey M, et al. Bier block regional anesthesia and casting for forearm fractures: safety in the pediatric emergency department setting. *J Pediatr Orthop.* 2014;34:45–49.
2. Akbar M, Bresch B, Raiss P, et al. Fractures in myelomeningocele. *J Orthop Traumatol.* 2010;11:175–182.
3. Ansari MZ, Swarup S, Ghani R, Tovey P. Oscillating saw injuries during removal of plaster. *Eur J Emerg Med.* 1998;5:37–39.
4. Bashyal RK, Chu JY, Schoenecker PL, et al. Complications after pinning of supracondylar distal humerus fractures. *J Pediatr Orthop.* 2009;29:704–708.
5. Bear DM, Friel NA, Lupo CL, et al. Hematoma block versus sedation for the reduction of distal radius fractures in children. *J Hand Surg Am.* 2015;40:57–61.
6. Bebbington A, Lewis P, Savage R. Cast wedging for orthopaedic surgeons! *Injury.* 2005;36:71–72.
7. Bernthal NM, Hoshino CM, Dichter D, et al. Recovery of elbow motion following pediatric lateral condylar fractures of the humerus. *J Bone Joint Surg Am.* 2011;93:871–877.
8. Borland M, Esson A, Babl F, Krieser D. Procedural sedation in children in the emergency department: a PREDICT study. *Emerg Med Australas.* 2009;21:71–79.
9. Boyle PK, Badal JJ, Boeve JW. Severe cast burn after bunionectomy in a patient who received peripheral nerve blocks for postoperative analgesia. *Local Reg Anesth.* 2011;4:11–13.
10. Brewster MB, Gupta M, Pattison GTR, Dunn-van der Ploeg ID. Ponseti casting: a new soft option. *J Bone Joint Surg Br.* 2008;90:1512–1515.
11. Carmichael KD, Goucher NR. Cast abscess: a case report. *Orthop Nurs.* 2006;25:137–139.
12. Carmichael KD, Westmoreland J. Effectiveness of ear protection in reducing anxiety during cast removal in children. *Am J Orthop (Belle Mead NJ).* 2005;34:43–46.
13. Ceroni D, Martin X, Delhumeau C, et al. Effects of cast-mediated immobilization on bone mineral mass at various sites in adolescents with lower-extremity fracture. *J Bone Joint Surg Am.* 2012;94:208–216.
14. Ceroni D, Martin XE, Farpour-Lambert NJ, et al. Assessment of muscular performance in teenagers after a lower extremity fracture. *J Pediatr Orthop.* 2010;30:807–812.
15. Chambers CT, Taddio A, Uman LS, McMurtry CM; HELPinKIDS Team. Psychological interventions for reducing pain and distress during routine childhood immunizations: a systematic review. *Clin Ther.* 2009;31(Suppl 2):S77–S103.
16. Chambers H, Becker RE, Hoffman MT, et al. Managing behavior for a child with autism in a body cast. *J Dev Behav Pediatr.* 2012;33:506–508.
17. Constantine E, Steele DW, Eberson C, et al. The use of local anesthetic techniques for closed forearm fracture reduction in children: a survey of academic pediatric emergency departments. *Pediatr Emerg Care.* 2007;23:209–211.
18. Cudny ME, Wang NE, Bardas SL, Nguyen CN. Adverse events associated with procedural sedation in pediatric patients in the emergency department. *Hosp Pharm.* 2013;48:134–142.
19. Davids JR, Frick SL, Skewes E, Blackhurst DW. Skin surface pressure beneath an above-the-knee cast: plaster casts compared with fiberglass casts. *J Bone Joint Surg Am.* 1997;79(4):565–569.
20. Delasobera BE, Place R, Howell J, Davis JE. Serious infectious complications related to extremity cast/splint placement in children. *J Emerg Med.* 2011;41:47–50.
21. Deshpande SV. An experimental study of pressure-volume dynamics of casting materials. *Injury.* 2005;36:1067–1074.
22. DiFazio R, Vessey J, Zurakowski D, et al. Incidence of skin complications and associated charges in children treated with hip spica casts for femur fractures. *J Pediatr Orthop.* 2011;31:17–22.
23. Dwyer AJ, John B, Mam MK, et al. Relation of nutritional status to healing of compound fractures of long bones of the lower limbs. *Orthopedics.* 2007;30:709–712.
24. Fletcher ND, Schiller JR, Garg S, et al. Increased severity of type III supracondylar humerus fractures in the preteen population. *J Pediatr Orthop.* 2012;32:567–572.
25. Flynn JM, Bashyal RK, Yeger-McKeever M, et al. Acute traumatic compartment syndrome of the leg in children: diagnosis and outcome. *J Bone Joint Surg Am.* 2011;93:937–941.
26. Forni C, Loro L, Tremosini M, et al. Use of polyurethane foam inside plaster casts to prevent the onset of heel sores in the population at risk. A controlled clinical study. *J Clin Nurs.* 2011;20(5–6):675–680.
27. Gannaway JK, Hunter JR. Thermal effects of casting materials. *Clin Orthop Relat Res.* 1983;181:191–195.
28. Garfin SR, Mubarak SJ, Evans KL, et al. Quantification of intracompartmental pressure and volume under plaster casts. *J Bone Joint Surg Am.* 1981;63:449–453.
29. Grottkau BE, Epps HR, Di Scala C. Compartment syndrome in children and adolescents. *J Pediatr Orthop.* 2005;40:678–682.
30. Gulati A, Dixit A, Taylor GJ. Pediatric fractures: temporal trends and cost implications of treatment under general anesthesia. *Eur J Trauma Emerg Surg.* 2012;38:59–64.
31. Guyton GP. An analysis of iatrogenic complications from the total contact cast. *Foot Ankle Int.* 2005;26:903–907.
32. Haapala J, Arokoski J, Pirttimäki J, et al. Incomplete restoration of immobilization induced softening of young beagle knee articular cartilage after 50-week remobilization. *Int J Sports Med.* 2000;21:76–81.
33. Halanski M, Noonan KJ. Cast and splint immobilization: complications. *J Am Acad Orthop Surg.* 2008;16:30–40.
34. Halanski MA. How to avoid cast saw complication. *J Pediatr Orthop.* 2016;36:S1–S5.
35. Halanski MA, Halanski AD, Oza A, et al. Thermal injury with contemporary cast-application techniques and methods to circumvent morbidity. *J Bone Joint Surg Am.* 2007;89:2369–2377.
36. Hang JR, Hutchinson AF, Hau RC. Risk factors associated with loss of position after closed reduction of distal radial fractures in children. *J Pediatr Orthop.* 2011;31:501–506.
37. Hossieny P, Carey Smith R, Yates P, Carroll G. Efficacy of patient information concerning casts applied post-fracture. *ANZ J Surg.* 2012;82:151–155.
38. Kannikeswaran N, Lieh-Lai M, Malian M, et al. Optimal dosing of intravenous ketamine for procedural sedation in children in the ED: a randomized controlled trial. *Am J Emerg Med.* 2016;34:1347–1353.
39. Killian JT, White S, Lenning L. Cast-saw burns: comparison of technique versus material versus saws. *J Pediatr Orthop.* 1999;19:683–687.
40. Kim JK, Kook SH, Kim YK. Comparison of forearm rotation allowed by different types of upper extremity immobilization. *J Bone Joint Surg Am.* 2012;94:455–460.
41. Kowalski KL, Pitcher JD Jr, Bickley B. Evaluation of fiberglass versus plaster of Paris for immobilization of fractures of the arm and leg. *Mil Med.* 2002;167(8):657–661.
42. Large TM, Frick SL. Compartment syndrome of the leg after treatment of a femoral fracture with an early sitting spica cast. A report of two cases. *J Bone Joint Surg Am.* 2003;85:2207–2210.
43. Larson JE, Nicolay RW. Cast saw burn prevention: an evidence based review. *J Am Acad Orthop Surg.* 2021;29:380–385.
44. Lee TG, Chung S, Chung YK. A retrospective review of iatrogenic skin and soft tissue injuries. *Arch Plast Surg.* 2012;39:412–416.
45. Leet AI, Mesfin A, Pichard C, et al. Fractures in children with cerebral palsy. *J Pediatr Orthop.* 2006;26:624–627.
46. Leet AI, Pichard CP, Ain MC. Surgical treatment of femoral fractures in obese children: does excessive body weight increase the rate of complications? *J Bone Joint Surg Am.* 2005;87:2609–2613.
47. Liddo LD, D'Angelo A, Nguyen B, et al. Etomidate versus midazolam for procedural sedation in pediatric outpatients: a randomized controlled trial. *Ann Emerg Med.* 2006;48:433–440.
48. Liu RW, Mehta P, Fortuna S, et al. A randomized prospective study of music therapy for reducing anxiety during cast room procedures. *J Pediatr Orthop.* 2007;27:831–833.
49. Lock TR, Aronson DD. Fractures in patients who have myelomeningocele. *J Bone Joint Surg Am.* 1989;71:1153–1157.
50. Marson BM, Keenan MA. Skin surface pressures under short leg casts. *J Orthop Trauma.* 1993;7:275–278.
51. McKenna P, Leonard M, Connolly P, et al. A comparison of pediatric forearm fracture reduction between conscious sedation and general anesthesia. *J Orthop Trauma.* 2012;26:550–555.
52. Monument M, Fick G, Buckley R. Quantifying the amount of padding improves the comfort and function of a fibreglass below-elbow cast. *Injury.* 2009;40:257–261.
53. Mubarak SJ, Frick S, Sink E, et al. Volkmann contracture and compartment syndromes after femur fractures in children treated with 90/90 spica casts. *J Pediatr Orthop.* 2006;26:567–572.
54. Netzer G, Fuchs BD. Necrotizing fasciitis in a plaster-casted limb: case report. *Am J Crit Care.* 2009;18:288–287.
55. Podeszwa DA, Mooney JF III, Cramer KE, Mendelow MJ. Comparison of Pavlik harness application and immediate spica casting for femur fractures in infants. *J Pediatr Orthop.* 2004;24:460–462.
56. Presedo A, Dabney KW, Miller F. Fractures in patients with cerebral palsy. *J Pediatr Orthop.* 2007;27:147–153.
57. Rana AR, Michalsky MP, Teich S, et al. Childhood obesity: a risk factor for injuries observed at a level-1 trauma center. *J Pediatr Surg.* 2009;44:1601–1605.
58. Rusy LM, Weisman SJ. Complementary therapies for acute pediatric pain management. *Pediatr Clin North Am.* 2000;47:589–599.
59. Sawyer JR, Ivie CB, Huff AL, et al. Emergency room visits by pediatric fracture patients treated with cast immobilization. *J Pediatr Orthop.* 2010;30:248–252.
60. Scheier E, Gadot C, Leiba R, Shavit I. Sedation with the combination of ketamine and propofol in a pediatric ED: a retrospective case series analysis. *Am J Emerg Med.* 2015;33:815–817.
61. Schofield S, Schutz J, Babl F; Paediatric Research in Emergency Departments International Collaborative (PREDICT). Procedural sedation and analgesia for reduction of distal forearm fractures in the paediatric emergency department: a clinic survey. *Emerg Med Australas.* 2013;25:241–247.
62. Shuler FD, Grisafi FN. Cast-saw burns: evaluation of skin, cast, and blade temperatures generated during cast removal. *J Bone Joint Surg Am.* 2008;90:2626–2630.
63. Singh A, Khalil P. Point-of-care ultrasound-guided hematoma block for forearm fracture reduction. *Pediatr Emerg Care.* 2021;37(10):534–535.
64. Sobel M, Lyden JP. Long bone fracture in a spinal-cord-injured patient: complication of treatment—a case report and review of the literature. *J Trauma.* 1991;31:1440–1444.
65. Stevens JE, Walter GA, Okereke E, et al. Muscle adaptations with immobilization and rehabilitation after ankle fracture. *Med Sci Sports Exerc.* 2004;36:1695–1701.
66. Terzioğlu A, Aslan G, Sarifakioğlu N, Ciğşar B. Pressure sore from a fruit seed under a hip spica cast. *Ann Plast Surg.* 2002;48:103–104.
67. Tseng PT, Leu TH, Chen YW, Chen YP. Hematoma block or procedural sedation and analgesia, which is the most effective method of anesthesia in reduction of displaced distal radius fracture? *J Orthop Surg Res.* 2018;13:62.
68. Warrington SE, Kuhn RJ. Use of intranasal medications in pediatric patients. *Orthopedics.* 2011;34:456.
69. Weisberg MD, Vingan P, Gordon AM, Lee MC. Having patience with out patients: a key technique in cast saw burn prevention. *J Am Acad Orthop Surg.* 2022;30:e1025-e1032.
70. Weiss JM, Choi P, Ghatan C, et al. Complications with flexible nailing of femur fractures more than double with child obesity and weight >50 kg. *J Child Orthop.* 2009;3:53–58.
71. Wenger D, Pring ME, Rang M. *Rang's Children's Fractures.* 3rd ed. Lippincott Williams & Wilkins; 2005.

5

Management of the Severely Injured Child

Jonas K. Owen and Robert M. Kay

ROLE OF THE PEDIATRIC TRAUMA CENTER

Role of the Pediatric Trauma Center: KEY CONCEPTS

- ❏ The American College of Surgeons has established specific criteria for pediatric trauma centers mirroring those in adult trauma centers, including the principles of rapid transport and rapid treatment by an in-house surgical team.
- ❏ Timely assessment and treatment during the "golden hour" decreases mortality.
- ❏ Pediatric trauma centers can provide improved outcomes for severely injured children, but there are relatively few such centers, and many children are stabilized or treated definitively at adult trauma centers.

Trauma centers have been established based on the premise that the first hour (the "golden hour") after injury is the most critical in influencing the rates of survival from the injuries.

The first trauma centers focused on adult patients, though pediatric trauma centers have recently been created due to differences between pediatric and adult polytrauma.[71] The American College of Surgeons has established comparable criteria for pediatric and adult trauma centers based on the principles of rapid transport and rapid treatment by an in-house surgical team. A pediatric general surgeon is always in the hospital and heads the pediatric trauma team with other surgical specialists immediately available. General radiographic services and computed tomography (CT) capability must be always available for patient evaluation, and an operating room must be immediately available.

There is increasing evidence that survival rates and outcomes for severely injured children are improved at trauma centers compared to community hospitals, with the best results often reported at pediatric trauma centers.[4,6,23,35,44,46,54,93,109,119,163] Data from adult trauma centers show significantly lower mortality rates in pediatric polytrauma patients treated at centers with added pediatric qualifications, specifically in the more severely injured patients.[128,138,139] Another recent study which queried the National Trauma Data Bank showed lower rates of complications, but no significant difference in mortality, in pediatric patients treated at hospitals verified as trauma centers by American College of Surgeons compared to those which were not.[66] Although adolescent trauma patients admitted to an adult surgical intensive care unit (SICU) have been reported to have similar outcomes to comparable patients admitted to a pediatric intensive care unit (PICU) in a single institution, those admitted to the SICU were more likely to be intubated and to have a Swan–Ganz catheter placed and had longer intensive care unit (ICU) stays and longer hospital stays.[152]

In conclusion, the most ideal hospital setting for caring for a severely injured child is a pediatric trauma center. These centers, established based on the concept of the "golden hour," prioritize rapid transport and treatment by an in-house surgical team led by a pediatric general surgeon. Having access to general radiographic services, CT capability, and an operating room is crucial for patient evaluation and immediate intervention. Evidence suggests that survival rates and outcomes for severely injured children are improved at trauma centers, particularly pediatric trauma centers. Studies have shown lower mortality rates and fewer complications in pediatric patients treated at centers with added pediatric qualifications. While running pediatric trauma centers can be costly, leading to limited availability, stabilizing pediatric trauma patients at other hospitals before transfer to a pediatric trauma center or treatment at an adult trauma center can be an acceptable alternative when a separate pediatric trauma center is not feasible.

INITIAL RESUSCITATION AND EVALUATION

 Initial Resuscitation and Evaluation:
KEY CONCEPTS

- ❑ Following polytrauma, the initial medical management focuses on the life-threatening, nonorthopaedic injuries.[88,112,162,174]
- ❑ Initial resuscitation follows the Advanced Trauma Life Support (ATLS) or Pediatric Advanced Life Support (PALS) protocols.
- ❑ The primary survey comprises the "ABCDEs": Airway, Breathing, Circulation and hemorrhage control, Disability (neurologic), and Exposure and screening radiographs (cervical spine, chest, and pelvis).
- ❑ Hypovolemia is the most common cause of shock in pediatric trauma patients, so early and adequate fluid resuscitation is critical.

INITIAL EVALUATION

The initial steps in resuscitation of a child are essentially the same as those used for an adult.[88,99,112,162,174] The primary survey begins with assessment of the "ABCDEs"—airway, breathing, circulation and hemorrhage control, disability (neurologic), and exposure—followed by the secondary survey and screening radiographs (cervical spine, chest, and pelvis). Each of these steps must be addressed in order before moving to another element. In severe injuries, the establishment of an adequate airway immediately at the accident site often means the difference between life and death. The cervical spine needs to be stabilized for transport if the child is unconscious or in those with facial

Figure 5-1. Temporary cervical spine stabilization is imperative in any child with multitrauma, especially those who are unconscious or complain of neck pain.

trauma and/or neck pain (Fig. 5-1). A special transport board with an occipital cutout is recommended for children younger than 6 years because head size is large, relative to body size, in young patients. If a young child is placed on a traditional transport board, the cervical spine is flexed, which may cause neurologic injury.[80]

FLUID REPLACEMENT

Once an adequate airway is established and breathing has been assessed and stabilized, circulation and the amount of hemorrhage from the injury, either internally or externally, is assessed. Because of the prevalence of blunt trauma in pediatric polytrauma patients, most of the blood loss is internal and is easily underestimated. The first step is to identify hemorrhage and control blood loss. This blood loss is replaced initially with intravenous (IV) crystalloid solution. Access should be obtained with two large-bore IV catheters. However, in younger children, rapid IV access may be difficult. In this situation, a large-bore intraosseous needle can typically be inserted into the tibial metaphysis within 1 to 2 minutes and then used to deliver both fluids and drugs during resuscitation.[12,125] Bielski et al.,[15] in a rabbit tibia model, demonstrated no adverse effects on the histology of bone or the adjacent physis with intraosseous injection of various resuscitation drugs and fluids.

In severe hemorrhage that does not respond to crystalloid alone, massive transfusion with balanced packed red blood cells, plasma, and platelets is given. A ratio of 1:1:1 is accepted in adults but may not be adequate in children, given physiologic differences.[141]

Because death is common if hypovolemic shock is not rapidly reversed, the child's blood pressure must be maintained at an adequate level for organ perfusion. A urinary catheter is used during the resuscitation to monitor urine output as a means of assessing organ perfusion. In some instances, a central venous catheter is used to monitor fluid resuscitation more precisely. In children with traumatic brain injuries, care is exercised during initial fluid resuscitation since overhydration can exacerbate cerebral edema. Excessive fluid resuscitation can also lead to fluid shifts and interstitial pulmonary edema, with potential drops in arterial oxygenation, particularly following thoracic trauma.

The "triad of death," consisting of acidosis, hypothermia, and coagulopathy, has been described in trauma patients as a result of hypovolemia and the systemic response to trauma.[190]

EVALUATION AND ASSESSMENT

 Evaluation and Assessment: KEY CONCEPTS

❏ Trauma rating systems have two functions: to aid in triage and to predict outcomes.
❏ Of the commonly used systems, the Injury Severity Score (ISS), Pediatric Trauma Score (PTS), and Glasgow Coma Scale (GCS) have prognostic value.
❏ The secondary survey is a systematic examination of the patient from head to toe and is performed after primary survey. It includes a complete history, physical examination, focused radiographs, and adjunctive imaging studies such as CT and magnetic resonance imaging (MRI) scans.
❏ Because of many distracting injuries, serial examinations of the child may reveal initially undiagnosed injuries in the ensuing days to weeks.

TRAUMA RATING SYSTEMS

After initial resuscitation has stabilized the injured child's condition, it is essential to perform a quick but thorough check for other injuries. At this point in the evaluation, a trauma rating is often performed. The purpose of the trauma rating is twofold: to aid in triage and to predict outcomes. Several trauma rating systems have been validated for the pediatric population,[18,30,31,43,52,53,73,90,102,121,126] but the most commonly used are the GCS, the ISS, and the PTS. Each of the scoring systems has strengths and weaknesses. The ISS is a valid, reproducible rating system that can be widely applied in the pediatric polytrauma setting (Table 5-1).[189] It is an ordinal, not a linear, scale (i.e., a score of 40 is not twice as bad as a score of 20). It has been found to be a valid predictor of mortality, length of hospital stay, and cost of care.[21] Another injury rating system for children that has been shown to be valid and reproducible is the PTS (Table 5-2).[189] It has good predictive value for injury severity, mortality, and the need for transport to a pediatric trauma center. However, it is a poor predictor of internal injury in children with blunt abdominal trauma.[150] Age-specific parameters for the PTS are more predictive of mortality than general PTS.[118,138] The BIG score has been advocated by some centers for its prognostic value and ease of use.[18,43,53,118]

Trauma Quality Improvement Program (TQIP) is used by many trauma centers treating pediatric trauma patients.[76,77] It uses the National Trauma Data Bank and allows for stratification of risk. It is in its nascency and there are only limited data available.

Head injury is most often evaluated and rated by the GCS, which evaluates eye opening (1–4 points), motor function (1–6

TABLE 5-1. Injury Severity Scoring

Abbreviated Injury Scale (AIS)

The AIS classifies injuries as moderate, severe, serious, critical, and fatal for each of the five major body systems. The criteria for each system into the various categories are listed in a series of charts for each level of severity. Each level of severity is given a numerical code (1–5). The criteria for severe level (code 4) are listed below.

Severity Code	Severity Category/ Injury Description	Policy Code
4	Severe (life-threatening, survival probable)	B

General
Severe lacerations and/or avulsions with dangerous hemorrhage; 30–50% surface second- or third-degree burns.

Head and Neck
Cerebral injury with or without skull fracture, with unconsciousness >15 minutes, with definite abnormal neurologic signs; posttraumatic amnesia 3–12 hours; compound skull fracture.

Chest
Open-chest wounds; flail chest; pneumomediastinum; myocardial contusion without circulatory embarrassment; pericardial injuries.

Abdomen
Minor laceration of intra-abdominal contents (ruptured spleen, kidney, and injuries to tail of pancreas); intraperitoneal bladder rupture; avulsion of the genitals.
Thoracic and/or lumbar spine fractures with paraplegia.

Extremities
Multiple closed long-bone fractures; amputation of limbs.

Injury Severity Score (ISS)
The ISS is a combination of values obtained from the AIS. The ISS is the sum of the squares of the highest AIS grade in each of the three most severely injured areas. For example, a person with a laceration of the aorta (AIS = 5), multiple closed long-bone fractures (AIS = 4), and retroperitoneal hemorrhage (AIS = 3) would have an ISS of 50 (25 + 16 + 9). The highest possible score for a person with trauma to a single area is 25. The use of the ISS has dramatically increased the correlation between the severity and mortality. The range of severity is from 0 to 75.

Adapted from Committee on Medical Aspects of Automotive Safety. Rating the severity of tissue damage. I. The abbreviated scale. *JAMA.* 1971;215(2):277–280; and Baker SP, et al. The Injury Severity Score: a method for describing patients with multiple injuries and evaluating emergency care. *J Trauma.* 1974;4:187–196.

points), and verbal function (1–5 points) on a total scale of 3 to 15 points (Table 5-3). GCS is of limited use in children who are preverbal or in the early stages of verbal development, but in other children, this rating system has been a useful guide for predicting early mortality and later disability.[17,30,31,73,118,193,196] Some authors have advocated a pediatric GCS for these younger children, though it has not yet proven to be as reliable as the GCS in older children.[17] Recent authors have reported predictive value in the motor component of the GCS, even without using other components of GCS, though it was not as predictive as was use of the entire GCS score.[31] A GCS score below eight

TABLE 5-2. Pediatric Trauma Score

Component	Category		
	+2	+1	−1
Size	≥20 kg	10–20 kg	<10 kg
Airway	Normal	Maintainable	Unmaintainable
Systolic blood pressure	≥90 mm Hg	90–50 mm Hg	<50 mm Hg
Central nervous system	Awake	Obtunded/ Loss of consciousness	Coma/decerebrate
Open wound	None	Minor	Major/penetrating
Skeletal	None	Closed fracture	Open/multiple fractures

This scoring system includes six common determinants of the clinical condition in the injured child. Each of the six determinants is assigned a grade: +2, minimal or no injury; +1, minor or potentially major injury; −1, major, or immediate life-threatening injury. The scoring system is arranged in a manner standard with advanced trauma life support protocol and thereby provides a quick assessment scheme. The ranges are from −6 for a severely traumatized child to +12 for a least traumatized child. This system has been confirmed in its reliability as a predictor of injury severity.

Adapted from Tepas JJ III, et al. The Pediatric Trauma Score as a predictor of injury severity in the injured child, *J Pediatr Surg.* 1987;22(1):14–18. Copyright © 1987, with permission from Elsevier.

TABLE 5-3. Glasgow Coma Scale

Response	Action	Score
Best motor response	Obeys	M6
	Localizes	5
	Withdraws	4
	Abnormal flexion	3
	Extensor response	2
	Nil	1
Verbal response	Oriented	V5
	Confused conversation	4
	Inappropriate words	3
	Incomprehensible sounds	2
	Nil	1
Eye opening	Spontaneous	E4
	To speech	3
	To pain	2
	Nil	1

This scale is used to measure the level of consciousness using the eye-opening, best verbal, and best motor responses. The range of scores is from 3 for the most severe to 15 for the least severe. This is a measure of level and progression of changes in consciousness.

Reproduced from Jennett B, et al. Severe head injuries in three countries. *J Neurol Neurosurg Psychiatry.* 1977;40(3):291–298, with permission from BMJ Publishing Group Ltd.

points indicates a significantly worse chance of survival than does a GCS above eight. The GCS should be noted on arrival in the trauma center and repeated 1 hour later. Serial changes in the GCS correlate with improvement or worsening of the neurologic injury. Repeated GCS assessments over the initial 72 hours after injury may be of prognostic significance.

PHYSICAL ASSESSMENT

The secondary survey starts with a full history and physical examination. A careful abdominal examination allows early detection of injuries to the liver, spleen, pancreas, or kidneys. When present, ecchymosis on the abdominal wall must be noted, as it is often a sign of significant visceral or spinal injury.[26,48,89]

The extremities are checked for swelling, deformity, or crepitus. If extremity deformity is present, it is important to determine whether the fracture is open or closed. Sites of external bleeding are examined, and sterile pressure dressings are applied if necessary to prevent further blood loss. Imaging studies facilitate surgical planning.

Pelvic fractures are high-energy injuries and often associated with significant morbidity and mortality.[45,130,155,161,165,184] A pelvic fracture combined with one or more other skeletal injuries has been suggested to be a marker for the presence of head and abdominal injuries.[183] Major arterial injuries associated with fractures of the extremity are usually diagnosed early by the lack of or diminished peripheral pulse. In contrast, abdominal venous injuries caused by blunt trauma—half of which are fatal—are rare and often remain undiagnosed before exploratory laparotomy. Consequently, in children who continue to require substantial blood volume support after the initial resuscitation has been completed, abdominal venous injury should be considered.[60]

Initial splinting of suspected extremity fractures is routinely done in the field. However, once the injured child is in the hospital, the orthopaedist should inspect the extremities to assess the injuries and determine the urgency of definitive treatment.

Any neurologic deficit is noted, and extremity function is documented prior to treatment. The inability to obtain a reliable examination due to the child's age, mental status, or pain from distracting injuries should be documented.

Head injuries and pain in other locations can result in injuries being missed initially. In a series of 149 pediatric polytrauma patients, 13 injuries were diagnosed an average of 15 days following the initial accident, including 5 fractures (1 involving the spine), 4 abdominal injuries, 2 aneurysms, 1 head injury, and 1 facial fracture.[102] Given this 9% incidence of delayed diagnosis, serial examinations should be performed on polytrauma patients once they are more comfortable to reassess for potential sites of injury. Despite careful inpatient examinations, some pediatric injuries escape detection until follow-up visits. Children with head injuries need to be reassessed once they awaken enough to cooperate with reexamination. Families and patients should be informed of the frequency of delayed diagnosis of some injuries in polytrauma patients so that they can help identify additional injuries and are not surprised in the event of later diagnoses.

IMAGING STUDIES

Radiographs

Primary screening radiographs classically consist of a cross-table lateral cervical spine, anteroposterior chest, and anteroposterior pelvis. In some centers, a lateral cervical spine radiograph is obtained only if the child has a head injury or if neck pain is noted on physical examination.

The lateral cervical spine radiograph detects 80% of C-spine injuries.[99] They are more accurate for osseous injuries but can miss purely ligamentous cervical spine injuries.[106] If there is suspicion of a cervical spine injury on the neutral lateral view, a lateral flexion radiograph of the cervical spine taken in an awake patient will help detect cervical instability safely. Radiographs should be followed by a CT scan as they are more accurate at identifying fracture patterns. Further workup with cervical spine MRI is necessary before cervical spine clearance in those who have persistent neck pain or tenderness despite normal plain films and CT and should be considered in patients who remain obtunded.

The cervical spine of a young child is much more flexible than the cervical spine of an adult. Under the age of 12 years, the movement of C1 on C2 during flexion of the neck can normally be up to 5 mm, whereas in adults, this distance should be less than 3 mm. Likewise, in this young age group, the distance between C2 and C3 is up to 3 mm. No forward movement of C2 on C3 should be present in a skeletally mature patient when the neck is flexed. Pseudosubluxation of C2 on C3 in a child should not be diagnosed as instability that requires treatment because this is a normal finding in young children.[29,50] Because it is difficult to detect a fracture of the thoracic or lumbar spine clinically, radiographs of this area, primarily a lateral view, should be carefully evaluated, particularly in a comatose child.

Biplanar imaging studies of any site of suspected musculoskeletal injury should be obtained as quickly as possible after the initial resuscitation and physical examination.

Computed Tomography

CT is essential in evaluating a child with multiple injuries and often provides useful information regarding injuries to the head, chest, abdomen, and pelvis.

CT of the pelvis is more sensitive for pelvic fractures than is a screening pelvic radiograph (Fig. 5-2). Pelvic CT is useful for thoroughly evaluating fracture pattern and determining appropriate treatment options, both surgical and nonsurgical. In one study, a screening pelvic radiograph demonstrated only 54% of pelvic fractures identified on CT scan.[67] A more recent study showed that CT scan resulted in a change in diagnosis of the pelvic fracture (compared to plain radiograph findings) in 38% of cases, though treatment was not changed, as none of their 30 patients required surgery.[14] If abdominal CT is being done to evaluate visceral injury, the CT should be extended distally to include the pelvis. Abdominal CT is required to classify and grade the severity of abdominal solid organ injury.[74]

CT of a fractured vertebra will provide the information needed to classify the fracture as stable or unstable and

Figure 5-2. CT is more sensitive and specific for the identification and classification of pediatric pelvic fractures.

determine whether operative treatment is needed. Some centers evaluate the cervical spine with a CT scan in children with polytrauma who have neck pain, a traumatic brain injury (TBI), or who have been drinking alcohol.[151]

Intravenous Pyelography

There is a strong correlation of urologic injury with anterior pelvic fractures, as well as with liver and spleen injury. Although CT and ultrasonography are used to evaluate renal injuries, the IV pyelogram still has a role in helping to diagnose bladder and urethral injuries (Fig. 5-3).[124]

Magnetic Resonance Imaging

MRI is used primarily for the detection of injury to the brain, spine, and spinal cord. In young children, the bony spine

Figure 5-3. Genitourinary injuries typically involve the urethra and/or bladder, are more common in males than females, and are associated with anterior pelvic ring fractures.

is more elastic than the spinal cord and spinal cord injury can occur without an obvious spinal fracture, particularly in automobile accidents.[8,20,50,54,58,194] In the spinal cord injury without radiographic abnormality (SCIWORA) syndrome, MRI is valuable in demonstrating the site and extent of spinal cord injury and in defining the level of injury to the disks or vertebral apophysis. A fracture through the vertebral apophysis is similar to a fracture through the physis of a long bone and may not be obvious on plain radiographs. MRI is useful in C-spine clearance in nonresponsive patients, abnormal neurologic examinations, or when radiographs and CT are inconclusive.

Ultrasonography

Ultrasound evaluation can detect hemopericardium and intraperitoneal fluid following injury.[24,81,144] The Focused Assessment with Sonography for Trauma (FAST) consists of a rapid ultrasound examination of four areas: the right upper abdominal quadrant, the left upper abdominal quadrant, the subxiphoid area, and the pelvis. Though FAST has been used as a rapid screening tool in pediatric polytrauma patients, it frequently misses intra-abdominal injuries following blunt trauma.[25,56,82,83,120,153] The extended FAST (eFAST) adds bilateral lung views to evaluate for pneumothorax and has replaced FAST as the screening tool in pediatric trauma patients.[122] Typically, eFAST has a higher specificity than sensitivity for intra-abdominal and intrathoracic injuries, making it a useful "rule-in" tool. As a result, CT is more often used for assessment and monitoring of visceral injury in children sustaining multiple injuries. Despite these limitations, hemodynamically unstable children with a positive eFAST are often taken for laparotomy rather than for CT scanning.

NONORTHOPAEDIC CONDITIONS IN THE MULTIPLY INJURED CHILD

Nonorthopaedic Conditions in the Multiply Injured Child: KEY CONCEPTS

- ❏ Head injury severity is the principle determinant of morbidity and mortality in a multiply injured child.
- ❏ Children often make substantial recovery from even severe head trauma.
- ❏ Management of orthopaedic injuries in children with head trauma should be based on the presumption of full recovery from the head injury.
- ❏ Spasticity and contracture are common sequelae of brain injury and should be addressed early.
- ❏ There is an association between pediatric pelvic fractures and both intra-abdominal and genitourinary injuries.
- ❏ Motion at the site of a long-bone fracture results in increased intracranial pressure (ICP). To control ICP, it is imperative that long-bone fractures are immobilized until definitive fracture care is provided.

TRAUMA-INDUCED COAGULOPATHY

A balance of procoagulant, anticoagulant, and fibrinolytic factors within the coagulation system is important to obtain hemostasis without developing thromboembolic events. Trauma-induced coagulopathy (TIC) is an imbalance in the coagulation system that has a negative prognostic factor. Patients presenting with TIC have an increased mortality, longer ICU stays, and more days ventilated.[108a] After significant trauma and blood loss, there is an initial hypocoagulable state that can lead to worsening hemorrhage. While the exact etiology is not understood, it is most likely due to loss of procoagulant factors and platelets as well as consumption of clotting factors without replacing them. This initial hypocoagulable state lasts approximately 24 hours and is followed by a longer period of hypercoagulable state which increases chances of thromboembolic events.[162a] Abnormal laboratory values of PT, aPTT, and international normalized ratio are poor markers for TIC. Viscoelastic hemostatic assays, such as thromboelastography, are better indicators of coagulation status in injured children.[51a] Use of balanced resuscitation (discussed previously) is a key to combat TIC.

Tranexamic acid (TXA) is a lysine analog that blocks the binding site of plasminogen, reducing breakdown of fibrin blood clots. It has been shown to be effective in decreasing surgical bleeding and need for blood transfusions in multiple elective pediatric orthopaedic procedures including posterior spinal fusions and hip reconstructions.[37,198,199] In adult trauma patients, TXA administration within 3 hours from injury decreases mortality, improves 30-day survival, and shows improved outcomes in TBI.[39,40,140,192] These studies showed benefits without an increase in thrombotic events. While there is robust literature for TXA use in adult trauma, data for pediatric patients are limited.[19] A TXA dose of 15 mg/kg and up to 1 g in pediatric trauma patients has a good safety profile and has an association with improved mortality.[19] The consensus recommendation is TXA may be used in children with hemorrhagic shock within 3 hours of injury.[148] Optimal dosing, timing, and overall effectiveness of TXA remain to be seen.

Deep venous thrombosis and pulmonary thromboembolism are much rarer in pediatric trauma patients than in adults, with rates between 0.02% and 1.2%.[2,7,9,10,41,42,100,104,146,149,175,182,195] Cunningham et al. reported an overall rate of 0.36% in over 8,000 pediatric trauma patients, with pulmonary thromboembolism in 0.04%.[41] The risk of deep venous thrombosis and pulmonary embolism is increased in older children, those with higher ISS scores, low GCS scores, and pelvic and/or lower extremity fractures.[41,42,146,195] One recent study reported a 9% rate of DVT in pediatric trauma patients admitted to the ICU, with the greatest risk following TBI.[100] Another recent study showed a 24% yield (11/47 patients) using a program of risk-stratified ultrasonography in medium- and high-risk pediatric trauma patients, with 82% (9/11) of patients with thromboembolism being asymptomatic, and 54% (6/11) of the VTE being associated with central venous catheters.[170] The role of prophylaxis for pediatric deep venous thrombosis and pulmonary thromboembolism is unclear and recommendations vary among surgeons and institutions.[2]

TRAUMATIC BRAIN INJURY

Prognosis for Recovery

Children recover more quickly and fully from significant head injuries than do adults, but head injuries remain the most common cause of ongoing disability in children following polytrauma.[51,55,103,193] The goal for management of patients with severe TBI is to maintain cerebral perfusion pressure while minimizing hypoxemia, hypercarbia, hypotension, and increased ICPs.[94,95] Mild cognitive, problem-solving, and/or learning deficits may persist, so educational testing needs to be considered for children who have had significant head injury.[185]

The severity of TBI is the single most important determinant of long-term outcome in polytraumatized children.[88] A recent study showed that severity of the brain injury based on CT scoring systems accurately predicted early mortality following TBI in children.[114] Better functional outcomes are reported at pediatric trauma centers than at adult trauma centers following pediatric TBI, regardless of whether or not the adult trauma center has added qualification in pediatric trauma.[138] The resiliency of children in the face of TBI was evident in one recent series, with approximately 15% of children who presented with an initial GCS of 3 or 4 having a good outcome 10 years after injury.[63]

Since children with brain injuries recover more fully than do adults, orthopaedic care is based on the assumption of full neurologic recovery. Without optimal orthopaedic care, the primary functional deficit may well result from ill-managed orthopaedic injuries rather than from the initial neurologic injury.

Intracranial Pressure

After a head injury, ICP is commonly monitored. Elevated ICP may exacerbate the sequelae of TBI, leading to further permanent disability or death. ICP can be controlled by elevating the head of the bed, lowering the PCO_2 (via mechanical ventilation), restricting IV fluids, or giving a hyperosmolar solution. External ventricular drains can also be placed. An ICP <20 mm Hg is the goal to improve overall outcomes.[94,95]

Since motion at the site of a long-bone fracture results in increased ICP, it is imperative that long-bone fractures are immobilized until definitive fracture is provided.[171]

Secondary Orthopaedic Effects of Head Injuries

A head injury can have direct impact on the musculoskeletal system. Head injury can lead to spasticity, contractures, and heterotopic ossification (HO), and can lead to accelerated fracture healing.

Spasticity

Spasticity may develop within a few days of head injury. An early effect of this spasticity is to cause shortening at the sites of long-bone fractures, despite traction or external immobilization. Fracture displacement or shortening in a cast may cause skin breakdown and increase the risk of infection. Operative stabilization should be done as soon as possible because fracture healing is accelerated by a head injury.[171]

Contractures

Contractures commonly develop after polytrauma and TBI. The persistence of spasticity in the extremities often leads to contractures of the joints spanned by the spastic muscles, but attention to appropriate positioning and splinting in the trauma center can decrease contracture frequency and severity. If the child lies in bed with the hips and knees extended, this extensor positioning will usually result in plantarflexion of the ankles. Part-time positioning with the hips and knees flexed helps prevent early equinus contractures from developing. Early physical therapy for range of motion, stretching, and splinting can often be effective in preventing contractures; casting may be needed if contractures develop. If these measures are not successful and are interfering with rehabilitation, the contractures may need to be released surgically.

Heterotopic Bone Formation

Heterotopic bone may form in the soft tissues within weeks after a significant head injury with persistent coma.[92,164] Although any joint can be affected, the most common sites are the hip and the elbow. There is some evidence that HO can be stimulated by surgical incisions and can form at the insertion site in head-injured children who undergo antegrade femoral intramedullary nailing.[91] HO should be considered in the differential diagnosis (along with a new fracture and deep vein thrombosis) if new swelling is noted in the extremity of a comatose child.[160] Technetium-99 bone scans show increased isotope uptake in the soft tissue where heterotopic bone forms.

The two primary approaches to managing HO are observation and excision.[92,164] Observation is the mainstay of treatment if the child remains comatose or if the child has recovered from the head injury, but the HO does not interfere with rehabilitation. Excision is chosen if there is significant restriction of joint motion from the heterotopic bone which interferes with rehabilitation. The timing of the heterotopic bone excision is controversial, but resection should be considered whenever heterotopic bone significantly interferes with rehabilitation, rather than waiting 12 to 18 months for the bone to mature. Recurrence of HO following excision does not appear to be affected by timing of excision, extent of HO, or the cognitive or functional level of the patient.[3] After surgical excision, early postoperative prophylaxis with local low-dose radiation therapy or medications (salicylates or nonsteroidal anti-inflammatory drugs, including indomethacin) decreases the risk of recurrence. Mital et al.[113] reported success in preventing recurrence of heterotopic bone after excision by use of salicylates at a dosage of 40 mg/kg/day in divided doses for 6 weeks postoperatively.

Fracture Healing Rates

Long-bone fractures heal more quickly in children and adults who have associated head injuries related to changes to posttraumatic alterations in the inflammatory and immune sytems.[70,115,201] Delay in treatment of acute fractures can make reduction more difficult due to the often early, exuberant callus formation.

PERIPHERAL NERVE INJURIES

Although TBI most often accounts for persistent neurologic deficits in a child with multiple injuries, one clinical review of brain-injured children reported that 7% had evidence of an associated peripheral nerve injury documented by electrodiagnostic testing.[135] For closed injuries, the peripheral nerve injury is typically associated with an adjacent fracture or with a stretching injury of the extremity and observation is indicated in most cases because these injuries often recover spontaneously. However, if the nerve injury is at the level of an open fracture, then exploration of the nerve is indicated at the time of the initial surgery. If function does not return within 2 to 3 months following observation of a closed injury, then electrodiagnostic testing is indicated. If peripheral nerve injury is present, surgical repair with nerve grafts offers an excellent chance of functional recovery in children and adolescents.

THORACIC INJURIES AND PULMONARY CONTUSIONS

Thoracic injuries encompass a wide spectrum of injuries and account for 14% of trauma-related deaths.[132] Many are more limited with blunt trauma and associated pulmonary contusion, while others involve damage to the great vessels, with very high associated mortality. Isolated thoracic injuries in children typically have quite good outcomes. On the other end of the spectrum, children with combined thoracic and brain and/or abdominal injuries have reported mortality rates of 20% to 40%.[132,142]

Pulmonary contusions have much better outcomes in the pediatric population than in adults.[65,72] However, if the lungs have been severely contused, protein leaks into the alveolar spaces, making ventilation more difficult. This may be exacerbated by the systemic inflammatory response syndrome, which is commonly seen following severe trauma.[190] Surfactant dysfunction follows and is most abnormal in patients with the most severe respiratory failure. As the time from the injury increases, pulmonary function can deteriorate and general anesthesia becomes riskier. Orthopaedic surgical treatment before such pulmonary deterioration limits the anesthetic risks in these patients. Bruises on the chest or rib fractures should alert the orthopaedist to potential pulmonary contusions as a part of the injury complex. Initial chest radiographs may not clearly demonstrate the degree of pulmonary parenchymal injury, and oxygen saturation (and arterial blood gas measurements) is more useful in estimating the anesthetic risk of these patients during operative fracture care. Previous authors have reported that operative stabilization of fractures within the first 2 or 3 days after injury led to fewer complications, shorter hospital and ICU stays, and a shorter time on ventilator assistance in children with multiple injuries.[96,97] Pneumothorax and hemothorax are more life-threatening injuries that may require emergent treatment to decompress the thoracic cavity.[173]

ABDOMINAL INJURIES

Abdominal injuries occur in approximately 10% to 30% of pediatric polytrauma patients and are usually from blunt trauma.[25,47,102] Abdominal swelling, tenderness, and bruising are all signs of injury. Abdominal injury is common if a child in a motor vehicle accident (MVA) has been wearing a lap seat belt, regardless of whether a contusion is evident.[26,89,157,176] Sivit et al. noted that over half of their 61 patients with abdominal ecchymosis had spine fracture and/or abdominal viscus injury, including 21% with fracture, 23% with viscus injury, and 8% with both fracture and viscus injury.[157] Bond et al.[16] noted that the presence of multiple pelvic fractures strongly correlated (80%) with the presence of abdominal or genitourinary injury, whereas the child's age or mechanism of injury had no correlation with abdominal injury rates.

Most hepatic and splenic lacerations are treated nonoperatively, by monitoring the hematocrit, by performing serial abdominal examinations, and by serial CT.[27,32,33,44,87,119,139,168,179] Hemodynamically unstable children with splenic lacerations or other solid organ injuries require angioembolization or laparotomy.[34] Addition of a pediatric trauma center to a regional trauma system has been reported to decrease the rate of splenectomy following blunt abdominal trauma in children.[119] Once the child's overall condition has stabilized, the presence of nonoperative abdominal injuries should not delay fracture care.

GENITOURINARY INJURIES

Genitourinary system injuries are rare in the pediatric polytrauma population, though they have been reported in 9% to 24% of children with pelvic fractures.[124,156,167,172]

Injuries to the bladder and urethra are more common in males and are associated with fractures of the anterior pelvic ring.[11] Although less common following pelvic fracture in girls, such injuries are often associated with injury to the vagina and rectum, with long-term concerns regarding continence, stricture formation, and childbearing.[49,137,147] If the iliac wings are displaced or the pelvic ring shape is changed, it may be necessary to reduce these fractures to reconstitute the birth canal in female patients. There are increased rates of cesarean section in young women who have had a pelvic fracture.[38] Adolescent females with displaced pelvic fractures should be informed of this potential problem with vaginal delivery. If the injury is severe, kidney injury may also occur, but most urologic injuries that occur with pelvic fractures are distal to the ureters.[1]

Kidney injury is the most common urinary tract injury caused by blunt trauma due to the relatively larger size of the kidney. Like other abdominal trauma, kidney injuries are usually treated nonoperatively, with operative treatment reserved for hemodynamic instability (Fig. 5-4).[110]

FAT EMBOLISM

Fat embolism and acute respiratory distress syndrome are rare in children.[57,105,136,143,188] When they do occur, the most common setting is an adolescent with two or more long-bone fractures.[136] Though hypoxemia likely develops in some children after multiple fractures, the full clinical picture of fat embolism seldom develops. When fat embolism occurs, the signs and symptoms are the same as in adults: axillary petechiae, hypoxemia, and radiograph changes of pulmonary infiltrates appearing within several hours of the fractures. If a child with multiple fractures without a head injury develops a change in sensorium and orientation, hypoxemia is the most likely cause. The other primary cause of mental status change after fracture is overmedication with narcotics.

If fat embolism is diagnosed, the treatment is the same as in adults, generally with endotracheal intubation, positive pressure ventilation, and hydration with IV fluid. The effect of early fracture stabilization, IV alcohol, or high-dose corticosteroids on fat embolism syndrome has not been studied well in children with multiple injuries.

NUTRITIONAL REQUIREMENTS

Pediatric polytrauma patients have high caloric demands. If an injured child requires ventilator support for several days, caloric intake through enteral or parenteral supplementation may help avoid catabolism, improve healing, and minimize complications. Children on mechanical ventilation in a PICU have been reported to require 150% of the basal energy or caloric requirements for age and weight.[169] The institution of nutritional support guidelines in a pediatric ICU has been shown to improve energy and protein intake in critically ill patients.[96]

Figure 5-4. Retrograde pyelogram showing extravasation suggestive of a grade 4 renal laceration. Patient was with stent placement and healed without issues.

ORTHOPAEDIC MANAGEMENT OF THE MULTIPLY INJURED CHILD

Orthopaedic Management of the Multiply Injured Child: KEY CONCEPTS

- ❏ Most fractures in multiply injured children can be splinted initially and undergo definitive treatment urgently, not emergently.
- ❏ Pelvic fractures in children can typically be treated nonoperatively, but some may require urgent external fixation or placement of a pelvic binder if the child is hemodynamically unstable.
- ❏ Prompt administration of IV antibiotics and appropriate irrigation and debridement are the most important steps in the treatment of open fractures.
- ❏ Tetanus status should be checked and updated in all patients with open fractures.
- ❏ Cultures should not routinely be performed for open fractures.
- ❏ Children will often heal open fractures that would necessitate amputation in an adult.
- ❏ If amputation is necessary, preserve as much residual limb length as possible.

TIMING

As noted, splinting is needed at the time of the initial resuscitation. In a child with multiple closed fractures, definitive treatment should proceed expeditiously once the child's condition has been stabilized. Loder[107] reported that operative stabilization of fractures within the first 2 or 3 days after injury led to fewer complications, shorter hospital and ICU stays, and a shorter time on ventilator assistance in children with multiple injuries. A more recent study by Loder et al.[108] reported a trend toward a

higher rate of complications in fractures treated after 72 hours. Although there appear to be other factors besides the timing of surgery that affect the eventual outcomes of polytrauma patients, the timing of surgery is a variable that can be controlled by the surgeon, and it seems prudent to complete fracture stabilization within 2 to 3 days of injury when possible. Loder also used the Modified Injury Severity Scale (MISS) to guide treatment timing. Those with a score of MISS of 3 or 4 should be stabilized within 2 to 3 days to prevent complications with immobilization.

PELVIC FRACTURES

Pelvic fractures occur in less than 1% of pediatric patients in the National Trauma Data bank but have been reported in up to 7% of children referred to level I regional trauma centers.[45,159,165,184] More than half of pelvic fractures involve a pedestrian struck by a motor vehicle and over 90% result from three mechanisms: pedestrian struck by motor vehicle, MVA, or fall from height.[156,161,165] Most pediatric pelvic fractures do not require surgery, though the frequency is higher in adolescents.

In a series of 166 pelvic fracture patients, associated substantial head trauma was reported in 39%, chest trauma in 20%, and visceral/abdominal injuries in 19%.[156] Mortality in children following pelvic fractures has been reported to occur in 3.6% to 10.5% of cases in some series.[45,156,165] Other authors reported that 62% of children (8/13) with pelvic fractures had additional orthopaedic injuries.[161]

Exsanguination may present an immediate threat to the life of a child following pelvic fracture, but death more frequently is due to other severe associated injuries.[45,86,161,165,177] Survival after pelvic fracture is related to ISS and type of hospital.[184]

Figure 5-5. A: AP radiograph showing vertical shear sacral fracture. **B:** Fluoroscopic view of a pelvis external fixator showing stabilization of the fracture. Note that the external fixator does not control the vertical shear component.

Most pelvic fractures in children are treated nonoperatively. However, in a child or preadolescent, an external fixator can be used to close a marked pubic diastasis or to control bleeding by stabilizing the pelvis for transport and other injury care. The external fixator will not reduce a displaced vertical shear fracture (Fig. 5-5), but the stability provided is helpful to control the hemorrhage while the child's condition is stabilized. Another option for acute pelvic stabilization in the emergency department is a simple pelvic binder. Injury to the sciatic nerve or the lumbosacral nerve roots may result from hemipelvis displacement through a vertical shear fracture.

OPEN FRACTURES

Background

Most serious open fractures in children result from high-velocity blunt injuries involving motorized vehicles. However, even low-energy blunt injuries can cause puncture wounds in the skin adjacent to fractures, especially displaced forearm and tibial fractures. In children with multiple injuries, approximately 10% of the fractures are open.[23,154] When open fractures are present, 25% to 50% of patients have additional injuries involving the head, chest, abdomen, and other extremities.[154]

Wound Classification

The classification used to describe the soft tissues adjacent to an open fracture is based on the system described by Gustilo and Anderson.[68,69] Primary factors that are considered and ranked in this classification system are the size of the wound, the degree of soft tissue damage and wound contamination, and the presence

or absence of an associated vascular injury (Table 5-4). Despite its widespread use, the Gustilo classification has only moderate interobserver reliability.[22,84,123]

Though type IIIC injuries are commonly associated with extensive soft tissue loss and contamination, a type IIIC injury may, in fact, be associated with even a small wound in some cases. Also, key distinguishing factors between types II and III fractures are the amount of periosteal stripping of the bone and the severity of the damage to the surrounding soft tissues, not simply the size of the skin laceration (Fig. 5-6).

TABLE 5-4. Gustilo Classification of Open Fractures

Type	Description
I	An open fracture with a wound <1 cm long and clean
II	An open fracture with a laceration >1 cm long without extensive soft tissue damage, flaps, or avulsions
III	Massive soft tissue damage, compromised vascularity, severe wound contamination, marked fracture instability
IIIA	Adequate soft tissue coverage of a fractured bone despite extensive soft tissue laceration or flaps, or high-energy trauma irrespective of the size of the wound
IIIB	Extensive soft tissue injury loss with periosteal stripping and bone exposure; usually associated with massive contamination
IIIC	Open fracture associated with arterial injury requiring repair

Data from Gustilo RB, Anderson JT. Prevention of infection in the treatment of one thousand and twenty-five open fractures of long bones: retrospective and prospective analyses. *J Bone Joint Surg Am.* 1976;58(4):453–458 and Gustilo RB, et al. Problems in the management of type III (severe) open fractures: a new classification of type III open fractures. *J Trauma.* 1984;24(8):742–746.

Figure 5-6. A: Type IIIC open tibia fracture in a 9-year-old boy hit by a bus. **B:** Appearance of the wound after several debridements. **C, D:** AP and lateral radiographs showing external fixation of the fracture. Note the vascular clips distally, where an autologous vein graft from the popliteal trifurcation was anastomosed to the posterior tibial artery.

Some of the factors that determine the correct classification of the open fracture may not be known until the time of surgery; as such, the grade the orthopaedic surgeon assigns to the open fracture may change at the time of surgery.

The final functional results of type III fractures in children appear to be superior to those in adults, likely because of their better peripheral vascular supply and the robust regenerative potential of pediatric periosteum.

Authors' Preferred Treatment of the Multiply Injured Child With Open Fractures (Algorithm 5-1)

Three Stages

The treatment of open fractures in children is like that for open fractures in adults. The primary goals are to prevent infection of the wound and fracture site, while allowing soft tissue healing, fracture union, and return of optimal function. Initial emergency care includes the ABCDEs of resuscitation, application of a sterile povidone–iodine dressing, and preliminary alignment and splinting of the fracture. If significant bleeding is present, a compression dressing is applied to limit blood loss. Tetanus toxoid is given for patients whose immunization status is unknown, or if more than 5 years have passed since their last dose. The initial dose of

IV antibiotics is given. All open fractures are treated with operative irrigation and debridement. The second stage of management is the primary surgical treatment, including initial and (if necessary) repeat debridement of the tissues in the open fracture until the entire wound appears viable. The fracture is reduced and stabilized at this time. If the bone ends are not covered with viable soft tissue, muscle or skin flap coverage is considered. Vacuum-assisted closure (VAC) therapy (Kinetic Concepts, Inc., San Antonio, TX) may be a useful adjunct to facilitate coverage and obviate the need for flaps in some patients.[79,101,117,123,186,187] VAC has been shown to shorten the time of healing of wounds associated with

Algorithm 5-1. Authors' preferred treatment of the multiply injured child with open fractures.

open fractures.[101] The third and final stage of management is bony reconstruction as needed if bone loss has occurred, followed by rehabilitation of the child.

Cultures

Previous studies have demonstrated poor correlation of growth on routine cultures with wound infections.[75,98,131,180]

Open fractures do not need to be routinely cultured. Cultures should be obtained only at the time of reoperation in patients with clinical evidence of infection.[149]

Antibiotic Therapy

Antibiotic therapy decreases the risk of infection in children with open fractures. Wilkins and Patzakis[191] reported a 13.9% infection rate in 79 patients who received no antibiotics after open fractures and a 5.5% rate in 815 patients with similar injuries who had antibiotic prophylaxis. Bacterial contamination has been noted in 70% of open fractures in children, including both gram-positive and gram-negative organisms, depending on the degree of wound contamination and adjacent soft tissue injury.

For all type I and some type II fractures, we use a first-generation cephalosporin (cefazolin 100 mg/kg/day divided q8h, maximal daily dose 6 g). For more severe type II fractures and for type III fractures, we use a combination of cephalosporin and aminoglycoside (gentamicin 5–7.5 mg/kg/day divided every 8 hours).[97] For farm injuries or grossly contaminated fractures, penicillin (150,000 units/kg/day divided q6h, maximal daily dose 24 million units) is added to the cephalosporin and aminoglycoside. Ceftriaxone has been used for type III fractures in adults but has little evidence in children.[145] Recent authors showed that a care pathway was able to decrease the delay in antibiotic administration for children with open fractures.[111]

All antibiotics are given intravenously for 24 after wound closure or 72 hours, whichever is shorter. Although there is a trend toward a shorter duration (24 hours) of antibiotic prophylaxis, there is currently a lack of evidence-based medicine to support specific regimens of duration of antibiotic prophylaxis in children.

Surgical Management

After the initial dose(s) of antibiotics are given, debridement and irrigation of the open fracture in the operating room is the next critical step in the primary management of open fractures in children. A multicenter study demonstrated an overall infection rate of 1% to 2% after open long-bone fractures, with no difference in infection rates between groups of patients treated with irrigation and debridement within 6 hours of injury and those treated between 6 and 24 hours following injury.[158] The debridement needs to be performed carefully and systematically to remove all foreign and nonviable materials from the wound. The order of debridement typically is (1) excision of the necrotic tissue from the wound edges, (2) extension of the wound to adequately explore the fracture ends, (3) debridement of the wound edges to bleeding tissue, (4) resection of necrotic skin, fat, muscle, and contaminated fascia, (5) fasciotomies as needed, and (6) thorough irrigation of the fracture ends and wound.

Emerging evidence supports "nonoperative" management of noncontaminated type I open fractures in children without an increased risk of infection. Such nonoperative treatment typically entails superficial debridement and irrigation in the emergency department, coupled with timely administration of IV antibiotics.[64,85,129,200] While such nonoperative treatment may suffice for noncontaminated type I fractures, operative debridement is absolutely required for any fracture with evident or suspected contamination.

For type II and III fractures, since children generally heal better and have less comorbidity than adults, it is often possible to do a less aggressive debridement at the initial surgery and wait until questionable tissue declares itself at a second look to determine the definitive necessary extent of debridement.

For wound irrigation, we routinely use 3 to 9 L of low-pressure normal saline lavage for the lower extremities and 2 to 6 L in the upper extremities because of the smaller compartment size. Several recent studies, including the multicenter, randomized, blinded Fluid Lavage of Open Wound (FLOW) study have found that low-pressure lavage is safer and more effective than high-pressure lavage.[61,62,127,133] Based on the most recent data, it appears that using a soap solution to irrigate has a higher infection rate than irrigation with saline.[61]

Fracture stabilization in children with open fractures decreases pain, protects the soft tissue envelope from further injury, decreases the spread of bacteria, allows stability important for early soft tissue coverage, decreases cerebral pressure, and improves the fracture union rate. The goals are to allow access for wound management, preserve motion, and early weight bearing when appropriate. Fractures may be stabilized temporarily with external fixation if patient is not stable enough to undergo definitive fixation.

The concept of "damage control" orthopaedics, in which an external fixator is used to temporarily stabilize a long-bone fracture until the patient is systemically stable enough to undergo definitive fracture fixation, is well studied and accepted in adults[166,178] but has not been as well studied in the pediatric population.[5,116,134]

Fracture management for specific anatomic locations is discussed throughout the other chapters of this book and will not be addressed here.

After debridement, irrigation, and fracture fixation are complete, local soft tissue is used to cover the neurovascular structures, tendons, and bone ends. If local soft tissue coverage is inadequate, consideration should be given to local muscle flaps or other coverage methods, including wound VAC. Serial debridements are done every 2 to 3 days until wounds are clean. For some wounds where there is good soft tissue coverage but inadequate skin coverage, delayed split-thickness grafting is used with VAC changes until tissue is ready to accept the graft. If flap coverage is necessary, this is optimally accomplished within 1 week of injury or at time of definitive fixation. The location of the soft tissue defect dictates the type of flap that is used whether it be a rotational flap or a free tissue flap. Occasionally, wound VAC can convert wounds that need free tissue transfers to ones that need splint-thickness skin grafts or can heal completely.[28,79,117,123]

For the rare case of significant bone defect in a child, we rely on the healing capacity of young periosteum and bone and the vascular supply of a child's extremity (Fig. 5-7). An external fixator is used to hold the bone shortened about 1 to 2 cm to decrease the size of the bone loss. In a growing child,

A   **B**

Figure 5-7. **A:** AP radiograph of a 6-year-old boy with bilateral open tibia fractures, fixed with external fixators. Despite the bone loss on the left, his periosteum was preserved. **B:** One year later, there is healing and hypertrophy of the cortical bone, without bone grafting.

1 to 2 cm of overgrowth can be expected in the subsequent 2 years after these severe injuries, so the final leg length will be satisfactory. Autogenous bone graft can be used early, but if there is surviving periosteum at this site, spontaneous bone formation often is surprisingly robust and may preclude the need for bone grafting. In teenagers with bone loss, once the soft tissue has healed, bone transport using either a uniplanar lengthening device or a circular external fixator with thin wire or cable transport is our preferred method of reconstruction, although use of an allograft or vascularized fibular graft may be considered.

In children, attempts should generally be made to preserve all extremities, but in rare circumstances, damage is so severe that the injured limb requires amputation. Wounds and fractures that do not heal in adults often heal satisfactorily in children, and preservation of limb length and physes are important in young children. Although the Mangled Extremity Severity Score (MESS) correlates well with the need for amputation in adults, the correlation is poor in children, and many limbs are salvageable despite a MESS of 7 or higher.[59] In one series,[59] the MESS predicted limb amputation or salvage correctly in 86% (31/36) of children, with 93% accuracy in salvaged limbs but only 63% in amputated limbs. Another study reported MESS of at least 6.5 had a sensitivity of only 73% and specificity of only 54% in children with open fractures due to polytrauma who underwent posttraumatic amputation.[13]

If amputation is absolutely necessary, as much length as possible should be preserved. For example, if the proximal tibial physis is preserved in a male with a below-knee amputation at age 7 years, 6 to 8 cm more growth of the tibial residual limb can be expected by skeletal maturity. Thus, even a very short tibial limb in a skeletally immature child may grow to an appropriate length by skeletal maturity. As a result, a short below-knee amputation at the time of injury would likely be superior to a knee disarticulation in final function.

STABILIZATION OF FRACTURES

 Stabilization of Fractures:
KEY CONCEPTS

❏ Fracture stabilization aids in the overall care of the multiply injured child.
❏ Although many children who sustain polytrauma have some residual disability, optimal and timely treatment of their orthopaedic injuries decreases their burden of musculoskeletal disability.

BENEFICIAL EFFECTS

Fracture stabilization provides a number of nonorthopaedic benefits to a child with multiple injuries, including ease of patient mobilization and nursing care, decreased risks of pressure sores, and better wound access. Criteria for early appropriate care versus damage control orthopaedics in children have not been completely described; however, open communication between the orthopaedic surgery and trauma surgery and neurosurgical teams can facilitate the decision.[5,116,134] Some markers include hemodynamic stability, normalized lactate (<4.0 mmol/L), and base excess (>5.5 mmol/L) as well as controlled ICPs.

Operative Fixation

Operative stabilization of fractures is needed to facilitate and hasten patient mobilization and to decrease complications in the pediatric polytrauma patient. It appears that operative fracture fixation for multiply injured children within 3 days of injury leads to fewer complications, shorter stays in the hospital and ICU and less time on a ventilator, shorter hospital and ICU stays, and a shorter time on a ventilator, though such surgery does not appear to be requisite within the first 24 hours of injury.[78,107,108] The type of operative stabilization used in multiply injured children commonly depends on the training, experience, and personal preference of the orthopaedist. The most common methods used are intramedullary rod fixation, external fixation, compression plating, and locking plating; Kirschner wires or Steinmann pins may be used in conjunction with casts. Optimal methods for various anatomic sites and fracture configurations are discussed in other chapters throughout this book.

OUTCOMES OF TREATMENT OF THE MULTIPLY INJURED CHILD

Though the vast majority of children survive following polytrauma, a large proportion remain disabled at follow-up. In one review of 74 children with multiple injuries, 59 (80%) survived, but after 1 year, 22% were disabled, mainly from a brain injury.[181] At 9 years after the injuries, 12% had significant physical disability, whereas 42% had cognitive impairment. In this group, however, the SF-36 or functional outcome survey did not differ from the control population. The best predictor of long-term disability was the GCS 6 weeks after injury and later.[181] Letts et al.[102] reported that 71.6% of multiply injured children made a full recovery, with a mean of 28 weeks until full recovery. Of the 53 residual deficits in their 48 patients, the common deficits were neurologic (38%), psychosocial (34%), and musculoskeletal (24%). Outcomes of children with pelvic fractures were near normal at 6 months.[155] Because of the obviously vital impact of central nervous system function on human performance, initial (including those made in the field by first responders) and follow-up measures of the GCS are excellent predictors of long-term disability in pediatric polytrauma patients.[17,30,31,52,121,197]

Whether operative or nonoperative fracture treatment is chosen for a child with multiple injuries, it is important that an orthopaedist be involved in the care of the child from the start. Although recognizing the need to care for the other organ system injuries, it is important to advocate for expeditious treatment of the orthopaedic injuries. Failure to do so will leave the multiply injured child with musculoskeletal disability once healing of the other injuries occurs.

ACKNOWLEDGMENTS

The authors gratefully acknowledge Vernon T. Tolo, MD, Frances Farley, MD, and Susan A. Scherl, MD, for their past contributions to this chapter.

Annotated References

Reference	Annotation
Bielski RJ, Bassett GS, Fideler B, Tolo VT. Intraosseous infusions: effects on the immature physis—an experimental model in rabbits. *J Pediatr Orthop.* 1993;13:511–515.	A rabbit study showing that intraosseous infusions did not result in physeal damage, thus supporting their potential use in young children requiring emergent fluid resuscitation in the setting of poor venous access.
Cattell HS, Filtzer DL. Pseudosubluxation and other normal variations in the cervical spine in children. A study of one hundred and sixty children. *J Bone Joint Surg Am.* 1965;47:1295–1309.	Classic work describing radiographic findings in the pediatric cervical spine, including pseudosubluxation.
FLOW Investigators; Petrisor B, Sun X, Bhandari M, et al. Fluid lavage of open wounds (FLOW): a multicenter, blinded, factorial pilot trial comparing alternative irrigating solutions and pressures in patients with open fractures. *J Trauma.* 2011;71:596–606.	A randomized, blinded, multicenter trial that showed that low-pressure lavage with normal saline is the safest, most effective irrigation method.
Gustilo RB, Anderson JT. Prevention of infection in the treatment of one thousand and twenty-five open fractures of long bones: retrospective and prospective analyses. *J Bone Joint Surg Am.* 1976;58:453–458.	The first description of the Gustilo–Anderson classification system for open fractures.
Haller JA Jr, Shorter N, Miller D, et al. Organization and function of a regional pediatric trauma center: does a system of management improve outcome? *J Trauma.* 1983;23:691–696.	One of the earliest reports on the establishment, function, and outcomes at a dedicated pediatric trauma center.
Herscovici D Jr, Sanders RW, Scaduto JM, et al. Vacuum-assisted wound closure (VAC therapy) for the management of patients with high-energy soft tissue injuries. *J Orthop Trauma.* 2003;17:683–688.	Consecutive, nonrandomized clinical series. Determined that VAC therapy does not obviate need for adequate debridement but can decrease need for free tissue transfer.
Herzenberg JE, Hensinger RN, Dedrick DK, Phillips WA. Emergency transport and positioning of young children who have an injury of the cervical spine. The standard backboard may be hazardous. *J Bone Joint Surg Am.* 1989;71:15–22.	Describes the anatomic characteristics that cause increased cervical spine flexion in young children on a standard backboard, along with recommendations for alternatives for safe transport.

Annotated References

Reference	Annotation
Lee J. Efficacy of cultures in the management of open fractures. *Clin Orthop Relat Res.* 1997(339):71–75.	A study of 245 consecutive open fractures reported that pre- and postdebridement cultures were not useful in predicting later infection and infecting organisms.
Lindholm EB, Malik A, Parikh D, et al. Single-lateral cervical radiograph in pediatric trauma is equivalent to multiple views. *J Trauma Acute Care Surg.* 2019;87(4):813–817.	A study showing that screening lateral cervical spine x-rays are able to detect osseous injuries but miss a significant proportion of ligamentous injuries.
Loder RT. Pediatric polytrauma: orthopaedic care and hospital course. *J Orthop Trauma.* 1987;1:48–54.	A study of 78 polytrauma patients showing decreased duration of stays in the ICU and hospital, along with less need for ventilator support in polytrauma patients undergoing orthopaedic surgery within 72 hours of injury compared to those operated on more than 72 hours after injury.
Sivit CJ, Taylor GA, Newman KD, et al. Safety-belt injuries in children with lap-belt ecchymosis: CT findings in 61 patients. *AJR Am J Roentgenol.* 1991;157:111–114.	A study showing that more than 50% of children (32/61) with lap-belt bruising had spine fracture and/or abdominal viscus injury, including 21% with spine fracture, 23% with viscus injury, and 8% with both.
Skaggs DL, Friend L, Alman B, et al. The effect of surgical delay on acute infection following 554 open fractures in children. *J Bone Joint Surg Am.* 2005;87:8–12.	A multicenter, retrospective study of 554 children with open fractures reporting comparable infection rates for those undergoing surgery within 6 hours and those undergoing surgery 7 to 24 hours after injury.

REFERENCES

1. Abou-Jaoude WA, Sugarman JM, Fallat ME, Casale AJ. Indicators of genitourinary tract injury or anomaly in cases of pediatric blunt trauma. *J Pediatr Surg.* 1996;31(1):86–89.
2. Allen CJ, Murray CR, Meizoso JP, et al. Risk factors for venous thromboembolism after pediatric trauma. *J Pediatr Surg.* 2016;51(1):168–171.
3. Almangour W, Schnitzler A, Salga M, et al. Recurrence of heterotopic ossification after removal in patients with traumatic brain injury: a systematic review. *Ann Phys Rehabil Med.* 2016;59(4):263–269.
4. Amini R, Lavoie A, Moore L, et al. Pediatric trauma mortality by type of designated hospital in a mature inclusive trauma system. *J Emerg Trauma Shock.* 2011;4(1):12–19.
5. Anari JB, Hosseinzadeh P, Herman MJ, et al. Pediatric polytrauma: what is the role of damage control orthopaedics in the pediatric population? *Instr Course Lect.* 2019;68:337–346.
6. Anders JF, Adelgais K, Hoyle JD Jr, et al; Pediatric Emergency Care Applied Research Network (PECARN). Comparison of outcomes for children with cervical spine injury based on destination hospital from scene of injury. *Acad Emerg Med.* 2014;21(1):55–64.
7. Askegard-Giesmann JR, O'Brien SH, Wang W, Kenney BD. Increased use of enoxaparin in pediatric trauma patients. *J Pediatr Surg.* 2012;47(5):980–983.
8. Aufdermaur M. Spinal injuries in juveniles. Necropsy findings in twelve cases. *J Bone Joint Surg Br.* 1974;56B(3):513–519.
9. Azu MC, McCormack JE, Scriven RJ, et al. Venous thromboembolic events in pediatric trauma patients: is prophylaxis necessary? *J Trauma.* 2005;59(6):1345–1349.
10. Babyn PS, Gahunia HK, Massicotte P. Pulmonary thromboembolism in children. *Pediatr Radiol.* 2005;35(3):258–274.
11. Batislam E, Ateş Y, Germiyanoğlu C, et al. Role of Tile classification in predicting urethral injuries in pediatric pelvic fractures. *J Trauma.* 1997;42(2):285–287.
12. Beaudin M, Daugherty M, Geis G, et al. Assessment of factors associated with the delayed transfer of pediatric trauma patients: an emergency physician survey. *Pediatr Emerg Care.* 2012;28(8):758–763.
13. Behdad S, Rafiei MH, Taheri H, et al. Evaluation of Mangled Extremity Severity Score (MESS) as a predictor of lower limb amputation in children with trauma. *Eur J Pediatr Surg.* 2012;22(6):465–469.
14. Bent MA, Hennrikus WL, Latorre JE, et al. Role of computed tomography in the classification of pediatric pelvic fractures—revisited. *J Orthop Trauma.* 2017;31(7):e200–e204.
15. Bielski RJ, Bassett GS, Fideler B, Tolo VT. Intraosseous infusions: effects on the immature physis—an experimental model in rabbits. *J Pediatr Orthop.* 1993;13(4):511–515.
16. Bond SJ, Gotschall CS, Eichelberger MR. Predictors of abdominal injury in children with pelvic fracture. *J Trauma.* 1991;31(8):1169–1173.
17. Borgialli DA, Mahajan P, Hoyle JD Jr, et al; Pediatric Emergency Care Applied Research Network (PECARN). Performance of the pediatric Glasgow Coma Scale score in the evaluation of children with blunt head trauma. *Acad Emerg Med.* 2016;23(8):878–884.
18. Borgman MA, Maegele M, Wade CE, et al. Pediatric trauma BIG score: predicting mortality in children after military and civilian trauma. *Pediatrics.* 2011;127(4):e892–e897.
19. Borgman MA, Nishijima DK. Tranexamic acid in pediatric hemorrhagic trauma. *J Trauma Acute Care Surg.* 2023;94(1S Suppl 1):S36–S40.
20. Bosch PP, Vogt MT, Ward WT. Pediatric spinal cord injury without radiographic abnormality (SCIWORA): the absence of occult instability and lack of indication for bracing. *Spine (Phila Pa 1976).* 2002;27(24):2788–2800.
21. Brazelton T, Gosain A. Classification of trauma in children. In: *UpToDate.* 2017.
22. Brumback RJ, Jones AL. Interobserver agreement in the classification of open fractures of the tibia. The results of a survey of two hundred and forty-five orthopaedic surgeons. *J Bone Joint Surg Am.* 1994;76(8):1162–1166.
23. Buckley SL, Gotschall C, Robertson W Jr, et al. The relationships of skeletal injuries with trauma score, injury severity score, length of hospital stay, hospital charges, and mortality in children admitted to a regional pediatric trauma center. *J Pediatr Orthop.* 1994;14(4):449–453.
24. Buess E, Illi OE, Soder C, Hanimann B. Ruptured spleen in children—15-year evolution in therapeutic concepts. *Eur J Pediatr Surg.* 1992;2(3):157–161.
25. Calder BW, Vogel AM, Zhang J, et al. Focused assessment with sonography for trauma in children after blunt abdominal trauma: a multi-institutional analysis. *J Trauma Acute Care Surg.* 2017;83(2):218–224.
26. Campbell DJ, Sprouse LR II, Smith LA, et al. Injuries in pediatric patients with seatbelt contusions. *Am Surg.* 2003;69(6):1095–1099.
27. Canarelli JP, Boboyono JM, Ricard J, et al. Management of abdominal contusion in polytraumatized children. *Int Surg.* 1991;76(2):119–121.
28. Caniano DA, Ruth B, Teich S. Wound management with vacuum-assisted closure: experience in 51 pediatric patients. *J Pediatr Surg.* 2005;40(1):128–132.
29. Cattell HS, Filtzer DL. Pseudosubluxation and other normal variations in the cervical spine in children: a study of one hundred and sixty children. *J Bone Joint Surg Am.* 1965;47(7):1295–1309.
30. Chung CY, Chen CL, Cheng PT, et al. Critical score of glasgow coma scale for pediatric traumatic brain injury. *Pediatr Neurol.* 2006;34(5):379–387.
31. Cicero MX, Cross KP. Predictive value of initial Glasgow coma scale score in pediatric trauma patients. *Pediatr Emerg Care.* 2013;29(1):43–48.
32. Cloutier DR, Baird TB, Gormley P, et al. Pediatric splenic injuries with a contrast blush: successful nonoperative management without angiography and embolization. *J Pediatr Surg.* 2004;39(6):969–971.
33. Coburn MC, Pfeifer J, DeLuca FG. Nonoperative management of splenic and hepatic trauma in the multiply injured pediatric and adolescent patient. *Arch Surg.* 1995;130(3):332–338.
34. Coccolini F, Montori G, Catena F, et al. Splenic trauma: WSES classification and guidelines for adult and pediatric patients. *World J Emerg Surg.* 2017;12:40.
35. Cochran A, Mann NC, Dean JM, et al. Resource utilization and its management in splenic trauma. *Am J Surg.* 2004;187(6):713–719.
36. Colombani PM, Buck JR, Dudgeon DL, et al. One-year experience in a regional pediatric trauma center. *J Pediatr Surg.* 1985;20(1):8–13.
37. Compton E, Goldstein RY, Nazareth A, et al. Tranexamic acid use decreases transfusion rate in children with cerebral palsy undergoing proximal femoral varus derotational osteotomy. *Medicine (Baltimore).* 2022;101(2):e28506.
38. Copeland CE, Bosse MJ, McCarthy ML, et al. Effect of trauma and pelvic fracture on female genitourinary, sexual, and reproductive function. *J Orthop Trauma.* 1997;11(2):73–81.
39. CRASH-2 trail collaborators; Shakur H, Roberts I, Bautista R, et al. Effects of tranexamic acid on death, vascular occlusive events, and blood transfusion in

trauma patients with significant haemorrhage (CRASH-2): a randomised, placebo-controlled trial. *Lancet.* 2010;376(9734):23–32.

40. CRASH-3 trail collaborators. Effects of tranexamic acid on death, disability, vascular occlusive events and other morbidities in patients with acute traumatic brain injury (CRASH-3): a randomised, placebo-controlled trial. *Lancet.* 2019; 394(10210):1713–1723.

41. Cunningham AJ, Dewey E, Lin S, et al. Pediatric trauma venous thromboembolism prediction algorithm outperforms current anticoagulation prophylaxis guidelines: a pilot study. *Pediatr Surg Int.* 2020;36(3):373–381.

42. Cyr C, Michon B, Pettersen G, et al. Venous thromboembolism after severe injury in children. *Acta Haematol.* 2006;115(3-4):198–200.

43. Davis AL, Wales PW, Malik T, et al. The BIG score and prediction of mortality in pediatric blunt trauma. *J Pediatr.* 2015;167(3):593–598.e1.

44. Davis DH, Localio AR, Stafford PW, et al. Trends in operative management of pediatric splenic injury in a regional trauma system. *Pediatrics.* 2005;115(1):89–94.

45. Demetriades D, Karaiskakis M, Velmahos GC, et al. Pelvic fractures in pediatric and adult trauma patients: are they different injuries? *J Trauma.* 2003;54(6):1146–1151.

46. Densmore JC, Lim HJ, Oldham KT, Guice KS. Outcomes and delivery of care in pediatric injury. *J Pediatr Surg.* 2006;41(1):92–98; discussion 92–98.

47. Dereeper E, Ciardelli R, Vincent JL. Fatal outcome after polytrauma: multiple organ failure or cerebral damage? *Resuscitation.* 1998;36(1):15–18.

48. Deutsch RJ, Badawy MK. Pediatric cervical spine fracture caused by an adult 3-point seatbelt. *Pediatr Emerg Care.* 2008;24(2):105–108.

49. Dorairajan LN, Gupta H, Kumar S. Pelvic fracture-associated urethral injuries in girls: experience with primary repair. *BJU Int.* 2004;94(1):134–136.

50. Dormans JP. Evaluation of children with suspected cervical spine injury. *J Bone Joint Surg Am.* 2002;84(1):124–132.

51. Doud AN, Schoell SL, Weaver AA, et al. Disability risk in pediatric motor vehicle crash occupants. *J Trauma Acute Care Surg.* 2017;82(5):933–938.

51a. Drucker NA, Wang SK, Newton C. Pediatric trauma-related coagulopathy: balanced resuscitation, goal-directed therapy and viscoelastic assays. *Semin Pediatr Surg.* 2019;28(1):61–66.

52. Ehrlich PF, Brown JK, Sochor MR, et al. Factors influencing pediatric injury severity score and Glasgow Coma Scale in pediatric automobile crashes: results from the Crash Injury Research Engineering Network. *J Pediatr Surg.* 2006;41(11):1854–1858.

53. El-Gamasy MAEA, Elezz AAEBA, Basuni ASM, Elrazek MESSA. Pediatric trauma BIG score: predicting mortality in polytraumatized pediatric patients. *Indian J Crit Care Med.* 2016;20(11):640–646.

54. Elgamal EA, Elwatidy S, Zakaria AM, Abdel-Raouf AA. Spinal cord injury without radiological abnormality (SCIWORA): a diagnosis that is missed in unconscious children. *Neurosciences (Riyadh).* 2008;13(4):437–440.

55. Emami P, Czorlich P, Fritzsche FS, et al. Impact of Glasgow Coma Scale score and pupil parameters on mortality rate and outcome in pediatric and adult severe traumatic brain injury: a retrospective, multicenter cohort study. *J Neurosurg.* 2017;126(3):760–767.

56. Eppich WJ, Zonfrillo MR. Emergency department evaluation and management of blunt abdominal trauma in children. *Curr Opin Pediatr.* 2007;19(3):265–269.

57. Eriksson EA, Rickey J, Leon SM, et al. Fat embolism in pediatric patients: an autopsy evaluation of incidence and etiology. *J Crit Care.* 2015;30(1):221.e1–e5.

58. Evans DL, Bethem D. Cervical spine injuries in children. *J Pediatr Orthop.* 1989; 9(5):563–568.

59. Fagelman MF, Epps HR, Rang M. Mangled extremity severity score in children. *J Pediatr Orthop.* 2002;22(2):182–184.

60. Fayiga YJ, Valentine RJ, Myers SI, et al. Blunt pediatric vascular trauma: analysis of forty-one consecutive patients undergoing operative intervention. *J Vasc Surg.* 1994;20(3):419–424.

61. FLOW Investigators; Bhandari M, Jeray KJ, Petrisor BA, et al. A trial of wound irrigation in the initial management of open fracture wounds. *N Engl J Med.* 2015; 373(27):2629–2641.

62. FLOW Investigators; Petrisor B, Sun X, Bhandari M, et al. Fluid lavage of open wounds (FLOW): a multicenter, blinded, factorial pilot trial comparing alternative irrigating solutions and pressures in patients with open fractures. *J Trauma.* 2011; 71(3):596–606.

63. Fulkerson DH, White IK, Rees JM, et al. Analysis of long-term (median 10.5 years) outcomes in children presenting with traumatic brain injury and an initial Glasgow Coma Scale score of 3 or 4. *J Neurosurg Pediatr.* 2015;16(4):410–419.

64. Godfrey J, Choi PD, Shabtai L, et al. Management of pediatric type I open fractures in the emergency department or operating room: a multicenter perspective. *J Pediatr Orthop.* 2019;39(7):372–376.

65. Goedeke J, Boehm R, Dietz HG. Multiply trauma in children: pulmonary contusion does not necessarily lead to a worsening of the treatment success. *Eur J Pediatr Surg.* 2014;24(6):508–513.

66. Grossman MD, Yelon JA, Szydiak L. Effect of American College of Surgeons Trauma Center designation on outcomes: measurable benefit at the extremes of age and injury. *J Am Coll Surg.* 2017;225(2):194–199.

67. Guillamondegui OD, Mahboubi S, Stafford PW, Nance ML. The utility of the pelvic radiograph in the assessment of pediatric pelvic fractures. *J Trauma.* 2003;55(2):236–239.

68. Gustilo RB, Anderson JT. Prevention of infection in the treatment of one thousand and twenty-five open fractures of long bones: retrospective and prospective analyses. *J Bone Joint Surg Am.* 1976;58(4):453–458.

69. Gustilo RB, Mendoza RM, Williams DN. Problems in the management of type III (severe) open fractures: a new classification of type III open fractures. *J Trauma.* 1984;24(8):742–746.

70. Haffner-Luntzer M, Weber B, Morioka K, et al. Altered early immune response after fracture and traumatic brain injury. *Front Immunol.* 2023;14:1074207.

71. Haller JA Jr, Shorter N, Miller D, et al. Organization and function of a regional pediatric trauma center: does a system of management improve outcome? *J Trauma.* 1983;23(8):691–696.

72. Hamrick MC, Duhn RD, Carney DE, et al. Pulmonary contusion in the pediatric population. *Am Surg.* 2010;76(7):721–724.

73. Hannan EL, Farrell LS, Meaker PS, Cooper A. Predicting inpatient mortality for pediatric trauma patients with blunt injuries: a better alternative. *J Pediatr Surg.* 2000;35(2):155–159.

74. Hannon MM, Middelberg LK, Lee LK. the initial approach to the multisystem pediatric trauma patient. *Pediatr Emerg Care.* 2022;38(6):290–298.

75. Hao M, Peng AQ. Comparison of bacteria isolated from open fractures following debridement and subsequent infection. *J Orthop Sci.* 2021;26(2):243–246.

76. Heaney JB, Guidry C, Simms E, et al. To TQIP or not to TQIP? That is the question. *Am Surg.* 2014;80(4):386–390.

77. Heaney JB, Schroll R, Turney J, et al. Implications of the Trauma Quality Improvement Project inclusion of nonsurvivable injuries in performance benchmarking. *J Trauma Acute Care Surg.* 2017;83(4):617–621.

78. Hedequist D, Starr AJ, Wilson P, Walker J. Early versus delayed stabilization of pediatric femur fractures: analysis of 387 patients. *J Orthop Trauma.* 1999;13(7):490–493.

79. Herscovici D Jr, Sanders RW, Scaduto JM, et al. Vacuum-assisted wound closure (VAC therapy) for the management of patients with high-energy soft tissue injuries. *J Orthop Trauma.* 2003;17(10):683–688.

80. Herzenberg JE, Hensinger RN, Dedrick DK, Phillips WA. Emergency transport and positioning of young children who have an injury of the cervical spine: the standard backboard may be hazardous. *J Bone Joint Surg Am.* 1989;71(1):15–22.

81. Hoffmann R, Nerlich M, Muggia-Sullam M, et al. Blunt abdominal trauma in cases of multiple trauma evaluated by ultrasonography: a prospective analysis of 291 patients. *J Trauma.* 1992;32(4):452–458.

82. Holmes JF, Brant WE, Bond WF, et al. Emergency department ultrasonography in the evaluation of hypotensive and normotensive children with blunt abdominal trauma. *J Pediatr Surg.* 2001;36(7):968–973.

83. Holmes JF, Gladman A, Chang CH. Performance of abdominal ultrasonography in pediatric blunt trauma patients: a meta-analysis. *J Pediatr Surg.* 2007;42(9):1588–1594.

84. Horn BD, Rettig ME. Interobserver reliability in the Gustilo and Anderson classification of open fractures. *J Orthop Trauma.* 1993;7(4):357–360.

85. Iobst CA, Tidwell MA, King WF. Nonoperative management of pediatric type I open fractures. *J Pediatr Orthop.* 2005;25(4):513–517.

86. Ismail N, Bellemare JF, Mollitt DL, et al. Death from pelvic fracture: children are different. *J Pediatr Surg.* 1996;31(1):82–85.

87. Jacobs IA, Kelly K, Valenziano C, et al. Nonoperative management of blunt splenic and hepatic trauma in the pediatric population: significant differences between adult and pediatric surgeons? *Am Surg.* 2001;67(2):149–154.

88. Jakob H, Lustenberger T, Schneidmuller D, et al. Pediatric polytrauma management. *Eur J Trauma Emerg Surg.* 2010;36(4):325–338.

89. Jordan B. Lap belt complex. Recognition and assessment of seatbelt injuries in pediatric trauma patients. *JEMS.* 2001;26(5):36–43.

90. Kaufmann CR, Maier RV, Rivara FP, Carrico CJ. Evaluation of the pediatric trauma score. *JAMA.* 1990;263(1):69–72.

91. Keret D, Harcke HT, Mendez AA, Bowen JR. Heterotopic ossification in central nervous system-injured patients following closed nailing of femoral fractures. *Clin Orthop Relat Res.* 1990(256):254–259.

92. Kluger G, Kochs A, Holthausen H. Heterotopic ossification in childhood and adolescence. *J Child Neurol.* 2000;15(6):406–413.

93. Knudson MM, Shagoury C, Lewis FR. Can adult trauma surgeons care for injured children? *J Trauma.* 1992;32(6):729–737.

94. Kochanek PM, Jackson TC, Jha RM, et al. Paths to successful translation of new therapies for severe traumatic brain injury in the golden age of traumatic brain injury research: a Pittsburgh vision. *J Neurotrauma.* 2020;37(22):2353–2371.

95. Kochanek PM, Tasker RC, Carney N, et al. Guidelines for the management of pediatric severe traumatic brain injury, third edition: update of the brain trauma foundation guidelines, executive summary. *Neurosurgery.* 2019;84(6):1169–1178.

96. Kyle UG, Lucas LA, Mackey G, et al. Implementation of nutrition support guidelines may affect energy and protein intake in the pediatric intensive care unit. *J Acad Nutr Diet.* 2016;116(5):844–851.e4.

97. Lavelle WF, Uhl R, Krieves M, Drvaric DM. Management of open fractures in pediatric patients: current teaching in Accreditation Council for Graduate Medical Education (ACGME) accredited residency programs. *J Pediatr Orthop B.* 2008;17(1):1–6.

98. Lee J. Efficacy of cultures in the management of open fractures. *Clin Orthop Relat Res.* 1997;(339):71–75.

99. Lee LK, Fleisher GR. Trauma management: approach to the unstable child. In: *UpToDate.* 2017.

100. Leeper CM, Neal MD, McKenna C, et al. Abnormalities in fibrinolysis at the time of admission are associated with deep vein thrombosis, mortality, and disability in a pediatric trauma population. *J Trauma Acute Care Surg.* 2017;82(1):27–34.

101. Leininger BE, Rasmussen TE, Smith DL, et al. Experience with wound VAC and delayed primary closure of contaminated soft tissue injuries in Iraq. *J Trauma.* 2006;61(5):1207–1211.

102. Letts M, Davidson D, Lapner P. Multiple trauma in children: predicting outcome and long-term results. *Can J Surg.* 2002;45(2):126–131.

103. Levin HS, High WM Jr, Ewing-Cobbs L, et al. Memory functioning during the first year after closed head injury in children and adolescents. *Neurosurgery.* 1988;22(6 Pt 1):1043–1052.

104. Levy ML, Granville RC, Hart D, Meltzer H. Deep venous thrombosis in children and adolescents. *J Neurosurg.* 2004;101(1 Suppl):32–37.

105. Limbird TJ, Ruderman RJ. Fat embolism in children. *Clin Orthop Relat Res.* 1978;(136):267–269.
106. Lindholm EB, Malik A, Parikh D, et al. Single-lateral cervical radiograph in pediatric trauma is equivalent to multiple views. *J Trauma Acute Care Surg.* 2019;87(4):813–817.
107. Loder RT. Pediatric polytrauma: orthopaedic care and hospital course. *J Orthop Trauma.* 1987;1(1):48–54.
108. Loder RT, Gullahorn LJ, Yian EH, et al. Factors predictive of immobilization complications in pediatric polytrauma. *J Orthop Trauma.* 2001;15(5):338–341.
108a. Lucisano AC, Leeper CM, Gaines BA. Trauma-induced coagulopathy in children. *Semin Thromb Hemost.* 2020;46(2):147–154.
109. MacKenzie EJ, Rivara FP, Jurkovich GJ, et al. A national evaluation of the effect of trauma-center care on mortality. *N Engl J Med.* 2006;354(4):366–378.
110. Mahran A, Fernstrum A, Swindle M, et al. Impact of trauma center designation in pediatric renal trauma: National Trauma Data Bank analysis. *J Pediatr Urol.* 2020;16(5):658.e1–658.e9.
111. Makarewich CA, McNeely LW, Gohel S, Baldwin KD. Open fractures in pediatric orthopaedics-can pathways improve care? A 1-year pre and postimplementation analysis. *J Pediatr Orthop.* 2022;42(9):e937–e942.
112. Maksoud JG Jr, Moront ML, Eichelberger MR. Resuscitation of the injured child. *Semin Pediatr Surg.* 1995;4(2):93–99.
113. Mital MA, Garber JE, Stinson JT. Ectopic bone formation in children and adolescents with head injuries: its management. *J Pediatr Orthop.* 1987;7(1):83–90.
114. Mohamed Hussein N, Zhu P, Meng S, et al. Early death prediction in children with traumatic brain injury using computed tomography scoring systems. *J Clin Neurosci.* 2022;95:164–171.
115. Mollahosseini M, Ahmadirad H, Goujani R, Khorramdelazad H. The association between traumatic brain injury and accelerated fracture healing: a study on the effects of growth factors and cytokines. *J Mol Neurosci.* 2021;71(1):162–168.
116. Mooney JF. The use of 'damage control orTHOPAEDics' techniques in children with segmental open femur fractures. *J Pediatr Orthop B.* 2012;21(5):400–403.
117. Mooney JF III, Argenta LC, Marks MW, et al. Treatment of soft tissue defects in pediatric patients using the V.A.C. system. *Clin Orthop Relat Res.* 2000;(376):26–31.
118. Mora MC, Veras L, Burke RV, et al. Pediatric trauma triage: a Pediatric Trauma Society Research Committee systematic review. *J Trauma Acute Care Surg.* 2020;89(4):623–630.
119. Murphy EE, Murphy SG, Cipolle MD, Tinkoff GH. The pediatric trauma center and the inclusive trauma system: impact on splenectomy rates. *J Trauma Acute Care Surg.* 2015;78(5):930–933.
120. Mutabagani KH, Coley BD, Zumberge N, et al. Preliminary experience with focused abdominal sonography for trauma (FAST) in children: is it useful? *J Pediatr Surg.* 1999;34(1):48–52.
121. Nesiama JAO, Pirallo RG, Lerner EB, Hennes H. Does a prehospital Glasgow Coma Scale score predict pediatric outcomes? *Pediatr Emerg Care.* 2012;28(10):1027–1032.
122. Netherton S, Milenkovic V, Taylor M, Davis PJ. Diagnostic accuracy of eFAST in the trauma patient: a systematic review and meta-analysis. *CJEM.* 2019;21(6):727–738.
123. Okike K, Bhattacharyya T. Trends in the management of open fractures: a critical analysis. *J Bone Joint Surg Am.* 2006;88(12):2739–2748.
124. Onuora VC, Patil MG, al-Jasser AN. Missed urological injuries in children with polytrauma. *Injury.* 1993;24(9):619–621.
125. Orlowski JP, Porembka DT, Gallagher JM, et al. Comparison study of intraosseous, central intravenous, and peripheral intravenous infusions of emergency drugs. *Am J Dis Child.* 1990;144(1):112–117.
126. Ott R, Krämer R, Martus P, et al. Prognostic value of trauma scores in pediatric patients with multiple injuries. *J Trauma.* 2000;49(4):729–736.
127. Owens BD, White DW, Wenke JC. Comparison of irrigation solutions and devices in a contaminated musculoskeletal wound survival model. *J Bone Joint Surg Am.* 2009;91(1):92–98.
128. Oyetunji TA, Haider AH, Downing SR, et al. Treatment outcomes of injured children at adult level 1 trauma centers: are there benefits from added specialized care? *Am J Surg.* 2011;201(4):445–449.
129. Padgett AM, Torrez TW, Kothari EA, et al. Comparison of nonoperative versus operative management in pediatric Gustilo-Anderson type I open tibia fractures. *Injury.* 2023;54(2):552–556.
130. Pascarella R, Bettuzzi C, Digennaro V. Surgical treatment for pelvic ring fractures in pediatric and adolescence age. *Musculoskelet Surg.* 2013;97(3):217–222.
131. Patzakis MJ, Bains RS, Lee J, et al. Prospective, randomized, double-blind study comparing single-agent antibiotic therapy, ciprofloxacin, to combination antibiotic therapy in open fracture wounds. *J Orthop Trauma.* 2000;14(8):529–533.
132. Peclet MH, Newman KD, Eichelberger MR, et al. Thoracic trauma in children: an indicator of increased mortality. *J Pediatr Surg.* 1990;25(9):961–965.
133. Petrisor B, Jeray K, Schemitsch E, et al; FLOW Investigators. Fluid lavage in patients with open fracture wounds (FLOW): an international survey of 984 surgeons. *BMC Musculoskelet Disord.* 2008;9:7.
134. Pfeifle VA, Schreiner S, Trachsel D, et al. Damage control orthopaedics applied in an 8-year-old child with life-threatening multiple injuries: a CARE-compliant case report. *Medicine (Baltimore).* 2019;98(16):e15294.
135. Philip PA, Philip M. Peripheral nerve injuries in children with traumatic brain injury. *Brain Inj.* 1992;6(1):53–58.
136. Piastra M, Picconi E, Morena TC, et al. Multisystemic involvement of post-traumatic fat embolism at a pediatric trauma center: a clinical series and literature review. *Eur J Pediatr.* 2023;182(4):1811–1821.
137. Podesta ML, Jordan GH. Pelvic fracture urethral injuries in girls. *J Urol.* 2001;165(5):1660–1665.
138. Potoka DA, Schall LC, Ford HR. Improved functional outcome for severely injured children treated at pediatric trauma centers. *J Trauma.* 2001;51(5):824–832.
139. Potoka DA, Schall LC, Ford HR. Risk factors for splenectomy in children with blunt splenic trauma. *J Pediatr Surg.* 2002;37(3):294–299.
140. Ramirez RJ, Spinella PC, Bochicchio GV. Tranexamic acid update in trauma. *Crit Care Clin.* 2017;33(1):85–99.
141. Reppucci ML, Pickett K, Stevens J, et al. Massive transfusion in pediatric trauma-does more blood predict mortality? *J Pediatr Surg.* 2022;57(2):308–313.
142. Reynolds SL. Pediatric thoracic trauma: recognition and management. *Emerg Med Clin North Am.* 2018;36(2):473–483.
143. Robinson CM. Current concepts of respiratory insufficiency syndromes after fracture. *J Bone Joint Surg Br.* 2001;83(6):781–791.
144. Roche BG, Bugmann P, Le Coultre C. Blunt injuries to liver, spleen, kidney and pancreas in pediatric patients. *Eur J Pediatr Surg.* 1992;2(3):154–156.
145. Rodriguez L, Jung HS, Goulet JA, et al. Evidence-based protocol for prophylactic antibiotics in open fractures: improved antibiotic stewardship with no increase in infection rates. *J Trauma Acute Care Surg.* 2014;77(3):400–407.
146. Rohrer MJ, Cutler BS, MacDougall E, et al. A prospective study of the incidence of deep venous thrombosis in hospitalized children. *J Vasc Surg.* 1996;24(1):46–49.
147. Rourke KF, McCammon KA, Sumfest JM, et al. Open reconstruction of pediatric and adolescent urethral strictures: long-term followup. *J Urol.* 2003;169(5):1818–1821; discussion 1821.
148. Russell RT, Bembea MM, Borgman MA, et al. Pediatric traumatic hemorrhagic shock consensus conference research priorities. *J Trauma Acute Care Surg.* 2023;94(1S Suppl 1):S11–S18.
149. Ryan SP, Pugliano V. Controversies in initial management of open fractures. *Scand J Surg.* 2014;103(2):132–137.
150. Saladino R, Lund D, Fleisher G. The spectrum of liver and spleen injuries in children: failure of the pediatric trauma score and clinical signs to predict isolated injuries. *Ann Emerg Med.* 1991;20(6):636–640.
151. Sanchez B, Waxman K, Jones T, et al. Cervical spine clearance in blunt trauma: evaluation of a computed tomography-based protocol. *J Trauma.* 2005;59(1):179–183.
152. Sanchez JL, Lucas J, Feustel PJ. Outcome of adolescent trauma admitted to an adult surgical intensive care unit versus a pediatric intensive care unit. *J Trauma.* 2001;51(3):478–480.
153. Scaife ER, Rollins MD, Barnhart DC, et al. The role of focused abdominal sonography for trauma (FAST) in pediatric trauma evaluation. *J Pediatr Surg.* 2013;48(6):1377–1383.
154. Schalamon J, von Bismarck S, Schober PH, Hollwarth ME. Multiple trauma in pediatric patients. *Pediatr Surg Int.* 2003;19(6):417–423.
155. Signorino PR, Densmore J, Werner M, et al. Pediatric pelvic injury: functional outcome at 6-month follow-up. *J Pediatr Surg.* 2005;40(1):107–112.
156. Silber JS, Flynn JM, Koffler KM, et al. Analysis of the cause, classification, and associated injuries of 166 consecutive pediatric pelvic fractures. *J Pediatr Orthop.* 2001;21(4):446–450.
157. Sivit CJ, Taylor GA, Newman KD, et al. Safety-belt injuries in children with lap-belt ecchymosis: CT findings in 61 patients. *AJR Am J Roentgenol.* 1991;157(1):111–114.
158. Skaggs DL, Friend L, Alman B, et al. The effect of surgical delay on acute infection following 554 open fractures in children. *J Bone Joint Surg Am.* 2005;87(1):8–12.
159. Smith WR, Oakley M, Morgan SJ. Pediatric pelvic fractures. *J Pediatr Orthop.* 2004;24(1):130–135.
160. Sobus KM, Sherman N, Alexander MA. Coexistence of deep venous thrombosis and heterotopic ossification in the pediatric patient. *Arch Phys Med Rehabil.* 1993;74(5):547–551.
161. Spiguel L, Glynn L, Liu D, Statter M. Pediatric pelvic fractures: a marker for injury severity. *Am Surg.* 2006;72(6):481–484.
162. Stafford PW, Blinman TA, Nance ML. Practical points in evaluation and resuscitation of the injured child. *Surg Clin North Am.* 2002;82(2):273–301.
162a. Stutz CM, O'Rear LD, O'Neill KR, et al. Coagulopathies in orthopaedics: links to inflammation and the potential of individualizing treatment strategies. *J Orthop Trauma.* 2013;27(4):236–241.
163. Stylianos S, Egorova N, Guice KS, et al. Variation in treatment of pediatric spleen injury at trauma centers versus nontrauma centers: a call for dissemination of American Pediatric Surgical Association benchmarks and guidelines. *J Am Coll Surg.* 2006;202(2):247–251.
164. Sullivan MP, Torres SJ, Mehta S, Ahn J. Heterotopic ossification after central nervous system trauma: a current review. *Bone Joint Res.* 2013;2(3):51–57.
165. Swaid F, Peleg K, Alfici R, et al; Israel Trauma Group. A comparison study of pelvic fractures and associated abdominal injuries between pediatric and adult blunt trauma patients. *J Pediatr Surg.* 2017;52(3):386–389.
166. Taeger G, Ruchholtz S, Waydhas C, et al. Damage control orthopaedics in patients with multiple injuries is effective, time saving, and safe. *J Trauma.* 2005;59(2):409–416.
167. Tarman GJ, Kaplan GW, Lerman SL, et al. Lower genitourinary injury and pelvic fractures in pediatric patients. *Urology.* 2002;59(1):123–126.
168. Tataria M, Nance ML, Holmes JH IV, et al. Pediatric blunt abdominal injury: age is irrelevant and delayed operation is not detrimental. *J Trauma.* 2007;63(3):608–614.
169. Tilden SJ, Watkins S, Tong TK, Jeevanandam M. Measured energy expenditure in pediatric intensive care patients. *Am J Dis Child.* 1989;143(4):490–492.
170. Tobias J, Labuz DF, Cunningham A, et al. Venous thromboembolic screening in pediatric trauma: a prospective cohort study of risk-stratified ultrasonography. *J Trauma Acute Care Surg.* 2023;94(1):107–112.
171. Tolo VT. Orthopaedic treatment of fractures of the long bones and pelvis in children who have multiple injuries. In: Price CT, ed. *Instructional Course Lectures.* Vol 49. American Academy of Orthopaedic Surgeons; 2000:415–423.
172. Torode I, Zieg D. Pelvic fractures in children. *J Pediatr Orthop.* 1985;5(1):76–84.
173. Tovar JA. The lung and pediatric trauma. *Semin Pediatr Surg.* 2008;17(1):53–59.
174. Tran A, Campbell BT. The art and science of pediatric damage control. *Semin Pediatr Surg.* 2017;26(1):21–26.

175. Truitt AK, Sorrells DL, Halvorson E, et al. Pulmonary embolism: which pediatric trauma patients are at risk? *J Pediatr Surg*. 2005;40(1):124–127.
176. Tso EL, Beaver BL, Haller JA Jr. Abdominal injuries in restrained pediatric passengers. *J Pediatr Surg*. 1993;28(7):915–919.
177. Tuovinen H, Soderlund T, Lindahl J, et al. Severe pelvic fracture-related bleeding in pediatric patients: does it occur? *Eur J Trauma Emerg Surg*. 2012;38(2):163–169.
178. Tuttle MS, Smith WR, Williams AE, et al. Safety and efficacy of damage control external fixation versus early definitive stabilization for femoral shaft fractures in the multiple-injured patient. *J Trauma*. 2009;67(3):602–605.
179. Uranus S, Pfeifer J. Nonoperative treatment of blunt splenic injury. *World J Surg*. 2001;25(11):1405–1407.
180. Valenziano CP, Chattar-Cora D, O'Neill A, et al. Efficacy of primary wound cultures in long bone open extremity fractures: are they of any value? *Arch Orthop Trauma Surg*. 2002;122(5):259–261.
181. van der Sluis CK, Kingma J, Eisma WH, ten Duis HJ. Pediatric polytrauma: short-term and long-term outcomes. *J Trauma*. 1997;43(3):501–506.
182. Van Haren RM, Valle EJ, Thorson CM, et al. Hypercoagulability and other risk factors in trauma intensive care unit patients with venous thromboembolism. *J Trauma Acute Care Surg*. 2014;76(2):443–449.
183. Vazquez WD, Garcia VF. Pediatric pelvic fractures combined with an additional skeletal injury is an indicator of significant injury. *Surg Gynecol Obstet*. 1993;177(5):468–472.
184. Vitale MG, Kessler MW, Choe JC, et al. Pelvic fractures in children: an exploration of practice patterns and patient outcomes. *J Pediatr Orthop*. 2005;25(5):581–587.
185. Wade SL, Cassedy AE, Fulks LE, et al. Problem-solving after traumatic brain injury in adolescence: associations with functional outcomes. *Arch Phys Med Rehabil*. 2017;98(8):1614–1621.
186. Webb LX. New techniques in wound management: vacuum-assisted wound closure. *J Am Acad Orthop Surg*. 2002;10(5):303–311.
187. Webb LX, Laver D, DeFranzo A. Negative pressure wound therapy in the management of orthopaedics wounds. *Ostomy Wound Manage*. 2004;50(4A Suppl):26–27.
188. Weisz GM, Rang M, Salter RB. Posttraumatic fat embolism in children: review of the literature and of experience in the hospital for sick children, Toronto. *J Trauma*. 1973;13(6):529–534.
189. Wesson DE, Spence LJ, Williams JI, Armstrong PF. Injury scoring systems in children. *Can J Surg*. 1987;30(6):398–400.
190. Wetzel RC, Burns RC. Multiple trauma in children: critical care overview. *Crit Care Med*. 2002;30(11 Suppl):S468–S477.
191. Wilkins J, Patzakis M. Choice and duration of antibiotics in open fractures. *Orthop Clin North Am*. 1991;22(3):433–437.
192. Williams-Johnson JA, McDonald AH, Strachan GG, Williams EW. Effects of tranexamic acid on death, vascular occlusive events, and blood transfusion in trauma patients with significant haemorrhage (CRASH-2): a randomised, placebo-controlled trial. *West Indian Med J*. 2010;59(6):612–624.
193. Winogron HW, Knights RM, Bawden HN. Neuropsychological deficits following head injury in children. *J Clin Neuropsychol*. 1984;6(3):267–286.
194. Yalcin N, Dede O, Alanay A, Yazici M. Surgical management of post-SCIWORA spinal deformities in children. *J Child Orthop*. 2011;5(1):27–33.
195. Yen J, Van Arendonk KJ, Streiff MB, et al. Risk factors for venous thromboembolism in pediatric trauma patients and validation of a novel scoring system: the risk of clots in kids with trauma score. *Pediatr Crit Care Med*. 2016;17(5):391–399.
196. Young B, Rapp RP, Norton JA, et al. Early prediction of outcome in head-injured patients. *J Neurosurg*. 1981;54(3):300–303.
197. Yousefzadeh-Chabok S, Kazemnejad-Leili E, Kouchakinejad-Eramsadati L, et al. Comparing pediatric trauma, glasgow coma scale and injury severity scores for mortality prediction in traumatic children. *Ulus Travma Acil Cerrahi Derg*. 2016;22(4):328–332.
198. Yuan QM, Zhao ZH, Xu BS. Efficacy and safety of tranexamic acid in reducing blood loss in scoliosis surgery: a systematic review and meta-analysis. *Eur Spine J*. 2017;26(1):131–139.
199. Yuan X, Li B, Wang Q, Zhang X. Comparison of 3 routes of administration of tranexamic acid on primary unilateral total knee arthroplasty: a prospective, randomized, controlled study. *J Arthroplasty*. 2017;32(9):2738–2743.
200. Zhang H, Fanelli M, Adams C, et al. The emerging trend of non-operative treatment in paediatric type I open forearm fractures. *J Child Orthop*. 2017;11(4):306–309.
201. Zhao XG, Zhao GF, Ma YF, Jiang GY. Research progress in mechanism of traumatic brain injury affecting speed of fracture healing. *Chin J Traumatol*. 2007;10(6):376–380.

6

Compartment Syndrome in Children

Haleh Badkoobehi, John M. Flynn, and Milan V. Stevanovic

INTRODUCTION

Compartment syndrome in children is caused by sustained increased pressures within an osteofascial compartment resulting in circulatory compromise, ischemia, and ultimately tissue death. Acute compartment syndrome is rapidly progressive and is a surgical emergency. The importance of timely diagnosis and surgical intervention is critical to optimize clinical outcomes. Sometimes, compartment syndrome may have progressed before surgical intervention, in which case the surgeon will need to take care of compartment syndrome sequelae. Failure to address compartment syndrome in an expeditious manner can lead to permanent disability in the affected limb. There is also chronic compartment syndrome, or exertional compartment syndrome, which is triggered by activity and is reversible.

DIAGNOSIS

A variety of injuries and medical conditions, including fractures, external compression by tight dressings or casts, excessive flexion in a long-arm cast, elective orthopaedic procedures such as osteotomies, soft tissue injuries, burn eschar, animal and insect bites, intravenous (IV) infiltration, antishock garments, infection (group B *Streptococcus*), and bleeding disorders can lead to compartment syndrome and can involve the forearm, hand, thigh, leg, and foot (Table 6-1). The most common cause of compartment syndrome is trauma, motor vehicle accidents, falls, and sports.[12,19] Similar to adults, compartment syndrome is up to four times more prevalent in boys than in girls.[2]

The pathophysiology of compartment syndrome is increased pressure in a noncompliant compartment from fluid, which then occludes microvasculature of the compartment. This occlusion reduces or blocks oxygen delivery to tissues and can lead to ischemic necrosis.

There is currently no gold standard diagnostic tool for compartment syndrome, so clinical judgment is paramount. The diagnosis of compartment syndrome can be made by measuring the absolute pressure *or* the differential pressure of a compartment. The absolute pressure for diagnosis of compartment syndrome is generally accepted to be a pressure of 30 mm Hg or higher in the affected compartment. Alternatively, delta pressure can be diagnostic. Differential pressure, or "delta pressure" is the absolute pressure of the compartment minus the diastolic blood pressure. The delta pressure is diagnostic of compartment syndrome if it is less than 30 mm Hg. Early diagnosis of compartment syndrome may be better predicted when using delta pressure over absolute pressure.[28] Pressure thresholds for diagnosis of compartment syndrome are controversial, as pressure is an indirect measure of oxygenation and can be variable depending on the operator and device used.

A Federal Drug Administration (FDA) Investigational Devise Exemption study found that near-infrared spectroscopy is a noninvasive compartment syndrome monitor that reliably measures oxygenation in at-risk tissues. In this FDA study, continuous near-infrared spectroscopy monitoring was performed on patients' injured and uninjured limbs for control. A difference in perfusion between the injured and control limb was diagnostic of ischemic insult to the injured limb. Although near-infrared spectroscopy shows promise in diagnosing compartment

TABLE 6-1. Causes of Compartment Syndrome

Intrinsic	Extrinsic
Fracture	Compressive casts, dressings
Soft tissue trauma without fracture	Pneumatic antishock garments
Vascular injury	
Penetrating trauma	
Burns	Burn eschar
Animal + insect bites	
Fluid infusion secondary to intravenous (or intraosseous) extravasation (also arthroscopy)	
Bleeding disorders	
Reperfusion injury following prolonged ischemia	
Elective orthopaedic procedure— osteotomy	

syndrome, the FDA recommended validation with further interventional studies.[39] The diagnosis of compartment syndrome is challenging and can be more difficult in children, and particularly in infants. In addition, a high index of suspicion must be maintained in obtunded or sedated patients.

The six Ps—*pain, pressure, pallor, paresthesia, paralysis,* and *pulselessness*—have been described as clinical markers of compartment syndrome. The reliability of these clinical findings is questionable, however, as they may be difficult to obtain in the pediatric or obtunded patient or in a patient with delayed presentation in whom irreversible tissue damage has already occurred. In younger children, the three As are more useful in making a diagnosis of compartment syndrome, and they are *anxiety* (or restlessness), *agitation* (or crying), and an increasing *analgesia* requirement.[2,6]

Pain out of proportion to the injury, especially aggravated by passive motion of the compartment, is a sensitive and early physical finding of compartment syndrome.[26] An increasing analgesia requirement, both in dose and frequency, is also a helpful early marker in children.[2] A retrospective review of 21 pediatric compartment syndrome patients demonstrated that swelling and worsening pain were presenting signs in 100% of cases and paresthesias were seen in 75%.[19]

A systematic review investigating if regional anesthesia or patient-controlled analgesia masked the pain of compartment syndrome in children reported mixed results, with 75% of studies after 2009 demonstrating that regional anesthesia and patient-controlled analgesia can safely be used in children without masking compartment syndrome. Authors postulate that modernized ultrasound-guided techniques for regional blocks allow for better targeting and thus lower volumes of injected anesthetic into a given compartment. Authors also argue that

regional anesthesia with complete motor and sensory blockade masked nociceptive pain, *not* ischemic pain, and therefore does not affect compartment syndrome evaluation.[16] Despite this, there is currently not a strong recommendation for or against the use of regional anesthesia or patient-controlled analgesia in children when there is a concern for development of compartment syndrome.[9] The American and European Society on Regional Anesthesia have established guidelines for dosing of peripheral nerve blocks in children to reduce variability in practice.[43] Further data are needed in this area.

In the case of "silent compartment syndrome," there is an absence of pain.[1,26] Agitation and anxiety may be present instead. Pressure, swelling, and tenseness of the affected compartment may be objective but often unreliable findings of early compartment syndrome.[26,38] Paralysis is a late and insensitive finding of compartment syndrome. One retrospective study at a pediatric tertiary care center reviewed 10 years of data and identified five cases of silent compartment syndrome.[17] Three were associated with upper extremity fractures and two with lower extremity fractures. At the time of diagnosis, silent compartment syndrome patients demonstrated no pulselessness, no pain with range of motion (ROM), no anxiety, and all had compressible compartments. Four out of five had paralysis. This atypical presentation may be due to sensory deficits.[17]

In unclear clinical presentations, compartment pressure measurements are recommended. In the pediatric setting, compartment pressures are best measured under conscious sedation or anesthesia. Multiple measurements at different sites and depths within each compartment are recommended. Compartment pressure measurements close to the level of fracture may be most accurate.

Historically, the threshold for lower leg fasciotomies in both adults and children was an absolute pressure greater than 30 mm Hg or pressures within 30 mm Hg of either the diastolic blood pressure or the mean arterial pressure. Application of this threshold to children may not be appropriate. Baseline compartment pressures have been shown to be higher in children compared to adults: normal adult leg compartment pressures are between 5.2 and 9.7 mm Hg, whereas in children they are 13.3 to 16.6 mm Hg.[41] Also, children have been shown to tolerate compartment pressures above traditional thresholds for fasciotomies, and many do not develop compartment syndrome without surgical treatment. A prospective study identified 41 children with fractured forearms. Of these patients, 15 had needle manometry compartment pressure readings above 30 mm Hg in the injured extremity. Only 1 in 15 went on to develop compartment syndrome. All the remaining children tolerated pressures greater than 30 mm Hg without developing compartment syndrome. Authors argue that traditional surgical cutoff pressure measurements may not apply to children and that children may be closely observed and may ultimately avoid the need for fasciotomies.[44] We recommend serial evaluation of the at-risk extremity and decompressive fasciotomy when there are clinical signs of compartment syndrome development and elevated compartment pressure readings. The 2020 American Academy of Orthopaedic Surgery Clinical Practice Guideline on Management of Acute Compartment Syndrome noted that overtreatment may be the result of operating based on pressure thresholds alone.[27]

Risk factors that may delay diagnosis are altered level of consciousness, associated nerve injury, polytrauma, and altered pain perception. Delay in diagnosis may also be related to longer elapsed time between the initial injury and peak compartment pressures in the pediatric setting.[11] Extended close monitoring after injury is recommended when there is concern for development of compartment syndrome in children.

CLASSIFICATION

COMPARTMENT SYNDROME

Compartment syndrome occurs when tissue pressures rise high enough within a fascial compartment to cause tissue ischemia.

IMPENDING COMPARTMENT SYNDROME

Impending compartment syndrome is when pressures are rising in a compartment but the tissue is not yet ischemic. In these at-risk cases, the clinical indicators do not yet meet the threshold for diagnosis of compartment syndrome. The exact time of conversion to compartment syndrome from impending compartment syndrome is difficult to determine and varies by patient. Patients with impending compartment syndrome necessitate vigilant monitoring.

FRACTURE COMPARTMENT SYNDROME

Most cases of compartment syndrome are associated with a fracture. Both high- and low-energy injuries can result in compartment syndrome. Open fractures are associated with a higher incidence of compartment syndrome than closed injuries.[12] Open fractures are generally associated with higher-energy injuries. Fascial disruption in these cases does not result in adequate decompression of all compartments.

NONFRACTURE COMPARTMENT SYNDROME

Soft tissue injury without fracture can also lead to compartment syndrome, especially in the setting of an underlying bleeding disorder or with the use of anticoagulants. Compartment syndrome in this setting has been associated with a high rate of disability.[13] A retrospective review over 16 years evaluating nonfracture compartment syndrome identified 39 cases of which 29 of 39 (74%) involved the leg. In this series, compartment syndrome was most commonly caused by vascular injury, followed by trauma and postoperative changes. Pain and swelling were the most common symptoms. Delay in diagnosis up to 48 hours was commonly seen and 21 of 39 (54%) had evidence of myonecrosis at time of surgery.[20] Muscle recovery is rare once myonecrosis has occurred. Rarely, IV infiltration can cause compartment syndrome. A retrospective review of compartment syndrome caused by IV infiltration found that pediatric patients constituted 40% of cases.[30] Other rare reported causes of nonfracture compartment syndrome includes acute hematogenous

osteomyelitis and ruptured subperiosteal abscess[37] as well as a severe ankle sprain with injury to a branch of the peroneal artery.[31]

EXERCISE-INDUCED OR EXERTIONAL COMPARTMENT SYNDROME

Exercise-induced compartment syndrome, or chronic compartment syndrome, is a transient increased compartment pressure and reversible tissue ischemia caused by a noncompliant fascial compartment that does not accommodate muscle expansion occurring during a repetitive exercise such as running. It has been described in both the upper and lower extremities.[3,50] Exertional compartment syndrome can be relieved with cessation of the offending activity or fasciotomies of affected compartments for refractory cases. A case series of 155 patients and 250 legs with chronic exertional compartment syndrome found that adolescent female running athletes were at highest risk. Fasciotomy allowed for return to play in 79.5%. Significantly, when compared to four-compartment release, anterior and lateral (two) compartment release increased the odds of reoperation by 3.4 times.[3]

NEONATAL COMPARTMENT SYNDROME

Neonatal compartment syndrome is caused by limb ischemia presenting at birth or in the postnatal period. It is characterized by skin lesions that can be confused with other diagnoses. Because of this, diagnosis is usually delayed and patients develop contractures, as well as bone and nerve disturbances.[6,32] Early recognition and treatment can improve the functional outcome and growth; however, established neonatal contractures cannot be improved by emergent intervention.

TREATMENT

Potentially devastating complications of compartment syndrome may be avoidable with early recognition and prompt intervention. The goal of treatment is to prevent tissue necrosis, neurovascular compromise, and permanent functional deficits.

The first step is to remove all possible extrinsic causes of pressure on the affected limb, including circumferential dressings, cast padding, and casts. A study simulating compartment syndrome in the anterior leg compartment in healthy patients was performed using a pneumatic thigh cuff to elevate pressures in the studied leg, with the contralateral leg as control. Compartment pressures, microvascular blood flow, perfusion pressure, pH, and oxygenation were evaluated with the leg at heart level and 12 cm above heart level. Authors found that tissue oxygenation, blood flow, perfusion pressure, and pH, all decrease as compartment pressure was increased, and leg elevation caused further decreases in all outcome variables.[7] Authors argue that in patients with compartment syndrome, the affected extremity should not be dependent but also should not be elevated higher than the patient's heart to maximize perfusion while minimizing swelling. Optimizing overall medical management is also recommended, as shock and hypoxia may lower tissue pressure tolerance.[12]

If the diagnosis of compartment syndrome is made, emergent fasciotomy should be performed. At times, release of the epimysium is also necessary. Necrotic tissue should be excised. If in doubt as to the viability of soft tissue, questionable tissue should *not* be debrided at the index procedure because the potential for tissue recovery in a child is substantial.[10] Viable tissue will be pink and perfused and muscle will conduct electric current. If tissue is obviously not perfused and is gray, brown, or black, malodorous, and does not conduct current, it may be necrotic and should be debrided to avoid becoming colonized with bacteria. If unsure of viability, allow time for the tissue to declare itself. The patient should subsequently return to the operating room for serial assessments, debridements, and ultimately, closure. Late fibrosis of necrotic muscle can lead to compression of the adjacent nerves and result in disability of the extremity. Other procedures may be indicated based on the etiology of the compartment syndrome, including fracture reduction and stabilization, vascular thrombectomy, repair, or grafting and nerve exploration. Nerve repair or reconstruction should be performed at the time of definitive wound closure.

In the case of a delayed compartment syndrome where there is no demonstrable muscle function in any segment of the involved limb, the limb can be splinted in a functional position. Fasciotomy is not indicated. For the upper extremity, if resources are available for immediate reconstruction with functional free muscle transfer, then early debridement and reconstruction can reduce the incidence of late contracture and can improve neurologic recovery.[36,42] Supportive care, usually in the form of vigorous IV hydration, should be given for the potential risk of myoglobinuria. Myoglobinuria, as well as metabolic acidosis and hyperkalemia, can also occur during reperfusion and requires medical management to prevent sequelae such as renal failure, shock, hypothermia, and cardiac arrhythmias and/or failure.

UPPER EXTREMITY

In the upper extremity, compartment syndrome most commonly involves the forearm and is typically associated with both bone fracture of the forearm and supracondylar humerus (SCH) fracture.[5,14] The incidence of forearm compartment syndrome following upper extremity injuries has been estimated at 1%.[12] One national study identified 31,167 patients with SCH fractures of whom 0.2% (67/31,167) developed compartment syndrome. Neurovascular injury was associated with compartment syndrome in 4.5% (24/530).[33] For example, SCH fractures with a median nerve injury are at high risk for compartment syndrome, as the pain of compartment syndrome is masked.[24] High-risk fracture patterns include displaced SCH fractures with concomitant ipsilateral forearm fractures, known as the floating elbow. In this case, the rate of compartment syndrome is as high as 33%.[5] Operatively managed Monteggia and Monteggia fracture equivalents had a higher rate of compartment syndrome

at 15.3% (9/59) when compared to operatively managed type three SCH fractures where compartment syndrome occurred in 0.9% (2/230).[15] Other risk factors for developing compartment syndrome include longer intraoperative and fluoroscopic times and male sex. Some studies have suggested younger age is a risk factor for compartment syndrome, while a national study has reported older pediatric patients are at higher risk.[5,23,33,51]

Intraoperative examination and pressure measurements should be used to determine what compartment is affected and where to do a fasciotomy. For example, if the arm is affected, decompression of the volar forearm may adequately decompress the arm so that the dorsal forearm does not require a fasciotomy as well.

The surgical incision for fasciotomy of the arm and forearm is extensile from the brachium to the carpal tunnel. The extent of the release performed is tailored to the clinical and intraoperative findings. Release of the dorsal forearm and compartments of the hand requires separate incisions when indicated (Table 6-2). Separate incisions for dermatomes of each finger may also be added to prevent skin necrosis and loss of fingers.

ARM

The anterior and posterior compartments of the arm can be decompressed through a single medial incision. This allows access to the neurovascular structures of the arm, the medial fascia of the biceps and brachialis in the anterior compartment, and the fascia of the triceps. Excision of the medial intermuscular septum will provide additional decompression of both compartments (Fig. 6-1). The incision can be extended to the elbow crease and incorporated with the incision for decompression of the forearm. This also allows release of the lacertus fibrosus and evaluation of the distal portion of the brachial artery. When there is no need to evaluate and decompress the neurovascular structures or extend the incision into the forearm, straight midline anterior and posterior fasciotomies may be performed to decompress the flexor and extensor compartments, respectively.

FOREARM

Several skin incisions have been described for the forearm. Since the surgical incisions are long and extensile. Almost any incision can be used to decompress the forearm compartments (Fig. 6-2). Because the incisions are left open, we prefer the incision described in Figure 6-3C,D over the incision seen in Figure 6-3A,B, as this minimizes exposure of neurovascular structures and can be extended proximally into the medial arm and distally into the carpal tunnel. After the skin incision is made, the antebrachial fascia is opened longitudinally from lacertus fibrosus to the wrist flexion crease. This decompresses the superficial flexor compartment. The deep flexor compartment is most easily and safely exposed through the ulnar side of the forearm.[34] Start at the mid- to distal forearm and identify the interval between flexor carpi ulnaris and flexor digitorum superficialis. The flexor digitorum profundus and flexor pollicis longus fascia are exposed and released through this interval. This is the most important component of this procedure, as the deep flexor compartment is usually the first and most affected

TABLE 6-2. Compartments of the Upper Extremity

Compartments			Contents
Arm	Anterior		Biceps and brachialis, brachial artery, and median nerve
	Posterior		Triceps, ulnar nerve, and radial nerve
Forearm	Volar	Superficial	FCR, PL, pronator teres, FCU, and FDS
		Deep	FDP, FPL, and pronator quadratus
			Anterior interosseous nerve and artery
	Dorsal	Mobile wad	Brachioradialis, ECRL, ECRB
		Extensor	EDC, ECU, EPL, APL, EPB, EIP, EDM, supinator,[a] posterior interosseous nerve
		Anconeus[b]	Anconeus
Hand	Thenar		Abductor pollicis brevis, opponens pollicis, and flexor pollicis brevis
	Hypothenar		Abductor digiti minimi, flexor digiti minimi, and opponens digiti minimi
	Adductor pollicis		Adductor pollicis (two heads)
	Dorsal interossei (4)		Each separate compartments
	Volar interossei (3)		Each separate compartments
Fingers			Cleland and Grayson ligaments[c]

[a]The supinator is not typically a component of extensor compartment syndrome, but decompression can be done through the brachioradialis/ECRL interval.
[b]Not typically listed as a separate compartment, but should be assessed.
[c]Not technically a compartment, but compression of the neurovascular structures by rigid Cleland and Grayson ligaments can lead to skin necrosis and/or loss of the finger.
APL, abductor pollicis longus muscle; BR, brachioradialis muscle; ECRB, extensor carpi radialis brevis muscle; ECRL, extensor carpi radialis longus muscle; ECU, extensor carpi ulnaris; ED, extensor digitorum muscle; EDM, extensor digiti minimi muscle; EPB, extensor pollicis brevis muscle; EPL, extensor pollicis longus muscle; FCR, flexor carpi radialis muscle; FCU, flexor carpi ulnaris muscle; FDP, flexor digitorum profundus muscle; FDS, flexor digitorum superficialis muscle; FPL, flexor pollicis longus muscle; PL, palmaris longus muscle.

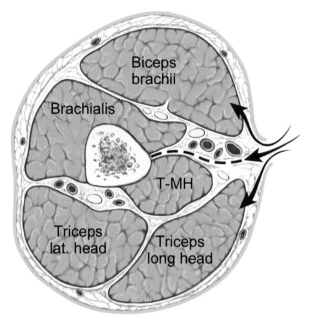

Figure 6-1. Cross-sectional anatomy of the arm is shown. The *dotted line* represents the plane of dissection for decompression of the anterior and posterior compartments through a medial incision. The intermuscular septum can be excised, which further decompresses both compartments. Alternatively, a straight anterior and posterior incision may be used to separately decompress the anterior and posterior compartments. (Courtesy of Dr. M. Stevanovic.)

by increased compartmental pressure. Through the same interval, the fascia overlying the pronator quadratus is also released.

During the dissection, if the muscles appear pale after release of the fascia, then additional release of the epimysium of the pale muscle should be performed. For these muscles, reperfusion injury will lead to more swelling in the muscle which will lead to further muscle injury if the epimysium is not released.

Clinical evaluation at this time of the remaining tension in the dorsal forearm compartment and/or hand should be done to determine whether additional release of the extensor compartments and hand should be added. The extensor compartments are released through a midline longitudinal dorsal incision

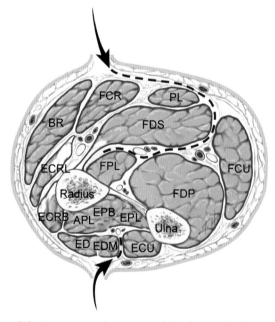

Figure 6-2. Cross-sectional anatomy of the forearm is shown. The *dotted lines* represent the plane of dissection for dorsal and volar compartments. The superficial flexor compartment can be released in the midline or any location, trying to avoid an incision over the radial or ulnar artery or median nerve. The deep flexor compartment is best released by opening the interval between flexor carpi ulnaris and the flexor digitorum superficialis. (Courtesy of Dr. M. Stevanovic.)

Figure 6-3. A: Dorsal (extensor) incision for forearm fasciotomy. **B:** Release of the extensor compartment. **C:** Volar (flexor) incision for forearm fasciotomy. This incision can be extended proximally into the medial arm and distally into the carpal tunnel as indicated by intraoperative findings. **D:** Release of the flexor compartment and carpal tunnel. (Courtesy of Dr. M. Stevanovic.)

extending from the lateral epicondyle to the distal radioulnar joint. This will allow release of the mobile wad and the extensor compartment (see Fig. 6-3A). Figure 6-4 is an example of a patient with an SCH fracture and compartment syndrome after the above-described fasciotomy. The following figure is another example of a patient with SCH and distal radius fractures and compartment syndrome, including excellent functional clinical outcomes (Fig. 6-5).

Figure 6-4. Intraoperative photograph of a patient with a SCH fracture and compartment syndrome after forearm fasciotomy. (Courtesy of Dr. M. Stevanovic.)

HAND

The hand has 10 separate compartments. It is rarely necessary to release all the 10 compartments. Intraoperative assessment and/or measurement of compartment pressures should be used to determine the extent of release needed (Figs. 6-6 and 6-7).

Volar Release

Decompression should start with an extended carpal tunnel release. This will usually adequately release Guyon canal without formally opening and decompressing the ulnar neurovascular structures. The carpal tunnel incision can be extended to the volar second web space. In the distal portion of the incision, the volar fascia of the adductor pollicis muscle can be released. Also, the fascia tracking to the long finger metacarpal (separating the deep radial and ulnar midpalmar space) can be decompressed. This will help decompress the volar interosseous muscles. The thenar and hypothenar muscles are decompressed through separate incisions as needed (Fig. 6-8A,C).

Dorsal Release

The dorsal interosseous muscles (and volar interosseous muscles) are decompressed through dorsal incisions between the second and third metacarpals and the fourth and fifth metacarpals. The first dorsal interosseous muscle is decompressed through an incision placed in the first dorsal web space. The dorsal fascia of the adductor pollicis can also be released through this incision (see Fig. 6-7B,D).

Fingers

Tense swollen fingers can result in skin and subcutaneous tissue necrosis. The tight fibers of Cleland and Grayson ligaments can compress and obstruct the digital arteries and veins. Dermotomy of all involved fingers reduces the risk of necrosis of the skin and possible loss of the digit. Dermotomies should be done in the midaxial plane to prevent subsequent contracture. When possible, the dermotomy should be performed on the side that will cause the least amount of scar irritation. The preferred locations for finger and thumb dermotomies are shown in Figure 6-7A,B.

POSTOPERATIVE CARE

All surgical incisions are left open. We do not like the use of retention sutures in children because even if there is minimal swelling of the muscle(s) during the primary release, muscle swelling will usually increase after perfusion has improved. If nerves and arteries are not exposed, a negative pressure wound vacuum can be used. If nerves or arteries are exposed, we prefer to use a moist gauze dressing. Dressing changes should be done in the operating room at 24 to 48 hours. Partial delayed primary wound closure can be performed at that time if swelling is decreased and/or to provide coverage over open neurovascular

Figure 6-5. This 7-year-old patient fell while riding a bicycle, sustaining an ipsilateral displaced SCH fracture and distal radius fracture. He was seen about 4 hours after his initial injury. He was diagnosed with a compartment syndrome on presentation and taken emergently to the operating room for surgical stabilization and fasciotomy. **A:** Injury films showing displaced SCH fracture and distal radius fracture. **B:** Postoperative reduction and stabilization. **C:** Volar fasciotomy. **D:** Dorsal fasciotomy. **E:** Finger flexion at 1-year postinjury. **F:** Wrist and finger extension at 1-year postinjury. (Courtesy of Dr. M. Stevanovic.)

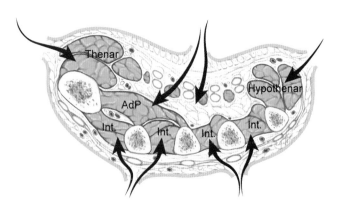

Figure 6-6. Cross-sectional anatomy of the hand. The *arrows* show the planes of dissection for decompression of the compartments of the hand. (Courtesy of Dr. M. Stevanovic.)

structures. Definitive wound closure should be performed only after swelling has considerably decreased. In the hand, only the incision for the carpal tunnel release should be considered for delayed primary wound closure. The other palmar and dorsal incisions as well as the dermotomy incisions will close quickly by secondary intention. If the skin cannot be closed without tension, then split-thickness skin grafting with or without dermal substitutes should be used.

Therapy should be started immediately postoperatively to maintain maximum active and passive ROM of the fingers. Splinting should be done as long as needed for soft tissue stabilization or for treatment of other associated injuries. Therapy may need to be temporarily discontinued during healing of skin grafts but should be resumed as soon as tissue healing allows. Once the soft tissues are adequately healed, continue nighttime splinting to prevent contractures of the wrist and fingers. Splinting is continued until scars and soft tissues are mature and supple.

Figure 6-7. A, B: Dorsal incisions for fasciotomy of the hand and dermotomies of the fingers. **C, D:** Volar incisions for release of the thenar and hypothenar compartments, carpal tunnel release, and dermotomy of the thumb. (Courtesy of Dr. M. Stevanovic.)

LOWER EXTREMITY

THIGH

Compartment syndrome involving the thigh is rare but has been reported in the pediatric population after blunt trauma, external compression with antishock trousers, and vascular injury with or without fracture of the femur. Children with femoral shaft fractures treated by skin or skeletal traction may also be at risk for compartment syndrome of the thigh.

The thigh has three compartments; anterior, medial, and posterior (Table 6-3). A long single lateral incision on the thigh can adequately decompress the anterior and posterior compartments (Fig. 6-9). Occasionally, a medial adductor incision is required as well.[35]

LEG

The most common presentation of compartment syndrome in children involves the lower leg following a tibia and/or fibula fracture.[11,12] A retrospective review over 13 years identified 1,407 patients with tibial fractures. Of these patients, 160 (11%) developed compartment syndrome. In another retrospective review of 517 tibial shaft fractures, only 10 fractures

TABLE 6-3. Compartments of the Thigh

Compartment	Contents
Anterior	Quadriceps muscle
	Femoral artery, vein, and nerve
Medial	Adductor muscles
	Obturator nerve
Posterior	Hamstring muscles
	Sciatic nerve

(1.9%) developed compartment syndrome, significantly less than the former report. In the same study, age 14 or older, higher body mass index, comminuted tibia fractures, and ipsilateral fibula fracture were associated with compartment syndrome.[47] In another retrospective study, 50,640 patients with tibia fractures were identified, 309 of whom had compartment syndrome. The incidence of compartment syndrome was 0.6% in all tibia fractures and 5.5% in open tibia fractures. Of note, compartment syndrome developed in 23 of 309 (7.4%) patients *after* discharge and was most common in nonoperatively managed tibia fractures. Age over 13 quadrupled the risk of compartment syndrome in this population.[25] Treatment of tibia fractures with flexible nails has been shown to be associated with compartment syndrome. Other risk factors include comminuted fractures, weight greater than 50 kg, and a neurologic deficit.[29] Compartment syndrome is also a well-known complication following tibial osteotomies for deformity correction.

In the lower leg, a one- or two-incision technique can be employed for decompressive fasciotomy of all four compartments, including the anterior, lateral, superficial posterior, and deep posterior compartment (Table 6-4). Both one- and two-incision techniques are appropriate if adequate decompression of all compartments is performed.[27] In the two-incision technique, the anterolateral incision provides access to the anterior and lateral compartments. Two- (Fig. 6-10A) and one-incision techniques are illustrated here (Fig. 6-10B). The posteromedial incision must be lengthy enough to allow for decompression of the superficial posterior compartment (more proximal) and deep posterior compartment (more distal). The soleus origin should be detached from the medial aspect of the tibia. The long lateral incision typically extends 3 to 5 cm within either end of the fibula. Identification of the septum between anterior and lateral compartments allows access to these compartments. Next, by elevating the lateral compartment musculature, the posterior intermuscular septum is visualized and access to the superficial and deep posterior compartments is possible.

FOOT

Foot compartment syndrome in children is rare and usually caused by crush injuries, such as a car tire running over the foot. It is associated with Lisfranc fracture–dislocations and

Figure 6-8. This 4-year-old girl placed a rubber band around her wrist before going to bed. She was brought to the emergency room the following morning because of swelling of her hand. She was taken immediately to the operating room for compartment release. **A:** Volar hand prior to fasciotomy. **B:** Dorsal hand prior to fasciotomy. **C:** Volar release. **D:** Dorsal release. **E:** Finger flexion at 6 months. **F:** Finger extension at 6 months. (Courtesy of Dr. M. Stevanovic.)

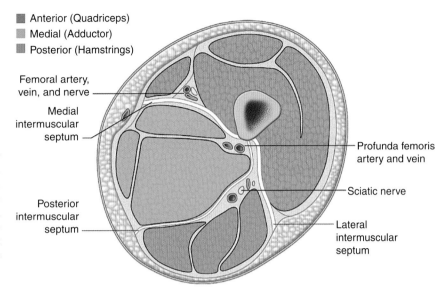

Anterior (Quadriceps)
Medial (Adductor)
Posterior (Hamstrings)

Femoral artery, vein, and nerve

Medial intermuscular septum

Posterior intermuscular septum

Profunda femoris artery and vein

Sciatic nerve

Lateral intermuscular septum

Figure 6-9. Cross-sectional anatomy of the thigh. Note the anterior (quadriceps), posterior (hamstrings), and medial (adductor) compartments. Entry sites for compartment pressure measurements should take into consideration the relationship between the intermuscular septa and the neurovascular structures of each compartment. (Modified with permission from Schwartz JT, et al. Acute compartment syndrome of the thigh. A spectrum of injury. *J Bone Joint Surg Am.* 1989;71(3):392–400.)

has been reported with fractures of the metatarsals and phalanges but may occur in the absence of a fracture.[40] There are also reports of compartment syndrome occurring following IV extravasation and with hemangioma of the foot.[49]

The foot has nine compartments—the interosseous (four), adductor, central (two), medial, and lateral (Table 6-5). A dorsal approach through two longitudinal incisions centered over the second and fourth metatarsals allows for adequate decompression of all nine compartments, though many authors recommend a third incision for the medial compartment (Fig. 6-11).

In a systematic review of pediatric foot compartment syndrome spanning 12 years, 62 patients aged 7 months to

18 years with foot compartment syndrome were reported on and all patients had fasciotomies.[49] There is a controversial trend toward not performing fasciotomies in adult foot compartment syndrome because the main complication associated with untreated adult compartment syndrome, that is, contractures leading to hammertoes, is viewed as less morbid than potential sequelae of performing fasciotomies. While this practice may apply to management of foot compartment syndrome in skeletally mature adolescents, it may not be appropriate in children with significant growth remaining, as sustained compartment pressures may cause physeal arrest. There are also case reports of fluid extravasation in the ankle causing growth arrest. Authors speculate that this could be due to compression of the perichondrial vessels and damage to the perichondrium, which leads to a bar formation, or from a physeal tether formed by scarring of soft tissue.[48] Given the limited data available, a low threshold for fasciotomies should be maintained especially in children with significant growth remaining, as long-term functional issues may develop if not treated.[49]

TABLE 6-4. Compartments of the Lower Leg

Compartment	Contents
Anterior	Tibialis anterior
	Extensor digitorum longus
	Extensor hallucis longus
	Peroneus tertius
	Deep peroneal (anterior tibial) vessels and nerve
Lateral	Peroneus longus
	Peroneus brevis
	Superficial peroneal nerve
Superficial posterior	Gastrocnemius
	Soleus
	Plantaris
	Sural nerve
Deep posterior	Tibialis posterior
	Flexor digitorum longus
	Flexor hallucis longus
	Posterior tibial nerve

TABLE 6-5. Compartments of the Foot

Compartments	Contents
Interosseous (4)	Interosseous muscles
	Digital nerves
Adductor	Adductor hallucis
Central (superficial)	Flexor digitorum brevis
Central (deep [or calcaneal])	Quadratus plantae
Medial	Abductor hallucis brevis
	Flexor hallucis brevis
Lateral	Flexor digiti minimi
	Abductor digiti minimi

A - Anterior compartment
B - Lateral compartment
C - T posterior
D - Posterior compartment
E - Superficial posterior compartment

Figure 6-10. Decompressive fasciotomy of the lower leg. **A:** Two-incision approach. The anterolateral incision allows decompression of the anterior and lateral compartments. The medial incision allows decompression of the superficial posterior and the deep posterior compartments. The *arrows* are indicating the compartments that are released with each incision. **B:** One-incision approach. A single lateral incision allows decompression of all four compartments in the lower leg. (Courtesy of Paul Choi, MD.)

Figure 6-11. Decompressive fasciotomy of the foot. Through a dorsal approach, two longitudinal skin incisions over the second and fourth metatarsals can be utilized to decompress all nine compartments of the foot. The superficial fascia is divided over each interspace to decompress the interosseous (*I*) compartments (×4). (Caution: Interosseous veins and the distal dorsalis pedis arterial branches are in the first interspace.) Next, the adductor, central (superficial and deep), medial, and lateral compartments are decompressed through each interspace. Many authors, however, recommend a third medial incision to decompress the medial/calcaneal compartment.

ESTABLISHED CONTRACTURE (VOLKMANN CONTRACTURE)

Volkmann ischemic contracture is the end result of prolonged ischemia with irreversible tissue necrosis. The most commonly used classification system is that of Tsuge, who classified Volkmann contracture into mild, moderate, and severe types, according to the extent of the muscle involvement.

The *mild type,* also described as the localized type, involves the muscles of the deep flexor compartment of the forearm. It can involve all the flexor digitorum profundus and the flexor pollicis longus, although usually only involves the flexor digitorum profundus of the ring or middle fingers. Nerve involvement is absent or mild, typically involving sensory changes that resolve spontaneously. With wrist flexion, the fingers can be fully extended. The majority of mild types result from direct trauma either from crush injury or forearm fractures and are typically seen in young adults.

In the *moderate type,* muscle degeneration includes most or all of the flexor digitorum profundus and flexor pollicis longus with partial involvement of the flexor superficialis muscles. Neurologic impairment is always present. Sensory impairment is generally more severe in the median than in the ulnar nerve distribution, and the hand demonstrates an intrinsic minus posture. Moderate-type Volkmann contracture is most commonly the result of SCH fractures in children between ages 5 and 10.

The *severe type* involves degeneration of all the flexor muscles of the fingers and of the wrist. There is central muscle necrosis and varying involvement of the extensor compartment. Neurologic deficits are severe, including complete palsy of all the intrinsic muscles of the hand. Hallmarks of the severe type include fixed joint contractures, scarred soft tissue, or previously failed surgeries. As with the moderate cases, the severe cases were most commonly the result of SCH fractures in children.[45]

Treatment of established Volkmann contracture depends on the severity of the contracture and neurologic deficits and the resultant functional losses.

Nonoperative management should be instituted early in most cases of established Volkmann contracture. In children, there may be more recovery of nerve and muscle function over time than in adults, so we do not advocate immediate surgical intervention. A formal program of splinting and therapy can improve the outcome of later surgical intervention and may result in less extensive surgical corrections. Therapy should be directed toward maintenance of passive joint motion, preservation and strengthening of remaining muscle function, and correction of deformity through a program of splinting. We prefer the use of static progressive splinting or serial casting for fixed contractures of the wrist, fingers, and thumb web space. Mild contractures with minimal to no nerve involvement can often be treated only with a comprehensive program of hand therapy and rehabilitation. For moderate to severe involvement where surgery is anticipated, therapy is indicated only as long as necessary to achieve supple passive motion of the fingers.

Preoperative therapy is also helpful in establishing a good patient and parent rapport with the therapist and in gaining an understanding of the postsurgical therapy program.

A variety of surgical procedures have been used to treat Volkmann ischemic contracture. These have included both bone and soft tissue procedures. Surgical treatment should not be undertaken before soft tissue equilibrium is present. We do not recommend a shortening osteotomy of the radius and ulna and proximal row carpectomy to match the skeletal length to the shortened fibrotic muscle because the bones are already relatively shortened by the initial ischemic insult to the growth plates. Further, the principal contracture is usually on the flexor surface. Shortening the forearm indiscriminately lengthens the muscle resting length of both the flexor and extensor muscles, neglecting the predominant involvement of the contracture within the flexor compartment. Bony reconstructive procedures for long-standing contractures or for distal reconstruction required for neurologic injury include wrist fusion, trapeziometacarpal joint fusion, or thumb metacarpophalangeal joint fusion, which should be done after skeletal maturity. These may be considered in conjunction with some of the soft tissue procedures listed below.

Soft tissue procedures have included excision of the infarcted muscle, fractional or z-lengthening of the affected muscles, muscle sliding operations (flexor origin muscle slide), neurolysis, tendon transfers, and functional free tissue transfers, as well as combinations of the above procedures. Excision of scarred fibrotic nerves without distal function followed by nerve grafting has been described to try and establish some protective sensation in the hand. Fixed contractures of the joints can be addressed with soft tissue release including capsulectomy and collateral ligament recession or excision depending on the joints involved.

OUTCOMES

Full functional recovery within 6 months has been reported with timely management of compartment syndrome in the pediatric population.[2] Functional outcomes are good to excellent in over 90% of patients. Of all compartment syndrome, upper extremity compartment syndrome and nonfracture compartment syndrome may have poorer outcomes.[21] Late diagnosis of compartment syndrome may increase the risk of severe complications, including infection, neurologic injury, need for amputation, and death. The duration of elevated tissue pressures before definitive surgical decompression may be the most important factor in determining outcome. In adults, prolonged ischemic insult to compartment musculature greater than 8 hours increases the risk of permanent sequelae.[11] Some studies have shown that after traumatic upper extremity injury in pediatric patients, delayed presentation and decompression of forearm compartment syndrome after 48 hours results in significant morbidity and can result in forearm muscle necrosis necessitating reconstructive surgery with a free gracilis muscle flap or long-term casting for long flexor tightness.[52] Despite this, good outcomes have been demonstrated even with delayed diagnosis of compartment syndrome, and authors postulate that the potential for recovery of muscle function may be greater in a child than in an adult.[18] This is consistent with the increased potential for recovery observed from other types of injuries in children, such as fractures, traumatic brain injuries, and articular cartilage injuries. Full recovery has been reported following compartment syndrome of the lower leg in children even after delayed presentation.[8] Good results may be possible in children even when fasciotomy is performed as late as 72 hours after the injury.[11] A multicenter study spanning 15 years showed that compartment syndrome in infants and toddlers is often delayed greater than 24 hours. Interestingly, even when fasciotomy is delayed by 48 to 72 hours, functional outcomes are excellent in most patients.[6] This should not encourage delay in treatment of compartment syndrome but rather demonstrate that some pediatric patients may still have good outcomes with unintentional delay.

Children may have a delayed *development* rather than delayed *diagnosis* of compartment syndrome after the initial injury. Clinicians may diagnose and treat this late-developing compartment syndrome acutely, which may result in good outcomes noted in studies. This is why it is imperative to continuously monitor children at risk for developing compartment syndrome. If muscle ischemia persists for longer than 6 to 8 hours, children are at risk for functional muscle loss, contracture, neurologic deficit (both motor and sensory distal to the level of injury), cosmetic deformity, growth arrest, and infection. Less commonly, loss of limb, rhabdomyolysis, multiorgan system failure, and death can be seen, especially in the setting of crush injury with severe large-volume muscle necrosis.

Delayed or missed diagnosis of compartment syndrome is one of the most common causes of successful litigation against medical professionals in North America.[4] Of 66 closed cases involving compartment syndrome, 73% (48/66) were ruled in favor of the patient, with an average payment of $574,680.[22]

Patients who develop Volkmann contracture of the upper extremity during childhood may have a permanently shortened extremity thereafter. After limb ischemia, muscles are generally more affected than bone, and thus muscles grow at a slower rate than the bone, which may lead to relative tightening of the muscles. Splinting the extremity in the functional position until age 18 may help mitigate contractures. Tendon lengthening alone often results in recurrence of contracture. Substantial improvements in hand function are noted in patients who undergo functional free muscle transfer.

Finally, in patients who have sufficient remaining muscle, procedures that combine infarct excision, tenolysis, neurolysis, and tendon transfer when necessary produce good hand function.[46] Improvement in sensory function in conjunction with neurolysis has been noted. In our experience, mild and moderate contractures can have significant functional improvement following flexor muscle slide and nerve reconstruction when indicated. Normal function is not anticipated, but a hand with protective sensation and functional grasp can often be achieved. Functional free muscle transfers can also restore gross grasp and have a much better outcome in patients with good intrinsic function.

Annotated References

Reference	Annotation
Bae DS, Kadiyala RK, Waters PM. Acute compartment syndrome in children: contemporary diagnosis, treatment, and outcome. *J Pediatr Orthop.* 2001;21(5):680–688.	This article examines 36 cases of compartment syndrome in children over 6 years at one institution. In this cohort, 75% of children who developed compartment syndrome had fractures. The authors demonstrated that previously used indicators of compartment syndrome, such as pain, pallor, paresthesias, etc., were not reliable. Increasing analgesia requirement was a more reliable predictor of compartment syndrome in the children studied.
Beck JJ, Tepolt FA, Miller PE, et al. Surgical treatment of chronic exertional compartment syndrome in pediatric patients. *Am J Sports Med.* 2016;44(10):2644–2650.	This is a retrospective review of 155 patients with chronic exertional compartment syndrome. Chronic exertional compartment syndrome was found most often in adolescent female running athletes. Anterior and lateral release as opposed to four-compartment release resulted in a recurrence in 18.8%.
Broom A, Schur MD, Arkader A, et al. Compartment syndrome in infants and toddlers. *J Child Orthop.* 2016;10(5):453–460.	This article distinguishes the diagnosis of compartment syndrome in infants and toddlers from compartment syndrome in older children. Fifteen infants and toddlers who developed compartment syndrome were studied. In infants and toddlers, diagnosis was delayed compared to older children (>24 hours after injury), but regardless, outcomes were generally good even when fasciotomy was not performed for 48 to 72 hours after injury.
Flynn JM, Bashyal RK, Yeger-McKeever M, et al. Acute traumatic compartment syndrome of the leg in children: diagnosis and outcome. *J Bone Joint Surg Am.* 2011;93(10):937–941.	This article examines 43 cases of compartment syndrome of the leg in children. These children had an overall delay in the time between injury and fasciotomy. The authors raise awareness for late presentation and late development of compartment syndrome of the leg in children and encourage monitoring of compartments in the days following injury.

Annotated References

Reference	Annotation
Kalyani BS, Fisher BE, Roberts CS, Giannoudis PV. Compartment syndrome of the forearm: a systematic review. *J Hand Surg Am.* 2011;36(3):535–543.	This is a systematic review evaluating evidence on compartment syndrome of the forearm in children. This review provides information on the causes, diagnosis, treatment, and outcomes of compartment syndrome in the forearm of children.
Lin J, Samora WP, Samora JB. Acute compartment syndrome in pediatric patients: a case series. *J Pediatr Orthop B.* 2022;31(2):e236–e240.	This is a retrospective review of pediatric compartment syndrome from 2009 to 2018. Twenty-one patients were included. Swelling and worsening pain were presenting signs in all patients and paresthesias in 75%. Fasciotomies were performed in all within 20 hours of injury. Postoperatively, 10% had complications, most commonly involving strength and ROM.
Obey MR, Shlykov MA, Nickel KB, et al. Incidence and risk factors for acute compartment syndrome in pediatric tibia fractures. *J Pediatr Orthop B.* 2023;32(4):401–404.	A national retrospective study was performed, which included 50,640 patients with tibia fractures. The incidence of compartment syndrome in this population was 0.6% in all tibia fractures and 5.5% in open tibia fractures. Compartment syndrome developed in 7.4% of teenagers who were discharged and most commonly involved tibia fractures that were managed nonoperatively.
Robertson AK, Snow E, Browne TS, et al. Who gets compartment syndrome? A retrospective analysis of the national and local incidence of compartment syndrome in patients with supracondylar humerus fractures. *J Pediatr Orthop.* 2018;38(5):e252–e256.	This is a retrospective review of SCH fractures from a level one pediatric trauma center and the National Trauma Data Bank (NTDB). The NTDB included 31,167 isolated SCH fractures. Compartment syndrome was seen in 0.2% (67/31,167) of isolated SCH fractures. 530 patients were noted to have neurovascular injury. Of those, 4.5% developed ACS (24/530).
Villarreal ED, Wrenn JO, Sheffer BW, et al. Do patient-specific or fracture-specific factors predict the development of acute compartment syndrome after pediatric tibial shaft fractures? *J Pediatr Orthop.* 2020;40(3):e193–e197.	This is a retrospective review of 517 pediatric tibial shaft fractures. Compartment syndrome developed in 1.9% of fractures (10/517). Risk factors for the development of compartment syndrome included higher BMI, age greater than 14, motor vehicle accidents, segmental tibia fractures, and ipsilateral fibular fracture.

REFERENCES

1. Badhe S, Baiju D, Elliot R, et al. The 'silent' compartment syndrome. *Injury.* 2009;40(2):220–222.
2. Bae DS, Kadiyala RK, Waters PM. Acute compartment syndrome in children: contemporary diagnosis, treatment, and outcome. *J Pediatr Orthop.* 2001;21(5):680–688.
3. Beck JJ, Tepolt FA, Miller PE, et al. Surgical treatment of chronic exertional compartment syndrome in pediatric patients. *Am J Sports Med.* 2016;44(10):2644–2650.
4. Bhattacharyya T, Vrahas MS. The medical-legal aspects of compartment syndrome. *J Bone Joint Surg Am.* 2004;86(4):864–868.
5. Blakemore LC, Cooperman DR, Thompson GH, et al. Compartment syndrome in ipsilateral humerus and forearm fractures in children. *Clin Orthop Relat Res.* 2000;(376):32–38.
6. Broom A, Schur MD, Arkader A, et al. Compartment syndrome in infants and toddlers. *J Child Orthop.* 2016;10(5):453–460.
7. Challa ST, Hargens AR, Uzosike A, Macias BR. Muscle microvascular blood flow, oxygenation, pH, and perfusion pressure decrease in simulated acute compartment syndrome. *J Bone Joint Surg Am.* 2017;99(17):1453–1459.
8. Choi PD, Rose RKT, Kay RM, Skaggs DL. Compartment syndrome of the thigh in an infant: a case report. *J Orthop Trauma.* 2007;21(8):587–590.
9. Driscoll EB, Maleki AH, Jahromi L, et al. Regional anesthesia or patient-controlled analgesia and compartment syndrome in orthopedic surgical procedures: a systematic review. *Local Reg Anesth.* 2016;9:65–81.
10. Erdos J, Dlaska C, Szatmary P, et al. Acute compartment syndrome in children: a case series in 24 patients and review of the literature. *Int Orthop.* 2011;35(4):569–575.
11. Flynn JM, Bashyal RK, Yeger-McKeever M, et al. Acute traumatic compartment syndrome of the leg in children: diagnosis and outcome. *J Bone Joint Surg Am.* 2011;93(10):937–941.
12. Grottkau BE, Epps HR, Di Scala C. Compartment syndrome in children and adolescents. *J Pediatr Surg.* 2005;40(4):678–682.
13. Hope MJ, McQueen MM. Acute compartment syndrome in the absence of fracture. *J Orthop Trauma.* 2004;18(4):220–224.
14. Kalyani BS, Fisher BE, Roberts CS, Giannoudis PV. Compartment syndrome of the forearm: a systematic review. *J Hand Surg Am.* 2011;36(3):535–543.
15. Kopriva J, Awowale J, Whiting P, et.al. Compartment syndrome in operatively managed pediatric Monteggia fractures and equivalents. *J Pediatr Orthop.* 2020;40(8):387–395.
16. Kucera TJ, Boezaart AP. Regional anesthesia does not consistently block ischemic pain: two further cases and a review of the literature. *Pain Med.* 2014;15(2):316–319.
17. Lee C, Lightdale-Miric N, Chang E, Kay R. Silent compartment syndrome in children: a report of five cases. *J Pediatr Orthop B.* 2014;23(5):467–471.
18. Lin J, Samora WP, Samora JB. Acute compartment syndrome in pediatric patients: a case series. *J Pediatr Orthop B.* 2022;31(2):e236–e240.
19. Lin JS, Samora JB. Pediatric acute compartment syndrome: a systematic review and meta-analysis. *J Pediatr Orthop B.* 2020;29(1):90–96.
20. Livingston K, Glotzbecker M, Miller PE, et al. Pediatric nonfracture acute compartment syndrome: a review of 39 cases. *J Pediatr Orthop.* 2016;36(7):685–690.
21. Livingston KS, Glotzbecker MP, Shore BJ. Pediatric acute compartment syndrome. *J Am Acad Orthop Surg.* 2017;25(5):358–364.
22. Marchesi M, Marchesi A, Calori GM, et al. A sneaky surgical emergency: acute compartment syndrome. Retrospective analysis of 66 closed claims, medico-legal pitfalls and damages evaluation. *Injury.* 2014;45(Suppl 6):S16–S20.
23. Martus JE, Preston RK, Schoenecker JG, et al. Complications and outcomes of diaphyseal forearm fracture intramedullary nailing: a comparison of pediatric and adolescent age groups. *J Pediatr Orthop.* 2013;33(6):598–607.
24. Mubarak SJ, Carroll NC. Volkmann's contracture in children: aetiology and prevention. *J Bone Joint Surg Br.* 1979;61-B(3):285–293.
25. Obey MR, Shlykov MA, Nickel KB, et al. Incidence and risk factors for acute compartment syndrome in pediatric tibia fractures. *J Pediatr Orthop B.* 2023;32(4):401–404.
26. Olson SA, Glasgow RR. Acute compartment syndrome in lower extremity musculoskeletal trauma. *J Am Acad Orthop Surg.* 2005;13(7):436–444.
27. Osborn CPM, Schmidt AH. Management of acute compartment syndrome. *J Am Acad Orthop Surg* 2020;28(3):e108–e114.
28. Ozkayin N, Aktuglu K. Absolute compartment pressure versus differential pressure for the diagnosis of compartment syndrome in tibial fractures. *Int Orthop.* 2005;29(6):396–401.
29. Pandya NK, Edmonds EW, Mubarak SJ. The incidence of compartment syndrome after flexible nailing of pediatric tibial shaft fractures. *J Child Orthop.* 2011;5(6):439–447.
30. Pare JR, Moore CL. Intravenous infiltration resulting in compartment syndrome: a systematic review. *J Patient Saf.* 2018;14(2):e6–e8.
31. Raad M, Anugraha A. Acute compartment syndrome of the leg following injury to perforating branch of peroneal artery after a severe ankle sprain in a pediatric patient: a case and a review of literature. *J Orthop Case Rep.* 2020;10(8):68–71.
32. Ragland R III, Moukoko D, Ezaki M, et al. Forearm compartment syndrome in the newborn: report of 24 cases. *J Hand Surg Am.* 2005;30(5):997–1003.
33. Robertson AK, Snow E, Browne TS, et al. Who gets compartment syndrome? A retrospective analysis of the national and local incidence of compartment syndrome

in patients with supracondylar humerus fractures. *J Pediatr Orthop*. 2018;38(5): e252–e256.

34. Ronel DN, Mtui E, Nolan WB III. Forearm compartment syndrome: anatomical analysis of surgical approaches to the deep space. *Plast Reconstr Surg*. 2004;114(3):697–705.

35. Schwartz JT Jr, Brumback RJ, Lakatos R, et al. Acute compartment syndrome of the thigh: a spectrum of injury. *J Bone Joint Surg Am*. 1989;71(3):392–400.

36. Seal A, Stevanovic M. Free functional muscle transfer for the upper extremity. *Clin Plast Surg*. 2011;38(4):561–575.

37. Shaw NM, Kish A, Pensy R. Acute hematogenous osteomyelitis resulting in atraumatic pediatric forearm compartment syndrome. *J Am Acad Orthop Surg Glob Res Rev*. 2022;6(6):e21.00228.

38. Shuler MS, Reisman WM, Kinsey TL, et al. Correlation between muscle oxygenation and compartment pressures in acute compartment syndrome of the leg. *J Bone Joint Surg Am*. 2010;92(4):863–870.

39. Shuler MS, Roskosky M, Kinsey T, et al. Continual near-infrared spectroscopy monitoring in the injured lower limb and acute compartment syndrome: an FDA-IDE trial. *Bone Joint J*. 2018;100-B(6):787–797.

40. Silas SI, Herzenberg JE, Myerson MS, Sponseller PD. Compartment syndrome of the foot in children. *J Bone Joint Surg Am*. 1995;77(3):356–361.

41. Staudt JM, Smeulders MJC, van der Horst CMAM. Normal compartment pressures of the lower leg in children. *J Bone Joint Surg Br*. 2008;90(2):215–219.

42. Stevanovic M, Sharpe F. Management of established Volkmann's contracture of the forearm in children. *Hand Clin*. 2006;22(1):99–111.

43. Suresh S, Ecoffey C, Bosenberg A, et al. The European Society of Regional Anaesthesia and Pain Therapy/American Society of Regional Anesthesia and Pain Medicine recommendations on local anesthetics and adjuvants dosage in pediatric regional anesthesia. *Reg Anesth Pain Med*. 2018;43(2):211–216.

44. Tharakan SJ, Subotic U, Kalisch M, et al. Compartment pressures in children with normal and fractured forearms: a preliminary report. *J Pediatr Orthop*. 2016;36(4): 410–415.

45. Tsuge K. Treatment of established Volkmann's contracture. *J Bone Joint Surg Am*. 1975;57(7):925–929.

46. Ultee J, Hovius SER. Functional results after treatment of Volkmann's ischemic contracture: a long-term followup study. *Clin Orthop Relat Res.*2005;(431):42–49.

47. Villarreal ED, Wrenn JO, Sheffer BW, et al. Do patient-specific or fracture-specific factors predict the development of acute compartment syndrome after pediatric tibial shaft fractures? *J Pediatr Orthop*. 2020;40(3):e193–e197.

48. Wada A, Fujii T, Takamura K, et al. Physeal arrest of the ankle secondary to extravasation in a neonate and its treatment by the Gruca operation: a modern application of an old technique. *J Pediatr Orthop B*. 2003;12(2):129–132.

49. Wallin K, Nguyen H, Russell L, Lee DK. Acute traumatic compartment syndrome in pediatric foot: a systematic review and case report. *J Foot Ankle Surg*. 2016;55(4): 817–820.

50. Wilder RP, Magrum E. Exertional compartment syndrome. *Clin Sports Med*. 2010; 29(3):429–435.

51. Yuan PS, Pring ME, Gaynor TP, et al. Compartment syndrome following intramedullary fixation of pediatric forearm fractures. *J Pediatr Orthop*. 2004;24(4):370–375.

52. Ziolkowski NI, Zive L, Ho ES, Zuker RM. Timing of presentation of pediatric compartment syndrome and its microsurgical implication: a retrospective review. *Plast Reconstr Surg*. 2017;139(3):663–670.

7

Pathologic Fractures and Nonaccidental Injuries

Alexandre Arkader and Karim Masrouha

Pathologic Fractures

The definition of a pathologic fracture is one that occurs through abnormal bone. Pathologic fractures may result from a localized or generalized bone weakness, either from an intrinsic or extrinsic process, such as tumors or tumor-like lesions, osteopenia, or osteoporosis of different etiologies.

The evaluation of a child with a pathologic fracture includes obtaining a detailed history, physical examination, and appropriate imaging. The past medical history, use of medications, and prodromal symptoms, such as pain, may assist with the diagnosis. Physical examination should include a complete neurologic and vascular evaluation that helps in differentiating between localized and generalized processes and, if a bone lesion is identified, they can frequently determine whether the lesion appears benign or malignant.

An important concept is that the fracture is a result of the underlying cause for bone weakness, therefore any attempt at "fixing" the fracture needs to be carried out with adequate assessment and management of the underlying pathology. For that reason, the treatment of these fractures may deviate from the classic principles of pediatric fracture management. An understanding of the natural history and prognosis related to the primary pathology will help guide treatment and the anticipation of outcomes, while preventing further complications. In the absence of an obvious diagnosis, temporizing methods, such as cast, brace, and traction, are highly recommended to avoid further complicating the management of the underlying condition. Below, we will discuss the most common causes of pathologic fractures in children and highlight some of the issues associated with the treatment of these diagnoses.

TUMORS OR TUMOR-LIKE PROCESSES

UNICAMERAL BONE CYST

Unicameral bone cyst (UBC) is a benign, active or latent solitary cystic lesion that involves the metaphysis or metadiaphysis of long bones.[10] The most common locations include the proximal humerus, proximal femur, and proximal tibia. Although the etiology is unknown, it is thought that UBC is caused by an obstruction of interstitial fluid drainage.

Most patients with this condition are in their first two decades of life, with a male-to-female ratio of 2:1.[37] UBCs are often asymptomatic, and in approximately 80% of cases, the initial presentation is with a pathologic fracture.[61,202] The fractures

Figure 7-1. A 6-year-old boy presented with shoulder pain after a fall. AP (**A**) and lateral (**B**) radiographs of the right proximal humerus show a pathologic fracture through a well-defined, lytic lesion in the proximal humeral metaphysis. The fracture presented some comminution that gave the appearance of fallen leaf sign (*arrow*). This lesion was consistent with unicameral bone cyst and conservative treatment with a fracture brace and sling was initiated. Six weeks after the injury, radiographs (**C, D**) show consolidation of the fracture and healing of the cyst. The patient was symptom free and returned to full physical activities. (Reproduced with permission from The Children's Orthopaedic Center, Los Angeles, CA.)

A

B

C

D

are usually incomplete or minimally displaced and tend to heal uneventfully, with an approximately 10% chance of cyst healing (partial or complete) (Fig. 7-1). However, complications such as malunion, growth arrest, and avascular necrosis have been reported.[181]

On imaging, UBCs are a well-defined, centrally located, radiolucent/lytic cystic lesion. Cortical thinning and mild expansion are common. When a pathologic fracture occurs, there is a periosteal reaction and the typical "fallen fragment" sign may be visualized (fragment of bone "floating" inside the fluid-filled cavity). Advanced imaging may be useful for lesions of the axial skeleton to rule out minimally displaced fractures, evaluate the adjacent physis, or to assist with the differential diagnosis (Fig. 7-2).

Figure 7-2. A 10-year-old boy presented with arm pain after low-energy trauma, 5 days prior. Anteroposterior (**A**) and lateral (**B**) radiographs of the right humerus show a nondisplaced pathologic fracture (*arrow* in **A**) through a lytic lesion in the proximal humerus. The lesion is difficult to visualize and the periosteal reaction is also of concern (*arrow* in **B**). T2-weighted coronal (**C**) and axial (**D**) MRI images show a well-defined, fluid-filled cystic lesion, with fluid–fluid levels (*arrow* in **D**) and no soft tissue mass or other worrisome signs cuts. The diagnosis was consistent with unicameral bone cyst and conservative treatment was recommended. (Reproduced with permission from The Children's Orthopaedic Center, Los Angeles, CA.)

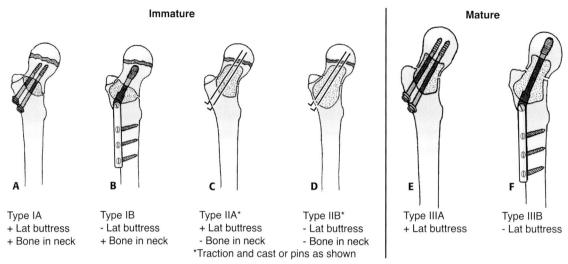

Immature

A | B | C | D | E | F

Type IA
+ Lat buttress
+ Bone in neck

Type IB
- Lat buttress
+ Bone in neck

Type IIA*
+ Lat buttress
- Bone in neck
*Traction and cast or pins as shown

Type IIB*
- Lat buttress
- Bone in neck

Mature

Type IIIA
+ Lat buttress

Type IIIB
- Lat buttress

For all: Curettage (with biopsy) and bone grafting with stabilization (as shown above) and spica cast

Figure 7-3. Classification system for the treatment of pathologic fractures of the proximal femur associated with bone cysts in children. **A:** In type IA, a moderately sized cyst is present in the middle of the femoral neck. There is enough bone in the femoral neck and lateral proximal femur (lateral buttress) to allow fixation with cannulated screws, avoiding the physis, after curettage and bone grafting. **B:** In type IB, a large cyst is present at the base of the femoral neck. There is enough bone proximally in the femoral neck but there is loss of lateral buttress, so a pediatric hip screw and a side plate should be considered rather than cannulated screws after curettage and bone grafting. **C, D:** In type IIA–B, a large lesion is present in the femoral neck, so there is not enough bone beneath the physis to accept screws. There are two options for treatment of these bone cysts: (1) after curettage and bone grafting, parallel smooth pins across the physis can be used in combination with spica cast; (2) the patient can be treated in traction until the fracture heals (with subsequent spica cast), followed by curettage and bone grafting. **E, F:** In type IIIA–B, the physis is closing or closed. The lateral buttress is present in type IIIA hips, so cannulated screws can be used to stabilize the fracture after curettage and bone grafting. In type IIIB hips, the loss of lateral buttress makes it necessary to use a pediatric hip screw and a side plate following curettage and bone grafting. In all types, we recommend spica cast immobilization after surgery.

Most pathologic fractures through UBC, especially of upper extremities, should be treated conservatively. The main reasons are to potentially allow for spontaneous regression or healing of the cyst and to treat the cyst within a stable, healed bone. While minimally or nondisplaced fractures of the lower extremities can also be treated conservatively, displaced fractures or fractures around the hip often need surgical intervention including treatment of the cyst and internal fixation. Large lesions involving more than 50% to 80% of the bone circumference, associated with cortical thinning, and pain are at a high risk of fracture and may warrant prophylactic treatment (Figs. 7-3 and 7-4).[87] A computed tomography (CT) model using a computerized regression system has been used to predict the likelihood of fracture.[128]

There have been several described treatment strategies for UBCs, and a detailed discussion of all available techniques is beyond the scope of this chapter; however, our preferred approach when surgery is indicated is via a formal open curettage and bone grafting or utilizing a minimally invasive technique for decompression, curettage, and grafting[61,143]; complete cyst healing can be achieved in over 80% of the cases after one treatment.

Operative Treatment of Unicameral Bone Cyst

 Surgical Technique for Unicameral Bone Cyst:
KEY SURGICAL STEPS

❑ Under fluoroscopic guidance, a Jamshidi trocar needle (Cardinal Health, Dublin, OH) is percutaneously inserted into the cyst cavity, preferably in the middle of the cyst.
❑ The cyst is aspirated to confirm the presence of straw-colored fluid.
❑ Three to 10 mL of 50% diluted Renografin dye (E.R. Squibb, Princeton, NJ) is injected to perform a cystogram and confirm the single fluid-filled cavity.
❑ A 0.5-cm longitudinal incision is then made over the site of the aspiration and a 6-mm arthroscopy trocar is advanced into the cyst cavity through the same cortical hole. The cortical entry is then enlarged manually.
❑ Under fluoroscopic guidance, percutaneous removal of the cyst lining is done with curved curettes and a pituitary rongeur.
❑ An angled curette and/or flexible intramedullary nail is used to perform the intramedullary decompression in one direction (toward diaphysis) or in both directions (if the growth plate is far enough to avoid injury).
❑ Bone grafting is done with medical-grade bone substitute inserted through the same cortical hole and deployed to completely fill the cavity. This acts as scaffolding for new bone formation and cyst healing. Angled curettes can be used to advance pellets into the medullary canal, which also confirms adequate decompression. Tight packing of the cyst is preferred.
❑ The wound is closed in a layered fashion.

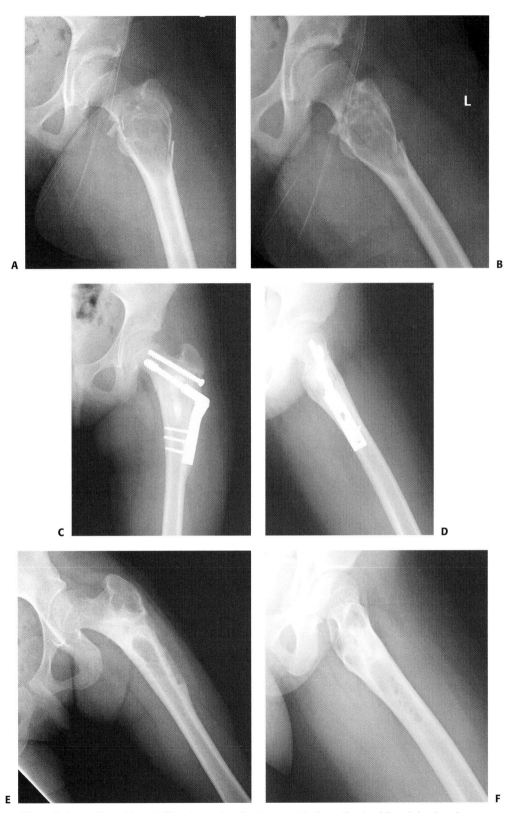

Figure 7-4. AP (**A**) and lateral (**B**) radiographs of a 12 year old who suffered a fall and developed acute left hip pain and inability to ambulate. There is a pathologic fracture through a well-defined, lytic, and loculated lesion in the proximal femur, with cortical thinning, no soft tissue mass or periosteal reaction. The patient underwent biopsy confirming the diagnosis of aneurysmal bone cyst, followed by curettage and allografting, supplemented by internal fixation with a variable hip screw and a cannulated antirotational screw (**C, D**). The 4-year follow-up, short after hardware removal, shows no signs of recurrence or persistence of the lesion (**E, F**). AP and lateral views show no evidence of recurrence. (Figures reproduced with permission from The Children's Orthopaedic Center, Los Angeles, CA.)

ANEURYSMAL BONE CYST

Aneurysmal bone cyst (ABC) is a benign but locally aggressive lesion, with an estimated incidence of approximately 1.4 cases per 100,000. The neoplastic basis of primary ABCs has been in part demonstrated by the chromosomal translocation t(16; 17)(q22; p13), resulting in the upregulation of ubiquitin-specific protease 6 (USP6), which blocks osteoblast cell maturation.[154]

These lesions are well defined, eccentric (early on), expansile (often beyond adjacent growth plate), osteolytic, septated, and are most often seen in the metaphyseal region of long bones (~65%). The most common locations include the femur, tibia, humerus, and posterior elements of the spine (~25%).[37,54]

Approximately a third of ABCs are associated with other benign and/or malignant tumors.

Differentiating between ABC and UBC in the setting of a pathologic fracture can be challenging. There are some radiographic features, such as the septations, eccentric location, and expansion beyond the width of the physis, which are more likely to be seen in ABCs. In addition, obtaining an adequate intraoperative sample for frozen section to be read by an experienced bone and soft tissue pathologist to confirm the diagnosis would be helpful. Ultimately, the open treatment of these fractures is quite similar; however, a correct diagnosis will help guide expectations during the follow-up period.

Pathologic fractures occur at a lower frequency than with UBC (11%–35% of long bone lesions; <20% of spinal lesions)

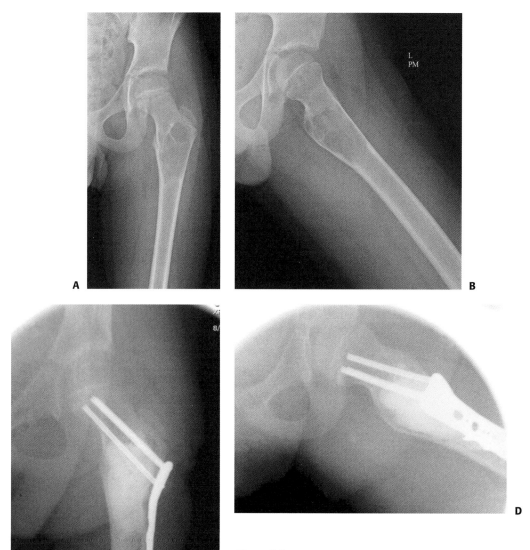

Figure 7-5. AP (**A**) and lateral (**B**) radiographs of a 10 year old who came in with chronic hip pain of several weeks duration. There is a well-defined, lytic lesion in the proximal femur, presenting with cortical thinning and some periosteal reaction, suggesting a healing stress pathologic fracture through a unicameral bone cyst. The patient underwent biopsy to confirm the diagnosis, followed by curettage and bone grafting, supplemented by internal fixation to improve the lateral buttress (**C, D**). (Reproduced with permission from The Children's Orthopaedic Center, Los Angeles, CA.)

and most lesions present with localized pain and/or swelling, while spinal lesions may also present with radicular symptoms.[31,74,77,124] The humerus and femur are the most common sites of pathologic fracture (Fig. 7-5).[74,123] Magnetic resonance imaging (MRI) is helpful, especially for axial lesions, and demonstrates the characteristic double-density fluid levels, septations, low signal intensity on T1-weighted images, and high signal intensity on T2-weighted images.[186]

Operative Treatment of Aneurysmal Bone Cyst

While conservative treatment of the fracture may be indicated, these lesions do not spontaneously heal and delayed surgical intervention is needed. Recurrence rates following intralesional curettage and bone grafting can be as high as 30%.[80] Several authors have shown that the recurrence is higher among younger children.[18,51,74] Serial embolization treatment utilizing n-butyl cyanoacrylate, concentrated bone marrow, doxycycline, or other substances has demonstrated adequate results but may require several treatment sessions.[15,188] A four-step approach to resection has been previously described with a reported recurrence rate for appendicular lesions of around 8%. We recommend the use of a headlamp for enhanced illumination and loupes for magnification. An image intensifier should be available for intraoperative confirmation of complete tumor excision and appropriate bone grafting. Diagnostic tissue confirmation is an essential part of this technique. For

large spinal tumors, preoperative embolization may be recommended (Fig. 7-6). If instrumentation is needed after spine tumor resection, we recommend titanium or cobalt chrome instrumentation that gives a much better visualization of the spine on future MRIs (less artifact) than stainless steel (Fig. 7-7).

✔ Four-Step Resection of Aneurysmal Bone Cyst: KEY SURGICAL STEPS

- ❏ Small incision over the cyst, respecting oncologic principles
- ❏ Lesional tissue is then retrieved and sent for frozen section for diagnostic confirmation; be prepared for possible excessive bleeding once cavity is opened
- ❏ A cortical window is enlarged to allow appropriate visualization and intralesional resection/curettage
- ❏ A high-speed burr is used, when possible, to extend the intralesional margins
- ❏ Electrocautery is used to help identify residual tumor pockets, to potentially kill residual tumor cells, and to coagulate the bleeding bone surface
- ❏ Adjuvants such as phenol solution 5%, or liquid nitrogen may be used
- ❏ Bone grafting is done with either a synthetic bone substitute or allograft
- ❏ Internal fixation is indicated on case-by-case basis; lesions of weight-bearing bones, particularly of the proximal femur, and some large vertebral lesions may warrant internal fixation/instrumentation

Figure 7-6. A 9-year-old boy presented with low back pain and abdominal discomfort. **A:** On plain radiographs of the abdomen, an expansile lesion (*arrow*) involving the left posterior elements of L1 was visualized. Axial T2-weighted MRI (**B**) and an axial CT scan (**C**) show the microfractures at the pedicle and lamina level (*arrow*) and the fluid–fluid levels. The patient underwent open biopsy that confirmed the diagnosis of aneurysmal bone cyst, followed by a four-step approach excision and bone grafting. **D:** Limited instrumentation of the spine was performed because of stability compromise. Nowadays, the author's preferred technique is pedicle screw fixation and fusion one level above and below the involved vertebra.

Figure 7-7. When dealing with pathologic fractures secondary to tumors or tumor-like processes of the spine, if instrumentation is needed, titanium instrumentation allows much better postoperative visualization with both CT and MRI for the detection of tumor recurrence as compared with standard stainless-steel instrumentation. **A:** Postoperative MRI of the spine with standard stainless-steel instrumentation showing a large degree of artifact that makes interpretation difficult. **B:** Preoperative CT scan of a patient with an ABC of the spine. **C:** Postoperative CT scan of the same patient showing an adequate view of the surgical area. **D:** Postoperative MRI of a patient with a previous spinal tumor again adequately showing the surgical site to monitor for recurrence or persistent tumor.

FIBROUS CORTICAL DEFECTS AND NONOSSIFYING FIBROMAS

Fibrous cortical defects (FCDs) and nonossifying fibromas (NOFs) are the most common bone tumor or tumor-like conditions seen in the growing child, with an estimated incidence of 20%. Most of these lesions are asymptomatic and incidentally found. Pathologic fractures may occur, especially through lesions involving more than 50% of the cortical diameter, early Ritschl stages associated with pain, in the lower extremity, and particularly among boys between 6 and 14 years of age.[149]

These lesions present as a well-defined, eccentric or cortical-based, lytic lesion in the metaphyseal region of long bones, surrounded by a sharp sclerotic border. FCDs are small, usually under 2 cm, while NOFs are larger and can present as multiple lesions (one-third of patients).[86]

The natural history of these lesions is that they generally spontaneously heal over time. Pathologic fractures heal uneventfully but the lesion usually persists, and refracture may occur.[67,86]

Fractures are usually treated with immobilization until there is evidence of radiographic healing. Surgery may be necessary due to persistent high risk of further pathologic fractures or chronic pain; however, it is best performed after fracture healing. Although absolute size parameters may be useful in predicting pathologic fracture, they do not imply a requirement for prophylactic curettage and bone grafting. A retrospective epidemiologic study found that the size of the lesion was not associated with pain.[68] The appearance or stage of the lesion has been used as a predictor of pathologic fracture.[165] This was studied in a group of patients with NOF of the distal tibia and it was found that Ritschl stage B, with greater than 50% involvement of the diameter on anteroposterior (AP) and lateral radiographs, and thinning of the cortex increased the risk of pathologic fractures.[14] The authors of that study created a treatment algorithm based on their findings. Another study used CT-based measurements, adding cortical breach and lack of neocortex formation as risks for pathologic fracture.[82] Most patients with large NOFs can be monitored without surgical intervention. Although we cannot readily identify an accurate denominator, we infer that many large NOFs remain unidentified and are not problematic (Fig. 7-8).

ENCHONDROMA

Enchondromas are benign latent or active cartilaginous tumors. These lesions are often found incidentally but can present with

Figure 7-8. An 11-year-old boy fell while playing baseball and developed acute pain over the right distal leg/ankle area. AP (**A**) and lateral (**B**) radiographs of the right ankle show a spiral fracture through a well-defined, eccentric lesion in the lateral distal aspect of the tibia metaphysis. There is narrow zone of transition and a sclerotic border. **C, D:** The lesion was thought to be consistent with a nonossifying fibroma, and the fracture was allowed to heal for 5 weeks. The patient then underwent biopsy confirming the diagnosis, followed by curettage and bone grafting. **E, F:** Four months postoperatively, the lesion is completely healed and the patient resumed normal physical activities. (Figures reproduced with permission from The Children's Orthopaedic Center, Los Angeles, CA.)

A, B

C

Figure 7-9. An 8-year-old boy presented with pain and swelling of the ulnar border of his right hand. **A:** Radiographic studies showed an expansile, lucent lesion of the diaphysis of the patient's right fifth metacarpal with microfractures. The patient had an open incisional biopsy with frozen section, which was consistent with enchondroma with subsequent curettage and bone grafting. **B:** Gross appearance of material removed at the time of surgery, which is consistent with enchondroma. **C:** At 6-month follow-up, the fracture is well healed, and there is no sign of recurrent tumor.

pain or pathologic fracture (more often with lesions in the phalanges of the hands or feet) (Fig. 7-9). The most common sites of involvement in decreasing order are the phalanges, metacarpals, metatarsals, humerus, and femur.[78] Children may present with multiple enchondromas or enchondromatosis (Ollier disease), which is usually diagnosed between 2 and 10 years of age. Although the lesion itself is similar to a solitary enchondroma, it can be more extensive, leading to deformity and shortening of the extremity due to growth disturbance (Fig. 7-10).[196]

On plain radiographs, enchondromas are intramedullary lesions with stippled calcification; however, in the hands and feet, they may appear as purely lytic lesions, extending from the metaphysis to the diaphysis.[163] Larger lesions may cause cortical thinning and endosteal scalloping, uneven expansion, and pathologic fractures.

For asymptomatic patients with small lesions and classic radiographic findings, biopsy is not necessary. Younger patients, with lesions in the fifth finger, and those in the distal phalanx are at a higher risk for fractures. Curettage and bone grafting are necessary for those lesions with recurrent or impending pathologic fracture or in cases of persistent pain.[163] Fixation is not necessary for lesions of the short tubular bones but may be necessary for lesions of the proximal femur or long bones of the lower extremity. Standard fracture care is adequate to treat most pathologic fractures, but bone quality may be compromised by

the tumor making fixation challenging. Load-sharing fixation with intramedullary devices is preferred.

OSTEOCHONDROMA

Osteochondromas are the most common benign bone tumor in children, and clinical symptoms are usually related to irritation of the surrounding soft-tissue structures. The radiographic appearance is pathognomonic, with continuity of the host bone cortex with the outer cortex of the lesion and intramedullary cavities. Although fractures associated with osteochondromas are rare, they may occur through the base or stalk of a pedunculated tumor (Fig. 7-11).[39] Fractures through osteochondromas can be treated conservatively; however, excision in the acute phase may be considered because the fragment is "floating free" in the soft tissues.

FIBROUS DYSPLASIA

Fibrous dysplasia (FD) is a benign bone abnormality characterized by replacement of normal bone and marrow by fibro-osseous tissue (woven bone formed by metaplasia with poorly oriented bone trabeculae) resulting in decreased strength, deformity, and pathologic fracture. The disease may involve a single bone (monostotic FD) or multiple bones (polyostotic FD). When polyostotic FD is associated with skin hyperpigmentation (referred to

Figure 7-10. Multiple enchondromatosis. **A:** A 10-year-old girl with multiple enchondromas sustained a spontaneous pathologic fracture of the femur while running. The lateral radiograph shows overriding of the fracture. **B:** At 3-year follow-up, the fracture is well healed. **C:** The anteroposterior radiograph of the hand in this patient demonstrated multiple expansile enchondromas of the small bones. **D:** A radiograph of the humerus shows the streaked-mud appearance of the lateral humerus (*arrow*).

as café-au-lait spots) and endocrine dysfunction (e.g., hyperthyroidism, precocious puberty, and increased growth hormone), it is referred to as McCune–Albright syndrome.[153]

Most often, the lesions are asymptomatic and pathologic fracture may be the presenting symptom. Fractures of long bones can be minimally displaced or incomplete; many being microfractures presenting with pain and swelling.[125] The bones most affected are the femur, tibia, and humerus. The age of first fracture, number of fractures, and fracture rate are related to the severity of the metabolic derangement and type of dysplasia (monostotic vs. polyostotic). The incidence of fractures in monostotic disease is around 5%.[83] The presence of an endocrinopathy may lead to phosphaturia, causing a rickets-type effect on the normal skeleton, leading to increased incidence of fractures.[38] Although the fractures heal rapidly, endosteal callus is poorly formed while periosteal callus is normal. With mild deformity, the cortex thickens on the concave side of long bones, and a progressive deformity can ensue.

On plain radiographs, FD is seen as well-defined, mostly lytic and central lesion, located in the diaphysis of long bones. The metaplastic woven bone comprising the lesion creates the classic "ground-glass" appearance, while those lesions that undergo cystic degeneration may appear purely lytic (Fig. 7-12). Bowing and/or angular deformity of tibia and femur are often seen. The differential diagnosis can include UBC and differentiating the two can be challenging, but MRI is helpful.

Conservative treatment (at least at first) with immobilization is indicated for most, except for fractures through severely deformed long bones (especially in the lower extremities), and those through large cystic areas. Fractures in polyostotic disease often require more aggressive treatment. Proximal femoral pathologic fractures are especially troublesome because of the propensity for malunion or progressive deformity leading to coxa vara and *shepherd's crook* deformity.[60]

Curettage and grafting are usually not indicated since the bone graft is reabsorbed and replaced by FD bone, though

Figure 7-11. A 13-year-old girl presented with right knee pain following direct trauma to that area 10 days prior. On AP (**A**) and lateral (**B**) radiographs, there was a pathologic fracture through the base of a pedunculated osteochondroma (*arrow*). The patient was very tender around that area and elected surgical excision. **C, D:** Immediately after excision, there was improvement of the symptoms. Four weeks later, she returned to full activities. (Figures reproduced with permission from The Children's Orthopaedic Center, Los Angeles, CA.)

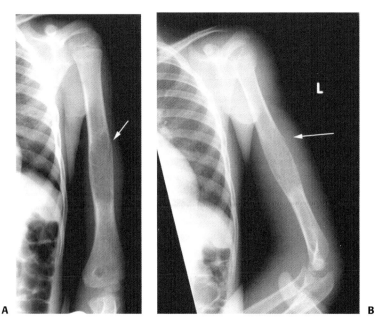

Figure 7-12. A 6-year-old girl presented with right arm acute pain after hitting the elbow in the bathtub. **A, B:** Radiographs of the humerus show a nondisplaced pathologic fracture through a humeral diaphyseal lesion (*arrows*). The lesion is well defined, mostly lytic but with definite matrix, cortical thinning, no periosteal reaction.

Figure 7-12. (*Continued*) MRI T1- (**C**) and T2-weighted (**D**) coronal images demonstrate absence of soft tissue mass or other aggressiveness signs. Bone scan shows increased activity at the lesion and fracture site (*arrow*). **E:** The patient underwent open incisional biopsy that confirmed the diagnosis of fibrous dysplasia. (Reproduced with permission from The Children's Orthopaedic Center, Los Angeles, CA.)

C   **D, E**

the use of cortical allograft seems to be the most resistant graft.[60] The use of bisphosphonates may prevent the occurrence and frequency of pathologic fractures in patients with severe or polyostotic FD. Pamidronate is a potent inhibitor of bone resorption and has a lasting effect on bone turnover. The drug is most effective at decreasing bone pain at the site of disease.[153] When pathologic fractures are managed surgically, internal fixation is key and intramedullary load-sharing fixation is preferred to decrease the metal–bone interface stress and preferably provide "total bone fixation" (Fig. 7-13). This frequently is combined with deformity correction to limit the risk of further fractures.[13]

MALIGNANT BONE TUMORS AND METASTASIS

The two most common primary bone malignancies in children are osteosarcoma and Ewing sarcoma. Malignant bone tumors can sometimes present with pathologic fractures (Fig. 7-14). Destructive bone lesions can also be caused by metastasis, being more common than primary bone tumors in certain age groups. Careful staging and biopsy are critical in the approach to children with bone tumors.[121] However, biopsy is not without risks. One of the complications following open biopsies is pathologic fracture caused by a decrease in torsional strength of the bone following cortical drilling. To prevent a pathologic fracture, an oval hole with smooth edges should be used, preferably in areas of less stress for weight-bearing bones. Sometimes, the biopsy hole can be filled with bone cement or other grafting material. Because most bone sarcomas are associated with a large soft tissue mass that can be sampled, drilling of the bone may be avoided. Nowadays, most biopsies can be safely performed by percutaneous means with image guidance, with high accuracy and lower risk of secondary fracture.[198] Lytic lesions, especially larger ones, have the highest accuracy rate.[198]

One of the major advances in the care of children with extremity sarcoma has been the development of limb-sparing surgical techniques for local control of the tumor. Pathologic fracture has previously been thought to be a contraindication to limb salvage because of concerns about tumor dissemination

Figure 7-13. A 10-year-old boy with McCune–Albright syndrome fell during a soccer match. An attempt at an AP (**A**) view of the femur shows a pathologic fracture through the subtrochanteric region. AP (**B**) and lateral (**C**) of the femur after open reduction and internal fixation with a reamed intramedullary blocked nail, and an orthoroentogram (**D**) showing "total bone fixation" and good alignment. (Reproduced with permission from CHOP Orthopaedics, Philadelphia, PA.)

(*continues*)   **A**   **B**

Figure 7-13. (*Continued*)

Figure 7-14. A 13-year-old boy presented with several months' history of right arm pain and recent increase in pain following minor trauma. AP (**A**) and lateral (**B**) radiographs show a minimally displaced midshaft humeral pathologic fracture (*arrows*) through a poorly defined, permeative, aggressive-looking diaphyseal lesion. **C:** T2-weighted axial MRI shows a huge soft tissue mass associated with the bone lesion and involvement of the neurovascular bundle. The patient was diagnosed with Ewing sarcoma, received neoadjuvant chemotherapy, and had a shoulder disarticulation (**D**), followed by postoperative chemotherapy. (Reproduced with permission from The Children's Orthopaedic Center, Los Angeles, CA.)

by fracture hematoma, leading to high local recurrence rates. Several studies, however, have shown that with adequate fracture care and modern neoadjuvant chemotherapy, free margin resection is achievable with no increased risk for local recurrence.[57] Some studies, however, have shown a possible negative effect of pathologic fractures on survival rates, though a recent analysis of 2,193 pediatric patients with osteosarcoma found that the presence of a pathologic fracture did not influence overall 5-year survival (Fig. 7-15).[71,105] Pathologic fracture after limb-sparing surgery is another major complication, occurring

Figure 7-15. An 8-year-old girl sustained a pathologic fracture of the femur after falling off her bicycle. She denied symptoms prior to this injury. **A, B:** The radiographs showed a grossly displaced fracture through a poorly defined, mixed lesion in the midshaft of the femur (*arrow*); there is disorganized periosteal reaction with sunburst sign. T2-weighted coronal (**C**) and axial (**D**) MRIs showed extensive soft tissue mass; the neurovascular bundle (*arrow*) does not seem to be involved by the tumor mass. The patient underwent biopsy that confirmed osteogenic sarcoma and fracture stabilization with an external fixator at a referring institute. **E:** Note that the external fixator pins were inappropriately placed too far from the tumor and fracture site postoperative appearance following Van Ness rotationplasty. The patient was continuously free of disease 5 years after surgery. **F, G:** Flexion and extension of the ankle, now used as a knee. (Reproduced with permission from The Children's Orthopaedic Center, Los Angeles, CA.)

most commonly after allograft reconstruction but also after limb salvage with endoprosthetic reconstruction.[195] Pathologic fractures in children because of metastatic disease tend to be mostly in the form of microfractures that can be successfully managed conservatively.

DISEASES OF THE BONE MARROW

GAUCHER DISEASE

Gaucher disease is a hereditary disorder of lipid metabolism. It is the most common lysosomal storage disease and is caused by deficient production and activity of the lysosomal enzyme beta-glucosidase (glucocerebrosidase), resulting in progressive accumulation of glucosylceramide (glucocerebroside) in macrophages of the reticuloendothelial system in the spleen, liver, and bone marrow. The most common sphingolipidosis is inherited as an autosomal recessive trait,[103] with most cases noted in Ashkenazi Jews of eastern European origin. There are three types of Gaucher disease: Type I represents more than 90% of all cases and is the most common type seen by orthopaedic surgeons; it presents as a chronic nonneuropathic disease with visceral (spleen and liver) and osseous involvement, also known as the adult form, although patients present during childhood.[103] Type II is an acute, neuropathic disease with central nervous system (CNS) involvement and early infantile death. Type III is a subacute nonneuropathic type with chronic CNS involvement. Types II and III are both characterized as either infantile or juvenile and are notable for severe progressive neurologic disease, usually being fatal.

Bone lesions are a result of marrow accumulation, and are most common in the femur, but they also occur in the pelvis, vertebra, humerus, and other locations. Infiltration of bone by Gaucher cells leads to vessel thrombosis, compromising the medullary vascular supply, leading to localized osteonecrosis of the long bones. Other radiographic findings include the Erlenmeyer flask appearance of the metaphyseal bone and pathologic fractures, especially of the spine and femoral neck.

Katz et al.[103] reported 23 pathologic fractures in nine children with Gaucher disease; seven had multiple fractures. In decreasing order of frequency, these involved the distal femur, femoral neck, spine, and proximal tibia. Fractures of the long bones were transverse and usually in the metaphysis. Fractures of the spine were either wedge shaped or centrally depressed at the end plate. The factors predisposing these children to fracture included significant medullary space infiltration, cortical bone erosion, osteonecrosis, and associated disuse osteoporosis. In another report of 53 patients with Gaucher disease aged 9 to 18 years, 11 children had vertebral fractures, usually at two or three sites in each patient, with either anterior wedging, central vertebral collapse, or total rectangular collapse.[104]

Conservative treatment with immobilization and non–weight bearing is recommended for long bone fractures when appropriate. Stable fractures of the femoral neck should be treated by immobilization with frequent follow-up radiographs, as varus

malunion often occurs; internal fixation should be performed for unstable femoral neck fractures. Preoperative planning is important, and the anesthesiologist must recognize that patients with Gaucher disease may be prone to upper airway obstruction because of infiltration of the upper airway with glycolipids and abnormal clotting function, even when clotting tests are normal.[192] Both delayed union and nonunion have been reported in older patients with Gaucher disease.

SICKLE CELL DISEASE

Sickle cell disease (SCD) is caused by the presence of sickle cell hemoglobin (HbS). The presence of the abnormal hemoglobin in red blood cells in SCD causes them to be mechanically fragile, and when they are deoxygenated, the cells assume a sickle shape, which makes them prone to clumping with blockage of the small vessels of the spleen, kidneys, and bones. The most common type of SCD, HbS-S, is a homozygous recessive condition in which individuals inherit the HbS globin gene from each parent. SCD affects approximately 1 in 400 African Americans. Chronic hemolytic anemia is present in most severely affected patients, and marrow hyperplasia is found in both the long bones and the short tubular bones. Sickle cell *trait* affects 8% to 10% of the African American population and other groups less frequently but usually has no apparent clinical manifestations. These disorders are diagnosed by hemoglobin electrophoresis.

Fractures may be a presenting symptom of the disorder.[24] Marrow hyperplasia may be a major contributing factor; not only does the hypercellular bone marrow expand the medullary canal with thinning of both trabecular and cortical bone, but it also extends into widened Haversian and Volkmann canals. This process may weaken the bone, leading to fractures.[34] The prevalence of osteopenia and osteoporosis in young adults with SCD is extremely high, which can also predispose to pathologic fractures (Fig. 7-16).[144] In a series of 81 patients with 198 long bone infarcts with occasional concurrent osteomyelitis, Bohrer[29] found a 25% incidence of fractures associated with femoral lesions, and 20% with humeral lesions. The most common pattern was transverse diaphyseal fractures, especially of the femur.[29]

Pathologic fractures in patients with SCD usually heal with conservative treatment. Furthermore, operative management may be hazardous. Extreme care must be taken to oxygenate the patient's tissues adequately during the procedure and, ideally, elective procedures should be preceded by a transfusion regimen to raise hemoglobin levels to 10 g/dL, which may help limit perioperative complications. Intravenous hydration is very important, with one and a half to two times the daily fluid requirements needed in addition to routine replacement of fluid losses. The use of a tourniquet during surgery for patients with SCD is controversial due to the risk of thrombosis.

LEUKEMIA

Leukemia accounts for over 30% of cases of childhood cancer. Acute lymphocytic leukemia accounts for 80% of pediatric leukemias. There is an increased occurrence of lymphoid leukemias in patients with Down syndrome, immunodeficiencies,

Figure 7-16. A 4-year-old boy with sickle cell disease presented with acute onset of right arm pain, swelling, increased warmth, and low-grade fever. **A, B:** The initial radiographs show a poorly defined area of lucency in the proximal humeral metaphysis (*arrows*). T2-weighted sagittal (**C**) and axial (**D**) MRIs show intramedullary changes (enhancement) and periosteal reaction/abscess with no soft tissue mass. The clinical diagnosis of osteomyelitis was initially made and the patient was started on intravenous antibiotics. **E, F:** Three weeks later, there was little clinical improvement and new radiographs showed pathologic fracture/insufficiency fracture through the proximal humeral metaphysis (*arrows*). The patient underwent a biopsy that showed that this was an infarct with no superimposed infection. After clinical treatment, the patient's symptoms improved. **G:** At 6-month follow-up, he was completely asymptomatic, and the radiographs showed remodeling and continued growth.

and ataxic telangiectasia. The peak incidence occurs at 4 years of age.

Approximately 50% to 75% of children with acute leukemia develop musculoskeletal signs and symptoms.[166,121] Skeletal lesions occur more frequently in leukemic children than in adults because leukemic cells can quickly replace the smaller marrow reserves in children. Diffuse osteopenia is the most frequent radiographic finding (Fig. 7-17).[103] Nonspecific juxtaepiphyseal lucent lines are often seen and are a result of generalized metabolic dysfunction[166,121]; these are usually bilateral and vary from 2 to 15 mm in width. Sclerotic bands of bone trabeculae are more typical in older children. Periosteal reaction is often present with osteolytic lesions and is most common in the posterior cortex of the distal femoral metaphysis, the medial neck of the femur (Fig. 7-18), and the diaphysis of the tibia and

fibula.[121] Most bone lesions in leukemia improve after adequate response to treatment.

Pathologic fracture risk is around 20%.[5,120,121,166] The risk of pathologic fractures is higher for children with lower bone density at presentation and tends to decrease with treatment. Fracture is most commonly associated with osteoporosis of the spine, particularly the thoracic region, resulting in mild vertebral collapse (compression fracture).[141] Prompt diagnosis and initiation of chemotherapy is the main step in the treatment of pathologic fractures associated with leukemia. Most fractures are stable microfractures and can be treated with conservative treatment and symptomatic support, with emphasis on early ambulation to avoid further osteopenia. For vertebral fractures, a back brace or thoracolumbosacral orthosis (TLSO) may be used to alleviate symptoms.[5]

Figure 7-17. An 8-year-old girl presented with back pain, fever, malaise, and weight loss. **A:** Lateral radiographs of the spine showed diffuse osteopenia and compression/insufficiency fractures of the vertebral body (*arrows*). **B:** T1-weighted sagittal MRI confirms disease process within the vertebral body (*arrow*) and no soft tissue mass or intraspinal involvement. She was diagnosed with acute lymphoblastic leukemia. (Reproduced with permission from The Children's Orthopaedic Center, Los Angeles, CA.)

OSTEOMYELITIS

The pattern of pediatric osteomyelitis in North America has changed during the past several decades. Although the typical clinical picture of acute onset of pain, associated with fever and inability, or refusal to bear weight is still seen, subtle presentations and more aggressive ones have become frequent. Among the potential reasons for these changes are the increased use of empiric antibiotics and the increased number of aggressive community-acquired pathogens such as methicillin-resistant *Staphylococcus aureus* (MRSA). Osteomyelitis can be classified according to the age of onset (neonatal, childhood, and adult osteomyelitis); causative organism (pyogenic and granulomatous infections); onset (acute, subacute, and chronic); and routes of infection (hematogenous and direct inoculation). Although the acute form is still the most common, subacute osteomyelitis, or Brodie abscess, and chronic recurrent multifocal nonbacterial osteomyelitis are seen more frequently. Chronic osteomyelitis is defined as symptoms that have been present for longer than 1 month (Fig. 7-19; Table 7-1).

At first, radiographs may be normal and the earliest finding is soft tissue swelling/loss of defined deep soft tissue planes. MRI is the most useful and has up to 98% sensitivity and 100% specificity for early detection of osteomyelitis.[123]

With early recognition and appropriate treatment, acute osteomyelitis rarely leads to a pathologic fracture. Pathologic fractures are more often associated with neglected or chronic osteomyelitis, neonatal osteomyelitis, or septic arthritis. During acute osteomyelitis, transitory osteopenia and surgical intervention can potentially predispose to fractures (Fig. 7-20). The presence of large subperiosteal abscess on MRI at the time of admission can lead to greater incidence of fractures.[22] These

Figure 7-18. A 4-year-old boy who presented with left hip pain and refusal to bear weight. He had a low-grade fever. Infectious workup was nonrevealing. However, the hip radiograph (**A**) demonstrated a metaphyseal linear lucency along the inferomedial femoral neck, and the MRI (**B**) revealed diffusely abnormal bone marrow and signal intensity concerning for a marrow infiltrative process. The patient underwent a bone marrow biopsy and was diagnosed with acute lymphoblastic leukemia. (Reproduced with permission from NYU Langone Health, New York, NY.)

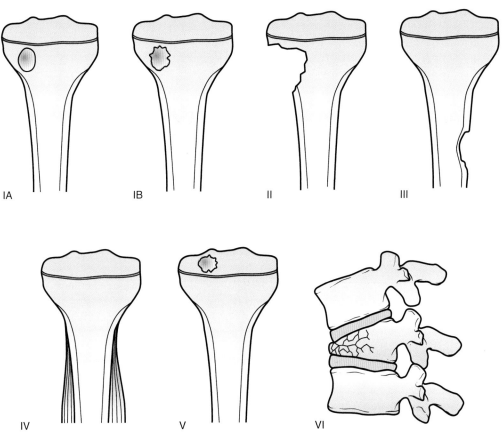

Figure 7-19. Classification of subacute osteomyelitis. Type IA, punched-out radiolucency suggestive of eosinophilic granuloma. Type IB, similar but with sclerotic margin; classic Brodie abscess. Type II, metaphyseal lesion with loss of cortical bone. Type III, diaphyseal lesion with excessive cortical reaction. Type IV, lesion with onionskin layering of subperiosteal bone. Type V, concentric epiphyseal radiolucency. Type VI, osteomyelitic lesion of vertebral body. (Adapted with permission from Dormans JP, Drummond DS. Pediatric hematogenous osteomyelitis: new trends in presentation, diagnosis, and treatment. *J Am Acad Orthop Surg.* 1994;2(6):333–341.)

TABLE 7-1. Comparison of Acute and Subacute Hematogenous Osteomyelitis

Presentation	Subacute	Acute
Pain	Mild	Severe
Fever	Few patients	Majority
Loss of function	Minimal	Marked
Prior antibiotics	Often (30–40%)	Occasional
Elevated white blood cell count	Few	Majority
Elevated erythrocyte sedimentation rate	Majority	Majority
Blood cultures	Few positive	50% positive
Bone cultures	60% positive	85% positive
Initial x-ray study	Frequently abnormal	Often normal
Site	Any location (may cross physis)	Usually metaphysis

Reprinted with permission from Dormans JP, Drummond DS. Pediatric hematogenous osteomyelitis: new trends in presentation, diagnosis, and treatment. *J Am Acad Orthop Surg.* 1994;2(6):333–341.

Figure 7-20. An 8-year-old girl sustained a fall from standing height and developed acute pain and deformity at the right knee. **A, B:** Radiographs at presentation demonstrated a pathologic fracture of the distal femur through a poorly defined, destructive lesion of the femur. **C:** MRI demonstrated soft tissue involvement abscess versus mass. **D:** A bone scan also showed increased uptake in the left proximal humerus. The patient underwent an open biopsy (**E**) of the lesion and was placed in a spanning external fixator until bone healing was evident (**F**). The final diagnosis was consistent with a multifocal methicillin-sensitive *Staphylococcus aureus* infection, and the patient responded to adequate antibiotics. **G:** The fracture healed in good alignment. (Reproduced with permission from The Children's Orthopaedic Center, Los Angeles, CA.)

fractures may be difficult to treat and be associated with complications, such as malunion and growth disturbance (Fig. 7-21).

The most important step in the treatment of a fracture associated with osteomyelitis is to control the underlying infection. This requires biopsy for culture and sensitivities, drainage and debridement of the infection (in the setting of an abscess) with appropriate immobilization, and antibiotic therapy (Table 7-2).

In advanced/chronic infections, sequestrectomy is necessary prior to fixation/immobilization of the fracture as the bone is likely nonviable. It is worth noting that fractures through the sequestrum are not necessarily a sign of recurrent infection but rather a fracture through nonviable bone which does not have the capacity to remodel. MRI is useful in identifying the sequestrum; an attempt should be made to leave as much supporting

Figure 7-21. Lateral radiograph of the humeral shaft of a 17-year-old boy showing a pathologic fracture through chronic osteomyelitis of the humerus. (Courtesy of B. David Horn, MD.)

involucrum as possible at the time of sequestrectomy. Prolonged immobilization with either cast application or external fixation devices may be needed, and segmental bone loss can be treated with bone transport or grafting.

PATHOLOGIC FRACTURES AFTER LIMB LENGTHENING

Limb lengthening has evolved dramatically in recent years; while the original Wagner method had a complication rate of over 90%, the use of gradual lengthening techniques, the combination of internal and external fixation techniques,[95] and the use of electromagnetic intramedullary devices has decreased these rates significantly.[91] Most lengthening procedures are performed through the metaphysis, which has a larger bone diameter and better blood supply than the diaphysis. This decreases the incidence of fractures post device removal to around 3% to 10%.[35,177]

Pathologic fractures can occur during, or after, limb lengthening. The regenerate, which is bone that is formed by distraction osteogenesis, must be subjected to normal weight-bearing forces over a period of time before normal bony architecture is established. Fractures through the regenerate can occur either soon after removal of the fixator or years later (Fig. 7-22), but most often they occur within the first 4 weeks, especially following lengthening of more than 5 cm.[35] Some of the causes include disuse osteopenia, adjacent joint contracture, and a stress riser from the pin tracts. Protective early weight bearing postoperatively, continued range of motion throughout treatment, and the use

TABLE 7-2. Initial Antibiotic Therapy for Osteomyelitis

Patient Type	Probable Organism	Initial Antibiotic
Neonate	Group B Streptococcus, *Staphylococcus aureus*, gram-negative rods (*Haemophilus influenzae*)	Cefotaxime (100–120 mg/kg/24 hr) or oxacillin and gentamicin (5–7.5 mg/kg/24 hr)
Infants and children	*S. aureus* (90%) if allergic to penicillin[a]	Oxacillin (150 mg/kg/24 hr), cefazolin (100 mg/kg/24 hr), clindamycin (25–40 mg/kg/24 hr), or vancomycin (40 mg/kg/24 hr)
Sickle cell disease	*S. aureus* or Salmonella	Oxacillin and ampicillin or chloramphenicol or cefotaxime (100–120 mg/kg/24 hr)

[a]Overall 80% because of *S. aureus.*

of smaller screw diameter are some of the preventive measures employed to limit the risk of fracture.[177] These fractures often lead to loss of correction, inadequate alignment, and risk for further joint contracture. Therefore, most patients who develop pathologic fractures following lengthening need surgical treatment with internal or external fixation and early mobilization.

OSTEOGENESIS IMPERFECTA

Osteogenesis imperfecta (OI) is an inherited disorder in which the structure and function of type I collagen is altered or deficient. The fragile bone is susceptible to frequent fractures and progressive deformity. OI incidence is 1 in 20,000 total births, with an overall prevalence of approximately 16 per 1,000,000.[51] The wide spectrum of clinical severity—from perinatal lethal forms to clinically silent forms—reflects the tremendous genotypic heterogeneity (>150 different mutations of the type I procollagen genes COL1A1 and COL1A2 have been described). Most forms (total of 13) of OI are the result of mutations in the genes that encode the pro alpha1 and pro alpha2 polypeptide chains of type I collagen.[151] Histologic findings reveal a predominance of woven bone, an absence of lamellar bone, and thinning of the cortical bone with osteopenia. From a practical viewpoint of orthopaedic care, patients with OI can be divided into two groups. One group of patients with severe disease who develop long bone deformity through repetitive fractures often needing surgical treatment, and another group of patients with mild disease and frequent fractures that tend to respond well to closed treatment.

Children with severe OI may present with a short trunk, marked deformity of the lower extremities, prominence of the sternum, triangular facies, thin skin, muscle atrophy, and ligamentous laxity. Some may develop kyphoscoliosis, basilar

Figure 7-22. Radiograph of a 15-year-old boy with achondroplasia (**A**) who underwent femoral lengthening with a monolateral external fixator for limb-length discrepancy (**B**). **C, D:** The procedure and the lengthening were uneventful, and the device was removed after four cortices were visualized on radiographs. **E:** Less than 2 months after external fixator removal, the patient fell and had a pathologic femoral fracture through the regenerated bone. **F, G:** He underwent ORIF with an intramedullary device and the fracture healed in approximately 3 months. (Reproduced with permission from The Children's Orthopaedic Center, Los Angeles, CA.)

invagination, and hearing loss (caused by otosclerosis). Children with OI usually have normal intelligence. Blue sclera, a classic finding in certain forms of OI, can also be present in normal infants, as well as in children with hypophosphatasia, osteopetrosis, Marfan syndrome, and Ehlers–Danlos syndrome. Children with OI also have a greater incidence of airway anomalies, thoracic anatomy abnormalities, coagulation dysfunction, hyperthyroidism, and an increased tendency to develop perioperative malignant hyperthermia.[135]

Pathologic fractures may present with swelling of the extremity, pain, low-grade fever, and a radiograph showing exuberant, hyperplastic, callus formation. The callus may occur without

Figure 7-23. This 10-month-old boy with a history of osteogenesis imperfecta presented with a right thigh pain and swelling and refusal to bear weight. AP (**A**) and lateral (**B**) radiographs of the right femur show the extraordinarily abundant, hyperplastic callus—with the characteristic butterfly shape—that can occur in osteogenesis imperfecta. This appearance may be mistaken for an infection or a neoplastic process.

obvious fracture and can have a distinct butterfly shape, as opposed to the usual fusiform callus of most healing fractures. The femur is the most common site of pathologic fractures.

The radiographic findings vary (Fig. 7-23). In severe OI, there is marked osteoporosis, thin cortical bone, and evidence

of past fractures with angular malunion. Both anterior and lateral bowing of the femur and anterior bowing of the tibia are common. Spinal radiographs may show compression of the vertebrae between the cartilaginous disc spaces (so-called codfish vertebra).

When the diagnosis of OI is suspected, but cannot be made on classic clinical grounds, the diagnosis may be made by biochemical assay. Genetic testing of individuals with typical features of OI typically has disease-causing mutations in 98% of patients.[16] The more severe the OI, the more genetic variety beyond collagen type I encoding genes are involved. If OI is suspected but there are no classic or typical signs, DNA sequencing of COL1A1, COL1A2, and IFITM5, including duplication/deletion testing is recommended; however, no additional genetic testing is needed if a variant is not identified.[156] It is crucial, but often difficult, to distinguish OI from nonaccidental injury (NAI). Before the diagnosis of OI is made, the parents may be presumed to be the cause of the fractures, with temporary removal of a child in 70% of cases.

Fractures tend to occur before skeletal maturity. Most pathologic fractures are transverse, diaphyseal, minimally displaced, and heal at a relatively normal rate. Although nonunion may occur, they seem to be associated with inadequate fixation after osteotomies and fractures. Recurrent fractures may result in angular deformities due to malunion leading to coxa vara, genu valgum, anterior bowing, and limb-length discrepancy. Olecranon sleeve (apophysis) avulsion fractures are essentially pathognomonic of OI (Fig. 7-24).[135,184]

The role of medical therapy in the prevention of fractures associated with OI has evolved; Bisphosphonates are a potent inhibitor of bone resorption and have been used for severe cases with the goal to reduce chronic bone pain and the rate of fractures, gain muscle force, increase bone density, thicken bone

Figure 7-24. A 13-year-old boy with mild osteogenesis imperfecta presented after a fall on an outstretched arm, with inability to move his elbow, pain, and swelling. **A:** Radiographs showed a displaced olecranon fracture. This fracture pattern is commonly seen in children with osteogenesis imperfecta and is quite uncommon in healthy children. The patient underwent open reduction and internal fixation. **B:** The fracture healed after 6 weeks. (Reproduced with permission from The Children's Orthopaedic Center, Los Angeles, CA.)

cortex, and increase growth rate.[27,66,81,201] Some of the reported negative effects include decrease in bone remodeling rate, growth plate abnormalities, and delayed osteotomy healing.[66,81] New therapies with other antiresorptive medications as well as anabolic agents and transforming growth factor (TGF)-β antibodies are currently in development.

The orthopaedist caring for children with OI must balance standard fracture care with the goal of minimizing immobilization to avoid a vicious cycle: immobilization leading to weakness and osteopenia, leading to refracture. Protected weight bearing is the goal for patients with severe OI. Close follow-up is necessary in the first few years of life, with protective splinting or soft cast for fractures. Orthoses are constructed for bracing of the lower extremities to aid in both standing and ambulation. Once ambulatory, the child is advanced to the use of a walker or independent ambulation. Severe bowing of the extremities especially after recurrent fractures is an indication for osteotomy and intramedullary

Figure 7-25. This 8-year-old girl presented with pain and deformity around the right hip after minor trauma. The patient had a known history of osteogenesis imperfecta. Initial radiographs (**A, B**) showed grossly displaced fracture of the proximal femur in the subtrochanteric area. The patient underwent closed reduction and internal fixation with titanium elastic nails, and the fracture healed after 5 weeks, with good alignment in both anteroposterior (**C**) and lateral (**D**) views. The nails were slightly prominent and the family elected removal of the hardware (**E, F**).

Figure 7-25. (*Continued*) Three months after removal of the hardware, the patient presented with new trauma to that region, followed by pain. Radiographs showed a min imally displaced transverse fracture in the subtrochanteric region (*arrow*) associated with varus and anterior angulation of the proximal femur (**G, H**). The patient underwent a Sofield procedure with Rush rods as the internal fixation. Ten weeks after the procedure, there was complete healing at the osteotomy/fracture site and adequate femoral alignment (**I, J**). (Reproduced with permission from The Children's Orthopaedic Center, Los Angeles, CA.)

rodding. Whenever possible, surgery is delayed until 6 or 7 years of age to allow for better fixation and to decrease the chance of recurrent deformities and fractures. Load-sharing devices (such as intramedullary rods) are used for internal fixation of long bone fractures or osteotomies in children with OI (Fig. 7-25).[170] It is important to perform fixation without the intent of hardware removal. Skeletally mature patients and patients with very small medullary canals are best treated with standard rods, whereas skeletally immature patients with adequate width of the medullary canal are best treated with extendible rods. Complications after internal fixation of fractures or osteotomies and intramedullary fixation include fracture at the rod tip, migration of the fixation device, joint or cortical penetration, loosening of components of extensible rods, and fractures through the area of uncoupled rods.[170]

OSTEOPETROSIS

Osteopetrosis is a condition in which excessive density of bone occurs as a result of abnormal function of osteoclasts.[9,160,182,199] The resultant bone of these children is dense, brittle, and highly susceptible to pathologic fracture. The incidence of osteopetrosis is approximately 1 per 200,000 births. The inherent problem is a failure of bone resorption with continued bone formation and persistent primary spongiosa. Osteopetrosis is classified into three main forms (malignant autosomal recessive, intermediate autosomal recessive, or benign autosomal dominant), leading to a severe infantile type or a milder form that presents later in life.[173,182]

Radiographically, the bones have a dense, chalk-like appearance. The spinal column may have a sandwich or "rugger jersey"

Figure 7-26. This 2 year old with osteopetrosis presented with forearm pain. An anteroposterior radiograph shows the characteristic increased bone density and absence of a medullary canal, especially in the distal radius and ulna. There is a typical transverse, nondisplaced fracture (*arrow*) in the distal ulnar diaphysis.

appearance because of dense, sclerotic bone at each end plate of the vertebrae and less involvement of the central portion. The long bones tend to have a dense, marble-like appearance and may have an Erlenmeyer flask shape at their ends owing to deficient cutback remodeling. There may be bowing of the bones because of multiple fractures, spondylolysis, or coxa vara.[160] The small bones of the hands and feet may show a bone-within-bone appearance with increased density around the periphery. The unusual radiographic appearance may initially obscure occult nondisplaced fractures (Fig. 7-26).[160,173,182] Patients with a severe form of the disease have more fractures than those with presentation later in childhood.

Patients with the severe, congenital disease have transverse or short oblique fractures of the diaphysis, particularly the femur. Distal physeal fractures with exuberant callus may be confused with osteomyelitis. Common locations for fractures include the inferior neck of the femur, the proximal third of the femoral shaft, and the proximal tibia. Upper extremity fractures are also frequent.[9] The onset of callus formation after fracture in osteopetrosis is variable.[61]

The orthopeadist treating fractures in children with osteopetrosis should follow the principles of standard pediatric fracture care, with additional vigilance for possible delayed union (Fig. 7-27).[173] Armstrong et al.[9] surveyed the membership of the Pediatric Orthopaedic Society of North America and compiled the combined experience of 58 pediatric orthopaedic surgeons with experience treating pathologic fractures in osteopetrosis. In this comprehensive review, they concluded that nonoperative treatment should be strongly considered for most diaphyseal fractures of the upper and lower limbs in children, but surgical management is recommended for femoral neck fractures and coxa vara. Open treatment of osteopetrotic fractures with fixation is technically difficult because of bone rigidity/density, and absence of intramedullary canal/sclerosis (leading to the use of multiple drill bits intraoperatively).

Figure 7-27. A: This 9-year-old girl with osteopetrosis sustained similar bilateral subtrochanteric fractures of the femur over a 2-year period. Anteroposterior (**A**) and lateral (**B**) femoral radiographs show a healing transverse subtrochanteric fracture of the left femoral.

Figure 7-27. (*Continued*) **C:** One year later, at age 10, she sustained a similar right transverse minimally displaced subtrochanteric femur fracture, which was treated with reduction and a spica cast. **D:** This anteroposterior radiograph taken at age 14 years shows that both proximal and femoral fractures have healed and there is mild residual coxa vara, especially on the right side.

In addition to these technical difficulties, patients with osteopetrosis are at risk for excessive bleeding and infection, related to the hematopoietic dysfunction caused by obliteration of the marrow cavity.[173,182]

In the past, primary medical treatment for osteopetrosis included transfusions, splenectomy, and adrenal corticosteroids, but these techniques have proved ineffective. Stimulation of host osteoclasts has been attempted with calcium restriction, calcitriol, steroids, parathyroid hormone, and interferon. Bone marrow transplantation for severe infantile osteopetrosis has proved to be an effective means of treatment for some patients; however, it does not guarantee survival, and those due to deficiency of the pro-osteoclastogenic cytokine, RANKL, are not suitable for this.[45,79,182]

RICKETS

Rickets is a disease of the growing skeleton caused by either a deficiency of vitamin D or an abnormality of its metabolism. In this condition, the osteoid of bone is not mineralized and broad, unossified osteoid seams form on the trabeculae. With failure of physeal mineralization, the zone of provisional calcification widens and the ingrowth of blood vessels into the zone is disrupted. In the rickets of renal failure, the effects of secondary hyperparathyroidism (bone erosion and cyst formation) are also present. Regardless of the underlying cause, the various types of rickets share similar clinical and radiographic features (Fig. 7-28).

Both pathologic fractures and epiphyseal displacement can occur in rickets.[8,44,134] The treatment of rickets depends on identification of the underlying cause.

Recognition and treatment of the underlying metabolic abnormalities is the most important aspect in the care of pathologic fractures in rickets. In addition to nutritional rickets and

lack of exposure to sunlight, many other diseases can affect vitamin D metabolism (Table 7-3). Most fractures of long bones respond readily to cast or splint immobilization, with concurrent aggressive medical treatment of the underlying metabolic disease. Slipped capital femoral epiphysis may be the first presenting sign of renal osteodystrophy and renal failure. The slip is bilateral in up to 95% of the patients and it is usually stable

Figure 7-28. This 12-year-old girl with rickets associated with chronic kidney disease presented with complaints of knocked knees and wrist pain. Hip to ankle radiographs (**A**) showed typical rickets changes with valgus deformity at the knee level. Looser lines around the distal femur, and physeal widening. Wrist images (**B, C**) demonstrated marked physeal widening and metaphyseal flare of the distal radius and ulna. (Reproduced with permission from The Children's Orthopaedic Center, Los Angeles, CA.)

TABLE 7-3. Rickets: Metabolic Abnormalities

Disorder	Cause	1,25(OH)₂ Vitamin D	Parathyroid Hormone	Calcium	P	Alkaline Phosphate
Vitamin D deficiency rickets	Lack of vitamin D in the diet	↓	↑	↓ or →	↓	↑
Gastrointestinal rickets	Decreased gastrointestinal absorption of vitamin D or calcium	↓ or →	↑	↓	↓	↑
Vitamin D-dependent rickets	Reduced 1,25(OH)₂ vitamin D production	↓↓	↑	↓	↓	↑
Vitamin D-resistant rickets—end-organ insensitivity	Intestinal cell insensitivity to vitamin D causing decreased calcium absorption	↑ or →	↑	↓	↓	↑
Renal osteodystrophy	Renal failure causing decreased vitamin D synthesis, phosphate retention, hypocalcemia, and secondary hyperparathyroidism	↓↓	↑↑	↓	↑	↑

(Fig. 7-29).[134] The aggressive medical treatment of renal osteo-dystrophy, including administration of vitamin D, calcitriol, hemodialysis, renal transplantation, and parathyroidectomy, has improved the long-term survival and quality of life for these patients. A slipped capital femoral epiphysis should be stabilized with in situ screw fixation in older children, and multiple screws should be considered because the underlying metaphyseal bone is quite soft. Contralateral prophylactic fixation should be considered as well. Significant cysts should be treated with curettage and bone grafting. Angular deformities of the long bones should be corrected when the patient is close to maturity.

IDIOPATHIC OSTEOPOROSIS

Idiopathic osteoporosis is a rare cause of pathologic fractures in children. The etiology is likely multifactorial and incompletely understood; however, poor calcium intake during the adolescent growth spurt may play some role. Symptoms can persist for 1 to 4 years after diagnosis, with spontaneous resolution in most patients after the onset of puberty. The only consistent metabolic abnormality is a negative calcium balance with high rates of fecal excretion of calcium.

Figure 7-29. This 13-year-old boy with renal osteodystrophy presented with bilateral hip and thigh pain. **A:** Anteroposterior pelvic radiograph shows widening of the proximal femoral physes with sclerosis. Slipped capital femoral epiphyses were diagnosed. **B:** This anteroposterior pelvic radiograph taken 9 months after surgery shows narrowing of the physis and no evidence of further displacement of the capital femoral epiphyses. (Reproduced with permission from The Children's Orthopaedic Center, Los Angeles, CA.)

Idiopathic osteoporosis usually presents with bone pain, deformities, and fractures, most often of the spine.[11,47] Although many children present with back pain as the only complaint, the most severely affected present with generalized skeletal pain. Patients may have difficulty walking, and their symptoms may be initiated by mild trauma. Metaphyseal impaction/insufficiency fractures are a hallmark of this disorder.[47]

Serum calcium, phosphorus, and alkaline phosphatase levels are usually normal. Low plasma calcitriol, a vitamin D metabolite that aids calcium absorption in the gut, has been observed in juvenile osteoporosis.[47]

Lower extremity and vertebral fractures are the most common (Fig. 7-30). While there is no definitive treatment, many patients have been treated by both vitamin D and calcium supplements with equivocal benefit, and usually mineralization of the skeleton does not improve until puberty, when the disease spontaneously resolves. Low-dose pamidronate may be indicated in patients with persistent bone pain.[76]

IATROGENIC OSTEOPOROSIS

OSTEOPOROSIS ASSOCIATED WITH CANCER TREATMENT

Osteoporosis is commonly seen in children who are undergoing cancer therapy. The cause of reduced bone mineral density is multifactorial. The disease itself may play a role (e.g., acute lymphoblastic leukemia, malignant bone tumors), but also the treatment including corticosteroids, chemotherapy (e.g., methotrexate, ifosfamide), and radiation (such as brain radiation that

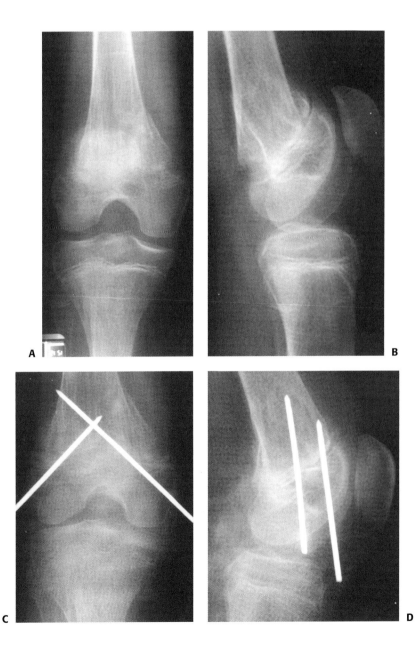

Figure 7-30. **A:** Multiple pathologic fractures in a previously healthy teenage boy who developed idiopathic osteoporosis. This anteroposterior radiograph of the right knee and this lateral radiograph (**B**) demonstrate a displaced distal femoral metaphyseal fracture with apex posterior angulation. **C:** This was treated with closed reduction and percutaneous pinning and application of a cast. **D:** This lateral radiograph shows satisfactory alignment with the pins in place.   *(continues)*

Figure 7-30. (*Continued*) **E:** A few months later, he sustained a left proximal femoral fracture, which was treated with a spica cast. **F:** This anteroposterior pelvic radiograph taken 3 years later shows healed proximal femoral fractures with varus angulation and severe osteopenia of the pelvis and femora with profusion of both acetabuli.

can reduce growth hormone secretion and cause hypogonadotropic hypogonadism) can contribute to the development of osteoporosis.[167] Methotrexate, for example, is believed to inhibit osteogenesis, causing both delayed union and nonunion of fractures.[101] The incidence of pathologic fractures after methotrexate use ranges from 19% to 57%.[142]

Generalized demineralization of the skeleton is seen with marked radiolucency of the metaphyseal regions of the long bones. Radiographic changes in the metaphysis and epiphysis resemble those seen in scurvy. Minimally displaced transverse fractures or insufficiency-type fractures occur in the long bones of both the upper and lower extremities and the small bones of the feet[142,160] (Fig. 7-31). Prevention is key to avoid pathologic fractures, with physical activity, adequate vitamin D intake, and bisphosphonates as some of the therapeutic options.[167]

IMMOBILIZATION OSTEOPOROSIS

Immobilization of an extremity for fracture treatment can result in loss of as much as a 44% of mineralization of trabecular bone. Immobilization leads to bone resorption, especially in unstressed areas.[183] Osteoporosis may persist for 6 months after an injury, but bone density returns to normal in most by 1 year. Persistent osteoporosis after cast immobilization for fracture can also contribute to refracture.[183]

CUSHING SYNDROME

Endogenous Cushing syndrome in children is a rare disorder that is most frequently caused by pituitary or adrenocortical tumors, resulting in excessive production of cortisol and its related compounds. If the hyperactivity of the adrenal cortex is caused by pituitary gland stimulation, the syndrome is known as Cushing disease. Exogenous Cushing occurs as a result of

corticosteroid therapy. The elevated adrenal corticosteroids inhibit the formation of osteoblasts, resulting in increased resorption of the bone matrix and decreased bone formation.

Presenting symptoms include failure to thrive, short stature with excessive weight gain, moon facies, presence of a buffalo hump, hirsutism, weakness, and hypertension, in addition to increased mortality.[127,137] In older children, the clinical picture is somewhat different: Truncal obesity, short stature, lowered hairline, acne, hirsutism, cutaneous striae, ecchymosis, weakness, emotional lability, and hypertension.

Radiographic findings may include severe osteopenia and a delayed bone age. Fractures of the ribs, vertebrae, and long bones have been reported in children with Cushing syndrome.[137] Single cortisol value at midnight followed by overnight high-dosage dexamethasone test leads to rapid and accurate confirmation, and diagnostic differentiation, respectively, of hypercortisolemia caused by pituitary and adrenal tumors.[19]

The primary treatment of Cushing syndrome of childhood is total adrenalectomy.[137] The associated fractures usually can be treated with standard immobilization techniques, but care should be taken not to increase the extent of osteopenia through excessive immobilization. In patients taking steroids, dose modification is attempted when possible. Also, children and adolescents who have Cushing syndrome may have significant alterations in body composition that result in a small but significant decrease in bone mass and increase in visceral adiposity. Long-term monitoring of body fat and bone mass should be instituted following treatment.[127]

SCURVY

Scurvy occurs in children who eat inadequate amounts of fresh fruit or vegetables leading to depletion in vitamin C. It takes up to 6 to 12 months before symptoms arise, and those may include

Figure 7-31. **A:** An 8-year-old boy who was diagnosed with a large alveolar rhabdomyosarcoma of the calf (*arrow*), as shown in the axial T1 MRI, was treated with chemotherapy, radiation, and surgical resection. **B, C:** At the end of treatment, he presented with increasing pain in the affected ankle and foot area, and MRI showed increased signal changes and edema consistent with an insufficiency fracture of the distal tibia and calcaneus. (Reproduced with permission from CHOP Orthopaedics, Philadelphia, PA.)

asthenia, vascular purpura, bleeding, and gum abnormalities. In 80% of cases, the manifestations of scurvy include musculoskeletal symptoms consisting of arthralgia, myalgia, hemarthrosis, and muscular hematomas.[70] Because vitamin C is essential for normal collagen formation, deficiency results in defective osteogenesis, vascular breakdown, delayed healing, and wound dehiscence. Children may experience severe lower limb pain related to subperiosteal bleeding. Although scurvy is often caused by a dietary deficiency of vitamin C, both aspirin and phenytoin are associated with decreased plasma levels of ascorbic acid. Vitamin C deficiency may also be present in myelomeningocele, although its contribution to fracture in that population is unclear. Infants with scurvy may present with irritability, lower extremity tenderness, weakness, pseudoparalysis, and possibly bleeding gums (if teeth have erupted). Subperiosteal hemorrhages may exist as well as hemorrhage into the subcutaneous tissues, muscles, urinary system, and gastrointestinal tract.

Radiographs may show osteolysis, joint space loss, osteonecrosis, osteopenia, and/or periosteal proliferation. Trabecular and cortical osteoporosis is common.[70] Profound demineralization is evident. In advanced disease, the long bones become almost transparent with a ground-glass appearance and extreme thinning of the cortex. Calcium accumulates in the zone of provisional calcification adjacent to the physis and becomes densely white (Fränkel line). Fractures generally occur in the scurvy line (Trummerfeld zone)—the radiolucent juxtaepiphyseal area above Fränkel line where the matrix is not converted to bone. Dense lateral spurs, known as the Pelken sign, may be seen. A characteristic finding of scurvy is the corner sign in which a peripheral metaphyseal defect exists where fibrous tissue replaces absorbed cortex and cartilage. The epiphysis becomes ringed with a thin, dense line (Wimberger sign). The periosteal elevation caused by hemorrhage calcifies within 10 days of treatment with vitamin C (Fig. 7-32).

The most common sites of fracture, in the order of frequency, are the distal femur, proximal humerus, costochondral junction of the ribs, and distal tibia. Fractures of the long bones generally are nondisplaced metaphyseal buckle fractures

Figure 7-32. Scurvy. **A:** A 10-month-old boy presented with a 2-week history of refusal to walk with tenderness of the lower extremities. He had a history of milk and cereal intake only. There are signs of scurvy in the metaphysis (*large arrow*). The dense white line in the zone of the provisional calcification of the distal femur is known as the Fränkel line. The radiolucent juxtaepiphyseal line above the white line is known as the scurvy line. The peripheral metaphyseal defect, where fibrous tissue replaces absorbed cortex in cartilage, is known as the corner sign. Wimberger sign is a thin, dense line surrounding the epiphysis (*small arrow*). **B:** This is a child with healing scurvy. There is marked periosteal calcification around the distal tibia (*arrowheads*). **C:** A newborn with scurvy. Periosteal hemorrhage has become calcified in the bones of the lower extremity (*arrows*). (Courtesy of Bruce Mewborne, MD.)

with mild angulation. In contrast, marked epiphyseal displacement occurs with a moderate amount of callus present even in untreated patients. Exuberant callus forms once vitamin C is administered. Standard immobilization, with administration of vitamin C, is adequate for most fractures. Remodeling potential is high in these patients. For infants who are older than 12 months of age and have begun weight bearing, spine films are recommended to rule out vertebral fractures.

FRACTURES IN NEUROMUSCULAR DISEASE

Pathologic fractures occur with frequency in children with neuromuscular diseases. While different diagnoses may come with different predisposing factors, most neuromuscular diseases share a few characteristics that may lead to osteopenia, osteoporosis, and pathologic fractures. Among these are decreased ambulation, joint contractures, and comorbidities such as seizures, nutritional depletion, kidney disease, etc.

The main goal of treating pathologic fractures in this group of patients is to return them to their prefracture level of activity, minimize further osteopenia, and recover motion and ambulation (if applicable). The second goal is to prevent further fractures. After surgical intervention for deformities or contractures, minimizing cast immobilization is important. Foam abduction pillows, knee immobilizers, and an intensive therapy program in the immediate postoperative period may avoid the deconditioning, osteopenia, and joint stiffness. For example, in ambulatory children who need hip osteotomies, use of rigid internal fixation allows for standing and gait training and prevents not only osteopenia but also the risk that the child may never regain the full level of preoperative function after a prolonged period of cast immobilization.

CEREBRAL PALSY

The main causes of low bone density and osteoporosis in children and adolescents with cerebral palsy (CP) are lack of activity, nutritional (e.g., low vitamin D), and pharmacologic treatments (e.g., anticonvulsant medications).[159,161,193] The diagnosis may be delayed because patients are often nonverbal.

The literature points to several predisposing factors, namely Gross Motor Function Classification System (GMFCS) 4 and 5, the presence of hip and knee contractures, a history of seizures, and spasticity. The incidence of fractures varies from 4% to 14%.[161,193] Most fractures involve the lower extremities, especially the midshaft femur.[126,161]

While fractures in patients with CP heal quickly with abundant callus, the challenges include a high rate of malunion (better tolerated in nonambulators) and around 20% risk of refracture. Closed treatment of these fractures is often preferred, but it can be complicated by the development of decubitus ulcers, or other skin issues. If a long-leg cast is used for a fracture of the lower extremity and the joint of the involved side is dislocated, the rigid cast may function as a lever arm, resulting in a proximal fracture femur above the cast.

If the patient is ambulatory, conventional forms of fracture treatment may be used (Fig. 7-33). When indicated, fixation with titanium elastic intramedullary nails can be an effective way to treat femoral shaft fractures (Fig. 7-34).

Fractures of the distal pole of the patella may occur in spastic ambulators with flexion contractures of the knees, patella alta, and a history of falls. If conservative treatment with extension casting is unsatisfactory, hamstring lengthening with correction of the knee flexion contracture can result in both healing of the fracture and relief of symptoms.

In a randomized controlled trial that studied the impact of a standing program on bone mineral density in GMFCS 5 patients, participation in 50% longer periods of standing improved vertebral but not tibia bone density. The authors concluded that such intervention might reduce the risk of vertebral fractures but is unlikely to reduce the risk of lower limb fractures in children with CP.[41] The use of pamidronate has been shown to decrease the incidence of fractures in this population, but a recent Cochrane review on the use of bisphosphonates in patients with CP found that there was very limited evidence that they might improve bone density.[93,171]

MYELOMENINGOCELE

Children with myelomeningocele are at a high risk of pathologic fractures of the lower extremities due to decreased bone mineral density from disuse, immobilization after reconstructive surgery, altered gait mechanics, decreased sensation (including protective sensation), and nephropathy (increased urinary calcium loss).[62,133] The incidence of fractures ranges from 12% to 31%.[63] An important risk factor is the level of disease; thoracic myelomeningocele has a higher incidence (around 40%) than lower levels (10% for low lumbar or sacral levels).[133] A retrospective review found that there was a bimodal age distribution of fractures at 1

Figure 7-33. A, B: An 11-year-old boy with total body involvement cerebral palsy was receiving physical therapy when he developed pain and swelling around the left knee. Radiographs showed displaced femoral supracondylar fracture.

(continues)

Figure 7-33. (*Continued*) **C, D:** To be able to fit to the brace adequately, closed reduction and percutaneous pinning were performed. **E, F:** The fracture healed in good alignment and the pins were removed after 6 weeks. (Reproduced with permission from The Children's Orthopaedic Center, Los Angeles, CA.)

to 5 years and then at 10 to 12 years, with fractures rarely occurring after 13 years of age.[3] The location of these fractures, in the order of decreasing frequency, are midshaft of the femur, distal femur, midshaft of the tibia, proximal femur, femoral neck, distal femoral physis, and proximal tibia. Fractures tend to heal rapidly, except for physeal fractures, and nonunion is rare.

Physeal fractures in patients with myelomeningocele may mimic infection, with elevated temperature, swelling, redness, and local warmth at the fracture site.[62] Both the white blood cell count and erythrocyte sedimentation rate are often elevated. Immobilization of these injuries usually results in a dramatic decrease in swelling and redness of the extremity within a few days. With healing, the radiographic picture can be alarming, with epiphyseal plate widening, metaphyseal fracture, and periosteal elevation. The radiographic differential diagnoses should include osteomyelitis, sarcoma, leukemia, and Charcot joint. Recurrent trauma to the physis, from either continued walking or passive joint motion after injury, results in an exuberant

Figure 7-34. A 12-year-old girl with cerebral palsy and in-house walking capabilities had an unwitnessed trauma to the right thigh, developing pain and deformity. **A, B:** Radiographs showed a displaced fracture of the femoral shaft. The patient underwent closed reduction, followed by titanium elastic nail fixation. **C, D:** At 6-week follow-up, there was abundant callus formation. (Reproduced with permission from The Children's Orthopaedic Center, Los Angeles, CA.)

healing reaction (Fig. 7-35). Physeal fractures require lengthy immobilization with strict avoidance of weight bearing to avoid destructive repetitive trauma to the physis.

Conservative treatment is best undertaken with well-padded immobilization to avoid pressure sores, and limited length to avoid further osteopenia.[133] In nonambulatory patients, mild malunion and shortening can be tolerated, and stable or minimally angulated fractures can be treated with either polyurethane splints or bulky soft dressings. In children who walk, fractures should be carefully aligned with heavily padded casts that allow continued protective weight bearing, if possible. Operative fixation may be associated with increased morbidity due to the higher risk of infection and development

of malignant hyperthermia.[133] In addition, between 18% and 40% of children with myelomeningocele are allergic to latex, so all patients considered for surgery should be operated on in a latex-free environment.[4]

MUSCULAR DYSTROPHY

The main treatment goal for fractures of the lower extremity in children with Duchenne muscular dystrophy (DMD) is to avoid premature loss of ambulation and/or ability to transfer.[96,139] In patients 9 to 10 years of age, increasing muscle weakness and joint contractures contribute to falls, in addition to the loss of normal muscle bulk and fat, which limit cushioning on impact.

Figure 7-35. A 10-year-old boy with low-lumbar spina bifida and community ambulation (with braces) presented with chronic bilateral leg/ankle pain. Anteroposterior (**A, C**) and lateral (**B, D**) radiographs of both tibia and fibula show stress/insufficiency fracture of the distal tibial physis associated with extensive periosteal bone formation, characteristic of myelomeningocele.

Patients in lower extremity braces seem to sustain fewer fractures from falls, probably because the overlying orthoses provide some protection. Patients confined to a wheelchair can fall because they have poor sitting balance, and fractures are frequent because these patients are more osteoporotic than ambulatory individuals.[96]

While corticosteroid therapy has improved longevity, walking ability, and the quality of life of children with DMD, it also increases the rate of osteoporosis and risk of fracture.[21,109] Fractures, when they occur, tend to heal rapidly. The most commonly fractured bone is the femur followed by the proximal humerus.

When ambulatory ability is tenuous, even minor bruises or ankle sprains may significantly limit walking ability. As little as 1 week in a wheelchair can prematurely end ambulation; patients on bed rest for more than 2 weeks will likely lose the ability to ambulate.[139] The patient should, therefore, be mobilized as soon as possible in a lightweight cast or orthosis. Load-sharing devices, such as intramedullary nails, allow earlier weight bearing and are preferred over other methods of internal fixation (Fig. 7-36). Aggressive physical therapy should be used to maintain functional status.

ARTHROGRYPOSIS

Arthrogryposis is a group of rare and heterogeneous disorders affecting children in whom there are at least two or more joint contractures in multiple body areas, with an incidence of 3 in

Figure 7-36. A, B: This 15-year-old domiciliary–ambulatory boy with Duchenne muscular dystrophy who sustained a fall at home had this displaced femoral shaft fracture. **C–E:** Because of his prefracture ambulatory status, he underwent closed reduction and intramedullary fixation of his fracture.

10,000 live births.[197] Although the etiology is unknown and likely multifactorial, there is a lack of fetal joint movement after initially normal development, leading to collagen proliferation, fibrotic replacement of muscle, a marked thickening of joint capsules, taut ligaments, and capsular tightness resulting in joint stiffness. Dislocations can occur with severe shortening of the involved muscles.

Fractures may occur in 25% of infants with arthrogryposis.[59] Clinical symptoms include poor feeding, irritability, and fussiness when handled. The involved extremity is generally swollen, and there is often an increased white blood cell count. Short-term immobilization is adequate to treat nondisplaced fractures in these patients (Fig. 7-37). Postnatal fractures are most common in patients with either knee contracture or dislocation of

the hip, and they could possibly be reduced by avoidance of forceful manipulation of these extremities. Older patients with lower extremity contractures do not seem to have increased risk for pathologic fractures.

Nonaccidental Injuries

Child maltreatment is any act or failure to act on the part of a parent or caretaker which results in death, serious physical or emotional harm, sexual abuse or exploitation, or an act or failure to act which presents an imminent risk of serious harm.[46]

Figure 7-37. **A, B:** A 4-year-old boy with arthrogryposis and bilateral knee extension contracture presented with swelling and pain around the knee. Initial films show minimally displaced transverse fracture through the distal femoral metaphysis (*arrows*). **C, D:** After 4 weeks in a long-leg cast, radiographs show new bone formation (*arrows*) and good alignment of the fracture in both views.

Child maltreatment includes all types of abuse and neglect that occur among children under the age of 18 years.[162] The four common types of maltreatment include physical, sexual, and emotional abuse as well as child neglect.[98] Maltreatment can be acute or chronic, with worse outcomes when inflicted over a number of years with multiple events.[100] Neglect is the most frequently encountered type of child maltreatment. Psychological maltreatment is increasingly recognized to be as harmful as other types of maltreatment.[88] Recent terminology for a battered child, physical abuse, or child abuse include child maltreatment, NAI, inflicted injury, or nonaccidental trauma (NAT).[73]

Child abuse has been recognized as a legitimate medical and social issue for many decades. In 1974, the United States Congress acknowledged the national importance of the prevention of child abuse by the passage of the Child Abuse Prevention and Treatment Act.[46] Because all health care professionals must be aware of reporting requirements for child maltreatment, there are recommendations for the establishment and management of hospital-based child multidiscipline collegial protection teams.[110] Ranade et al. have reviewed the role of the orthopaedic surgeon in the identification and management of NAT.[164]

EPIDEMIOLOGY

The National Child Abuse and Neglect Data System (NCANDS) was initiated in response to Public Law 93–247 to collect and analyze child abuse statistics.[46] NCANDS documents that the epidemic of child abuse continues to worsen in the United States, with approximately 3.4 million reports filed in the federal fiscal year 2015 compared to 1.2 million in 1982, and almost 4 million reports filed in 2021.[194] Over 17% of children who received an investigation were confirmed to have been abused or neglected. This represents a victim rate of 9.2 per 1,000. Approximately 60% of confirmed cases are neglect, 16% physical abuse, 10% sexual abuse, and 7% psychological abuse.[162] While children under the age of 4 years are at greatest risk for maltreatment, the victim rate is highest for infants, 24.2 per infant children. Abuse is second only to sudden infant death syndrome (SIDS) for mortality in infants 1 to 6 months of age and second only to accidental injury in children older than 1 year. Up to 11% of infants treated in the emergency room for apparent life-threatening events are later confirmed to be victims of child abuse.[30] A threefold increased mortality rate was noted in children who have been listed on a state abuse registry for all types of abuse.[99] The mortality rate is highest for those who are physically abused, especially infants.[99]

RISK FACTORS FOR CHILD ABUSE

THE HOME AT RISK

In assessing where child abuse may occur, households in turmoil from marital separation, job loss, divorce, family death, housing difficulties, or financial difficulties are more likely to have abusive episodes.[64,169] Compared to single-parent families, death caused by child abuse was noted to be 50 times higher in households that had unrelated adults; the perpetrator was the unrelated adult in 83.9% of these cases. Parental substance abuse, whether alcohol or other drugs, makes child abuse more likely. Although the youngest, poorest, most socially isolated, and economically frustrated caretakers are the most likely to act violently toward their children, any adult from any social or economic level may abuse a child. Day care may be an at-risk environment in situations in which there is poor supervision of the child caregivers. Primary parental predictors of child abuse are listed in Table 7-4.

THE CHILD AT RISK

Most reported cases of child abuse involve children less than 3 years of age.[20,75] In one report of abused children, 78% of all fractures reported were in children younger than 3 years of age and 50% of all fractures occurred in children younger than 1 year of age.[20] Infants younger than 1 year are especially at risk for infant homicide, the most severe form of child abuse.[115] An infant may present to the emergency room dead on arrival or death after an apparent "brief resolved unexplained events" which were previously termed, "life-threatening event."[203,204] In these cases, it is important to be open to all diagnostic possibilities and use a multidisciplinary team approach to evaluate the child.[148] Possible explanations for these events include SIDS, metabolic disease, cardiac disease, infection, as well as accidental or nonaccidental suffocation. Firstborn children, premature infants, stepchildren, and disabled children are at a

TABLE 7-4. Parental Predictors of Child Abuse

General

- Unrelated adult living in the home[a]
- Parent history of child abuse
- Divorce or separation of mother's parents
- Maternal history of being separated from mother, parental alcohol, or drug abuse
- Maternal history of depression
- Child attends a home day care

Mother

- Age <20 years
- Lower educational achievement
- History of sexual abuse
- Child guidance issues
- Absent father during childhood
- History of psychiatric illness

Father

- Age <20 years
- Lower educational achievement
- Child guidance issues
- History of psychiatric illness

[a]Fifty times the risk of death during infancy because of nonaccidental trauma.
Adapted from Sidebotham P, Golding J; The ALSPAC Study Team. Child maltreatment in the "Children of the Nineties"—a longitudinal study of parental risk factors. *Child Abuse Negl.* 2001;25(9):1177–1200. Copyright © 2001, With permission from Elsevier Science Inc.

greater risk for child abuse, as are twins and children of multiple births.[20] Some 25% to 83% of children with a disability have been reported to be abused. Physically abused children have a one in six chance of being sexually abused, whereas sexually abused children have a one in seven risk of being physically abused.[89] Children who have experienced neglect or abuse or have been exposed to toxic stress, frequently have major health or behavior problems later in life, into adulthood.[172]

ORTHOPAEDIC RECOGNITION OF CHILD MALTREATMENT

Orthopaedists become involved in the care of 30% to 50% of abused children. Early recognition by the orthopaedist is critical because children returned to their homes after an unrecognized episode of child abuse have a 25% risk of serious reinjury and a 5% risk of death.[168] However, it has been found that orthopaedic surgeons, especially those with more experience, do not always try to determine the underlying cause of the child's symptoms.[187]

OBTAINING THE HISTORY

The history is critical in the diagnosis of child abuse, which is a multidisciplinary effort, involving the consulting pediatrician, social worker, and other personnel from the hospital's child protective team, child protective services worker, law enforcement, and the appropriate consulting services. It is critical to inquire of the parent or caretaker if the information being provided is firsthand observation or secondhand recollection of another person. Physicians infrequently inquire about basic historical information such as the timing of the injury and who were the witnesses.[7]

When involved, the orthopaedic surgeon performs a detailed musculoskeletal history and physical examination to characterize the features and mechanism of the obvious injury and to discover evidence of additional undocumented injuries. A delay in seeking medical care for an injured child is very suggestive of child abuse.[64] An infant who has sustained abusive head trauma (AHT) typically will develop immediate neurologic change and will invariably show symptoms within a few hours.

To make the diagnosis of child abuse, the orthopaedic surgeon or child abuse team must determine if the history of trauma is adequate to explain the severity of injury.[43] This should be based on their experience in the care of fractures with knowledge of the mechanisms of injury and special insight into the types of trauma most likely to cause significant injury. We advise consultation with child abuse pediatricians for assistance in matching the mechanism of injury to the child's developmental level and family situation. A finite element study found that rolling, as a mechanism for humerus fractures in nonambulatory infants, was not a plausible explanation and should be approached with caution when such a mechanism is proposed.[6]

Details given as the reason for the injury should be carefully considered. Although it is not unusual for a young child to sustain an accidental fall, it is unusual to sustain a serious injury from that fall alone. Infants fall from a bed or a raised surface during a diaper change fairly frequently. A major injury or cluster of injuries in such falls is, however, extremely rare. A much higher rate of fracture is seen in older children "falling" from furniture, with 98% sustaining fractures, mostly of the upper extremity, from catapulting during play activity rather than sustaining a simple short-height fall.[85] More severe injuries occur with falls from greater heights. Stairway falls usually result in low-energy injuries, but there is an increased risk of injury if the child is being carried by the caregiver. In a report of 363 stairway injuries,[10] were infants dropped by their caretakers, and 4 of those sustained skull fractures. In patients 6 months to 1 year of age, 60% were using walkers at the time of the stairway injury. Only 4% of patients had extremity fractures and 1% had skull fractures. Reported short-height falls (<1.5 m) rarely result in death,[42] and fatally injured child from a reported short-height fall at home must receive an expert postmortem investigation to rule out child abuse.[52]

PHYSICAL EXAMINATION

After the initial musculoskeletal evaluation for acute fracture assessment, a detailed physical examination should follow, systematically evaluating from head to toe, to detect any signs of additional acute or chronic injury. Careful evaluation for signs of previous injury is useful because 50% of verified abuse cases

show evidence of prior abuse. Acute and subacute fractures may cause local tenderness and swelling, whereas chronic fractures may produce swelling from the presence of callus and clinical deformity from malunion. Radiographs should be obtained to confirm clinically suspected fractures. A skeletal survey must be performed in children under 2 years of age when there is reasonable suspicion of abuse, and it should be considered an extension of the physical examination in this age group. A thorough examination should focus on the body areas commonly involved in child abuse, including the skin, CNS, abdomen, and genitalia.

Soft Tissue Injuries

The child's entire body should be systematically evaluated to detect acute and chronic soft tissue trauma and is one of the most important physical findings to observe and to document. Sentinel injuries to observe and to document include the external ear for bruising, the eye for subconjunctival hemorrhage, and the tongue for tearing of the frenulum. Identification of sentinel injuries, such as rib fractures, abdominal trauma, or intracranial hemorrhage indicate abuse in more than 20% of cases.[131] Soft tissue injuries are present in 81% to 92% of abused patients,[75,140] making them the most common abuse-related physical examination finding. The types of skin lesions commonly encountered include bruises, welts, abrasions, lacerations, scars, and burns.

Approximately 17% of ambulatory infants, 53% of toddlers, and most school children have bruises that are not related to abuse.[136] Infants under 5 months of age have a much lower prevalence of accidental bruising (1.3%) compared to older infants (6.4%) or ambulatory toddlers.[136] Accidental bruises in babies are also typically noted over bony prominences.[38] Toddlers may have multiple accidental bruises over bony prominences such as the chin, brow, knees, and shins.[168,185] Bruises on the back of the head, neck, arms, legs, buttocks, abdomen, cheeks, or genitalia may be suspicious for abuse. Although any number of bruises may be present in children, the location and configuration of the bruises and the ambulatory status of the child, taken together with the rest of the medical and social history determines the suspicion for abuse (Fig. 7-38; Table 7-5). Photographs must be taken to document skin lesions prior to cast application, especially when applying large spica casts.

Burns

Burns are found in approximately 20% of abused patients[75] and are most likely to occur in patients younger than 3 years of age.[140] Scalds are the most frequent type of abusive burns and are caused either by a spill or an immersion.[122] Accidental spill burns are generally located on the trunk and proximal upper extremities (Fig. 7-39). Most accidental pour or spill burns occur on the front of the child, but accidental burns can also occur on the back as well. In accidental flowing liquid burns, the injury usually has an arrowhead configuration in which the burn becomes shallower and more narrow as it moves downward, and there may be splash marks surrounding the lesion.[94] The pattern in accidental burns may also be indicative of flowing water.[174] Abuse should

Figure 7-38. Schematic illustrates distribution of abusive versus accidental bruising. (Redrawn from original, courtesy of Samir Abedin, MD.)

Figure 7-39. Schematic illustrates location of accidental versus abusive burns. Note the buttock and lower extremity distribution of nonaccidental immersion burns compared to thoracic distribution accidental burns. (Redrawn from original, courtesy of Samir Abedin, MD.)

be suspected when deep second- or third-degree burns are well demarcated with circumferential definition. Since burns are frequently intentional and are associated with evidence of previous abuse such as rib fractures, skeletal survey should be obtained on burned children less than 2 years of age.[69]

In accidental hot water immersion, an indistinct stocking or glove configuration may be seen with varying burn depths

and indistinct margins. In deliberate immersion burns such as occurs when a child's buttocks are immersed in hot water, the burn demarcation has uniform depth and a well-demarcated water line.[94] The gluteal crease of the buttocks may be spared, giving a doughnut-like appearance to the burn. In accidental hot water immersion, the child is uniformly scalded about the lower extremities as the legs are quickly extended by the child to climb out of the water, but in deliberate, abusive immersion, the child is lowered into the water and instinctively flexes the hips and knees, thus sparing the popliteal area.[75]

Fractures

After skin lesions, fractures are the second most common physical presentation of abuse. The child abuse literature shows varying incidence of abuse-related fractures, depending on the age of the study population, institution, study entry criteria, selection bias, and time period when the study was published.[129] The younger the child with a fracture, especially under 18 months of age, the more likely abuse is the cause.[49,50,107] Particularly concerning is a bone that fractures under tension with torsion, rather than the physiologic loading of compression of normal childhood activity or falls. Pierce et al.[159] recommend that the clinician determine if the observed injury of a long bone and the stated mechanism are consistent (Tables 7-6 and 7-7).

Kleinman ranked the specificity of skeletal fractures for abuse based on the location and type of fracture (Table 7-8).[111]

TABLE 7-5. Evaluating Bruising in a Child: Implications for Practice

A bruise must never be interpreted in isolation and must always be assessed in the context of medical and social history, developmental stage, explanation given, full clinical examination, and relevant investigations.

Patterns of bruising that are suggestive of physical child abuse:
- Bruising in children who are not independently mobile
- Bruising in infants under 1 year of age
- Bruises that are seen away from bony prominences
- Bruises to the face, back, abdomen, arms, buttocks, ears, hands
- Multiple bruises in clusters
- Multiple bruises of uniform shape
- Bruises that carry the imprint of implement used or a ligature

---

Adapted from Maguire S, et al. Are there patterns of bruising in childhood which are diagnostic or suggestive of abuse? A systematic review. *Arch Dis Child.* 2005;90(2): 182–186, with permission from BMJ Publishing Group Ltd.

TABLE 7-6. Considerations When Evaluating a Child With a Long Bone Fracture

1. What are the biodynamics of the injury event, the energies generated by the event, and how could certain factors of the injury environment contribute to the likelihood of injury?

2. What injuries are expected, and what is the likelihood that the event generated the specific load required to cause each and all of the injuries?

3. Did the energy of the event exceed the injury threshold, or was there a biologic abnormality such as decreased bone density that resulted in a lowering of the actual threshold for injury? Is there evidence of bone weakness or disease?

4. Is the fracture morphology consistent with the direction, magnitude, and rate of loading of the described mechanism?

5. Is the fracture pattern unusual, and one that requires an extremely unusual loading condition, as is the case with a classic metaphyseal lesion (also termed corner or bucket-handle fracture)?

6. What are the child's developmental capabilities, and could the child have generated the necessary energy independent of "outside" forces to cause the observed injury?

7. Does the fracture reflect a high-energy fracture? Did the event generate enough energy to cause a high-energy fracture? Or is the fracture a small cortical defect, or hairline crack, reflecting a smaller amount of energy required for propagation of the fracture type?

8. What regions of the bone have been injured and what are the structural components that affect the ultimate pattern of fracture that is being observed? Were there structural factors that contributed to the likelihood of fracture?

Adapted from Pierce MC, et al. Evaluating long bone fractures in children: a biomechanical approach with illustrative cases. *Child Abuse Negl.* 2004;28(5):505–524.

TABLE 7-7. Specificity of Skeletal Trauma for Abuse

High Specificity

- Classic metaphyseal lesions
- Posterior rib fracture
- Scapular fracture
- Spinous process fracture
- Sternal fracture

Moderate Specificity

- Multiple fractures, especially bilateral
- Fractures in various stages of healing
- Epiphyseal separation
- Vertebral body fracture or subluxation
- Digital fracture
- Complex skull fracture

Low Specificity

- Clavicular fracture
- Long bone shaft fracture
- Linear skull fracture

Adapted from O'Connor JF, Cohen J. Dating fractures. In: Kleinman PK, ed. *Diagnostic Imaging of Child Abuse*. Williams & Wilkins; 1987:6. Permission courtesy of Cambridge University Press. Copyright © 2004 Elsevier Ltd. With permission.

TABLE 7-8. Pearls and Pitfalls of Nonaccidental Trauma

- Be particularly cautious of a young infant with an injury.
- It is unusual for a young child to sustain a life-threatening injury from a fall alone, and they are highly unlikely to die from a short-height fall.
- Ask to describe in detail the mechanism of the injury and make sure that it is consistent with the observed injury. However, a parent may not have witnessed the injury or was distracted while it was occurring.
- Multiple rib fractures, fractures in various stages of healing, and classic metaphyseal fractures are highly specific.
- Injury mechanism stated by the parents should agree with the type and energy of the fracture.
- Failure to diagnose child abuse may result in 25% risk of repeat abuse and 5% chance of death.
- Concerning bruises and skin lesions are the most common presentation of abuse. However, the child with such bruises should receive a proper evaluation for bleeding disorder.
- Unexplained fractures are much more likely to represent abuse and not a rare disease such as osteogenesis imperfecta (OI). Always consider OI when multiple fractures are seen.
- Obtain skeletal survey in all children younger than 2 years old, and individualize for 2–5 year old when child abuse is suspected. Repeat in 2 weeks.
- Involve the hospital child protective team early in the evaluation.
- Prepare records as though everything will be reviewed and read in court.

He emphasized that both moderate- and low-specificity radiographic findings become more specific when there is an inadequate or inconsistent explanation for the injury. The location and the type of fracture can aid in distinguishing between an accident and child abuse but is only one piece of information.

All types of fractures have been reported in the child abuse literature, and it is often the presence of multiple fractures that indicates NAT (Fig. 7-40). King et al.[108] reported 429 fractures in 189 abused children. Fifty percent of these patients had a single fracture, and 17% had more than three fractures. Approximately 60% of fractures were found in roughly equal numbers in the humerus, femur, and tibia. Fractures also occurred in the radius, skull, spine, ribs, ulna, and fibula, in order of decreasing frequency. Another study found a similar incidence of fractures of the humerus, femur, and tibia in abused children, with skull fractures seen in 14%.[152] In contrast, Akbarnia et al.[1] found that rib fractures in abused patients were twice as prevalent as fractures of any one long bone; the next most frequently fractured bone was the humerus, followed by the femur and the tibia. Nearly a third of these patients had skull fractures. In a classic study of 31 postmortem infants, the fracture pattern was very different from clinical studies in living children, with metaphyseal and rib fractures being the most common.[116]

The Skeletal Survey

In addition to standard radiographic studies of the acute injury, a complete skeletal survey should be used to screen for additional

Figure 7-40. Multiple fractures in a 3-month-old female victim of inflicted injury. **A:** Frontal radiograph of the humerus shows proximal metaphyseal irregularity consistent with a corner fracture (*arrow*) and an oblique diaphyseal fracture with extensive periosteal reaction and healing (*arrowhead*). **B:** Axial CT image reveals a depressed left calvarial fracture (*arrow*). **C:** Lateral thoracolumbar radiograph suggests a T12 compression fracture (*arrow*), which is confirmed on nuclear bone scintigraphy (**D**) as a region of increased uptake (*arrow*). Bone scan also confirms left parietal (*arrowhead*) and humeral (*curved arrow*) fractures.

fractures in all children younger than age 2 years when abuse is suspected.[106] Use of the skeletal survey in children suspected of abuse yielded positive findings in 10.8% of cases, most commonly in children with AHT, a life-threatening event, and in infants under 6 months of age in which the physical examination is less reliable.[65] Besides the index child, children under the age of 2 years in the same household of the injured, abused child have an 11.9% risk of a positive skeletal survey, so it is also recommended that they undergo a skeletal survey.[132] A suspected metaphyseal lesion of the extremity is more likely to be detected when a lateral view is done in addition to the AP view.[102] Lateral views coned to the joints may help in diagnosing classic metaphyseal lesions (CMLs). Lateral views of the entire spine must always be included in the skeletal survey. Bilateral oblique views of the thorax are important for the diagnosis of subtle rib fractures.[106] A "baby gram" has no place in diagnosing fractures of child abuse because the obliquity of the angle at which the radiographs traverse the skeleton may obscure many subtle fractures.

The standard views obtained on a skeletal survey recommended by the American College of Radiology for imaging suspected child abuse in children less than 2 years of age with a low effective radiation dose of only 0.2 mSv[25,179] are listed in Table 7-9. Follow-up skeletal survey at 2 weeks increases the diagnostic yield when occult fractures are present, because some fractures, especially of the ribs, may not be seen until a callus appears at 10 to 14 days. The second look skeletal survey better defines the fracture seen on the original survey and may help determine the age of the fracture.[106] Kleinman et al.[117] reported that a follow-up skeletal survey 2 weeks after the initial series detected 27% more fractures and provided assistance in dating 20% of previously detected fractures. Fractures or questionable fractures diagnosed on the initial screening skeletal survey should be reimaged on the follow-up survey. Almost 10% of children who sustained suspected abuse have a normal initial skeletal survey but have significant findings on the 2-week follow-up survey.[23,84] The sensitivity of skeletal surveys diminishes in patients older than

TABLE 7-9. Complete Skeletal Survey Table

Appendicular Skeleton
- Humeri (AP)
- Forearms (AP)
- Hands (PA)
- Femurs (AP)
- Lower legs (AP)
- Feet (AP)

Axial Skeleton
- Thorax (AP, lateral, right and left obliques), to include ribs, thoracic and upper lumbar spine
- Pelvis (AP), to include the midlumbar spine
- Lumbosacral spine (lateral)
- Cervical spine (lateral)
- Skull (frontal and lateral)

Adapted with permission from Clinical practice guideline: diagnosis and evaluation of the child with attention-deficit/hyperactivity disorder. American Academy of Pediatrics. *Pediatrics.* 105(6):1345–1348, Copyright © 2000 by the AAP.

2 years of age. They have less value for children older than age 5 years because the older child can describe where the pain is located. For children between the ages of 2 and 5 years, the test should be individualized.

Dating Fractures

Radiographic proof of unexplained fractures in various stages of healing is believed to be strong evidence of child abuse (Fig. 7-41).[1] The orthopaedist often is asked to determine the age of fractures with some certainty to corroborate a history of injury given by caretakers. Experienced orthopaedists and radiologists can roughly estimate the age range of fractures by their radiographic appearance and their experience reading

Figure 7-41. Rib fractures in multiple stages of healing in a 4-month-old female victim of nonaccidental injury. Frontal chest radiograph reveals acute (no periosteal reaction or healing) and subacute/healing (positive periosteal reaction) rib fractures (*arrows*).

many radiographs of known dated injuries. There is limited evidence-based data for accurately predicting the age of healing fractures.[162] In a review of studies that met minimal evidence-based inclusion criteria, the following conclusions were reached: The science of fracture dating is inexact and periosteal reaction is seen as early as 4 days and is present in at least 50% of cases by 2 weeks with remodeling peaking at 8 weeks after the fracture. The most difficult fractures to date are those that are completely healed, with substantial remodeling, and often the only sign of a healed fracture is a thickened cortex.

Extremity Fractures

There is no predominant pattern of diaphyseal fracture in child abuse. Traditionally, a midshaft spiral fracture such as in the femur was believed to be caused by a violent abusive twisting injury. However, this is not typically the case, and it has been found that 71% of diaphyseal fractures were transverse in abused children, indicating a different plausible mechanism.[75] Transverse fractures are most commonly associated with either a violent bending force or a direct blow to the extremities, whereas spiral or oblique fractures of the long bones are caused by axial-loaded, twisting injuries, such as in a fall. Humeral shaft fractures in children under 3 years of age have an 18% risk of being due to probable abuse.[174] In delayed medical care, long bone fractures may show exuberant callus because of lack of immobilization, and multiple fractures may be present at different stages of healing.

Femur fractures in infants are especially suspicious for NAT; whereas children old enough to run can fall and accidentally fracture their femurs if there is a significant twisting motion at the time of injury.[191] Despite a high likelihood of NAT in an infant with a femoral fracture, accidental trauma may still be a plausible cause if the parent's reported mechanism is consistent with the injury. In a recent case series from Alberta, Canada, only 17% of femoral fractures in infants less than 1 year of age were from abuse, whereas the author's review of eight previous reports showed that NAT was the cause in 42% to 93% of cases.[92] As children get older and more active, a femur fracture is more likely to be from accidental injury than from abuse. Schwend et al.[170] reported that femoral fractures were related to NAT in 42% of nonambulatory infants and only 2.6% of ambulatory toddlers. Blakemore et al.[28] noted that only 2% of femoral fractures in patients aged 1 to 5 years were caused by abuse. Risk factors for abuse were age younger than 12 months, the child not yet walking, a questionable mechanism, and other associated injuries.

Humeral shaft fractures are frequently seen in NAT. Fractures in unusual locations such as the distal clavicle, scapula, acromial tip, proximal humeral metaphysis, or distal humeral physis may result from violent blows or upper extremity traction injury and are suggestive of abuse in young children. Infants may normally have a separate ossification center adjacent to the tip of the acromion, simulating a fracture, but a true fracture has sharp, demarcated edges, may be positive on bone scan, and will show callus or healing.

Fractures of the hands and feet are commonly due to accidental trauma in older children but are suggestive of abuse in

Figure 7-42. Humeral fracture in a 3-week-old boy after a difficult delivery. Radiograph shows a transverse middiaphyseal fracture with extensive callus (*arrow*).

infants. Nimkin et al.[150] reviewed 11 hand and foot fractures in abused children younger than 10 months of age and found mostly torus fractures either of the metacarpals or the proximal phalanges of the hand and similar fractures of the first metatarsals of the feet (Fig. 7-42). These injuries are best seen on the oblique views, which are standard in the skeletal survey.

Metaphyseal and epiphyseal fractures of the long bones are classically associated with child abuse.[36,176] In infants and toddlers, these fractures can occur when the child is violently shaken by the extremities with traction or rotation of the extremity (see Fig. 7-43). Buckle fractures may occur at multiple sites, seldom producing exuberant callus. Repeated injury may cause irregular metaphyseal deformities. Periosteal avulsion typically produces new bone formation within 2 to 3 weeks of injury and may be confused with osteomyelitis. New bone formation may be delayed, particularly in children with malnutrition or rickets.

The almost pathognomonic fracture of child abuse is the CML commonly termed the "corner" or "bucket-handle fracture."

These fractures are almost exclusively seen in NAT but are not the most common fractures in abused children. The incidence of CML in large series ranges from 15% to 32%.[75,108] Radiographs show a corner fracture at the edge of the ossified portion of the zone of provisional calcification, *which is the metaphyseal side of the physis as opposed to the epiphyseal side.* If a significant portion of the metaphyseal rim is involved, a bucket-handle fracture pattern is produced. Based on their histopathologic autopsy study of metaphyseal fractures in abused infants, Kleinman et al.[114,115] found that bucket-handle or corner fractures are actually a full-thickness metaphyseal fracture extending through the primary spongiosa of bone just above the zone of provisional calcification (Fig. 7-44). Centrally, the amount of metaphysis remaining attached to the physis was thin, but peripherally the fracture line curved away from the physis so that a substantial metaphyseal rim remained attached to the physis (Fig. 7-45). On radiographic study, this metaphyseal rim formed the basis for both corner and bucket-handle fractures. In healing fractures, biopsy specimens showed metaphyseal extension of hypertrophied chondrocytes. Metaphyseal corner fractures are most likely caused by either violent shaking or traction injuries to the extremity. Even one CML noted on a skeletal survey is highly suspicious and specific for child abuse.[118,189] Subepiphyseal–metaphyseal lucency can also be caused by systematic diseases such as rickets and leukemia, but there is evidence that CML is caused by rickets.[157,158] Lesions resembling corner fractures of the distal radius, ulna, tibia, and proximal humerus also have

Figure 7-43. Metatarsal fractures in a 2-month-old female victim of nonaccidental trauma. Radiographic image from a skeletal survey shows multiple healing, bilateral, and symmetric proximal and distal metatarsal fractures (*arrows*).

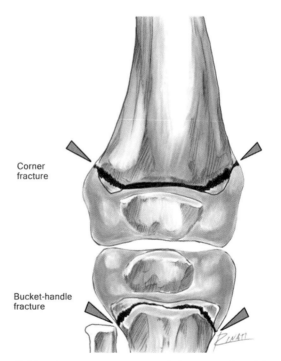

Figure 7-44. Schematic representation of classic metaphyseal lesions (CMLs). Illustration demonstrates the path of the CML. Depending on the angle at which the CML is viewed from, it may appear to extend across the width of the ossified physis (tibia illustrating a bucket-handle fracture) or only the margins of the physis (femur, illustrating a corner fracture). (Artwork courtesy of Gholamreza Zinati, MD.)

A   **B**

Figure 7-45. Classic metaphyseal fracture in a 2.5-month-old male victim of nonaccidental injury. **A:** Frontal radiograph of the tibia and fibula demonstrates transmetaphyseal lucencies or bucket-handle fractures (*arrows*). **B:** A lateral ankle radiograph reveals lucency at the tibial and fibular metaphyseal margins indicating corner fractures (*arrows*).

Figure 7-46. Schematic representation of rib fracture mechanism. Anterior chest compression causes the posterior ribs to be levered over the transverse processes of the vertebra (*arrows*) causing posterior and lateral rib fractures (*arrowheads*). (Artwork courtesy of Samir Abedin, MD.)

been reported with one variant of spondylometaphyseal dysplasia.[55] Because fracture callus does not reliably occur, dating the CML lesion is unreliable. The presence of callus suggests that the fracture is probably greater than 10 to 14 days.

Rib Fractures

Rib fractures are uncommon in childhood accidents, especially when located posteriorly and associated with other long bone fractures. Although no single fracture is specific for abuse, rib fractures are highly suggestive of abuse if there is no plausible trauma or medical explanation.[106] Abusive rib fractures may be caused by squeezing of the chest by a caretaker,[36] hitting the child from behind, or stepping on the chest.[117,180] Kleinman et al. postulated that severe shaking of an infant can cause front-to-back chest compression, which levers the posterior rib over the transverse process of the vertebral body, causing fractures of the posterior rib shaft at the transverse process and of the rib head adjacent to the vertebra (Fig. 7-46). One series showed that fractures of the first rib in children were seen only in abuse.[117] Barsness et al.[17] reported that rib fractures had a positive predictive value of NAT of 95% in children younger than 3 years of age. In this study, rib fractures were the only skeletal manifestation of NAT in 29% of the children. Posterior rib fractures are difficult to diagnose acutely because they lack callus and are rarely displaced. Even with healing, the callus on radiography may be obscured by the overlying transverse process.[113] Oblique views of the chest are included in skeletal surveys because they better show these fractures. Posterior rib fractures are the most common location in child abuse, but fractures may occur anywhere along the arc of the rib, including disruption of the anterior costochondral junction (Fig. 7-47). Posterior rib fractures tend to occur between T4 and T9. Rib fractures may be discovered in abused infants who have undergone resuscitation for cardiac arrest; in which case, there may be confusion about the

etiology of the fractures. Older fractures of the ribs in NAT may form lytic, expansile lesions.

In infant fatalities of suspicious origin, postmortem high-detailed preautopsy skeletal surveys and specimen radiographs are helpful in fully evaluating and diagnosing child abuse.[111] In a postmortem study of 31 infants who died of inflicted skeletal injury,[116] there were a total of 165 fractures (51% rib fractures, 39% metaphyseal long bone fractures, 5% long bone shaft fractures, 4% fractures of the hands and feet, 1% clavicular fractures, and less than 1% spinal fractures). Postmortem thoracic CT is more sensitive than radiography for pediatric anterior and posterior rib fractures.[90] If an abdominal CT is being performed for evaluation of NAT, inclusion of the chest may yield additional information about rib fractures, but with additional radiation of approximately 3 mSv.

Spinal Fractures

Spinal fractures in abused children are infrequent but important to recognize. Based on autopsy findings, spinal fractures of fatally abused children generally involve 25% or less compression of the vertebrae.[112] In a report of 103 children with cervical spine injury, only 3 patients had injury because of abuse and all had spinal cord injury without radiographic abnormality (SCIWORA).[33] Hangman-type fractures of the posterior elements have been described in infants as a result of child abuse.[119] CT is helpful in evaluating pediatric cervical spine trauma. Vertebral compression fractures can occur when a child's buttocks are forcibly slammed onto a flat surface with hyperflexion of the spine.[2] Carrion et al.[40] reported circumferential physeal fractures of the thoracolumbar spine associated with child abuse that required open reduction. Thoracolumbar fracture dislocations may occur in abused children with or without neurologic injury.[175] Flexion–distraction Chance fractures and synchondroses injuries (Fig. 7-48) may also be seen in NAT. Although neurologic injury in spinal fractures resulting

Figure 7-47. Rib fractures in a 9-month-old male victim of nonaccidental trauma. **A:** Chest radiograph reveals left lateral sixth and seventh rib fractures (*arrows*). **B:** Nuclear medicine bone scan confirms foci of increased uptake within the left lateral ribs as well as revealing additional hot foci in multiple right posterior lateral ribs.

from child abuse is uncommon, any patient with abusive spinal injury should undergo thorough neurologic examination. As previously discussed, the skeletal survey must include a lateral view of the cervical, thoracic, and lumbar spine. For children younger than 36 months, the cervical spine injury incidence is as high as 15%, so children suspected of AHT should also have

cervical spine imaging.[12] Because of the potentially serious consequences of a spinal injury in an infant or young child, clinical or radiographic suggestion of a spinal injury should be further evaluated with MRI. If a patient has evidence of AHT to require MRI, it should include the entire spine.[107]

Laboratory Studies

An abused child should have a complete blood cell count with erythrocyte sedimentation rate, liver function studies, and urinalysis. When abdominal trauma is suspected, liver and pancreatic enzymes and a urinalysis should be obtained; if abnormal, a CT of the abdomen and pelvis with intravenous contrast should be ordered.[48] Clotting studies, including prothrombin time and activated partial thromboplastin time, thrombin time, fibrinogen, factor VIII, factor IX, and von Willebrand factor antigen and activity should be performed in patients with bleeding or ecchymosis to evaluate for bleeding diathesis. If bruising is the only finding of possible abuse, consultation with a hematologist may be necessary to fully evaluate for an unusual bleeding disorder.[190] Infants born prematurely are at risk for rickets and low bone density. Therefore, evaluation of calcium, phosphorous, alkaline phosphatase, and 25-OH vitamin D may be useful in such infants, particularly in the setting of a fracture.

If there is suspicion of substance abuse by any family member, and the child has symptoms, a toxicology screen should also be performed on the patient.[75]

Figure 7-48. Lumbar spine fracture in a 16-month-old male victim of nonaccidental trauma. **A:** Lateral lumbar radiograph shows lucency through the L3 synchondrosis (*arrow*) with anterolisthesis of L3 body on L4. **B:** Sagittal T2-weighted MRI reveals hyperintense signal within the bone marrow of the fractured L3. Slight compression fractures of T10 and T11 are also noted (*arrows*).

THE DIFFERENTIAL DIAGNOSIS

The most important consultation to request for a child with suspected inflicted injury is the child protective services team. In many major pediatric centers, a child abuse pediatrician, who has received specialty training in this field, is the leader of the team. Any suspected abuse should initiate a minimum evaluation that includes an appropriate radiographic evaluation with a skeletal survey in the younger child and consultation by a child abuse specialist. Any significant nonorthopaedic injury should prompt consultation by the appropriate subspecialty: neurosurgery, general surgery, plastic surgery, ophthalmology, or urology.

Although it is extremely important not to miss the diagnosis of child abuse, it is equally important to maintain an objective, critical view and not to make the diagnosis in error.[97] Overdiagnosing child abuse can be harmful to the family, with the parents being placed at risk of losing custody of their children and also facing criminal charges. Patients or family friends may make

false statements about an abuse situation through misinterpretation, confabulation, fantasy, delusions, and other situations.[26]

Normal metaphyseal variations are seen occasionally and should not be confused with corner fractures of child abuse. These variants are seen most commonly in the proximal tibia, distal femur, proximal fibula, distal radius, and distal ulna. A bony beak may be seen medially in the proximal humerus or tibia and is usually bilateral. Cortical irregularity in the medial proximal tibia may also be seen in 4% of normal infants and young toddlers and is bilateral in 25%.

The signs of child abuse found on radiographs can overlap with the findings of systemic diseases such as Caffey disease (infantile cortical hyperostosis), osteomyelitis, septic arthritis, insufficiency fracture, hypophosphatasia (Fig. 7-49), leukemia,

Figure 7-49. Hypophosphatasia in a 2-month-old female with multiple fractures. **A:** Chest radiograph shows severe osteopenia and multiple bilateral healing rib fractures. **B:** Lateral spine radiograph reveals multiple compressed vertebra. **C:** Lower extremity radiographs demonstrate multiple, bilateral healing femoral and lower leg fractures.

metastatic neuroblastoma, OI, scurvy, vitamin D deficient and drug-induced rickets, congenital insensitivity to pain, osteopetrosis, kinky hair syndrome, prostaglandin therapy, osteoid osteoma, and other benign bone tumors. Children with biliary atresia may present with osteopenia and fractures without history of significant injury, which should not be mistaken for child abuse.[58] There has been an increase in the incidence of syphilis in females of childbearing age, and, although extremely rare, congenital syphilis can mimic fractures of child abuse with diaphysitis, metaphysitis, and multiple pathologic fractures in different stages of healing.[130] Physiologic periostitis, in contrast to lesions from child abuse, is seen in young infants of about 6 months of age, is usually bilateral, symmetric, diaphyseal, located on the long bones—humerus, femur, and tibia—and has no periostitis of the metaphysis.[53] Insufficiency rib fractures may be seen in rickets of prematurity as well as rickets of low birth weight. The presence of metabolic disease and pathologic fractures does not exclude the possibility of child abuse.

Several diseases are commonly brought up in custodial hearings as alternative possibilities to NAT injuries, and these diseases should be objectively considered in the differential diagnosis. Leukemia should always be considered in a child with diffuse osteopenia or metaphyseal lucency. McClain et al.[138] reported a 2-year-old child who died of undiagnosed acute lymphoblastic leukemia, having been earlier reported as a possible victim of child abuse. Clinical signs of leukemia, including fever, pallor, petechia, purpura, adenopathy, hepatosplenomegaly, and bone pain, should be sought in children with bruising of unknown origin. Factor XIII deficiency may cause unexplained bleeding from minor trauma and be mistaken for child abuse because the standard coagulation profile may be negative and factor-specific tests may be negative if performed posttransfusion.[147]

Undiagnosed OI should always be considered when a child presents with multiple fractures of unknown etiology but maybe a difficult diagnosis to make. Before the diagnosis of OI is made, the parents may be presumed to be the cause of the fractures, with temporary removal of the child in 70% of cases.[178] Thoughtful review of the medical history and clinical evaluation identify most children with OI, without the need for genetic testing, which has low yield when there are no clinical findings.[200] However, when the diagnosis of OI is suspected, but cannot be made on classic clinical grounds, the diagnosis may be made by biochemical assay.[156] Genetic testing of individuals with typical features of OI typically have disease-causing mutations in 98%.[16] OI was further discussed earlier in this chapter, a more complete review of this topic is beyond the scope of this chapter.

POST–EMERGENCY DEPARTMENT TREATMENT AND LEGAL REPORTING REQUIREMENTS

Once NAT is recognized, the first step in treatment is hospital admission.[146] This is therapeutic in that it places the child in a safe, protected environment, provides the opportunity for additional diagnostic workup, and, more importantly, investigation of the family's social situation by appropriate personnel.

In tertiary centers, multidisciplinary teams are available to evaluate and treat such children, but in other circumstances, the orthopaedist may be primarily responsible for coordinating both evaluation and treatment. Mandatory reporting functions as a screening test for suspected abuse. False positives are much preferred to a false negative, which could be fatal. Court custody may be required for children of uncooperative families who refuse admission, and hospitalization should be continued until a full investigation is completed by the appropriate child protective services and a safe disposition is established. In the United States, the physician is required by law to report all suspected abuse to appropriate child protective services or legal authorities. Although physicians have better reporting rates than most other professionals, 27% of injuries considered likely to be caused by abuse, and 76% of injuries that were considered possibly related to child abuse were not reported.[72] When the reporting is done in good faith, the physician has immunity against criminal or civil liability for these actions. The granting of absolute immunity, even for physicians, is not encouraged by the American legal system because, in theory, it would protect individuals who make false reports of child abuse to harass families and would deprive the injured parties of their legal right to seek damages for harmful actions. In contrast, physician immunity based on good faith reporting of suspected child abuse is contingent on the physician having a reasonable belief that abuse or neglect has occurred. Since the stakes for failure to report suspected child abuse are so high, physicians should always report suspicions of abuse.

THE ORTHOPAEDIC SURGEON'S LEGAL ROLE IN NONACCIDENTAL INJURY

The orthopaedist may fill a dual role in the courtroom in child abuse proceedings. First, the physician serves as a material witness whose testimony is confined to their personal involvement in the legal matter of the child's evaluation and treatment. The testimony may include clarification to the court of information contained in the medical record. As a material witness, the physician cannot render opinions about the facts as stated during their testimony. However, the physician may also be requested to be an expert witness.[145,155] An expert witness is an individual considered by the court to have special knowledge and experience that qualifies them to render opinions about certain facts presented in the courtroom. The limits of the physician's expertise usually are defined by the attorneys in court before the testimony of the expert witness.

Physicians may be reluctant to testify in court for many reasons. The courtroom is an unfamiliar setting for most physicians and the adversarial nature of the American legal system may be perceived as a hostile environment. In the courtroom, opposing attorneys are likely to search for inconsistencies in the testimony or unfamiliarity with the record to discredit the physician witness, which can be very uncomfortable for the physician not used to this behavior. When a physician is asked to be an expert witness or a material witness, consultation with the child's attorney is essential. Principles of testimony include a meticulous preparation of the case, an understanding of what to expect in a deposition, and thorough instruction by the attorney about what to expect in court. The key to deposition or court testimony is to understand and honestly answer the defense attorney's questions as succinctly as possible. Testimony should be objective, honest, and thorough. In child abuse cases, in particular, the testimony will lead to the fact that the abuse has occurred and that it has been appropriately diagnosed. In addition, the physician expert witness may be asked to give an opinion of the risk for subsequent abuse if the child returns to the home where the alleged abuse occurred. Questions regarding medical findings often will be prefaced in the courtroom by the words "reasonable medical certainty," a term that is poorly understood by most physicians. Chadwick[42] offered a definition of reasonable medical certainty as "certain as a physician should be in order to recommend and carry out treatment for a given medical condition."

During testimony, the orthopaedist's words should be carefully chosen and understandable by a lay jury. Attorneys may frame questions in ways that are difficult to understand, and the orthopaedist should not hesitate to ask the attorney to clarify a question.[42] Language should be straightforward, and visual aids may be used in providing clear testimony. The expert witness should use testimony as an educational process for the court, in which the common experience and knowledge of the jury is used to build understanding with common sense explanations of medical findings.[42] The material witness should provide answers that are brief, without volunteering extra information. The child's attorney should prepare the orthopaedic surgeon for the rigors of cross-examination by the defense attorneys, which often works to question the physician's credibility. A strategy of aggressive cross-examination is to provoke the physician into arguments or unprofessional behavior that could discredit their testimony before the court. The physician witnesses are always expected to respond professionally, even under extreme duress.[56] Brent[32] assembled an excellent series of vignettes of expert medical witness case studies in court and provided detailed instructions with regard to the responsibilities of such experts.

Annotated References

Reference	Annotation
Belthur MV, Birchansky SB, Verdugo AA, et al. Pathologic fractures in children with acute *Staphylococcus aureus* osteomyelitis. *J Bone Joint Surg Am.* 2012;94(1):34–42.	The authors report on 17 children with acute osteomyelitis who developed pathologic fracture. MRI studies at the time of admission demonstrated a significantly greater prevalence and size of subperiosteal abscess in the pathologic fracture group.
Christian CW; Committee on Child Abuse and Neglect, American Academy of Pediatrics. The evaluation of suspected child physical abuse. *Pediatrics.* 2015;135(5):e1337–e1354.	Comprehensive article describing the role of the physician in suspecting, reporting, and evaluating physical abuse.
Deng ZP, Ding Y, Puri A, et al. The surgical treatment and outcome of nonmetastatic extremity osteosarcoma with pathological fractures. *Chin Med J (Engl).* 2015;128(19):2605–2608.	In this retrospective review of a large Asian database, the authors demonstrate that patients with osteosarcoma and associated pathologic fracture can safely be treated with limb salvage, achieving comparable results to nonfracture group.
James KA, Cunniff C, Apkon SD, et al. Risk factors for first fractures among males with Duchenne or Becker muscular dystrophy. *J Pediatr Orthop.* 2015;35(6):640–644.	Retrospective review of 747 children with muscular dystrophy aiming to identify risk factors for first fracture. Incidence of fractures was 33% and full-time wheelchair use increased the risk of first fracture by 75%; corticosteroid use, bisphosphonate use, and calcium/vitamin D use did not significantly affect incidence of fractures.
Kocher MS, Kasser JR. Orthopaedic aspects of child abuse. *J Am Acad Orthop Surg.* 2000;8:10–20.	A concise review of the orthopaedic detection of child abuse.
Laposata ME, Laposata M. Children with signs of abuse: when is it not child abuse? *Am J Clin Pathol.* 2005;123(Suppl 1):S119–S124.	Illustrates the need to keep an open mind regarding other diagnoses and the mimics of child abuse.
Leong NL, Anderson ME, Gebhardt MC, Snyder BD. Computed tomography-based structural analysis for predicting fracture risk in children with benign skeletal neoplasms: comparison of specificity with that of plain radiographs. *J Bone Joint Surg Am.* 2010;92(9):1827–1833.	The authors report on the use of quantitative computed tomography-based rigidity analysis for predicting the risk of fractures through UBCs.
Lindberg DM, Shapiro RA, Laskey AL, et al; ExSTRA Investigators. Prevalence of abusive injuries in siblings and household contacts of physically abused children. *Pediatrics.* 2012;130(2):193–201.	Recommendation to obtain a skeletal survey in siblings and other contacts under age 2 years when a child is found to be abused.
Pierce MC, Bertocci GE, Vogeley E, Moreland MS. Evaluating long bone fractures in children: a biomechanical approach with illustrative cases. *Child Abuse Negl.* 2004;28(5):505–524.	Highly recommended for the orthopaedic surgeon to develop a clearer understanding of underlying biomechanical plausible injury mechanisms.

Annotated References

Reference	Annotation
Ranade SC, Allen AK, Deutsch SA. The role of the orthopaedic surgeon in the identification and management of nonaccidental trauma. *J Am Acad Orthop Surg.* 2020;28:53–65.	Summary of the role of the orthopaedic surgeon in child maltreatment.
Sees JP, Sitoula P, Dabney K, et al. Pamidronate treatment to prevent reoccurring fractures in children with cerebral palsy. *J Pediatr Orthop.* 2016;36(2):193–197.	This is a retrospective review of children with cerebral palsy GMFCS 3, 4, and 5 who underwent pamidronate treatment aiming to reduce the incidence of fractures. The posttreatment group showed 0.10 fracture/yr rate, compared to 2.4 fractures/yr in the pretreatment group.
Sheets LK, Leach ME, Koszewski IJ, et al. Sentinel injuries in infants evaluated for child physical abuse. *Pediatrics.* 2013;131(4):701–707.	27.5% of abused infants were noted to have a previous sentinel injury.
Sugar NF, Taylor JA, Feldman KW. Bruises in infants and toddlers: those who don't cruise rarely bruise. Puget Sound Pediatric Research Network. *Arch Pediatr Adolesc Med.* 1999;153(4):399–403.	Bruising in infants under 9 months of age or atypical bruises in toddlers (trunk, hands, buttocks) are unusual and causes for concern.

REFERENCES

1. Akbarnia B, Torg JS, Kirkpatrick J, Sussman S. Manifestations of the battered-child syndrome. *J Bone Joint Surg Am.* 1974;56(6):1159–1166.
2. Akbarnia BA. Pediatric spine fractures. *Orthop Clin North Am.* 1999;30(3):521–536.
3. Aliatakis N, Schneider J, Spors B, et al. Age-specific occurrence of pathological fractures in patients with spina bifida. *Eur J Pediatr.* 2020;179(5):773–779.
4. Allergic reactions to latex containing medical devices: FDA Medical Alert. DHHS (NIOSH). 1997;97–135.
5. Alos N, Grant RM, Ramsay T, et al. High incidence of vertebral fractures in children with acute lymphoblastic leukemia 12 months after the initiation of therapy. *J Clin Oncol.* 2012;30(22):2760–2767.
6. Altai Z, Viceconti M, Li X, Offiah AC. Investigating rolling as mechanism for humeral fractures in non-ambulant infants: a preliminary finite element study. *Clin Radiol.* 2020;75:78.e9–78.e16.
7. Anderst JD. Assessment of factors resulting in abuse evaluations in young children with minor head trauma. *Child Abuse Negl.* 2008;32(3):405–413.
8. Arkader A, Woon RP, Gilsanz V. Can subclinical rickets cause SCFE? A prospective, pilot study. *J Pediatr Orthop.* 2015;35(7):e72–e75.
9. Armstrong DG, Newfield JT, Gillespie R. Orthopedic management of osteopetrosis: results of a survey and review of the literature. *J Pediatr Orthop.* 1999;19(1):122–132.
10. Aycan OE, Çamurcu IY, Özer D, et al. Unusual localizations of unicameral bone cysts and aneurysmal bone cysts: a retrospective review of 451 cases. *Acta Orthop Belg.* 2015;81(2):209–212.
11. Bacchetta J, Wesseling-Perry K, Gilsanz V, et al. Idiopathic juvenile osteoporosis: a cross-sectional single-centre experience with bone histomorphometry and quantitative computed tomography. *Pediatr Rheumatol Online J.* 2013;11:6.
12. Baerg J, Thirumoorthi A, Vannix R, et al. Cervical spine imaging for young children with inflicted trauma: expanding the injury pattern. *J Pediatr Surg.* 2017;52(5):816–821.
13. Baghdadi S, Arkader A. Fibrous dysplasia: recent developments and modern management alternatives: current concept review. *J Pediatr Orthop Soc North Am.* 2020;2(2).
14. Baghdadi S, Nguyen JC, Arkader A. Nonossifying fibroma of the distal tibia: predictors of fracture and management algorithm. *J Pediatr Orthop.* 2021;41:e671–e679.
15. Barbanti-Brodano G, Girolami M, Ghermandi R, et al. Aneurysmal bone cyst of the spine treated by concentrated bone marrow: clinical cases and review of the literature. *Eur Spine J.* 2017;26(Suppl 1):158–166.
16. Bardai G, Moffatt P, Glorieux FH, Rauch F. DNA sequence analysis in 598 individuals with a clinical diagnosis of osteogenesis imperfecta: diagnostic yield and mutation spectrum. *Osteoporos Int.* 2016;27(12):3607–3613.
17. Barsness KA, Cha ES, Bensard DD, et al. The positive predictive value of rib fractures as an indicator of nonaccidental trauma in children. *J Trauma.* 2003;54(6):1107–1110.
18. Basarir K, Pişkin A, Güçlü B, et al. Aneurysmal bone cyst recurrence in children: a review of 56 patients. *J Pediatr Orthop.* 2007;27(8):938–943.
19. Batista DL, Riar J, Keil M, Stratakis CA. Diagnostic tests for children who are referred for the investigation of Cushing syndrome. *Pediatrics.* 2007;120(3):e575–e586.
20. Beals RK, Tufts E. Fractured femur in infancy: the role of child abuse. *J Pediatr Orthop.* 1983;3(5):583–586.
21. Bell JM, Shields MD, Watters J, et al. Interventions to prevent and treat corticosteroid-induced osteoporosis and prevent osteoporotic fractures in Duchenne muscular dystrophy. *Cochrane Database Syst Rev.* 2017;1:CD010899.
22. Belthur MV, Birchansky SB, Verdugo AA, et al. Pathologic fractures in children with acute Staphylococcus aureus osteomyelitis. *J Bone Joint Surg Am.* 2012;94(1):34–42.
23. Bennett BL, Chua MS, Care M, et al. Retrospective review to determine the utility of follow-up skeletal surveys in child abuse evaluations when the initial skeletal survey is normal. *BMC Res Notes.* 2011;4:354.
24. Bennett OM, Namnyak SS. Bone and joint manifestations of sickle cell anaemia. *J Bone Joint Surg Br.* 1990;72(3):494–499.
25. Berger RP, Panigrahy A, Gottschalk S, Sheetz M. Effective radiation dose in a skeletal survey performed for suspected child abuse. *J Pediatr.* 2016;171:310–312.
26. Bernet W. False statements and the differential diagnosis of abuse allegations. *J Am Acad Child Adolesc Psychiatry.* 1993;32(5):903–910.
27. Biggin A, Munns CF. Long-term bisphosphonate therapy in osteogenesis imperfecta. *Curr Osteoporos Rep.* 2017;15(5):412–418.
28. Blakemore LC, Loder RT, Hensinger RN. Role of intentional abuse in children 1 to 5 years old with isolated femoral shaft fractures. *J Pediatr Orthop.* 1996;16(5):585–588.
29. Bohrer SP. Acute long bone diaphyseal infarcts in sickle cell disease. *Br J Radiol.* 1970;43(514):685–697.
30. Bonkowsky JL, Guenther E, Filloux FM, Srivastava R. Death, child abuse, and adverse neurological outcome of infants after an apparent life-threatening event. *Pediatrics.* 2008;122(1):125–131.
31. Boriani S, De Iure F, Campanacci L, et al. Aneurysmal bone cyst of the mobile spine: report on 41 cases. *Spine (Phila Pa 1976).* 2001;26(1):27–35.
32. Brent RL. The irresponsible expert witness: a failure of biomedical graduate education and professional accountability. *Pediatrics.* 1982;70(5):754–762.
33. Brown RL, Brunn MA, Garcia VF. Cervical spine injuries in children: a review of 103 patients treated consecutively at a level 1 pediatric trauma center. *J Pediatr Surg.* 2001;36(8):1107–1114.
34. Buison AM, Kawchak DA, Schall JI, et al. Bone area and bone mineral content deficits in children with sickle cell disease. *Pediatrics.* 2005;116(4):943–949.
35. Burke NG, Cassar-Gheiti AJ, Tan J, et al. Regenerate bone fracture rate following femoral lengthening in paediatric patients. *J Child Orthop.* 2017;11(3):210–215.
36. Caffey J. Multiple fractures in the long bones of infants suffering from chronic subdural hematoma. *Am J Roentgenol Radium Ther.* 1946;56(2):163–173.
37. Campanacci M, Capanna R, Picci P. Unicameral and aneurysmal bone cysts. *Clin Orthop Relat Res.* 1986;(204):25–36.
38. Carpenter RF. The prevalence and distribution of bruising in babies. *Arch Dis Child.* 1999;80(4):363–366.
39. Carpintero P, León F, Zafra M, et al. Fractures of osteochondroma during physical exercise. *Am J Sports Med.* 2003;31(6):1003–1006.
40. Carrion WV, Dormans JP, Drummond DS, Christofersen MR. Circumferential growth plate fracture of the thoracolumbar spine from child abuse. *J Pediatr Orthop.* 1996;16(2):210–214.
41. Caulton JM, Ward KA, Alsop CW, et al. A randomised controlled trial of standing programme on bone mineral density in non-ambulant children with cerebral palsy. *Arch Dis Child.* 2004;89(2):131–135.
42. Chadwick DL. Preparation for court testimony in child abuse cases. *Pediatr Clin North Am.* 1990;37(4):955–970.
43. Chadwick DL, Bertocci G, Castillo E, et al. Annual risk of death resulting from short falls among young children: less than 1 in 1 million. *Pediatrics.* 2008;121(6):1213–1224.
44. Chapman T, Sugar N, Done S, et al. Fractures in infants and toddlers with rickets. *Pediatr Radiol.* 2010;40(7):1184–1189.
45. Chen CJ, Chao TY, Chu DM, et al. Osteoblast and osteoclast activity in a malignant infantile osteopetrosis patient following bone marrow transplantation. *J Pediatr Hematol Oncol.* 2004;26(1):5–8.
46. Children's Bureau. *The Child Abuse Prevention and Treatment Act (CAPTA).* US Department of Health and Human Services; 2003.
47. Chlebna-Sokol D, Loba-Jakubowska E, Sikora A. Clinical evaluation of patients with idiopathic juvenile osteoporosis. *J Pediatr Orthop B.* 2001;10(3):259–263.
48. Christian CW; Committee on child abuse and neglect, American Academy of Pediatrics. The evaluation of suspected child physical abuse. *Pediatrics.* 2015; 135(5):e1337–e1354.
49. Clarke NMP, Shelton FRM, Taylor CC, et al. The incidence of fractures in children under the age of 24 months—in relation to non-accidental injury. *Injury.* 2012;43(6):762–765.

50. Coffey C, Haley K, Hayes J, Groner JI. The risk of child abuse in infants and toddlers with lower extremity injuries. *J Pediatr Surg*. 2005;40(1):120–123.

51. Cole WG. The Nicholas Andry Award—1996. The molecular pathology of osteogenesis imperfecta. *Clin Orthop Relat Res*. 1997;(343):235–248.

52. Committee on Child Abuse and Neglect, Committee on Injury, Violence, and Poison Prevention, Council on Community Pediatrics. American Academy of Pediatrics. Policy statement—child fatality review. *Pediatrics*. 2010;126(3):592–596.

53. Conway JJ, Collins M, Tanz RR, et al. The role of bone scintigraphy in detecting child abuse. *Semin Nucl Med*. 1993;23(4):321–333.

54. Cottalorda J, Kohler R, Sales de Gauzy J, et al. Epidemiology of aneurysmal bone cyst in children: a multicenter study and literature review. *J Pediatr Orthop B*. 2004;13(6):389–394.

55. Currarino G, Birch JG, Herring JA. Developmental coxa vara associated with spondylometaphyseal dysplasia (DCV/SMD): "SMD-corner fracture type" (DCV/SMD-CF) demonstrated in most reported cases. *Pediatr Radiol*. 2000;30(1):14–24.

56. Dalton HJ, Slovis T, Helfer RE, et al. Undiagnosed abuse in children younger than 3 years with femoral fracture. *Am J Dis Child*. 1990;144(8):875–878.

57. Deng ZP, Ding Y, Puri A, et al. The surgical treatment and outcome of nonmetastatic extremity osteosarcoma with pathological fractures. *Chin Med J (Engl)*. 2015;128(19):2605–2608.

58. DeRusso PA, Spevak MR, Schwarz KB. Fractures in biliary atresia misinterpreted as child abuse. *Pediatrics*. 2003;112(1 Pt 1):185–188.

59. Diamond LS, Alegado R. Perinatal fractures in arthrogryposis multiplex congenita. *J Pediatr Orthop*. 1981;1(2):189–192.

60. DiCaprio MR, Enneking WF. Fibrous dysplasia. Pathophysiology, evaluation, and treatment. *J Bone Joint Surg Am*. 2005;87(8):1848–1864.

61. Dormans JP, Sankar WN, Moroz L, Erol B. Percutaneous intramedullary decompression, curettage, and grafting with medical-grade calcium sulfate pellets for unicameral bone cysts in children: a new minimally invasive technique. *J Pediatr Orthop*. 2005;25(6):804–811.

62. Dosa NP, Eckrich M, Katz DA, et al. Incidence, prevalence, and characteristics of fractures in children, adolescents, and adults with spina bifida. *J Spinal Cord Med*. 2007;30(Suppl 1):S5–S9.

63. Drummond DS, Moreau M, Cruess RL. Post-operative neuropathic fractures in patients with myelomeningocele. *Dev Med Child Neurol*. 1981;23(2):147–150.

64. Dubowitz H, Bross DC. The pediatrician's documentation of child maltreatment. *Am J Dis Child*. 1992;146(5):596–599.

65. Duffy SO, Squires J, Fromkin JB, Berger RP. Use of skeletal surveys to evaluate for physical abuse: analysis of 703 consecutive skeletal surveys. *Pediatrics*. 2011;127(1):e47–e52.

66. Dwan K, Phillipi CA, Steiner RD, Basel D. Bisphosphonate therapy for osteogenesis imperfecta. *Cochrane Database Syst Rev*. 2016;10:CD005088.

67. Easley ME, Kneisl JS. Pathologic fractures through nonossifying fibromas: is prophylactic treatment warranted? *J Pediatr Orthop*. 1997;17(6):808–813.

68. Emori M, Tsuchie H, Teramoto A, et al. Non-ossifying fibromas and fibrous cortical defects around the knee: an epidemiologic survey in a Japanese pediatric population. *BMC Musculoskelet Disord*. 2022;23:378.

69. Fagen KE, Shalaby-Rana E, Jackson AM. Frequency of skeletal injuries in children with inflicted burns. *Pediatr Radiol*. 2015;45(3):396–401.

70. Fain O. Musculoskeletal manifestations of scurvy. *Joint Bone Spine*. 2005;72(2):124–128.

71. Ferguson PC, McLaughlin CE, Griffin AM, et al. Clinical and functional outcomes of patients with a pathologic fracture in high-grade osteosarcoma. *J Surg Oncol*. 2010;102(2):120–124.

72. Flaherty EG, Sege RD, Griffith J, et al; PROS network, NMAPedsNet. From suspicion of physical child abuse to reporting: primary care clinician decision-making. *Pediatrics*. 2008;122(3):611–619.

73. Frasier L, Alexander R, Parrish R, et al. *Abusive Head Trauma in Infants and Children: A Medical, Legal and Forensic Reference*. GW Medical Publishing; 2006.

74. Freiberg AA, Loder RT, Heidelberger KP, Hensinger RN. Aneurysmal bone cysts in young children. *J Pediatr Orthop*. 1994;14(1):86–91.

75. Galleno H, Oppenheim WL. The battered child syndrome revisited. *Clin Orthop Relat Res*. 1982;(162):11–19.

76. Gandrud LM, Cheung JC, Daniels MW, Bachrach LK. Low-dose intravenous pamidronate reduces fractures in childhood osteoporosis. *J Pediatr Endocrinol Metab*. 2003;16(6):887–892.

77. Garg S, Mehta S, Dormans JP. Modern surgical treatment of primary aneurysmal bone cyst of the spine in children and adolescents. *J Pediatr Orthop*. 2005;25(3):387–392.

78. Gaulke R, Suppelna G. Solitary enchondroma at the hand. Long-term follow-up study after operative treatment. *J Hand Surg Br*. 2004;29(1):64–66.

79. Gerritsen EJ, Vossen JM, van Loo IH, et al. Autosomal recessive osteopetrosis: variability of findings at diagnosis and during the natural course. *Pediatrics*. 1994;93(2):247–253.

80. Gibbs CP Jr, Hefele MC, Peabody TD, et al. Aneurysmal bone cyst of the extremities. Factors related to local recurrence after curettage with a high-speed burr. *J Bone Joint Surg Am*. 1999;81(12):1671–1678.

81. Glorieux FH. Experience with bisphosphonates in osteogenesis imperfecta. *Pediatrics*. 2007;119(Suppl 2):S163–S165.

82. Goldin AN, Muzykewicz DA, Mubarak SJ. Nonossifying fibromas: a computed tomography–based criteria to predict fracture risk. *J Pediatr Orthop*. 2020; 40:e149–e154.

83. Han I, Choi ES, Kim HS. Monostotic fibrous dysplasia of the proximal femur: natural history and predisposing factors for disease progression. *Bone Joint J*. 2014;96-B(5):673–676.

84. Harper NS, Eddleman S, Lindberg DM; ExSTRA Investigators. The utility of follow-up skeletal surveys in child abuse. *Pediatrics*. 2013;131(3):e672–e678.

85. Hennrikus WL, Shaw BA, Gerardi JA. Injuries when children reportedly fall from a bed or couch. *Clin Orthop Relat Res*. 2003;(407):148–151.

86. Herget GW, Mauer D, Krauß T, et al. Non-ossifying fibroma: natural history with an emphasis on a stage-related growth, fracture risk and the need for follow-up. *BMC Musculoskelet Disord*. 2016;17:147.

87. Herring JA, Peterson HA. Simple bone cyst with growth arrest. *J Pediatr Orthop*. 1987;7(2):231–235.

88. Hibbard R, Barlow J, Macmillan H; Child Abuse and Neglect, American Academy of Child and Adolescent Psychiatry, Child Maltreatment and Violence. Psychological maltreatment. *Pediatrics*. 2012;130(2):372–378.

89. Hobbs CJ, Wynne JM. The sexually abused battered child. *Arch Dis Child*. 1990;65(4):423–427.

90. Hong TS, Reyes JA, Moineddin R, et al. Value of postmortem thoracic CT over radiography in imaging of pediatric rib fractures. *Pediatr Radiol*. 2011;41(6):736–748.

91. Hood RW, Riseborough EJ. Lengthening of the lower extremity by the Wagner method: a review of the Boston Children's Hospital Experience. *J Bone Joint Surg Am*. 1981;63(7):1122–1131.

92. Hui C, Joughin E, Goldstein S, et al. Femoral fractures in children younger than three years: the role of nonaccidental injury. *J Pediatr Orthop*. 2008;28(3):297–302.

93. Hurley T, Zareen Z, Stewart P, et al. Bisphosphonate use in children with cerebral palsy. *Cochrane Database Syst Rev*. 2021;7(7):CD012756.

94. Hyden PW, Gallagher TA. Child abuse intervention in the emergency room. *Pediatr Clin North Am*. 1992;39(5):1053–1081.

95. Iobst CA, Dahl MT. Limb lengthening with submuscular plate stabilization: a case series and description of the technique. *J Pediatr Orthop*. 2007;27(5):504–509.

96. James KA, Cunniff C, Apkon SD, et al. Risk factors for first fractures among males with Duchenne or Becker muscular dystrophy. *J Pediatr Orthop*. 2015;35(6):640–644.

97. Jenny C; Committee on Child Abuse and Neglect. Evaluating infants and young children with multiple fractures. *Pediatrics*. 2006;118(3):1299–1303.

98. Jenny C; Committee on Child Abuse and Neglect, American Academy of Pediatrics. Recognizing and responding to medical neglect. *Pediatrics*. 2007;120(6):1385–1389.

99. Jenny C, Isaac R. The relation between child death and child maltreatment. *Arch Dis Child*. 2006;91(3):265–269.

100. Jonson-Reid M, Kohl PL, Drake B. Child and adult outcomes of chronic child maltreatment. *Pediatrics*. 2012;129(5):839–845.

101. Kanagawa H, Masuyama R, Morita M, et al. Methotrexate inhibits osteoclastogenesis by decreasing RANKL-induced calcium influx into osteoclast progenitors. *J Bone Miner Metab*. 2016;34(5):526–531.

102. Karmazyn B, Duhn RD, Jennings SG, et al. Long bone fracture detection in suspected child abuse: contribution of lateral views. *Pediatr Radiol*. 2012;42(4):463–469.

103. Katz K, Cohen IJ, Ziv N, et al. Fractures in children who have Gaucher disease. *J Bone Joint Surg Am*. 1987;69(9):1361–1370.

104. Katz K, Sabato S, Horev G, et al. Spinal involvement in children and adolescents with Gaucher disease. *Spine (Phila Pa 1976)*. 1993;18(3):332–335.

105. Kelley LM, Schlegel M, Hecker-Nolting S, et al. Pathological fracture and prognosis of high-grade osteosarcoma of the extremities: an analysis of 2,847 consecutive Cooperative Osteosarcoma Study Group (COSS) patients. *J Clin Oncol*. 2020;38(8):823–833.

106. Kemp AM, Butler A, Morris S, et al. Which radiological investigations should be performed to identify fractures in suspected child abuse? *Clin Radiol*. 2006;61(9):723–736.

107. Kemp AM, Joshi AH, Mann M, et al. What are the clinical and radiological characteristics of spinal injuries from physical abuse: a systematic review. *Arch Dis Child*. 2010;95(5):355–360.

108. King J, Diefendorf D, Apthorp J, et al. Analysis of 429 fractures in 189 battered children. *J Pediatr Orthop*. 1988;8(5):585–589.

109. King WM, Ruttencutter R, Nagaraja HN, et al. Orthopedic outcomes of long-term daily corticosteroid treatment in Duchenne muscular dystrophy. *Neurology*. 2007;68(19):1607–1613.

110. Kistin CJ, Tien I, Bauchner H, et al. Factors that influence the effectiveness of child protection teams. *Pediatrics*. 2010;126(1):94–100.

111. Kleinman PK, Blackbourne BD, Marks SC, et al. Radiologic contributions to the investigation and prosecution of cases of fatal infant abuse. *N Engl J Med*. 1989; 320(8):507–511.

112. Kleinman PK, Marks SC. Vertebral body fractures in child abuse. Radiologic-histopathologic correlates. *Invest Radiol*. 1992;27(9):715–722.

113. Kleinman PK, Marks SC, Adams VI, Blackbourne BD. Factors affecting visualization of posterior rib fractures in abused infants. *AJR Am J Roentgenol*. 1988;150(3):635–638.

114. Kleinman PK, Marks SC, Blackbourne B. The metaphyseal lesion in abused infants: a radiologic-histopathologic study. *AJR Am J Roentgenol*. 1986;146(5):895–905.

115. Kleinman PK, Marks SC Jr. Relationship of the subperiosteal bone collar to metaphyseal lesions in abused infants. *J Bone Joint Surg Am*. 1995;77(10):1471 1476.

116. Kleinman PK, Marks SC Jr, Richmond JM, Blackbourne BD. Inflicted skeletal injury: a postmortem radiologic-histopathologic study in 31 infants. *AJR Am J Roentgenol*. 1995;165(3):647–650.

117. Kleinman PK, Nimkin K, Spevak MR, et al. Follow-up skeletal surveys in suspected child abuse. *AJR Am J Roentgenol*. 1996;167(4):893–896.

118. Kleinman PK, Perez-Rossello JM, Newton AW, et al. Prevalence of the classic metaphyseal lesion in infants at low versus high risk for abuse. *AJR Am J Roentgenol*. 2011;197(4):1005–1008.

119. Kleinman PK, Shelton YA. Hangman's fracture in an abused infant: imaging features. *Pediatr Radiol*. 1997;27(9):776–777.

120. Kobayashi D, Satsuma S, Kamegaya M, et al. Musculoskeletal conditions of acute leukemia and malignant lymphoma in children. *J Pediatr Orthop B*. 2005;14(3):156–161.

121. Kocher MS, Dichtel L. Osteogenesis imperfecta misdiagnosed as child abuse. *J Pediatr Orthop B.* 2011;20(6):440–443.

122. Kos L, Shwayder T. Cutaneous manifestations of child abuse. *Pediatr Dermatol.* 2006;23(4):311–320.

123. Kothari NA, Pelchovitz DJ, Meyer JS. Imaging of musculoskeletal infections. *Radiol Clin North Am.* 2001;39(4):653–671.

124. Kransdorf MJ, Sweet DE. Aneurysmal bone cyst: concept, controversy, clinical presentation, and imaging. *AJR Am J Roentgenol.* 1995;164(3):573–580.

125. Leet AI, Chebli C, Kushner H, et al. Fracture incidence in polyostotic fibrous dysplasia and the McCune-Albright syndrome. *J Bone Miner Res.* 2004;19(4):571–577.

126. Leet AI, Mesfin A, Pichard C, et al. Fractures in children with cerebral palsy. *J Pediatr Orthop.* 2006;26(5):624–627.

127. Leong GM, Abad V, Charmandari E, et al. Effects of child- and adolescent-onset endogenous Cushing syndrome on bone mass, body composition, and growth: a 7-year prospective study into young adulthood. *J Bone Miner Res.* 2007;22(1):110–118.

128. Leong NL, Anderson ME, Gebhardt MC, Snyder BD. Computed tomography-based structural analysis for predicting fracture risk in children with benign skeletal neoplasms: comparison of specificity with that of plain radiographs. *J Bone Joint Surg Am.* 2010;92(9):1827–1833.

129. Leventhal JM, Larson IA, Abdoo D, et al. Are abusive fractures in young children becoming less common? Changes over 24 years. *Child Abuse Negl.* 2007;31(3):311–322.

130. Lim HK, Smith WL, Sato Y, Choi J. Congenital syphilis mimicking child abuse. *Pediatr Radiol.* 1995;25(7):560–561.

131. Lindberg DM, Beaty B, Juarez-Colunga E, et al. Testing for abuse in children with sentinel injuries. *Pediatrics.* 2015;136(5):831–838.

132. Lindberg DM, Harper NS, Laskey AL, et al. Prevalence of abusive fractures of the hands, feet, spine, or pelvis on skeletal survey: perhaps "uncommon" is more common than suggested. *Pediatr Emerg Care.* 2013;29(1):26–29.

133. Lock TR, Aronson DD. Fractures in patients who have myelomeningocele. *J Bone Joint Surg Am.* 1989;71(8):1153–1157.

134. Loder RT, Hensinger RN. Slipped capital femoral epiphysis associated with renal failure osteodystrophy. *J Pediatr Orthop.* 1997;17(2):205–211.

135. Lundgren SS, Rosengren BE, Dencker M, et al. Low physical activity is related to clustering of risk factors for fracture—a 2-year prospective study in children. *Osteoporos Int.* 2017;28(12):3373–3378.

136. Maguire S, Mann MK, Sibert J, Kemp A. Are there patterns of bruising in childhood which are diagnostic or suggestive of abuse? A systematic review. *Arch Dis Child.* 2005;90(2):182–186.

137. McArthur RG, Cloutier MD, Hayles AB, Sprague RG. Cushing's disease in children. Findings in 13 cases. *Mayo Clin Proc.* 1972;47(5):318–326.

138. McClain JL, Clark MA, Sandusky GE. Undiagnosed, untreated acute lymphoblastic leukemia presenting as suspected child abuse. *J Forensic Sci.* 1990;35(3):735–739.

139. McDonald DGM, Kinali M, Gallagher AC, et al. Fracture prevalence in Duchenne muscular dystrophy. *Dev Med Child Neurol.* 2002;44(10):695–698.

140. McMahon P, Grossman W, Gaffney M, Stanitski C. Soft-tissue injury as an indication of child abuse. *J Bone Joint Surg Am.* 1995;77(8):1179–1183.

141. Meehan PL, Viroslav S, Schmitt EW Jr. Vertebral collapse in childhood leukemia. *J Pediatr Orthop.* 1995;15(5):592–595.

142. Meier R, van Tuyll van Sersooskerken AM, Liberton E, et al. Fractures of the proximal tibia associated with longterm use of methotrexate: 3 case reports and a review of literature. *J Rheumatol.* 2010;37(11):2434–2438.

143. Mik G, Arkader A, Manteghi A, Dormans JP. Results of a minimally invasive technique for treatment of unicameral bone cysts. *Clin Orthop Relat Res.* 2009;467(11):2949–2954.

144. Miller RG, Segal JB, Ashar BH, et al. High prevalence and correlates of low bone mineral density in young adults with sickle cell disease. *Am J Hematol.* 2006;81(4):236–241.

145. Narang SK, Paul SR; Committee on Medical Liability and Risk Management. Expert witness participation in civil and criminal proceedings. *Pediatrics.* 2017;139(3):e20164122.

146. National Association of Children's Hospitals and Related Institutions. *Defining the Children's Hospital Role in Child Maltreatment.* Author; 2006.

147. Newman RS, Jalili M, Kolls BJ, Dietrich R. Factor XIII deficiency mistaken for battered child syndrome: case of "correct" test ordering negated by a commonly accepted qualitative test with limited negative predictive value. *Am J Hematol.* 2002;71(4):328–330.

148. Newton AW, Vandeven AM. Unexplained infant and child death: a review of sudden infant death syndrome, sudden unexplained infant death, and child maltreatment fatalities including shaken baby syndrome. *Curr Opin Pediatr.* 2006;18(2):196–200.

149. Nielsen G, Kyriakos M. Fibrohistiocytic tumours. In: Fletcher CDM, Bridge J, Hogendom PCW, et al., eds. *WHO Classifications of Tumours of Bone and Soft Tissue.* IARC Press; 2013:301–304.

150. Nimkin K, Spevak MR, Kleinman PK. Fractures of the hands and feet in child abuse: imaging and pathologic features. *Radiology.* 1997;203(1):233–236.

151. Niyibizi C, Smith P, Mi Z, et al. Potential of gene therapy for treating osteogenesis imperfecta. *Clin Orthop Relat Res.* 2000;(379 Suppl):S126–S133.

152. O'Neill JA Jr, Meacham WF, Griffin JP, Sawyers JL. Patterns of injury in the battered child syndrome. *J Trauma.* 1973;13(4):332–339.

153. O'Sullivan M, Zacharin M. Intramedullary rodding and bisphosphonate treatment of polyostotic fibrous dysplasia associated with the McCune-Albright syndrome. *J Pediatr Orthop.* 2002;22(2):255–260.

154. Oliveira AM, Hsi BL, Weremowicz S, et al. USP6 (Tre2) fusion oncogenes in aneurysmal bone cyst. *Cancer Res.* 2004;64(6):1920–1923.

155. Paul SR, Narang SK; Committee on Medical Liability and Risk Management. Expert witness participation in civil and criminal proceedings. *Pediatrics.* 2017;139(3):e20164122.

156. Pepin MG, Byers PH. What every clinical geneticist should know about testing for osteogenesis imperfecta in suspected child abuse cases. *Am J Med Genet C Semin Med Genet.* 2015;169(4):307–313.

157. Pereira EM. Clinical perspectives on osteogenesis imperfecta versus non-accidental injury. *Am J Med Genet C Semin Med Genet.* 2015;169(4):302–306.

158. Perez-Rossello JM, McDonald AG, Rosenberg AE, et al. Absence of rickets in infants with fatal abusive head trauma and classic metaphyseal lesions. *Radiology.* 2015;275(3):810–821.

159. Pierce MC, Bertocci GE, Vogeley E, Moreland MS. Evaluating long bone fractures in children: a biomechanical approach with illustrative cases. *Child Abuse Negl.* 2004;28(5):505–524.

160. Plotkin H, Sueiro R. Osteoporosis in children with neuromuscular diseases and inborn errors of metabolism. *Minerva Pediatr.* 2007;59(2):129–135.

161. Popoff SN, Marks SC Jr. The heterogeneity of the osteopetroses reflects the diversity of cellular influences during skeletal development. *Bone.* 1995;17(5):437–445.

162. Presedo A, Dabney KW, Miller F. Fractures in patients with cerebral palsy. *J Pediatr Orthop.* 2007;27(2):147–153.

163. Prosser I, Maguire S, Harrison SK, et al. How old is this fracture? Radiologic dating of fractures in children: a systematic review. *AJR Am J Roentgenol.* 2005;184(4):1282–1286.

164. Ranade SC, Allen AK, Deutsch SA. The role of the orthopaedic surgeon in the identification and management of nonaccidental trauma. *J Am Acad Orthop Surg.* 2020;28:53–65.

165. Riester S, Ramaesch R, Wenger D, et al. Predicting fracture risk for enchondroma of the hand. *Hand (N Y).* 2016;11(2):206–210.

166. Rodgers WB, Schwend RM, Jaramillo D, et al. Chronic physeal fractures in myelodysplasia: magnetic resonance analysis, histologic description, treatment, and outcome. *J Pediatr Orthop.* 1997;17(5):615–621.

167. Ruck J, Dahan-Oliel N, Montpetit K, et al. Fassier-Duval femoral rodding in children with osteogenesis imperfecta receiving bisphosphonates: functional outcomes at one year. *J Child Orthop.* 2011;5(3):217–224.

168. Sala A, Barr RD. Osteopenia and cancer in children and adolescents: the fragility of success. *Cancer.* 2007;109(7):1420–1431.

169. Schnitzer PG, Ewigman BG. Child deaths resulting from inflicted injuries: household risk factors and perpetrator characteristics. *Pediatrics.* 2005;116(5):e687–e693.

170. Schwend RM, Werth C, Johnston A. Femur shaft fractures in toddlers and young children: rarely from child abuse. *J Pediatr Orthop.* 2000;20(4):475–481.

171. Scollan JP, Jauregui JJ, Jacobsen CM, Abzug JM. The outcomes of nonelongating intramedullary fixation of the lower extremity for pediatric osteogenesis imperfecta patients: a meta-analysis. *J Pediatr Orthop.* 2017;37(5):e313–e316.

172. Sees JP, Sitoula P, Dabney K, et al. Pamidronate treatment to prevent reoccurring fractures in children with cerebral palsy. *J Pediatr Orthop.* 2016;36(2):193–197.

173. Sege RD, Amaya-Jackson L. Clinical considerations related to the behavioral manifestations of child maltreatment. *Pediatrics.* 2017;139(4):e20170100.

174. Shapiro F, Glimcher MJ, Holtrop ME, et al. Human osteopetrosis: a histological, ultrastructural, and biochemical study. *J Bone Joint Surg Am.* 1980;62(3):384–399.

175. Shoenfeld Y. Osteogenesis imperfecta. Review of the literature with presentation of 29 cases. *Am J Dis Child.* 1975;129(6):679–687.

176. Sieradzki JP, Sarwark JF. Thoracolumbar fracture-dislocation in child abuse: case report, closed reduction technique and review of the literature. *Pediatr Neurosurg.* 2008;44(3):253–257.

177. Silverman FN. The roentgen manifestations of unrecognized skeletal trauma in infants. *Am J Roentgenol Radium Ther Nucl Med.* 1953;69(3):413–427.

178. Simpson AH, Kenwright J. Fracture after distraction osteogenesis. *J Bone Joint Surg Br.* 2000;82(5):659–665.

179. Sinigaglia R, Gigante C, Bisinella G, et al. Musculoskeletal manifestations in pediatric acute leukemia. *J Pediatr Orthop.* 2008;28(1):20–28.

180. Slovis TL, Strouse PJ, Strauss KJ. Radiation exposure in imaging of suspected child abuse: benefits versus risks. *J Pediatr.* 2015;167(5):963–968.

181. Smith FW, Gilday DL, Ash JM, Green MD. Unsuspected costo-vertebral fractures demonstrated by bone scanning in the child abuse syndrome. *Pediatr Radiol.* 1980;10(2):103–106.

182. Stanton RP, Abdel-Mota'al MM. Growth arrest resulting from unicameral bone cyst. *J Pediatr Orthop.* 1998;18(2):198–201.

183. Stark Z, Savarirayan R. Osteopetrosis. *Orphanet J Rare Dis.* 2009;4:5.

184. Stott NS, Zionts LE. Displaced fractures of the apophysis of the olecranon in children who have osteogenesis imperfecta. *J Bone Joint Surg Am.* 1993;75(7):1026–1033.

185. Strouse PJ, Owings CL. Fractures of the first rib in child abuse. *Radiology.* 1995;197(3):763–765.

186. Sullivan PM, Brookhouser PE, Scanlan JM, et al. Patterns of physical and sexual abuse of communicatively handicapped children. *Ann Otol Rhinol Laryngol.* 1991;100(3):188–194.

187. te Winkel ML, Pieters R, Hop WCJ, et al. Bone mineral density at diagnosis determines fracture rate in children with acute lymphoblastic leukemia treated according to the DCOG-ALL9 protocol. *Bone.* 2014;59:223–228.

188. Tenenbaum S, Thein R, Herman A, et al. Pediatric nonaccidental injury: are orthopedic surgeons vigilant enough? *J Pediatr Orthop.* 2013;33(2):145–151.

189. Terzi S, Gasbarrini A, Fuiano M, et al. Efficacy and safety of selective arterial embolization in the treatment of aneurysmal bone cyst of the mobile spine: a retrospective observational study. *Spine (Phila Pa 1976).* 2017;42(15):1130–1138.

190. Thackeray JD, Wannemacher J, Adler BH, Lindberg DM. The classic metaphyseal lesion and traumatic injury. *Pediatr Radiol.* 2016;46(8):1128–1133.

191. Thomas AE. The bleeding child; is it NAI? *Arch Dis Child.* 2004;89(12):1163–1167.

192. Thomas SA, Rosenfield NS, Leventhal JM, Markowitz RI. Long-bone fractures in young children: distinguishing accidental injuries from child abuse. *Pediatrics.* 1991;88(3):471–476.

193. Trinh A, Wong P, Brown J, et al. Fractures in spina bifida from childhood to young adulthood. *Osteoporos Int.* 2017;28(1):399–406.

194. US Department of Health & Human Services Administration for Children and Families Administration on Children, Youth and Families, Children's Bureau. *Child Maltreatment 2021*. February 9, 2023. https://www.acf.hhs.gov/cb/data-research/child-maltreatment

195. Waguespack SG, Hui SL, Dimeglio LA, Econs MJ. Autosomal dominant osteopetrosis: clinical severity and natural history of 94 subjects with a chloride channel 7 gene mutation. *J Clin Endocrinol Metab*. 2007;92(3):771–778.

196. Wang J, Temple HT, Pitcher JD, et al. Salvage of failed massive allograft reconstruction with endoprosthesis. *Clin Orthop Relat Res*. 2006;443:296–301.

197. Watanabe K, Tsuchiya H, Sakurakichi K, et al. Treatment of lower limb deformities and limb-length discrepancies with the external fixator in Ollier's disease. *J Orthop Sci*. 2007;12(5):471–475.

198. Williams P. The management of arthrogryposis. *Orthop Clin North Am*. 1978;9(1):67–88.

199. Wort UU, Nordmark E, Wagner P, et al. Fractures in children with cerebral palsy: a total population study. *Dev Med Child Neurol*. 2013;55(9):821–826.

200. Wu JS, Goldsmith JD, Horwich PJ, et al. Bone and soft-tissue lesions: what factors affect diagnostic yield of image-guided core-needle biopsy? *Radiology*. 2008;248(3):962–970.

201. Zarate YA, Clingenpeel R, Sellars EA, et al. COL1A1 and COL1A2 sequencing results in cohort of patients undergoing evaluation for potential child abuse. *Am J Med Genet A*. 2016;170(7):1858–1862.

202. Zeitlin L, Fassier F, Glorieux FH. Modern approach to children with osteogenesis imperfecta. *J Pediatr Orthop B*. 2003;12(2):77–87.

203. Zhao JG, Wang J, Huang WJ, et al. Interventions for treating simple bone cysts in the long bones of children. *Cochrane Database Syst Rev*. 2017;2:CD010847.

204. Zwemer E, Claudius I, Tieder J. Update on the evaluation and management of brief resolved unexplained events (previously apparent life-threatening events). *Rev Recent Clin Trials*. 2017;12(4):233–239.

Fractures and Dislocations of the Hand and Carpal Bones in Children

Lindley Wall and Andrea S. Bauer

Fractures of the Hand and Carpal Bones

INCIDENCE OF FRACTURES AND DISLOCATIONS OF THE HAND AND CARPAL BONES

The pediatric hand is exposed and vulnerable to injury during play as a curious child explores their surrounding world. Hand injuries account for up to 25% of pediatric fractures. The reported annual incidence in 5- to 14-year-olds is approximately 54.6 fractures per 10,000 children[10] (Table 8-1).

Pediatric hand fractures occur primarily in a *biphasic* age distribution: toddler and adolescent. In toddlers, the injury occurs most often secondary to a crush mechanism (e.g., a finger caught in a door). In contrast, in the teenage population,

TABLE 8-1. Incidence of Pediatric Hand Injuries

Peak age: 13 years

Annual incidence: 26.4 per 10,000 children

Proportion of all pediatric emergency patients: 1.7%

Right side incidence equals left

Male incidence is greater than female incidence

Most common fracture types
- Nonphyseal: Distal phalanx (crush)
- Physeal: Proximal phalanx
- Index and small fingers most commonly injured

Data from Chung KC, Spilson SV. The frequency and epidemiology of hand and forearm fractures in the United States. *J Hand Surg Am.* 2001;26:908–915.

the mechanism is more commonly a torque, twist, or axial load sustained during contact activities and athletics.[9,83]

Overweight adolescents can have poorer balance or increased body mass indices, which may explain their propensity for upper extremity fractures related to falls on an outstretched hand.[29] Hand fractures in children peak around age 13, coinciding with active participation in organized contact sports, random play, as well as punching.

The two most common pediatric hand fractures are distal phalanx crush injuries and Salter–Harris (S-H) type II fractures of the proximal phalanx.[53] The border digits (thumb and small fingers) are the most vulnerable to injury because of their location.[83] Dislocations and ligament injuries are relatively uncommon in children. The force at time of energy transmits through the physis because the physeal cells of the growth plate are biomechanically the path of least resistance, rather than the collateral ligaments. Additionally, avulsion fractures are more likely to occur than ligament injuries, as the ligament pulls off its bony attachment to the softer-growing bone. Proximal phalanx S-H type II fractures account for nearly 33% of all hand fractures in children. Although rare, the thumb metacarpophalangeal (MCP) joint is the most commonly dislocated joint in the skeletally immature hand.[54] The proximal interphalangeal (PIP) joint is the most commonly injured articular surface, often due to volar plate or collateral ligament avulsion fractures.

Fractures and dislocations about the child's carpus are rare compared to injuries of the adjacent, more vulnerable physis of the distal radius. The scaphoid is the most frequently injured carpal bone in children.[20] Pediatric scaphoid fractures have a peak incidence between the ages of 12 and 15 years. Scaphoid fractures are rare during the first decade of life, with only a few reported cases involving children younger than 8 years of age.[24]

Carpal ligament dissociation and tears of the triangular fibrocartilage complex (TFCC) do occur in children and adolescents, mostly common with athletic trauma, associated with skeletal trauma such as distal radial fractures, or as a consequence of radial growth arrest, positive ulnar variance, and ulnar carpal impaction.

APPLIED ANATOMY OF HAND AND CARPAL BONES

Children have distinct patterns of hand injury because of their underlying skeletal and soft tissue anatomy. Knowledge of the

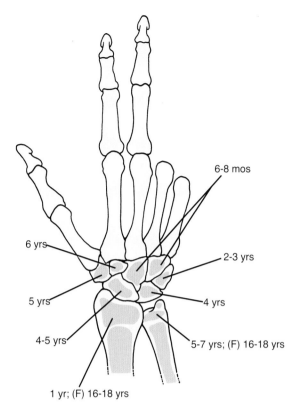

Figure 8-1. The age at the time of appearance of the ossific nucleus of the carpal bones and distal radius and ulna. The ossific nucleus of the pisiform (not shown) appears at about 6 to 8 years of age.

anatomy of the physes, the ligament and tendon origins and insertions, and the surrounding periosteum is essential for the diagnosis and treatment of children's hand fractures.

OSSEOUS ANATOMY

There is potential for epiphyses to exist at both the proximal and distal ends of all the tubular bones. Yet, secondary ossification centers typically develop at the distal ends of the metacarpals of the index, long, ring, and small rays and at the proximal end of the thumb. Conversely, the epiphyses are present only at the proximal ends of the phalanges in all digits.

Secondary Ossification Centers

The pattern of carpal bone ossification and the appearance of secondary ossification sites in the metacarpals and phalanges are often used to predict the skeletal bone age and years of remaining growth (Fig. 8-1). The fetal wrist begins as a single cartilaginous mass. By the 10th week of gestation, the carpus transforms into eight distinct entities with definable intercarpal separations. Although these precursors display minor differences in contour, the anatomic elements greatly resemble the individual carpal bones in their mature form.

In boys, the secondary ossification centers within the proximal phalanges appear at 15 to 24 months and fuse by bone age of 16 years (Fig. 8-2). In girls, the appearance and closure occur earlier, at 10 to 15 months and bone age of 14 years, respectively. The secondary ossification centers of the middle and distal phalanges

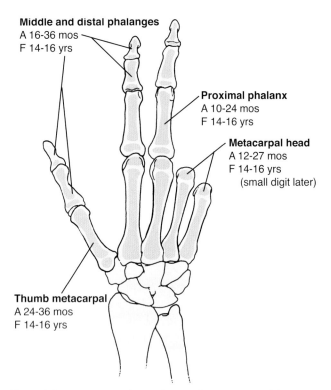

Figure 8-2. Appearance of secondary ossification centers (*A*). Fusion of secondary centers to the primary centers (*F*).

appear later in both girls and boys, usually by 6 to 8 months. Fusion of the secondary ossification centers, however, occurs first distally and then proceeds proximally with maturity. Within the metacarpal, the secondary ossification centers appear at 18 to 27 months in boys and at 12 to 17 months in girls. The proximal thumb metacarpal secondary ossification center appears 6 to 12 months after the fingers. The secondary centers within the metacarpals fuse between 14 and 16 years of age in girls and boys.

The capitate is the first carpal bone to ossify, usually within the first few months of life and uniformly by 1 year of age. The hamate appears next, usually at about 4 months of age. The pattern of ossification proceeds stepwise from the distal row to the proximal row moving counterclockwise in a circular fashion from a dorsal perspective of the left hand. The triquetrum appears during the second year, and the lunate begins to ossify around the fourth year. The scaphoid begins to ossify in the fifth year, usually slightly predating the appearance of the trapezium. Scaphoid ossification begins at the distal aspect and progresses in a proximal direction. The trapezium and trapezoid ossify in the fifth year, with the trapezoid slightly delayed. The ossification pattern usually concludes with the pisiform in the ninth or tenth year. The scaphoid, trapezoid, lunate, trapezium, and pisiform may demonstrate multiple centers of ossification. Although well recognized, variations in ossification may be confused with acute trauma or ligamentous rupture by the inexperienced observer. For example, since the scaphoid ossifies from proximal to distal, the distance between the scaphoid and lunate is greater in the immature wrist (pseudo-Terry Thomas sign). Contralateral x-rays or advanced imaging can clarify the anatomy and prevent misdiagnosis.

PHYSEAL ANATOMY

The physis of the long bones of the hand provides longitudinal growth. The physis is divided into four distinct zones: germinal, proliferative, hypertrophic, and provisional calcifications (zones I, II, III, and IV, respectively).[7] The zone of chondrocyte hypertrophy (zone III) is the least resistant to mechanical stresses. This zone is devoid of the collagen that provides inherent stabilizing properties. Collagen is dominant in zones I and II while the calcium in zone IV provides the most structural strength. Therefore, physeal fractures often propagate through zone III as the path of least resistance. High-energy injuries, however, may undulate through all four zones of the physis.

The irregularity of the physeal zones in the phalanges and metacarpals increases near skeletal maturity. Thus, a fracture line may be transmitted through several zones in adolescents. This variable path through irregular topography contributes to the increased risk of partial growth arrest following adolescent physeal fractures. Physeal irregularity also explains the differing patterns of physeal injuries dependent on age: S-H type I and II fractures tend to occur in younger patients compared to the S-H type III or IV fractures which are more prevalent in children close to skeletal maturity.

SOFT TISSUE ANATOMY

The tensile strength of a younger child's soft tissues usually exceeds that of the adjacent physis and epiphysis. For this reason, tendon or collateral ligament avulsions are less common compared to physeal or epiphyseal fractures in the skeletally immature hand.

Tendons

The terminal tendon of the digital extensor mechanism and the extensor pollicis longus insert on the epiphyses of the distal phalanx. The central slip of the extensor mechanism inserts into the epiphysis of the middle phalanx. The extensor pollicis brevis inserts onto the epiphysis of the proximal phalanx of the thumb. The abductor pollicis longus has a broad-based insertion onto both the radial epiphysis and metaphysis of the thumb metacarpal. These extensor tendinous insertions are broad to the thick periosteum, which predisposes bony avulsion injuries.

The long digital flexor tendons (flexor digitorum profundus [FDP] and the flexor pollicis longus [FPL]) insert along the metadiaphyseal, not epiphyseal, region of their respective terminal phalanges of the fingers and thumb. The flexor digitorum superficialis (FDS) inserts onto the central three-fifths of the middle phalanx.

Collateral Ligaments

The collateral ligaments at the interphalangeal joint originate from the collateral recesses of the phalangeal head, span the physis, and insert onto both the metaphysis and epiphysis of the middle and distal phalanges (Fig. 8-3). The collaterals also insert onto the volar plate to create a three-sided box that protects the physes and epiphyses of the interphalangeal joints from laterally directed forces. This configuration explains the rarity of S-H type III injuries at the interphalangeal joints.[31]

Figure 8-3. Anatomy of the collateral ligaments at the distal (**A**) and proximal (**B**) interphalangeal joints. The collateral ligaments at the interphalangeal joints originate in the collateral recesses and insert into both the metaphyses and epiphyses of their respective middle and distal phalanges. Additional insertion into the volar plane (*arrows*) is seen at the interphalangeal joints.

In contrast, the collateral ligaments about the MCP joints originate from the metacarpal epiphysis and insert almost exclusively onto the epiphysis of the proximal phalanx (Fig. 8-4). This anatomic arrangement accounts for the frequency of S-H type III injuries at the MCP joint level.

Figure 8-4. The collateral ligaments at the MCP joint originate and insert almost exclusively on the epiphyseal regions of the metacarpal and the proximal phalanges.

Volar Plate

The volar plate is a stout stabilizer of the interphalangeal joint and MCP joints and resists hyperextension forces. The volar plate originates from the metaphysis of the respective proximal digital segment and inserts onto the epiphysis of the distal segment (see Fig. 8-3B). The plate receives insertional fibers from the accessory collateral ligaments to create a three-sided box that protects the joint. Hyperextension of the finger joints often results in avulsion injuries of the epiphysis or more rarely S-H type III at the volar plate insertion site.

Periosteum

The periosteum is robust in a child's hand and can act as a considerable asset or liability in fracture management. On the positive side, the periosteal sleeve can minimize fracture displacement and aid in fracture reduction. On the negative side, the periosteum can shear off, become interposed between displaced fracture fragments, and prevent reduction.

Nail Matrix

The skin, nail elements, soft tissues, and bone of the distal digit are closely related (Fig. 8-5). The dorsal periosteum of the distal phalanx is the underlying nutritional and structural support for the sterile matrix and nail bed. The germinal matrix is responsible for generating the nail plate. The sterile matrix has a role in nail plate adherence as well as in adding strength and thickness to the plate.

Triangular Fibrocartilage Complex

The TFCC is a soft tissue structure in the wrist that provides connection between the carpal bones and the distal radius and ulna. The TFCC provides stability to the wrist and distal radioulnar joint and supports loading of the proximal carpal row

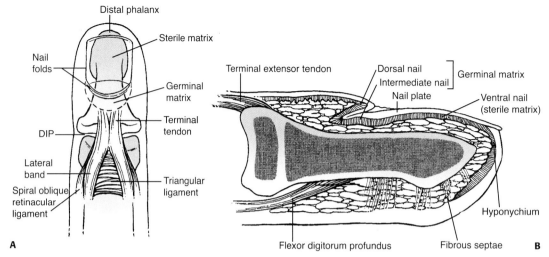

Figure 8-5. Anatomy of the distal phalanx. **A:** The skin, nail, and extensor apparatus share a close relationship with the bone of the distal phalanx. Specific anatomic structures at the terminal aspect of the digit are labeled. **B:** This lateral view of the nail demonstrates the tendon insertions and the anatomy of the specialized nail tissues.

on the head of the ulna. The structure of the TFCC consists of a meniscus homologue, an articular disc, ulnocarpal ligament, dorsal and volar radiocarpal ligaments, and ECU subsheath. The TFCC has a deep foveal attachment to the ulnar head in addition to its lateral ligamentous attachments (Fig. 8-6).

REMODELING OF HAND AND CARPAL BONES

A young child's ability to remodel displaced fractures in the hand and carpus must be incorporated into the treatment algorithm. Factors that influence remodeling potential include the patient's age, the proximity of the fracture to the physis, direction of displacement, and the plane of motion of the adjacent joint. The

remodeling capacity is greater in younger children, fractures that are closer to the physis, and deformity in the plane of motion. Remodeling potential in the coronal or adduction–abduction plane is rarely quantified but is likely less than or equal to 50% of the remodeling potential in the sagittal plane. Rotational deformity remodeling rarely occurs unless there is rotatory joint motion (carpometacarpal [CMC] joint thumb) and therefore, rotational malalignment is an indication of fracture reduction.

The speed of healing in the skeletally immature is remarkable, with most fractures becoming clinically stable within 2 weeks. This rapid healing allows earlier motion and decreased stiffness; however, a delay in treatment of just 7 to 10 days may negate the possibility of closed reduction without osteoclasis.

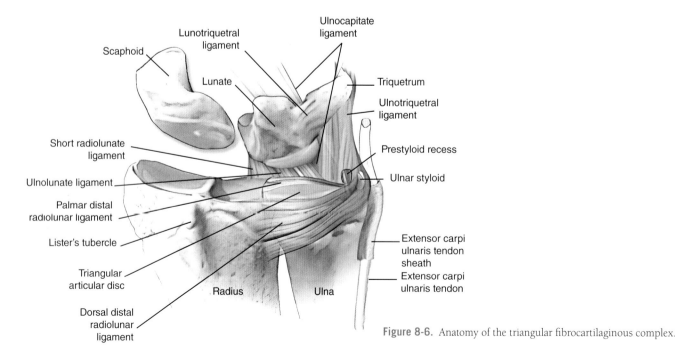

Figure 8-6. Anatomy of the triangular fibrocartilaginous complex.

MECHANISMS OF INJURY FOR HAND AND CARPAL BONE FRACTURES

Assessment of a child with a hand fracture should begin with a detailed description of the injury itself, timing of the injury, treatment prior to presentation, history of previous injuries to the same hand, and identification of potential penetrating or embedded materials such as glass, metal, or teeth.

Axial load injuries, such as punching, yield injury primarily to the metacarpals or CMC joints. Digital torsion or lateral bending forces most often propagate through the physis of the phalanx. Hyperextension injuries cause volar plate avulsion fractures.

INJURIES ASSOCIATED WITH CARPAL BONE FRACTURES

Pediatric carpal bone fractures and dislocations are relatively uncommon and associated with higher-velocity trauma. Motor vehicle accidents, contact sports, and falls from a height can cause carpal injury. Additional injuries to the head, cervical spine, wrist, elbow, or shoulder girdle may be present. In these polytrauma cases, treatment decision making may be driven by a need for earlier stabilization to allow mobilization of the child or to prevent fracture displacement during rehabilitation of concomitant injuries. However, it is important to note that children can make remarkable recoveries following high-energy injuries, so even "minor" hand injuries should not be neglected in the polytrauma setting.

Children who have sustained carpal bone fractures and dislocations from crush injuries, penetrating trauma, mechanical equipment entrapment, or motor vehicle accidents may also have injuries to the soft tissue envelope of the fingers and hand. Nerve, artery, and tendon repair as well as flap or skin graft coverage may dictate the need for hand fracture stabilization.

SIGNS AND SYMPTOMS OF HAND AND CARPAL BONE FRACTURES

The evaluation of a child's hand, especially of traumatized infants and toddlers, is more challenging than that of an adult. The child may be anxious, unable to understand instructions, and fearful of the physician. The examiner must be patient, engage the child, and often employ the parents to comfort the child. Observation and play are the tricks of the trade. The child's hand use, posture, and movements provide clues about the location and severity of the injury as the child interacts with toys, parents, and the environment in the examining area. A hurried examination or a frightened child can lead to an erroneous or missed diagnosis.

Fractures should be suspected when there is swelling, ecchymosis, deformity, or limited movement of the fingers or hand. Fracture malrotation is noted by digital scissoring during active grasp or passive tenodesis. Tendon integrity is observed by digital posture at rest and during active grasp around objects of varying size. Passive wrist extension with finger flexion

Figure 8-7. Clinical photograph of a malrotated digit. (Courtesy of Children's Orthopaedic Surgery Foundation.)

tenodesis is a critical part of the evaluation to accurately diagnose fracture malrotation (Fig. 8-7).

The history, physical examination, and clinical suspicion are the essential elements to diagnosis of a scaphoid and carpus fracture. The relative infrequency of this injury and the difficulty in interpreting radiographs of the immature wrist increase the likelihood of missing a pediatric scaphoid fracture. The complete physical examination of the scaphoid consists of palpation of the anatomic snuffbox as well as the volar scaphoid tubercle, and axial load of the thumb. A positive response to all three examination maneuvers is highly sensitive for the detection of a scaphoid fracture, even in the presence of normal radiographs.[61]

For TFCC and distal radioulnar joint ligamentous injuries, pain is localized to the distal ulna, fovea, and ulnar carpal region. Forearm rotation may be limited and usually reproduces the pain, particularly at the extremes of supination and/or pronation. Compression and ulnar deviation of the carpus against the ulna may reproduce the pain with associated crepitus at times. The stability of the distal radioulnar joint should be compared to the contralateral side.

In the relaxed child, the physician may palpate areas of tenderness and move injured joints to assess their integrity. Gentle comparative stress testing and joint stability should be recorded in the anteroposterior (AP) and lateral directions. Repeat examination may be needed after the pain and swelling subside. Reexamination in 5 to 7 days allows a better examination with ample time to intervene.

Neurovascular injuries are especially difficult to detect in a young child. The proper digital artery is dorsal to the proper digital nerve within the finger. Therefore, pulsatile bleeding is indicative of a digital artery injury and usually indicates a concomitant digital nerve laceration. Discriminatory sensibility testing is not

Figure 8-8. Clinical photograph of the wrinkle test. (Courtesy of Children's Orthopaedic Surgery Foundation.)

reliable until 5 to 7 years of age. Therefore, meaningful objective data are difficult to obtain in the very young. A clinical clue to sensory impairment is that children often bypass a painful or anesthetic digit during grasp and pinch. A helpful examination maneuver is the wrinkle test (Fig. 8-8). Immersion of an innervated digit in warm water for 5 minutes usually results in corrugation or wrinkling of the volar skin of the pulp. Wrinkling is absent in a digit without nerve innervation. If there is doubt about the integrity of the nerve, operative exploration is indicated.

IMAGING AND OTHER DIAGNOSTIC STUDIES OF HAND AND CARPAL BONE FRACTURES

A careful clinical evaluation directs a focused radiographic assessment. Several pediatric imaging factors complicate interpretation of plain radiographs, including unossified segments and normal variations. Lack of understanding of normal ossification pattern of the immature hand creates problems with the detection of fractures and also promotes false interpretation of ligamentous injuries. Accurate interpretation may require comparison to the uninjured hand or consultation with a pediatric atlas of child development and normal radiographic variants.[78]

Complete evaluation of the injured hand or digit requires AP, lateral, and oblique views (Fig. 8-9). Oblique views are particularly useful for assessing displacement and intra-articular extension. A common radiographic pitfall is failure to obtain a true lateral radiograph of the injured digit. Isolation of the affected digit on the film or splaying of the fingers (cascade lateral) projects a true lateral view. Stress views are rarely used for pediatric fracture evaluation. If the injury can be clinically isolated to a single digit, individual finger x-rays will demonstrate more detail than a zoomed-out image of the entire hand.

Ultrasound, although operator dependent, is increasingly used in emergency departments and clinical triage centers to diagnose a fracture of the upper extremity. Advanced imaging studies are rarely used for finger injuries, although they may provide additional detail in distal radius and carpal bone fractures.

Scaphoid fractures may or may not be evident on initial radiographs; however, sclerosis may appear after a few weeks. A

scaphoid view places the scaphoid parallel to the film and reveals the scaphoid in its full size. If the clinical picture is consistent with a scaphoid fracture but the radiographs are negative, the patient should be immobilized. The child should either be instructed to return in 2 weeks for repeat examination and radiographs, or advanced imaging studies may be ordered. MRI can detect scaphoid fractures that are not visualized on the initial radiographs.[8,12,18,39,52,55] Johnson et al. evaluated 56 children (57 injuries) with MRI within 10 days of injury.[39] All children had a suspected scaphoid injury but negative radiographs. In 33 (58%) of the 57 injuries, the MRI was normal, and the patients were discharged from care. In 16 cases (28%), a fractured scaphoid was diagnosed, and treatment was initiated. Sedation is required for a young child having MRI, and the modality may be overly sensitive in identifying bone edema without cortical disruption. CT images of the scaphoid can be useful to assess fracture displacement and fracture union. CT images must be made along the longitudinal axis of the scaphoid, which is out of plane to the radiocarpal joint.[11]

OUTCOMES OF HAND AND CARPAL BONE FRACTURES

Outcomes assessment following pediatric hand and carpal bone fractures include subjective and objective measures. Patient-reported outcomes are important to consider alongside clinician-derived measures of motion and strength. Outcome instruments such as the Disabilities of the Arm, Shoulder and Hand (DASH), Pediatric Outcomes Data Collection Instrument (PODCI), and Michigan Hand Outcomes Questionnaire (MHQ) can be completed by parents or adolescent children to survey a broad spectrum of long- and short-term results. Functional evaluations such as pinch and grip strength, pegboard test, dexterity, in-hand manipulation, and Jebsen–Taylor timed testing are examples of validated outcome instruments in the assessment of hand function in children.

Fractures of the Distal Phalanx

Classification of Distal Phalangeal Fractures

Extraphyseal

- Transverse diaphysis
- Longitudinal splitting
- Comminuted separations
- Avulsion of FDP tendon with bone (bony Jersey finger)

Physeal

- S-H type I or II including Seymour fracture
- S-H type III with or without extensor tendon displacement "bony mallet finger"
- S-H type IV with articular extension

Mechanism

- Crush
- Hyperflexion
- Hyperextension

A

B

C

Figure 8-9. The straight method of assessing alignment about the MCP joint. The long axes of the metacarpal and proximal phalanx should align, as they do in this normal hand (**A**). If there is a fracture in the proximal phalanges, as in this patient's opposite or injured hand (**B, C**), the axes will not be colinear (*arrows*). (Courtesy of Robert M. Campbell Jr, MD.)

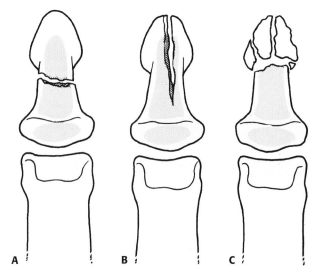

Figure 8-10. Three types of extraphyseal fractures of the distal phalanx. **A:** Transverse diaphyseal fracture. **B:** Cloven-hoof longitudinal splitting fracture. **C:** Comminuted distal tuft fracture with radial fracture lines.

Fractures of the distal phalanx in children can be classified into extraphyseal and physeal injuries. Extraphyseal fractures range from a simple distal tuft fracture to an unstable diaphyseal fracture underlying a nail bed laceration. The extraphyseal fracture pattern can be divided into three types: transverse, longitudinal split, or comminuted. A transverse fracture (Fig. 8-10A) may occur either at the distal extent of the terminal phalanx or through the diaphysis. Displaced transverse fractures through the diaphysis are almost always associated with a considerable nail bed injury that requires repair. A longitudinal splitting-type fracture, much less common, is the result of excessive hoop stress within the tubular distal phalanx at the time of a crush injury (Fig. 8-10B). Comminuted or stellate fractures of the distal diaphysis also can occur and usually are often accompanied by extensive nail and soft tissue injury (Fig. 8-11).

Physeal fractures clinically can resemble a mallet finger. There are four basic fracture patterns, and most result in a flexed

Figure 8-12. Mallet-equivalent fracture types.

posture of the distal interphalangeal (DIP) joint (Fig. 8-12). An S-H type I or II fracture with flexion of the distal fragment, known as a Seymour fracture,[73] occurs predominantly in young patients less than 12 years of age. Because the extensor tendon attaches to the epiphysis dorsally while the FDP attaches to the metaphysis volarly, the unopposed FDP flexes the distal fragment. The fracture is open through what is typically a very proximal nail bed injury. The proximal nail plate may lie on top of the dorsal nail fold, whereas the distal nail plate remains intact

Figure 8-11. Stellate or comminuted extraphyseal fractures shown radiographically (**A**) and clinically (**B**).

Figure 8-13. Clinical photograph (**A**) and lateral radiograph (**B**) of a displaced Seymour fracture. (Courtesy of Children's Orthopaedic Surgery Foundation.)

(Fig. 8-13). This open fracture exposes the underlying bone to bacterial contamination and osteomyelitis. Closed reduction may be blocked by interposition of the nail bed in the dorsal physis deep into the nail plate. Rarely, an S-H type I or II fracture causes extrusion of the epiphyseal fragment.[85] This "epiphyseal dislocation" is challenging to diagnose if the epiphysis is not yet ossified. A dorsal S-H type III or IV fracture of the distal phalanx, "bony mallet finger," occurs in teenagers and results in an extension lag at the DIP joint and joint incongruity. Very rarely, the epiphysis may also separate from the terminal extensor tendon.[70]

Distal phalanx fractures can also be described by mechanism of injury including crush, hyperflexion, and hyperextension.

A crush injury creates a spectrum of damage from minor tissue disruption with little need for intervention to severe tissue trauma that requires bony fixation, meticulous nail bed repair, and skin coverage (Fig. 8-14). A hyperflexion injury results in a malletlike injury to the terminal tendon insertion or physeal separation with nail bed injury as described above. A hyperextension force can produce a bony avulsion injury of the volar articular surface or rupture of the insertion of the FDP tendon (Jersey finger) (Fig. 8-15).

Figure 8-14. Crush injury to the fingers of an 18-month-old child with multiple lacerations requiring meticulous repair with absorbable suture.

Figure 8-15. An FDP avulsion fracture of the distal phalanx (Jersey finger). This bony avulsion is apparent on radiograph, indicating the extent of proximal migration.

TREATMENT OPTIONS FOR FRACTURES OF THE DISTAL PHALANX

NONOPERATIVE TREATMENT OF FRACTURES OF THE DISTAL PHALANX

Indications/Contraindications

Nonoperative Treatment of Distal Phalanx Fractures in Children:
INDICATIONS AND CONTRAINDICATIONS

Indications

- Stable
- Closed
- Low risk of infection, nail deformity, joint instability, or growth plate arrest

Contraindications

- Unstable
- Open
- High risk of infection, nail deformity, joint instability, or growth plate arrest

Figure 8-16. A: Lateral radiograph demonstrating bony mallet injury with small avulsion fragment and congruent DIP joint. **B:** Lateral radiograph demonstrating healing and remodeling of the DIP joint 2 years after initial injury. (Courtesy of Children's Orthopaedic Surgery Foundation.)

Distal phalanx fractures in children are frequently associated with nail bed lacerations. The soft tissue repair may be at the bedside or in the operating room, depending on the emergency room facilities, operating room availability, and surgeon's preference. Distal phalanx fractures associated with 100% subungual hematomas are treated with nail removal irrigation, debridement, and repair to decrease the risk of nail deformity and osteomyelitis.

Immobilization

Most distal phalangeal fractures can be treated with nonoperative measures using a splint or cast. Mild and moderate displacement of extraphyseal fractures will heal in days to weeks. Clinical union precedes complete radiographic healing by about 1 month. Physeal injuries with mild displacement of the dorsal epiphyseal fragment and joint congruity, "bony mallet finger," have favorable results with hyperextension splinting (Fig. 8-16). Extreme hyperextension is avoided because dorsal skin hypoperfusion and necrosis may result.

Hematoma Evacuation

Indications for a hematoma evacuation, or trephination, have typically been described for subungual hematoma involving more than 50% of the nail plate or painful pressure under the nail in adults, although pediatric-specific indications are unknown. Decompression can be done with a sterile hypodermic needle, heated paper clip, or electrocautery, but the heat can cause further nail bed injury if penetration is too deep. After 12 to 24 hours, the effectiveness of trephination decreases as the blood coagulates. The use of oral antibiotics in the setting of trephination, although theoretically protective against infection, has not been proven.[14,68]

Nail Bed Repair

A nail bed repair can be performed at bedside, in a clinical procedure room, in the emergency department under digital block and/or conscious sedation, or in the operating room. A digital tourniquet is often used but care has to be taken to remove the digital tourniquet at the end of the repair procedure. Nail bed repair is recommended for substantial nail bed lacerations and potentially for subungual hematomas that involve more than 50% of the nail plate. After adequate anesthesia, a blunt Freer elevator is used to remove the nail plate, avoiding additional nail bed injury. Curved clamps should not be used as they can cause further nail matrix injury. Proximal exposure of the germinal matrix may require incisions along the eponychial folds and proximal retraction of the eponychial flap. The nail bed is repaired with an interrupted 6-0 chromic gut or equivalent absorbable sutures under loupe magnification. Following repair, the nail bed is supported and the dorsal nail fold is kept open typically using the previously removed nail plate. Other substitutes are possible, such as petrolatum gauze, the foil from the suture pack, or a cut portion of a plastic culture tube.[30] Nail plate replacement surgeries are typically unnecessary in children and can lead to limited benefits and more complications. Always remember to remove the digital tourniquet.

OPERATIVE TREATMENT OF FRACTURES OF THE DISTAL PHALANX

Unstable extraphyseal fractures with wide displacement require stabilization.[37] Open injuries with severe displacement or irreducible fractures require reduction and stabilization[6] (Fig. 8-17). The Seymour fracture represents an open and potentially irreducible fracture that requires open reduction.[3,45,66] The sterile matrix must be extricated from the fracture site and repaired beneath the eponychium. Epiphyseal dislocations also require operative intervention to both restore growth potential and

A   **B**

Figure 8-17. A: An irreducible distal phalangeal fracture that required extrication of the nail bed from within the fracture site. **B:** Stabilization of the fracture fragments with a longitudinal K-wire across the DIP joint.

reestablish extensor tendon continuity. Physeal fractures with a dorsal fragment larger than 50% of the epiphysis or considerable DIP joint subluxation may require operative intervention.[47] Volar distal phalanx fractures associated with avulsion of the FDP require repair with tendon reinsertion.

Fingertip amputations often involve the distal phalanx. The injury may involve skin, nail tissue, and bone. Support for nail growth is a primary consideration. Minimal loss of tissue can be treated with local wound care and healing through secondary intention. A small amount of exposed bone does not preclude spontaneous healing in children. Debridement of minimally exposed bone will not negatively impact digital length and can expedite healing. The likelihood of nail deformity (hook nail or "parrot's beak") is high for amputations that involve more than 50% of the distal phalanx. Primary nail ablation may be indicated in children with loss of the majority of the distal phalanx to avoid a hook-nail deformity.

Soft tissue coverage varies depending on the degree of tissue loss, direction of injury, and amount of bone exposed or at risk. When the amputated part is available, composite grafting of the part as a biologic dressing can have surprisingly good results even in older children. Eberlin and colleagues reviewed 39 subjects who underwent composite grafting after fingertip injuries at an average age of 5.9 years. While only three subjects had complete take of the graft, 90% did not require any additional surgery, suggesting that the partial coverage achieved was enough to allow satisfactory results.[19] Local flaps are another option for coverage of large volar or dorsal oblique amputations. Options include a variety of flaps, such as a V-Y volar advancement, a thenar flap, a cross-finger flap, a pedicled flap, or a neurovascular island flap (Figs. 8-18 and 8-19). Fortunately, coverage issues are rare in children as most heal with local wound care without flap reconstruction. The choice of coverage depends on the degree and direction of soft tissue loss, age of the patient, amount of bone exposed, long-term outcome risks, and preference of the surgeon and family.

Preoperative Planning

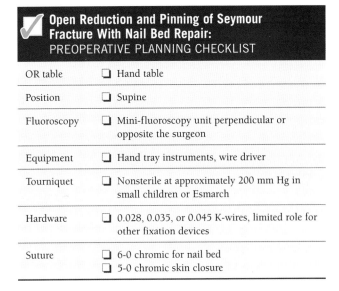

✔	**Open Reduction and Pinning of Seymour Fracture With Nail Bed Repair:** PREOPERATIVE PLANNING CHECKLIST	
OR table	❏ Hand table	
Position	❏ Supine	
Fluoroscopy	❏ Mini-fluoroscopy unit perpendicular or opposite the surgeon	
Equipment	❏ Hand tray instruments, wire driver	
Tourniquet	❏ Nonsterile at approximately 200 mm Hg in small children or Esmarch	
Hardware	❏ 0.028, 0.035, or 0.045 K-wires, limited role for other fixation devices	
Suture	❏ 6-0 chromic for nail bed ❏ 5-0 chromic skin closure	

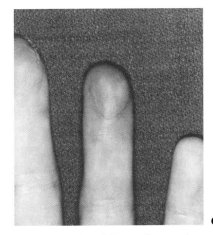

A, B   **C**

Figure 8-18. Volar V-Y advancement flap for coverage. **A:** A volar oblique tissue loss of the ring finger with intact nail bed. **B:** Flap designed with apex at the DIP joint and mobilized to cover the fingertip. The defect is closed proximal to the flap creating the Y. **C:** Satisfactory result with good durability and sensibility.

Figure 8-19. Cross-finger flap in an 18-year-old male with open distal phalangeal injury and tissue loss. **A:** Extensive volar and distal soft tissue loss with preservation of the bone and nail bed. **B:** A cross-finger flap of skin and subcutaneous tissue is elevated from the dorsal aspect of the adjacent donor digit based on the side of the index finger. **C:** The vascular epitenon is preserved on the donor digit to support a skin graft. The flap is transferred to the volar aspect of the index finger to recreate the tuft. **D:** Satisfactory coverage and functional result.

While nonoperative management is appropriate for most pediatric bony mallet injuries, fractures associated with DIP subluxation may require operative management. Closed manipulation with percutaneous K-wire fixation is usually effective in these cases. One or two smooth 0.35 or 0.45 K-wires can be inserted retrograde through the tip of the finger and across the fracture for stabilization. A cast is used for most children and teenagers after surgery, although a DIP-immobilizing splint alone may be adequate in older teenagers.

Jersey Finger

Bony and soft tissue FDP avulsions typically require operative management (Fig. 8-20). An extensile volar approach to the finger is required. For soft tissue injuries, tendon fixation to bone is preferred using pull-out wires or suture. Suture anchors generally cannot be used due to the small size of the child's phalanx. For bony injuries, pins or screws may be used in addition to soft tissue repair. Fragments that are too small for fixation require bone removal and repair of the tendon directly to the fracture bed.

Technique

Seymour Fracture:
KEY SURGICAL STEPS

- ❑ Remove nail plate using Freer elevator
- ❑ Make back-cuts at medial and lateral edges of proximal eponychial fold to expose underlying germinal matrix
- ❑ Perform thorough irrigation and debridement of foreign bodies or contamination, taking care not to damage the physeal cartilage
- ❑ Remove any interposed nail bed from fracture site and reduce fracture
- ❑ If alignment is adequate, place one or two K-wires from fingertip, across fracture, and across DIP joint
- ❑ In case of a difficult reduction, K-wire can be started from inside the fracture site, driven out through fingertip, and then passed back across fracture site and DIP joint
- ❑ Repair nail bed laceration and replace nail plate under proximal eponychial fold

A, B   **C**

Figure 8-20. **A:** Lateral radiograph of an avulsion fracture from the FDP tendon in a 14-year-old boy. **B:** Clinical photograph demonstrating a volar exposure and screw placement, with intraosseous sutures tied over a button on the nail dorsally. **C:** Postoperative appearance after healing.

Authors' Preferred Treatment for Fractures of the Distal Phalanx (Algorithm 8-1)

Algorithm 8-1. Authors' preferred treatment for distal phalanx fractures.

Extraphyseal Fractures

Simple closed stable fractures are treated with immobilization in a splint or cast for 1 to 2 weeks, reevaluated, and converted to early mobilization when healing is evident. Distal phalanx fractures with a substantial nail bed laceration or avulsion are treated with removal of the nail plate, fracture reduction, and nail bed repair. It takes several cycles of nail growth (3–6 months) before the final morphology of the nail is known. An unstable, displaced distal extraphyseal phalangeal fracture that penetrated through the nail bed or is irreducible requires open reduction and percutaneous pinning with a smooth K-wire across the DIP joint and physis (with or without nail bed repair). The pin is removed 3 to 4 weeks after injury, followed by early protected range of motion.

Physeal Fractures

Most closed pediatric S-H type III physeal fractures, or bony mallet fingers, are treated with splinting of the DIP joint into neutral or mild hyperextension. Adequate healing requires full-time splinting for 4 to 6 weeks depending on the age of the child, size of the fracture fragment, and amount of bony apposition. Adolescent mallet fingers that are acute or chronic with soft tissue terminal tendon disruption are treated similarly to adults with 4 to 6 weeks of dorsal DIP joint splint immobilization. Operative repair of soft tissue or bony mallet fingers is rarely indicated, even for a delay in presentation. The loss of digital flexion associated with surgery can be more disabling than a minor extension lag. Surgery is reserved for fractures that are open, grossly unstable, irreducible, or have unacceptable alignment (Fig. 8-21). Even in these cases, closed reduction and longitudinal percutaneous fixation are preferred.

Seymour fractures are open physeal fractures with disruption of the nail bed. These require urgent nail plate removal, irrigation and debridement, fracture alignment, pinning, and nail bed repair.

Amputations

Mild to moderate loss of skin, subcutaneous tissue, and bone is best treated by wound cleansing, dressing changes, and healing by secondary intention. Acceptable functional and aesthetic results are uniform. Skin or composite grafts are rarely necessary for coverage in children. Extensive soft tissue loss with exposed bone requires more innovative coverage (see Figs. 8-18 and 8-19).

Dorsal tissue loss is more difficult to reconstruct. The nail bed injury adds additional complexity. Mild loss can be treated by local wound care. Moderate to severe loss may require a reverse cross-finger flap or a more distant flap. Unfortunately, nail bed replacement techniques, such as partial-thickness grafting from the toe, often result in considerable nail deformity.

Postoperative Care and Rehabilitation

Children younger than 4 or 5 years of age are immobilized with long-arm mitten strapping, soft casts (3M, St. Paul, Minnesota), or rigid casts. As the child ages, the degree of immobilization may be decreased, but even adolescents are tolerant of rigid casts for 3 to 4 weeks without prolonged stiffness. The use of adjunctive antibiotics and tetanus prophylaxis should be utilized in contaminated cases. Nonabsorbable suture should be removed after 2 weeks, but, whenever possible, absorbable suture is used in a child to avoid the trauma of suture removal. Percutaneous skeletal fixation (K-wire fixation) is removed in the office 3 to 4 weeks after surgery. Formal hand therapy is usually not required, though a home exercise program (HEP) with an emphasis on DIP joint motion is useful. Formal therapy is reserved for patients who fail to regain motion and strength after 3 to 4 weeks on a home program.

A

B

Figure 8-21. A: Displaced mallet fracture with considerable articular involvement and DIP joint subluxation. **B:** Placement of extension blocking pin under fluoroscopic guidance.

Figure 8-21. *(Continued)* **C:** The fracture is reduced using the extension block pin. **D:** Final intraoperative appearance after pinning of the DIP joint.

Potential Pitfalls and Preventive Measures

Distal Phalanx Fracture: PITFALLS AND PREVENTIONS	
Pitfall	**Prevention**
Osteomyelitis	• Irrigation and debridement • Nail bed laceration repair • Monitor and treat infection signs early with repeat irrigations and antibiotic coverage
Premature physeal closure	• Smooth wires • Minimize reduction attempts
Hook nail	• Ablate nail matrix when majority distal phalanx amputated, avoid advancing nail matrix pulp during repair, and use thenar flap closure to support nail
Quadrigia	• Do not sew extensors or flexors to tip of amputated finger
Extensor lag	• Neutral or 10-degree extension splint or pin fixation • Continue night, school, and sports splint use for additional 4 to 6 weeks after full-time day splint use discontinued to prevent recurrence
Osteomyelitis	• Irrigation, debridement

Outcomes

There are few studies that assess outcomes following distal phalanx fractures. The cost-effectiveness of observation with

or without trephination versus removal of the nail plate in nail bed lacerations over distal phalanx fractures has been studied in several case series.[30] These studies concluded that osteomyelitis and nail deformity were equivalent; however, trephination and observation were more cost-effective than nail bed repair. In a series of 200 children, S-H type IV, bony mallet, and Seymour fracture patterns were shown to be associated with a higher risk of complications.[47] Identification of these high-risk injuries and early intervention can improve outcomes. A recent retrospective review of 35 Seymour fractures attempted to identify ways to diminish complications. The authors defined "appropriate" treatment as irrigation and debridement, fracture reduction, and antibiotic administration, and "acute" treatment as within 24 hours of injury. They found an infection rate of 0% in the acute, appropriate treatment group, while the infection rate was 15% in the acute, incompletely treated group and 45% in the delayed treatment group.[66]

MANAGEMENT OF EXPECTED ADVERSE OUTCOMES AND UNEXPECTED COMPLICATIONS RELATED TO DISTAL PHALANX FRACTURES

Distal Phalanx Fractures: COMMON ADVERSE OUTCOMES AND COMPLICATIONS

• Osseous: Nonunion, malunion, osteomyelitis
• Soft tissue: Scar, stiffness, extensor tendon insufficiency with extensor lag
• Nail: Split or hook-nail deformity, rides, ingrown lateral or dorsal nail fold

The overall results following distal phalangeal fractures are favorable. A small loss of motion has negligible functional impact. A small extensor lag or minor longitudinal nail ridge is well tolerated by most patients. Considerable nail irregularity or deformity is a source of dissatisfaction.

Bony complications from distal phalangeal fractures are uncommon. Potential problems include nonunion, malunion, and osteomyelitis. Nonunion and malunion are exceedingly rare, except in open injuries that result in avascular fracture fragments. Osteomyelitis can result from open fractures and requires application of the basic tenets for the treatment of infected bone. Debridement, removal of any sequestrum, and intravenous antibiotics are required to resolve the infection. Diagnosis of osteomyelitis requires careful attention to the clinical exam, as inflammatory markers are typically normal and clinical indicators such as fever may be absent.

Soft tissue complications are more prevalent than bony problems. Difficulties may involve the skin, subcutaneous tissue, nail, and tendons. An inadequate soft tissue envelope can be reconstructed with replacement using a variety of local flaps. Severe DIP joint deformities are uncommon but may result in swan-neck positioning of the finger. Reconstruction options are similar to methods used in adults, such as a spiral oblique retinacular ligament reconstruction or central slip tenotomy. In a young child, untreated lacerations proximal to the terminal tendon insertion may result in an extensor lag that can be repaired successfully with a tenodermodesis reconstruction.[41] Nail problems depend on the location and degree of nail bed injury. Damage to the germinal matrix produces deficient nail growth and nail ridging. Injury to the sterile matrix causes poor nail adherence or nail ridging. Treatment options are limited and usually involve resection of the damaged segment and replacement with a full- or split-thickness skin or nail bed graft.[90] Adjacent digits or toes are potential sources of nail bed transfers. The results in children have been superior to those in adults, although not uniformly satisfying. The hook nail or "parrot's beak" nail is a nail plate complication related to the underlying bony and soft tissue deficit. The nail plate curves over the abbreviated end of the distal phalanx (Fig. 8-22). Treatment requires restoring length to the shortened distal phalanx and creation of an adequate soft tissue envelope to support the nail plate (Fig. 8-23). In these situations, a thenar flap or composite graft is typically used to provide improved support for the nail bed.

Middle and Proximal Phalangeal Fractures in Children

CLASSIFICATION OF MIDDLE AND PROXIMAL PHALANGEAL FRACTURES

Classification of Proximal and Middle Phalangeal Fractures

Physeal

- S-H types I, II, III, IV

Extraphyseal

- Shaft
- Phalangeal neck
- Intra-articular (condylar)

Classification of middle and proximal phalangeal fractures in children is based primarily on anatomic location. There are four locations: physeal, shaft, neck, and condyles. The fracture pattern varies with the direction and amount of force incurred. Most fractures of the proximal and middle phalanges result from a torsional or angular force combined with an axial load, such as catching a ball, falling on an outstretched hand, or colliding in sports. In young children, fractures of the middle and proximal phalanx occur when the fingers get caught in a door and the finger twists as the child pulls away. Crush injuries are less common in the proximal and middle phalanges than in the distal phalanx.

Every fracture must be carefully examined for rotational deformity regardless of classification, mechanism of injury, or radiographic appearance. Active finger flexion will produce deviation of the plane of the nails or overt digital scissoring (Fig. 8-24). Passive wrist extension produces tenodesis, and malrotation will manifest with an abnormal digital cascade or crossover. Examining the dorsal aspect of the hand with the digits in midflexion is very good for evaluating any rotation of the nail plates as well as deviation and overlap of the digits.

Figure 8-22. A hook-nail deformity of the small finger after a distal fingertip amputation.

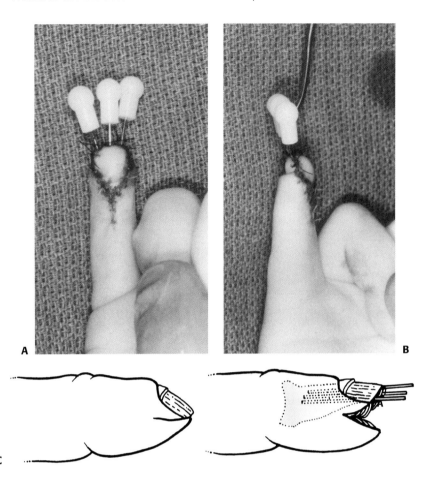

Figure 8-23. A, B: Postoperative photographs of the patient shown in Figure 8-22 after the antenna procedure. The procedure involved the optional technique of a volar V-Y advancement flap to cover the distal tip, elevation of the sterile matrix, and the nail supported using three K-wires. **C:** Line drawings demonstrating technique of elevation and support of the sterile matrix with wires. (**A, B:** Courtesy of William B. Kleinman, MD. **C:** Reprinted from Atasoy E, Godfrey A, Kalisman M. The "antenna" procedure for the "hook-nail" deformity. *J Hand Surg Am.* 1983;8(1):55–58. Copyright © 1983 American Society for Surgery of the Hand. With permission.)

Figure 8-24. A: An AP radiograph of an S-H type II fracture at the index finger proximal phalanx. The radiograph reveals slight angulation and can appear benign. Clinical examination must be done to assess the digital cascade for malrotation. **B:** Tenodesis of the wrist with passive extension reveals unacceptable malrotation as evident by the spread between the index finger and middle finger.

A **B**

Figure 8-25. **A:** An extra-octave fracture in a 12-year-old girl. **B:** The fracture was reduced with the MCP joint in full flexion.

PHYSEAL FRACTURES

Physeal fractures of the proximal phalanx are among the most common pediatric hand fractures.[9] Extra-articular S-H type II fractures are more prevalent, and intra-articular S-H type III and IV fractures are less common. A common fracture pattern is the S-H type II fracture along the ulnar aspect of the proximal phalanx of the small digit. The small digit is angulated in an ulnar direction. This fracture has been termed the "extra-octave" fracture to denote its potential benefit to the span of a pianist's hand[4] (Fig. 8-25). Physeal fractures about the middle phalanx are much less common and can involve the lateral, dorsal, or volar aspects of the physis. A lateral force across the PIP joint may cause an S-H type III or IV fracture. Similarly, a flexion force may produce a dorsal S-H type III fracture, indicative of a central slip avulsion fracture (pediatric boutonnière injury). A hyperextension injury produces small avulsion fragments from the middle phalangeal epiphysis associated with damage to the volar plate.

The thumb proximal phalanx is particularly susceptible to physeal fractures. An ulnar collateral ligament (UCL) avulsion injury at the base of the thumb proximal phalanx is the pediatric equivalent of the adult gamekeeper's or skier's thumb. The mechanisms of injury, clinical findings of UCL laxity at the MCP joint and physical symptoms of instability with grip and pinch will be similar to the adult soft tissue UCL injury. However, the fracture pattern is usually an S-H type III injury, as the ligament typically remains attached to the epiphyseal fracture fragment (Fig. 8-26). Displaced injuries with articular incongruity or joint instability require open reduction and internal fixation (ORIF) to restore articular alignment and joint stability. Similar to the adult counterpart, the epiphyseal fracture with the attached UCL can be displaced outside the adductor aponeurosis ("Stener lesion").[76] This location prohibits healing and requires open reduction.

Children rarely sustain comminuted intra-articular fractures of the PIP joint, the so-called "pilon" fractures of the middle phalanx or fracture–dislocations. These injuries can occur in adolescent athletes and result from an axial load sustained while attempting to catch a ball or contacting an opponent. The fracture fragment from the volar side may have the volar

Figure 8-26. Bony gamekeeper's or skier's thumb is an S-H type III fracture of the base of the thumb proximal phalanx attached to the UCL of the MCP joint.

plate attached, whereas the dorsal fragment is likely to have the central slip attached. The central aspect of the joint may be depressed and comminuted. The joint can be unstable and incongruent, requiring careful treatment.

SHAFT FRACTURES

Extraphyseal middle and proximal phalanx shaft fractures in children are less common. The fracture configuration may be transverse, spiral, or spiral oblique. The fracture may be comminuted. Proximal and middle phalangeal fractures are usually angulated in an apex volar pattern because the distal fragment is extended by the central slip and lateral band, and the proximal fragment is flexed by the FDS in the middle phalanx and by the intrinsic musculature in the proximal phalanx (Fig. 8-27). Oblique fractures often rotate and shorten. Careful clinical evaluation of rotational alignment is critical. Comminution is most often secondary to a high-energy injury or crush mechanism (Fig. 8-28).

NECK FRACTURES

Neck fractures of the phalanx are problematic with regard to diagnosis, with suboptimal outcomes if the fracture is not appropriately identified and treated in a timely manner. Displaced neck fractures are also referred to as subcondylar fractures or "door jam fracture" as they often occur in young children as a result of finger entrapment (Fig. 8-29). The head fragment remains attached to the collateral ligaments and tends to rotate into extension.[5] This displacement disrupts the architecture of the subcondylar fossa, which normally accommodates the volar plate and base of the adjacent phalanx during interphalangeal joint flexion. Malunited neck fractures typically result in a mechanical block to interphalangeal joint flexion and may

Figure 8-27. Radiographs of transverse middle and proximal phalangeal fractures, respectively, which demonstrate the characteristic apex volar deformity.

have coronal deviation as well. Because these fractures are as far as possible from the physis, remodeling potential is limited, even in young children, so anatomic reduction and fixation are important.

INTRA-ARTICULAR (CONDYLAR) FRACTURES

Condylar fractures involve the joint and represent a constellation of fracture patterns, including small lateral avulsion fractures, unicondylar or intracondylar fractures, bicondylar or transcondylar fractures (Fig. 8-30). Condylar fractures can be associated with subluxations or dislocations of the joint. Many

Figure 8-28. Comminuted fractures secondary to a crush injury with longitudinal splitting into the physis.

of these fractures are initially misdiagnosed as sprains and too often present late with an articular malunion. Restoration of articular alignment and joint stability is critical to a successful outcome (Fig. 8-31).

Figure 8-29. A: Phalangeal neck fractures are often unstable and rotated. These fractures are difficult to reduce and control by closed means because of the forces imparted by the volar plate and ligaments. **B, C:** Fixed with a closed reduction and hyperextension maneuver across the DIP joint as well as a derotational wire.

Figure 8-30. A: An AP radiograph reveals an intra-articular fracture of the small finger. **B:** Lateral view demonstrates the double-density sign indicative of displacement (*arrows*).

TREATMENT OPTIONS FOR MIDDLE AND PROXIMAL PHALANX FRACTURES

The treatment of middle and proximal phalangeal fractures varies greatly with the type of injury. Nonoperative treatment is overwhelmingly the most common management for most physeal fractures as well as nondisplaced fractures of the shaft. Operative treatment is utilized most for displaced shaft fractures, and neck and condylar fractures, given the high risk of displacement and instability.

NONOPERATIVE AND OPERATIVE TREATMENT OF MIDDLE AND PROXIMAL PHALANGEAL FRACTURES

Indications/Contraindications

Nonoperative Treatment of Middle and Proximal Phalangeal Fractures: INDICATIONS AND CONTRAINDICATIONS
Nonoperative Indications
• Stable initially or after closed reduction • Closed, isolated • Normal tenodesis (no malrotation) • Joint congruity and stability
Operative Indications
• Unstable • Open, polytrauma • Malrotation (scissoring) • Joint incongruity (S-H type III, neck, or condylar fractures)

Physeal Fractures

Nondisplaced physeal fractures of the proximal and middle phalanges are treated by nonoperative management. Minimal displacement is treated with splinting or functional casting in the intrinsic plus or safe position for 3 weeks.

Moderate displacement in the sagittal or coronal plane of more than 10 degrees or any rotational malalignment requires closed reduction with local anesthesia or conscious sedation. Placing the MCP joint into flexion tightens the collateral ligaments and facilitates fracture manipulation and reduction. In the "extra-octave" fifth proximal phalanx fracture, a pencil or digit in the fourth web space as a fulcrum may assist in reduction. Buddy tape and cast immobilization will maintain alignment until healing (see Fig. 8-24). The age and compliance of

Figure 8-31. A 15-year-old male baseball player who injured his left small finger sliding into first base. **A:** Oblique x-ray with displaced unicondylar fracture small finger distal interphalangeal joint. **B:** Postoperative x-ray with restoration of joint congruity after closed reduction and pinning with K-wires.

Figure 8-33. AP radiograph of base of proximal phalanx S-H type III fracture. (Courtesy of Children's Orthopaedic Surgery Foundation.)

Figure 8-32. Displaced S-H type II fracture of the proximal phalanx that was irreducible. The distal fragment was herniated through a rent in the periosteum and extensor mechanism that prohibited reduction.

the patient determine if buddy tape alone or combined with casting is necessary. Minimally displaced S-H type III epiphyseal fractures at the base of the middle phalanx associated with volar plate avulsion are treated with early buddy tape or extension block splint. "Pediatric boutonnière" fractures or dorsal S-H type III epiphyseal fractures can be treated with a PIP extension splint and early DIP range-of-motion exercises similar to the adult paradigm.

Irreducible fractures of the physis may be caused by any surrounding soft tissue structures, including periosteum and tendon.[67] Open treatment with removal of the impeding tissue and fracture reduction is required for these rare injuries (Fig. 8-32). Some S-H type II fractures may be reducible but unstable after reduction. These fractures require insertion of a smooth K-wire after reduction is required to maintain fracture alignment.[4] Another indication for operative management is to restore articular congruity after a displaced S-H type III fracture of the proximal phalangeal base with a sizable (>25%) epiphyseal fragment (Fig. 8-33). Operative exposure and fixation techniques are challenging with nonborder digit proximal phalangeal S-H type III fractures.

A bony gamekeeper's or skier's thumb is an S-H type III fracture of the proximal phalanx that requires closed reduction and percutaneous pinning (CRPP) or ORIF with K-wires or compression screw fixation if the fragment is large enough. Open visualization is typically necessary to ensure anatomic articular reduction. The approach is similar to the operative steps of an adult gamekeeper's thumb surgery with incision of the adductor

aponeurosis for exposure, followed by later repair after fracture reduction (Fig. 8-34).

Beware of the "flipped physis" of the middle or proximal phalanx in younger children. The findings on x-ray may be subtle and only visible on the lateral view. Treatment most often requires open "flipping" of the physis, attempting to keep any collateral ligaments or capsule intact. Surprisingly, appropriate management rarely results in growth arrest (Fig. 8-35).

Shaft Fractures

Nondisplaced shaft fractures are treated with simple immobilization. Splinting in the intrinsic plus position for 3 to 4 weeks should be adequate for clinical union. Displaced or angulated fractures require reduction. The amount of acceptable angulation in the plane of motion is controversial. In children less than 10 years of age, 20 to 30 degrees may be acceptable in the sagittal plane. In children older than 10 years, 10 to 20 degrees of angulation is acceptable in the sagittal plane. Less angulation is acceptable in the coronal plane. Malrotation is unacceptable.

Fractures that are unstable after reduction or irreducible by closed methods require operative intervention. A shaft fracture that is unstable after reduction is managed primarily by closed reduction and percutaneous K-wire fixation in either a longitudinal or horizontal direction, depending on the obliquity of the fracture (Fig. 8-36). Open reduction is indicated for fractures that cannot be reduced. A dorsal approach is usually used for exposure. The extensor tendon is split for proximal phalangeal fractures and elevated for middle phalangeal fractures. The choice of implant depends on the age of the patient and the fracture configuration. Smooth wires, tension bands, or modular set screws are preferable to plates to avoid extensor mechanism adherence.[34] All malrotated fractures require reduction and fixation.

Figure 8-34. **A:** AP radiograph demonstrating displaced bony gamekeeper injury. **B:** Clinical photo demonstrating valgus instability of the thumb MCP joint. **C–G:** Open reduction and k-wire fixation of the bony fragment with the UCL attached, taking care to align the articular surface and repair the adductor aponeurosis. **H:** Postoperative radiograph demonstrating articular reduction with k-wire in place.

Phalangeal Neck Fractures

Closed treatment of fractures of the phalangeal neck is difficult because these fractures are typically unstable (see Fig. 8-29A). For fractures that are truly nondisplaced, cast immobilization can be attempted, but repeat radiographs should be obtained out of cast after 1 week of immobilization to ensure that the fracture has not displaced. Closed manipulation is done with digital distraction, a volar-directed pressure on the distal

A, B   C, D

Figure 8-35. Beware of the "flipped" epiphysis. Requires open reduction and fixation, but in younger children may not even cause growth arrest. Higher risk of infection and growth arrest than other epiphyseal fractures. (Courtesy of Children's Hospital, Los Angeles, CA.)

fragment, and hyperflexion of the DIP or PIP joint depending on the phalanx fractured. Percutaneous pinning is necessary to maintain the reduced position.[42] Under fluoroscopy, K-wires are inserted from distal to proximal obliquely across the fracture. These wires should engage the contralateral cortex proximal to the fracture site.

Remodeling potential has been demonstrated in phalangeal neck fractures displaced in extension in very young children.

A   B

Figure 8-36. Closed reduction, percutaneous pinning of a proximal phalanx spiral oblique shaft fracture. (Courtesy of Children's Hospital, Los Angeles, CA.)

Remarkable reforming of the anatomic condyles can occur despite being so far from the epiphysis. If very young children present late, allowing time for remodeling may obviate the need for any management (Fig. 8-37).

Intra-Articular Fractures

Nondisplaced intra-articular fractures can be treated by immobilization. Weekly radiographs, often out of cast to gain acceptable visualization, are necessary to ensure maintenance of reduction. Displaced intra-articular fractures require closed or open reduction.[68] Closed or percutaneous reduction can be accomplished with traction and use of a percutaneous towel clip or reduction clamp to obtain provisional fracture reduction. Percutaneous fixation is used for definitive fracture fixation. Fractures not appropriate for closed manipulation require ORIF (Fig. 8-38). A dorsal, lateral, or rare volar incision is used for direct inspection of the fracture and articular surface. Care is taken to preserve the blood supply of the fracture fragments entering through the collateral ligaments. Fracture stabilization is either by K-wires (preferred) or mini-screws.

Certain unusual intra-articular fractures are especially difficult to treat. Shear fractures and osteochondral slice fractures are difficult to recognize. Treatment is by open reduction and smooth wire fixation. Osteonecrosis, especially of small fragments, is a concern. Some of these fractures require a volar surgical approach. Avoidance of extensive soft tissue dissection lessens the risk of osteonecrosis.

Comminuted pilon fracture–dislocations of the PIP joint are uncommon in children. Operative intervention is usually required to restore articular congruity. Anatomic reduction is preferred whenever possible (Fig. 8-39). Bone grafting may be necessary to support the articular surface. Extreme joint comminution may preclude anatomic reduction, and alternative treatment options, such as dynamic traction, may be necessary.

A, B   **C**

Figure 8-37. Remodeling potential of the subcondylar fracture in a very young child.

OPERATIVE TREATMENT OF MIDDLE AND PROXIMAL PHALANGEAL FRACTURES

CRPP Versus ORIF of Middle and Proximal Phalangeal Fractures

Preoperative Planning

> ✓ **CRPP Versus ORIF of Middle and Proximal Phalangeal Fractures:**
> PREOPERATIVE PLANNING CHECKLIST

OR table	❏ Hand table
Position	❏ Supine
Fluoroscopy	❏ Perpendicular or opposite the surgeon
Equipment	❏ Hand tray instruments, wire driver
Tourniquet	❏ Nonsterile at approximately 200 mm Hg in small children or Esmarch elastic bandage placed in the proximal forearm; not needed for CRPP
Hardware	❏ 0.028-, 0.035-, or 0.045-inch K-wires; modular screw set with 1.1-, 1.5-, or 2.0-mm screws
Suture	❏ Absorbable suture for incision closure

Technique

> ✓ **CRPP Versus ORIF of Middle and Proximal Phalangeal Fractures:**
> KEY SURGICAL STEPS

❏ Attempt closed reduction first
❏ If alignment is adequate, place one or two K-wires parallel or crossed at fracture site, across physeal or extraphyseal fracture. Limit crossing of PIP joint
❏ Use "joystick" smaller K-wires, Freer elevator, dental pick, towel clip, or small fragment reduction forceps to enhance the closed reduction, osteoclasis for partially healed fractures
❏ If necessary, open skin through a dorsal (between central slip and lateral band) or midlateral approach or expose the articular surface through the open fracture wound
❏ Preserve extensor and collateral soft tissue attachments
❏ Avoid dissection of smaller bone fragments
❏ Reduce incarcerated, rotated, or extruded fragments and proceed with K-wire or lag screw fixation.

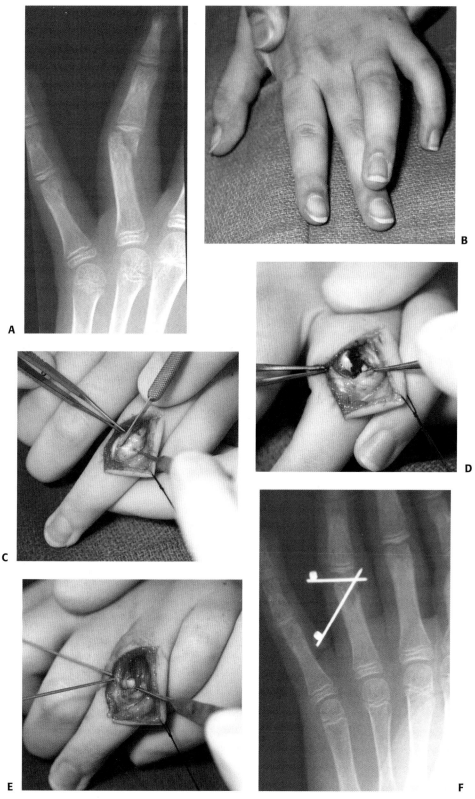

Figure 8-38. **A:** A 10-year-old girl with a displaced unicondylar fracture of the ring finger proximal phalanx. **B:** Clinical examination reveals malrotation of the digit. **C:** Dorsal exposure with incision between lateral band and central slip. **D:** Exposure of displaced fracture fragment. **E:** Fracture reduced with K-wire fixation. **F:** Postoperative radiograph shows restoration of articular surface. (Courtesy of Shriners Hospitals for Children, Philadelphia, PA.)

Figure 8-39. A: A 16-year-old girl with a severe intra-articular pilon fracture of the small finger PIP joint. **B:** Traction radiograph helps define fracture components. **C:** Dorsal exposure reveals ulnar condyle outside of joint requiring incision of extensor tendon for reduction. **D:** Reduction of joint surface and K-wire fixation. **E:** Postoperative AP radiograph shows restoration of articular surface. **F:** Lateral radiograph shows sagittal alignment of condyles. (Courtesy of Shriners Hospitals for Children, Philadelphia, PA.)

Authors' Preferred Treatment for Middle and Proximal Phalangeal Fractures (Algorithm 8-2)

Physeal Fractures

Nondisplaced stable fractures are generally treated with immobilization for 3 weeks but can be treated with early range of motion and buddy tape in adolescents. Displaced S-H type I and II fractures are treated with closed reduction (Fig. 8-40). Alignment and rotation are verified by clinical examination and reduction is assessed with radiographs. Even subtle fractures can result in malrotation and digital scissoring, so all fractures need to be assessed

with tenodesis out of cast before immobilization treatment is chosen or continued (Fig. 8-41). Physeal fractures that are open or unstable after closed reduction require smooth percutaneous pin fixation. Irreducible fractures require open reduction, removal of any interposed tissue, and fixation.

Dorsal S-H type III or IV fractures that fail closed reduction of the middle phalangeal base often require open reduction and fixation to avoid the development of a boutonnière

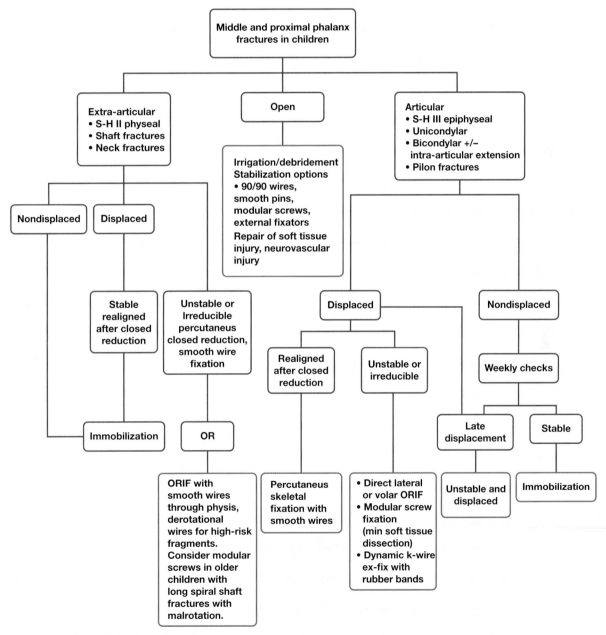

Algorithm 8-2. Authors' preferred treatment for middle and proximal phalangeal fractures.

deformity (Fig. 8-42). Lateral S-H type III fractures that are displaced more than 1.5 mm or involve more than 25% of the articular surface may also require ORIF.

Shaft Fractures

Nondisplaced fractures are treated with immobilization for 3 to 4 weeks. Displaced fractures are treated with CRPP fixation (Fig. 8-43). For a proximal phalangeal fracture, the MCP joint is flexed to relax the intrinsic muscle pull and stabilize the proximal fragment. Open reduction is reserved for open or irreducible fractures.

Neck Fractures

Phalangeal neck fractures usually require CRPP. The pins are placed through the collateral recesses to engage the proximal fragment in a crossed fashion or directly across the displaced fragment with the joint flexed. Open reduction should be avoided due to the risk of avascular necrosis. Late presentation of a neck fracture requires consideration of the time from injury, age of the patient, and fracture displacement. Considerable displacement requires treatment to regain joint flexion (Fig. 8-44). If the fracture line is still visible, a percutaneous pin osteoclasis is used.[87] The fracture is then stabilized with

additional percutaneous pins. A nascent or established malunion that cannot be reduced by osteoclasis can be treated by late open reduction or subcondylar fossa reconstruction. Mild loss of the condylar recess can be treated with recession of the prominent volar bone rather than risk osteonecrosis associated with extensive fracture mobilization by osteotomy.[74,80] In addition, slow remodeling is feasible in very young children without rotational malalignment and with a family that is willing to wait up to 2 years for remodeling and restoration of normal motion.[32,62]

Intra-Articular Fractures

Intra-articular fractures of the phalanges typically require percutaneous or open reduction. Unicondylar fractures that are mildly displaced can be treated with CRPP. Widely displaced unicondylar and bicondylar fractures require open reduction (see Fig. 8-37).

Pilon fractures or intra-articular fracture–dislocations present a management dilemma.[77] Open reduction is worthwhile when the fragments are large and the joint surface can be reconstructed. Bone grafting may be necessary to support the reduction. Severe articular damage and comminution are best treated with dynamic traction.[71]

Postoperative Care

The duration of immobilization after surgical intervention for phalangeal fractures is usually 3 to 4 weeks. Percutaneous pins are removed at the time and motion instituted. Formal hand therapy usually is not required, though the child must be encouraged to reestablish a normal usage pattern to improve

motion and flexibility. Periarticular fractures are monitored closely for persistent loss of motion that would benefit from formal hand therapy. Patients with complex fractures or replantation are more prone to develop stiffness. In these instances, therapy is routinely prescribed to regain motion. Therapy is directed at both flexion and extension of the injured digit. Static or dynamic splinting may be required after fracture healing.

A

B

Figure 8-40. A: An S-H type II fracture of the proximal phalanx of the thumb. **B:** Gentle closed reduction under fluoroscopic control obtained an anatomic reduction.

Figure 8-41. An 8-year-old girl was in a bouncy ball doing cartwheels when she felt a crack in her left ring finger. **A:** Innocuous fracture of the left finger proximal phalanx. **B:** Lateral x-ray with fracture difficult to recognize. **C:** Clinical examination benign with fingers in extension. **D:** Examination using wrist tenodesis for finger flexion demonstrated malrotation. (Courtesy of Shriners Hospital for Children, Philadelphia, PA.)

Figure 8-42. A, B: A 16-year-old boy sustained a dorsal S-H type IV fracture of the middle phalanx. **C:** Open reduction and internal screw fixation was accomplished through a dorsal approach. Radiographs show reduction of joint subluxation and fixation of fracture fragment. **D–F:** Postoperative extension and flexion with near-normal motion. (Courtesy of Shriners Hospitals for Children, Philadelphia, PA.)

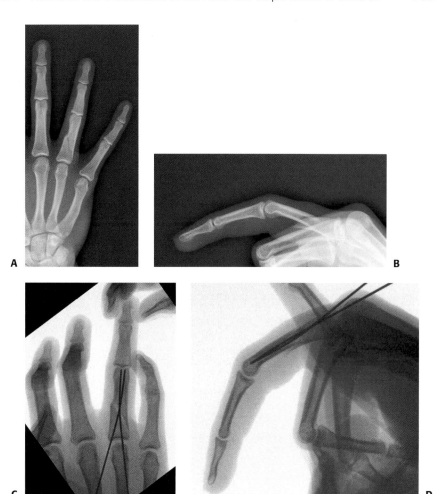

Figure 8-43. An 18-year-old young man injured his right finger 2 weeks earlier while tubing at camp. **A:** Anteroposterior x-ray with spiral fracture right ring finger proximal phalanx. **B:** Lateral x-ray with apex volar angulation. **C:** Anteroposterior fluoroscopic imaging demonstrating longitudinal traction and fracture reduction following intramedullary Kirschner-wire fixation. **D:** Fluoroscopic imaging demonstrating fracture reduction in the lateral plane. (Courtesy of Shriners Hospital for Children, Philadelphia, PA.)

Figure 8-44. Displaced phalangeal neck fracture of the proximal phalanx revealing loss of subchondral fossa at the PIP joint. If this is not corrected to anatomic alignment, there will be a mechanical block to flexion.

Potential Pitfalls and Preventive Measures

Middle and Proximal Phalanx Fractures: SURGICAL PITFALLS AND PREVENTIONS	
Pitfall	**Prevention**
Malrotation	• Check tenodesis intraoperatively • Use true lateral x-ray view to establish if radial and ulnar condyles of middle or proximal phalanx are overlapping
Osteonecrosis	• Minimize open procedures and soft tissue stripping of fragile blood supply to condyles
Pin-tract infection	• Bicortical fixation, relax any tension between the wire and skin, utilize dressings and immobilization to decrease motion between wire and skin
Stiffness	• Allow early range of motion as soon as clinically stable; radiographic union will lag behind clinical union

Outcomes

The overall results following proximal and middle phalangeal fractures are positive. Considering the frequency of these fractures, the occurrence of complications and functional impairment is low. Despite appropriate treatment, however, some children have permanent loss of motion, malunion, or growth disturbance. The major concern is to avoid rotational, articular, or periarticular malunion caused by the inappropriate diagnosis or treatment.

MANAGEMENT OF EXPECTED ADVERSE OUTCOMES AND UNEXPECTED COMPLICATIONS OF MIDDLE AND PROXIMAL PHALANGEAL FRACTURES

Middle and Proximal Phalangeal Fractures: COMMON ADVERSE OUTCOMES AND COMPLICATIONS

- Malunion, malrotation, finger deformity
- Growth arrest
- Stiffness
- Osteonecrosis
- Degenerative joint changes
- Pin-tract infection, osteomyelitis

Complications associated with proximal and middle phalangeal fractures begin with failure to recognize the injury (Fig. 8-45). AP and true lateral x-ray views of the injured digit must be made orthogonal and scrutinized for subtle abnormalities. Questionable findings warrant additional views or advanced imaging studies. A common misdiagnosis is failure to recognize a displaced phalangeal neck fracture because of inadequate lateral radiographs of the finger.

Another early complication is false interpretation of a "nondisplaced" fracture that is malrotated. All children with phalangeal fractures require careful examination for rotational alignment. The clinical examination is the mainstay for determining fracture rotation. Digital scissoring is indicative of fracture malrotation and requires reduction. Regardless of radiographic appearance, rotational alignment should be evaluated by active finger flexion and passive finger tenodesis via wrist extension.

Most phalangeal fractures can be maintained in satisfactory alignment after closed reduction. Certain fractures, however, have a propensity for redisplacement (Fig. 8-46). Oblique shaft fractures, unicondylar articular fractures, and neck fractures are prime examples of fractures that are best treated with closed reduction and pin fixation rather than manipulation alone.

Late complications include rare nonunion, malunion, osteonecrosis, growth disturbance, and arthritis. Nonunion is rare except in combined injuries with devascularization of the fracture fragments. Bone grafting is usually successful for union. Malunion can result in angulation or limited motion. Extraarticular malunion can cause angulation or rotational abnormalities. The treatment depends on the child's age and ability to remodel according to fracture location, plane of malunion, and degree of deformity (Fig. 8-47). Considerable deformity may require osteotomy to realign the bone.[27] A subcondylar or intra-articular malunion is particularly difficult to treat. Early diagnosis within the first month offers the possibility of fracture realignment through the site of deformity. Treatment of a late diagnosis must include consideration of the risks and benefits associated with extensive surgery. Successful late osteotomies can restore normal digital alignment and functional recovery, but risk nonunion, stiffness, and pain (Fig. 8-48).

Osteonecrosis is usually related to extensive fracture comminution, soft tissue injury, or surgical dissection of an intraarticular fracture. In severe cases, reconstruction is limited to some form of joint transfer or fusion of the joint (Fig. 8-49). Growth disturbance can result from any injury that involves the

Figure 8-45. A: A 3-year-old girl sustained a fracture of the neck of the proximal phalanx of the index and middle fingers. The displaced fracture in the middle finger appears similar to an epiphysis at the distal end of the phalanx. **B:** No true lateral radiograph of the injured finger was obtained. Close scrutiny of this lateral view shows a dorsally displaced neck fracture, rotated almost 90 degrees (*arrow*). **C:** A lateral radiograph taken 18 months later reveals malunion with hyperextension of the PIP joint and loss of flexion.

Figure 8-46. **A, B:** An 8-year-old girl with a mildly displaced fracture of the neck of the middle phalanx. **C:** Closed reduction was successful on the day of injury and a plaster splint was applied. **D:** Two weeks later, the fracture had markedly redisplaced.

A

B

C

D

Figure 8-47. **A:** A 13-year-old boy with malunion of the ring finger middle phalanx articular surface. **B, C:** Radiographs reveal slight malunion of the radial condyle with mild intra-articular incongruity. The lateral view suggests a double-density shadow (*arrow*). The flexion and extension motion of the digit was normal, and reconstruction was not recommended.   **A, B**

C

Figure 8-50. A: An S-H type II fracture of the metacarpal head. **B:** Head-splitting fracture of the metacarpal epiphysis.

subcondylar fossa is relatively thin, making it vulnerable to injury. Neck fractures in children are analogous to boxer's fractures in adults (Fig. 8-51). Neck fractures are more common in the small and ring fingers. Fortunately, these injuries are juxtaphyseal and have considerable remodeling potential.

METACARPAL SHAFT FRACTURES

Metacarpal shaft fractures are relatively common. Torsional forces combined with axial load cause long oblique and spiral fractures whereas direct trauma (being stepped on or a heavy object dropping onto the hand) produces short oblique or transverse fractures. An isolated shaft fracture of a central ray is suspended by the intermetacarpal ligaments, which limit displacement and shortening. In contrast, the border digits (index and small) displace more readily.

METACARPAL BASE FRACTURES

Metacarpal base fractures are less common in children than in adults. The base is protected from injury by its proximal location in the hand and the stability afforded by the bony congruence and soft tissue restraints. The small finger CMC joint is the most prone to injury. Fracture–dislocations of the small finger CMC joint are often unstable because of the proximal pull of the extensor carpi ulnaris (reverse Bennett fracture).

TREATMENT OPTIONS FOR METACARPAL FRACTURES

The treatment of metacarpal fractures varies with the location, extent, and configuration of the fracture. Nonoperative or closed treatment is the primary mode of management for most fractures. Operative intervention is used for extensive soft tissue injury, intra-articular head-splitting fractures, malrotated fractures, and irreducible fractures. While multiple metacarpal fractures in an indication for surgery in skeletally mature, in children these injuries can often times be treated successfully if minimally displaced and acceptable clinical digit alignment. Attempts at

Figure 8-51. A: A true boxer's fracture of the metacarpal neck of the fifth ray. **B:** This fracture is more in the diaphysis and should not be considered a boxer's fracture.

CRPP should be utilized before proceeding with open reduction and fixation to minimize invasiveness of treatment.

INDICATIONS/CONTRAINDICATIONS

Metacarpal Fractures:
INDICATIONS FOR NONOPERATIVE VERSUS OPERATIVE TREATMENT

Nonoperative Indications

- Nondisplaced
- Closed
- Reducible
- Stable

Operative Indications

- Multiple metacarpals (Not a strict indication. Some injuries with multiple metacarpal fractures with minimal displacement can heal without operative fixation)
- Open or extensive soft tissue injury
- Displaced articular
- Unstable
- Irreducible
- Malrotation
- Excessive shortening

OPERATIVE TREATMENT OF METACARPAL FRACTURES

ORIF of Metacarpal Fractures

Preoperative Planning

Technique

 ORIF of Metacarpal Fractures:
KEY SURGICAL STEPS

- ❑ Expose longitudinally and dorsally with incision directly over metacarpal or in the case of multiple fractures, in the interval between the two fractured metacarpals
- ❑ Protect the extensor tendons and their juncturae. Handle with care, as increased manipulation may lead to postoperative adhesions
- ❑ Split the periosteum over the metacarpal shaft
- ❑ Use towel clips, bone clamps, or tenaculums to reduce fracture and pin with longitudinal crossed pattern, proximal to distal or distal to proximal
- ❑ Definitive fixation can be accomplished with K-wires, screws, or plates and screws depending on fracture configuration
- ❑ In Bennett fractures, reduce displaced lateral metacarpal to intact ulnar fragment that is attached to the volar beak ligament
- ❑ Metacarpal neck fractures are amenable to closed reduction and percutaneous stabilization with K-wires
- ❑ Always check digit rotation and alignment after fracture fixation by assessing tenodesis

Metacarpal Head Fractures

A metacarpal head-splitting fracture may be difficult to detect and requires special x-ray views. The Brewerton view is helpful and is performed with the dorsum of the hand against the cassette and the MCP joints flexed about 65 degrees. The central beam is angled 15 degrees to the ulnar side of the hand.[46] This projection focuses on the metacarpal heads and may highlight subtle bony abnormalities. An MRI or CT scan to assess articular alignment is diagnostic in complex injuries; however, advanced imaging is reserved for difficult cases.

Displaced intra-articular head-splitting fractures require fixation to restore articular congruity. Many of these fractures have unrecognized comminution that complicates internal fixation. Closed reduction with percutaneous fixation can be utilized if articular alignment is able to be obtained. Utilizing live fluoroscopy is helpful in these cases to ensure anatomic alignment. When open reduction is necessary, K-wire or screw fixation is used depending on the age of the patient and size of the fragments. Transosseous suture repair may be necessary for small fragments. Bone grafting may be necessary to support the articular reduction. The primary goal of surgical treatment is anatomic reduction of the joint. A secondary goal is stable fixation to allow early motion. Open approach is performed dorsally by dividing the extensor tendon or sagittal band longitudinally to allow full visualization of the head fracture.

Metacarpal Neck Fractures

Metacarpal neck fractures are usually treated by closed methods. The amount of acceptable apex dorsal angulation in children as in adults is controversial. Greater angulation is allowable in the mobile ring and small rays compared to the index and long. Another consideration is the effect of remodeling over time, which is dependent on the age of the child. In general, 10 to 30 degrees of angulation greater than the corresponding CMC joint motion is acceptable. AP and lateral x-ray views may be supplemented by an oblique view to assess fracture configuration. Two additional reduction indications include an extensor lag of the involved digit or notable prominence of the metacarpal head in the palm in racquet and batting athletes, where the head would block function of grasping.

Considerable angulation can be treated with attempted closed reduction with local anesthesia or conscious sedation and splint or cast application, although attempts at reduction may not ultimately affect the final angulation.[48] The Jahss maneuver is commonly recommended and involves initial flexion of the MCP joint to 90 degrees to relax the deforming force of the intrinsic muscles and tighten the collateral ligaments.[38] Subsequently, upward pressure is applied along the proximal phalanx to push the metacarpal head in a dorsal direction whereas counterpressure is applied along the dorsal aspect of the proximal metacarpal fracture. Immobilization with a plaster splint or cast with three-point molding over the volar metacarpal head and proximal dorsal shaft is recommended. In addition, immobilization with the fingers more extended to maintain the fracture reduction is acceptable as MCP joint stiffness is less problematic in young patients in comparison to adults.[79] The PIP joints may or may not be included in the immobilization depending on the status of the reduction and reliability of the patient.

Uncommonly, a neck fracture may be unstable or notably flexed and require percutaneous pinning. Pins can be inserted in a variety of configurations. Extramedullary techniques include crossed pinning or pinning to the adjacent stable metacarpal. Intramedullary techniques can also be used, similar to those used for metacarpal shaft and neck fractures in adults.[28,69] Intramedullary techniques are reserved for patients near physeal closure. Pre-bent K-wires or commercially available implants are inserted through the metacarpal base in an antegrade fashion. The wires can be used to assist in fracture reduction. Stability is obtained by stacking several wires within the canal and across the fracture site.

Open reduction of metacarpal neck fractures is seldom required in children and is reserved for irreducible fractures, unstable fractures in skeletally mature children, and combination injuries that require a stable bony platform.

Metacarpal Shaft Fractures

An isolated long or ring metacarpal fracture is often minimally displaced because the metacarpals are suspended by the intermetacarpal ligaments. Immobilization for 4 weeks in a cast or metacarpal cuff brace is typically all that is necessary. In contrast, the index and small digits may require additional treatment, such as closed reduction and immobilization. Unstable shaft fractures can require fixation, such as percutaneous pinning or intramedullary screw fixation (Fig. 8-52). Pins can be inserted with extramedullary or intramedullary techniques. Intramedullary screws are placed through the dorsal articular surface of the head of the metacarpal and down the shaft. Care must be taken to ensure no malrotation with placement. Diaphyseal fractures are slower to heal and more prone to malunion than neck fractures.

An ORIF approach to a metacarpal shaft fracture is rarely indicated in children unless there are multiple unstable fractures or extensive soft tissue damage. However, a long spiral–oblique fracture with substantial malrotation and shortening may benefit from mini-screw fixation to reestablish anatomic alignment and normal digit cascade.

Metacarpal Base Fractures

Fractures of the metacarpal base or fracture–dislocations at the CMC joint are usually high-energy injuries with substantial tissue disruption. Assessment for signs of hand compartment syndrome and careful neurovascular assessment are mandatory. Isolated fracture–dislocations of the small ray CMC joint are the most common metacarpal base fractures. A CT scan may better define articular congruity and comminution. A CRPP approach is usually sufficient to restore alignment and resist the deforming force of the extensor carpi ulnaris. The reduction is performed with longitudinal traction of the metacarpal and dorsal pressure on the metacarpal base. The pins can be placed transversely between the small and ring metacarpals and/or across the fifth CMC joint.

Open reduction may be necessary to achieve reduction and ensure stable fixation in high-energy injuries. A transverse or longitudinal incision can be used for exposure. Longitudinal incisions are recommended in patients with concomitant compartment syndrome to allow for simultaneous decompression. Fixation options are numerous, depending on the fracture configuration. Oftentimes there is a sufficiently large hamate avulsion fragment, which can be fixed independently with screw or wire fixation. Supplemental bone graft may be necessary for substantial comminution. Late presentation is especially difficult. Treatment often requires open reduction or CMC arthrodesis (Fig. 8-53).

Figure 8-52. A: Midshaft fifth metacarpal fracture in a skeletally immature patient fixed with crossing K-wires. **B:** Skeletally mature teenage athlete with a fifth metacarpal fracture treated with an intramedullary screw. (Courtesy of Dr. Charles A. Goldfarb.)

Figure 8-53. A 15-year-old boy with crush injury of the right hand requiring compartment release. He presented 6 weeks later with persistent pain and limited motion. **A:** An AP radiograph shows overlapping long, ring, and small CMC joints. **B:** Lateral radiographs reveal fracture–dislocations of long, ring, and small CMC joints. **C:** Postoperative AP radiograph after reduction and CMC fusion using miniplates. **D:** Lateral radiograph after reduction and CMC fusion. (Courtesy of Shriners Hospitals for Children, Philadelphia, PA.)

Authors' Preferred Treatment for Metacarpal Fractures (Algorithm 8-3)

Metacarpal Head Fractures

Metacarpal head-splitting fractures need anatomic reduction at the articular surface, obtained either open or closed and stabilized with K-wire or screw fixation.

Metacarpal Neck Fractures

Nonoperative and closed methods are the mainstays of treatment. Small and ring fingers can accept more flexion deformity then index and ring fingers. Reduction is indicated for those with extensor lag or rotation of the involved digit, or notable prominence in the palm of the metacarpal head. Pin fixation is used for unstable fractures, and open reduction is rarely necessary.

Metacarpal Shaft Fractures

Isolated fractures that are minimally displaced require only immobilization. Isolated fractures that are displaced or malrotated require reduction and fixation. An irreducible fracture or multiple unstable fractures usually require open reduction. The operative approach and internal fixation principles are similar in children and adults.

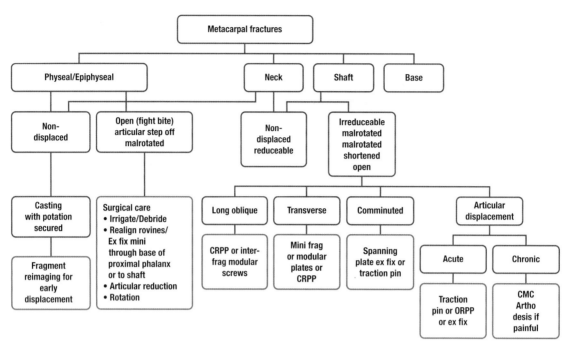

Algorithm 8-3. Authors' preferred treatment for metacarpal fractures.

Metacarpal Base Fractures

Extra-articular metacarpal base fractures can be treated by closed reduction with or without percutaneous pinning. Intra-articular fracture–dislocations are more challenging. Percutaneous pinning is often required to stabilize the fracture and to reduce CMC joint subluxation (Fig. 8-54). Irreducible or multiple fracture–dislocations require open reduction. Late presentation with symptomatic degenerative changes requires CMC arthrodesis (see Fig. 8-53).

Figure 8-54. A 12-year-old boy fell off a scooter, injuring his left hand. **A:** Anteroposterior x-ray with comminuted fracture at the base of the small metacarpal. **B:** Longitudinal traction resulted in anatomic reduction, followed by percutaneous pin fixation. (Courtesy of Shriners Hospital for Children, Philadelphia, PA.)

A

B

Postoperative Care

Most metacarpal fractures managed by closed treatment are immobilized for 4 weeks. Subsequently, a home program of range-of-motion exercises is started and formal therapy is not needed. In active children and young athletes, a light splint can be worn for protection and as a reminder for the patient and others that the hand is still healing for an additional few weeks. If percutaneous pin fixation is used, the wires are removed in the office 4 weeks after surgery.

Rehabilitation of open fracture reduction depends on the stability of the fixation and the reliability of the patient to postoperative recommendations. Older and reliable patients with stable internal fixation are mobilized earlier, usually 5 to 7 days after surgery. A removable splint for protection between exercise sessions is used for 4 to 6 weeks.

Potential Pitfalls and Preventive Measures

Metacarpal Fractures:
SURGICAL PITFALLS AND PREVENTIONS

Pitfall	Prevention
Malrotation/malunion	• Check tenodesis • After each K-wire or reduction maneuver, recheck tenodesis
Osteonecrosis of metacarpal head	• Avoid dissection of fragments during open repair

MANAGEMENT OF EXPECTED ADVERSE OUTCOMES AND UNEXPECTED COMPLICATIONS RELATED TO METACARPAL FRACTURES

Metacarpal Fractures:
COMMON ADVERSE OUTCOMES AND COMPLICATIONS

• Epiphyseal and physeal fractures: osteonecrosis, malreduction/malunion
• Neck fractures: Excessive apex dorsal angulation, malrotation
• Shaft fractures: Malrotation, soft tissue interposition, nonunion
• Metacarpal base fractures: Loss of reduction, malreduction of articular fragments, late instability, arthritis

Most metacarpal fractures heal without sequelae. Mild deformity in the plane of motion is tolerated and may correct with remodeling. Considerable angulation or rotation creates a functional impairment that requires treatment.

Bony complications include malunion and osteonecrosis. Nonunion is rare.[36] Even a small amount (less than 10 degrees) of rotational malalignment may create overlap of the digits during flexion and a functional disturbance requiring corrective osteotomy. The osteotomy for rotational correction can be made at the site of fracture or anywhere along the metacarpal. The proximal shaft or base is advantageous because it provides ample bone for healing and offers the opportunity for internal

fixation using wires or a plate. Diaphyseal malunions with symptomatic flexion deformity into the palm require a dorsal wedge osteotomy and internal fixation.

Osteonecrosis of the metacarpal head may occur after an intra-articular fracture. Factors include the degree of injury and the intracapsular pressure caused by the hemarthrosis. Theoretically, early joint aspiration may diminish the intra-articular pressure. Fortunately, partial osteonecrosis in a growing child incites remarkable remodeling of the adjacent articular surface and often results in a functional joint. Part-time splint protection during the remodeling phase is recommended. Considerable joint incongruity is rare and reconstruction options are limited. However, recent experience with osteochondral autograft transplant surgery (OATS) transfer from the knee has been successful.[44]

Thumb Metacarpal Fractures in Children

CLASSIFICATION OF THUMB METACARPAL FRACTURES

Classification of Thumb Metacarpal Fractures

• Fractures of the head
• Fractures of the shaft
• Intra-articular S-H type III or IV fractures of the thumb metacarpal base/epiphysis
• Physeal/epiphyseal S-H type II fractures—types A, B, C, D
• Thumb metacarpal shaft fractures
• Thumb metacarpal neck fractures
• Thumb metacarpal head fractures

Fractures of the thumb metacarpal can occur at the epiphysis, physis, neck, shaft, or base. Fractures of the neck and shaft and their treatment principles are similar to those of the fingers. Thumb metacarpal base fractures that involve the physis or epiphysis require unique considerations (Fig. 8-55).

The adductor pollicis, abductor pollicis longus, and thenar muscles play a role in fracture mechanics and can displace thumb

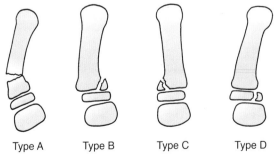

Type A   Type B   Type C   Type D

Figure 8-55. Classification of thumb metacarpal fractures. **Type A:** Metaphyseal fracture. **Types B and C:** S-H type II physeal fractures with lateral or medial angulation. **Type D:** An S-H type III fracture (pediatric Bennett fracture).

metacarpal fractures. The muscles' directions of pull dictate the direction of fracture displacement and deformity. The adductor pollicis inserts onto the proximal phalanx and into the extensor apparatus through the adductor aponeurosis. The abductor pollicis longus inserts onto the metacarpal base and is the primary deforming force in most fracture–dislocations about the thumb CMC joint (Bennett fractures or pediatric equivalents).

Direct trauma, rotational forces, and axial loading may all cause thumb metacarpal fractures. Sporting endeavors are the prime events causing fractures. Skiing, biking, and playing baseball catcher are specific activities that place the thumb MCP joint and metacarpal shaft in a vulnerable position. Adduction forces, such as direct trauma to a soccer goalie or basketball player during a fall or ball injury, place the thumb CMC joint and base of thumb metacarpal at risk.

THUMB METACARPAL BASE FRACTURES

Fractures of the base of the thumb metacarpal are subdivided according to their location. Type A fractures occur between the physis and the junction of the proximal and middle thirds of the bone. The fractures are often transverse or slightly oblique. There is often an element of medial impaction, and the fracture is angulated in an apex lateral direction (Fig. 8-56).

Figure 8-56. Metaphyseal thumb metacarpal fracture that does not involve the physis. Treatment consisted of closed reduction and cast immobilization.

Type B and C fractures are S-H type II fractures at the thumb metacarpal base. Most patterns have the metaphyseal fragment on the medial side (type B) (Fig. 8-56). The shaft fragment is adducted by the pull of the adductor pollicis and shifted in a proximal direction by the pull of the abductor pollicis longus. Although this pattern resembles a Bennett fracture with respect to the deforming forces, there is no intra-articular extension. Type C fractures are the least common and have the reverse pattern, with the metaphyseal fragment on the lateral side and the proximal shaft displacement in a medial direction. This pattern often results from more substantial trauma and does not lend itself to closed treatment.

A type D fracture is an S-H type III or IV fracture that most closely resembles the adult Bennett fracture. The deforming forces are similar to a type B injury with resultant adduction and proximal migration of the base-shaft fragment.

Biplanar x-rays including a hyperpronated view of the thumb accentuate the view of the CMC joint. Examination under live fluoroscopy or CT scan may also be helpful for preoperative planning and classification of fracture severity.

TREATMENT OPTIONS FOR THUMB METACARPAL BASE FRACTURES

Thumb Metacarpal Fractures: INDICATIONS FOR NONOPERATIVE VERSUS OPERATIVE TREATMENT

Nonoperative Indications

- Nondisplaced
- Closed
- Reducible
- Stable

Operative Indications

- Displaced articular
- Open or extensive soft tissue injury
- Irreducible
- Unstable

Type A Fractures

Type A fractures can usually be treated by closed methods. Although swelling about the thenar eminence limits manipulation of the fracture and diminishes the effectiveness of immobilization, most fractures can still be treated successfully by closed reduction and immobilization. Because the CMC joint has near-universal motion and the physis is proximal in the metacarpal, remodeling is extensive in young patients. The multiplanar motion of the CMC joint combined with the potential for remodeling makes less than 20 to 30 degrees of angulation inconsequential. If reduction is attempted, pressure is applied to the apex of the fracture to effect reduction. Anatomic reduction is not required because remodeling is plentiful. Unstable fractures with marked displacement require percutaneous pin fixation to maintain alignment (Fig. 8-57).

Figure 8-57. A 13-year-old boy fell downstairs and injured his right thumb. **A:** An AP radiograph shows displaced fracture base of the thumb metacarpal. **B:** Lateral radiograph shows considerable angulation. **C:** At time of reduction, fracture was very unstable. **D:** Closed reduction under fluoroscopy. **E:** Percutaneous pin fixation to maintain alignment. (Courtesy of Shriners Hospitals for Children, Philadelphia, PA.)

Type B and C Fractures

Closed reduction is more difficult for type B and C fractures. The mobility of the metacarpal and the swelling make closed reduction difficult.[63] Comminution, soft tissue interposition, or transperiosteal "buttonholing" in type C fractures may further complicate reduction. If closed reduction is accomplished and stable, then short-arm thumb spica splint or cast immobilization is possible. Repeat radiographic evaluation should be obtained 5 to 7 days later to ensure maintenance of reduction.

If closed reduction is possible but the reduction is unstable, percutaneous pinning is recommended (Fig. 8-58). There are multiple options for pin configuration including direct fixation across the fracture, pinning across the reduced CMC joint, and pinning between the first and second metacarpals. Open reduction is indicated for irreducible fractures. Type C fractures more often require open reduction to remove potential interposed periosteum that blocks reduction (Fig. 8-59).

Type D Fractures

Type D fractures are unstable and require closed or open reduction to restore physeal and articular alignment. An acceptable closed reduction is maintained by percutaneous pin fixation.

Figure 8-58. A: An 8-year-old boy with reducible, but unstable, fracture. **B:** A single percutaneous pin was placed to maintain alignment.

An unacceptable closed reduction is rare but when it occurs, it requires open reduction and fixation. The choice of implant must be individualized, though smooth wires are favored to minimize potential injury to the physis and articular cartilage. These injuries nearly all require fixation across the CMC joint to maintain the reduction.

Figure 8-59. A: Fracture of the thumb metacarpal base with a small lateral metaphyseal flag that appears innocuous on radiograph (*arrow*). **B:** However, additional images revealed marked displacement of the distal fragment. **C:** Closed reduction was unsuccessful because of interposed tissue. After open reduction, K-wires were used to stabilize the fracture.

Authors' Preferred Treatment of Thumb Metacarpal Fractures (Algorithm 8-4)

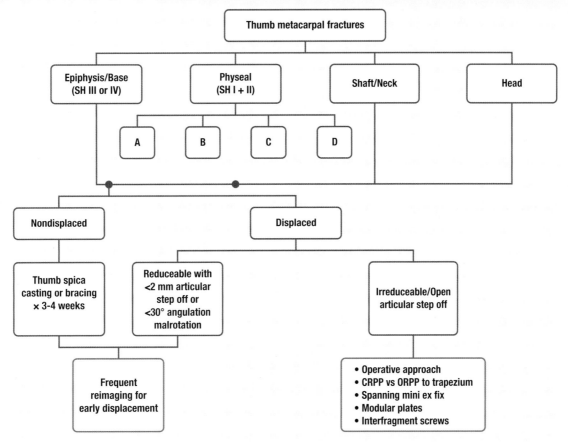

Algorithm 8-4. Authors' preferred treatment for thumb metacarpal fractures.

POSTOPERATIVE CARE

Closed treatment requires immobilization for 4 to 6 weeks depending on the fracture severity and degree of soft tissue damage. A home program for range of motion is started thereafter. A removable custom splint is fabricated for protection for a few additional weeks after initial immobilization. Formal therapy is not instituted unless considerable soft tissue injury occurred.

Open reduction and fixation postoperative management depends on the stability of the fixation and the reliability of the patient. Young children or marginal fracture fixations require 4 to 6 weeks of immobilization. Fracture union with mild stiffness takes precedence over fracture nonunion with excessive motion. Typically K-wires can be removed at 4 weeks a removable splint fabricated and range of motion begun. If any question of stability, then K-wires are removed at 5 to 6 weeks. A removable splint is used for protection between exercise sessions until union. Strengthening is typically started, if necessary at 6 to 8 weeks.

MANAGEMENT OF EXPECTED ADVERSE OUTCOMES AND UNEXPECTED COMPLICATIONS RELATED TO THUMB METACARPAL FRACTURES

Thumb metacarpal fractures usually heal without altering hand function. The remodeling capabilities of fractures near or involving the physis are extensive. The basilar thumb joint also allows multiplanar motion and can accommodate moderate fracture malunion. Residual deformity along the thumb metacarpal can be concealed through CMC joint motion, and the thumb tolerates malrotation better than the fingers (Fig. 8-60).

Complications are uncommon. Nonunion, malunion, and articular incongruity are potential problems. Intra-articular incongruity may occur after incomplete reduction of an intra-articular fracture or inadequate fixation after an initial satisfactory reduction. Sequelae include pain, diminished motion, and arthrosis. Available treatment options include intra-articular osteotomy, fusion, or interposition arthroplasty.

Figure 8-60. A 14-year-old boy presents 3 weeks after injury with mild pain and deformity at the base of right thumb. **A:** An AP radiograph shows a moderately displaced fracture at the base of the thumb metacarpal. **B:** Lateral radiograph shows mild angulation. **C:** Follow-up motion after splinting for an additional 2 weeks, and home therapy reveals excellent opposition. **D:** The thumb is able to touch the base of the small finger. (Courtesy of Shriners Hospitals for Children, Philadelphia, PA.)

Fractures of the Carpal Bones

INTRODUCTION TO FRACTURES OF THE CARPAL BONES

SCAPHOID FRACTURES

The low incidence of scaphoid fractures in children is most likely related to the thick peripheral cartilage that covers and protects the ossification center. Therefore, fracture requires a considerable force to disrupt this cartilaginous shell and injure the underlying bone. The pattern of scaphoid injury in young children differs from that of adults because of the evolving ossification center. During early stages of ossification, the scaphoid is more susceptible to avulsion fractures about the distal pole fracture. As the ossification progresses from distal to proximal, the fracture pattern mirrors the adult forms by early adolescence[13,21,81] (Fig. 8-61).

In children, fractures of the distal third of the scaphoid have traditionally been the most common injury pattern and often result from direct trauma. However, scaphoid waist fractures are increasing in frequency in younger children as participation in contact athletics begins earlier.[26] Proximal pole fractures are rare in children and often represent an avulsion fracture of the scapholunate ligament. Proximal pole fractures are at higher risk for nonunion and osteonecrosis. The scaphoid can also be fractured as a component of a greater arc perilunate injury[2,33] (Fig. 8-62).

Classification of Scaphoid Fractures

Figure 8-61. Three types of scaphoid fractures. **A:** Distal third. **B:** Middle third. **C:** Proximal pole.

Classification of Scaphoid Fractures	
Type	**Description**
A	Fractures of the distal pole
A1	Extra-articular distal pole fractures
A2	Intra-articular distal pole fractures
B	Fractures of the middle third (waist fractures)
C	Fractures of the proximal third

Type A: Fractures of the Distal Pole

Distal pole fractures are often secondary to direct trauma or avulsion with a dorsoradial or dorsovolar fragment. The strong scaphotrapezial ligaments and capsular attachments produce

Figure 8-62. A 13-year-old boy was playing tag at night when he jumped over a wall, falling 5 feet onto his outstretched left wrist. A closed reduction and CT scan were performed at an outside institution. **A:** Lateral x-rays with volar perilunate and multiple carpal fractures. **B:** Semisupinated lateral x-ray with markedly displaced carpal fractures. **C:** 3D CT scan demonstrated fractures of the radial styloid, lunate, and triquetrum. **D:** Postoperative anteroposterior x-ray status post open reduction and internal fixation radial styloid, scaphoid fracture, and lunate fracture. **E:** Postoperative lateral x-ray after fixation of carpal fractures. (Courtesy of Shriners Hospital for Children, Philadelphia, PA.)

A

B

C, D

E

Figure 8-63. A 13-year-old boy girl onto an outstretched hand and was tender over scaphoid tubercle. Radiograph reveals a small avulsion fracture of the distal scaphoid that might easily be overlooked.

Figure 8-64. A 12-year-old boy fell playing ice hockey and complained of right wrist pain. Radiograph reveals an extra-articular distal pole scaphoid fracture with slight comminution. (Courtesy of Shriners Hospitals for Children, Philadelphia, PA.)

mechanical failure through the bone (Fig. 8-63). The fracture line and size of the avulsion fragment vary from an isolated chondral injury that is barely visible on radiographs to a large osteochondral fragment.

Type A1: Extra-Articular Distal Pole Fractures

Extra-articular fractures may be either volar or dorsal avulsions (Fig. 8-64). A volar pattern is more common and is attributed to the stout scaphotrapezial ligaments. A dorsal fracture configuration is less common and is attributed to the dorsal intercarpal ligament. The fragments vary in size, and the radiographic appearance is age-dependent.

Type A2: Intra-Articular Distal Pole Fractures

This type of fracture may be a variation of a type A1 fracture with an intra-articular extension. Similar types (i.e., volar and dorsal) and mechanisms of injury are possible.

Type B: Fractures of the Middle Third (Waist Fractures)

Middle-third fractures do occur in skeletally immature patients. The mechanism of injury is usually a fall onto the outstretched hand and pronated forearm, which exerts tensile forces acting across the volar portion of the scaphoid as the wrist extends. Bony comminution may be present (Fig. 8-65). A careful scrutiny for other injuries about the carpus is mandatory.

Dividing the bone into thirds or delineating the area bounded by the radioscaphocapitate ligament defines the waist of the scaphoid. Waist fractures occur in many forms. Pediatric fractures may be incomplete, minimally displaced, or complete with or without displacement. Comminuted fractures are rare and are associated with higher-energy injuries.

Type C: Fractures of the Proximal Third

Proximal pole fractures are rare in children but not infrequent in adolescent athletes. A proximal pole fracture may propagate through the interface between newly ossified tissue and the cartilaginous anlage, or the injury may be strictly through the cartilage. Proximal fractures may cause destabilization of the scapholunate joint, as the scapholunate interosseous ligament remains attached to the avulsed fragment (Fig. 8-66).

Proximal third fractures present diagnostic and therapeutic dilemmas. The proximal pole is the last to ossify, which further complicates diagnosis. The tenuous blood supply of this region presents the same problems in children as adults in terms of nonunion and risks of osteonecrosis.

Bipartite Scaphoid Controversy: Traumatic Versus Developmental

A bipartite scaphoid probably exists but is uncommon and may be associated with Down syndrome.[16,51] Criteria that must be met to diagnose a congenital bipartite scaphoid include the following: (1) similar bilateral appearance, (2) absence of historical or clinical evidence of antecedent trauma, (3) equal size and

A   B

Figure 8-65. **A:** A displaced midwaist scaphoid fracture with comminution, including a butterfly fragment from the volar radial aspect (*arrow*). **B:** A CT scan demonstrates the comminution.

uniform density of each component, (4) absence of degenerative change between the scaphoid components or elsewhere in the carpus, and (5) smooth, rounded architecture of each scaphoid component. A unilateral "bipartite scaphoid" should be viewed as a post-traumatic scaphoid nonunion (Fig. 8-67).

CAPITATE FRACTURES

Isolated fractures of the capitate are rare and usually result from high-energy trauma. Capitate fractures may represent a form of greater arc perilunar injury (Fig. 8-68). The force can propagate completely around the lunate and cause a perilunate or lunate dislocation. The injury can also halt within the capitate and produce a scaphocapitate syndrome, a trans-scaphoid, transcapitate perilunar injury.[2,33,84]

Excessive dorsiflexion of the wrist is the most common mechanism. The waist of the capitate abuts the lunate or dorsal

aspect of the radius. The fracture occurs through the waist with variable displacement. The wrist is usually markedly swollen and painful to palpation. The clinical presentation varies with the associated carpal injuries. Median nerve paresthesias may be present secondary to swelling within the carpal tunnel.

Standard AP and lateral views are usually adequate (Fig. 8-69). Careful scrutiny of the radiographs is necessary. The capitate fracture can be subtle, or the proximal capitate fragment can rotate 180 degrees. Either scenario can create a confusing image that often results in misinterpretation. Incomplete ossification further complicates radiographic diagnosis and degree of displacement. Small osteochondral fragments in the midcarpal region may indicate a greater arc injury or isolated capitate fracture. In these cases, advanced imaging studies, such as MRI or CT, may be useful[59] (Fig. 8-70).

TRIQUETRUM FRACTURES

Dorsal avulsion fractures of the triquetrum are more common in adults than in children. The injury may occur in adolescents as carpal ossification nears completion. A fracture through the body of the triquetrum is rare and may occur with a perilunar injury as the path of the greater arc injury passes through the triquetrum (see Fig. 8-62). A fall on an outstretched wrist is the common event. The probable mechanism for a dorsal triquetrum fracture is a pulling force through the dorsal ligaments or abutment of the ulnar styloid. The wrist is mildly swollen and painful to palpation directly over the dorsal triquetrum. The clinical presentation is more severe with associated carpal injuries. Radiologic AP and lateral views may not show the avulsion fracture. A pronated oblique view highlights the dorsum of the triquetrum and can reveal the avulsed fragment (Fig. 8-71). At times, a CT scan is necessary for accurate diagnosis.

Figure 8-66. An AP radiograph of an 18-year-old male football player with a proximal one-third scaphoid fracture.

A, B   C

Figure 8-67. A: A 9-year-old boy who fell on an outstretched wrist and had radial-sided pain and tenderness; original radiographs failed to reveal any bony abnormalities. **B:** About 1.5 years later, he had persistent radial-sided wrist pain, and radiographs revealed a midwaist scaphoid nonunion. This would *not* be considered a bipartite scaphoid but instead, an injury that was sustained when the cartilaginous anlage was present. **C:** After 2 months of casting, early fracture union is present.

HAMATE, PISIFORM, LUNATE, AND TRAPEZIUM FRACTURES

Pediatric fractures of the hamate, pisiform, lunate, and trapezium are rare. Hamate fractures are classified by their location in the hook, type I, or in the body, type II. Hook of the hamate fractures may occur in adolescents who play baseball or golf or following a fall, usually bicycle related. If the fracture involves the distal third of the hook, it may have occurred from an avulsion injury secondary to pull from the transverse carpal ligament. A CT scan or MRI may be necessary for diagnosis if the fracture is not visible on the carpal tunnel view (Fig. 8-72).

Figure 8-68. Progressive perilunar instability. The greater arc (*black arrow*) is associated with fractures of the carpal bones, which may include the scaphoid, lunate, capitate, hamate, and triquetrum. The *red arrow* depicts the lesser arc, in which forces are transmitted only through soft tissue structures. (Reprinted from Mayfield JK, et al. Carpal dislocations: pathomechanics and progressive perilunar instability. *J Hand Surg Am.* 1980;5(3):226–241. Copyright © 1980 American Society for Surgery of the Hand. With permission.)

Figure 8-69. A 12-year-old boy sustained multiple carpal fractures attributed to a crushing injury. An established nonunion of the capitate is present 16 months later, which required bone grafting to obtain union. (Courtesy of James H. Dobyns, MD.)

Figure 8-70. A 13-year-old boy with persistent midcarpal pain after a fall. An MRI scan shows a capitate fracture. (Courtesy of Shriners Hospitals for Children, Philadelphia, PA.)

Figure 8-71. A minimally displaced dorsal triquetral avulsion fracture (*arrow*) that was treated with short-term immobilization.

Figure 8-72. A: A 15-year-old baseball player with chronic pain over hypothenar eminence while batting. **B:** A CT scan coronal view demonstrated a base of the hook of the hamate fracture. **C:** After 3 months of immobilization and rest from baseball, the patient is elected for fragment removal. Returned to baseball wearing a silicone gel patch in his batting glove over the hypothenar area.

Dorsal or body hamate fractures can occur with axial load or punching injuries, as the bases of the fourth and fifth metacarpals act like pistons and shear off large or small pieces of the hamate.

Pisiform fractures are the result of direct trauma. Lunate fractures are associated with Kienböck disease, which is relatively uncommon in children. Trapezium fractures can occur with CMC joint injuries about the thumb.

ASSESSMENT AND TREATMENT OPTIONS FOR FRACTURES OF THE CARPAL BONES

INDICATIONS/CONTRAINDICATIONS

Fractures of the Carpal Bones:
NONOPERATIVE AND OPERATIVE INDICATIONS

Nonoperative Indications

- Nondisplaced
- Avulsion fractures

Operative Indications

- Displaced
- Fractures with high risk of avascular necrosis or nonunion (proximal scaphoid and displaced capitate)

SCAPHOID FRACTURES

Nondisplaced Scaphoid Fractures

Normal radiographs do not preclude the presence of a scaphoid fracture. Clinical suspicion in the presence of normal radiographs warrants immobilization and reevaluation in 2 weeks. The cast is removed, the wrist is examined, and repeat radiographs are obtained. Pain resolution and negative radiographs warrant discontinuation of immobilization and return to normal activities. Persistent pain with normal radiographs requires continued immobilization, with or without advanced imaging studies. In this clinical setting, MRI scans have been shown to be diagnostically useful in avoiding both misdiagnosis and overtreatment (Fig. 8-73).[8,12,18,39,52,55] However, MRI may be overly sensitive in identifying bone edema that fails to develop into a fracture, and overimmobilization is less of a concern in children than in adults.

If radiographs reveal a fracture, immediate treatment is required. Most pediatric scaphoid fractures can be treated with cast immobilization because children possess a great ability to heal. Therefore, cast immobilization is the standard of treatment for most nondisplaced or minimally displaced (<1-mm) pediatric scaphoid fractures, but prompt treatment is imperative to avoid nonunion. For distal pole and occult fractures, a short-arm thumb spica cast for 4 to 6 weeks is recommended. In young children, a long-arm cast is appropriate to prevent the cast from sliding off the arm, but this is not typically necessary in children over 10 years old. For complete, stable distal third

Figure 8-73. A CT scan of a minimally displaced healing scaphoid fracture not seen on radiographs.

and waist fractures, immobilization consisting of up to 6 to 8 weeks of casting is recommended until healing.

A longer period of immobilization (8–12 weeks) is recommended for proximal pole fractures. The exact cast position and the joints immobilized are a matter of surgeon preference.[25]

Percutaneous Screw Fixation

In adults, percutaneous screw fixation for displaced fractures has been advocated.[65,89] This technique can be applied to adolescent patients with proximal pole and waist fractures, particularly high-level athletes who are concerned about a more rapid return to sports.[58] Screws can be placed under fluoroscopic control either volarly (distal to proximal) or dorsally (proximal to distal) depending on fracture patterns and surgeon preference (Fig. 8-74). This procedure is challenging in displaced scaphoid fractures.

Displaced Scaphoid Fractures

Open Reduction and Internal Fixation

Displacement of more than 1 mm or intrascaphoid angulation of more than 10 degrees on any image warrants ORIF. Fractures that present initially as a nonunion are also best treated with ORIF. A volar or dorsal approach can be used depending on the fracture configuration and surgeon preference. The implant choice is individualized according to the fracture and patient. Scaphoid screws are the primary fixation techniques, though K-wires can be used. Smaller screws (2.0 or 2.4 mm) may be necessary in the pediatric patient. Modern compression screws have been shown to speed up healing.[1] For fracture nonunions with humpback deformity of the scaphoid, a volar approach with interposed structural graft can successfully restore the scaphoid shape and therefore, carpal alignment. Iliac crest structural graft in this setting has been shown to have low morbidity in the pediatric population[72] (Fig. 8-75).

Figure 8-74. A: Nondisplaced proximal pole scaphoid fracture in a skeletally mature adolescent athlete. **B:** Treatment by percutaneous screw fixation led to healing.

Figure 8-75. A: A 16-year-old male with a right scaphoid nonunion with resorption at the fracture site. **B:** Volar approach and exposure of the fracture site. **C:** The fracture site was debrided of fibrous material, and the humpback deformity was corrected.

(continues)

Figure 8-75. (*Continued*) **D:** The fracture site was packed with bone graft and a guidewire was placed for screw fixation. **E:** The screw was inserted over the guidewire. **F, G:** Radiographic AP and lateral views after fracture reduction, bone grafting, and screw placement. (Courtesy of Shriners Hospitals for Children, Philadelphia, PA.)

CAPITATE FRACTURES

Treatment depends on the capitate fracture pattern, degree of displacement, and associated injuries. Distraction radiographs, MRI, or CT scans may be necessary to determine the exact pattern of injury. Nondisplaced fractures of the capitate can be treated with cast immobilization for 6 to 8 weeks. Closed reduction of displaced fractures is not feasible. Displaced fractures require open reduction to rotate the proximal capitate pole into anatomic position. Associated perilunar injuries also require internal fixation and ligamentous repair. The anatomic

relationships within the carpus must be restored. Wire or osseous screw fixation can both be appropriate stabilization after open reduction.

TRIQUETRAL FRACTURES

An avulsion fracture is treated with a short period of immobilization (3–6 weeks) followed by motion and return to activities. A fracture through the body of the triquetrum with a perilunar injury requires ORIF.

Figure 8-76. Clinical photograph during open excision of a hamate hook fracture nonunion. Yellow loops are placed around the ulnar nerve as well as its deep and superficial branches in Guyon canal. The red loop is placed around the ulnar artery. (Courtesy of Children's Orthopaedic Surgery Foundation.)

HAMATE FRACTURES

Hook of the hamate, type I, fractures are often missed in the acute setting unless a carpal tunnel view is ordered or a CT scan of the wrist is obtained. Immobilization and avoidance of baseball batting, gymnastics, or golf may lead to complete union in children when the injury is recognized acutely. After a period of casting, if imaging is consistent with a delayed union and the child is symptomatic, surgical fragment excision may be pursued (Fig. 8-76). Careful protection of the ulnar nerve motor branch and ulnar artery is required. Subperiosteal dissection and wide exposure can minimize chances of neurovascular injury. Most young patients are able to return to sports by 6 weeks after surgery.[15] However, postoperative return to sports that requires direct pressure on the hypothenar eminence may be slow because of scar hypersensitivity or transient ulnar neurapraxias. Silicone patches or glove padding may facilitate return to sporting activity.

Dorsal body hamate, type II, fractures may be part of a CMC dislocation or isolated. Reduction of the hamate fracture usually reduces the CMC dislocation. If the fragment is large enough, ORIF with a headless screw may be performed (Fig. 8-77).

CARPAL LIGAMENTOUS INJURY

Treatment recommendations for traumatic dislocation injuries are lacking as the injury is rare. Decisive factors include the child's age, and extent of injury. Minor injuries are treated with immobilization for 3 to 6 weeks and reexamination. Resolution of symptoms and signs allows return to normal activities. Persistent pain warrants further clinical and radiographic evaluation. Overt ligamentous injuries with static instability and malalignment require accurate diagnosis and appropriate treatment. A complete ligament tear (e.g., an adolescent with a scapholunate injury) is treated according to principles similar to those for adults. Open reduction, anatomic reduction, and ligament repair are the basic tenets of treatment.

OPERATIVE TREATMENT OF FRACTURES OF THE SCAPHOID

ORIF of Fractures of the Scaphoid

Preoperative Planning

✓ ORIF of Fractures of the Scaphoid: PREOPERATIVE PLANNING CHECKLIST

OR table	❏ Hand table, radiolucent preferable
Position	❏ Supine. A skilled wrist arthroscopic may perform an arthroscopic-assisted reduction and fixation in which case a tower or wrist distraction system may be utilized
Fluoroscopy	❏ Mini-fluoroscopy in the small child or C-arm in adult-sized limbs
Equipment	❏ Headless conical or compression screw, K-wires
Tourniquet	❏ Nonsterile

Technique

✓ ORIF of Fractures of the Scaphoid: KEY SURGICAL STEPS

Dorsal Approach

❏ Use fluoroscopy to plan small incision. Spread soft tissue to avoid dorsal radial sensory nerve and extensor pollicis longus during pin or screw placement
❏ Flex the wrist to identify screw starting point on the scaphoid, adjacent to scapholunate ligament (need 90 degrees or greater for dorsal percutaneous screw placement)
❏ Aim guidewire down the thumb axis
❏ Verify guidewire placement in 1:1 position, centered in the proximal fragment
❏ Follow standard sequence of steps to insert headless screw

Volar Approach

❏ Hockey stick incision over flexor carpi radialis and scaphoid tubercle
❏ Open sheath of flexor carpi radialis, protect radial artery, incision between the radiocapitate and radiotriquetral palmar radiocarpal ligaments
❏ Expose fracture and clear of fibrous debris or loose fragments
❏ Aim guidewire toward Lister tubercle; use angiocatheter as guide
❏ If guidewire placement is difficult, can remove proximal volar corner of trapezium with rongeur
❏ Place pins or screws distal to proximal angled volar to dorsal

Joysticks

❏ In fractures with substantial dorsal intercalated segmental instability (DISI), consider reducing the lunate and driving a K-wire from the radius into the lunate to hold the lunate and the proximal pole in neutral position during fixation. This will open up the space volarly that needs to be filled to correct the deformity.
❏ Joysticks can also be inserted in the proximal and distal poles to help open the volar surface and allow for adequate debridement.

Figure 8-77. A: A 16-year-old male sustained a large dorsal hamate fracture from punching a wall. **B–E:** Dorsal exposure of fragment with cannulated headless screw fixation. **F:** Postoperative radiographs of healed fracture.

Authors' Preferred Treatment for Fractures of the Carpal Bones (Algorithm 8-5)

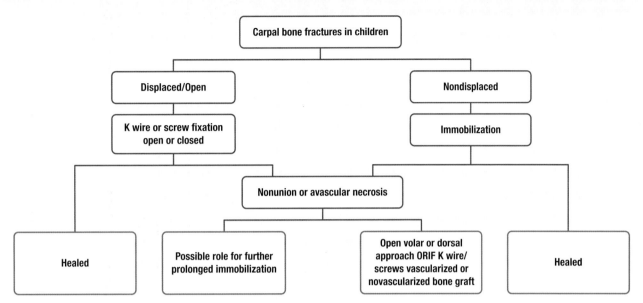

Algorithm 8-5. Authors' preferred treatment for carpal fractures.

Almost all nondisplaced scaphoid fractures are treated with cast immobilization. The preferred immobilization is a short arm thumb spica cast until clinical and radiographic union. Radiographs are obtained in the first 7 to 10 days to ensure alignment and then monthly until union. If there is doubt regarding anatomic alignment or subsequent union, a CT oriented in the plane of the scaphoid is obtained.

Proximal pole fractures are at high risk for osteonecrosis and nonunion. Percutaneous or mini-open screw fixation is preferred to stabilize the fracture and promote union. Ideally,

this is a dorsal proximal to distal screw placement to compress the fracture site and tighten the scapholunate ligament.

Indications for open reduction and fracture fixation are a waist fracture with more than 1 mm of displacement or an angular deformity of more than 10 degrees. Greater arc injuries, such as trans-scaphoid perilunate injuries, require operative management, as do fracture nonunions. Fractures of the middle and distal thirds are exposed through a volar approach. Proximal third fractures are exposed through a dorsal approach.

Postoperative Care and Rehabilitation

Nondisplaced fractures are treated with immobilization until union. After the cast is removed, a home therapy program is started. Formal therapy usually is not necessary. Displaced fractures and nonunions treated with ORIF require variable periods of immobilization. Fixation with K-wires necessitates prolonged immobilization and may involve formal therapy for the recovery of motion. Stable screw fixation in an acute fracture may early motion 10 to 14 days after surgery with a short-arm thumb spica splint worn for protection during vigorous activity until union. However, many adolescents will not wear the splint dependably and require longer periods of nonremovable immobilization to ensure compliance and prevent loss of screw fixation and nonunion.

Potential Pitfalls and Preventive Measures

Fractures of the Carpal Bones: POTENTIAL PITFALLS AND PREVENTIONS

Pitfall	Prevention
Nonunion	• Early diagnosis and treatment • Cast immobilization • Identify displaced fractures
Malunion	• Early recognition of lunate extension and DISI deformity • Three-dimensional advanced imaging, such as CT scan
Avascular necrosis	• Early treatment of high-risk fractures, such as proximal pole of the scaphoid • Knowledge of the vascular supply to each carpal bone to avoid injury during dissection
Intercarpal instability	• Static and dynamic examination of entire wrist to identify greater or lesser arc injuries

Scaphoid Fractures

Prompt treatment of a nondisplaced scaphoid fracture allows healing in most patients. Nondisplaced pediatric scaphoid fractures have a better than 95% healing rate. A delay in treatment impedes healing and increases the possibility of displacement. Displaced fractures require prompt recognition and open reduction because adequate reduction and fixation result in predictable union.[26]

Capitate Fractures

The rarity of this injury prevents broad generalizations. Early recognition and appropriate treatment lead to an acceptable outcome. Nonunion is rare and requires bone grafting[57] (see Fig. 8-68). Despite the considerable rotation of the proximal pole in displaced fractures, osteonecrosis of the capitate is rare.

Triquetral Fractures

Avulsion fractures are relatively minor injuries. Treatment results in expedient and complete recovery. Body fractures associated with perilunate injuries have a guarded prognosis depending on the extent of concomitant injuries and treatment employed.

MANAGEMENT OF EXPECTED ADVERSE OUTCOMES AND UNEXPECTED COMPLICATIONS OF SCAPHOID FRACTURES

Scaphoid Fractures: COMMON ADVERSE OUTCOMES AND COMPLICATIONS

- Nonunion
- Malunion
- Avascular necrosis
- Intercarpal instability

The most common complications are missed diagnosis and late presentation. Scaphoid nonunions do occur in children and adolescents with the incidence as 20% to 25% due to late presentation.[22,50,56,86] Late presentation occurs for a number of reasons, including children's reluctance to tell their parents about a mechanism of injury, moderate symptoms seemingly not severe enough to warrant medical attention, and a child's fear of losing his or her position on a sporting team. Open reduction, bone grafting, and internal fixation are the standard procedures for treatment of scaphoid nonunions (Fig. 8-78). The approach varies according to the location of fracture and vascularity of the fracture fragments. The principles of operative scaphoid nonunion treatment in children are similar to those in adults, although results with nonvascularized bone grafts are better in children. Persistent scaphoid nonunion results in altered kinematics within the wrist and produces degenerative changes over time. The goal is to obtain union to prevent long-term arthrosis.

The long-term outcomes of treatment of nonunions of the scaphoid have been reported following treatment using both

screws and K-wires. Masquijo and Willis reviewed 23 children, mean age 15.1 years old with scaphoid nonunions after bone grafting and fixation with a follow-up over 5 years. Scaphoid outcome scores were excellent in 66% and good in 33%.[56] Reigstad et al. reported 8-year outcomes in 11 adolescents with scaphoid waist nonunions treated with bone graft and K-wire fixation only.[64] Range of motion, grip strength, key pinch strength, and subjective outcome scores were all excellent. No evidence of persistent nonunion or degenerative changes was evident on radiographs or from CT evaluation.

Osteonecrosis may result from a scaphoid fracture. The proximal fragment is more prone to avascular changes. Avascular changes within the proximal fragment do not preclude union after internal fixation. The size of the fragment and the extent of avascularity dictate management. The treatment principles are similar in adults and children. Options to obtain union include nonvascularized or vascularized bone grafting.[75] With nonunion and osteonecrosis of the proximal pole, vascularized bone grafting from the distal radius has been successful, although the distal radial physis must be avoided.

Triangular Fibrocartilage Complex Tears in Children

CLASSIFICATION OF TRIANGULAR FIBROCARTILAGE COMPLEX TEARS

The TFCC consists of the triangular fibrocartilage (TFC) and the volar ulnocarpal ligaments. The location of TFCC injury determines the classification of TFCC tears.[60] TFCC tears can be traumatic or degenerative, with traumatic being the most common in the younger population. Ulnar peripheral tears (type B) are most common in adolescents. Tears from the radial insertion (type D) are next in frequency, whereas central (type A) and volar (type C) tears are rare.

TREATMENT OF TRIANGULAR FIBROCARTILAGE COMPLEX TEARS

The initial approach to adolescents with chronic wrist pain without instability incorporates rest until symptoms subside, followed by a strengthening program.[17] If pain persists after regaining symmetric pinch and grip strength, then further evaluation is appropriate. If clinical examination is consistent with a TFCC tear or ulnar–carpal impaction, radiographs and MRI are the next appropriate evaluation. A single-shot intra-articular steroid injection can help with inflammation and should be considered when there is pain and no instability. If these methods fail to yield symptom relief, then a surgical is recommended. Wrist arthroscopy provides the best technique to fully evaluate the intra-articular structures of the wrist (Fig. 8-79). One should be systematic and consistent in evaluation. The articular surfaces, volar ligaments, dorsal capsule, intrinsic

Figure 8-78. A–C: Radiographs of a 12-year-old boy with scaphoid nonunion and lunate extension through the fracture seen on the lateral view. **D:** Volar approach through the wrist to correct the mild humpback and flexion deformity. **E:** Iliac crest bone graft in place and headless screw fixation. **F–H:** Final radiographs after integration of graft, demonstrating correction of flexion deformity seen by lunate position on lateral. (Courtesy of Shriners Hospitals for Children, Philadelphia, PA.)

Figure 8-79. Arthroscopic image of a 15-year-old girl with ulnar-sided wrist pain after traumatic injury. There is visualization of a central TFCC tear with foveal detachment, seen by elevation of the TFCC off the head of the ulnar with the probe.

ligaments, and TFCC should all be evaluated. With regard to the TFCC in particular, a trampoline test helps to assess TFCC tension and can be suggestive of a peripheral tear. The hook test allows for assessment of the deep foveal attachment to the head of the ulna. Central tears can also be seen with concomitant foveal detachment tears and should not be overlooked.

Authors' Preferred Treatment of TFCC Tears

In treatment of type A or D tears, arthroscopic debridement is used to trim the TFCC back to a stable rim. In type B tears, a peripheral repair is performed by an outside-in approach utilizing a horizontal suture repair of the TFCC to the peripheral capsule. Type C tears can be debrided if stable and can be repaired if large. Foveal detachment, seen by a positive hook test, require fixation for DRUJ stability. This is performed through an ulnar transosseous tunnel approach, suturing the TFCC down to the head of the ulnar. If a central tear is seen in the setting of a foveal detachment, the central tear should be debrided first and then the foveal repair performed.

The adolescent patient should also be evaluated for ulnar variance when being assessed for ulnar-sided pain. Frequently, a past distal radius fracture or activities of chronic loading of the wrist will yield a positive ulnar variance. In this setting, when seen with a TFCC tear, it is the authors' recommendation to perform an ulnar epiphysiodesis (if open physis and enough growth remaining to yield an ulnar negative variance) or an ulnar shortening osteotomy at the same surgical setting.

Postoperative Care

When only arthroscopic debridement is performed, the patient is placed into a short arm plaster splint for two weeks and then transitioned into a short arm cast for an additional 3 to 4 weeks. At 6 weeks postoperatively, a custom volar wrist splint is fabricated, and wrist and forearm range of motion is begun. Strengthening starts at 10 weeks. If a foveal repair is performed, a sugar-tong plaster splint is used for the first 2 weeks. At 2 weeks, the patient is transitioned into a Munster cast for an additional 3 to 4 weeks. At 6 weeks, the rehabilitation is the same as debridement only. If an ulnar shortening osteotomy is performed, then the strengthening will be dependent on radiographic healing of the osteotomy.

Outcomes

Outcomes in TFCC in skeletally immature patients are typically good. Adolescents return to preinjury level of sport at 3 to 6 months.[23,88] Though while most have favorable outcomes and satisfaction, not all patients decide to return to sport, and some change positions.[82]

MANAGEMENT OF EXPECTED ADVERSE OUTCOMES AND UNEXPECTED COMPLICATIONS OF TFCC TREATMENT

There are some notable complications that can occur after surgical treatment of TFCC tears. Forearm supination and pronation can be limited. Neuropraxia of the ulnar dorsal sensory nerve can occur, but typically resolves over time. The nerve is also at risk for laceration given its position is in line with the incision for foveal repairs and outside-in TFCC repairs. If concern for laceration, then exploration and repair are recommended. Painful hardware can occur with ulnar shortening osteotomy, necessitating implant removal. Lastly, continued or recurrent (if additional trauma) DRUJ instability can occur. Ensuring complete and accurate assessment of the TFCC injury type and addressing ulnar positive variance minimizes this risk and avoids the need for secondary surgery.

TFCC Injuries:
TREATMENT PITFALLS AND PREVENTIONS

Pitfall	Prevention
In accurate TFCC injury diagnosis	• Perform trampoline and hook test
Missing positive ulnar variance	• Assess variance and perform ulnar epiphysiodesis or ulnar shortening when ulnar positive

Dislocations of the Hand and Carpus

DISLOCATIONS OF THE INTERPHALANGEAL JOINTS

In children, the soft tissue stabilizers about the interphalangeal joints are stronger than the physis, which explains the propensity for fracture rather than dislocation. Occasionally, dislocations

Figure 8-80. A dorsal dislocation of the PIP joint with an S-H type II fracture of the middle phalanx in a 15-year-old boy.

and fracture–dislocations occur about the interphalangeal and MCP joints, especially in adolescents as they skeletally mature and engage in higher-impact activities (Fig. 8-80).

DISTAL INTERPHALANGEAL JOINT

A hyperextension or lateral force may result in dorsal or lateral DIP joint dislocation. The collateral ligaments and volar plate typically detach from the middle phalanx. Most dislocations can be reduced by longitudinal traction, recreation of the dislocation force, and reduction of the distal phalanx. The DIP joint reduction and congruity are confirmed by clinical motion and radiographs. Splinting of DIP joint for 2 to 3 weeks is sufficient, followed by a home program that focuses on DIP joint motion.

Irreducible or complex dislocations of the DIP occur primarily in adults but can occur in pediatric patients. Open reduction through a dorsal approach is required for removal of the interposed tissue. The volar plate is often the offending agent, though the collateral ligaments and the FDP can block reduction. A stable DIP joint is treated with DIP joint immobilization for 4 weeks. An unstable DIP joint requires pin fixation for 4 weeks.

PROXIMAL INTERPHALANGEAL JOINT

Dislocation of the PIP joint may occur in a variety of directions. Dorsal dislocations are the most common, though lateral and volar dislocations also occur. The differential diagnosis includes adjacent bony and tendon injuries.[40] Radiographs are required to assess the physis and to confirm joint alignment. The postreduction lateral radiograph must confirm concentric joint reduction. Persistent joint subluxation is unacceptable and detected by a slight offset between the proximal and middle phalanges along with a dorsal V-shaped space instead of smooth concentric articular congruity.

Dorsal Proximal Interphalangeal Joint Dislocations

The middle phalanx is displaced dorsal to the proximal phalanx. The collateral ligaments and volar plate are disrupted. Many dorsal dislocations are probably joint subluxations that retain some of the collateral ligament or volar plate integrity. Some subluxations are reduced by the patient or trainer on the field and never receive medical evaluation.

Unreduced dorsal dislocations cause pain and obvious deformity. If necessary, anesthesia can usually be accomplished with a digital block. The dislocation is reduced with longitudinal traction, hyperextension, and palmar translation of the middle phalanx onto the proximal phalanx. The quality of the reduction and the stability of the joint must be assessed. Asking

the patient to flex and extend the digit evaluates active motion. Most dislocations are stable throughout the normal range of motion, and radiographs confirm a concentric reduction. A stable joint requires a brief period (3–5 days) of splinting for comfort, followed by range of motion and buddy tape to an adjacent uninjured digit. Immediate motion may be started, though pain often prohibits movement and exacerbates swelling. Prolonged immobilization (>1 week) leads to PIP joint stiffness.

An unstable reduction tends to subluxate or dislocate during PIP joint extension. The radiographs must be scrutinized for subtle dorsal subluxation and concomitant fracture of the middle phalangeal base. Unstable PIP joint dislocations, with or without small fractures of the middle phalangeal base, have a stable arc of motion that must be defined. The stable arc is typically from full flexion to about 30 degrees of flexion. This arc is used to determine the confines of extension block splinting. Dynamic fluoroscopic imaging is an optimal tool to assess the degree of stability, visualizing joint alignment with live motion. Once the degree of stability is understood, a custom dorsal blocking splint that positions the MCP joint in flexion and the PIP joint in 10 degrees less than the maximal extension that leads to joint subluxation should be fashioned. Reduction is verified by lateral radiographs or fluoroscopic imaging. The splint is modified every week to increase PIP joint extension by 10 degrees. A lateral view or dynamic fluoroscopy is used to confirm concentric reduction. This process is continued over 4 to 5 weeks until full extension is reached. The splint is then discontinued and a home therapy program is instituted.

Extremely unstable injuries that dislocate in more than 30 degrees of flexion almost always involve considerable fracture of the middle phalanx. Treatment presents a management dilemma as discussed earlier. Options range from open reduction to dynamic traction. Long-term subluxation, stiffness, and arthrosis are concerns. Aggressive surgical care has the best chance for but does not guarantee, a good outcome. Bone and articular alignment should be established first and then motion secondary. In these difficult situations, families should be made aware of the possible need for a secondary surgery to improve motion such as tenolysis and joint release.

Volar Proximal Interphalangeal Joint Dislocations

Volar PIP joint dislocations are uncommon in children, and the diagnosis is often delayed. Interposition of soft tissues or bony fragments can render the dislocation irreducible. The proximal phalangeal head may herniate between the lateral band and the central tendon. Long-term results are often suboptimal if anatomic alignment is not restored. This outcome may be related to a delay in treatment or the degree of soft tissue involvement, especially the central slip.

Volar dislocations require closed or open reduction. Reducible dislocations are treated with 4 weeks of full-time PIP joint extension splinting to promote healing of the central slip. Radiographs are necessary to confirm concentric reduction. An unstable reduction may require temporary pin fixation across the PIP joint. Irreducible dislocations require open reduction through a dorsal approach to extricate any interposed tissue. The central slip can be repaired to the middle phalanx. Postoperative immobilization consists of 4 weeks of full-time PIP joint extension splinting. During this time, DIP joint motion should be encouraged.

Lateral Proximal Interphalangeal Joint Dislocations

Pure lateral dislocations are uncommon, though dorsal dislocations may have a lateral component. An isolated lateral dislocation represents severe disruption of the collateral ligament complex. The injury represents a spectrum of damage, beginning with the proper and accessory collateral ligaments and culminating in volar plate disruption. Bony avulsion fragments may accompany the ligamentous failure. Closed reduction is uniformly successful. A brief period (5–7 days) of immobilization followed by buddy tape to protect the healing collateral ligament complex is the customary treatment.

Authors' Preferred Treatment of Proximal Interphalangeal Joint Dislocations (Algorithm 8-6)

Algorithm 8-6. Authors' preferred treatment for proximal interphalangeal joint dislocations.

The initial treatment of almost all PIP dislocations is an attempt at closed reduction followed by a stability assessment. If stable, a brief period of immobilization lessens pain and swelling. Subsequent mobilization prevents PIP joint stiffness.

Dorsal Dislocation

A stable reduction is treated with brief immobilization followed by early motion. An unstable reduction that can be held reduced in more than 30 to 40 degrees of flexion is treated with extension block splinting. Extremely unstable fracture–dislocations require open treatment, external fixation, or dynamic traction depending on the size of the fracture fragments.

Volar Dislocation

A stable congruent reduction is treated with immobilization for 4 weeks with the PIP joint in extension. Unstable reductions are treated with percutaneous pin fixation to maintain a concentric reduction. Irreducible dislocations require open reduction with repair of the central slip.

Lateral Dislocations

Closed reduction is usually obtainable, followed by a brief period of immobilization. Irreducible dislocations require open reduction with or without collateral ligament repair.

Figure 8-81. A: A 3-year-old boy with a complete complex dislocation of the index finger metacarpal joint. **B:** Note the parallelism in this lateral view. Open reduction was done through a volar approach.

DISLOCATIONS OF THE METACARPOPHALANGEAL JOINT

The MCP joint is an uncommon site for dislocation in the child's hand. While rare, the dislocation may involve a finger or thumb. The gamekeeper's or skier's thumb can be considered a subset of subluxation or dislocation.

DORSAL METACARPOPHALANGEAL JOINT

The most frequent dislocation of the MCP joint is dorsal dislocation of the index digit or thumb (Fig. 8-81), which results from a hyperextension force that ruptures the volar plate. The proximal phalanx is displaced dorsal to the metacarpal head. The diagnosis is readily apparent because the digit is shortened, supinated, and deviated in an ulnar direction. The interphalangeal joints are slightly flexed because of the digital flexor tendon tension. The volar skin is taut over the prominent metacarpal head.

Dislocations of the MCP joint are classified as simple or complex. Complex dislocations are irreducible because of volar plate interposition in the joint. The injury can be open with the metacarpal head penetrating the palmar skin (Fig. 8-82). Simple dislocations are in a position of hyperextension on radiographs. Irreducible dislocations have bayonet apposition of the proximal phalanx dorsal to the metacarpal head. The sesamoid bone(s) of the index finger or thumb may be seen within the joint. The position of the sesamoid bones is indicative of the site of the volar plate. The most common irreducible dislocation is at the index MCP joint. In these injuries, the metacarpal head becomes "picture-framed" by the flexor tendon on the ulnar side and the lumbrical on the radial side. The superficial transverse metacarpal ligament and the natatory ligaments can also entrap the metacarpal neck. The collar of the restraining tissue is tightened by longitudinal traction, and this reduction maneuver may convert a dislocation from reducible to irreducible.

Most simple dislocations can be reduced with distraction and volar manipulation of the proximal phalanx over the metacarpal head. Avoidance of hyperextension during reduction is important to prevent conversion of a simple to a complex dislocation. These reductions are usually stable. Reduction of a complex dislocation is problematic at best and usually not possible. The maneuver involves further hyperextension of the joint and palmar translation of the proximal phalanx. The goal is to extricate the volar plate with the proximal phalanx during palmar translation. The success rate for conversion of

Figure 8-82. An 18-year-old male after a fall from height, with open index and middle finger dorsal dislocations. (Courtesy of Joshua Ratner, MD.)

an irreducible dislocation to a reducible dislocation is low; open reduction is necessary for almost all patients.[43]

Open Reduction

Open Reduction of Dorsal Metacarpophalangeal Joint Dislocations:
KEY SURGICAL STEPS

☐ Volar or dorsal approach: Volar more at risk of NV injury; dorsal allows visualization of associated metacarpal head fracture if present. Both are effective
☐ Protect neurovascular structures
☐ Remove interposed soft tissue, usually volar plate
☐ Pin fractures or ORIF if present
☐ Early motion after brief postoperative immobilization

Open reduction can be accomplished through a volar or dorsal approach. The volar approach provides excellent exposure to the metacarpal head and the incarcerated structures. However, the digital nerves are draped over the articular surface of the metacarpal head and precariously close to the skin. A deep skin incision can cut these nerves. The skin is gently incised and soft tissue is dissected. The first annular pulley is incised. The metacarpal head is extricated from between the flexor tendon and the lumbrical. The joint is evaluated for interposed structures, such as the volar plate, and then reduced under direct observation.

The dorsal approach offers a less extensive exposure but avoids the risk of digital nerve injury. Through a dorsal incision, the extensor tendon is longitudinally split over the MCP joint. A transverse or longitudinal capsulotomy is made if the injury has not torn the capsule. A Freer elevator is placed within the joint to clear it of any interposed tissue. Often, the interposed volar plate needs to be split longitudinally to reduce the joint. If the flexor tendon is wrapped around the metacarpal, the Freer is used to extricate the metacarpal head. If there is an impacted or displaced intra-articular metacarpal head fracture, it can be reduced and stabilized through this approach.

Regardless of the approach used, early motion as appropriate is best to optimize outcome. The postoperative regimen is a 3- to 5-day immobilization period, followed by active motion. Rarely, a dorsal blocking splint is needed to prevent hyperextension that may foster repeat dislocation.

Dorsal dislocations of the other fingers are uncommon (Fig. 8-83). Lateral fracture–dislocations are often S-H type III fractures involving the base of the proximal phalanx (Fig. 8-84) and require ORIF of the displaced physeal fracture.

NEGLECTED METACARPOPHALANGEAL JOINT DISLOCATIONS

Early treatment is preferred for MCP joint dislocations, but delay of a few months may still result in an acceptable outcome. A delay of more than 6 months is associated with joint degeneration and a less predictable result. Late reduction may require a combined dorsal and volar approach for adequate exposure. Collateral ligament release and temporary MCP joint pin fixation may be necessary.

Figure 8-83. A rare dorsal dislocation of the long finger that was irreducible by closed means. A dorsal approach permitted inspection of the joint and extrication of the volar plate.

DORSAL DISLOCATION OF THE THUMB RAY

Thumb MCP joint dislocations are similar to those of the fingers, and hyperextension is the common mechanism. Thumb dislocations are classified according to the integrity and position of the volar plate, the status of the collateral ligaments, and the relative position of the metacarpal and proximal phalanx. The components of the classification are incomplete dislocation, simple complete dislocation, and complex complete dislocation (Fig. 8-85).

INCOMPLETE THUMB METACARPOPHALANGEAL JOINT DISLOCATION

An incomplete dislocation implies rupture of the volar plate with partial preservation of the collateral ligament integrity. The proximal phalanx perches on the dorsum of the metacarpal. Closed reduction is easily accomplished, and a 3-week course of immobilization is adequate. Return to sports requires protection for an additional 3 weeks.

SIMPLE COMPLETE THUMB METACARPOPHALANGEAL DISLOCATION

A simple complete dislocation implies volar plate and collateral ligament disruption. The proximal phalanx is displaced in a dorsal direction and is angulated 90 degrees to the long axis of the thumb metacarpal. Many of these dislocations can be reduced by closed means, though unnecessary longitudinal

Figure 8-84. A: A 9-year-old girl sustained this radial fracture–dislocation of the middle fingers. **B:** Closed reduction restored joint and fracture alignment.

traction may convert a reducible condition into an irreducible situation (Fig. 8-86). A successful reduction requires thumb spica immobilization for 3 to 4 weeks to allow healing of the volar plate and collateral ligaments.

Figure 8-85. Simple and complex dorsal dislocations of the thumb MCP joint. Simple dislocations (**A**) are in extension and reducible. Complex dislocations (**B**) are in bayonet apposition and are irreducible because of the interposed volar plate.

COMPLEX COMPLETE THUMB METACARPOPHALANGEAL JOINT DISLOCATION

A complete or irreducible dislocation is the most severe form of this injury. The long axes of both the proximal phalanx and metacarpal are often parallel. Open reduction is usually required to extricate the volar plate from within the joint (Fig. 8-87). A dorsal or volar approach is suitable and raises concerns similar to those for irreducible index MCP joint dislocations discussed above.

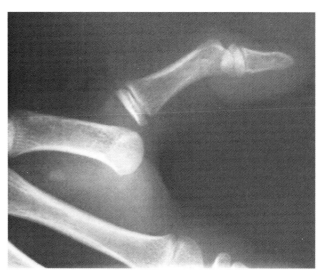

Figure 8-86. A 9-year-old boy with a complete simple dorsal dislocation of the thumb MCP joint.

A   **B**

Figure 8-87. **A:** Irreducible dorsal MCP dislocation in an 8-year-old boy. **B:** After open reduction through a volar incision.

THUMB METACARPOPHALANGEAL ULNAR COLLATERAL LIGAMENT INJURY (GAMEKEEPER'S THUMB)

Injuries of the UCL are less prevalent in children than in adults. Forced abduction stress at a child's thumb MCP joint results in four types of injuries: (1) a simple sprain of the UCL, (2) a rupture or avulsion of the insertion or origin of the ligament, (3) an S-H type I or II fracture of the proximal physis, or (4) an S-H type III avulsion fracture that involves one-fourth to one-third of the epiphysis of the proximal phalanx (Figs. 8-88 and 8-89).

The injury is most common in preadolescents and adolescents and occurs from a direct trauma to the thumb. The thumb is swollen about the MCP joint with ecchymosis, and tenderness to palpation is well localized over the UCL. Pain is exacerbated by abduction stress. A complete rupture or displaced fracture lacks a discrete endpoint during stress testing. Radiographic AP and lateral views are used to diagnose and delineate

A, B   **C, D**

Figure 8-88. Ulnar instability of the thumb metacarpal joint. **A:** Simple sprain. **B:** Rupture of the ligament. **C:** Avulsion fracture (S-H type III). **D:** Pseudo-gamekeeper's injury resulting from an S-H type I or II fracture of the proximal phalanx.

A, B   **C**

Figure 8-89. Spectrum of UCL injuries of the thumb. **A, B:** On stress examination, a widening of the physis is seen. Varying sizes of fragments (**B, C**) may be associated with UCL avulsion fractures (*arrows*). The size of the fragment is important with respect to the congruity of the MCP joint.

fracture configuration. Stress views may be needed if no fracture and the diagnosis is questionable. An MRI scan can be used to evaluate ligament disruption in complicated injuries, although rarely necessary.

Cast immobilization for 4 to 6 weeks is adequate for simple sprains, incomplete injuries, and nondisplaced fractures. A major concern is displacement of the ligament or fracture fragment outside the adductor aponeurosis, or Stener lesion, which prohibits healing.[76] Complete ruptures, Stener lesion, or displaced fractures usually require operative intervention. Distal insertion avulsion without bony fracture will require suture anchor fixation for repair (Fig. 8-90).

An S-H type III fracture of the ulnar corner of the epiphysis of the proximal phalanx is the most common childhood gamekeeper's injury. A displaced fracture (fragment rotated or displaced more) may require open reduction and fixation (screw or K-wire) to restore the integrity of the UCL and to obtain a congruous joint surface[35] (see Fig. 8-34).

Figure 8-90. An 11-year-old boy with a Stener lesion. It is uncommon for young patients to have a purely ligamentous avulsion of the ulnar collateral ligament as seen here.

Authors' Preferred Treatment of Metacarpophalangeal Joint Dislocation (Algorithm 8-7)

Algorithm 8-7. Authors' preferred treatment for metacarpophalangeal joint dislocations.

Chronic UCL injuries are more difficult to manage. Treatment depends on the length of time since original injury, age of the patient, and current level of function. Options range from UCL reconstruction to MCP joint fusion.

The initial treatment for simple dislocations is closed reduction. Irreducible dislocations require open reduction. A dorsal or volar approach is used with removal of any interposed structure(s). The advantages and disadvantages of both approaches were discussed previously. Postoperative immobilization is used for 7 to 10 days, followed by active motion with splint protection.

Injuries of the UCL of the thumb are treated according to stability and displacement. Stable ligamentous injuries or minimally displaced fractures are treated with cast immobilization with reduced stress on fracture or ligament injury. Unstable complete ligamentous injuries or displaced fractures are treated with open reduction.

ACKNOWLEDGMENTS

The authors would like to acknowledge Nina Lightdale-Miric and Scott Kozin for their work on the previous edition of this chapter.

Annotated References

Reference	Annotation
Abzug JM, Dua K, Bauer AS, et al. Pediatric phalanx fractures. *J Am Acad Orthop Surg*. 2016;24(11):e174–e183.	Review article that discusses pediatric phalanx fractures with an emphasis on diagnosis and treatment.
Gholson JJ, Bae DS, Zurakowski D, Waters PM. Scaphoid fractures in children and adolescents: contemporary injury patterns and factors influencing time to union. *J Bone Joint Surg Am*. 2011;93(13):1210–1219.	Update on scaphoid fracture in children that notes changing trends in fracture patterns. Reconfirms that nonoperative treatment will heal nondisplaced fractures, although casting may be prolonged. Highlights the factors that directly affect treatment, healing, and outcome.
Godfrey J, Cornwall R. Pediatric metacarpal fractures. *Instr Course Lect*. 2017;66:437–445.	Review article on pediatric metacarpal fractures. Finger and thumb metacarpal fractures are discussed with an emphasis on clinical evaluation and management.
Matzon JL, Cornwall R. A stepwise algorithm for surgical treatment of type II displaced pediatric phalangeal neck fractures. *J Hand Surg Am*. 2014;39(3):467–473.	Stepwise algorithm presented for surgical treatment of type II displaced pediatric phalangeal neck fractures. Algorithm produced 92% good to excellent results while minimizing the need for open reduction even in late-presenting fractures.
Ramavath AL, Unnikrishnan PN, George HL, et al. Wrist arthroscopy in children and adolescent with chronic wrist pain: arthroscopic findings compared with MRI. *J Pediatr Orthop*. 2017;37(5):e321–e325.	Retrospective review of 32 pediatric and adolescent patients who underwent wrist arthroscopy after failing at least 4 months of conservative management. Pathology was identified in 32 of the 33 wrists at arthroscopy.
Ting B, Sesko Bauer A, Abzug JM, et al. Pediatric scaphoid fractures. *Instr Course Lect*. 2017;66:429–436.	Excellent review article covering pediatric scaphoid fractures. Diagnosis including the use of advanced imaging studies is discussed. Treatment algorithm is presented.

REFERENCES

1. Adolfsson L, Lindau T, Arner M. Acutrak screw fixation versus cast immobilization for undisplaced scaphoid waist fractures. *J Hand Surg Br*. 2001;26:192–195.
2. Aggarwal AK, Sangwan SS, Siwach RC. Transscaphoid perilunate dislocation in a child. *Contemp Orthop*. 1993;26:172–174.
3. Al-Qattan MM. Extra-articular transverse fractures of the base of the distal phalanx (Seymour's fracture) in children and adults. *J Hand Surg Br*. 2001;26:201–206.
4. Al-Qattan MM. Juxta-epiphyseal fractures of the base of the proximal phalanx of the fingers in children and adolescents. *J Hand Surg Br*. 2002;27:24–30.
5. Al-Qattan MM. Phalangeal neck fractures in children: classification and outcome in 66 cases. *J Hand Surg Br*. 2001;26(2):112–121.
6. Al-Qattan MM, Hashem F, Helmi A. Irreducible tuft fractures of the distal phalanx. *J Hand Surg Br*. 2003;28(1):18–20.
7. Brian JM, Choi DH, Moore MM. The primary physis. *Semin Musculoskelet Radiol*. 2018;22(1):95–103.
8. Brydie A, Raby N. Early MRI in the management of clinical scaphoid fracture. *Br J Radiol*. 2003;76:296–300.
9. Chew EM, Chong AK. Hand fractures in children: epidemiology and misdiagnosis in a tertiary referral hospital. *J Hand Surg Am*. 2012;37(8):1686.
10. Chung KC, Spilson SV. The frequency and epidemiology of hand and forearm fractures in the United States. *J Hand Surg Am*. 2001;26:908–915.
11. Clementson M, Björkman A, Thomsen NOB. Acute scaphoid fractures: guidelines for diagnosis and treatment. *EFORT Open Rev*. 2020;5(2):96-103.
12. Cook PA, Yu JS, Wiand W, et al. Suspected scaphoid fractures in skeletally immature patients: application of MRI. *J Comput Assist Tomogr*. 1997;21(4):511–515.
13. D'Arienzo M. Scaphoid fractures in children. *J Hand Surg Br*. 2002;27(5):424–426.
14. Dean B, Becker G, Little C. The management of the acute traumatic subungual haematoma: a systematic review. *Hand Surg*. 2012;17(1):151–154.
15. Devers BN, Douglas KC, Naik RD, et al. Outcomes of hook of hamate fracture excision in high-level amateur athletes. *J Hand Surg Am*. 2013;38(1):72–76.
16. Doman AN, Marcus NW. Congenital bipartite scaphoid. *J Hand Surg Am*. 1990;15:869–873.
17. Dorich JM, Cornwall R. Evaluation of a grip-strengthening algorithm for the initial treatment of chronic, nonspecific wrist pain in adolescents. *J Hand Surg Glob Online*. 2021;4(1):8–13.
18. Dorsay TA, Major NM, Helms CA. Cost-effectiveness of immediate MR imaging versus traditional follow-up for revealing radiographically occult scaphoid fractures. *AJR Am J Roentgenol*. 2001;177:1257–1263.
19. Eberlin KR, Busa K, Bae DS, et al. Composite grafting for pediatric fingertip injuries. *Hand (NY)*. 2015;10(1):28-33.
20. Elhassan BT, Shin A. Scaphoid fracture in children. *Hand Clin*. 2006;22(1):31–41.
21. Elhassan BT, Shin AY, Kozin SH. Scaphoid fractures in children. In: Shin AY, ed. *Scaphoid Fractures*. American Academy of Orthopaedic Surgeons Monograph Series; 2007:85–95.
22. Fabre O, De Boeck H, Haentjens P. Fractures and nonunions of the carpal scaphoid in children. *Acta Orthop Belg*. 2001;67(2):121–125.
23. Fishman FG, Barber J, Lourie GM, Peljovich AE. Outcomes of operative treatment of triangular fibrocartilage complex tears in pediatric and adolescent athletes. *J Pediatr Orthop*. 2018;38(10):e618–622.

24. Gause TM II, Moran TE, Carr JB, Deal DN. Scaphoid waist nonunion in an 8-year-old: a rare occurrence. *Case Rep Orthop.* 2019;2019:4701585.
25. Gellman H, Caputo RJ, Carter V, et al. Comparison of short and long thumb-spica casts for nondisplaced fractures of the carpal scaphoid. *J Bone Joint Surg Am.* 1989;71(3):354–357.
26. Gholson JJ, Bae DS, Zurakowski D, Waters PM. Scaphoid fractures in children and adolescents: contemporary injury patterns and factors influencing time to union. *J Bone Joint Surg Am.* 2011;93:1210–1219.
27. Gollamudi S, Jones WA. Corrective osteotomy of malunited fractures of phalanges and metacarpals. *J Hand Surg Br.* 2000;25:439–441.
28. Gonzalez MH, Ingram CM, Hall RF Jr. Flexible intramedullary nailing for metacarpal fractures. *J Hand Surg Am.* 1995;20(3):382–387.
29. Goulding A, Jones IE, Taylor RW, et al. Dynamic and static tests of balance and postural sway in boys: effects of previous wrist bone fractures and high adiposity. *Gait Posture.* 2003;17(2):136–141.
30. Greig A, Gardiner MD, Sierakowski A, et al. Randomized feasibility trial of replacing or discarding the nail plate after nail-bed repair in children. *Br J Surg.* 2017;104(12):1634–1639.
31. Hankin FM, Janda DH. Tendon and ligament attachments in relationship to growth plate in a child's hand. *J Hand Surg Br.* 1989;14:315–318.
32. Hennrikus WL, Cohen MR. Complete remodeling of displaced fractures of the neck of the phalanx. *J Bone Joint Surg Br.* 2003;85:273–274.
33. Hildebrand KA, Ross DC, Patterson SD, et al. Dorsal perilunate dislocations and fracture-dislocations: questionnaire, clinical, and radiographic evaluation. *J Hand Surg Am.* 2000;25(6):1069–1079.
34. Horton TC, Hatton M, Davis TR. A prospective, randomized controlled study of fixation of long oblique and spiral shaft fractures of the proximal phalanx: closed reduction and percutaneous Kirschner-wiring versus open reduction and lag screw fixation. *J Hand Surg Br.* 2003;28:5–9.
35. Huynh MNQ, Tang K, Cheung K. A comparison of conservative and operative management of thumb ulnar collateral ligament avulsion fractures in children. *Hand (N Y).* 2020;15(6):812–817.
36. Ireland ML, Taleisnik J. Nonunion of metacarpal extraarticular fractures in children: report of two cases and review of the literature. *J Pediatr Orthop.* 1986;6(3):352–355.
37. Jagodzinski N, Bavan L, McNab IS. Intraosseous suture fixation of a sagittal fracture of the distal phalanx. *J Hand Surg Eur.* 2016;41(4):458–459.
38. Jahss SA. Fractures of the metacarpals: a new method of reduction and immobilization. *J Bone Joint Surg.* 1938;20:178–186.
39. Johnson KJ, Haigh SF, Symonds KE. MRI in the management of scaphoid fractures in skeletally immature patients. *Pediatr Radiol.* 2000;30(10):685–688.
40. Jones NF, Jupiter JB. Irreducible palmar dislocation of the proximal interphalangeal joint associated with an epiphyseal fracture of the middle phalanx. *J Hand Surg Am.* 1985;10:261–264.
41. Kardestuncer T, Bae DS, Waters PM. The results of tenodermodesis for severe chronic mallet finger deformity in children. *J Pediatr Orthop.* 2008;28(1):81–85.
42. Karl JW, White NJ, Strauch RJ. Percutaneous reduction and fixation of displaced phalangeal neck fractures in children. *J Pediatr Orthop.* 2012;32(2):156–161.
43. Khursheed O, Haq A, Rashid S, et al. Clinical outcome of metacarpophalangeal joint dislocation of the thumb in children: case series of 10 patients. *J Hand Microsurg.* 2016;8(1):13–16.
44. Kitay A, Waters PM, Bae DS. Osteochondral autograft transplantation surgery for metacarpal head defects. *J Hand Surg Am.* 2016;41(3):457–463.
45. Krusche-Mandl I, Köttstorfer J, Thalhammer G, et al. Seymour fractures: retrospective analysis and therapeutic considerations. *J Hand Surg Am.* 2013;38(2):258–264.
46. Lane CS. Detecting occult fractures of the metacarpal head: the Brewerton view. *J Hand Surg Am.* 1977;2:131–133.
47. Lankachandra M, Wells CR, Cheng CJ, Hutchison RL. Complications of distal phalanx fractures in children. *J Hand Surg Am.* 2017;42(7):574.
48. Lee SJ, Merrison H, Williams KA, et al. Closed reduction and immobilization of pediatric fifth metacarpal neck fractures. *Hand (NY).* 2022;17(3):416–421.
49. Light TR, Ogden JA. Metacarpal epiphyseal fractures. *J Hand Surg Am.* 1987;12:460–464.
50. Littlefield WG, Friedman RL, Urbaniak JR. Bilateral nonunion of the carpal scaphoid in a child: a case report. *J Bone Joint Surg Am.* 1995;77(1):124–126.
51. Louis DS, Calhoun TP, Gam SM, et al. Congenital bipartite scaphoid—fact or fiction? *J Bone Joint Surg Am.* 1976;58(8):1108–1112.
52. Mack MG, Keim S, Balzer JO, et al. Clinical impact of MRI in acute wrist fractures. *Eur Radiol.* 2003;13(3):612–617.
53. Mahabir RC, Kazemi A, Cannon WG, Courtemanche DJ. Pediatric hand fractures: a review. *Pediatr Emerg Care.* 2001;17(3):153–156.
54. Maheshwari R, Sharma H, Duncan RD. Metacarpophalangeal joint dislocation of the thumb in children. *J Bone Joint Surg.* 2007;89(2):227–229.
55. Mallee W, Doornberg JN, Ring D, et al. Comparison of CT and MRI for diagnosis of suspected scaphoid fractures. *J Bone Joint Surg.* 2011;93:20–28.
56. Masquijo JJ, Willis BR. Scaphoid nonunions in children and adolescents: surgical treatment with bone grafting and internal fixation. *J Pediatr Orthop.* 2010;30(2):119–124.
57. Minami M, Yamazaki J, Chisaka N, et al. Nonunion of the capitate. *J Hand Surg Am.* 1987;12(6):1089–1091.
58. Muramatsu K, Doi K, Kuwata N, et al. Scaphoid fracture in the young athlete—therapeutic outcome of internal fixation using the Herbert screw. *Arch Orthop Trauma Surg.* 2002;122(9–10):510–513.
59. Obdeijn MC, van der Vlies CH, van Rijn RR. Capitate and hamate fracture in a child: the value of MRI imaging. *Emerg Radiol.* 2010;17(2):157–159.
60. Palmer AK. Triangular fibrocartilage complex lesions: a classification. *J Hand Sur Am* 1989;14:594–606.
61. Parvizi J, Wayman J, Kelly P, Moran CG. Combining the clinical signs improves diagnosis of scaphoid fractures: a prospective study with follow-up. *J Hand Surg Br.* 1998;23(3):324–327.
62. Puckett BN, Gaston RG, Peljovich AE, et al. Remodeling potential of phalangeal distal condylar malunions in children. *J Hand Surg Am.* 2012;37(1):34–41.
63. Qiao F, Qu D, Cheng L, Jiang F. Closed reduction of severely angulated Rockwood and Wilkins' type C thumb metacarpal base fractures in children: case series. *BMC Musculoskelet Disord.* 2021;22(1):775.
64. Reigstad O, Thorkildsen R, Grimsgaard C, et al. Excellent results after bone grafting and K-wire fixation for scaphoid non-union surgery in skeletally immature: a mid-term follow-up study of 11 adolescents after 6.9 years. *J Orthop Trauma.* 2012;27:285–289.
65. Rettig ME, Raskin KB. Retrograde compression screw fixation of acute proximal pole scaphoid fractures. *J Hand Surg Am.* 1999;24:1206–1210.
66. Reyes BA, Ho CA. The high risk of infection with delayed treatment of open Seymour fractures: Salter-Harris I/II or juxta-epiphyseal fractures of the distal phalanx with associated nailbed laceration. *J Pediatr Orthop.* 2017;37(4):247–253.
67. Rodríguez-Vega V, Pretell-Mazzini J, Marti-Ciruelos R, et al. Simultaneous juxta-epiphyseal proximal phalanx fracture with flexor tendon entrapment in a child: a case report and review of literature. *J Pediatr Orthop B.* 2013;22(2):148–152.
68. Roser SE, Gellman H. Comparison of nail bed repair versus nail trephination for subungual hematomas in children. *J Hand Surg Am.* 1999;24(6):1166–1170.
69. Ruchelsman DE, Puri S, Feinberg-Zadek N, et al. Clinical outcomes of limited-open retrograde intramedullary headless screw fixation of metacarpal fractures. *J Hand Surg Am.* 2014;39(12):2390–2395.
70. Savage R. Complete detachment of the epiphysis of the distal phalanx. *J Hand Surg Br.* 1990;15:126–128.
71. Schenck RR. Dynamic traction and early passive movement for fractures of the proximal interphalangeal joint. *J Hand Surg Am.* 1986;11:850–858.
72. Schott T, Eisenberg KA, Vuillermin CB, et al. Donor-site morbidity for iliac crest harvesting for pediatric scaphoid nonunion. *J Hand Surg Am.* 2022;S0363–5023(22):00122-8.
73. Seymour N. Juxta-epiphysial fracture of the terminal phalanx of the finger. *J Bone Joint Surg Br.* 1966;48:347–349.
74. Simmons BP, Peters TT. Subcondylar fossa reconstruction for malunion of fractures of the proximal phalanx in children. *J Hand Surg Am.* 1987;12(6):1079–1082.
75. Steinmann SP, Bishop AT, Berger RA. Use of the 1,2 intercompartmental suprareti-nacular artery as a vascularized pedicle bone graft for difficult scaphoid nonunion. *J Hand Surg Am.* 2002;27:391–401.
76. Stener B. Displacement of the ruptured ulnar collateral ligament of the MCP joint of the thumb: a clinical and anatomical study. *J Bone Joint Surg Br.* 1962;44:869–879.
77. Stern PJ, Roman RJ, Kiefhaber TR, McDonough JJ. Pilon fractures of the proximal interphalangeal joint. *J Hand Surg Am.* 1991;16(5):844–850.
78. Stuart HC, Pyle SI, Cornoni J, Reed RB. Onsets, completions, and spans of ossification in the 29 bone growth centers of the hand and wrist. *Pediatrics.* 1962;29:237–249.
79. Tavassoli J, Ruland RT, Hogan CJ, Cannon DL. Three cast techniques for the treatment of extra-articular metacarpal fractures: comparison of short-term outcomes and final fracture alignments. *J Bone Joint Surg.* 2005;87A:2196–2201.
80. Teoh LC, Yong FC, Chong KC. Condylar advancement osteotomy for correcting condylar malunion of the finger. *J Hand Surg Br.* 2002;27:31–35.
81. Toh S, Miura H, Arai K, et al. Scaphoid fractures in children: problems and treatment. *J Pediatr Orthop.* 2003;23(2):216–221.
82. Trehan SK, Schimizzi G, Shen TS, et al. Arthroscopic treatment of triangular fibrocartilage complex injuries in paediatric and adolescent patients. *J Hand Surg Eur Vol.* 2019;44(6):582–586.
83. Vadivelu R, Dias JJ, Burke FD, Stanton J. Hand injuries in children: a prospective study. *J Pediatr Orthop.* 2006;26(1):29–35.
84. Vance RM, Gelberman RH, Evans EF. Scaphocapitate fractures: patterns of dislocation, mechanisms of injury, and preliminary results of treatment. *J Bone Joint Surg Am.* 1980;62(2):271–276.
85. Waters PM, Benson LS. Dislocation of the distal phalanx epiphysis in toddlers. *J Hand Surg Am.* 1993;18(4):581–585.
86. Waters PM, Stewart SL. Surgical treatment of nonunion and avascular necrosis of the proximal part of the scaphoid in adolescents. *J Bone Joint Surg Am.* 2002;84(6):915–920.
87. Waters PM, Taylor BA, Kuo AY. Percutaneous reduction of incipient malunion of phalangeal neck fractures in children. *J Hand Surg Am.* 2004;29:707–711.
88. Wu M, Miller PE, Waters PM, Bae DS. Early results surgical treatment of triangular fibrocartilage complex tears in children and adolescence. *J Hand Surg.* 2020;45(5):449.e1–9.
89. Yip HS, Wu WC, Chang RY, So TY. Percutaneous cannulated screw fixation of acute scaphoid waist fracture. *J Hand Surg Br.* 2002;27(1):42–46.
90. Zook EG. Reconstruction of a functional and aesthetic nail. *Hand Clin.* 2002;18(4):577–594.

9

Fractures of the Distal Radius and Ulna

Apurva S. Shah

INTRODUCTION TO FRACTURES OF THE DISTAL RADIUS AND ULNA

Forearm fractures are the most common long-bone fractures in children, occurring with an annual incidence of approximately 0.5 to 1.7 per 100 children per year[75] and comprising approximately 35% of all pediatric fractures.[33,128,149] Among all forearm fractures, the distal radius and ulna are most commonly affected and represent nearly one-third of all pediatric fractures.[149] The peak incidence of distal radius and ulna fractures occurs during preadolescence and these injuries occur more commonly in males than females, with the largest difference between sexes occurring during adolescence.[128,162] Several recent studies suggest that the frequency of pediatric distal radius fractures may be rising, possibly due to epidemiologic trends toward diminished bone density, increased childhood obesity, and greater sports participation.[67,68,98,144,155,163]

In regions with seasonal temperature variation, the incidence of pediatric distal radius fractures demonstrates considerable variation over the year.[128,162] In a report that used the Swedish National Patient Register, the risk of pediatric distal radius fractures was found to be lowest during the winter months and highest during the spring and summer months. The highest seasonal variation was seen in preschool children and the lowest in adolescents.[128]

Because of the greater forces borne and imparted to the radius, as well as the increased porosity of the distal radial metaphysis, distal radial fractures are far more common than distal ulna fractures, and therefore, isolated distal radius fractures are regularly observed. However, approximately 50% of distal radius fractures occur in association with a distal ulna fracture, most commonly involving the distal ulnar metaphysis or styloid.[162] Complex fracture patterns can occur. Notably, the pediatric Galeazzi injury usually involves a distal radial metaphyseal diaphyseal fracture and a distal ulnar physeal fracture that

A, B   C, D

Figure 9-1. A: Greenstick fracture in a 9-year-old girl with tension failure of the volar cortex (*black arrows*) and plastic deformation of the dorsal cortex (*white arrow*). **B:** Torus fracture with compression of the dorsal cortex in a 20-month-old boy. **C:** Complete fracture with dorsal bayonet position in a 4-year-old girl. **D:** Salter–Harris type II physeal fracture with dorsal translation and angulation in a 12-year-old boy.

result in a displaced distal radioulnar joint (DRUJ). Galeazzi fracture–dislocations are relatively rare injuries in children with a cited occurrence of 3% of pediatric distal radial fractures.[177]

Given the high frequency of distal radius and ulna fractures in children, the evaluation and management of these injuries remain a fundamental element of pediatric orthopaedics. Despite established treatment principles, however, care of these injuries remains challenging due to the spectrum of injury patterns, issues of skeletal growth and remodeling, diversity of nonoperative and surgical techniques, evolving patient/family expectations, and increasing emphasis on cost-effective care.

ASSESSMENT OF FRACTURES OF THE DISTAL RADIUS AND ULNA

MECHANISMS OF INJURY OF FRACTURES OF THE DISTAL RADIUS AND ULNA

Distal Radius and Ulna Fractures

The mechanism of injury is generally a fall on an outstretched hand, often during sports or playground activities.[149,162] Typically, the extended position of the wrist at the time of loading leads to tensile failure on the volar cortex of the distal radius, compression of the dorsal cortex, or both, with dorsal translation and

angulation of the distal fragment (Fig. 9-1). Conversely, and far less commonly, axial loading on the flexed wrist will produce a volar translation and angulation of the distal fragment (Fig. 9-2). More rarely, distal radius fractures can occur from direct blows or motor vehicle collisions. In addition to the angular deformity caused by axial and bending loads applied to the distal forearm, rotational displacement may also occur, based on the position of the forearm and torsional forces sustained at the time of injury.

Fracture type and degree of displacement are also dependent on the height and force of the fall or injury mechanism. Indeed, the spectrum of injury may range from incomplete torus (or "buckle") fractures (common in younger children with low-energy falls) or complete dorsally displaced fractures with apex volar angulation (more common in older children with higher-velocity injuries). Displacement may be severe enough to cause foreshortening and bayonet apposition. A large multicenter registry in the United States demonstrated that approximately 44% of distal radius fractures are torus fractures, 31% are complete or bicortical metaphyseal fractures, 21% are physeal fractures, and 2% to 3% are greenstick fractures.[162] Adult-type injuries with intra-articular extension do uncommonly occur. Rarely, a mechanism such as a fall from a height can cause a distal radial fracture associated with a more proximal fracture of the forearm or elbow.[13,151] These "floating elbow" situations connote higher-energy trauma and may be associated with risks of neurovascular compromise and compartment syndrome.[151]

A

B

Figure 9-2. Reverse bayonet. **A:** Typical volar bayonet fracture. Often the distal end of the proximal fragment is buttonholed through the extensor tendons (*arrows*). (Reproduced with permission from Wilkins KE, ed. *Operative Management of Upper Extremity Fractures in Children.* American Academy of Orthopaedic Surgeons; 1994.) **B:** Intact volar periosteum and disrupted dorsal periosteum (*arrows*). The extensor tendons are displaced to either side of the proximal fragment.

Fractures of the distal forearm in children typically occur when the radius and/or ulna are more susceptible to fracture secondary to biomechanical changes during skeletal development. Work based on load-to-strength ratio and other measures of bone quality has identified specific times during skeletal development when the biologic properties of the distal upper extremity produce relatively weaker bone, making a child more susceptible to fracture.[55,89,99,129] In these studies, preadolescent boys and girls were found to have lower estimates of bone strength compared to same-sex postpubertal peers. From these studies, it can be concluded that children are uniquely susceptible for fracture when longitudinal growth outpaces mineral accrual during rapid growth.[14] As 90% of the radius growth is from the distal physis and accounts for 70% of the loading across the wrist, the radius is more prone to fracture than the ulna during rapid growth.[178] Fractures occur at the biomechanically weakest anatomic location of bone, which also varies over time. As the metaphyseal cortex of the radius is relatively thin and porous, fractures of the metaphysis are most common, followed by physeal fractures, as noted above.[162] Usually, fractures occur during falls or sports-related activities. Indeed, the trend toward increased sports participation in children appears to have led to a substantial increase in the incidence of distal radius and ulna fractures.[186] Certain sports, such as soccer, football, rugby, basketball, ice hockey, and snowboarding have been associated with an increased risk of distal radial fracture, though a fall or injury of sufficient severity may occur in any recreational activity.[162,186] Protective wrist guards have been shown to decrease the injury rate in snowboarders by approximately 50%.[154]

As cited above, there is seasonal variation, with an increase in both incidence and severity of fractures in the spring and summer.[128,162,179] Children who are overweight, have poor postural balance, ligamentous laxity, or less bone mineralization are at increased risk for distal radial fractures. Although bone quality measures predict that boys had lower risk of fracture than girls at every stage except during early puberty,[129] these fractures have been reported to be three times more common in boys. This may be due to relative risk-taking behaviors or participation in higher risk of injury activities. However, the increased participation in athletics by girls at a young age may change this ratio in the future.

Distal Radial Physeal Stress Injury

Repetitive axial loading of the wrist may lead to physeal stress injuries, almost always involving the distal radius (Fig. 9-3). These physeal stress injuries are most commonly seen in competitive gymnasts and are often termed "gymnast wrist."[41,119,173] Factors that predispose to this injury include excessive training, poor techniques, and attempts to advance too quickly in competitive level. Stress injuries have been also observed sports such as wrestling, break dancing, and cheerleading. In children with gymnast wrist, continued sports participation and repetitive axial loading without rest can lead to premature physeal arrest, ulnar positive variance, and development of ulnar impaction syndrome with pain.

Galeazzi Fracture

Axial loading of the wrist in combination with extremes of forearm rotation (Fig. 9-4) may result in distal radius fractures with

Figure 9-3. Radiographic images of the gymnast's wrist. **A:** AP radiograph of the left wrist in a 12-year-old girl demonstrates physeal widening, cystic changes, and metaphyseal sclerosis. **B:** AP radiograph of the same wrist after 3 months of rest from gymnastics, demonstrating partial resolution of the physeal changes.

associated disruption of the DRUJ, the so-called Galeazzi fracture.[50,103,109,177] In adults, the mechanism of injury usually is an axially loading fall with hyperpronation. This results in a distal radial fracture with DRUJ ligament disruption and dorsal dislocation of the distal ulna. However, in children, both supination (apex volar) and pronation (apex dorsal) deforming forces have been described.[109,177] The mechanism of injury is most obvious when the radial fracture is incomplete. With an apex volar (supination) radial fracture, the distal ulna is displaced volarly; whereas with an apex dorsal (pronation) radial fracture, the distal ulna is displaced dorsally. This is evident both on clinical and radiographic examinations. In addition, the radius is foreshortened in a complete fracture, causing more radial deviation of the hand and wrist. In children, this injury may involve either true dislocation of the distal ulna with disruption of the DRUJ ligaments or, more commonly, a distal ulnar physeal fracture (Fig. 9-5).[1]

INJURIES ASSOCIATED WITH FRACTURES OF THE DISTAL RADIUS AND ULNA

The risk of associated injuries is significantly less in the skeletally immature as compared to skeletally mature patients. The entire ipsilateral extremity should be carefully examined for concomitant fractures of the carpus, forearm, or elbow, particularly the supracondylar humerus. Associated fractures of the elbow region need to be assessed because their presence implies more severe trauma. The incidence of a compartment syndrome is theoretically higher with a "floating elbow" combination of radial, ulnar, and elbow fractures.[151] However, the risk of acute compartment syndrome was recently reported to be lower than previously suspected, with an incidence of approximately 2% in pediatric floating elbows.[13]

With marked radial or ulnar fracture displacement, neurovascular compromise can occur.[17,181] Median neuropathy may be

Figure 9-4. Supination-type Galeazzi fracture. **A:** View of the entire forearm of an 11-year-old boy with a Galeazzi fracture–dislocation. **B:** Close-up of the distal forearm shows that there has been disruption of the distal radioulnar joint (*arrows*). The distal radial fragment is dorsally displaced (apex volar), making this a supination type of mechanism. Note that the distal ulna is volar to the distal radius. **C, D:** The fracture was reduced by flexing and pronating the distal fragment. Because the distal radius was partially intact by its greenstick nature, the length was easily maintained, reestablishing the congruity of the distal radioulnar joint. The patient was immobilized in supination for 6 weeks, after which full forearm rotation and function returned.

seen in severely displaced distal radius fractures, due to direct nerve contusion sustained at the time of fracture displacement, persistent pressure or traction from an unreduced fracture, or an acute compartment syndrome (Fig. 9-6). Ulnar neuropathy has been described with similar mechanisms, as well as entrapment or incarceration of the ulnar nerve within the fracture site.

Wrist ligamentous and articular cartilage injuries have been described in association with distal radial and ulna fractures in adults and less commonly in children. Concomitant scaphoid fractures have occurred (Fig. 9-7). Associated wrist injuries need to be treated both in the acute setting and in the patient with persistent pain after fracture healing. Approximately 50% of distal radial physeal fractures have an associated ulnar fracture. This usually is an ulnar metaphyseal or styloid fracture but can also be a physeal or diaphyseal fracture.[162] Some patients with distal radial and ulna fractures are multitrauma victims. Care of the distal forearm fracture in these situations must be provided within the context of concomitant systemic injuries.

Ulnar fractures are most commonly metaphyseal fractures or styloid fractures. Isolated ulnar physeal fractures are rare.[1] Most ulnar physeal fractures occur in association with distal radial metaphyseal or physeal fractures. Physeal fractures represent less than 5% of all distal ulnar injuries and are classified by

Figure 9-5. Galeazzi fracture–dislocation variant. Interposed periosteum can block reduction of the distal ulnar physis (*arrow*). This destabilizes the distal radial metaphyseal fracture. (Reprinted with permission from Lanfried MJ, et al. Variant of Galeazzi fracture–dislocation in children. *J Pediatr Orthop.* 1991;11(3):333–335.)

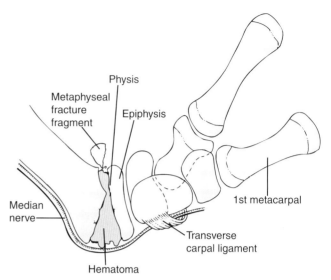

Figure 9-6. Volar forearm anatomy outlining the potential compression of the median nerve between the metaphysis of the radius and dorsally displaced physeal fracture. The taut volar transverse carpal ligament and fracture hematoma also are contributing factors. (Redrawn with permission from Waters PM, et al. Acute median neuropathy following physeal fractures of the distal radius. *J Pediatr Orthop.* 1994;14(2):173–177.)

Figure 9-7. Radiographs (**A**) and coronal computer tomography (CT) image (**B**) of ipsilateral comminuted Salter–Harris type IV distal radius fracture and distal pole scaphoid fracture in a 14-year-old boy. Coronal CT image (**C**) of another patient with a more subtle presentation of an associated scaphoid waist fracture. (Courtesy of Children's Orthopaedic Surgery Foundation.)

the standard Salter–Harris system.[162] An ulnar styloid fracture is typically an epiphyseal avulsion and can be associated with soft tissue injuries of the triangular fibrocartilage complex (TFCC) and ulnocarpal joint. Ulnar styloid fractures do not typically cause growth-related complications unless the styloid fracture represents a Salter–Harris type III or IV fracture pattern. The rare pediatric Galeazzi injury usually involves an ulnar physeal fracture rather than a soft tissue disruption of the DRUJ.

SIGNS AND SYMPTOMS OF FRACTURES OF THE DISTAL RADIUS AND ULNA

Traumatic Fractures

Children with distal radial and/or ulna fractures present with pain, swelling, and deformity of the wrist (Fig. 9-8). The clinical signs depend on the degree of fracture displacement. With a nondisplaced torus fracture in a young child, medical attention may not be sought until several days after injury; the intact periosteum and biomechanical stability are protective in these injuries, resulting in minimal pain and guarding. Similarly, many of the physeal injuries are nondisplaced and present only with pain and tenderness at the physis. With displaced fractures, the typical dorsal displacement and apex volar angulation create an extension deformity that is usually clinically apparent. Careful inspection of the forearm is critical to evaluate for possible skin lacerations, wounds, and open fractures.

With greater displacement, physical examination is often limited by the patient's pain and anxiety, but it is imperative to obtain an accurate examination of the motor and sensory components of the radial, median, and ulnar nerves before treatment is initiated. Neurovascular compromise is uncommon but can occur.[17,181] Median nerve irritability or dysfunction is most common, caused by direct trauma to the nerve at the time of injury or ongoing ischemic compression from the displaced fracture. Median nerve motor function is evaluated by testing the abductor pollicis brevis (intrinsic) and flexor pollicis longus

(extrinsic) muscles. Ulnar nerve motor evaluation includes testing the first dorsal interosseous (intrinsic), abductor digiti quinti (intrinsic), and flexor digitorum profundus to the small finger (extrinsic) muscles. Radial nerve evaluation involves testing the common digital extensors for metacarpophalangeal joint extension as well as thumb extensor pollicis longus. Sensibility to light touch and objective sensory testing can be tested. Normal two-point discrimination is less than 4 mm but may not be reliably tested in children younger than 6 or 7 years of age.[47] In contrast, monofilament testing has been found to be reliable in the majority of 4- and 5-year-old children.[47] Pinprick sensibility testing is likely to increase anxiety in the injured child and should be avoided.

Distal Radial Physeal Stress Injury

In contrast to the child with an acute, traumatic distal radius fracture, patients with distal radial physeal stress injuries typically report recurrent activity-related wrist pain. This condition is often referred to as "gymnast wrist" and is seen most commonly in gymnasts and cheerleaders. Characteristically, this pain is described as diffuse "aching" and "soreness" in the region of the distal radial metaphysis and physis. Pain may be reproduced in the extremes of wrist extension and flexion, and usually there is focal tenderness over the distal radial physis. Resistive strength testing of the wrist extensors may also reproduce the pain. The differential diagnosis includes physeal stress injury, ganglion cyst, dorsal wrist impingement, juvenile inflammatory arthritis, ligamentous or TFCC injury, tendinosis or musculotendinous strain, carpal fracture, and osteonecrosis of the scaphoid (Preiser disease) or lunate (Kienbock disease). Diagnosis is made radiographically in the context of the clinical presentation.

Radiographs are also usually diagnostic in cases of suspected distal radial physeal stress injuries. Physeal widening, cystic and sclerotic changes in the metaphyseal aspect of the distal radial physis, beaking of the distal radial epiphysis, and reactive bone formation are highly suggestive of chronic physeal stress fracture. In advanced cases, premature physeal closure or physeal bar formation may be seen, indicating long-standing stress.[41,153,173,188] In these situations, continued ulnar growth leads to an ulnar positive variance with resulting pain from ulnocarpal impaction and/or TFCC tearing.[11,153] Plain radiographs may not reveal early physeal stress injury. If the diagnosis is suggested clinically, additional studies may be indicated. Technetium bone scanning is sensitive but nonspecific. Magnetic resonance imaging (MRI) is usually diagnostic, demonstrating physeal thickening, particularly on the volar side in symptomatic children.[101]

Galeazzi Fracture-Dislocation

Children with Galeazzi injuries present with pain, limited forearm rotation, and limited wrist flexion and extension. Neurovascular impairment is rare. The radial deformity usually is clinically evident. Prominence of the ulnar head is seen with DRUJ disruption. Ligamentous disruption is often subtle and may be evident only by local tenderness and instability to testing of the DRUJ.

Figure 9-8. Dorsal bayonet deformity. **A:** Typical distal metaphyseal fracture with dorsal bayonet showing a dorsal angulation of the distal forearm. **B:** Usually, the periosteum is intact on the dorsal side and disrupted on the volar side.

IMAGING AND OTHER DIAGNOSTIC STUDIES
FRACTURES OF THE DISTAL RADIUS AND ULNA

Plain radiographs are diagnostic of the fracture type and degree of displacement. Standard posteroanterior (PA) and lateral radiographs usually are sufficient. Oblique views are more useful with intraarticular injuries. Complete wrist, forearm, and elbow views are recommended in cases of high-energy injuries or when there is clinical suspicion for a concomitant ipsilateral fracture of the hand, wrist, or elbow. Cross-sectional radiographic evaluation (e.g., computed tomography [CT], MRI) is typically reserved for evaluation of suspected or known intraarticular fractures or associated carpal injuries (e.g., scaphoid fractures, hook of hamate fractures, perilunate instability); these situations are most commonly encountered in older adolescents. Cross-sectional imaging may be particularly useful in assessing Salter–Harris type III and IV fractures of the distal radius in order to assess the degree of displacement and need for surgery.

Radiographic evaluation should be performed not only to confirm the diagnosis but also to quantify the degree of displacement, angulation, malrotation, and comminution (Fig. 9-9). Understanding of the normal radiographic parameters is essential in quantifying displacement. In adults, the normal distal radial inclination averages 22 degrees on the AP view and 11 degrees of volar tilt on the lateral projection. Radial inclination refers to the angle between the distal radial articular surface and a line perpendicular to the radial shaft on the AP radiograph. Volar tilt is measured by a line across the distal articular surface and a line perpendicular to the radial shaft on the lateral view. Pediatric values for radial inclination and volar tilt may vary from adult

normative values, depending on the degree of skeletal maturity and the ossification of the epiphysis.[81,156] Indeed, radial inclination and radial height increase steadily during growth and reach the adult range at the beginning of the pubertal growth spurt.[156] Volar tilt does not visibly appear until approximately 11 years of age but typically reaches adult values by 14 years of age.[156]

As noted above, advanced imaging may be helpful in cases of intra-articular extension to characterize fracture pattern and joint congruity. This may be done by CT or MRI. Dynamic motion studies with fluoroscopy can provide important information on fracture stability and the success of various treatment options. Dynamic fluoroscopy requires adequate pain relief and is used more often in adult patients with distal radial fractures.

In Galeazzi fractures, the radial fracture is readily apparent on plain radiographs. Careful systematic evaluation of the radiographs will reveal concurrent injuries to the ulna and/or DRUJ (Fig. 9-10). A true lateral radiograph is essential to identify the direction of displacement and thus to determine the method of reduction. Rarely are advanced imaging studies, such as CT or MRI scan, necessary.

CLASSIFICATION OF FRACTURES OF
THE DISTAL RADIUS AND ULNA

Distal Radius and Ulna Fractures

Distal Forearm Fractures: GENERAL CLASSIFICATION

Physeal fractures
    Distal radius
    Distal ulna

Distal metaphyseal (radius or ulna)
    Torus
    Greenstick
    Complete/bicortical fractures

Galeazzi fracture-dislocations
    Dorsally displaced
    Volarly displaced

Distal radius and ulna fractures are classified according to fracture pattern, type of associated ulnar fracture, and direction of displacement, angulation, and rotation. Most distal radial metaphyseal fractures are displaced dorsally with apex volar angulation. Volar displacement with apex dorsal angulation occurs less commonly, typically following falls on a flexed wrist.

Distal radial and ulna fractures are then defined by their anatomic relationship to the physis. Physeal fractures are classified by the widely accepted Salter–Harris system (see below). Metaphyseal injuries are often different from their adult equivalents, due to the thick periosteum surrounding the relatively thin metaphyseal cortex. Metaphyseal fractures are generally classified according to fracture pattern and may be torus fractures, greenstick fractures, or complete bicortical injuries. This system of classification (torus, greenstick, bicortical, physeal) has been shown to have good intra- and inter-observer reliability, both of which increase with provider experience.[147] A more recent study

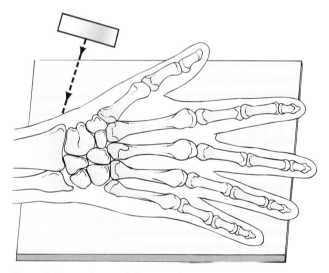

Figure 9-9. Angulation of the x-ray beam tangential to the articular surface, providing the optimal lateral view of the distal radius. The wrist is positioned as for the standard lateral radiograph, but the x-ray beam is directed 15 degrees cephalad. (Reprinted by permission from Springer Nature: Johnson PG, Szabo RM. Angle measurements of the distal radius: a cadaver study. *Skel Radiol.* 1993;22(4):243–246. Copyright © 1993 International Skeletal Society.)

Figure 9-10. Lateral radiograph depicting volar subluxation of the distal ulna in relation to the distal radius, a pediatric Galeazzi equivalent. Careful inspection reveals a distal ulnar physeal fracture.

Figure 9-11. Dorsally displaced physeal fracture (type A). The distal epiphysis with a small metaphyseal fragment is displaced dorsally (*curved arrow*) in relation to the proximal metaphyseal fragment.

demonstrated only fair agreement on classifying distal radius fractures using a similar system.[48] This study suggests poor provider ability to distinguish torus fractures from greenstick fractures and offers opportunity for improved orthopaedic education. Pediatric equivalents of adult Galeazzi fracture–dislocations involve a distal radial fracture and either a soft tissue disruption of the DRUJ or a physeal fracture of the distal ulna.

Physeal Injuries

The Salter–Harris system is the basis for classification of physeal fractures.[157] Most distal radial physeal injuries (nearly 85%) are Salter–Harris type II fractures.[162] In the more common apex volar injuries, dorsal displacement of the distal epiphysis and the dorsal Thurston–Holland metaphyseal fragment is evident on the lateral view (Fig. 9-11). Salter–Harris type I fractures also usually displaced dorsally. Volar displacement of either a Salter–Harris type I or II fracture is less common (Fig. 9-12). Nondisplaced Salter–Harris type I fractures may be indicated only by a displaced pronator hematoma sign on a lateral radiograph or tenderness over the involved physis. Point-of-care ultrasound appears to have high sensitivity in detecting hematoma adjacent to the pronator quadratus when there is cortical breaching.[164] A scaphoid fat pad sign may indicate a concomitant scaphoid fracture (Fig. 9-13).[78]

Salter–Harris type III and IV fractures are rare and represent less than 1% of all distal radius fractures in children.[92,162] Salter–Harris type III fractures may be caused by a compression, shear, or avulsion of the radial origin of the volar radiocarpal ligaments (Fig. 9-14).[107] Salter–Harris type IV fractures can present as triplane-equivalent fractures, appearing like a Salter–Harris type II

on a lateral radiograph and a type III fracture on the PA radiograph. CT scans may be necessary to define the fracture pattern and degree of intra-articular displacement in deciding best treatment options for Salter–Harris type III and IV fractures.

Metaphyseal Injuries

Distal Radial Metaphyseal Fractures: CLASSIFICATION

Directional displacement
  Dorsal
  Volar

Fracture combinations
  Isolated radius
  Radius with ulna
    Ulnar styloid
    Ulnar physis
    Ulnar metaphysis, incomplete
    Ulnar metaphysis, complete

Biomechanical patterns
  One cortex
    Torus
    Greenstick
  Two cortices
  Complete bicortical fracture
    Length maintained
    Bayonet apposition

Metaphyseal fracture patterns are classified as torus, greenstick, and complete fractures (Fig. 9-15). This system of classification has been shown to have good agreement between experienced observers.[147] Torus fractures are incomplete fractures resulting from axial compression. The site of cortical failure is often the transition from metaphysis to diaphysis.[111] As the mode of failure is compression, these injuries are inherently stable and are further stabilized by the intact surrounding periosteum. Rarely, they may extend into the physis, putting them at risk for growth impairment.

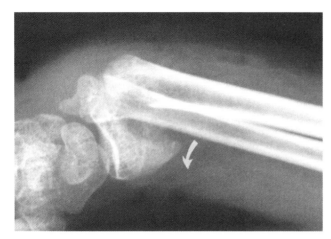

Figure 9-12. Volarly displaced physeal fracture (type B). Distal epiphysis with a large volar metaphyseal fragment is displaced in a volar direction (*curved arrow*). (Reproduced with permission from Wilkins KE, ed: *Operative Management of Upper Extremity Fractures in Children.* American Academy of Orthopaedic Surgeons; 1994.)

Greenstick fractures are incomplete fractures that occur with a combination of tensile, rotatory, and compressive forces, resulting in complete failure of one cortex and plastic deformation of the other cortex. Most commonly, the combined extension and supination forces lead to tensile failure of the volar cortex and dorsal compression injury. The degree of force determines the amount of plastic deformation, dorsal comminution, and fracture angulation and rotation. These fractures must be distinguished from torus fractures due to increased instability. There is typically tearing of the surrounding periosteum resulting in prolonged healing time.

With greater applied loads, complete bicortical fracture occurs with disruption of both the volar and dorsal cortices. Length may be maintained with apposition of the proximal and

Figure 9-13. Anatomic relationships of the navicular fat stripe (NFS). The NFS is located between the combined tendons of the abductor pollicis longus and extensor pollicis brevis, and the lateral surface of the carpal navicular. (Reproduced with permission of the American Roentgen Ray Society from Terry DW Jr, Ramin JE. The navicular fat stripe. *Am J Roentgenol Radium Ther Nucl Med.* 1975;124:25. Copyright© [1975] American Roentgen Ray Society.)

A   B

Figure 9-14. A: AP radiograph of Salter–Harris type III fracture of the distal radius. **B:** Series of AP, oblique and lateral radiographs of a Salter–Harris type IV fracture of the distal radius with ulnar styloid fracture.

A, B   **C**

Figure 9-15. Metaphyseal biomechanical fracture patterns. **A:** Torus fracture in a 3-year-old boy with simple bulging of the thin dorsal cortex from compression mechanism (*arrow*). **B:** Greenstick fracture in a 6-year-old girl with tension failure of the volar cortex (*small white arrow*) and secondary compression of the dorsal cortex (*curved arrow*). **C:** Bicortical fractures of the metaphyseal distal radius and ulna with maintenance of length in an 11-year-old girl.

distal fragments. Frequently, the distal fragment lies proximal and dorsal to the proximal fragment in bayonet apposition.

Ulna fractures often associated with radial metaphyseal injuries may occur in the metaphysis, physis, or through the ulnar styloid. Similar to radial metaphyseal fractures, the ulnar fracture can be complete or incomplete. These injuries are also characterized according to fracture pattern and displacement.

Distal radial fractures also can occur in conjunction with more proximal forearm fractures, Monteggia fracture–dislocations, supracondylar distal humeral fractures, or carpal fractures. The combination of a displaced supracondylar distal humeral fracture and a displaced distal radial metaphyseal fracture has been called the pediatric "floating elbow."

Distal Ulna Fractures

Isolated distal ulnar fractures are uncommon. Distal ulnar fractures most commonly occur in association with distal radial fractures and are most commonly metaphyseal fractures or styloid fractures. Distal ulnar physeal fractures are rare and occur with approximately 3% of distal radius fractures.[162] Physeal injuries are classified according to the Salter–Harris classification. Ulnar physeal fractures may also be seen with the pediatric Galeazzi injuries,[150] which usually involve an ulnar physeal fracture rather than a soft tissue disruption of the DRUJ.

Avulsion fractures of the ulnar styloid also represent epiphyseal avulsion injuries. Most commonly associated with distal radial fractures,[1] these styloid fractures typically represent avulsions of the ulnar insertion of the TFCC or ulnocarpal ligaments[11] and are rarely associated with growth-related complications.

Galeazzi Fracture

Galeazzi Fractures: CLASSIFICATION

Type I: Dorsal (apex volar) displacement of distal radius
    Radius fracture pattern
        Greenstick
        Complete
    Distal ulna dislocation
        True dislocation
        Physeal fracture (equivalent or variant)

Type II: Volar (apex dorsal) displacement of distal radius
    Radius fracture pattern
        Greenstick
        Complete
    Distal ulna dislocation
        True dislocation
        Physeal fracture (equivalent or variant)

Galeazzi fracture–dislocations are most commonly described by direction of displacement of either the distal ulnar dislocation or the radial fracture.[109] Letts preferred to describe the direction of the ulna, either volar or dorsal.[109] Others classified pediatric Galeazzi injuries by the direction of displacement of the distal radial fracture. Dorsally displaced or angulated (apex volar) fractures were more common than volarly displaced or angulated (apex dorsal) injuries in their series.[177] Wilkins and O'Brien[185] modified the Walsh and McLaren method by classifying distal radial fractures as incomplete and complete fractures and ulnar injuries as true dislocations versus physeal fractures. Distal radial fractures accompanied by DRUJ dislocations are called true Galeazzi lesions, and injuries accompanied by distal ulnar physeal fractures are called pediatric Galeazzi equivalents or variants.[91,103,109]

PATHOANATOMY AND APPLIED ANATOMY RELATING TO FRACTURES OF THE DISTAL RADIUS AND ULNA

The distal radial epiphysis normally appears between 0.5 and 2.3 years in boys and 0.4 and 1.7 years in girls.[124,133] Initially transverse in appearance, it rapidly becomes more adult-like with its triangular shape. The contour of the radial styloid progressively elongates with advancing skeletal maturity. The secondary center of ossification for the distal ulna appears at about age 7 years.[133] Similar to the radius, the ulnar styloid

appears with the adolescent growth spurt. It also becomes more elongated and adult-like until physeal closure. On average, the ulnar physis closes at age 16 in girls and age 17 in boys, whereas the distal radial physis closes on average 6 months later than the ulnar physis.[153,193] The distal radial and ulnar physes contribute approximately 75% to 80% of the growth of the forearm and 40% of the growth of the upper extremity (Fig. 9-16).[133]

The distal radius articulates with the distal ulna at the DRUJ.[160] Both the radius and ulna articulate with the carpus, serving as the platform for the carpus and hand. The radial joint surface has three concavities for its articulations: the scaphoid and lunate fossa for the carpus and the sigmoid notch for the ulnar head. These joints are stabilized by a complex series of volar and dorsal radiocarpal, ulnocarpal, and distal radioulnar ligaments. The volar ligaments are the major stabilizers. Starting

Figure 9-16. Ossification of the distal radius. **A:** Preossification of the distal radius in a 10-month-old boy. **B:** The triangular secondary ossification center of the distal radius in a 2-year-old girl. **C:** Initial ossification center of the ulnar styloid in a 7-year-old boy progresses radially (*arrow*). **D:** Extension of the ulnar ossification center into the styloid process in a 9-year-old girl.

Figure 9-16. (*Continued*) **E:** The ulnar styloid is fully ossified and the epiphyses have capped their relative metaphyses in this 12-year-old boy.

Figure 9-17. Diagrammatic drawing of the TFCC and the prestyloid recess. The meniscal reflection runs from the dorsoulnar radius to the ulno-volar carpus. The *arrow* denotes access under the reflection to the tip of the styloid, the so-called prestyloid recess. V, fifth metacarpal; S, scaphoid; C, capitate; H, hamate; L, lunate; TQ, triquetrum. (Redrawn with permission of Elsevier Science and Technology Journals from Bowers WH. *Green's Operative Hand Surgery.* Churchill-Livingstone; 1993, permission conveyed through Copyright Clearance Center Inc.)

radially at the radial styloid, the radial collateral, radioscapho-capitate, radiolunotriquetral (long radiolunate), and radios-capholunate (short radiolunate) ligaments volarly stabilize the radiocarpal joint. The dorsal radioscaphoid and radial triquetral ligaments are less important stabilizers. The complex structure of ligaments stabilize the radius, ulna, and carpus through the normal wrist motion of 120 degrees of flexion and extension, 50 degrees of radial and ulnar deviation, and 150 degrees of forearm rotation.[136]

The TFCC is the primary stabilizer of the ulnocarpal and radioulnar articulations.[136] It extends from the sigmoid notch of the radius across the DRUJ and inserts into the base of the ulnar styloid. The TFCC also extends distally as the ulnolunate, ulnotriquetral, and ulnar collateral ligaments and inserts into the ulnar carpus and base of the fifth metacarpal.[136] The volar ulnocarpal ligaments (V ligament) from the ulna to the lunate and triquetrum are important ulnocarpal stabilizers.[160] The central portion of the TFCC is the articular disk (Fig. 9-17). The interaction between the bony articulation and the soft tissue attachments accounts for stability of the DRUJ during prona-tion and supination.[136] At the extremes of rotation, the joint is most stable. The compression loads between the radius and ulna are aided by the tensile loads of the TFCC to maintain stability throughout rotation.

The interosseous membrane of the forearm (Fig. 9-18) helps stabilize the radius and ulna more proximally in the midpor-tion of the forearm. Throughout the mid-forearm, the inter-osseous membrane connects the radius to the ulna. It passes obliquely from the proximal radius to the distal ulna. The inter-osseous membrane has been traditionally described as having five components including a central band, accessory band, dis-tal oblique bundle, proximal oblique cord, and dorsal oblique accessory cord.[130] The central band is the most essential com-ponent and plays pivotal roles in longitudinal stability and load transfer from the radius to the ulna. However, the inter-osseous membrane does not extend to the distal radius. Moore et al.[127] found that injuries to the TFCC and interosseous

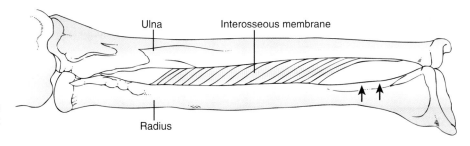

Figure 9-18. The attachment and the fibers of the interosseous membrane are such that there is no attachment to the distal radius.

Figure 9-19. Hafner's technique to measure ulnar variance. **A:** The distance from the most proximal point of the ulnar metaphysis to the most proximal point of the radial metaphysis. **B:** The distance from the most distal point of the ulnar metaphysis to the most distal point of the radial metaphysis. (Adapted by permission from Springer: Hafner R, et al. Ulnar variance in children. Standard measurements for evaluation of ulnar shortening in juvenile rheumatoid arthritis, hereditary multiple exostosis and other bone or joint disorders in childhood. *Skel Radiol.* 1989;18(4):513–516. Copyright © 1989 International Skeletal Society.)

ligament were responsible for progressive shortening of the radius with fracture in a cadaveric study. The soft tissue component to the injury is a major factor in the deformity and instability in a Galeazzi fracture–dislocation.

The length relationship between the distal radius and ulna at the wrist is defined as ulnar variance and is typically measured in millimeters. If the ulna and radius are of equal lengths at the wrist, there is ulnar neutral variance. If the ulna is longer, there is ulnar positive variance. If the ulna is shorter, there is ulnar negative variance. In adolescents or skeletally mature individuals, this is most reliably measured with the method of perpendiculars described by Steyers and Blair.[65,166] In this technique, the ulnar variance is defined as the distance between peak of the distal ulna cortical rim and a line drawn perpendicular to the longitudinal axis of the radius and through the distal corner of the sigmoid notch.[166] However, measurement of ulnar variance in younger children requires modifications of this technique as the epiphysis may not be visible or sufficiently ossified. Hafner et al.[73] described measuring from the distal metaphysis of the radius to the distal metaphysis of the ulna to lessen the measurement inaccuracies related to epiphyseal size and shape (Fig. 9-19). It should be recognized that this technique should be reserved for use in younger children. Although it provides a reliable point for comparison, the technique does not truly compare radius and ulna length. Instead, this measurement allows assessment in a single patient over time or allows comparison with the normative values established by Hafner et al.

Although not dependent on the length of the ulnar styloid, the measurement of ulnar variance is dependent on forearm position and radiographic technique.[53] Supination decreases ulnar variance and pronation increases ulnar variance. For this reason, radiographs of the wrist to determine ulnar variance should be standardized with the hand and wrist placed on the cassette, with the shoulder abducted 90 degrees, elbow flexed 90 degrees, and forearm in neutral rotation (Fig. 9-20). The importance of ulnar variance relates to the force transmission across the wrist with axial loading. Normally, the radiocarpal joint bears approximately 80% of the axial load across the wrist, and the ulnocarpal joint bears 20%. Changes in the length relationship of the radius and ulna alter respective load bearing. Indeed, 2.5 mm of ulnar positive variance has been

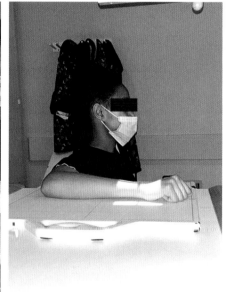

Figure 9-20. Technique for neutral rotation posteroanterior (PA) wrist radiograph. By abducting the shoulder to 90 degrees and flexing the elbow to 90 degrees the forearm is maintained in neutral pronation-supination.

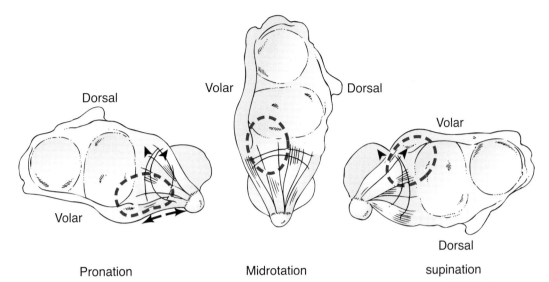

Dorsal   Volar   Dorsal

Volar

Volar

Dorsal

Pronation   Midrotation   supination

Figure 9-21. Distal radioulnar joint stability in pronation (**left**) is dependent on tension developed in the volar margin of the triangular fibrocartilage (TFCC, *small arrowheads*) and compression between the contact areas of the radius and ulna (volar surface of ulnar articular head and dorsal margin of the sigmoid notch, *large arrows*). Disruption of the volar TFCC would therefore allow dorsal displacement of the ulna in pronation. The reverse is true in supination, where disruption of the dorsal margin of the TFCC would allow volar displacement of the ulna relative to the radius as this rotational extreme is reached. The dark area of the TFCC emphasizes the portion of the TFCC that is not supported by the ulnar dome. The *dotted circle* is the arc of load transmission (lunate to TFCC) in that position. (Redrawn with permission of Elsevier Science and Technology Journals from Bowers WH. *Green's Operative Hand Surgery.* Churchill-Livingstone; 1993, permission conveyed through Copyright Clearance Center Inc.)

demonstrated to double the forces borne across the ulnocarpal articulation in adult biomechanical analyses.[86,136] Biomechanical and clinical studies have shown that this load distribution is important in fractures, TFCC tears (positive ulnar variance), and Kienbock disease (negative ulnar variance).[3,61]

The distal radius normally rotates around the relatively stationary ulna. The two bones of the forearm articulate at the proximal radioulnar joint and DRUJ. In addition, proximally the radius and ulna articulate with the distal humerus and distally with the carpus. These articulations are necessary for forearm pronation and supination. At the DRUJ, the concave sigmoid notch of the radius incompletely matches the convex, asymmetric, semicylindrical shape of the distal ulnar head.[136] This allows some translation at the DRUJ with rotatory movements. The ligamentous structures are critical in stabilizing the radius as it rotates about the ulna (Fig. 9-21).

TREATMENT OPTIONS FOR FRACTURES OF THE DISTAL RADIUS AND ULNA

NONOPERATIVE TREATMENT OF FRACTURES OF THE DISTAL RADIUS AND ULNA

The goal of pediatric distal radius fracture care is to achieve bony union within acceptable radiographic parameters to optimize long-term function and avoid late complications. Management is influenced tremendously by the remodeling potential

of the distal radius in growing children (Fig. 9-22). In general, remodeling potential is dependent on the amount of skeletal growth remaining, proximity of the injury to the physis, and relationship of the deformity to plane of adjacent joint motion. Fractures in very young children, close to the distal radial physis, with predominantly sagittal plane angulation have the greatest remodeling capacity. Acceptable sagittal plane angulation of acute distal radial metaphyseal fractures has been reported to be from 25 to 35 degrees in patients under 5 years of age, and 15 to 25 degrees in patients under 10 years of age[133,185] (Table 9-1).

Criteria for what constitutes acceptable coronal plane deformity have been more strict. The fracture tends to displace radially with an apex ulnar angulation. This deformity also has remodeling potential,[138,194] but less so than sagittal plane deformity. Most authorities agree that 10 degrees or less of acute malalignment in the frontal plane should be accepted. Historically, it has been suggested that greater magnitudes of coronal plane malalignment may not remodel and could result in limitations of forearm rotation.[36,49] This has been challenged by Lynch et al. who reported on coronal remodeling of the pediatric distal radius in children less than 12 years of age. In this investigation, mean coronal plane remodeling occurred at a rate of 2.3 degrees per month. The investigators suggested that up to 24 degrees of coronal plane malalignment can be accepted in children less than 12 years of age.[116]

In general, 10 to 30 degrees maximum of sagittal plane angulation, 10 to 20 degrees maximum of coronal plane angulation, and even complete bayonet apposition will reliably remodel in younger children with at least 2 years of significant growth remaining.[44,59,82,194]

Figure 9-22. **A:** AP and lateral fluoroscopy views of a distal radial physeal fracture at the time of closed reduction (CR) in a 10-year-old girl. **B:** Loss of reduction with impending malunion 1 month after CR. **C:** Continued bone healing and early fracture remodeling 2 months after CR. **D:** Significant remodeling without physeal arrest only 6 months from CR with residual ulnar positive variance and decreased radial inclination. Anticipated full remodeling with additional skeletal growth.

Indications/Contraindications

Nonoperative Treatment of Distal Radius Fractures: INDICATIONS AND CONTRAINDICATIONS

Indications

Torus fractures

Nondisplaced fractures

Displaced fractures within acceptable radiographic alignment

Displaced fractures amenable to closed reduction and immobilization

Late-presenting physeal fractures

Distal radial physeal stress fractures

Relative Contraindications

Open fractures

Neurovascular compromise or excessive swelling precluding circumferential cast immobilization

Irreducible fracture in unacceptable alignment

Unstable fractures failing initial reduction and cast immobilization

TABLE 9-1. Angular Corrections in Degrees

Age (Years)	Sagittal Plane		Coronal Plane
	Boys	Girls	
<5	35	35	25
5–10	25	25	25
10–13	15	10	10
13–15	5	0	0

Acceptable residual angulation is that which will result in total radiographic and functional correction based on the author's experience and the available literature.

Figure 9-23. Anteroposterior (**A**) and lateral (**B**) radiographs of a distal radius torus fracture in a 5-year-old boy.

For the reasons cited above, most pediatric distal radius fractures can be successfully treated with nonoperative means (no reduction or closed reduction, with splint or cast immobilization). General indications for nonoperative treatment include torus fractures, displaced physeal or metaphyseal fractures within acceptable parameters of expected skeletal remodeling, displaced fractures with unacceptable alignment amenable to closed reduction and immobilization, and late-presenting displaced physeal injuries in which late closed reduction has high risk of growth arrest.

Contraindications to nonoperative care include open fractures, fractures with excessive soft tissue injury or neurovascular compromise precluding circumferential cast immobilization, irreducible fractures in unacceptable alignment, unstable fractures failing initial nonoperative care, and fractures with displacement that will not remodel sufficiently to be acceptable long term.

Splint Immobilization of Torus Fractures

By definition, torus fractures are compression fractures of the distal radial metaphysis and are inherently stable (Fig. 9-23). There is typically minimal cortical disruption or displacement. As a result, treatment should consist of protected immobilization to prevent further injury and relieve pain. Multiple studies have compared the effectiveness and cost of casting, splinting, and simple soft bandage application in the treatment of torus fractures. As expected, there is little difference in outcome of the various immobilization techniques.[2,21,131,142,139] The preponderance of evidence suggesting that the type of immobilization does not affect outcome in pediatric distal radius torus fractures has gradually resulted in most orthopaedic surgeons limiting the use of cast immobilization.[110] In centers where casting continues to dominate, quality improvement initiatives may result in a substantial shift toward bracing in most patients.[112]

Davidson et al.[37] randomized 201 children with torus fractures to plaster cast or removable wrist splint immobilization for 3 weeks. All patients went on to successful healing without complications or need for follow-up clinical visits or radiographs. Similarly, Plint et al.[140] reported the results of a prospective randomized clinical trial in which 87 children were treated with either short-arm casts or removable splints for 3 weeks. Not only were there no differences in healing or pain, but also early wrist function was considerably better in the splinted patients.

Given the reliable healing seen with torus fracture healing, Symons et al.[168] performed a randomized trial of 87 patients treated with plaster splints to either hospital follow-up or home removal. No difference was seen in clinical results, and patient/families preferred home splint removal. A similar study by Khan et al.[97] confirmed these findings. No differences in outcomes were seen in 117 patients treated with either rigid cast removal in fracture clinic versus soft cast removal at home, and families preferred home removal of their immobilization. A meta-analysis of torus and minimally displaced fractures treated by removable splints instead of circumferential casts was found to have improved secondary outcomes for the patient and family and with equal position at healing.[10]

These findings were recently furthered by Perry et al. in a randomized controlled trial with 965 children that demonstrated that there was no difference in pain or function between children treated with soft bandages versus rigid immobilization (splint or cast) during the first 6 weeks.[139]

Therefore, soft bandages or simple splinting are both sufficient, and once the patient is comfortable, range-of-motion exercises and nontraumatic activities may begin. Fracture healing usually occurs in 3 to 4 weeks.[2,9] Although there has been a shift toward avoiding casting for distal radius torus fractures, Lawrence et al. demonstrated that some families prefer casting despite the higher cost.[106] Physicians must continue to emphasize that simple torus fractures heal without long-term sequelae or complications. Refractures are uncommon in children with distal radius torus fractures.

Cast Immobilization of Nondisplaced or Minimally Displaced Distal Radial Metaphyseal and Physeal Fractures

Nondisplaced fractures are treated with cast immobilization until appropriate bony healing and pain resolution have been achieved. Although these fractures are radiographically well aligned at the time of presentation, fracture stability is difficult to assess and a risk of late displacement exists (Fig. 9-24). Weekly serial radiographs are obtained in the first 2 weeks postreduction to confirm maintenance of acceptable radiographic alignment. In general, most fractures will heal within 4 to 6 weeks.

Simple immobilization without reduction may also be considered in minimally displaced fractures within acceptable alignment, based on patient age and remodeling potential. Hove

A, B
C
D

Figure 9-24. **A, B:** Anteroposterior (AP) and lateral radiographs of a distal radial metaphyseal fracture. This injury was initially assumed to be stable and was treated with cast immobilization with suboptimal mold. **C, D:** Subsequent radiographs taken 3 weeks after injury demonstrate loss of alignment and early bony healing. (Courtesy of Children's Orthopaedic Surgery Foundation.)

and Brudvik[83] evaluated a cohort of 88 patients treated nonoperatively for distal radius fractures. Though eight patients had early loss of reduction with greater than 15 to 20 degrees angulation, all demonstrated complete remodeling and restoration of normal function later. Al-Ansari et al. similarly evaluated 124 patients with "minimally angulated" distal radius fractures. Even patients who healed with 30 to 35 degrees angulation went on to complete fracture remodeling and normal function.[4] Finally, in a randomized clinical trial, 96 patients between 5 and 12 years of age with distal radius fractures with less than 15 degrees of sagittal plane angulation were treated with either cast or splint immobilization.[21] No difference was seen in fracture alignment at 6 weeks in the two treatment groups, and functional outcomes did not differ, as measured by the Activity Scale for Kids. Though the risk of late displacement and issues of compliance and comfort exist, this investigation supports the concept that splint immobilization may be considered in younger patients (age <10 years) with minimal displacement. The high potential for remodeling of a distal radial metaphyseal malunion has led some clinicians to recommend immobilization alone.[44]

Reduction and Immobilization of Incomplete Fractures of the Distal Radius and Ulna

Treatment of greenstick distal radial and ulna fractures is similarly dependent on patient age and remodeling potential, magnitude and direction of fracture displacement and angulation, and the biases of the care provider and patient/family regarding fracture remodeling and deformity. In cases of greenstick distal radius fractures—with or without ulnar involvement—with unacceptable deformity, closed reduction and cast immobilization are recommended.

The method of reduction for greenstick fractures depends on the pattern of displacement. With apex volar angulated fractures of the radius, the rotatory deformity is supination. Pronating the radius and applying a dorsal-to-volar reduction force is utilized to restore bony alignment. Conversely, fractures with apex dorsal angulation result from pronation mechanisms of injury. Supinating the distal forearm and applying a volar-to-dorsal force should reduce the incomplete fracture of the radius.[123] Though these fractures are incomplete and patients often present with minimal pain, adequate analgesia will facilitate bony reduction and quality of cast application. Typically, this is done with the assistance of conscious sedation, though there is emerging evidence that closed reductions can be performed effectively without anesthesia.[54,64,113]

Following reduction, repeat radiographs or portable fluoroscopy may be used to evaluate fracture alignment. Once acceptable alignment is achieved, a cast is applied with appropriate rotation and three-point molds, based on the initial pattern of injury. Long-arm casting is typically used for the first 4 weeks, and bony healing is achieved in 6 weeks in most patients. A short-arm cast with acceptable cast indices is equally effective if derotation was not a critical feature of the reduction technique.

As in the case of torus fractures,[175] there is a study indicating that soft bandages can be applied to treat incomplete greenstick forearm fractures[102]; however, as greenstick fractures are substantially more unstable than the torus fractures and can take considerably longer to heal,[146] the author does not advocate soft bandage treatment of greenstick fractures.

Closed Reduction and Cast Immobilization of Displaced Distal Radial Metaphyseal Fractures

Closed reduction and cast immobilization remain the standard of care for children with displaced distal radial metaphyseal

Figure 9-25. A, B: Use of the thumb to push the distal fragment hyperdorsiflexed 90 degrees (*solid arrow*) until length is reestablished. Countertraction is applied in the opposite direction (*open arrows*).

(continues)

C   D

Figure 9-25. *(Continued)* **C, D:** Once length has been reestablished, the distal fragment is flexed into the correct position. Alignment is checked by determining the position of the fragments with the thumb and forefingers of each hand.

fractures presenting with unacceptable alignment. Again, fracture reduction maneuvers are dependent on injury mechanism and fracture pattern. In patients with typical dorsal displacement of the distal epiphyseal fracture fragment with apex volar angulation, closed reduction is performed with appropriate analgesia, typically conscious sedation or general anesthesia. Finger traps applied to the ipsilateral digits may facilitate limb positioning and stabilization during fracture reduction but application of weights may hinder reduction by increasing dorsal periosteal tension. The lower extremity-aided fracture reduction maneuver (LEAFR) has been proposed as a simple, effective, reproducible, and mechanically advantageous technique of effectuating closed reductions in children with bayoneted distal radius fractures.[52] Given the stout, intact dorsal periosteum in these injuries, pure longitudinal traction is often insufficient to restore bony alignment, particularly in cases of bayonet apposition. Fracture reduction is performed first by hyperextension and exaggeration of the deformity, which relaxes the dorsal periosteal sleeve (Fig. 9-25). Longitudinal traction is then applied to restore adequate length. Finally, the distal fracture fragment is flexed to correct the translational and angular displacement, with rotational correction imparted as well. If available, fluoroscopy may be utilized to confirm adequacy of reduction, and a well-molded cast is applied.

The optimal type of cast immobilization remains controversial. Both long- and short-arm casts have been proposed following distal radial fracture reduction.[72,77,183] Long-arm casts have the advantage of restricting forearm rotation and theoretically reducing the deforming forces imparted to the distal radius. However, above-elbow immobilization is more inconvenient and has been associated with greater need for assistance with activities of daily living, as well as more days of school missed.[183] Prior randomized controlled trials have demonstrated that short-arm casts are as effective at maintaining reduction as long-arm casts, provided that acceptable alignment is achieved and an appropriate cast mold is applied.[20,183] A recent meta-analysis pooling the results of over 300 study subjects has further supported these findings.[77]

Perhaps more important than the length of the cast applied is the cast mold applied at the level of the fracture (Fig. 9-26). Avoidance of excess cast padding and appropriate use of three-point molds will assist in maintenance of alignment in bending injuries. Similarly, application of interosseous mold will help to maintain interosseous space between the radius and ulna as well as coronal plane alignment. A host of radiographic indices have been proposed to quantify and characterize the quality of the cast mold, including the cast index, three-point index, gap index, padding index, Canterbury index, and second

Figure 9-26. Three-point molding. **Top:** Three-point molding for dorsally angulated (apex volar) fractures, with the proximal and distal points on the dorsal aspect of the cast and the middle point on the volar aspect just proximal to the fracture site. **Bottom:** For volar angulated fractures, where the periosteum is intact volarly and disrupted on the dorsal surface, three-point molding is performed with the proximal and distal points on the volar surface of the cast and the middle point just proximal to the fracture site on the dorsal aspect of the cast.

Figure 9-27. Radiographic evaluation of cast mold. **A:** Cast index (x/y) is the ratio of the inner cast diameter at the level of the fracture on the lateral projection (x) to the inner cast diameter at the level of the fracture as seen on the anteroposterior (AP) view (y). **B:** The three-point index is the sum of the three critical gaps divided by the contact area of the fracture fragments. The anteroposterior 3-point index is (a + b + c)/d. The lateral 3-point index is (e + f + g)/h. (Courtesy of Children's Orthopaedic Surgery Foundation.)

metacarpal/distal radius angle (Fig. 9-27).[51,88,142,148] Although the three-point index has gained popularity, some authorities tout the cast index as the preferred index for assessment and prediction of redisplacement.[148] Although cast bivalving is not routinely necessary, Bae et al. demonstrated in a randomized controlled trial that this can be performed without increased risk for loss of reduction.[12] The author recommends that cast bivalving be performed on a case-by-case basis as needed for swelling or other concerns.

Complete fractures of the distal radius have a higher rate of loss of reduction after closed treatment than do incomplete fractures (Fig. 9-28). Indeed, prior investigations have demonstrated that 20% to 30% of patients will have radiographic loss of reduction following closed reduction and casting of displaced distal radius fractures.[105] Risk factors for loss of reduction include greater initial fracture displacement and/or comminution, suboptimal reduction especially in the sagittal plane, suboptimal cast mold, and associated distal ulna fractures.[7,9,51,74,105,125,142]

Given the risk of radiographic loss of reduction, serial radiographs are recommended in the early postinjury period. Weekly two-view radiographs are obtained in the first 2 weeks following reduction to confirm adequacy of alignment, since approximately 80% of loss of reductions occur in the first 2 weeks.[115] The author recommends that repeat radiographs in the third week should also be considered in older children closer to skeletal maturity given the limited remodeling potential. Failure to

Figure 9-28. Bicortical distal radius and ulna fractures status-post closed reduction and casting in a 7-year-old girl. Cast index (CI = X ÷ Y) measures 0.88 and there is no three-point molding. Serial radiographs at (**A**) 7 days and (**B**) 15 days postreduction revealing a loss of reduction in the second week.

identify and correct malalignment in the early postinjury period may lead to malunion and subsequent clinical loss of motion and upper limb function.

Malalignment of fractures during the development of soft tissue callus before bridging ossification (injury to 2–3 weeks after reduction) often can be realigned using cast wedging (Fig. 9-29).[16,18,184] Recently, this technique has been utilized less frequently given the advances in surgical management of fractures. Authors have advocated opening wedges, closing wedges, as well as a combination of each of these approaches. Most commonly we use open wedge techniques as closing wedges have the potential for pinching of the skin and causing accumulation of cast padding at the wedge site which may cause skin breakdown. In addition, closing wedges also may shorten and reduce the volume of the cast thus decreasing fracture stability. There have been multiple techniques proposed for predicting the size of a wedge. Bebbington et al.[16] suggested a technique

that involves tracing the angle of displacement onto the cast itself thus representing the fracture fragments. Wedges are then inserted until the malalignment is reduced as the traced line becomes straight. Wells et al. described a technique in which the wedge position and opening angle are determined from the radiographic displacement and center of rotational alignment.[184] Utilizing these methods on saw bones, they were able to reduce malalignment within 5 degrees with 90% success.[184] Regardless of the method, if utilized appropriately, cast wedging reduces the risk of additional anesthesia and potential surgery.

Separate consideration of overriding distal radius fractures in young children is warranted. Cast immobilization alone without fracture manipulation may even be effective in young patients with complete dorsal displacement and bayonet apposition with acceptable sagittal and coronal plane alignments. Crawford et al. prospectively evaluated 51 children under the age of 10 years treated without reduction and with

Figure 9-29. Lateral fluoroscopic projection of a distal radius fracture treated with dorsal cast wedging to correct loss of reduction. (Courtesy of Children's Orthopaedic Surgery Foundation.)

cast immobilization for shortened and bayoneted fractures of the distal radial metaphysis.[35] All patients went on to complete radiographic remodeling and full return of wrist motion, demonstrating the excellent remodeling potential of the pediatric distal radius. Bradley et al. reported on 49 children with a mean age of 4.7 years with overriding distal radius fractures that underwent closed reduction and cast immobilization. In comparing these children to the cohort reported on by Crawford et al., final sagittal and coronal plane alignment was significantly worse in the reduction cohort compared with the casting only cohort.[24] A prospective comparative study is warranted. Notably, a recent survey of Pediatric Orthopaedic Society of North America (POSNA) members demonstrated preference for closed reduction in completely displaced fractures.[62]

Displaced Distal Radial Physeal Fractures

Most displaced Salter–Harris type I and II fractures are treated with closed reduction and cast stabilization. Closed manipulation of the displaced fracture is similarly performed with appropriate conscious sedation, analgesia, or, rarely, anesthesia to achieve pain relief and an atraumatic reduction.[54,64] Forceful reduction without adequate analgesia may increase the risk for iatrogenic injury to the distal radial physis. Most of these fractures

A

B

Figure 9-30. A: Lateral radiograph of dorsally displaced Salter–Harris type II fracture. **B:** Lateral radiograph after closed reduction and cast application with three-point molding over the carpus and dorsal epiphysis, volar metaphysis, and dorsal proximal shaft (*white arrows*).

involve dorsal and proximal displacement of the epiphysis with an apex volar extension deformity. Manipulative reduction is by gentle distraction and flexion of the distal epiphysis, carpus, and hand over the proximal metaphysis (Fig. 9-30). The intact dorsal periosteum is used as a tension band to aid in reduction and stabilization of the fracture. Unlike similar fractures in adults, finger trap distraction with pulley weights is often counterproductive. However, finger traps can help stabilize the hand, wrist, and arm for manipulative reduction and casting by applying a few pounds of weight for balance. Otherwise, an assistant is helpful to support the extremity in the proper position for casting.

If portable fluoroscopy is available, immediate radiographic assessment of the reduction is obtained. Otherwise, a well-molded cast is applied and AP and lateral radiographs obtained to assess the reduction. The cast should provide three-point molding over the distal radius to lessen the risk of fracture displacement and should follow the contour of the normal forearm. The distal dorsal mold should not impair venous outflow from the hand, which can occur if the mold is placed too distal and too deep so as to obstruct the dorsal veins. Advocates of short-arm casting indicate at least equivalent results with proper casting techniques and more comfort during immobilization due to free elbow mobility. Instructions for elevation and close monitoring of swelling and the neurovascular status of the extremity are critical.

The fracture also should be monitored closely with serial radiographs to be certain that there is no loss of anatomic alignment (Fig. 9-31). Generally, these fractures are stable after closed reduction and cast immobilization. If there is loss of

Figure 9-31. A: AP and lateral radiographs of severely displaced Salter–Harris type II fracture of the distal radius. **B:** Closed reduction shows marked improvement but not anatomic reduction. The case had to be bivalved due to excess swelling. **C:** Unfortunately, the patient lost reduction after a new fiberglass cast was applied. **D:** Out-of-cast radiographs show a healed malunion in a similar position to the prereduction radiographs.

reduction after 7 days, the surgeon should be wary of repeat reduction, as forceful remanipulation may increase the risk of iatrogenic physeal arrest.[27,104] Fortunately, remodeling of an extension deformity with growth is common if the patient has more than 2 years of growth remaining and the deformity is less than 20 degrees.[92] More substantial deformity can remodel if there is sufficient growth remaining and the deformity is in the plane of motion of the wrist.

Galeazzi Fracture Repair

Nonoperative management remains the first-line treatment for pediatric Galeazzi fractures, distinguishing these injuries from their adult counterparts.[50,150,177] Indeed, the adult Galeazzi fracture has been often called a "fracture of necessity," given the near-universal need for surgical reduction and internal fixation to restore anatomic radial alignment and DRUJ congruity. In pediatric patients, however, the distal radial fracture often is a greenstick type that is stable after reduction; therefore, nonoperative treatment with closed reduction and cast immobilization is often sufficient.[91,150] Surgical treatment may be considered for adolescents with complete fractures and displacement, as their injury pattern, skeletal maturity, remodeling potential, and DRUJ instability concerns are more similar to the adult Galeazzi.

Incomplete fractures of the distal radius with either a true dislocation of the DRUJ or an ulnar physeal fracture are treated with closed reduction and long-arm cast immobilization. This can be done in the emergency room with conscious sedation or in the operating room with general anesthesia. Portable fluoroscopy is useful in these situations. If the radius fracture has apex volar angulation and dorsal displacement of the radius with associated volar dislocation of the ulnar head in relationship to the radius, pronation and volar-to-dorsal force on the radial fracture are used for reduction. Conversely, if the radius fracture is apex dorsal with volar displacement and dorsal dislocation of the distal ulna, supination and dorsal-to-volar force is utilized during reduction. The reduction and stability of the fracture and DRUJ dislocation may then be checked on dynamic fluoroscopy; if both are anatomically reduced and stable, a long-arm cast with the forearm in the appropriate rotatory position of stability (i.e., pronation or supination) is applied. Six weeks of long-arm casting is recommended to allow for sufficient bony and soft tissue healing.

In patients with Galeazzi-equivalent injuries characterized by complete distal radius fractures associated with ulnar physeal fractures, both bones should be reduced. Usually, this can be accomplished with the same methods of reduction as when the radial fracture is incomplete. If there is sufficient growth remaining and the distal ulnar physis remains open, remodeling of a nonanatomic distal ulnar physeal reduction may occur. As long as the DRUJ is reduced, malalignment of less than 10 degrees can remodel in a young child. DRUJ congruity and stability, however, are dependent on distal ulnar alignment, and great care should be taken in assessment of the DRUJ when accepting a nonanatomic distal ulnar reduction. Cha et al. reported that reduction of the distal ulnar physeal fracture in Galeazzi-equivalent injuries can be blocked by entrapped periosteum or an interposed extensor carpi ulnaris,

either of which could necessitate open reduction.[28] If the fracture is severely malaligned, the DRUJ or distal ulnar epiphysis cannot be adequately reduced, or the patient is older and remodeling is unlikely, open reduction and smooth pin fixation are indicated.[185] The risk of ulnar growth arrest after distal ulnar physeal fracture has been reported to be as high as 55%, though this is based on a small sample size of 18 patients.[66]

Distal Radial Physeal Stress Injury Treatment

Treatment of distal physeal stress injuries first and foremost involves rest. This activity restriction may be challenging in the pediatric athlete, depending on the level of the sports participation and the desires of the child, parents, and other stakeholders to continue athletic participation. Education regarding the long-term consequences of a growth arrest is important in these emotionally charged situations. Short-arm cast immobilization for several weeks may be the only way to restrict stress to the distal radial physis in some patients. Splint protection is appropriate in cooperative patients. Protection should continue until there is resolution of tenderness and pain with activity. In the author's experience, this takes at least 6 to 12 weeks. The young athlete can maintain cardiovascular fitness, strength, and flexibility while protecting the injured wrist. Once the acute physeal injury has healed, return to weight-bearing and open-chain activities should be gradual. The process of return to sports should be protective, often 3 to 6 months, and adjustment of techniques and training methods is necessary to prevent recurrence. The major concern is development of a radial growth arrest in a skeletally immature patient, and consideration should be given to serial clinical and radiographic follow-up in high-risk patients to confirm maintenance of growth. A radial growth arrest will result in ulnar overgrowth, with subsequent risk of ulnar carpal impaction and TFCC injury.

Distal Ulna Physeal Fracture Repair

Treatment options are similar to those for radial physeal fractures: immobilization alone, closed reduction and cast immobilization, closed reduction and percutaneous pinning, and open reduction. Often, these fractures are minimally displaced or nondisplaced. Immobilization until fracture healing at 3 to 6 weeks is standard treatment. Closed reduction is indicated for displaced fractures with more than 50% translation or 20 degrees of angulation. Most ulnar physeal fractures reduce to a near-anatomic alignment with reduction of the concomitant radius fracture due to the attachments of the DRUJ ligaments and TFCC. Failure to obtain a closed reduction of the ulnar fracture may indicate that there is soft tissue interposed in the fracture site, including periosteum or extensor carpi ulnaris, necessitating open reduction and fixation.[28]

Outcomes

Most of the published literature providing information on the short-term clinical and radiographic results of treatment for pediatric distal radius fractures indicates a positive outcome. With adherence to the principles and techniques described above, radiographic realignment, successful bony healing, and avoidance of complications are achieved in most cases. Given the high healing capacity and remodeling potential of these injuries, there is less concern regarding long-term outcomes of nonoperative treatment compared with adult patients. In general, concerns regarding long-term outcomes have focused on patients who sustain distal radial physeal fractures and thus are at risk for subsequent growth disturbance and skeletal imbalance of the distal forearm.

The risk of growth disturbance following extra-articular physeal fracture (Salter–Harris type I and II fractures) of the distal radius is approximately 4%. Cannata et al.[27] previously reported the long-term outcomes of 163 distal radial physeal fractures in 157 patients. Displaced fractures were treated with closed reduction and cast immobilization for 6 weeks. Mean follow-up was 25.5 years. Posttraumatic growth disturbance resulting in 1 cm or greater of length discrepancy was seen in 4.4% of distal radial and 50% of distal ulnar physeal fractures. In a similar prospective analysis of 290 children with distal radial physeal fractures, Bae and Waters[11] noted that 4% of patients went on to demonstrate clinical or radiographic distal radial growth disturbance. Kallini et al. reported on the more rare intra-articular distal radius physeal fractures (Salter–Harris type III and IV fractures). In this cohort of 28 patients, growth disturbance occurred in 43% of patients.[90] Consideration should be given for follow-up radiographic evaluation following distal radial physeal fractures to assess for possible physeal arrest. The author recommends routine screening radiographs 6 to 9 months after the initial injury. In symptomatic patients with posttraumatic growth disturbance and growth remaining, surgical interventions including distal ulnar epiphysiodeses, corrective osteotomies of the radius, ulnar shortening osteotomies, and associated soft tissue reconstructions have been demonstrated to improve clinical function and radiographic alignment.[26,180]

OPERATIVE TREATMENT OF FRACTURES OF THE DISTAL RADIUS AND ULNA

Indications/Contraindications

Operative Treatment of Fractures of the Distal Radius and Ulna:
INDICATIONS AND CONTRAINDICATIONS

Indications

Open fracture

Floating elbow injury

Displaced, intra-articular fracture

Distal radius fractures with median neuropathy

Adolescent patients with a complete Galeazzi fracture

Irreducible fracture

Loss of reduction with inadequate remodeling potential

Contraindications

Extra-articular fracture in child with >2 years of growth remaining, displaced <20 degrees in the plane of motion

Physeal fracture >5 to 7 days after initial reduction that has lost reduction, unless limited growth potential

Although surgical indications and techniques continue to evolve, in general surgical indications for pediatric distal radius and ulna fractures include open fractures, irreducible fractures, unstable fractures with loss of reduction, floating elbow injuries, and fractures with soft tissue or neurovascular compromise precluding circumferential cast immobilization. Surgical reduction and fixation is also indicated in cases of joint incongruity associated with intra-articular Salter–Harris type III or type IV fractures. In an investigation of 49 tertiary-care pediatric hospitals in the United States, Mahan et al. demonstrated that the aggregate rate for surgery in pediatric distal radius fractures is less than 3%.[117] The overall surgical rate is far lower than in the adult population.

Distal radial fracture stability has been more clearly defined in adults[182] than in children. At present, an unstable fracture in a child is often defined as one in which closed reduction cannot be maintained. Pediatric classification systems have yet to more precisely define fracture stability, but this issue is critical in determining proper treatment management. As noted above, distal radial metaphyseal fractures have been shown to have a high degree of recurrent displacement and, therefore, inherent instability.[6,9,74,142,182] For these reasons, pediatric distal radial metaphyseal fractures are not classified in the same manner as adults in regard to stability. Instead, unstable fractures have been predominantly defined by the failure to maintain a successful closed reduction. Irreducible fractures may be due to entrapped periosteum or pronator quadratus.

Surgical treatment is similarly recommended in patients with neurovascular compromise and severely displaced injuries. Operative stabilization serves both to maintain adequate bony alignment and more importantly, minimize the risk of compartment syndrome due to excessive swelling and circumferential immobilization. Perhaps the best indication is a displaced radial physeal fracture with median neuropathy and significant volar soft tissue swelling (Fig. 9-32).[181] These patients are at risk for development of an acute carpal tunnel syndrome or forearm compartment syndrome with closed reduction and well-molded cast immobilization.[17,181] Percutaneous pin fixation allows the application of a loose dressing, splint, or cast without the risk of loss of fracture reduction.

Internal fixation usually is with smooth, small-diameter pins to lessen the risk of growth arrest. Plates and screws rarely are used unless the patient is near skeletal maturity because of concerns about further physeal injury. In the rare displaced intra-articular Salter–Harris type III or IV fracture, internal fixation can be intraepiphyseal without violating the physis. If it is necessary to cross the physis, then smooth, small-diameter pins should be used to lessen the risk of iatrogenic physeal injury. In the author's opinion, arthroscopic guidance may be useful in these rare fractures to maximize the congruity of the articular surface and to limit residual physeal displacement.

Figure 9-32. A: Clinical photograph of patient with a displaced Salter–Harris type II fracture of the distal radius. The patient has marked swelling volarly with hematoma and fracture displacement. The patient had a median neuropathy upon presentation. **B:** Lateral radiograph of the displaced fracture. **C:** Lateral radiograph following closed reduction and cast application. Excessive flexion has been utilized to maintain fracture reduction, resulting in persistent median neuropathy and increasing pain. **D:** Radiographs following urgent closed reduction and percutaneous pinning. **E:** Follow-up radiograph depicting distal radial physeal arrest and increased ulnar variance. (Courtesy of Children's Orthopaedic Surgery Foundation.)

Closed Reduction and Pin Fixation of Displaced Distal Radial Fractures

Preoperative Planning

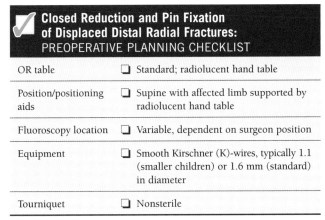

Closed Reduction and Pin Fixation of Displaced Distal Radial Fractures: PREOPERATIVE PLANNING CHECKLIST	
OR table	❏ Standard; radiolucent hand table
Position/positioning aids	❏ Supine with affected limb supported by radiolucent hand table
Fluoroscopy location	❏ Variable, dependent on surgeon position
Equipment	❏ Smooth Kirschner (K)-wires, typically 1.1 (smaller children) or 1.6 mm (standard) in diameter
Tourniquet	❏ Nonsterile

Preoperative planning begins with careful clinical and radiographic evaluation. Thorough neurovascular examination is performed to assess for signs and symptoms of nerve injury or impending compartment syndrome. Radiographs—both from the time of injury, after initial attempts at closed reduction, and any subsequent follow-up radiographs—are carefully evaluated to assess pattern of injury and direction of instability.

Given the relative simplicity of closed reduction and percutaneous fixation techniques, minimal equipment is required. Intraoperative fluoroscopy and surgical instrumentation for pin placement are typically sufficient.

Positioning

After adequate induction of general anesthesia, patients are positioned supine on a standard operating table, with the affected limb abducted and supported on a radiolucent hand table. While a nonsterile tourniquet may be applied to the proximal brachium, this is typically not utilized. Fluoroscopy may be brought in from the head, foot, or side of the patient, depending on surgeon position and preference. For example, as most pinning is performed from distal to proximal, the right-hand–dominant surgeon may wish to sit in the axilla and have the fluoroscopy unit come in from the head of the patients when pinning a left distal radius.

Surgical Approach

While percutaneous pinning may be performed without need for skin incision, placement of smooth C- or K-wires into the region of the radial styloid carries the risk of iatrogenic radial sensory nerve or extensor tendon injury.[123] For this reason, a small longitudinal incision over the radial styloid at the site of pin insertion may be utilized to identify and retract adjacent soft tissues, facilitating safe pin passage. Alternatively, smooth pins may be inserted using an oscillating technique.

Technique

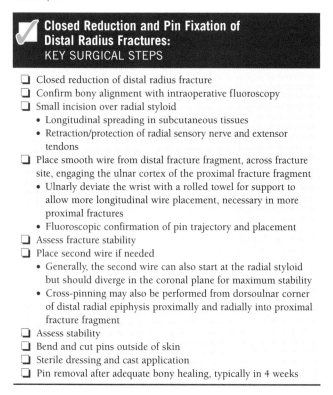

> ✓ **Closed Reduction and Pin Fixation of Distal Radius Fractures:**
> KEY SURGICAL STEPS

- ❑ Closed reduction of distal radius fracture
- ❑ Confirm bony alignment with intraoperative fluoroscopy
- ❑ Small incision over radial styloid
  - Longitudinal spreading in subcutaneous tissues
  - Retraction/protection of radial sensory nerve and extensor tendons
- ❑ Place smooth wire from distal fracture fragment, across fracture site, engaging the ulnar cortex of the proximal fracture fragment
  - Ulnarly deviate the wrist with a rolled towel for support to allow more longitudinal wire placement, necessary in more proximal fractures
  - Fluoroscopic confirmation of pin trajectory and placement
- ❑ Assess fracture stability
- ❑ Place second wire if needed
  - Generally, the second wire can also start at the radial styloid but should diverge in the coronal plane for maximum stability
  - Cross-pinning may also be performed from dorsoulnar corner of distal radial epiphysis proximally and radially into proximal fracture fragment
- ❑ Assess stability
- ❑ Bend and cut pins outside of skin
- ❑ Sterile dressing and cast application
- ❑ Pin removal after adequate bony healing, typically in 4 weeks

After appropriate anesthesia, closed reduction of the distal radius fracture into anatomic alignment is performed using the principles and techniques previously described. While maintaining fracture reduction, a skin incision is made over the radial styloid, long enough to ascertain there is no iatrogenic injury to the radial sensory nerve or extensor tendons (Fig. 9-33). Careful longitudinal spreading is performed in the subcutaneous tissues, and the radial sensory nerve and extensor tendons may be identified and carefully retracted. Pin fixation can be either single or double, though often a single pin will suffice (Fig. 9-34). A smooth pin is then inserted into the distal fracture fragment and passed obliquely in a proximal and ulnar fashion, crossing the fracture site and engaging

Figure 9-33. Small incision noted with pins left out of skin for removal at 4 weeks. (Courtesy of Children's Orthopaedic Surgery Foundation.)

the far ulnar cortex proximal to the fracture line. Fluoroscopy is used to guide proper fracture reduction and pin placement.

Pin(s) may be placed within the distal radial epiphysis and passed across the physis before engaging the more proximal metaphyseal fracture fragment. Alternatively, smooth pins may be placed just proximal to the distal radial physis; while theoretically decreasing the risk of physeal disturbance, this advantage has not been well demonstrated in the published literature.

Stability of the fracture should be evaluated with flexion and extension and rotatory stress under fluoroscopy. Often, in children and adolescents, a single pin and the reduced periosteum provide sufficient stability to prevent redisplacement of the fracture (Fig. 9-35). If fracture stability is questionable with a single pin, a second pin should be placed. The second pin can either parallel the first pin or, to create cross-pin stability, can be placed distally from the dorsal ulnar corner of the radial epiphysis between the fourth and fifth dorsal compartments and passed obliquely to the proximal radial portion of the metaphysis (Fig. 9-36). Again, the skin incisions for pin placement should be sufficient to avoid iatrogenic injury to the extensor tendons. In the author's experience, arthroscopic guidance may be useful when pinning Salter–Harris type III and IV fractures as visualization can help restore the alignment of the articular surface and by extension limit residual physeal displacement.

The pins are bent, left out of the skin, and covered with petroleum gauze and sterile dressing. Short-arm splint or cast immobilization is used but does not need to be tight, as fracture stability is conferred by the pins. The author prefers a short-arm thumb spica cast with the interphalangeal joint free to minimize thumb movement and skin irritation or surgical site infection at the pin site. The pins are left in until there is adequate fracture healing (usually 4 weeks). The pins can be removed in the office without sedation or anesthesia.

One of the arguments against pin fixation is the risk of additional injury to the physis by a pin.[22] The risk of physeal arrest is more from the displaced fracture than from a short-term, smooth pin. As a precaution, smooth, small-diameter pins should be used, insertion should be as atraumatic as

Figure 9-34. **A:** AP and lateral radiographs of a bicortical distal radius fracture pinned with a single pin placed proximal to the physis. **B:** A Salter–Harris type II distal radius fracture pinned with slightly divergent pins utilizing a transphyseal technique.

Figure 9-35. Severe swelling. **A, B:** Complete displacement and bayonet apposition of a distal radial fracture associated with severe swelling from a high-energy injury. **C:** Once reduced, the fragment is secured with an oblique percutaneous pin across the fracture site, sparing the distal radial physis.

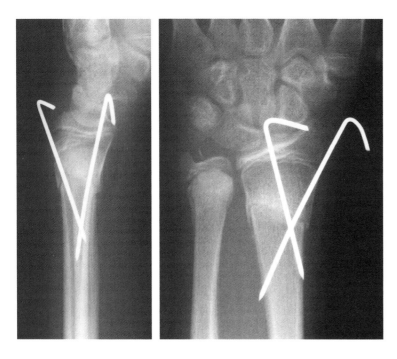

Figure 9-36. Crossed-pin technique for stabilization of distal radial metaphyseal fracture in a skeletally immature patient. (Courtesy of Children's Orthopaedic Surgery Foundation.)

possible, and removal should be done as soon as there is sufficient fracture healing for fracture stability in a cast or splint alone.

An alternative pinning technique involves intrafocal placement of multiple pins into the fracture site to lever the distal fragment into anatomic reduction (Fig. 9-37). The pins are then

Figure 9-37. Pin leverage. **A:** If a bayonet is irreducible, after sterile preparation, a chisel-point Steinmann pin can be inserted between the fracture fragments from a dorsal approach. Care must be taken not to penetrate too deeply past the dorsal cortex of the proximal fragment. **B:** Once the chisel is across the fracture site, it is levered into position and supplementary pressure is placed on the dorsum of the distal fragment (*arrow*) to slide it down the skid into place. This procedure is usually performed with an image intensifier.

passed through the opposing cortex for stability.[114,174] A supplemental, loose-fitting cast is applied.

Open Reduction and Fixation of Distal Radius Fractures

Preoperative Planning

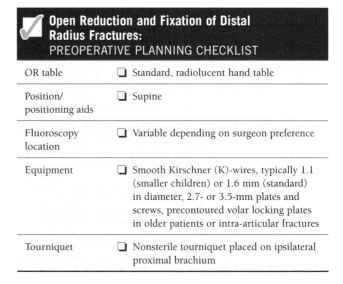

✓ Open Reduction and Fixation of Distal Radius Fractures: PREOPERATIVE PLANNING CHECKLIST	
OR table	❑ Standard, radiolucent hand table
Position/ positioning aids	❑ Supine
Fluoroscopy location	❑ Variable depending on surgeon preference
Equipment	❑ Smooth Kirschner (K)-wires, typically 1.1 (smaller children) or 1.6 mm (standard) in diameter, 2.7- or 3.5-mm plates and screws, precontoured volar locking plates in older patients or intra-articular fractures
Tourniquet	❑ Nonsterile tourniquet placed on ipsilateral proximal brachium

Open reduction is indicated for open fractures, irreducible fractures, or loss of reduction when repeat closed reduction is not feasible. Open fractures constitute approximately 1% of all distal radial metaphyseal fractures. Although treatment approaches to open fractures continue to evolve, at present the standard of care remains surgical irrigation and debridement, followed by appropriate fracture care (also see Controversies) regarding nonoperative management of open fractures.

Irreducible metaphyseal or physeal fractures are rare and generally are secondary to interposed soft tissues. With dorsally displaced fractures, the interposed structure usually is the volar periosteum or pronator quadratus[79] and rarely the flexor tendons or neurovascular structures.[79,94,189] In volarly displaced fractures, the periosteum or extensor tendons may be interposed. Open reduction could also be required for fractures with loss of reduction if an adequate repeat closed reduction cannot be achieved.

For acute fractures, closed reduction rarely fails if there is no interposed soft tissue. Occasionally, however, multiple attempts at reduction of a bayonet apposition fracture can lead to significant swelling that makes closed reduction impossible. If the patient is too old to remodel bayonet apposition, open reduction is appropriate.

Plate fixation can be used in more skeletally mature adolescents or in children with more proximal metaphyseal–diaphyseal fractures that are not amenable to pin fixation. Low-profile, fragment-specific fixation methods and locking plates also are now commonly used for internal fixation of distal radial fractures in adults. The utility of these anatomically contoured locking plates in children and skeletally immature adolescents is unknown, as is the deleterious effect, if any, on growth potential. Furthermore, the advantage of these more rigid constructs in younger patients in whom adequate stability may be achieved with pins is unclear, particularly given the reports of late tendon rupture and other soft tissue complications associated with fixed-angle volar plates.[145] Indications for skeletally mature adolescents are the same as for adults. Articular malalignment and comminution are assessed by CT preoperatively, and fracture-specific fixation is used as appropriate. These plates have proved to be quite useful in indicated cases.

Preoperative planning for open reduction and fixation is similar to the approach cited above, with a few additional considerations. Assessment of skeletal maturity and physeal status is important, particularly when considering use of implants which rigidly engage the distal radial epiphysis and when open reduction may potentially increase the risk of physeal disturbance. Secondly, children are not small adults, and care should be made to evaluate the width of the distal radial metaphysis and epiphysis. Use of precontoured volar locking plates typical of adult distal radius fractures may not be feasible, given size mismatch and/or presence of an open distal radial physis. With the numerous plate options available, it is quite feasible to match up sizes of plate and bone. Finally, care should be made to assess for articular extension of the fracture. Anatomic realignment of the distal radial joint surface is critical, even in the young child.

Positioning

Patients are positioned supine with the affected limb supported by a radiolucent hand table. Positioning of the fluoroscopic unit is similar to that in closed reduction and pinning techniques.

Surgical Approach

All open fractures, regardless of grade of soft tissue injury, should be irrigated and debrided in the operating room (Fig. 9-38).

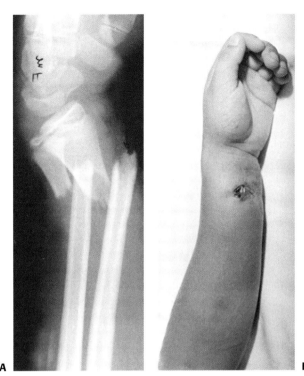

Figure 9-38. Open fractures. Radiograph (**A**) and clinical photo (**B**) of an open fracture of the distal radius. This patient needs formal irrigation and debridement in the operating room.

The open wound should be enlarged adequately to debride the contaminated and nonviable tissues and identify, protect, or if needed, repair the adjacent neurovascular structures. Judicious extension of the traumatic wound will allow for extensile exposure, facilitate fracture reduction, and allow for implant placement.

Open reduction for closed unstable or irreducible fractures is typically performed through a volar approach to the distal radius. A longitudinal incision overlying the flexor carpi radialis (FCR) tendon is created, centered on the fracture site with awareness of the location of the distal radial physis. Classically, superficial dissection is carried out in the interval between the radial artery and the FCR. In distal radius fractures, dissection may also be performed directly through the FCR sheath by incising the roof of the FCR sheath and retracting the tendon ulnarly; the intact radial FCR sheath, when retracted, will serve to protect the adjacent radial artery. Deep to the FCR, a fat plane will be encountered overlying the pronator quadratus. The pronator quadratus is incised along its distal and radial borders, leaving a small cuff of tissue for subsequent repair, and elevated in a subperiosteal fashion from radial to ulnar. Although this muscle can be interposed in the fracture site, the volar periosteum is more commonly interposed. This is evident only after elevation of the pronator quadratus. The periosteum is extracted from the physis with care to minimize further injury to the physis. Upon completion of pronator quadratus elevation, the fracture may be easily visualized.

Technique

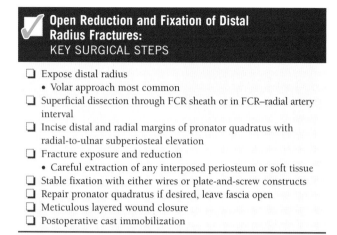

✓ **Open Reduction and Fixation of Distal Radius Fractures:**
KEY SURGICAL STEPS

❏ Expose distal radius
  • Volar approach most common
❏ Superficial dissection through FCR sheath or in FCR–radial artery interval
❏ Incise distal and radial margins of pronator quadratus with radial-to-ulnar subperiosteal elevation
❏ Fracture exposure and reduction
  • Careful extraction of any interposed periosteum or soft tissue
❏ Stable fixation with either wires or plate-and-screw constructs
❏ Repair pronator quadratus if desired, leave fascia open
❏ Meticulous layered wound closure
❏ Postoperative cast immobilization

After adequate fracture exposure is obtained, bony reduction is performed easily using similar maneuvers as during closed manipulations. Once anatomic fracture alignment is achieved, percutaneous smooth K-wires may be used for stabilization of the reduction. The method of pin insertion is the same as after closed reduction; use of a small incision during wire insertion will minimize risk to the radial sensory nerve and extensor tendons.

Similarly for open fracture care, fracture reduction and fixation are performed, usually with two smooth divergent or crossed wires, after thorough irrigation and debridement. In the uncommon open physeal fractures, care is taken with mechanical debridement to avoid injury to the physeal cartilage. If the soft tissue injury is severe, supplemental external fixation allows observation and treatment of the wound without jeopardizing the fracture reduction. The original open wound should not be closed primarily. Appropriate prophylactic antibiotics should be used depending on the severity of the open fracture.

Plate fixation may also be used for stabilization following open reduction. While the indications for plate fixation evolve and remain patient- and surgeon-dependent, plate fixation is more strongly considered in multitrauma patients, comminuted fractures, older patients nearing or at skeletal maturity, refractures, and fractures at the metaphyseal–diaphyseal junction in whom percutaneous pinning techniques are more challenging.

Following standard surgical exposure and fracture reduction, neutralization or dynamic compression plates are applied to the radius using techniques similar to adult fracture care, with a few caveats. Foremost, in patients with skeletal growth remaining, implants should be placed sparing the distal radial physis. Standard 3.5-mm implants may be too bulky for younger or smaller pediatric patients. In these situations, double-stacked one-third tubular plates, 2.7-mm plates, or even 2.4-mm plates may be used. In addition, given the rapid bony healing, stout periosteum, and postoperative cast immobilization characteristic of pediatric fracture care, four cortices of fixation may be sufficient distal to the fracture site though a T-shaped plate may allow for placement of multiple screws proximal to the physis

In older adolescents at skeletal maturity or those with intra-articular injuries, volar locking plates may be used for internal fixation. The physis can be ignored if the patient is within 6 months or at skeletal maturity. Although a host of commercially available plates are available, the principles are constant: meticulous exposure, anatomic fracture reduction, and stable fixation proximal and distal to the fracture site. Care should be made in anatomically contoured volar locking plates to avoid penetration of obliquely angled distal locking screws into the radiocarpal joint, as well as excessive dorsal prominence of screws, which may lead to late extensor tendon irritation or rupture (Fig. 9-39).

Following fixation, the pronator quadratus is repaired if desired and a layered skin closure is performed. In cases of stable plate fixation, short-arm cast immobilization is sufficient postoperatively but may not be required for as long as patients undergoing closed reduction and percutaneous pinning.

Fixation of Intra-Articular Fractures

Preoperative Planning

✓ **Open Reduction and Fixation of Intra-Articular Fractures:**
PREOPERATIVE PLANNING CHECKLIST

OR table	❏ Standard, radiolucent hand table
Position/ positioning aids	❏ Supine
Fluoroscopy location	❏ Variable depending on surgeon preference
Equipment	❏ K-wires, small fragment plating systems, anatomically precontoured volar locking plates, small joint arthroscope
Tourniquet	❏ Nonsterile tourniquet placed on proximal brachium
Other	❏ Adequate preoperative imaging, including CT or MRI

The rare Salter–Harris type III or IV fracture or "triplane" fracture may require open reduction if the joint or physis cannot be anatomically reduced via closed means. If anatomic alignment of the physis and articular surface is not present, the risk of growth arrest, long-term deformity, or limited function is greater (Fig. 9-40).[90] Even minimal displacement (more than 2 mm) should not be accepted in this situation.

Preoperatively, CT or MRI scans are invaluable in defining fracture pattern, assessing articular congruity, and planning definitive treatment (Fig. 9-41). Based on these images, appropriate preoperative planning may be performed. There is great variation in fracture patterns, and treatment and fixation must be individualized to restore bony alignment and stability. In addition to traditional percutaneous and open techniques, arthroscopically assisted reduction may be helpful to align and stabilize these uncommon intra-articular fractures.[46] Although equipment-intensive, anatomic reduction and stabilization of the physis and articular surface can be achieved with arthroscopy, fluoroscopy, and combinations

Figure 9-39. ORIF of distal radius with T plate and supplemental pin fixation. **A:** Injury CT scan revealing intra-articular displacement. **B:** ORIF with T buttress plate and supplemental styloid pin 1-month postoperative. **C:** One year after ORIF with anatomic alignment and asymptomatic hardware. (Courtesy of Children's Orthopaedic Surgery Foundation.)

Figure 9-40. A: A markedly displaced Salter–Harris type IV fracture of the distal radius in an 11-year-old boy who fell from a horse. **B:** Radiograph taken 3 weeks after closed reduction demonstrates displacement of the comminuted fragments. **C:** Eighteen months after injury, there was 15 mm of radial shortening, and the patient had a pronounced radial deviation deformity of the wrist.

Figure 9-41. A: Displaced distal radius metaphyseal and intra-articular fracture. **B:** Emergency department postreduction radiographs in cast. **C:** Representative postreduction CT scan images revealing joint displacement. **D:** Clinical appearance after decreased swelling over 5 days preoperatively.

Figure 9-41. *(Continued)* **E:** Planned plate for fracture-fragment–specific volar fixation. **F:** Volar approach via FCR tendon sheath. **G:** Exposed fracture site with reduction. **H:** Plate fixation of fracture anatomically. **I:** Radiographs of ORIF with volar plating system. (Courtesy of Children's Orthopaedic Surgery Foundation.)

of external fixation or transphyseal or all-epiphyseal fixation pins or screws (Fig. 9-42).

Positioning

Standard positioning is used, as described above. In cases where wrist arthroscopy is to be performed, use of a wrist traction tower with finger trap suspension applied to the index and long fingers will stabilize the wrist and provide appropriate traction for arthroscopic visualization.

Surgical Approach

The volar surgical approach remains the standard workhorse exposure for distal radius fractures requiring open reduction.

Often, more distal subperiosteal elevation is needed to visualize intra-articular fracture lines. This is more common in older, skeletally mature adolescents.

In many intra-articular fracture patterns, there are radial styloid and/or dorsal lunate facet fragments that necessitate exposure, reduction, and fixation. In these cases, supplemental dorsal approaches may need to be used. A longitudinal incision based over or ulnar to Lister tubercle is most commonly used and provides a utilitarian approach. Superficial dissection is performed to the extensor retinaculum, with preservation of the dorsal veins if possible. In dorsal lunate facet fractures, incision of the retinaculum over the third or fourth extensor compartment and subsequent retraction of the extensor pollicis longus or extensor digitorum communis tendons, respectively,

Figure 9-42. A: CT scan of displaced Salter–Harris type IV fracture. **B:** Surgical correction included external fixation distraction, arthroscopically assisted reduction, and smooth pin fixation. (Courtesy of Children's Orthopaedic Surgery Foundation.)

will provide access to the distal dorsal radius. Care is made to preserve the origins of the radiocarpal ligaments whenever possible.

Technique

 Fixation of Intra-Articular Fractures: SURGICAL PRINCIPLES

❏ Careful preoperative evaluation of fracture pattern, comminution, and displacement
❏ Fracture-specific surgical approaches
❏ Articular realignment
  • Use of traction, wrist arthroscopy, fluoroscopy, or arthrotomy to aid in visualization
❏ Stabilization of the articular surface to the proximal radius
❏ Fixation using K-wires, interfragmentary screws, or plate-and-screw constructs for maintenance of alignment

Given the spectrum of intra-articular distal radius fracture patterns, a sequential description of surgical steps is difficult; each patient must be treated in an individualized fashion according to fracture pattern, size of bony fragments, severity of displacement, and skeletal maturity. Universal surgical principles of adequate fracture reduction, anatomic realignment, and stable fixation will provide for optimal results. A few additional considerations are important.

Attempts should be made to achieve closed or minimally invasive reduction whenever possible. With adequate anesthesia, muscle relaxation, and traction, displaced articular fragments may often be anatomically realigned, facilitating percutaneous fixation or implant placement without violating the radiocarpal joint or physis. Furthermore, K-wires may be used to joystick-displaced fracture fragments or in an intrafocal fashion[174] to further assist in fracture reduction. Intraoperative fluoroscopy is invaluable in these cases.

Wrist arthroscopy may be a helpful adjunct for articular visualization.[32,46] With approximately 12 to 15 lb of distraction placed via finger traps to the index and long fingers, a small joint arthroscope (2.4–2.9 mm in diameter) may be inserted into the standard 3–4 wrist arthroscopy portal; this portal lies between the third and fourth extensor compartments and is typically 1 cm distal to Lister tubercle. Care should be taken to avoid excessive extravasation of arthroscopy fluid into the zone of injury during arthroscopy; expeditious arthroscopy and use of low pressure and flow rates are helpful in these situations. After evacuating hematoma from the joint, visualization can often be adequately maintained with the fluid inflow clamped.

Finally, a wide spectrum of internal fixation options is available. Percutaneous K-wires are effective when properly positioned, particularly in younger patients with open physes in whom efforts are made to minimize the risk of iatrogenic growth disturbance. Wires passed obliquely from distal to proximal are effective for radial styloid and dorsal lunate facet fracture fragments; similarly, transverse all-epiphyseal pins may impart stability to articular fracture fragments. In older patients nearing or at skeletal maturity, adult-like locking plate constructs may be used.

Reduction and Fixation of Distal Ulna Fractures

Open reduction is performed in cases where acceptable alignment is not achieved following radial reduction and attempted closed manipulation. This is an indication for open reduction.

Preoperative Planning

Preoperative planning and patient positioning are similar to that of displaced distal radius fractures.

Surgical Approach

Incisions for surgical exposure of the ulna are typically ulnar or dorsoulnar, though ideally, surgical exposure approaches the ulna from the side of periosteal disruption. In physeal fractures, the periosteum is typically torn opposite the Thurston–Holland fragment; in metaphyseal injuries, periosteal injury is opposite the direction of displacement. Deep dissection is most commonly made in the extensor carpi ulnaris—flexor carpi ulnaris interval ulnarly or the extensor digiti quinti—extensor carpi ulnaris intervals dorsally. Careful subperiosteal elevation may be performed in the zone of injury, which is typically already traumatized from the fracture. Interposed soft tissue (periosteum, extensor carpi ulnaris tendon, or flexor tendons) may then be identified and must be extracted from the fracture site.[1,66] During the surgical exposure, care should be taken to avoid injury to sensory branches of the dorsal cutaneous branch of the ulnar nerve, which typically pass obliquely from proximal volar to distal dorsal 1 to 4 cm distal to the ulnar articular surface.[152]

Technique

✓ **Fixation of Displaced Distal Ulna Fractures:**
KEY SURGICAL STEPS

❑ Expose distal ulna
  • Preserve distal ulnar physis, capsular attachments of DRUJ and ulnocarpal joint, and ulnar wrist ligaments whenever possible
❑ Anatomic reduction of ulnar fracture
❑ Stable fixation based on fracture pattern and patient age
  • K-wire fixation
  • K-wire with tension-band construct
  • Plate-and-screw fixation
❑ Assess DRUJ alignment and stability intraoperatively
❑ Postoperative cast immobilization

Following exposure, soft tissue extraction, and bony reduction, if fracture instability persists, internal fixation is performed. Often, a single small-diameter smooth K-wire can be used to maintain alignment. This K-wire may be passed obliquely from distal to proximal, crossing the fracture site. In older patients with larger bones and greater instability, two parallel K-wires may be used, and this may be further supplemented by tension-band fixation (Fig. 9-43). A small drill hole made proximal to the fracture site is created, and a nonabsorbable braided suture or small-caliber stainless steel wire is passed through the drill hole and around the previously placed K-wires in a figure-of-eight fashion. Pins are typically removed after 4 weeks following radiographic confirmation of bony healing. Plate-and-screw fixation may also be performed in distal metaphyseal fractures and/or older, skeletally mature patients. Use of smaller implants, distal locking screws, or mini-fragment blade plates will assist in obtaining adequate fixation in the often small distal ulnar fracture fragment. Further injury to the physis should be avoided during operative exposure and reduction because of the high risk of growth arrest.[66]

ORIF of Galeazzi Fractures

Open reduction of the radius is indicated in Galeazzi fractures or fracture equivalents in cases of failure to obtain or maintain fracture and DRUJ reduction. This most often occurs with unstable complete fractures in older adolescents.

Preoperative Planning

Preoperative planning and patient positioning are similar as described above. Unlike adult Galeazzi fracture dislocations, advanced imaging (e.g., CT or MRI) is rarely needed in pediatric patients.

Surgical Approach

Open reduction and internal fixation of complete radius fractures is performed through a standard volar approach, as described above. In most acute injuries, with anatomic reduction of the radius, restoration of radial length and alignment will allow for spontaneous reduction of the DRUJ. Occasionally, however, the DRUJ dislocation cannot be reduced via closed means (Fig. 9-44). In these situations, the first intraoperative step is to reassess the quality of radial fracture reduction and fixation. Following this, open reduction of the DRUJ may be performed to remove any interposed soft tissues blocking reduction (periosteum, extensor carpi ulnaris tendon, extensor digiti quinti tendon, other ligamentous structures).[70,109,134,150,177]

The easiest approach for open reduction of the DRUJ is an extended ulnar approach. Care should be taken to avoid injury to sensory branches of the dorsal cutaneous branch of the ulnar nerve, which typically pass obliquely from proximal volar to distal dorsal 1 to 4 cm distal to the ulnar articular surface.[152] This approach allows exposure both volarly and dorsally to extract the interposed soft tissues and repair the torn structures. Alternatively, Bowers' approach to the DRUJ may be used (Fig. 9-45). A linear or curvilinear incision is made over the DRUJ. The fifth dorsal extensor compartment is incised and the extensor digiti quinti is retracted. The DRUJ lies immediately deep to this interval, and the joint may be opened and inspected, facilitating reduction.

Figure 9-43. A: Plain radiographs depicting displaced distal radial metaphyseal and ulnar styloid fractures. Given the fracture and distal radioulnar joint instability, the injury was treated with closed reduction and percutaneous pinning of the distal radius as well as open reduction and tension-band fixation of the ulnar styloid. **B:** Follow-up radiograph following reduction and fixation demonstrates anatomic alignment. The prior radial pins have been removed, and the parallel smooth wires used for tension-band fixation of the ulnar styloid are seen. (Courtesy of Children's Orthopaedic Surgery Foundation.)

Figure 9-44. An adolescent girl presented 4 weeks after injury with a painful, stiff wrist. **A:** By examination, she was noted to have a volar distal radioulnar dislocation that was irreducible even under general anesthesia. **B:** At the time of surgery, the distal ulna was found to have buttonholed out of the capsule, and there was entrapped triangular fibrocartilage and periosteum in the joint. (Courtesy of Children's Orthopaedic Surgery Foundation.)

Figure 9-45. A: Clinical photograph depicting the dorsoulnar curvilinear incision used to approach the distal radioulnar joint in a patient with an irreducible Galeazzi fracture. **B:** Intraoperative photograph depicting the sigmoid notch of the distal radius. The ECU and EDQ tendons are seen retracted volarly and radially. The volarly displaced distal ulna remains dislocated. (Courtesy of Children's Orthopaedic Surgery Foundation.)

Technique

✓ ORIF of Galeazzi Fractures: SURGICAL STEPS

- ☐ Expose distal radius fracture
- ☐ Anatomic reduction and stabilization of radius
  - Plate fixation preferred
- ☐ Careful intraoperative assessment of forearm rotation and DRUJ stability
  - Intraoperative fluoroscopy to confirm DRUJ alignment
- ☐ If DRUJ not reducible, open reduction via ulnar or Bowers' approach
- ☐ If DRUJ not reducible in setting of distal ulnar physeal fracture, open reduction and stabilization of ulnar fracture or dislocation performed
- ☐ Radioulnar pinning in cases of reducible but unstable DRUJ reduction
- ☐ Long-arm cast immobilization for 6 weeks
  - If utilized, radioulnar pin removal 4–6 weeks postoperatively

Open reduction and internal fixation of the radius is done through an anterior approach. Standard compression plating is preferred to intramedullary nailing or pinning techniques (Fig. 9-46). Stable, anatomic reduction of the radius almost always leads to stable reduction of the DRUJ dislocation. A long-arm cast is used for 6 weeks to allow fracture and soft tissue healing.

If the DRUJ dislocation cannot be reduced, it is exposed as described above. After anatomic alignment of the radius and extraction of any soft tissues blocking DRUJ reduction, the joint is typically stable and no additional fixation is required. In cases of extreme instability and/or soft tissue compromise, smooth K-wire fixation of the DRUJ can be used to maintain reduction and allow application of a loose-fitting cast. The K-wire(s), typically 1.6 mm in diameter, are placed with the forearm in supination and passed transversely across from the reduced DRUJ from the ulna to the radius (usually all four cortices penetrated), and the pin(s) left exposed out of the skin. Pin removal is in the office at 4 weeks with continuation of the cast for 6 weeks.

Ulnar physeal fractures may also be irreducible in Galeazzi-equivalent injuries. This also has been reported to be secondary to interposed periosteum, extensor tendons, or joint capsule.[28,50,70,109,134,150,177] Open reduction must be executed with care to avoid further violating the physis.

External Fixation

External fixation rarely is indicated for fractures in skeletally immature patients. Though a viable treatment option,[161] the success rates of both closed reduction and percutaneous pinning techniques make external fixation unnecessary for uncomplicated distal radial fractures in children. Presently, indications for external fixation include distal radius fractures with severe associated soft tissue injuries. Major crush injuries, open fractures, or replantations after amputation requiring additional soft tissue coverage are all indications for external fixation. Supplemental external fixation also may be necessary for severely comminuted fractures to maintain length and provide additional stability to pin or plate constructs. Standard application of the specific fixator chosen is done with care to avoid injury to the adjacent sensory nerves and extensor tendons.

Preoperative Planning

Preoperative planning and patient positioning are similar to as described above. A host of commercially available external fixators may be utilized, with selection of pin diameter based on fracture location and patient size.

Surgical Approach

In general, external fixation for distal radius fractures in children spans the radiocarpal articulation. Although nonbridging

A   B

Figure 9-46. A: The patient with a pronation injury had a closed reduction and attempted fixation with pins placed percutaneously across the fracture site. However, this was inadequate in maintaining the alignment and length of the fracture of the distal radius. **B:** The length of the radius and the distal radioulnar relationship were best reestablished after internal fixation of the distal radius with a plate placed on the volar surface. The true amount of shortening present on the original injury film is not really appreciated until the fracture of the distal radius is fully reduced. (**A, B:** Reproduced with permission from Wilkins KE, ed: Operative Management of *Upper Extremity Fractures in Children*. American Academy of Orthopaedic Surgeons; 1994). **C:** Injury films of another patient with a Galeazzi fracture-dislocation. **D:** Radial length and distal radioulnar joint alignment are restored with closed reduction alone.

C

D

(or wrist joint sparing) constructs may be utilized, the small size of the distal radial epiphysis in young children often precludes the ability to obtain adequate purchase with external fixator pins. For this reason, typical constructs involve fixator pin placement through the index metacarpal and more proximal radial diaphysis.

Distally, a dorsoradial incision is made over the mid-diaphyseal region of the index metacarpal. Dissection is performed through the subcutaneous tissues. The periosteum may be incised via an open approach, and careful limited subperiosteal elevation will allow for the first dorsal interosseous and adductor pollicis muscles to retract safely. Percutaneous techniques may also be utilized, with care taken to avoid inadvertent injury to the radial sensory nerve, extensor tendons, or intrinsic muscles.

Proximally, a dorsoradial approach in the region of the distal radial metadiaphysis is made. Again, identification and retraction of the radial sensory nerve are performed. Deep dissection will allow visualization of the characteristic "bare area" between the musculotendinous units of the first and second extensor compartments. A longitudinal periosteal incision is created, facilitating safe and direct placement of external fixator pins.

Technique

External Fixation:
SURGICAL STEPS

- ❏ Perform an initial closed reduction under fluoroscopy
- ❏ Expose mid-diaphyseal index metacarpal down to bone via a dorsoradial incision
- ❏ Incise the periosteum longitudinally
- ❏ Limit subperiosteal elevation and retract the first dorsal interosseous and adductor pollicis muscles
- ❏ Place two terminally threaded parallel pins into the index metacarpal using a drill guide placed down to bone
- ❏ Expose the radial metadiaphysis down to bone via a dorsoradial approach
- ❏ Identify and retract the radial sensory nerves
- ❏ Expose the bare area between the first and second extensor compartments
- ❏ Incise the periosteum longitudinally
- ❏ Place two terminally threaded parallel pins into the radius proximal to the fracture site using a drill guide placed down to bone
- ❏ Perform traction and additional reduction under fluoroscopy
- ❏ Attach radiolucent bars to the pins
- ❏ Add a smooth percutaneous K-wire via the radial styloid dorsally if needed
- ❏ Close prior surgical incisions
- ❏ Place sterile bandages to the incisions and pin sites

Exposure and pin placement are described as above. Following placement of two terminally threaded pins distal and proximal to the fracture, appropriate traction and reduction may be performed. Use of double-stacked radiolucent bars will increase construct rigidity and facilitate radiographic evaluation.

After fluoroscopic confirmation of pin placement and acceptable fracture alignment, prior surgical incisions may be closed primarily and sterile bandages and/or petroleum gauze may be applied to the pin sites.

Authors' Preferred Method of Treatment for Fractures of the Distal Radius and Ulna (Algorithm 9-1)

Torus Fractures

Torus fractures may be safely and effectively treated with removable splint immobilization for 3 weeks. In children less than 3 or 4 years of age, cast immobilization can be considered due to anticipated difficulties with compliance. Patients can return to playground activities and sports 3–4 weeks after injury.

Incomplete Greenstick Fractures

Closed reduction and long-arm cast immobilization are performed for displaced greenstick fractures with greater than 10 degrees of angulation. With isolated distal radial fractures, it is imperative to reduce the DRUJ with appropriate forearm rotation. A long-arm cast with three-point molding is used for 3–4 weeks. Repeat wrist radiographs to assess alignment are obtained weekly for 1–2 weeks based on fracture instability. A short-arm cast or volar wrist splint is then used until full healing, generally at 5–6 weeks after fracture reduction. Therapy is generally not required. Patients can return to playground activities and sports 1–2 weeks after cast discontinuation, provided that pain has resolved and wrist motion has normalized.

Bicortical Complete Radial Metaphyseal Injuries

Nondisplaced bicortical metaphyseal fractures are treated with cast immobilization. A short-arm, well-molded cast is utilized. Radiographs are obtained for the first 2 weeks. Casts are discontinued at 6 weeks.

Displaced fractures with unacceptable alignment are treated with closed reduction and long-arm cast immobilization. This fracture can be reduced in the emergency room. Portable fluoroscopy is used. Loss of reduction with cast immobilization is more likely if the fracture is not well-reduced. A long-arm cast is applied with the elbow flexed 90 degrees, the wrist in slight palmar flexion, and the forearm in the desired rotation for stability and alignment. Rotational positioning and short- versus long-arm casting varies with each fracture and each surgeon. A three-point mold is applied at the fracture site as the cast hardens. In addition, molds are applied to maintain a straight ulnar border, the interosseous space, and straight posterior humeral line. This creates a "box" long-arm cast that lessens displacement risk rather than the "banana" cast that allows displacement. Portable fluoroscopy is used. The cast is bivalved and spread anytime there are signs of neurovascular compromise or excessive

swelling. The patient is instructed to maintain elevation for at least 48–72 hours after discharge and return immediately if excessive swelling or neurovascular compromise occurs. We inform our patients and parents that the risk of loss of reduction is approximately 30% during the first 3 weeks and that some children will need cast wedging, repeat reduction, or pinning under anesthesia.

If there is loss of reduction, we individualize treatment depending on the patient's age, degree of deformity, time since fracture, and remodeling potential. Closed reduction and percutaneous pinning is often used for the second reduction (Fig. 9-47). Occasionally, in pure bending injuries, loss of reduction can be corrected with cast wedging.

Cast immobilization usually is for 5–6 weeks. A protective volar splint is often used as needed after casting. Physical therapy rarely is indicated. Patients can return to playground activities and sports 1–2 weeks after cast discontinuation, provided that pain has resolved and wrist motion has normalized.

In cases of loss of reduction exceeding the limits of fracture remodeling, repeat closed reduction and pin fixation is considered. Percutaneous pinning is also performed in cases of excessive swelling or signs of neurologic injury. Similarly, concurrent displaced supracondylar and distal radial fractures are treated with percutaneous fixation of both fractures to lessen the risk of neurovascular compromise. Older patients near the end of growth with bayonet apposition fractures also are treated with percutaneous pin fixation. Finally, open fractures usually are treated with pin fixation after appropriate irrigation and debridement.

A small incision is made for the insertion of the pin to protect the radial sensory nerve and adjacent extensor tendons. Smooth pins are used and are removed in the office as soon as there is sufficient healing to make the fracture stable in a cast or splint (usually at 4 weeks).

Open reduction is typically reserved for open or irreducible fractures. Open fractures are irrigated and debrided in the operating room. The initial open wound is extended adequately to inspect and cleanse the open fracture site. After thorough irrigation and debridement, the fracture is reduced and stabilized. A cast rarely is applied in this situation because of concern about fracture stability, soft tissue care, and excessive swelling. Pin fixation often is used with Gustilo grade 1 or 2 open fractures. More severe soft tissue injuries may require external fixation. If flap coverage is necessary for the soft tissue wounds, the fixator pins should be placed in consultation with the microvascular surgeon

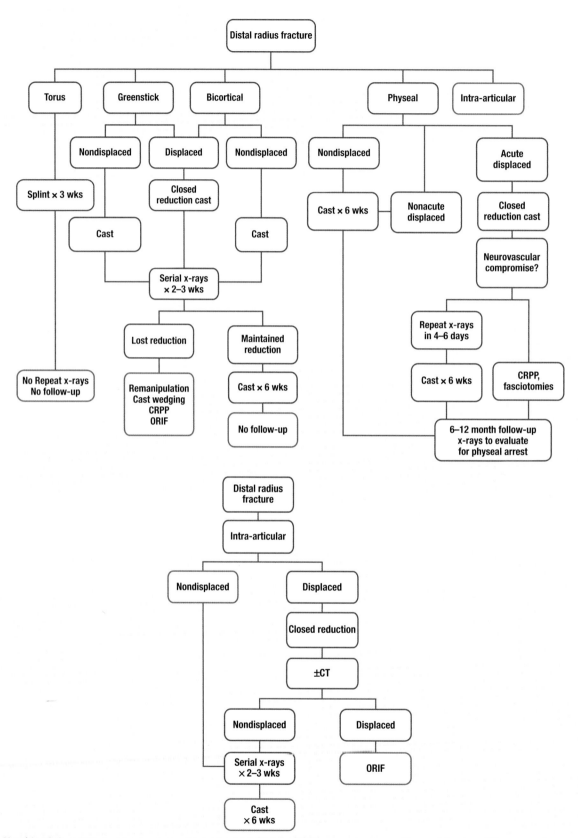

Algorithm 9-1. CRPP, closed reduction and percutaneous pinning; ORIF, open reduction and internal fixation; CT, computed tomography; MRI, magnetic resonance imaging.

Figure 9-47. Remanipulation. **A:** Displaced Salter–Harris type II distal radius fracture in a 14-year-old boy at time of injury. **B:** Near anatomic alignment achieved with closed reduction. **C:** Late loss of reduction at 2-week alignment check with excessive volar tilt (25 degrees). **D:** Since the patient was within 2 years of skeletal maturity, a repeat closed reduction and percutaneous pinning was performed, restoring volar tilt to 13 degrees.

planning the soft tissue coverage. In addition, open reduction internal fixation with volar plating is performed for unstable fractures in the skeletally mature adolescent.

Percutaneous pin fixation usually is used to stabilize the fracture in patients with open physes. If plate fixation is used, it should be placed proximally to avoid violation of the physis (Fig. 9-48). A T-shaped plate may allow improved screw fixation in the small segment of metaphyseal bone distal to the fracture and proximal to the physis. Displaced intra-articular injuries (Salter–Harris type III and IV

fractures) in skeletally immature adolescents are adult-like and require open reduction and internal fixation.

Physeal Injuries

A patient with a displaced Salter–Harris type I or II physeal fracture associated with significant volar soft tissue swelling, median neuropathy, or ipsilateral elbow and radial fractures (floating elbow) is treated with closed reduction and percutaneous pinning[11,27] (Fig. 9-49). This avoids the increased risk of compartment syndrome in the carpal canal or volar

Figure 9-48. A: Radiograph of an open humeral diaphyseal fracture in the setting of a "floating elbow injury." **B:** Radiograph depicting a displaced distal radial metaphyseal fracture. **C:** Plate fixation following irrigation and debridement of the humerus fracture. **D, E:** Radiographs following open reduction and plate fixation of the radius fracture, sparing the distal radial physis. (Courtesy of Children's Orthopaedic Surgery Foundation.)

forearm that is present if a well-molded, tight cast is applied. In addition, acute percutaneous pinning of the fracture prevents increased swelling, cast splitting, loss of reduction, and concerns about malunion or growth arrest with repeat reduction. The risk of growth arrest from a narrow-diameter, smooth pin left in place for 3–4 weeks is exceedingly small.[191]

Open reduction is reserved for irreducible Salter–Harris type I and II fractures, open fractures, fractures with associated acute carpal tunnel or forearm compartment syndrome, displaced (more than 1 mm) Salter–Harris type III or IV fractures, or triplane-equivalent fractures. For an irreducible Salter–Harris type I or II fracture, exposure is from the side of the torn periosteum. Because these fractures usually are displaced dorsally, a volar exposure is used. Smooth pins are used for stabilization and are left in for 3–4 weeks. Open fractures are exposed through the open wound with proximal and distal extension for adequate debridement. All open debridements are performed in the operating room under general anesthesia. Acute compartment syndromes are treated with immediate release of the transverse carpal ligament and/or forearm fascia. The transverse carpal ligament can be released in a Z-plasty fashion to lengthen the ligament and facilitate subsequent repair to prevent volar bow-stringing and scarring of the median nerve against the palmar skin.

Intra-Articular Fractures

Displaced intra-articular fractures (Salter–Harris type III or IV fractures) in the skeletally immature are best treated with arthroscopically assisted reduction and fixation. Distraction across the joint can be achieved with application of wrist arthroscopy traction devices and finger traps or with a temporary external fixator. Standard dorsal portals (3–4 and 4–5) are used for viewing the intra-articular aspect of the fracture and alignment of the reduction. In addition, direct observation through the arthroscope can aid in safe placement of the trans- or all-epiphyseal pins.[46,71,76] Fluoroscopy is used to evaluate the extra-articular aspects of the fracture (triplane-equivalent and type IV fractures), the reduction, and placement of fixation pins.

In older patients near or at skeletal maturity with intra-articular comminution, volar locking plate fixation is performed, similar to adults. Fixation and physeal preservation may be at odds in these situations and treatment should be individualized. Given the high risk of distal radial growth arrest in this cohort, concurrent distal ulnar epiphysiodesis can be considered to avoid downstream ulnar impaction.

Figure 9-49. A: Ipsilateral distal radial (*white arrow*) and ulnar bicortical fractures and associated supracondylar humerus fracture (*black arrows*) in a 6-year-old girl after a fall from monkey bars. **B:** Simultaneous cross-pinning of the distal radius and lateral-entry pinning of the supracondylar humerus fractures.

Potential Pitfalls and Preventative Measures

Distal Radius Fractures: POTENTIAL PITFALLS AND PREVENTIONS	
Pitfall	**Preventions**
• Loss of reduction	• Correct diagnosis of bicortical disruption • Optimal fracture reduction • Well-molded cast application • Serial radiographic evaluation
• Posttraumatic growth arrest	• Avoidance of repeated or forceful reduction maneuvers acutely • Avoidance of late manipulation for loss of reduction in children with considerable remaining growth
• Compartment syndrome	• Thorough neurovascular evaluation at time of initial presentation • Avoidance of excessive forceful manipulation during reduction maneuvers • Immediate pin fixation in patients with excessive soft tissue swelling or neurovascular compromise • Bivalve circumferential casts to avoid excessive external compression • Timely surgical stabilization with fasciotomies or carpal tunnel release in patients with impending compartment syndrome
• Radial sensory nerve injury	• Use of small incisions for nerve identification and retraction during pinning procedures • Pin placement using oscillating technique

MANAGEMENT OF EXPECTED ADVERSE OUTCOMES AND UNEXPECTED COMPLICATIONS IN FRACTURES OF THE DISTAL RADIUS AND ULNA

Distal Radial and Ulna Fractures:
COMMON ADVERSE OUTCOMES AND COMPLICATIONS

- Loss of reduction
- Malunion
- Nonunion
- Refracture
- Growth disturbance (radius or ulna)
- Ulnocarpal impaction
- TFCC tears
- Synostosis
- Neuropathy
- Infection

LOSS OF REDUCTION

Loss of reduction is a common occurrence after closed reduction and cast immobilization of displaced distal radius fractures (Fig. 9-50). Multiple studies demonstrate an incidence of loss of reduction of 20% to 30%.[6,7,9,51,74,84,105,121,126,142,192] From these studies, factors that have been identified as increasing the risk of loss of reduction with closed manipulation and casting include poor casting, bayonet apposition, age greater than 10 years, translation of more than 50% the diameter of the radius, apex volar angulation of more than 30 degrees, isolated radial fractures, and radial and ulnar metaphyseal fractures at the same level. More specifically, Mani et al.[118] concluded that initial displacement of the radial shaft of over 50% was the single most reliable predictor of failure of reduction. Proctor et al.[143] found that complete initial displacement resulted in a 52% incidence

of redisplacement of distal radial fractures in children and described remanipulation rates of 23%. Pretell et al.[142] found that postreduction translation of the radius greater than 10% in the sagittal plane resulted in 2.7 times more likely loss of reduction. LaValva et al. similarly demonstrated that fractures with residual sagittal plane translation have a 4.7 times higher risk of loss of reduction.[105] Alemdaroğlu et al.[6,7] suggested that radial fractures with greater than 30 degrees of obliquity have 11.7 times more likelihood to redisplace than a straight transverse fracture.

In addition to the initial and postreduction angulation, poor casting technique is often implicated as a cause of loss of reduction. It has become evident that casting alone is likely not sufficient to prevent loss of reduction for high-risk fractures. Miller et al.[123] reported that despite these optimal conditions, 30% of high-risk patients treated with cast immobilization alone sustained a loss of reduction that required remanipulation. These findings have generated enthusiasm for percutaneous pinning and casting as a preferable method to avoid loss of reduction.[63,191] Although the authors of these studies and others conclude that pinning is a safe, effective means of treating distal radial metaphyseal fractures (see Controversies), the results of casting versus pinning were equivalent after 2 years postfracture.[35,121]

In general, loss of reduction has been tolerated because of the remodeling potential of the distal radius.[59,138,194] However, given that remodeling can be incomplete leading to malunion (see Malunion section) with functional deficits, high rates of loss of reduction have led to considerable controversies regarding acceptable displacement, casting techniques, remanipulation, and need for initial percutaneous pinning. We prefer to reduce forearm fractures as near to perfect alignment as possible. No element of malrotation is accepted in the reduction. As indicated in the treatment sections, fractures at high risk of loss of reduction and malunion are treated with anatomic reduction and pin or, rarely, plate fixation. Fractures treated in a cast are followed closely and rereduced for any loss of alignment of

Figure 9-50. Results of angulation. **A:** Significant apex volar angulation of the distal fragment. **B:** The appearance was not as apparent cosmetically as in another patient with less angulation that was directed apex dorsally. **C:** Radial deviation constricts the interosseous space, which may decrease forearm rotation. (**B, C:** Reproduced with permission from Wilkins KE, ed: *Operative Management of Upper Extremity Fractures in Children.* American Academy of Orthopaedic Surgeons; 1994.)

more than 10 to 20 degrees. Although loss of forearm rotation can occur with anatomic healing, it is less likely than with a malunion.

MALUNION

While complications from metaphyseal and physeal fractures of the radius are relatively rare, malunions do occur.[10,34,35,44] De Courtivron[39] reported that of 602 distal radial fractures, 14% had an initial malunion of more than 5 degrees. In addition, as noted above, the rate of loss of reduction for distal radius fractures ranges from 20% to 30%, and although many of these fractures will be rereduced, inevitably surgeons will encounter malunion of the distal radius, most often due to decisions to avoid injury to the physis from remanipulation beyond 7 days of injury, to avoid unnecessary repeat reduction in a child with substantial remodeling potential, or a patient missed follow-up appointments before healing occurs. Fortunately, with significant growth remaining, many angular malunions of the distal radius will remodel,[39,44,59,89,138,194] probably because of asymmetric physeal growth (see Fig. 9-22).[93,104] The younger the patient, the less the deformity, and the closer the fracture is to the physis, the greater the potential for remodeling. Distal radial fractures are most often juxtaphyseal, the malunion typically is in the plane of motion of the wrist joint (dorsal displacement with apex volar angulation), and the distal radius accounts for 60% to 80% of the growth of the radius. All these factors favor remodeling of a malunion.

The malunited fracture should be monitored over the next 6 to 12 months for remodeling. If the fracture does not remodel, persistent extension deformity of the distal radial articular surface puts the patient at risk for developing midcarpal instability[170,171] and degenerative arthritis of the wrist, though a recent report has raised the question of whether imperfect final radiographic alignment necessarily leads to symptomatic arthrosis.[58] Some patients with apex volar malunion of the distal radius may have symptomatic volar instability of the DRUJ.[122] For malunion correction, an opening-wedge (dorsal or volar) osteotomy is made, iliac crest bone of appropriate trapezoidal shape to correct the deformity is inserted, and either a plate or external fixator is used to maintain correction until healing.[57]

As there are controversies as to what degree of deformity is either less likely to remodel or cause a functional loss (see Controversies), the degree and plane of loss of motion, as well as the individual affected, determine if this is functionally significant.[190] In cadaver studies, malangulation of more than 20 degrees of the radius or ulna caused loss of forearm rotation,[171] whereas less than 10 degrees of malangulation did not alter forearm rotation significantly. Distal third malunion affected rotation less than middle or proximal third malunion. Radioulnar malunion affected forearm rotation more than volar–dorsal malunion. Excessive angulation may lead to a loss of rotation at a 1:2 degree ratio, whereas malrotation may lead to rotational loss at only a 1:1 degree loss. The functional loss associated with rotational motion loss is difficult to predict. This has led some clinicians to recommend no treatment,[37] arguing that most of these fractures will remodel and those that do not remodel will

not cause a functional problem.[87] However, a significant functional problem is present if shoulder motion cannot compensate for loss of supination.

Intra-articular malunion is a potentially devastating complication, due to the risk of degenerative arthritis if the articular step-off is more than 2 mm.[100] MRI or CT scans can be useful in preoperative evaluations. Arthroscopy allows direct examination of the deformity and areas of impingement or potential degeneration. Intra-articular osteotomy with bone grafting in the metaphysis to support the reconstructed articular surface is controversial and risky; however, it has the potential to restore anatomic alignment to the joint and prevent serious long-term complications. This problem fortunately is uncommon in children because of the rarity of the injury and this type of malunion.

In Galeazzi fractures, malunion of the radius can lead to subluxation of the DRUJ, limited forearm rotation, and pain, usually secondary to persistent shortening and malrotation of the radial fracture. Most often, this occurs when complete fractures are treated with closed reduction and there is failure to either obtain or maintain reduction of the radial fracture. The ulna remains subluxed and heals with an incongruent joint. Treatment of this requires proper recognition and corrective osteotomy. If physical examination is not definitive for diagnosis, then a CT scan in pronation, neutral rotation, or supination may be helpful. MRI or wrist arthroscopy will aid in the diagnosis and management of associated ligamentous, chondral, or TFCC injuries that will benefit from debridement or repair. It is important to understand that if the DRUJ subluxation is caused by a radial malunion, a soft tissue reconstruction of the DRUJ alone will fail. Concurrent repair of the TFCC will further stabilize the DRUJ. If the TFCC is not repairable, soft tissue reconstruction of the DRUJ ligaments with imbrication of the extensor retinaculum (Herbert sling) at the sigmoid notch will greatly help in restoring stability to the DRUJ.[15]

NONUNION

Nonunion of a closed distal radial or ulnar fracture is rare. In children, nonunion has been generally related to a pathologic condition of the bone, open fractures, or compromised vascularity, but rare cases of distal radial nonunion in healthy children with closed fractures have been reported.[165] Congenital pseudarthrosis or neurofibromatosis (Fig. 9-51) should be suspected in a young patient with a nonunion after a benign fracture. This occurs most often after an isolated ulnar fracture. The distal bone is often narrowed, sclerotic, and plastically deformed. These fractures rarely heal with immobilization. Vascularized fibular bone grafting usually is necessary for healing of a nonunion associated with neurofibromatosis or congenital pseudarthrosis. If the patient is very young, this may include a vascularized epiphyseal transfer to restore distal growth.

Vascular impairment also can lead to nonunion. Distal radial nonunion has been reported in a child with an ipsilateral supracondylar fracture with brachial artery occlusion. Revascularization of the limb led to eventual union of the fracture. Nonunion

Figure 9-51. This 3-year-old presented to the emergency room with pain after an acute fall on his arm. The ulna is clearly pathologic with thinning and deformity before this injury. This represents neurofibromatosis. (Courtesy of Children's Orthopaedic Surgery Foundation.)

also can occur following open fractures in the setting of osteomyelitis or bone loss. Debridement of the necrotic bone and either traditional bone grafting, osteoclasis lengthening, vascularized bone grafting, or creation of a single-bone forearm are surgical options. The choice depends on the individual patient.

CROSS-UNION

Cross-union, or posttraumatic radioulnar synostosis, is a rare complication of pediatric distal radial and ulna fractures. It has been described after high-energy trauma and internal fixation.[176] A single pin crossing both bones increases the risk of cross-union.[176] Synostosis take-down can be performed, but the results usually are less than full restoration of motion. Interposition of a vascularized flap should be considered in these cases. It is important to determine if there is an element of rotational malunion with the cross-union because this will affect the surgical outcome.

Soft tissue contraction across both bones also has been described.[56] Contracture release resulted in restoration of forearm motion.

REFRACTURE

Fortunately, refractures after distal radial fractures are rare and much less common than after pediatric diaphyseal radial and ulna fractures and fractures in adults. This is likely due to the unique biology in children where, as opposed to adults,

remineralization after forearm fractures occurs rapidly with a transient elevation in bone mineral density.[60] Most commonly, refracture occurs with premature discontinuation of immobilization or early return to potentially traumatic activities. Although greenstick and torus fractures are both unicortical injuries, the treating provider must appreciate that greenstick fractures are more unstable, take longer to heal and have a higher risk of refracture. It is advisable to protectively immobilize the wrist until full radiograph and clinical healing (usually 5–7 weeks) and to restrict activities until full motion and comfort are regained (usually an additional 1–2 weeks). Individuals involved in high-risk activities, such as downhill ski racing, snowboarding, or skateboarding, should be protected with a splint during those activities for much longer.

PHYSEAL ARREST OF THE DISTAL RADIUS

Distal radial physeal arrest can occur from either the trauma of the original injury (Fig. 9-52)[8,80] or late reduction of a displaced fracture.[96] The incidence of radial growth arrest has been shown to be 4% to 7% of all displaced distal radial physeal fractures.[11,27,107] The trauma to the physeal cartilage from displacement and compression is a significant risk factor for growth arrest, particularly in Salter–Harris type III and IV fractures. Kallini et al. reported on 28 patients with these rarer intra-articular distal radius physeal fractures. In this cohort, growth disturbance occurred in 43% of patients.[90] Further research on risk factors for growth arrest is needed. Lee et al. demonstrated that multiple closed reduction attempts significantly increases the risk of physeal arrest.[107] The severity of initial fracture displacement and the quality of fracture reduction could portend higher risks of growth arrest, but this has not been carefully examined. Similarly, the risk of further compromising the physis with late reduction at various time intervals is still unclear. The current recommendation is for a single atraumatic reduction of a displaced physeal fracture less than 7 days after injury.

When a growth arrest develops, the consequences depend on the severity of the arrest and the amount of growth remaining. Surgical decision-making is multifactorial and should include the age and sex of the patient, the remaining growth potential, and the size and location of the physeal bar.[158] A complete arrest of the distal radial physis in a skeletally immature patient can be a serious problem. The continued growth of the ulna with cessation of radial growth can lead to incongruity of the DRUJ, ulnocarpal impaction, and development of a TFCC tear (Fig. 9-53).[11,180] The radial deviation deformity at the wrist can be severe enough to cause limitation of wrist and forearm motion. Pain and clicking can develop at the ulnocarpal or radioulnar joints, indicative of ulnocarpal impaction or a TFCC tear. The deformity will progress until the end of growth. Pain and limited motion and function will be present until forearm length is rebalanced, until the radiocarpal, ulnocarpal, and DRUJ are restored, and until the TFCC tear and areas of chondromalacia are repaired or debrided.[11]

Ideally, physeal arrest of the distal radius will be discovered early before the consequences of unbalanced growth develop. Radiographic screening 6 to 12 months after injury can identify

Figure 9-52. A: AP radiograph of growth arrest with open ulnar physis. **B:** MRI scan of large area of growth arrest that was not deemed respectable by mapping. Note is made of impaction of the distal ulna against the triquetrum and a secondary peripheral TFCC tear. **C:** Radiograph after ulnar shortening osteotomy, restoring neutral ulnar variance.

Figure 9-53. A: Coronal plane CT image demonstrating central distal radial growth arrest with physeal bar formation and associated ulnar positive variance. **B:** Clinical photograph of this patient's distal ulnar prominence and radial deviation deformity.

the early arrest. A small area of growth arrest in a patient near skeletal maturity may be clinically inconsequential. However, a large area of arrest in a patient with marked growth remaining can lead to ulnocarpal impaction and forearm deformity if intervention is delayed. MRI can map the area of arrest. If it is less than 45% of the physis, a bar resection with fat interposition can be attempted.[169] This may restore radial growth and prevent future problems (Fig. 9-54). If the bar is larger than 45% of the physis, bar resection is unlikely to be successful. In older children, an early ulnar epiphysiodesis will prevent growth imbalance of the forearm.[26,180] Campbell et al. recently reported that the success rate of ulnar epiphysiodesis exceeds 90%. The

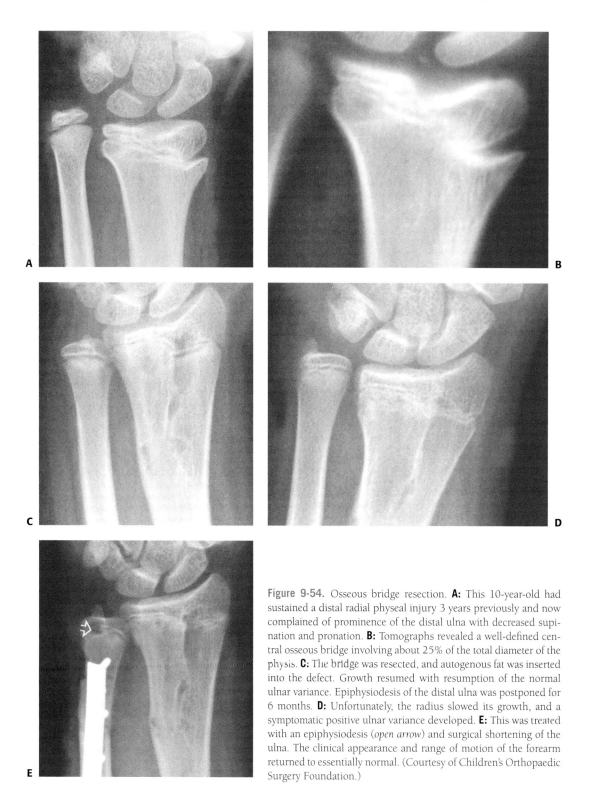

Figure 9-54. Osseous bridge resection. **A:** This 10-year-old had sustained a distal radial physeal injury 3 years previously and now complained of prominence of the distal ulna with decreased supination and pronation. **B:** Tomographs revealed a well-defined central osseous bridge involving about 25% of the total diameter of the physis. **C:** The bridge was resected, and autogenous fat was inserted into the defect. Growth resumed with resumption of the normal ulnar variance. Epiphysiodesis of the distal ulna was postponed for 6 months. **D:** Unfortunately, the radius slowed its growth, and a symptomatic positive ulnar variance developed. **E:** This was treated with an epiphysiodesis (*open arrow*) and surgical shortening of the ulna. The clinical appearance and range of motion of the forearm returned to essentially normal. (Courtesy of Children's Orthopaedic Surgery Foundation.)

growth discrepancy between forearm lengths in most patients is minor and does not require treatment. However, this is not the case for a patient with an arrest at a very young age, for whom complicated decisions regarding acute versus gradual distraction lengthening of the radius need to occur whether or not bar resection is feasible and successful. Many of these children may need an ulnar shortening osteotomy.

If a radial growth arrest occurs associated with a radial physeal stress injury, treatment depends on the degree of deformity and the patient's symptoms. Physeal bar resection often is not possible because the arrest is usually too diffuse in stress injuries. If there is no significant ulnar overgrowth, a distal ulnar epiphysiodesis will prevent the development of an ulnocarpal impaction syndrome. For ulnar overgrowth and ulnocarpal pain, an ulnar shortening osteotomy is indicated and appears to have a lower risk of nonunion than in the adult population.[29] Techniques include transverse, oblique, and Z-shortening osteotomies. Transverse osteotomy has a higher risk of nonunion than either oblique or Z-shortening and should be avoided. Even when oblique or Z-shortenings are used, making the osteotomy more distally in the metaphyseal region will lessen the risk of nonunion, owing to the more robust vascularity of the distal ulna. The status of the TFCC also should be evaluated by MRI or wrist arthroscopy. If there is an associated TFCC tear, it should be repaired as appropriate.

Growth arrest of the distal radius after metaphyseal fracture is extremely rare with only five cases reported in the literature. Wilkins and O'Brien[185] proposed that these arrests may be in fractures that extend from the metaphysis to the physis. This coincides with a Peterson type I fracture (Fig. 9-55) and in essence is a physeal fracture. These fractures should be monitored for growth arrest.

Rarely, patients present late with established deformity. Treatment involves rebalancing the length of the radius and ulna. The options include hemiphyseal arrest of the radius, corrective radial closing wedge osteotomy, and ulnar lengthening, or a combination of these procedures. The painful impingement of the radius and ulna with forearm rotation can be corrected with reconstitution of the DRUJ. If the radial physis has significant growth remaining, a complete radial physeal arrest should be done at the same time as the surgical rebalancing of the radius and ulna. Treatment is individualized depending on the age of the patient, degree of deformity, and level of pain and dysfunction.

Both undergrowth and overgrowth of the distal radius after fracture were described by de Pablos.[40] The average difference in growth was 3 mm, with a range of −5 to +10 mm of growth disturbance compared with the contralateral radius. Maximal overgrowth occurred in the 9- to 12-year-old age group. As long as the patient is asymptomatic, under- or overgrowth is not a problem. If ulnocarpal impaction or DRUJ disruption occurs, then surgical rebalancing of the radius and ulna may be necessary.

Physeal Arrest Distal Ulna

Physeal growth arrest is frequent with distal ulnar physeal fractures (Fig. 9-56), occurring in 10% to 55% of patients.[66] These figures may have limited accuracy due to the infrequency of scientific reports and the small sample sizes. It is unclear why the distal ulna has a higher incidence of growth arrest after fracture than does the radius, although this may be due to a higher incidence of intra-articular physeal fractures. Ulnar growth arrest in a young child leads to relative radial overgrowth and bowing. The most common complication of distal ulnar physeal fractures is growth arrest. Golz et al.[66] described 18 such fractures, with growth arrest in 55%. If the patient is young enough, continued growth of the radius will lead to deformity and dysfunction. The distal ulnar aspect of the radial physis and epiphysis appears to be tethered by the foreshortened ulna (Fig. 9-57). The radial articular surface develops increased inclination toward the foreshortened ulna. This is similar to the deformity Peinado[137] created experimentally with arrest of the distal ulna in rabbits' forelimbs. The distal ulna loses its normal articulation in the

Figure 9-55. Physeal arrest in a Peterson type I fracture. **A:** Injury film showing what appears to be a benign metaphyseal fracture. Fracture line extends into the physis (*arrows*). **B:** Two years postinjury, a central arrest (*open arrow*) has developed, with resultant shortening of the radius. (Reproduced with permission from Wilkins KE, ed: *Operative Management of Upper Extremity Fractures in Children*. American Academy of Orthopaedic Surgeons; 1994.)   **A**   **B**

Figure 9-56. A, B: A 10-year-old boy sustained a closed Salter–Harris type I separation of the distal ulnar physis (*arrows*) combined with a fracture of the distal radial metaphysis. **C:** An excellent closed reduction was achieved atraumatically. **D:** Long-term growth arrest of the distal ulna occurred.

sigmoid notch of the distal radius. The metaphyseal–diaphyseal region of the radius often becomes notched from its articulation with the distal ulna during forearm rotation. Frequently, these patients have pain and limitation of motion with pronation and supination.

Ideally, this problem is identified before the development of marked ulnar foreshortening and subsequent radial deformity. Because it is well known that distal ulnar physeal fractures have a high incidence of growth arrest, these patients should have follow-up radiographs at 6 to 12 months after fracture for early identification. Unfortunately, in the distal ulnar physis, physeal bar resection generally is unsuccessful. Surgical epiphysiodesis of the distal radius can prevent worsening deformity. In most children, distal ulnar physeal arrest occurs toward the end of growth so that the forearm length discrepancy is not a problem. In younger children, the foreshortened ulna can act as a tether, causing asymmetric growth of the radius. There will be increased radial articular inclination on the AP radiograph and subluxation of the DRUJ. Operative choices include ulnar lengthening, radial closing wedge osteotomy, radial epiphysiodesis, and a combination of the above procedures that is appropriate for the individual patient's age, deformity, and disability.

Ulnocarpal Impaction Syndrome

The growth discrepancy between the radius and ulna can lead to relative radial shortening and ulnar overgrowth. The distal ulna can impact upon the lunate and triquetrum and cause pain with ulnar deviation, extension, and compression activities. This is particularly true in repetitive wrist-loading sports such as field hockey, lacrosse, and gymnastics.[43] Physical examination loading the ulnocarpal joint in ulnar deviation and compression will recreate the pain. Radiographs show the radial arrest, ulnar overgrowth, and distal ulnocarpal impingement. The ulnocarpal impaction also may be caused by a hypertrophic ulnar styloid fracture union or an ulnar styloid nonunion.[25] MRI may reveal chondromalacia of the lunate or triquetrum, a tear of the TFCC, and the extent of the distal radial physeal arrest.

Treatment should correct all components of the problem. The ulnar overgrowth is corrected by either an ulnar shortening or radial lengthening osteotomy. Most often, a marked degree

Figure 9-57. **A:** The appearance of the distal ulna in the patient seen in Figure 9-42, 3 years after injury, demonstrating premature fusion of the distal ulnar physis with 3.2 cm of shortening. The distal radius is secondarily deformed, with tilting and translocation toward the ulna. **B:** Because of distal ulnar physeal arrest, a lengthening of the distal ulna was performed using a small unipolar distracting device. The ulna was slightly overlengthened to compensate for some subsequent growth of the distal radius. **C:** Six months after the lengthening osteotomy, there is some deformity of the distal ulna, but good restoration of length has been achieved. The distal radial epiphyseal tilt has corrected somewhat, and the patient has asymptomatic supination and pronation to 75 degrees. **D:** Different case than in **A–C,** showing more progressive distal radial deformity treated with corrective osteotomy and epiphysiodesis of the distal radius.

of positive ulnar variance requires ulnar shortening to neutral or negative variance (Fig. 9-58). If the ulnar physis is still open, a simultaneous distal ulnar epiphysiodesis should be done to prevent recurrent deformity. If the degree of radial deformity is marked, this should be corrected by a realignment or lengthening osteotomy. Criteria for radial correction are debatable, but radial inclination of less than 10 degrees on the AP radiograph may be an indication for correction.[180] In the rare case of complete arrest in a very young patient, radial lengthening is preferable to ulnar shortening to rebalance the forearm.

Triangular Fibrocartilage Complex Tears

Most TFCC tears in children occur following distal radius and ulna fractures.[108,187] The most common patterns are Palmer type 1B (approximately 50%) and 1D (approximately 20%) tears.[187] Peripheral traumatic TFCC tears should be repaired. The presence of an ulnar styloid nonunion at the base often is indicative of an associated peripheral tear of the TFCC.[1,11,135,172] The symptomatic ulnar styloid nonunion is excised,[25] and any TFCC tear is repaired. If physical examination or preoperative

MRI indicates a TFCC tear in the absence of an ulnar styloid nonunion, an initial arthroscopic examination can define the lesion and appropriate treatment. Peripheral tears are the most common TFCC tears in children and adolescents and can be repaired arthroscopically by an outside-in suture technique. Tears off the sigmoid notch are the next most common in adolescents and can be repaired with arthroscopic-assisted, transradial sutures. With Palmer type 1B and 1D tears, excellent pain relief and functional outcomes can be expected in the majority of children.[187] Central tears are rare in children and, as opposed to adults with degenerative central tears, arthroscopic debridement usually does not result in pain relief in children. Distal volar tears also are rare and are repaired open, at times with ligament reconstruction.[172]

Some ulnar styloid fractures result in nonunion or hypertrophic union.[1,11,25,135,172] Nonunion may be associated with TFCC tears. Hypertrophic healing represents a pseudoulnar positive variance with resultant ulnocarpal impaction. Both cause ulnar-sided wrist pain. Compression of the lunate or triquetrum on the distal ulna reproduces the pain. Clicking with ulnocarpal compression or forearm rotation represents either a TFCC tear

A

B

Figure 9-58. A: AP radiograph of distal radial growth arrest, ulnar overgrowth, and an ulnar styloid nonunion. Wrist arthroscopy revealed an intact triangular fibrocartilage complex. **B:** AP and lateral radiographs after ulnar shortening osteotomy. (Courtesy of Children's Orthopaedic Surgery Foundation.)

or chondromalacia of the lunate or triquetrum. Surgical excision of the nonunion or hypertrophic union with repair of the TFCC to the base of the styloid is the treatment of choice. Postoperative immobilization for 4 weeks in a long-arm cast followed by 2 weeks in a short-arm cast protects the TFCC repair.

Neuropathy

Median neuropathy can occur from direct trauma from the initial displacement of the fracture, traction ischemia from a persistently displaced fracture, or the development of a compartment syndrome in the carpal canal or volar forearm (see Fig. 9-6).[17,181] Median neuropathy and marked volar soft tissue swelling are indications for percutaneous pin stabilization of the fracture to lessen the risk of compartment syndrome in a cast. Median neuropathy caused by direct trauma or traction ischemia generally resolves after fracture reduction. The degree of neural injury determines the length of time to recovery. Recovery can be monitored with an advancing Tinel sign along the median nerve. Motor-sensory testing can define progressive return of neural function.

Median neuropathy caused by a carpal tunnel syndrome will not recover until the carpal tunnel is decompressed. After anatomic fracture reduction and pin stabilization, volar forearm and carpal tunnel pressures are measured. Before measuring pressures, wait at least 20 minutes to allow for pressure–volume equilibration. If the pressures are elevated beyond 40 mm Hg or the difference between the diastolic pressure and the compartment pressure is less than 30 mm Hg, an immediate release of the affected compartments should be performed. The carpal tunnel is released through a palmar incision in line with the fourth ray, with care to avoid injuring the palmar vascular arch and the ulnar nerves exiting the Guyon canal. The transverse carpal ligament can be released with subsequent Z-plasty closure of the ligament to prevent late bow-stringing of the nerve against the palmar skin. The volar forearm fascia is released in the standard fashion.

Both the median and ulnar nerves are less commonly injured in metaphyseal fractures than in physeal fractures.[31]

The mechanisms of neural injury in a metaphyseal fracture include direct contusion from the displaced fragment, traction ischemia from tenting of the nerve over the proximal fragment, entrapment of the nerve in the fracture site, rare laceration of the nerve, and the development of an acute compartment syndrome. If signs or symptoms of neuropathy are present, a prompt closed reduction should be performed. Extreme positions of immobilization should be avoided because this can lead to persistent traction or compression ischemia and increase the risk of compartment syndrome. If there is marked swelling, it is better to percutaneously pin the fracture than to apply a constrictive cast. If there is concern about compartment syndrome, the forearm and carpal canal pressures should be measured immediately. If pressures are markedly elevated, appropriate fasciotomies and compartment releases should be performed immediately. Finally, if the nerve was intact before reduction and is out after reduction, neural entrapment should be considered, and surgical exploration and decompression may be required. Fortunately, most median and ulnar nerve injuries recover after anatomic reduction of the fracture.

Injuries to the ulnar nerve and anterior interosseous nerve have been described with Galeazzi fracture–dislocations.[50,150,177] These reported injuries have had spontaneous recovery. Moore et al.[127] described an 8% rate of injury to the radial nerve with operative exposure of the radius for internal fixation in their series. Careful surgical exposure, dissection, and retraction can decrease this risk.

Infection

Infection after distal radial fractures is uncommon and is associated with open fractures or surgical intervention (also see Controversies).

Infections related to surgical intervention occur in less than 1% of cases and less commonly in children than in adults with distal radius fractures.[5] Superficial pin-site infections can occur and should be treated with pin removal and antibiotics. Less than 10% of infections require surgical debridement.[5] Deep-space infections from percutaneous pinning of the radius are exceedingly rare but could result in physeal trauma and arrest.

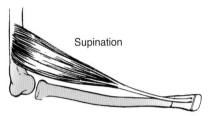

Figure 9-59. The brachioradialis is relaxed in supination but may become a deforming force in pronation.

CONTROVERSIES RELATED TO FRACTURES OF THE DISTAL RADIUS AND ULNA

ACCEPTABLE DEFORMITY

There is considerable controversy about what constitutes an acceptable reduction. This is clearly age dependent: the younger the patient, the greater the potential for remodeling. Volar–dorsal malalignment has the greatest potential for remodeling because this is in the plane of predominant motion of the joint. A 2012 prospective study found excellent long-term clinical and radiographic results, as well as reduced cost, with cast molding of displaced fractures in unsedated preteen children.[35] Marked coronal plane malalignment is less likely to remodel but may be more substantial than previously described.[116] Malrotation will not remodel. The ranges for acceptable reduction according to age are given in the immobilization section on incomplete fractures and apply to complete fractures as well.

GREENSTICK FRACTURES

Controversy exists regarding completion of greenstick fractures.[37,159] Although some researchers advocate completion of the fracture to reduce the risk of subsequent loss of reduction from the intact periosteum and concave deformity acting as a tension band to redisplace the fracture, completing the fracture increases the risk of instability and malunion.[185]

IMMOBILIZATION

The position and type of immobilization after reduction also have been controversial. Recommendations for the position of postreduction immobilization include supination, neutral, and pronation. The rationale for immobilization in pronation is that reduction of the more common apex volar fractures requires correction of the supination deformity. Following this rationale, apex dorsal fractures should be reduced and immobilized in supination. Pollen[141] believed that the brachioradialis was a deforming force in pronation and was relaxed in supination (Fig. 9-59) and advocated immobilization in supination for all displaced distal radial fractures. Kasser[95] recommended immobilization in slight supination to allow better molding of the volar distal radius. Some researchers advocate immobilization in a neutral position, believing this is best at maintaining the interosseous space and has the least risk of disabling loss of forearm rotation in the long term. Davis and Green[38] and Ogden[132] advocated that each fracture seek its own preferred position of stability. Gupta and Danielsson[72] randomized immobilization of distal radial metaphyseal greenstick fractures in neutral, supination, or pronation to try to determine the best position of immobilization. Their study showed a statistical improvement in final healing with immobilization in supination. More recently, Boyer et al.[23] prospectively randomized 109 distal third forearm fractures into long-arm casts with the forearm in neutral rotation,

supination, or pronation following closed reduction. No significant differences in final radiographic position were noted among the differing positions of forearm rotation.

Another area of controversy is whether long- or short-arm cast immobilization is better. Historically, most publications on pediatric distal radial fracture treatment advocated long-arm cast treatment for the first 3 to 4 weeks of healing.[20,77,131,140] The rationale is that elbow flexion reduces the muscle forces acting to displace the fracture. In addition, a long-arm cast may further restrict the child's activity and therefore decrease the risk of displacement. However, Chess et al.[30] reported redisplacement and reduction rates with well-molded short-arm casts similar to those with long-arm casts. They used a cast index (sagittal diameter divided by coronal diameter at the fracture site) of 0.7 or less to indicate a well-molded cast. In addition, two prospective studies have recapitulated these findings. The short-arm cast offers the advantage of elbow mobility and better patient acceptance of casting. Two randomized prospective clinical trials and a meta-analysis review compared the efficacy of short- and long-arm cast immobilization following closed reduction for pediatric distal radial fractures.[20,77] Bohm et al.[20] randomized 102 patients over the age of 4 years to either short- or long-arm casts following closed reduction of displaced distal radial metaphyseal fractures. No statistically significant difference was seen in loss of reduction rate between the two treatment groups. Webb et al.[183] similarly randomized 103 patients to short- or long-arm casts after reduction of distal radial fractures. No significant difference in rate of lost reduction was seen between the two cohorts. Patients in short-arm casts, however, missed fewer days of school and required less assistance with activities of daily living than those with long-arm casts. In both these studies, quality of fracture reduction and cast mold were influential factors in loss of reduction rates. These studies have challenged the traditional teaching regarding the need for elbow immobilization to control distal radial fracture alignment.

IMMEDIATE PINNING OF DISPLACED DISTAL RADIUS FRACTURES

In the past few decades, closed reduction and percutaneous pinning have become more common as the primary treatment of distal radial metaphyseal fractures in children and adolescents.[114,167,174,191] Despite this practice change, a meta-analysis review of the data comparing cast immobilization versus immediate pinning reveals equivalent long-term outcomes, despite more loss of reduction in the cast groups and more pin complications in the pin groups.[10] The indications cited include fracture instability and high risk of loss of reduction increasing the likelihood of the need for remanipulation,[7,42,51,74,84,118,121,125,142,143,192] excessive local swelling that increases the risk of neurovascular compromise,[17,38,181] and ipsilateral fractures of the distal radius and elbow region (floating elbow) that increase the risk of compartment syndrome.[19,151] In addition, surgeon's preference for pinning in a busy office practice has been considered an acceptable indication because of similar complication rates and long-term outcomes with pinning and casting[120,123] and the avoidance of remanipulation because alignment is secure.

OPEN FRACTURES

Multiple studies have demonstrated that the infection rate (2.5–4%) following nonoperative treatment of Gustilo grade 1 open fractures[45,85] is comparable to rates for operative treatment[69] (2.5%). However, these were retrospective studies and likely will not change the standard of care of these fractures until an appropriate prospective randomized study has been conducted. Even with prospective studies, it is unclear if the studies will be large enough to include the impact of rare deep infections.

CONCLUSIONS

Fractures of the distal forearm are common in the pediatric population. Given their proximity to the distal physes of the radius and ulna, these fractures have tremendous remodeling capacity and as a result, the majority may be effectively treated with appropriate nonoperative means. The future direction for management of these fractures is primarily focused on prognosticating which fractures would be better served through surgical reduction and fixation, considering the relatively high rate of loss of reduction of these fractures.

ACKNOWLEDGMENTS

The author acknowledges Drs. William Hennrikus and Donald Bae, who prepared this chapter in the previous edition.

Annotated References

Reference	Annotation
Chess DG, Hyman JC, Leahey JL, et al. Short arm plaster cast for distal pediatric forearm fracture. *J Pediatr Orthop.* 1994;14:211–213.	A forearm cast should be flat not round to maintain reduction. The "cast index"—the ratio of the cast diameter on the lateral compared to the AP radiograph—of less than or equal to 0.7 is a key cast-molding technique for successful maintenance of reduction of distal forearm fractures.
Crawford SN, Lee LS, Izuka BH. Closed reduction of overriding distal radius fractures without reduction in children. *J Bone Joint Surg.* 2012;94:246–252.	A simple, effective, cost- and time-efficient method of treatment for overriding distal radius fractures in children. Demonstrates the remarkable remodeling potential of the pediatric distal radius.
Do TT, Strub WM, Foad SL, et al. Reduction versus remodeling in pediatric distal forearm fractures: a preliminary cost analysis. *J Pediatr Orthop B.* 2003;12:109–115.	A study ahead of its time that predates the Michael Porter value revolution—Porter ME. What is value in health care? *NEJM.* 2010;363: 2477–2481.
Godambe SA, Elliot V, Matheny D, Pershad J. Comparison of propofol/fentanyl versus ketamine/midazolam for brief orthopaedic procedural sedation in the emergency department. *Pediatrics.* 2003;112:116–123.	A prospective, controlled trial evaluating the advantages and disadvantages of two commonly used methods of conscious sedation in children for fracture reduction.
Hang JR, Hutchinson AF, Hau RC. Risk factors associated with loss of position after closed reduction of distal radial fractures in children. *J Pediatr Orthop.* 2011;31:501–506.	Completely displaced distal radius fractures and an ipsilateral ulna fracture that cannot be anatomically reduced is the best predictor for redisplacement.
Iobst CA, Spurdel C, Baitner AC, et al. A protocol for the management of pediatric type 1 open fractures. *J Child Orthop.* 2014;8:71–76.	Forty-five consecutive patients treated with wound cleansing in the ED, closed reduction under conscious sedation in the ED, IV antibiotics, and no formal I and D in the operating room resulted in uncomplicated fracture healing and no infections.
Kallini JR, Fu EC, Shah AS, et al. Growth disturbance following intra-articular distal radius fractures in the skeletally immature patient. *J Pediatr Orthop.* 2020;40(10):e910–e915.	Demonstrates that the risk of distal radial growth arrest following Salter–Harris type III and IV fractures exceeds 40%.

Annotated References

Reference	Annotation
Lynch KA, Wesolowski M, Cappello T. Coronal Remodeling Potential of Pediatric Distal Radius Fractures. *J Pediatr Orthop.* 2020;40(10):556–561.	Establishes the degree of coronal plane remodeling that can be expected following pediatric distal radius fracture. In skeletally immature patients, 24 degrees of coronal plane remodeling can be expected in the first year after fracture.
McQuinn AG, Jaarsma RL. Risk factors for redisplacement of pediatric distal forearm and distal radius fractures. *J Pediatr Orthop.* 2012;32:687–692.	Initial displacement of >50% and inability to achieve an anatomic reduction are the major risk factors for redisplacement. The cast index is the most useful method to grade cast molding.
Plint AC, Perry JJ, Correll R, et al. A randomized, controlled trial of removable splinting versus casting for wrist buckle fractures in children. *Pediatrics.* 2006;117:691–697.	Removable splinting was superior to casting for function and bathing with equal outcomes noted for pain, healing, and reinjury.
Samora JB, Klingele KE, Beebe AC, et al. Is there still a place for cast wedging in pediatric forearm fractures? *J Pediatr Orthop.* 2014;34:246–252.	An update on the technique of cast wedging of the distal radius and ulna for the millennial generation.
Shah AS, Guzek RH, Miller ML, et al; Pediatric Distal Radius Fracture (PDRF) Study Group. Descriptive epidemiology of isolated distal radius fractures in children: results from a prospective multicenter registry. *J Pediatr Orthop.* 2023;43(1):e1–e8.	First registry and prospective study to describe the clinical presentation of pediatric distal radius fractures. Demonstrates the relative frequency of various distal radius and ulna fracture patterns. Shows that approximately 84% of physeal fractures are Salter–Harris type II injuries.
Voto SJ, Weiner DS, Leighley B. Redisplacement after closed reduction of forearm fractures in children. *J Pediatr Orthop.* 1990;10:79–84.	Redisplacement occurs in about 7% of cases and can usually be successfully treated with a second closed reduction and casting.
Waters PM, Bae DS, Montgomery KD. Surgical management of post-traumatic distal radial growth arrest in adolescents. *J Pediatr Orthop.* 2002;22:717–724.	Growth arrest occurs in about 4% of fractures. Surgical options and outcomes are well-outlined in this paper.

REFERENCES

1. Abid A, Accadbled F, Kany J, et al. Ulnar styloid fracture in children: a retrospective study of 46 cases. *J Pediatr Orthop B.* 2008;17(1):15–19.
2. Abraham A, Handoll HHG, Khan T. Interventions for treating wrist fractures in children. *Cochrane Database Syst Rev.* 2008;(2):CD004576.
3. af Ekenstam F. Anatomy of the distal radioulnar joint. *Clin Orthop Relat Res.* 1992;(275):14–18.
4. Al-Ansari K, Howard A, Seeto B, et al. Minimally angulated pediatric wrist fractures: is immobilization without manipulation enough? *CJEM.* 2007;9(1):9–15.
5. Albright JA, Meghani O, Rebello E, et al. A comparison of the rates of postoperative infection following distal radius fixation between pediatric and young adult populations: an analysis of 32 368 patients. *Hand (N Y).* 2022:15589447221142896.
6. Alemdaroğlu KB, Iltar S, Aydoğan NH. 3-point index in redisplacement of distal radial fractures in children: how should it be used? *J Hand Surg Am.* 2009;34(5):964.
7. Alemdaroğlu KB, Iltar S, Cimen O, et al. Risk factors in redisplacement of distal radial fractures in children. *J Bone Joint Surg Am.* 2008;90(6):1224–1230.
8. Aminian A, Schoenecker PL. Premature closure of the distal radial physis after fracture of the distal radial metaphysis. *J Pediatr Orthop.* 1995;15(4):495–498.
9. Bae DS. Pediatric distal radius and forearm fractures. *J Hand Surg Am.* 2008;33(10):1911–1923.
10. Bae DS, Howard AW. Distal radius fractures: what is the evidence? *J Pediatr Orthop.* 2012;32(Suppl 2):S128–S130.
11. Bae DS, Waters PM. Pediatric distal radius fractures and triangular fibrocartilage complex injuries. *Hand Clin.* 2006;22(1):43–53.
12. Bae DS, Valim C, Connell P, et al. Bivalved versus circumferential cast immobilization for displaced forearm fractures: a randomized clinical trial to assess efficacy and safety. *J Pediatr Orthop.* 2017;37(4):239–246.
13. Baghdadi S; CORTICES. Pediatric floating elbow injuries are not as problematic as they were once thought to be: a systematic review. *J Pediatr Orthop.* 2020;40(8):380–386.
14. Bailey DA, Wedge JH, McCulloch RG, et al. Epidemiology of fractures of the distal end of the radius in children as associated with growth. *J Bone Joint Surg Am.* 1989;71(8):1225–1231.
15. Bauer AS, Lee SJ, Smith MD, et al. Extensor retinaculum reconstruction of the distal radioulnar joint in adolescents. *Hand (N Y).* 2022;17(5):957–962.
16. Bebbington A, Lewis P, Savage R. Cast wedging for orthopaedic surgeons! *Injury.* 2005;36(1):71–72.
17. Bell CJ, Viswanathan S, Dass S, Donald G. The incidence of neurologic injury in paediatric forearm fractures requiring manipulation. *J Pediatr Orthop B.* 2010;19(4):294–297.
18. Berberich T, Reimann P, Steinacher M, et al. Evaluation of cast wedging in a forearm fracture model. *Clin Biomech (Bristol, Avon).* 2008;23(7):895–899.
19. Biyani A, Gupta SP, Sharma JC. Ipsilateral supracondylar fracture of humerus and forearm bones in children. *Injury.* 1989;20(4):203–207.
20. Bohm ER, Bubbar V, Yong Hing K, Dzus A. Above and below-the-elbow plaster casts for distal forearm fractures in children: a randomized controlled trial. *J Bone Joint Surg Am.* 2006;88(1):1–8.
21. Boutis K, Willan A, Babyn P, et al. Cast versus splint in children with minimally angulated fractures of the distal radius: a randomized controlled trial. *CMAJ.* 2010;182(14):1507–1512.
22. Boyden EM, Peterson HA. Partial premature closure of the distal radial physis associated with Kirschner wire fixation. *Orthopedics.* 1991;14(5):585–588.
23. Boyer BA, Overton B, Schrader W, et al. Position of immobilization for pediatric forearm fractures. *J Pediatr Orthop.* 2002;22(2):185–187.
24. Bradley H, Hartman CA, Crawford SE, Ramo BA. Outcomes and cost of reduction of overriding pediatric distal radius fractures. *J Pediatr Orthop.* 2022;42(6):307–313.
25. Burgess RC, Watson HK. Hypertrophic ulnar styloid nonunions. *Clin Orthop Relat Res.* 1988;(228):215–217.
26. Campbell T, Faulk LW, Vossler K, et al. Ulnar epiphysiodesis: success of the index procedure. *J Pediatr Orthop.* 2022;42(3):158–161.
27. Cannata G, De Maio F, Mancini F, Ippolito E. Physeal fractures of the distal radius and ulna: long-term prognosis. *J Orthop Trauma.* 2003;17(3):172–179.
28. Cha SM, Shin HD, Jeon JH. Long-term results of Galeazzi-equivalent injuries in adolescents–open reduction and internal fixation of the ulna. *J Pediatr Orthop B.* 2016;25(2):174–182.
29. Cha SM, Shin HD, Kim YK, Lee KW. Ulnar shortening osteotomy for posttraumatic ulnar impaction syndrome in adolescent (younger than 18 years)-Based on the Cha & Shin assessment. *Injury.* 2022;53(12):4038–4047.
30. Chess DG, Hyndman JC, Leahey JL, et al. Short arm plaster cast for distal pediatric forearm fractures. *J Pediatr Orthop.* 1994;14(2):211–213.
31. Clarke AC, Spencer RF. Ulnar nerve palsy following fractures of the distal radius: clinical and anatomical studies. *J Hand Surg Br.* 1991;16(4):438–440.
32. Cooney WP, Dobyns JH, Linscheid RL. Arthroscopy of the wrist: anatomy and classification of carpal instability. *Arthroscopy.* 1990;6(2):133–140.
33. Cooper C, Dennison EM, Leufkens HG, et al. Epidemiology of childhood fractures in Britain: a study using the general practice research database. *J Bone Miner Res.* 2004;19(12):1976–1981.
34. Crawford AH. Pitfalls and complications of fractures of the distal radius and ulna in childhood. *Hand Clin.* 1988;4(3):403–413.
35. Crawford SN, Lee LSK, Izuka BH. Closed treatment of overriding distal radial fractures without reduction in children. *J Bone Joint Surg Am.* 2012;94(3):246–252.
36. Daruwalla JS. A study of radioulnar movements following fractures of the forearm in children. *Clin Orthop Relat Res.* 1979;(139):114–120.
37. Davidson JS, Brown DJ, Barnes SN, Bruce CE. Simple treatment for torus fractures of the distal radius. *J Bone Joint Surg Br.* 2001;83(8):1173–1175.

38. Davis DR, Green DP. Forearm fractures in children: pitfalls and complications. *Clin Orthop Relat Res.* 1976;(120):172–183.
39. De Courtivron B. Spontaneous correction of the distal forearm fractures in children. *Presented at: European Pediatric Orthopaedic Society Annual Meeting.* Brussels, Belgium; 1995.
40. de Pablos J, Franzreb M, Barrios C. Longitudinal growth pattern of the radius after forearm fractures conservatively treated in children. *J Pediatr Orthop.* 1994;14(4):492–495.
41. De Smet L, Claessens A, Lefevre J, Beunen G. Gymnast wrist: an epidemiologic survey of ulnar variance and stress changes of the radial physis in elite female gymnasts. *Am J Sports Med.* 1994;22(6):846–850.
42. Devalia KL, Asaad SS, Kakkar R. Risk of redisplacement after first successful reduction in paediatric distal radius fractures: sensitivity assessment of casting indices. *J Pediatr Orthop B.* 2011;20(6):376–381.
43. DiFiori JP, Puffer JC, Aish B, Dorey F. Wrist pain, distal radial physeal injury, and ulnar variance in young gymnasts: does a relationship exist? *Am J Sports Med.* 2002;30(6):879–885.
44. Do TT, Strub WM, Foad SL, et al. Reduction versus remodeling in pediatric distal forearm fractures: a preliminary cost analysis. *J Pediatr Orthop B.* 2003;12(2):109–115.
45. Doak J, Ferrick M. Nonoperative management of pediatric grade 1 open fractures with less than a 24-hour admission. *J Pediatr Orthop.* 2009;29(1):49–51.
46. Doi K, Hattori Y, Otsuka K, et al. Intra-articular fractures of the distal aspect of the radius: arthroscopically assisted reduction compared with open reduction and internal fixation. *J Bone Joint Surg Am.* 1999;81(8):1093–1110.
47. Dua K, Lancaster TP, Abzug JM. Age-dependent reliability of Semmes-Weinstein and 2-point discrimination tests in children. *J Pediatr Orthop.* 2019;39(2):98–103.
48. Dua K, Stein MK, O'Hara NN, et al. Variation among pediatric orthopaedic surgeons when diagnosing and treating pediatric and adolescent distal radius fractures. *J Pediatr Orthop.* 2019;39(6):306–313.
49. Dumont CE, Thalmann R, Macy JC. The effect of rotational malunion of the radius and the ulna on supination and pronation. *J Bone Joint Surg Br.* 2002;84(7):1070–1074.
50. Eberl R, Singer G, Schalamon J, et al. Galeazzi lesions in children and adolescents: treatment and outcome. *Clin Orthop Relat Res.* 2008;466(7):1705–1709.
51. Edmonds EW, Capelo RM, Stearns P, et al. Predicting initial treatment failure of fiberglass casts in pediatric distal radius fractures: utility of the second metacarpal-radius angle. *J Child Orthop.* 2009;3(5):375–381.
52. Eichinger JK, Agochukwu U, Franklin J, et al. A new reduction technique for completely displaced forearm and wrist fractures in children: a biomechanical assessment and 4-year clinical evaluation. *J Pediatr Orthop.* 2011;31(7):e73–e79.
53. Epner RA, Bowers WH, Guilford WB. Ulnar variance—the effect of wrist positioning and roentgen filming technique. *J Hand Surg Am.* 1982;7(3):298–305.
54. Evans JK, Buckley SL, Alexander AH, Gilpin AT. Analgesia for the reduction of fractures in children: a comparison of nitrous oxide with intramuscular sedation. *J Pediatr Orthop.* 1995;15(1):73–77.
55. Farr JN, Tomas R, Chen Z, et al. Lower trabecular volumetric BMD at metaphyseal regions of weight-bearing bones is associated with prior fracture in young girls. *J Bone Miner Res.* 2011;26(2):380–387.
56. Fatti JF, Mosher JF. An unusual complication of fracture of both bones of the forearm in a child: a case report. *J Bone Joint Surg Am.* 1986;68(3):451–453.
57. Fernandez DL. Correction of post-traumatic wrist deformity in adults by osteotomy, bone-grafting, and internal fixation. *J Bone Joint Surg Am.* 1982;64(8):1164–1178.
58. Forward DP, Davis TR, Sithole JS. Do young patients with malunited fractures of the distal radius inevitably develop symptomatic post-traumatic osteoarthritis? *J Bone Joint Surg Br.* 2008;90(5):629–637.
59. Friberg KS. Remodelling after distal forearm fractures in children. III. Correction of residual angulation in fractures of the radius. *Acta Orthop Scand.* 1979;50(6 Pt 2):741–749.
60. Fung EB, Humphrey ML, Gildengorin G, et al. Rapid remineralization of the distal radius after forearm fracture in children. *J Pediatr Orthop.* 2011;31(2):138–143.
61. Gelberman RH, Salamon PB, Jurist JM, Posch JL. Ulnar variance in Kienbock's disease. *J Bone Joint Surg Am.* 1975;57(5):674–676.
62. Georgiadis AG, Burgess JK, Truong WH, Janicki JA. Displaced distal radius fracture treatment: a survey of POSNA membership. *J Pediatr Orthop.* 2020;40(9):e827–e832.
63. Gibbons CL, Woods DA, Pailthorpe C, et al. The management of isolated distal radius fractures in children. *J Pediatr Orthop.* 1994;14(2):207–210.
64. Godambe SA, Elliot V, Matheny D, Pershad J. Comparison of propofol/fentanyl versus ketamine/midazolam for brief orthopedic procedural sedation in a pediatric emergency department. *Pediatrics.* 2003;112(1 Pt 1):116–123.
65. Goldfarb CA, Strauss NL, Wall LB, Calfee RP. Defining ulnar variance in the adolescent wrist: measurement technique and interobserver reliability. *J Hand Surg Am.* 2011;36(2):272–277.
66. Golz RJ, Grogan DP, Greene TL, et al. Distal ulnar physeal injury. *J Pediatr Orthop.* 1991;11(3):318–326.
67. Goulding A, Jones IE, Taylor RW, et al. More broken bones: a 4-year double cohort study of young girls with and without distal forearm fractures. *J Bone Miner Res.* 2000;15(10):2011–2018.
68. Goulding A, Jones IE, Taylor RW, et al. Bone mineral density and body composition in boys with distal forearm fractures: a dual-energy x-ray absorptiometry study. *J Pediatr.* 2001;139(4):509–515.
69. Greenbaum B, Zionts LE, Ebramzadeh E. Open fractures of the forearm in children. *J Orthop Trauma.* 2001;15(2):111–118.
70. Gunes T, Erdem M, Sen C. Irreducible Galeazzi fracture-dislocation due to intra-articular fracture of the distal ulna. *J Hand Surg Eur Vol.* 2007;32(2):185–187.
71. Guofen C, Doi K, Hattori Y, Kitajima I. Arthroscopically assisted reduction and immobilization of intraarticular fracture of the distal end of the radius: several options of reduction and immobilization. *Tech Hand Up Extrem Surg.* 2005;9(2):84–90.
72. Gupta RP, Danielsson LG. Dorsally angulated solitary metaphyseal greenstick fractures in the distal radius: results after immobilization in pronated, neutral, and supinated position. *J Pediatr Orthop.* 1990;10(1):90–92.
73. Hafner R, Poznanski AK, Donovan JM. Ulnar variance in children—standard measurements for evaluation of ulnar shortening in juvenile rheumatoid arthritis, hereditary multiple exostosis and other bone or joint disorders in childhood. *Skeletal Radiol.* 1989;18(7):513–516.
74. Hang JR, Hutchinson AF, Hau RC. Risk factors associated with loss of position after closed reduction of distal radial fractures in children. *J Pediatr Orthop.* 2011;31(5):501–506.
75. Hansen RT, Borghegn NW, Gundtoft PH, et al. Change in treatment preferences in pediatric diaphyseal forearm fractures: a Danish nationwide register study of 36,244 fractures between 1997 and 2016. *Acta Orthop.* 2023;94:32–37.
76. Hattori Y, Doi K, Estrella EP, Chen G. Arthroscopically assisted reduction with volar plating or external fixation for displaced intra-articular fractures of the distal radius in the elderly patients. *Hand Surg.* 2007;12(1):1–12.
77. Hendrickx RP, Campo MM, van Lieshout AP, et al. Above- or below-elbow casts for distal third forearm fractures in children? A meta-analysis of the literature. *Arch Orthop Trauma Surg.* 2011;131(12):1663–1671.
78. Hernandez JA, Swischuk LE, Bathurst GJ, Hendrick EP. Scaphoid (navicular) fractures of the wrist in children: attention to the impacted buckle fracture. *Emerg Radiol.* 2002;9(6):305–308.
79. Holmes JR, Louis DS. Entrapment of pronator quadratus in pediatric distal-radius fractures: recognition and treatment. *J Pediatr Orthop.* 1994;14(4):498–500.
80. Horii E, Tamura Y, Nakamura R, Miura T. Premature closure of the distal radial physis. *J Hand Surg Br.* 1993;18(1):11–16.
81. Hosseinzadeh P, Olson D, Eads R, et al. Radiologic evaluation of the distal radius indices in early and late childhood. *Iowa Orthop J.* 2018;38:137–140.
82. Houshian S, Holst AK, Larsen MS, Torfing T. Remodeling of Salter-Harris type II epiphyseal plate injury of the distal radius. *J Pediatr Orthop.* 2004;24(5):472–476.
83. Hove LM, Brudvik C. Displaced paediatric fractures of the distal radius. *Arch Orthop Trauma Surg.* 2008;128(1):55–60.
84. Iltar S, Alemdaroglu KB, Say F, Aydoğan NH. The value of the three-point index in predicting redisplacement of diaphyseal fractures of the forearm in children. *Bone Joint J.* 2013;95-B(4):563–567.
85. Iobst CA, Tidwell MA, King WF. Nonoperative management of pediatric type I open fractures. *J Pediatr Orthop.* 2005;25(4):513–517.
86. Ishii S, Palmer AK, Werner FW, et al. Pressure distribution in the distal radioulnar joint. *J Hand Surg Am.* 1998;23(5):909–913.
87. Johari AN, Sinha M. Remodeling of forearm fractures in children. *J Pediatr Orthop B.* 1999;8(2):84–87.
88. Kahraman HÇ, Şibar K, Alemdaroğlu KB, et al. Is three-point index reliable in the follow-up of the distal radius metaphys fractures in the pediatric age group? *J Pediatr Orthop B.* 2023;32(4):369–377.
89. Kalkwarf HJ, Laor T, Bean JA. Fracture risk in children with a forearm injury is associated with volumetric bone density and cortical area (by peripheral QCT) and areal bone density (by DXA). *Osteoporos Int.* 2011;22(2):607–616.
90. Kallini JR, Fu EC, Shah AS, et al. Growth disturbance following intra-articular distal radius fractures in the skeletally immature patient. *J Pediatr Orthop.* 2020;40(10):e910–e915.
91. Kamano M, Honda Y. Galeazzi-equivalent lesions in adolescence. *J Orthop Trauma.* 2002;16(6):440–443.
92. Kannan S, Chong HH, Fadulelmola A, et al. A prediction model for treatment decisions in distal radial physeal injuries: a multicenter retrospective study. *J Child Orthop.* 2022;16(5):374–384.
93. Karaharju EO, Ryoppy SA, Mäkinen RJ. Remodelling by asymmetrical epiphyseal growth. An experimental study in dogs. *J Bone Joint Surg Br.* 1976;58(1):122–126.
94. Karlsson J, Appelqvist R. Irreducible fracture of the wrist in a child: entrapment of the extensor tendons. *Acta Orthop Scand.* 1987;58(3):280–281.
95. Kasser JR. *Forearm Fractures.* Lippincott Williams & Wilkins;1993.
96. Khan H, Green G, Arnander M, et al. What are the risk factors and presenting features of premature physeal arrest of the distal radius? A systematic review. *Eur J Orthop Surg Traumatol.* 2021;31(5):893–900.
97. Khan S, Sawyer J, Pershad J. Closed reduction of distal forearm fractures by pediatric emergency physicians. *Acad Emerg Med.* 2010;17(11):1169–1174.
98. Khosla S, Melton LJ 3rd, Dekutoski MB, et al. Incidence of childhood distal forearm fractures over 30 years: a population-based study. *JAMA.* 2003;290(11):1479–1485.
99. Kirmani S, Christen D, van Lenthe GH, et al. Bone structure at the distal radius during adolescent growth. *J Bone Miner Res.* 2009;24(6):1033–1042.
100. Knirk JL, Jupiter JB. Intra-articular fractures of the distal end of the radius in young adults. *J Bone Joint Surg Am.* 1986;68(5):647–659.
101. Kraan RBJ, Kox LS, Oostra RJ, et al. The distal radial physis: exploring normal anatomy on MRI enables interpretation of stress related changes in young gymnasts. *Eur J Sport Sci.* 2020;20(9):1197–1205.
102. Kropman RHJ, Bemelman M, Segers MJ, Hammacher ER. Treatment of impacted greenstick forearm fractures in children using bandage or cast therapy: a prospective randomized trial. *J Trauma.* 2010;68(2):425–428.
103. Landfried MJ, Stenclik M, Susi JG. Variant of Galeazzi fracture-dislocation in children. *J Pediatr Orthop.* 1991;11(3):332–335.
104. Larsen E, Vittas D, Torp-Pedersen S. Remodeling of angulated distal forearm fractures in children. *Clin Orthop Relat Res.* 1988;(237):190–195.
105. LaValva SM, Rogers BH, Arkader A, Shah AS. Risk factors for failed closed reduction of pediatric distal radius fractures. *J Hand Surg Glob Online.* 2020;2(4):196–202.

106. Lawrence JTR, MacAlpine EM, Buczek MJ, et al. Impact of cost information on parental decision making: a randomized clinical trial evaluating cast versus splint selection for pediatric distal radius buckle fractures. *J Pediatr Orthop.* 2022; 42(1):e15–e20.
107. Lee BS, Esterhai JL Jr, Das M. Fracture of the distal radial epiphysis: characteristics and surgical treatment of premature, post-traumatic epiphyseal closure. *Clin Orthop Relat Res.* 1984;(185):90–96.
108. Lee SJ, Bae DS. Triangular fibrocartilage complex injuries in children and adolescents. *Hand Clin.* 2021;37(4):517–526.
109. Letts M, Rowhani N. Galeazzi-equivalent injuries of the wrist in children. *J Pediatr Orthop.* 1993;13(5):561–566.
110. Lindsay SE, Holmes S, Swarup I, Halsey M. Trends in management of pediatric distal radius buckle fractures. *J Pediatr Orthop.* 2022;42(7):367–371.
111. Light TR, Ogden DA, Ogden JA. The anatomy of metaphyseal torus fractures. *Clin Orthop Relat Res.* 1984;(188):103–111.
112. Little KJ, Godfrey J, Cornwall R, et al. Increasing brace treatment for pediatric distal radius buckle fractures: using quality improvement methodology to implement evidence-based medicine. *J Pediatr Orthop.* 2019;39(8):e586–e591.
113. Livingstone J, Opanova M, Beaman A, et al. "You're O.K. Anesthesia": closed reduction of displaced pediatric forearm and wrist fractures in the office without anesthesia. *J Pediatr Orthop.* 2022;42(10):595–599.
114. Low CK, Liau KH, Chew WY. Results of distal radial fractures treated by intra-focal pin fixation. *Ann Acad Med Singapore.* 2001;30(6):573–576.
115. Luther G, Miller P, Waters PM, Bae DS. Radiographic evaluation during treatment of pediatric forearm fractures: implications on clinical care and cost. *J Pediatr Orthop.* 2016;36(5):465–471.
116. Lynch KA, Wesolowski M, Cappello T. Coronal remodeling potential of pediatric distal radius fractures. *J Pediatr Orthop.* 2020;40(10):556–561.
117. Mahan ST, Kalish LA, Shah AS, et al. Institutional variation in surgical rates and costs for pediatric distal radius fractures: analysis of the Pediatric Health Information System (PHIS) database. *Iowa Orthop J.* 2020;40(1):75–81.
118. Mani GV, Hui PW, Cheng JC. Translation of the radius as a predictor of outcome in distal radial fractures of children. *J Bone Joint Surg Br.* 1993;75(5):808–811.
119. Mauck B, Kelly D, Sheffer B, et al. Gymnast's wrist (distal radial physeal stress syndrome). *Orthop Clin North Am.* 2020;51(4):493–497.
120. McLauchlan GJ, Cowan B, Annan IH, Robb JE. Management of completely displaced metaphyseal fractures of the distal radius in children: a prospective, randomised controlled trial. *J Bone Joint Surg Br.* 2002;84(3):413–417.
121. McQuinn AG, Jaarsma RL. Risk factors for redisplacement of pediatric distal forearm and distal radius fractures. *J Pediatr Orthop.* 2012;32(7):687–692.
122. Miller A, Lightdale-Miric N, Eismann E, et al. Outcomes of isolated radial osteotomy for volar distal radioulnar joint instability following radial malunion in children. *J Hand Surg Am.* 2018;43(1):81.e1–81.e8.
123. Miller BS, Taylor B, Widmann RF, et al. Cast immobilization versus percutaneous pin fixation of displaced distal radius fractures in children: a prospective, randomized study. *J Pediatr Orthop.* 2005;25(4):490–494.
124. Mino DE, Palmer AK, Levinsohn EM. Radiography and computerized tomography in the diagnosis of incongruity of the distal radio-ulnar joint. A prospective study. *J Bone Joint Surg Am.* 1985;67(2):247–252.
125. Monga P, Raghupathy A, Courtman NH. Factors affecting remanipulation in paediatric forearm fractures. *J Pediatr Orthop B.* 2010;19(2):181–187.
126. Moore DC, Hogan KA, Crisco JJ 3rd, et al. Three-dimensional in vivo kinematics of the distal radioulnar joint in malunited distal radius fractures. *J Hand Surg Am.* 2002;27(2):233–242.
127. Moore TM, Lester DK, Sarmiento A. The stabilizing effect of soft-tissue constraints in artificial Galeazzi fractures. *Clin Orthop Relat Res.* 1985;(194):189–194.
128. Morohoshi A, Qureshi AR, Iseri K, et al. Secular trends in incidence and seasonal variation of distal radius fracture among children: a nationwide study based on the Swedish National Patient Register 2002–2016. *Bone.* 2022;162:116479.
129. Nishiyama KK, Macdonald HM, Moore SA, et al. Cortical porosity is higher in boys compared with girls at the distal radius and distal tibia during pubertal growth: an HR-pQCT study. *J Bone Miner Res.* 2012;27(2):273–282.
130. Noda K, Goto A, Murase T, et al. Interosseous membrane of the forearm: an anatomical study of ligament attachment locations. *J Hand Surg Am.* 2009;34(3):415–422.
131. Oakley EA, Ooi KS, Barnett PLJ. A randomized controlled trial of 2 methods of immobilizing torus fractures of the distal forearm. *Pediatr Emerg Care.* 2008; 24(2):65–70.
132. Ogden JA. *Skeletal Injury in the Child.* WB Saunders;1990.
133. Ogden JA, Beall JK, Conlogue GJ, Light TR. Radiology of postnatal skeletal development. IV. Distal radius and ulna. *Skeletal Radiol.* 1981;6(4):255–266.
134. Ooi LH, Toh CL. Galeazzi-equivalent fracture in children associated with tendon entrapment—report of two cases. *Ann Acad Med Singap.* 2001;30(1):51–54.
135. Palmer AK, Werner FW. The triangular fibrocartilage complex of the wrist—anatomy and function. *J Hand Surg Am.* 1981;6(2):153–162.
136. Palmer AK, Werner FW. Biomechanics of the distal radioulnar joint. *Clin Orthop Relat Res.* 1984;(187):26–35.
137. Peinado A. Distal radial epiphyseal displacement after impaired distal ulnar growth. *J Bone Joint Surg Am.* 1979;61(1):88–92.
138. Perona PG, Light TR. Remodeling of the skeletally immature distal radius. *J Orthop Trauma.* 1990;4(3):356–361.
139. Perry DC, Achten J, Knight R, et al; FORCE Collaborators in collaboration with PERUKI. Immobilisation of torus fractures of the wrist in children (FORCE): a randomised controlled equivalence trial in the UK. *Lancet.* 2022;400(10345):39–47. Erratum in: *Lancet.* 2022;400(10348):272. Erratum in: *Lancet.* 2022;400(10358):1102.
140. Plint AC, Perry JJ, Correll R, et al. A randomized, controlled trial of removable splinting versus casting for wrist buckle fractures in children. *Pediatrics.* 2006; 117(3):691–697.
141. Pollen AG. *Fractures and Dislocations in Children.* Lippincott Williams & Wilkins; 1973.
142. Pretell Mazzini J, Rodriguez Martin J. Paediatric forearm and distal radius fractures: risk factors and re-displacement—role of casting indices. *Int Orthop.* 2010;34(3):407–412.
143. Proctor MT, Moore DJ, Paterson JM. Redisplacement after manipulation of distal radial fractures in children. *J Bone Joint Surg Br.* 1993;75(3):453–454.
144. Pullagura M, Gopisetti S, Bateman B, van Kampen M. Are extremity musculoskeletal injuries in children related to obesity and social status? A prospective observational study in a district general hospital. *J Child Orthop.* 2011;5(2):97–100.
145. Rampoldi M, Marsico S. Complications of volar plating of distal radius fractures. *Acta Orthop Belg.* 2007;73(6):714–719.
146. Randsborg PH, Sivertsen EA. Distal radius fractures in children: substantial difference in stability between buckle and greenstick fractures. *Acta Orthop.* 2009;80(5):585–589.
147. Randsborg PH, Sivertsen EA. Classification of distal radius fractures in children: good inter- and intraobserver reliability, which improves with clinical experience. *BMC Musculoskelet Disord.* 2012;13:6.
148. Ravier D, Morelli I, Buscarino V, et al. Plaster cast treatment for distal forearm fractures in children: which index best predicts the loss of reduction? *J Pediatr Orthop B.* 2020;29(2):179–186.
149. Rennie L, Court-Brown CM, Mok JY, Beattie TF. The epidemiology of fractures in children. *Injury.* 2007;38(8):913–922.
150. Rettig ME, Raskin KB. Galeazzi fracture-dislocation: a new treatment-oriented classification. *J Hand Surg Am.* 2001;26(2):228–235.
151. Ring D, Waters PM, Hotchkiss RN, Kasser JR. Pediatric floating elbow. *J Pediatr Orthop.* 2001;21(4):456–459.
152. Root CG, London DA, Schroeder NS, Calfee RP. Anatomical relationships and branching patterns of the dorsal cutaneous branch of the ulnar nerve. *J Hand Surg Am.* 2013;38(6):1131–1136.
153. Roy S, Caine D, Singer KM. Stress changes of the distal radial epiphysis in young gymnasts: a report of twenty-one cases and a review of the literature. *Am J Sports Med.* 1985;13(5):301–308.
154. Russell K, Hagel B, Francescutti LH. The effect of wrist guards on wrist and arm injuries among snowboarders: a systematic review. *Clin J Sport Med.* 2007;17(2):145–150.
155. Ryan LM, Teach SJ, Singer SA, et al. Bone mineral density and vitamin D status among African American children with forearm fractures. *Pediatrics.* 2012;130(3):e553–e560.
156. Sallam AA, Briffa N, Mahmoud SS, Imam MA. Normal wrist development in children and adolescents: a geometrical observational analysis based on plain radiographs. *J Pediatr Orthop.* 2020;40(9):e860–e872.
157. Salter RHW. Injuries involving the epiphyseal plate. *J Bone Joint Surg Am.* 1963;45:587–622.
158. Samora JB. Distal radius physeal bar and ulnar overgrowth: indications for treatment. *J Pediatr Orthop.* 2021;41(Suppl 1):S6–S13.
159. Schranz PJ, Fagg PS. Undisplaced fractures of the distal third of the radius in children: an innocent fracture? *Injury.* 1992;23(3):165–167.
160. Schuind F, An KN, Berglund L, et al. The distal radioulnar ligaments: a biomechanical study. *J Hand Surg Am.* 1991;16(6):1106–1114.
161. Schuind F, Cooney WP 3rd, Burny F, An KN. Small external fixation devices for the hand and wrist. *Clin Orthop Relat Res.* 1993;(293):77–82.
162. Shah AS, Guzek RH, Miller ML, et al; Pediatric Distal Radius Fracture (PDRF) Study Group. Descriptive epidemiology of isolated distal radius fractures in children: results from a prospective multicenter registry. *J Pediatr Orthop.* 2023;43(1):e1–e8.
163. Skaggs DL, Loro ML, Pitukcheewanont P, et al. Increased body weight and decreased radial cross-sectional dimensions in girls with forearm fractures. *J Bone Miner Res.* 2001;16(7):1337–1342.
164. Snelling PJ, Keijzers G, Ware RS. Point-of-care ultrasound pronator quadratus hematoma sign for detection of clinically non-angulated pediatric distal forearm fractures: a prospective cohort study. *J Ultrasound Med.* 2022;41(1):193–205.
165. Song KS, Lee SW, Bae KC. Primary nonunion of the distal radius fractures in healthy children. *J Pediatr Orthop B.* 2016;25(2):165–169.
166. Steyers CM, Blair WF. Measuring ulnar variance: a comparison of techniques. *J Hand Surg Am.* 1989;14(4):607–612.
167. Subramanian P, Kantharuban S, Shilston S, Pearce OJ. Complications of Kirschner-wire fixation in distal radius fractures. *Tech Hand Up Extrem Surg.* 2012;16(3):120–123.
168. Symons S, Rowsell M, Bhowal B, Dias JJ. Hospital versus home management of children with buckle fractures of the distal radius: a prospective, randomised trial. *J Bone Joint Surg Br.* 2001;83(4):556–560.
169. Takemura Y, Kodama N, Ueba H, et al. Physeal bar resection under guidance with a navigation system and endoscopy for correction of distal radial deformities after partial growth plate arrest. *J Hand Surg Am.* 2018;43(10):953.e1–953.e7.
170. Taleisnik J, Watson HK. Midcarpal instability caused by malunited fractures of the distal radius. *J Hand Surg Am.* 1984;9(3):350–357.
171. Tarr RR, Garfinkel AI, Sarmiento A. The effects of angular and rotational deformities of both bones of the forearm: An in vitro study. *J Bone Joint Surg Am.* 1984;66(1):65–70.
172. Terry CL, Waters PM. Triangular fibrocartilage injuries in pediatric and adolescent patients. *J Hand Surg Am.* 1998;23(4):626–634.
173. Tolat AR, Sanderson PL, De Smet L, Stanley JK. The gymnast's wrist: acquired positive ulnar variance following chronic epiphyseal injury. *J Hand Surg Br.* 1992;17(6):678–681.
174. Trumble TE, Wagner W, Hanel DP, et al. Intrafocal (Kapandji) pinning of distal radius fractures with and without external fixation. *J Hand Surg Am.* 1998;23(3):381–394.
175. Vernooij CM, Vreeburg ME, Segers MJ, Hammacher ER. Treatment of torus fractures in the forearm in children using bandage therapy. *J Trauma Acute Care Surg.* 2012;72(4):1093–1097.
176. Vince KG, Miller JE. Cross-union complicating fracture of the forearm. Part II: Children. *J Bone Joint Surg Am.* 1987;69(5):654–661.
177. Walsh HP, McLaren CA, Owen R. Galeazzi fractures in children. *J Bone Joint Surg Br.* 1987;69(5):730–733.

178. Wang Q, Wang XF, Iuliano-Burns S, et al. Rapid growth produces transient cortical weakness: a risk factor for metaphyseal fractures during puberty. *J Bone Miner Res.* 2010;25(7):1521–1526.

179. Wareham K, Johansen A, Stone MD, et al. Seasonal variation in the incidence of wrist and forearm fractures, and its consequences. *Injury.* 2003;34(3): 219–222.

180. Waters PM, Bae DS, Montgomery KD. Surgical management of posttraumatic distal radial growth arrest in adolescents. *J Pediatr Orthop.* 2002;22(6):717–724.

181. Waters PM, Kolettis GJ, Schwend R. Acute median neuropathy following physeal fractures of the distal radius. *J Pediatr Orthop.* 1994;14(2):173–177.

182. Waters PM, Mintzer CM, Hipp JA, Snyder BD. Noninvasive measurement of distal radius instability. *J Hand Surg Am.* 1997;22(4):572–579.

183. Webb GR, Galpin RD, Armstrong DG. Comparison of short and long arm plaster casts for displaced fractures in the distal third of the forearm in children. *J Bone Joint Surg Am.* 2006;88(1):9–17.

184. Wells L, Avery A, Hosalkar HH, et al. Cast wedging: a "forgotten" yet predictable method for correcting fracture deformity. *UPOJ.* 2010;20:113–116.

185. Wilkins KE, O'Brien E. *Distal Radius and Ulnar Fractures.* Lippincott Williams & Wilkins;2002.

186. Wood AM, Robertson GA, Rennie L, et al. The epidemiology of sports-related fractures in adolescents. *Injury.* 2010;41(8):834–838.

187. Wu M, Miller PE, Waters PM, Bae DS. Early results of surgical treatment of triangular fibrocartilage complex tears in children and adolescents. *J Hand Surg Am.* 2020;45(5):449.e1–449.e9.

188. Yong-Hing K, Wedge JH, Bowen CV. Chronic injury to the distal ulnar and radial growth plates in an adolescent gymnast. A case report. *J Bone Joint Surg Am.* 1988;70(7):1087–1089.

189. Young TB. Irreducible displacement of the distal radial epiphysis complicating a fracture of the lower radius and ulna. *Injury.* 1984;16(3):166–168.

190. Younger AS, Tredwell SJ, Mackenzie WG, et al. Accurate prediction of outcome after pediatric forearm fracture. *J Pediatr Orthop.* 1994;14(2):200–206.

191. Yung PSH, Lam CY, Ng BKW, et al. Percutaneous transphyseal intramedullary Kirschner wire pinning: a safe and effective procedure for treatment of displaced diaphyseal forearm fracture in children. *J Pediatr Orthop.* 2004;24(1):7–12.

192. Zamzam MM, Khoshhal KI. Displaced fracture of the distal radius in children: factors responsible for redisplacement after closed reduction. *J Bone Joint Surg Br.* 2005;87(6):841–843.

193. Zerin JM, Hernandez RJ. Approach to skeletal maturation. *Hand Clin.* 1991;7(1): 53–62.

194. Zimmermann R, Gschwentner M, Pechlaner S, Gabl M. Remodeling capacity and functional outcome of palmarly versus dorsally displaced pediatric radius fractures in the distal one-third. *Arch Orthop Trauma Surg.* 2004;124(1):42–48.

10

Diaphyseal Radius and Ulna Fractures

Kevin J. Little and Eric J. Wall

INTRODUCTION TO DIAPHYSEAL RADIUS AND ULNA FRACTURES

Injuries to the shafts of the radius and ulna represent some of the most common reasons for children to receive orthopaedic care[39,41] and are among the most challenging for the orthopaedist because of their treatment complexity and risk of complications.[169,181] Because of numerous differences in both treatment and prognosis, shaft fractures are considered to be clinically distinct from fractures of the distal (metaphyseal fractures and physeal fractures) and proximal (radial neck fractures and physeal fractures) ends of the same bones.[45,97,215,216] Many shaft injuries in children are effectively treated with skillful closed fracture care,[107] but failures continue to occur despite good orthopaedic intentions.[26] Nonoperative care by reduction, splint/cast molding, remanipulation, and recasting, as well as the operative treatment of delayed union, malunion, and some refractures must be mastered.

Over the past 20 years, there has been a dramatic increase in surgical fixation of forearm shaft fractures,[92,201] primarily with elastic nails.[66] Shaft fractures of the forearm are also the most common reason for operative care of the upper extremity in children.[39,88] The evolving indications for surgical treatment of forearm shaft fractures and the resulting outcomes will be covered in detail in this chapter. Thus, it is very important for orthopaedic surgeons who treat children to skillfully manage the cognitive and technical aspects of both nonoperative and operative treatment for injuries to the shafts of the radius and ulna.

Risk is a central concept in clinical epidemiology.[153] Landin[129] has shown that the overall risk of fracture in children slowly increases for both males and females until they are 11 or 12 years old and then drops for females and increases further for males (Fig. 10-1). This risk difference is starkly illustrated by the fact that males who are 13 years or older have approximately double the fracture rate of their female peers.[129] Forearm fractures have been reported to be the most common pediatric fracture associated with backyard trampoline use[17] and the second most common one (supracondylar humeral fractures were first) associated with monkey bars.[225] Using a national database, Chung and Spilson[41] looked at the frequency of upper extremity fractures in the United States and found that the single largest demographic group was fractures of the radius and ulna in children aged 14 years or less, with a rate approaching 1 in 100. Two groups of researchers have recently evaluated the relationship between bone mineral density and forearm fractures in children. Using dual-energy X-ray absorptiometry (DXA or DEXA) scans, Kaelin and his coauthors in Geneva, Switzerland prospectively studied 50 teenagers presenting with their first forearm fracture and 50 healthy controls and found no significant differences between the groups.[37] These same authors suggested that forearm fractures in such teenagers do not appear to be related to osteopenia.[37] Similarly, Segal et al. in Cincinnati, United States showed no differences in vitamin D levels in obese pediatric patients with body mass index (BMI) >85%.[196] However, Tosi and her fellow researchers studied African American children (5–9 years of age) in Washington, DC and found that those who sustained forearm fractures did demonstrate lower bone mineral density and lower vitamin D levels.[189] Similarly, Assaf et al. showed a threefold risk for male patients and a fivefold increase in fracture risks in patients with hypovitaminosis.[7]

Large studies that distinguish distal radial fractures from forearm shaft fractures indicate that overall, radial shaft injuries rank as the third most common fracture of childhood, behind distal radial and supracondylar humeral fractures.[39] Open fractures in children are most often fractures of the shaft of the radius and ulna or tibial shaft fractures.[39] Among pediatric fractures, forearm shaft injuries are the most common site of refracture.[129] Forearm shaft fractures have been shown to occur most commonly in the 12- to 16-year-old age group, a challenging age group to treat.[39] The impact of increasing age on fracture incidence is further illustrated by Worlock and Stower,[232] who showed that the rate of forearm shaft fractures in school-aged children (>5 years old) is more than double than that in toddlers (1.5–5 years old). Age also may have an effect on injury severity. Many experienced clinicians have pointed out the increasing level of treatment difficulty as the level of forearm fracture moves proximally,[45,97,215,216] and more proximal fractures tend to occur in older patients.[45]

ASSESSMENT OF DIAPHYSEAL RADIUS AND ULNA FRACTURES

MECHANISMS OF INJURY FOR DIAPHYSEAL RADIUS AND ULNA FRACTURES

The primary mechanism of injury associated with radial and ulnar shaft fractures is a fall on an outstretched hand that transmits indirect force to the bones of the forearm.[3] Biomechanical studies have suggested that the junction of the middle and distal thirds of the radius and a substantial portion of the shaft of the ulna have an increased vulnerability to fracture.[101] Often, a significant rotational component is associated with the fall, causing the radius and ulna to fracture at different levels (Fig. 10-2).[150] If the radial and ulna fractures are near the same level, a minimal torsional component can be inferred (Fig. 10-3). If comminution is present, higher-energy trauma should be suspected. Significant hyperpronation forces are associated with isolated shaft

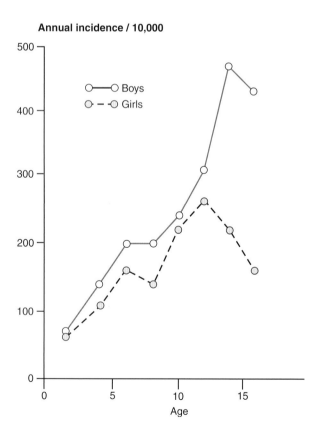

Annual incidence / 10,000

Figure 10-1. Annual incidence of all fractures in children. (Reprinted with permission from Landin LA. Epidemiology of children's fractures. *J Pediatr Orthop B.* 1997;6(2):79–83.)

Pronation
mechanism

No rotational
mechanism

Supination
mechanism

Figure 10-2. Radius and ulna shaft fractures occurring at different levels, implying rotational mechanism.

fractures of either the radius or the ulna and concomitant dislocation of either the distal (DRUJ) or the proximal radioulnar joint (PRUJ). Thus, in any single-bone forearm shaft fracture, these important joints need to be closely scrutinized. Galeazzi and Monteggia fracture-dislocations are discussed in Chapters 9 and 12, respectively.

A direct force to the arm (such as being hit by a baseball bat) can fracture a single bone (usually the ulna) without injury to the adjacent DRUJ or PRUJ. Isolated ulnar shaft fractures have been referred to as "nightstick fractures." Alignment of the radial head should be confirmed in any child with such a fracture to avoid a "missed Monteggia" injury. Isolated radial shaft fractures are rare but notoriously difficult to reduce with closed methods.[43]

The mechanisms of injury of two particular forearm fracture patterns, traumatic bowing (also known as bow fractures or plastic deformation) and greenstick fracture, also bear mentioning. The bone behaves differently based on the direction of the forces applied to it. This is the so-called anisotropic property of bone, and it can be simply explained as follows: Bone is more resistant to axial forces than to bending and rotational forces. Pediatric bone also is much more porous than its adult counterpart and behaves somewhat differently from a biomechanical standpoint. Because of its porosity, pediatric bone absorbs significantly more energy prior to failure than the adult bone does. When relatively slowly applied, longitudinal forces bend the immature bone beyond its elastic limits and into its plastic zone, resulting in traumatic bowing.[143] Thus, when a bending force is applied relatively slowly, many microfractures occur along the length of the bone, leading to macroscopic deformity without discernible radiographic fracture. This bending can usually be seen radiographically if suspected.

Greenstick fractures represent an intermediate step between plastic deformation and complete fractures.[35] On anteroposterior (AP) and lateral radiographs, greenstick fractures show cortical violation of one, two, or three of their radiographic cortices, and thus some bony continuity is preserved. Rotational deformity is considered to be intimately related to the clinical deformity seen with greenstick fractures of the forearm, and the analogy of a cardboard tube that tends to bend as it is twisted has been offered by Holdsworth.[97] Specifically, hyperpronation injuries usually are associated with apex-dorsal greenstick fractures of the forearm, and hypersupination injuries usually are associated with the opposite, apex-volar injuries.[161] The treatment of these greenstick fractures requires a derotation maneuver in addition to correction of any angulation.[35]

INJURIES ASSOCIATED WITH DIAPHYSEAL RADIUS AND ULNA FRACTURES

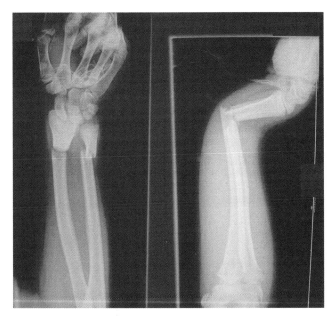

Figure 10-3. Radial and ulnar shaft fractures occurring at same level, implying no significant rotation.

Most fractures of the shafts of the radius and ulna occur as isolated injuries, but wrist and elbow fractures may occur in conjunction with forearm fractures, and the elbow and wrist region needs to be included on standard forearm radiographs.[236] If clinical suspicion is high, then dedicated wrist and elbow films are necessary. The so-called floating elbow injury (fracture of the bones of the forearm along with ipsilateral supracondylar humeral fracture) is a well-described entity that must not be missed.[188] Surgical stabilization of both the supracondylar fracture and the forearm fractures has been recommended by multiple authors in recent years[19,91,187,188,209] to avoid the risk of a compartment syndrome. Galeazzi and Monteggia fracture-dislocations also must be ruled out. Compartment syndrome can also occur in conjunction with any forearm shaft fracture.[46,241] This rare but potentially devastating complication can lead to a Volkmann ischemic contracture, which has been shown to occur after forearm shaft fractures almost as often as it does after supracondylar humeral fractures in children.[162] Patients with severe pain unrelieved by immobilization and mild narcotic medication should be reassessed for excessive swelling and tight forearm compartments. If loosening of the splint, cast, and underlying cast materials fails to relieve pain, then measurement of compartment pressures and subsequent fasciotomy may be necessary. The measurement of compartment pressures is difficult in pediatric patients, both due to anxiety in the patient and the low systolic and diastolic pressures seen in these patients. In patients where compartment syndrome is clinically suspected, there is usually an increase in the three As, anxiety, agitation, and analgesia requirements.[168]

Abrasions or seemingly small unimportant lacerations that occur in conjunction with forearm fractures must be carefully evaluated because they may be an indication of an open fracture. Clues to the presence of an open fracture include persistent slow bloody ooze from a small laceration near the fracture site and subcutaneous emphysema on injury films. Careful evaluation and, in some situations, sterile probing of suspicious wounds

will be necessary. Open forearm fractures are discussed later in this chapter.

Vascular or neurologic injuries can be associated with forearm shaft fractures, and the consequences of such injuries are far-reaching. Serial neurovascular examinations should be performed and documented. Radial and ulnar pulses along with distal digital capillary refill, in terms of number of seconds from blanching to return to full turgor, should be routinely evaluated. Davis and Green[50] reported nerve injuries in 1% (5/547) of their pediatric forearm fracture patients, with the most commonly injured nerve being the median nerve. Combined data from three large series of pediatric open forearm fractures reveal an overall nerve injury rate at presentation of 10% (17/173), with the median nerve once again being the one most commonly injured.[88,140] To screen for these rare but significant injuries, every child with a forearm fracture should routinely have evaluation of the radial, ulnar, and median nerves for both motor and sensory function.[43] Nerve injuries occurring at the time of injury must be differentiated from treatment-related or iatrogenic neurologic deficits, as nerve entrapment can occur during closed reduction or during operative fixation.

Davidson[49] suggested using the game of "rock–paper–scissors" for testing the median, radial, and ulnar nerves (Fig. 10-4). The pronated fist is the rock and tests median nerve function (pronator teres [PT], flexor digitorum profundus [FDP], flexor pollicis longus [FPL]). The extended fingers and wrist depict paper and test radial nerve function (extensor digitorum comminus [EDC], extensor pollicis longus [EPL], extensor carpi radialis brevis/longus [ECRB/L]). Fully flexed small and ring fingers, an adducted thumb, and spreading the index and ring fingers mimic scissors and test ulnar nerve function (intrinsics). Further focused testing should also be done on two important nerve branches: the anterior interosseous nerve (branch of median nerve) and the posterior interosseous nerve (PIN) (branch of radial nerve). The anterior

A

B

C

D

Figure 10-4. Upper extremity motor nerve physical examination. **A:** Rock position demonstrates median nerve motor function. **B:** Paper position demonstrates radial nerve motor function. **C:** Scissor position demonstrates ulnar nerve motor function. **D:** "OK" sign demonstrates function of anterior interosseous nerve.

interosseous nerve provides motor function to the index flexor digitorum profundus, the flexor pollicis longus, and pronator quadratus and is best tested by having the patient make an "OK" sign. The PIN typically innervates the extensor carpi ulnaris, extensor digitorum communis, extensor digiti minimi, extensor indicis, and the three outcropping muscles of the thumb (abductor pollicis longus, extensor pollicis brevis, and extensor pollicis longus).[28] Its function is best documented by full extension of the phalangeal and metacarpophalangeal joints. This is especially difficult to test in a patient in a cast or splint that partially covers the fingers. Most injuries that occur in association with forearm fractures are true neurapraxias and typically resolve over the course of days to weeks.[46,50] However, there are instances of entrapment of the nerve in the fracture site with open injuries or reduction maneuvers.

SIGNS AND SYMPTOMS OF DIAPHYSEAL RADIUS AND ULNA FRACTURES

The signs and symptoms indicating fracture of the shafts of the radius and ulna usually are not subtle. Deformity and pain are the classic findings. Patients typically experience exquisite pain emanating from the involved area. Decreased pronation and supination motion are also usually noted. Neither practitioners nor parents are always reliable assessors of children's pain, and ideally, patients should rate their own pain.[116,199] Significant anxiety and muscle spasm almost always amplify a child's painful experience.[32] It has been suggested that muscle spasm is a protective effort by the body to splint or otherwise protect the injured body part. When such muscle spasm occurs in association with certain fracture patterns (e.g., a radial shaft fracture proximal to the pronator teres insertion), it produces predictable fracture displacement (e.g., a pronated distal radial fragment and a supinated proximal fragment).

More subtle fractures present special diagnostic challenges. Certain pathologic fractures of the forearm may occur in the absence of overt trauma. Many minimally displaced fractures of the shafts of the radius and ulna can be mistaken for a "sprain" or "just a bruise" for several days to several weeks. This usually occurs in young children who continue to use the fractured arm during low-level play activities. As a general rule, a fracture should be suspected if the child has not resumed all normal arm function within 1 or 2 days of injury.

IMAGING AND OTHER DIAGNOSTIC STUDIES FOR DIAPHYSEAL RADIUS AND ULNA FRACTURES

Because important forearm fracture treatment decisions frequently are based on radiographic measurement of angular deformities, it must be remembered that these angles are projected shadows that are affected by rotation. If angulation is present on both AP and lateral views (commonly called two orthogonal views), the true deformity is out of the plane of the radiographs, and its true magnitude is greater than that measured on each individual view. Certain forearm shaft fracture deformities are clearly "two-plane deformities" whose maximal angular magnitude is in some plane other than the standard AP or lateral plane (Fig. 10-5). Bär and Breitfuss produced a table (based on the Pythagorean theorem) that predicts the true maximal angulation. Accurate deformity measurement can be made when angulation is seen on only one view and there is no angulation on the other orthogonal view.

Evans pointed out the importance of tracking the rotational alignment of the free-moving radial fragment by ascertaining the relative location of the bicipital tuberosity. This was a major step forward in refining the orthopaedic care of these forearm injuries. On a fully supinated AP radiograph of an unfractured forearm, the bicipital tuberosity points predominantly in a medial direction (nearly 180 degrees opposite of the radial tuberosity).[59] The radius and ulna are also nearly parallel to each other on such a view. On a fully pronated AP radiograph of an unfractured forearm, the bicipital tuberosity points in a lateral direction and the radial tuberosity is situated medially.[59] The radius also crosses over the ulna in a pronated AP view. In an unfractured limb, the bicipital tuberosity tended to align with a point near the thenar eminence (Fig. 10-6), more nearly a 165-degree relationship than a true 180-degree one. These relationships are best assessed on standard radiographs that include

Figure 10-5. Underestimation of true angulation. **A:** "Out of the AP and lateral plane" underestimates angulation at 30 degrees. **B:** True AP and lateral demonstrates that true maximal angulation is 45 degrees.

Figure 10-6. Rang's illustration depicting the position of the bicipital tuberosity on AP and lateral views with the forearm in pronation, supination, and neutral position. (Redrawn with permission from Rang M. *Children's Fractures*. Philadelphia, PA: JB Lippincott; 1974:96.)

the entire forearm on one film[181,216] rather than the specialized bicipital tuberosity view originally suggested by Evans.[59] A computed tomography (CT) scan of both forearms with cuts through the bicipital tuberosity and the radial styloid is probably the best way to accurately identify a rotational malunion after a fracture that could be causing a loss of forearm rotation. The ulna can be similarly assessed by comparing the distal ulnar styloid to the proximal coronoid process on orthogonal views (similar to bicipital tuberosity and radial styloid, the coronoid process and ulnar styloid should be 180 degrees apart). CT scan cuts of the coronoid process and the ulnar styloid on the fractured and nonfractured sides are most reliable for measuring the rotational alignment of the ulna.

CLASSIFICATION OF DIAPHYSEAL RADIUS AND ULNA FRACTURES

Fractures of the shafts of the radius and ulna often are described in rather imprecise terms such as "both-bone forearm fracture" and "greenstick fracture." Radiographs confirm the diagnosis of forearm shaft fracture and are the basis for most classification systems. The most comprehensive classification of forearm fractures is the one adopted by the Orthopaedic Trauma Association (OTA).[69] Although this system is sound in concept, its 36 discrete subtypes[69] make it impractical for everyday clinical use,

and it has not been widely used by clinical researchers. Despite its complexity, the OTA classification does not account for one of the most important prognostic factors in pediatric forearm shaft fracture: location of the fracture in the distal, middle, or proximal third of the shaft.

Clinicians and clinical researchers have favored simpler descriptions of forearm shaft fractures. An orderly and practical approach to forearm shaft fracture classification should provide information about the bone (single bone, both bones), the level (distal, middle, or proximal third), and the pattern (plastic deformation, greenstick, complete, comminuted). Bone involvement is important because it not only indicates the severity of injury but also influences suspicion regarding additional soft tissue injury (e.g., single-bone injury increases the likelihood of a Monteggia or Galeazzi injury) and affects reduction tactics (unique single-bone fracture reduction strategies can be used) (Fig. 10-7). Single-bone shaft fractures occur, but both-bone fractures are far more common. Level is important for anatomic reasons relative to muscle and interosseous ligament attachments, as well as differences in prognosis for distal-, middle-, and proximal-third shaft fractures. The pattern is important because it significantly alters the treatment approach. For example, the primary reduction strategy is very different for greenstick fractures (rotation) compared to that for complete fractures (vertical traction). Certain comminuted fractures (e.g.,

Figure 10-7. Isolated ulnar shaft reduction technique (Blount). Valgus force applied to fracture site and direct thumb pressure over distal ligament. **A:** Reductive force is applied as illustrated. **B:** The fracture is reduced.

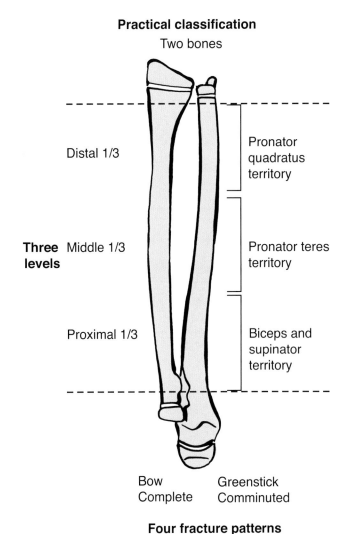

Practical classification
Two bones

Distal 1/3

Three levels   Middle 1/3

Proximal 1/3

Pronator quadratus territory

Pronator teres territory

Biceps and supinator territory

Bow / Complete

Greenstick / Comminuted

Four fracture patterns

Figure 10-8. Practical classification of forearm shaft fractures. (*Distal dotted line* defined by proximal extent of the Lister tubercle and *proximal dotted line* defined by proximal extent of bicipital tuberosity.)

comminution of both bones) may preclude reduction and casting and require surgical fixation.[65,67] Fortunately, comminuted fracture patterns are rare in children, but increasingly seen in high-risk sporting activities of adolescents. For all practical purposes, the buckle fracture pattern that is common in the distal radial metaphysis never occurs in isolation in the shaft region except in very young patients. The typical buckle fracture "speed bump" may accompany either plastic deformation or greenstick fractures. Thus, there are two bones, three levels, and four common fracture patterns (Fig. 10-8). We believe this is a practical and clinically relevant way to describe forearm shaft fractures.[154]

Once the forearm fracture has been described in the terms of this practical classification, fracture displacement must be evaluated. Fracture displacement can occur as angulation, rotation, shortening, or translation. Angulation is important in treatment decision making and can be measured with reasonable reliability.[133,210] Rotation is a simple concept, but it is difficult to assess clinically.[181] The best that usually can be done is to roughly estimate rotation within a 45-degree margin of error.[45,181] Based on available clinical studies, it appears that less than 1 cm of shortening should be accepted in either single- or both-bone fracture patterns.[34,54] It has also been suggested that the shortening that accompanies displaced fractures may help preserve future motion through interosseous membrane relaxation.[181] Completely (100%) translated fractures of the middle third[45,181] and distal third[54] of the forearm have been shown to reliably remodel. Certain situations may raise concern regarding complete translation, such as isolated middle-third radial fractures

with medial (ulnar) displacement that significantly narrows the interosseous space and translation in children who have less than 2 full years of growth remaining, because remodeling of the translated fracture site is less in older than in younger children.[169]

OUTCOMES OF DIAPHYSEAL RADIUS AND ULNA FRACTURES

The fundamental reason for treating fractures of the shafts of the radius and ulna relates to the likelihood of bad results in the absence of adequate care. Data from certain developing countries may be as close as we come to natural history studies of untreated fractures. Archibong and Onuba[6] reported on 102 pediatric fracture patients treated in Southeastern Nigeria. Their patients most commonly had upper extremity fractures, and they frequently experienced significant delays in seeking medical treatment, which led to high rates of malunion requiring surgical

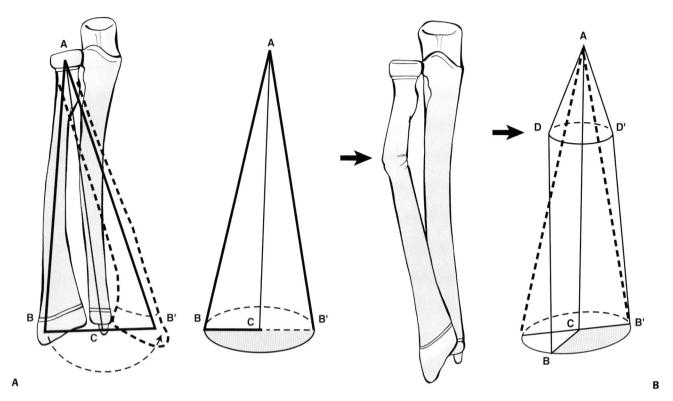

A   **B**

Figure 10-9. Effect of forearm malunion on forearm motion. **A:** Normal arc of forearm motion. **B:** Angulated radius leads to diminished arc of forearm motion. (Redrawn with permission from Ogden JA. *Skeletal Injury in the Child.* Lea & Febiger; 1982:56–57.)

treatment.[6] Other Nigerian authors have found that young age was not protective against fracture malunion (>50%) and nonunion (25%) following traditional bonesetter treatment.[172] It is unclear whether children treated in this fashion are better or worse off than if they had received no treatment at all. The rationale for treating pediatric forearm shaft fractures is thus based on the premise that the results of modern orthopaedic treatment will exceed "pseudonatural histories" such as these.

The consequences of excessively crooked (and malrotated) forearm bones are both aesthetic and functional (Fig. 10-9).[97,216] Limited forearm supination following a forearm shaft malunion is illustrated in Figure 10-10. Despite their great concern to parents, aesthetic issues have not been formally studied, and as a result, the practitioner must interpret forearm appearance issues on a case-by-case basis. Clinical experience has shown that the ulna appears to be less forgiving from an aesthetic standpoint because of its long subcutaneous border. Early and repeated involvement of the parents (or other legal guardians) in an informed and shared decision-making process is essential.

Bony malunion and soft tissue fibrosis have both been implicated as causes of limited forearm motion after forearm shaft fractures.[96] Limited forearm pronation and supination can have significant effects on upper extremity function.[181] Inability to properly pronate often can be compensated for with shoulder abduction (but can lead to fatigue with prolonged activities), and no easy compensatory mechanism exists for supination deficits.[43,97,181] Daruwalla identified a nearly 53% rate of limited forearm rotation (subtle in some, dramatic in others) in his series of 53 children with forearm fractures and attributed it to angular deformity and rotational malalignment. Several patients in Price's[181] classic series of pediatric forearm malunions had severe forearm range-of-motion losses that significantly limited vocational and recreational activities. Trousdale and Linscheid[216] reported range-of-motion losses severe enough to prompt corrective osteotomies in many of their predominantly pediatric (<14 years old at time of injury) patients with forearm malunions. Meier[155] also reported significant range-of-motion deficits in association with pediatric forearm malunion.

Range-of-motion losses caused by deformity have been studied by numerous authors using adult cadaveric forearm specimens. Matthews et al.[149] studied 10- and 20-degree midshaft angular deformities of the radius and ulna in 10 forearm specimens. They found that 10-degree deformities of either bone individually resulted in little or no measurable motion loss (in the range of 3 degrees or less). When both bones were angulated 10 degrees dorsal, volar, or toward the interosseous membrane, larger motion losses were documented (approximately 10-degree pronation and 20-degree supination). Significantly greater losses of motion occurred when one or both bones were angulated 20 degrees (approximately 40 degrees for both pronation and supination). Some of the 10-degree angulated specimens demonstrated "cosmetically unacceptable deformity."[149] Keep in mind that similar deformities in children will likely improve with time due to their remodeling potential.

Additional important information about the influence of fracture level on forearm motion was provided by a series of adult cadaver experiments conducted by Sarmiento et al.[193,211] They found that fracture angulation of 15 to 30 degrees led to greater supination losses when the deformity was in the middle third of the forearm (40–90 degrees) and greater pronation losses when in the distal third (30–80 degrees).[211] Fracture angulation of 10 degrees or less in the proximal or middle forearm rarely resulted in more than 15 degrees of motion loss,[193,211] but the same angulation in the distal third of the forearm was at times (usually with isolated radius fracture) associated with pronation losses of 20 degrees.[193,211] These findings challenge commonly held beliefs that the distal-third fracture of the forearm is the most forgiving. These same authors asserted that rotational malalignment led to rotational motion losses that usually were equal in magnitude and opposite in direction to the deformity (e.g., a 10-degree pronation deformity led to a 10-degree loss of supination).[211]

Figure 10-10. A 6-year-old male who suffered a right forearm shaft malunion. **A:** Radiograph 1 week after fracture showing complete midshaft ulnar and proximal third radial fractures. **B:** Healed fractures at 6-month follow-up. **C:** Twenty-month follow-up. **D:** Twenty-six–month follow-up.

(continues)

E, F   G

H   I

Figure 10-10. (*Continued*) **E:** Symmetrical pronation. **F:** Limited supination on the right. **G:** Axial alignment with palms together. **H:** An effort at supination. **I:** Axial alignment in pronation.

Rotational malalignment of the forearm has been studied in greater detail in recent years, mostly in adults and in the laboratory.[56,113,217] In isolated midshaft radial fractures, more than 30 degrees of malrotation was a threshold for significant losses in motion (approximately 15 degrees).[113] Isolated midshaft ulna fracture malrotation did not alter the total arc of forearm motion but did change the set point (e.g., a 30-degree pronation deformity took away 30 degrees of pronation and added 30 degrees of supination).[217] Larger ulnar axial malalignment of

45 degrees decreased overall forearm rotation by no more than 20 degrees.[217] Large residual ulnar shaft translation has similarly been found to have little impact on forearm rotation.[152] Simulated combined radial and ulnar midshaft rotational malunions resulted in the worst motion (>50% losses of pronation and supination when 60-degree rotational malunions were in opposite directions).[56] Rotational malunions that approximated recommended limits in the literature (45 degrees)[181] produced less extreme but real limitations of motion.[56] From these studies

and our clinical experience, it appears that the radius is more sensitive to rotational problems and less sensitive regarding aesthetic issues, whereas the ulna is exactly the opposite.

Several generations of orthopaedic surgeons have been taught that 50 degrees of pronation and 50 degrees of supination represent adequate forearm motion.[160] It must be remembered that this classic study performed by Morrey and his Mayo Clinic colleagues involving 33 normal subjects (18 female, 15 male) from 21 to 75 years of age is not the only study that addresses forearm motion. The average arc of normal forearm motion for the Mayo group (68-degree pronation to 74-degree supination)[160] was approximately 20 degrees less than that measured in 53 healthy male subjects who were not older than 19 years old (77-degree pronation to 83-degree supination) reported by Boone and Azen[21] and 35 degrees less than that reported by Rickert et al.[186] (75-degree pronation to 100-degree supination) in 141 subjects of both sexes between 20 and 30 years of age. Contemporary three-dimensional motion analysis has revealed that maximal pronation occurs when pouring liquid from a pitcher and maximal supination commonly occurs during personal hygiene activities.[184] Thus, it seems clear that the forearm motion "goals" reported by Morrey et al.[160] are not necessarily ideal or even optimal, but rather they may be considered as the minimal limits of forearm function. Stated another way, losing 20 degrees or 30 degrees of either pronation or supination carries the potential for significant functional impact on important activities of daily living (ADLs).

The goal of treatment is to achieve satisfactory healing of the forearm injury within the established anatomic and functional guidelines while also taking into account the reasonable degree of remodeling that can be expected in growing children.[103] Most of the time, these goals can be achieved with closed fracture care, and little or no radiographic or clinical abnormality can be detected following healing. A paradox exists in pediatric forearm fractures whereby anatomic radiographic alignment is not always associated with normal motion, and normal motion can be associated with nonanatomic radiographic healing.[96,166,211] Herein lies the inherent controversy between operative and nonoperative treatment approaches (Table 10-1). In patients with anatomic radiographs, range-of-motion problems usually have been attributed to scarring of the interosseous membrane.[181] With nonanatomic radiographs (incomplete remodeling), range-of-motion deficits usually are attributed to the radiographic abnormalities. Thus, treatment of forearm shaft fracture must balance the risk of allowing stiffness to occur secondary to malunion against the risk of creating stiffness secondary to surgical procedures. Thus, the goal of surgical intervention is to provide sufficient stability to fracture(s) to allow for early motion to lessen risk of soft tissue stiffness and fracture malunion.

The rationalization for the remodeling of pediatric forearm fractures has strong historical support,[14] but knowledge of the limits of remodeling must be taken into consideration. Established reduction criteria state that complete (100%) translation is acceptable,[181] as well as up to 15 degrees of angulation and up to 45 degrees of malrotation.[181] The fundamental reason for treating fractures of the shafts of the radius and ulna relates to

TABLE 10-1. Pros and Cons of Nonoperative Versus Operative Treatment

Treatment	Pros	Cons
Cast	Long track record	Stiffness may still occur
	Negligible infection risk	Frequent follow-up visits
	Fine-tuning possible	Anatomic reduction rare
Surgery	Anatomic reduction	Risk of infection
	Minimize immobilization	Need for implant removal
	Fewer follow-up visits	Stiffness from surgery

the likelihood of bad results in the absence of adequate care or acceptable remodeling. As noted earlier, data from certain developing countries may be as close as we come to natural history studies of untreated fractures. Nigerian[6,172] studies indicate high rates of malunion with untreated or bonesetter treatment of diaphyseal fractures.

Pediatric forearm shaft fractures in children less than about 8 years of age have great remodeling potential that occurs through several mechanisms. The distal radial epiphysis will redirect itself toward normal at about 10 degrees/yr. As long as the physis is open, this rate is relatively independent of age. Although the epiphysis will return to normal direction, it will have much less effect on correcting an angular deformity at the midshaft compared to fractures at the subphyseal level. Remodeling also occurs with lengthening of the bone through growth, which produces an apparent decrease in angulation, especially if measured as the difference between the proximal and distal ends of the bone. The bone also remodels by intramembranous apposition on the concave side and resorption on the convex side.[103] This occurs throughout life but more rapidly when driven by the thick periosteum found in young children. Larsen et al.[130] found that although the epiphyseal angle realigns quickly, children older than 11 years correct bone angulation less than the younger children. Thomas et al. stated the following regarding pediatric forearm remodeling potential: "We should not fail to recall that the remodeling capabilities of the bones of children have not changed in the last million years and that open reduction and internal fixation must be undertaken only after due deliberation."[212] Others such as Johari[104] would state that if one critically evaluates the limits of forearm shaft remodeling capacity, one will find a much higher rate (approximately 50%) of incomplete remodeling in children over 10 years of age.

The perfect (or nearly perfect) pediatric diaphyseal forearm fracture outcome study has not yet been performed, therefore scientific answers regarding optimal treatment are lacking.[70] However, there is a growing consensus among pediatric orthopaedic trauma surgeons that there are patient subsets (usually older patients with more proximal fractures) whose outcomes are clearly improved by flexible intramedullary nail surgical intervention.[228] A large retrospective cohort study focusing on radiographic outcomes has indicated that among pediatric forearm shaft fracture patients who underwent closed reduction treatment, most (51%) exceeded established radiographic criteria over the course of 2 to 4 weeks.[26] This is greatly concerning as a very clear relationship exists between radiographic and clinical outcomes for forearm shaft injuries in both adults and children.[22,55,111] For those patients deemed at higher risk, the risk–benefit ratio appears to be favorable as flexible nail surgical complications are mainly minor and in some respects, measurably lower than nonoperative forearm shaft fracture care.[190,200]

PATHOANATOMY AND APPLIED ANATOMY RELATING TO DIAPHYSEAL RADIUS AND ULNA FRACTURES

The forearm is a triarthrodial joint with nearly a 180-degree arc of motion encompassing two hyaline cartilage joints (PRUJ and DRUJ) and a membranous joint (interosseous membrane). Its bones, the radius and ulna, are not simple straight bony tubes. The shaft of the radius is a three-sided structure with two prominent curvatures. One major gradual convexity (approximately 10 degrees with its apex lateroradial) is present along its midportion; a second, more acute curve of approximately 15 degrees with its apex medial occurs proximally near the bicipital tuberosity.[63,87] The deviation along the midportion is commonly referred to as the radial bow, and maintenance of this normal contour is a goal of forearm shaft fracture care (the radius is bowed so it can "radiate" around the ulna).[182] The most important bony landmarks of the radius are the radial styloid (lateral prominence) and the bicipital tuberosity (anteromedial prominence), which are oriented about 160 degrees away from each other (Fig. 10-11).[227] Maintenance of this styloid–tuberosity rotational relationship is another forearm shaft fracture principle. The nutrient artery of the radius enters the bone in its proximal half and courses anterior to ulnar (medial).[78] Such nutrient vessels typically are seen on only one orthogonal view and should not be confused with fracture lines. In cross-section, most of the shaft of the ulna is also shaped like a classic three-sided prism, although its more distal and proximal portions are much more circular. The most important bony landmarks of the ulna are its styloid process (distally) and its coronoid process (proximally). These two landmarks are oriented nearly 180 degrees from one another, with the styloid aimed in a posterior (dorsal) direction and the coronoid in an anterior (volar) direction.[227] Tracking styloid–coronoid rotational alignment of the ulna is another part of forearm shaft fracture care. The ulnar shaft has mild curvatures in both its proximal (apex lateral/radial) and distal (apex medial/ulnar) portions but is otherwise relatively straight.[87] The nutrient artery to the ulna enters the bone in its proximal half and courses anterior to radial (lateral).[78]

The classic works of Evans helped focus attention on rotational deformity associated with fractures of both bones of the forearm.[59,150] Evans stated, "The orthodox position in which to immobilize these fractures is that of full supination for the upper third, and the midposition for fractures of the middle and lower thirds, these positions being based on the anatomical arrangement of the pronators and supinators of the forearm. However, it

Figure 10-11. Radial and ulnar anatomy.

is unreasonable to suppose that all fractures at a given level will present the same degree of rotational deformity."[59] The radius and ulna are joined by three major passive restraints: the PRUJ, DRUJ, and the interosseous membrane complex, all of which have important stabilizing and load-transferring functions in addition to their role in forearm rotation. These structures allow rotation of the radius about the ulna along an axis that runs approximately from the center of the radial head to the center of the distal ulna.[98] The PRUJ and DRUJ are discussed elsewhere in this book (Chapters 9 and 12). The structure and biomechanical function of the interosseous membrane have been studied extensively in recent years. Hotchkiss et al.[100] showed that the central band of the interosseous membrane (the interosseous ligament) courses from a point near the junction of the proximal and middle thirds of the radius to a point near the junction of the middle and distal thirds of the ulna. It is an important longitudinal stabilizer of the forearm in that 71% of forearm longitudinal stiffness is provided by the interosseous ligament after radial head excision.[100] Transverse vectors have also been identified[178] and reflect the stabilizing effect of the interosseous ligament during pronation and supination movements. The interosseous ligament demonstrates tensile properties comparable to the patellar tendon and the anterior cruciate ligament, indicative of the magnitude of the arm forces to which this structure is subjected.

Although some difference of opinion still exists,[51,73] multiple studies have shown that the most strain in the central band of the interosseous membrane is generated when the forearm is in the neutral position.[145,146] These findings of maximal strain in

Figure 10-12. Anatomy of interosseous ligament. **A:** Central oblique orientation of interosseous ligament. **B:** Interosseous ligament attachment in terms of percentage forearm length. (Reprinted from Skahen JR III, et al. Reconstruction of the interosseous membrane of the forearm in cadavers. *J Hand Surg Am.* 1997;22(6):986–994. Copyright © 1997 with permission from Elsevier.)

neutral in cadaver studies also are consistent with radiographic measurement studies[45] and dynamic magnetic resonance imaging studies of the forearm showing that the interosseous space is maximal near a neutral position.[167] This may help explain certain pathologic situations such as the fixed supination deformity of neonatal brachial plexus palsy[151] as well as limitations of pronation and supination because of encroachment on the interosseous space from malangulated fractures (Fig. 10-12).[237] The interosseous membrane also serves as an important anchoring point for several forearm muscles: the flexor digitorum profundus, flexor pollicis longus, extensor indicis, and the outcropping muscles (extensor digitorum brevis, abductor pollicis longus).

The paired and seemingly balanced radial and ulnar bones have an unbalanced number of muscular connections. The ulna typically has 14 attached muscles and the radius 10.[87] Powerful supinators attach to the proximal third of the forearm, whereas important pronators attach to its middle and distal thirds (Fig. 10-13). The accompanying vasculature of the forearm is complex: These muscles are supplied by more than 248 vascular pedicles arising from the brachial artery, its branches, or other collateral vessels. The radial, ulnar, and median nerves (or their branches) along with the musculocutaneous nerve provide all of the key innervations to the motors that attach to the forearm bones. As mentioned earlier, the median nerve is the most commonly injured nerve with forearm fractures.[49,50,88]

The radial nerve proceeds from a posterior-to-anterior direction and enters the forearm after passing the lateral epicondyle between the brachialis and brachioradialis muscles (BRBr). Near this same level, it divides into superficial and deep terminal branches. The deep motor branch of the radial nerve is also known as the PIN. In addition to its routine innervation of the brachioradialis and extensor carpi radialis longus, most commonly (55% of the time), a motor branch arises from the radial nerve proper or its superficial terminal branch to innervate

Figure 10-13. Muscle forces acting in proximal, middle, and distal thirds. **A:** Distal radial fragment significantly pronated by associated muscles while proximal fragment is flexed and supinated. **B:** The key involved muscles prior to significant displacement.

the extensor carpi radialis brevis, whereas the rest of the time (45%), this motor branch comes from the PIN.[2] The superficial branch travels along with and beneath the brachioradialis. The PIN enters the supinator muscle, passing the fibrous thickening called the arcade of Frohse shortly after branching from the radial nerve proper. It courses within the supinator past the proximal radius, later exiting this muscle dorsally (posteriorly) near the junction of the proximal and middle thirds of the radius. Following its emergence from the supinator, the PIN branches repetitively to the superficial extensors and the deeper outcropping muscles. The ulnar nerve enters the forearm between the two heads of the flexor carpi ulnaris.[81] It traverses the forearm between flexor carpi ulnaris and the flexor digitorum profundus. In the distal forearm, it lays just beneath the flexor carpi ulnaris. The median nerve enters the forearm as it passes between the two heads of the pronator teres. It next passes beneath the archway created by the two heads of the flexor digitorum superficialis. The median nerve then continues down the course of the forearm nestled between the flexor digitorum superficialis and the flexor digitorum profundus. It becomes much more superficial as it nears the level of the carpal tunnel. The anterior interosseous branch arises from the median nerve at the level of the pronator and travels deep with the anterior interosseous vessels. Abundant muscles shield the radial, ulnar, and median nerves from the shafts of the radius and ulna through most of the forearm except for the PIN near the proximal radius.

COMMON SURGICAL APPROACHES TO DIAPHYSEAL RADIUS AND ULNA FRACTURES

The large exposure required for plate fixation of pediatric forearm fractures can be achieved with the Henry (anterior) or Thompson (posterior) approaches to the radial shaft and the direct (medial) approach to the ulnar shaft. Compartment syndrome release usually requires the serpentine incision of McConnell's combined approach. These approaches and their variations are well described and illustrated in detail in the literature. For open reduction of both the radius and the ulna, most authors favor separate incisions to minimize the possibility of communicating hematomas and the development of a radioulnar synostosis.[128,182,218] The Thompson approach to the radius is generally used for fractures of its proximal third[235] but requires special care to protect the PIN.[53,156] Other authors have emphasized the utility of the Henry approach for plating of the entire radius including the proximal aspect.[156] When open reduction is done in conjunction with other internal fixation techniques (e.g., intramedullary fixation), limited versions of the same surgical approaches are used.

Indirect reduction and internal fixation of forearm fractures require knowledge of appropriate physeal-sparing entry portals about the distal and proximal forearm. Because of the relative inaccessibility of its proximal end, the radius usually is approached only distally through either a dorsal or radial entry point. The dorsal entry point is near the proximal base of the Lister tubercle or just lateral to it in a small bare area between the second and third dorsal compartments. This location is a short distance proximal to the physis of the distal radius. Another dorsal alternative is pin entry just medial to the Lister tubercle, between the third and fourth dorsal compartments,

but this entails greater risk to the extensor tendons, especially the extensor pollicis longus as it is tightly anchored in the retinaculum of the third compartment as it courses around the tubercle from ulnar to radial.[164] The most commonly used radial entry point is located in line with the styloid process just proximal to the physis. Entry in this area passes adjacent to the first dorsal compartment, and thus the tendons of abductor pollicis longus and extensor pollicis brevis (as well as branches of the superficial radial nerve) must be protected (Fig. 10-14). Because of its extensive branching pattern, portions of the superficial branch of the radial nerve may also be at risk when dorsal or radial intramedullary entry points are used.[1]

Both distal and proximal intramedullary entry sites for the ulna have been described.[135,139] In the distal portion of the ulna, an entry site can be made proximal to the physis and in the interval between the extensor carpi ulnaris and flexor carpi ulnaris tendons. Care must be taken to avoid branches of the dorsal cutaneous sensory nerve. Ulnar entry is most easily accomplished in the proximal portion of the bone either along its lateral metaphyseal border just distal to the olecranon apophysis, piercing peripheral fibers of the anconeus (Fig. 10-15),[31,132,137] or directly through the olecranon apophysis. The metaphyseal anconeus entry site described by the Nancy group avoids the physis and avoids the painful bursa that tends to form over the "tip of the olecranon" pins.

Transphyseal approaches to both the distal radius[242,243] and the proximal ulna[4,139] have been suggested by some authors. Significant growth potential exists at the distal radius (approximately 10 mm/yr), whereas there is proportionately less from the olecranon apophysis (approximately 2 mm/yr). There is an unnecessary risk to the radial physis and few, if any, technical advantages to transphyseal entry of the radius in diaphyseal-level fracture fixation. The ulna apophyseal entry site is used in many centers.

TREATMENT OPTIONS FOR DIAPHYSEAL RADIUS AND ULNA FRACTURES

NONOPERATIVE TREATMENT OF DIAPHYSEAL RADIUS AND ULNA FRACTURES

Indications/Contraindications

Nonoperative Treatment of Diaphyseal Radius and Ulna Fractures:
INDICATIONS AND CONTRAINDICATIONS

Indications
- Closed fractures
- Skeletally immature, displaced and nondisplaced
- Reducible by closed means

Relative Contraindications
- Open fractures
- Displaced and advanced skeletal maturity
- Unable to achieve reduction within accepted parameters
- Tense swelling/impending compartment syndrome

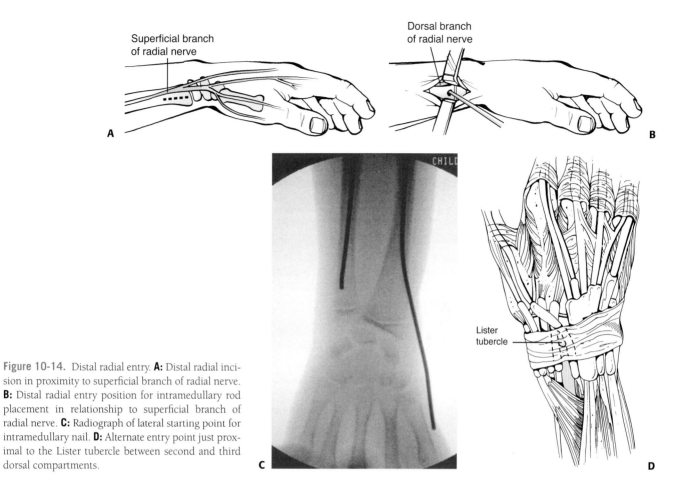

Figure 10-14. Distal radial entry. **A:** Distal radial incision in proximity to superficial branch of radial nerve. **B:** Distal radial entry position for intramedullary rod placement in relationship to superficial branch of radial nerve. **C:** Radiograph of lateral starting point for intramedullary nail. **D:** Alternate entry point just proximal to the Lister tubercle between second and third dorsal compartments.

Figure 10-15. Proximal ulnar entry. **A:** Anconeus entry point. **B:** Radiograph of proximal ulnar entry point.

Most pediatric radial and ulnar shaft fractures can be treated by nonoperative methods.[243] Low-energy, nondisplaced, and minimally displaced forearm fractures can be immediately immobilized in a properly molded (three-point mold concept of Charnley) above-elbow cast.[4] Above-elbow casts have a propensity to fall off in children, especially in those less than 4 years old and in the obese. This can be countered with a molded sharp, geometric right angle in the cast at the elbow. Avoid any curve in the outer edge of the cast at the elbow (create a straight ulnar border to your long arm cast). If posttraumatic tissue swelling is a concern, noncircumferential splint immobilization (e.g., sugar-tong splint) can be used initially.[43,240] For fractures in the distal third of the forearm, below-elbow casting has been shown to be as effective as above-elbow casting in maintenance of satisfactory fracture alignment.[40,75] Appropriate follow-up is important for these minimally displaced fractures (an initial follow-up radiograph usually is taken 7 to 14 days after injury) because displacement may still occur for a variety of reasons: new trauma to the extremity, male gender, and poor casting technique.[43,240]

Good casting technique is infrequently discussed in contemporary orthopaedic textbooks and sometimes is underemphasized during orthopaedic residency training. The principles of good forearm casting technique include (a) interosseous molding, (b) supracondylar above-elbow molding, (c) appropriate padding, (d) evenly distributed cast material, (e) straight ulnar border, and (f) three-point molding (Fig. 10-16). The risk of excessive cast tightness can be minimized through the use of the

Figure 10-16. Interosseous mold technique.

stretch–relax fiberglass casting technique described by Davids et al.[47] Chess et al.[40] described a cast index for distal radial fractures defined as the sagittal cast width divided by the coronal cast width at the level of the fracture site; a normal ratio is considered to be 0.70. The cast index has not been validated for forearm shaft fractures, but it embodies the sound concept of good interosseous molding. Techniques such as pins and plaster and cast wedging also have had a role in fracture care.[11,57] Cast wedging is almost always done with an opening wedge technique because this entails less risk of soft tissue impingement.[114]

Displaced fractures usually require reduction following appropriate analgesia.[54,219] Options include hematoma block,[71,94] regional intravenous (IV) anesthesia[29,48] and inhalational methods,[60,94] and IV sedation with propofol or ketamine. After informed consent for sedation and reduction is obtained, monitored sedation can be used in the emergency department with a combination of narcotics and anxiolytics.[119] This typically requires a dedicated nurse to administer oxygen and perform appropriate monitoring functions (vital signs, continuous electrocardiogram, and pulse oximetry).[42,95] Ketamine protocols are also being used with increased frequency.[79,119] Young children with less than 5 or 10 degrees of angulation in the plane of wrist and elbow motion probably do not require the additional trauma, time, expense, and sedation risk involved in a formal reduction because of the predictable remodeling in this age group as long as immobilization brings stability to the fracture and prevents late displacement.[6] It has been shown that the more displaced the fracture, the more likely that formal monitored sedation techniques will be used for pediatric forearm fracture reduction as opposed to other techniques.[219]

More specific closed treatment options are discussed for pediatric forearm injuries in terms of their common fracture patterns: bow (plastic deformation), greenstick, complete, and comminuted.

Traumatic Bowing/Plastic Deformation

Although traumatic bowing was described by Rauber in 1876, it was not widely recognized until Spencer Borden's classic paper was published in 1974. This injury occurs almost exclusively with children's forearm fractures. Bow fractures (Fig. 10-17) show no obvious macroscopic fracture line or cortical discontinuity, but they do demonstrate multiple microfractures (slip lines) along the length of the bow.[191] At times, a nearly classic buckle fracture (torus fracture) coexists with a bow fracture. The most common clinical scenario is a plastically deformed ulna along with a more typical fracture of the radius.[143]

Borden and subsequent authors stressed the importance of natural remodeling potential in these injuries but voiced concern about this approach in older children (especially those >10 years of age).[143,191] Vorlat and De Boeck[221] reported incomplete remodeling in 3 of 11 children at long-term follow-up (average 6.7 years) after traumatic bowing of the forearm. Because these three children were between the ages of 7 and 10 at the time of injury, the authors recommended more aggressive efforts at reduction in all patients with clinically significant deformity (>10 degrees) older than 6 years of age.[221] Traumatic bowing

Figure 10-17. Bow fracture: approximately 15 degrees of apex-dorsal bowing of radius and ulna shaft.

that causes aesthetically and/or functionally unacceptable angular deformity should be manipulated under general anesthesia or deep sedation because strong (20–30 kg) gradual force applied over 2 to 3 minutes is required to obtain acceptable alignment (Fig. 10-18).[191] Application of this reductive pressure over a rolled towel, block, or surgeon's knee fulcrum followed by a three-point molded cast can substantially (although at times still incompletely) correct the deformity (Fig. 10-19). Care must be taken to avoid direct pressure over adjacent epiphyses for fear of creating a physeal fracture.

Greenstick Fractures

Greenstick fractures present special issues in terms of diagnosis and treatment. Angulated greenstick fractures of the shafts of the radius and ulna at different levels indicate a significant rotational component to the injury (see Fig. 10-2). Evans, Rang, and others have stated that the apex-volar angulation pattern usually is associated with a supination-type injury mechanism, whereas most apex-dorsal greenstick fractures involve a pronation-type injury mechanism (Fig. 10-20),[59,169] although exceptions certainly occur. Often, the apparent angular deformity can be corrected by simply reversing the forearm rotational forces (e.g., reducing an apex-dorsal pronation-type injury with supination). Noonan and Price[169] observed that it is difficult to remember whether to use pronation or supination reductive forces and suggested that most fractures can be reduced by rotating the palm toward the deformity. They also noted that most greenstick fractures are supination injuries with apex-volar angulation and thus can be reduced by a pronation movement.[169] Pediatric orthopaedic researchers from the Arnold Palmer Hospital for Children have recently proposed the "radius crossover sign" as an indicator of significant angular and torsional deformity in greenstick fractures of the radial shaft.[233] Proper interpretation of this sign relies on full-length forearm films that include a good AP view of the distal humerus.

Greenstick fractures that occur near the same level probably have little to no rotational component and are best corrected by manipulative reduction and three-point molding techniques (see Fig. 10-3). Charnley believed that greenstick fractures of the forearm in children perfectly illustrated his dictum that "A curved plaster is necessary to make a straight limb."[38] He also stated that "The unsuspected recurrence of angular deformity in greenstick fractures of the forearm, while concealed in plaster, is an annoying event if it takes the surgeon by surprise and is not discovered until the plaster is removed. Parents, quite understandably, may be more annoyed about this happening to their children than if it had happened to themselves, and do not easily forgive the surgeon."[38] Despite these concerns, it is clear from large published reports that greenstick fractures can almost always be successfully treated with nonoperative manipulative reduction methods.[242]

Figure 10-18. Reduction technique of bow fracture over fulcrum. (Redrawn with permission from Sanders WE, Heckman JD. Traumatic plastic deformation of the radius and ulna: a closed method of correction of deformity. *Clin Orthop Relat Res.* 1984;188:58–67.)

A

C

D

E

B

F

G

Figure 10-19. Reduction technique for plastic deformation. **A:** 7-year-3-month-old female demonstrating clinical deformity of her plastically deformed right forearm. **B:** Injury radiograph that pretty much looks exactly like her arm (some lucency in radius but cortices intact). **C:** Beginning of slow steady reduction maneuver over soft but firm bolster (roll of medical tape). **D:** End-of-reduction maneuver showing how force has corrected forearm and flattened tape. **E:** Intraoperative fluoroscopic image showing improved radiographic alignment. **F, G:** Anteroposterior and lateral radiographs at 2-month follow-up showing satisfactory healing and alignment.

Figure 10-20. Shaft fractures at different levels imply rotational mechanism. **A:** Apex-volar angulation with supination deformity of the forearm. **B:** Apex-dorsal angulation with pronation deformity of the forearm.

Two philosophies are reflected in the literature regarding greenstick fracture reduction: one in which the greenstick fracture is purposely completed and another in which it is not. Those who favor completing the fracture (dating back at least to the 1859 work of Malgaigne) cite concerns about lost reduction and recurrent deformity that can be prevented only by converting the greenstick into a complete fracture.[65] Others prefer to maintain and perhaps exploit some of the inherent stability of the greenstick fracture.[40,50,212] In addition to the traditional view that loss of reduction is less likely if a greenstick fracture is completed, there also is the theoretical advantage of a lower refracture rate because of more exuberant callus formation.[40,169] To the best of our knowledge, these theories have not been validated in any controlled clinical studies. Davis and Green[50] advocated a derotational approach to greenstick fracture reduction and reported a 10% (16/151) reangulation rate in their series of patients with greenstick fracture. They compared this to the 25% (12/47) reangulation rate in patients with complete fractures and questioned the wisdom of routinely completing greenstick fractures.[50] In a prospective study, Boyer et al.[27] showed statistically that greenstick fractures maintain their reduction better than complete forearm fractures.

Complete Fractures

Complete fractures in different regions of the shaft of the forearm behave differently from a clinical perspective and have classically been divided into distal-, middle-, and proximal-third fractures. Single-bone complete fractures usually are caused by direct trauma (nightstick fracture) and are difficult to reduce. Blount described a reduction technique that may be effective for reduction of a displaced single-bone shaft fracture. The intact bone is used as a lever to reestablish the length of the fractured bone, and then transverse forces are applied to realign the bone

ends (see Fig. 10-7). Both-bone complete fractures (often with bayonet shortening) are common and are best treated with finger-trap or arm traction applied over 5 to 10 minutes. This stretches out the soft tissue envelope and aids in both reduction and cast or splint application. Traction allows complete fractures to "seek their own level of rotation" and allows correction of rotational malalignment.[50]

The position of immobilization for forearm fractures has been an area of debate since the days of Hippocrates. Theoretically, the position of forearm rotation in an above-elbow cast or splint affects rotational alignment of complete fractures at all levels; however, a study of distal third forearm fractures found no significant effect of forearm rotation position on ultimate alignment.[27] We are aware of no similar studies analyzing the effects of forearm position on middle- or proximal-third shaft fractures, and treatment is influenced by certain anatomic considerations. Because of the strong supination pull of the biceps, aided by the supinator, complete proximal radial fractures may be best immobilized in supination so that the distal forearm rotation matches that of the proximal forearm (see Fig. 10-13). The position of immobilization of fractures in the middle third of the forearm commonly is dictated by whether the radial fracture occurs distal or proximal to the insertion of the pronator teres. Fractures proximal to its insertion are best treated by fully supinating the distal fragment, whereas those distal to its insertion are probably best treated in a neutral position. Fractures at different levels in the midshaft that require pronation or supination as part of the reduction maneuver should be immobilized in the position of reduction.

Manipulated fractures should be evaluated weekly for the first 3 to 5 weeks because most position loss can be recognized and corrected during this time.[125] Any significant shift in position between visits necessitates cast wedging or a cast change, with remolding and possible fracture remanipulation if unacceptable displacement is present. Voto et al. found that, in general, 7% of forearm fractures redisplace; this can occur up to 24 days after the initial manipulation. Davis[50] reported a 25% reangulation rate in complete fractures. Remanipulation can be done in the office following administration of oral analgesics. Judicious use of benzodiazepines may also be valuable because of their anxiolytic effects.

Although in adults the above-elbow cast generally is changed to a below-elbow cast after 3 to 4 weeks, this is unnecessary in most children because they heal more quickly and permanent elbow stiffness is rare.[117] A cast change at week 3 or 4 also can be traumatic to a young child and carries the additional small risk of cast-saw injury. Once the fracture shows good callus formation, the cast can be removed. Because shaft fractures of the radius and ulna in children have a significant rate of refracture,[129] they should be splinted for an additional period of time. Parents should be warned that forearm shaft fractures have the highest risk of refracture of any pediatric fracture, which can occur even 6 to 12 months after the original injury. Refractures were most common within 6 weeks of clearance and noted more commonly in fractures with more than 15 degrees of residual angulation, and in the middle third of the forearm (72%).[214] In addition, some studies have shown that splint wear following cast discontinuation does not appear to alter the refracture rate.[207]

Above-elbow casting with the elbow in extension has been suggested for some complete fractures of the middle and proximal thirds.[197,224] The supination moment exerted by the biceps has been shown to be diminished when the elbow is extended.[165] Walker and Rang[224] reported successful treatment of 13 middle- or proximal-third forearm shaft fractures with this method (some following failed flexed-elbow casting). They suggested that the "short fat forearms" of some young children prevented successful flexed-elbow casting.[224] Shaer et al.[197] also reported 20 children treated with this method and emphasized full supination of the forearm. Three of their patients required cast wedging, but at final follow-up, 19 of the 20 patients had excellent results.[197] One patient who was lost to follow-up for 6 months (presumably removing their own cast) did suffer "mild residual deformity."[197] Walker and Rang[224] recommended that benzoin be applied to the skin, in addition to creation of an adequate supracondylar mold, to further secure the cast. Casting the thumb in abduction with extra padding may prevent the cast from sliding. Turco[197] suggested that reduction should be obtained with horizontal traction applied to the extended upper extremity, followed by additional steps outlined in the table above. Based on published clinical results, concerns related to cast slippage and elbow stiffness appear to have been overstated.[197,224] The main drawback of this technique is its awkwardness as compared to flexed-elbow casting (Fig. 10-21).[224]

Figure 10-21. A forearm fracture lost position while treated in an above-elbow cast with elbow at standard 90-degree elbow flexion. At 3 weeks postinjury, the arm was remanipulated and placed in an above-elbow cast with elbow extended down to only 45 degrees of flexion, with three-point mold placed. The fracture healed anatomically.

Because radius and ulna shaft fractures have the highest rate of childhood refracture, casting is generally recommended for 6 to 8 weeks. This is followed with a forearm splint until all four cortices of each bone are healed and there is no transverse lucency at the site of the original fracture (complete healing).

Comminuted Fractures

Although comminuted forearm fractures are less common in children than in adults,[212] they do occur.[15,65,67,128,235] Comminuted fractures tend to occur in conjunction with high-energy injuries, such as open fractures.[147] Comminuted forearm fractures deserve special attention because they often require specially tailored treatment approaches. If satisfactory reduction cannot be achieved or maintained by closed methods, then other treatment alternatives should be considered.

One option is to accept some shortening; according to Price,[181] this may help maintain motion through interosseous membrane slackening. Shortening of more than 1 cm is unacceptable in either single- or both-bone comminuted patterns. Standard closed fracture treatment generally is unsuccessful when both bones are comminuted, and surgical stabilization may be necessary.[65] Bellemans and Lamoureux[15] reported intramedullary nailing of all comminuted forearm fractures in their pediatric series. Other reported fixation methods for comminuted forearm fractures in children include plate-and-screw devices,[65,67] flexible intramedullary nailing for single-bone comminution, and pins-and-plaster techniques.[222] Bone grafting is rarely if ever indicated in acute comminuted forearm features in children.

OPERATIVE TREATMENT OF DIAPHYSEAL RADIUS AND ULNA FRACTURES

Indications/Contraindications

Operative Treatment of Diaphyseal Radius and Ulna Fractures:
INDICATIONS AND CONTRAINDICATIONS

Indications

- High-risk fracture patterns in older children
- Acceptable alignment not attained via casting (using age-adjusted criteria)
- Open fractures with significant instability
- Status post compartment releases to facilitate wound care
- Floating elbow injury pattern

Contraindications

- Active infection
- Suspected malignancy requiring further workup including biopsy
- No detectable clinical deformity in young child

Duncan and Weiner[57] cited an "aggressive surgical mentality" as the reason for frequent operative treatment of pediatric forearm fractures, and Wilkins[229] expressed concern about "impetuous" surgeons who are too eager to operate. Cheng et al.[39] and Flynn et al.[66] documented a 10-fold and 7-fold increase in the rate of operative treatment of forearm shaft fractures in children, but it is unclear as to whether this increase in operative treatment has led to a commensurate improvement in clinical outcomes.

Operative treatment of radial and ulnar shaft fractures usually is reserved for open fractures, those associated with compartment syndrome, floating elbow injuries, and fractures that develop unacceptable displacement during nonoperative management. Residual angulation after closed treatment is much better tolerated by younger children than older adolescents and adults because of the increased remodeling potential in the younger age group.[75] As a consequence, adolescents are more likely to benefit from surgical treatment of their forearm fractures than are younger children. Although internal fixation is the standard of care for displaced forearm fractures in adults, the success of nonoperative methods and the complications associated with internal fixation have tempered enthusiasm for its routine application to pediatric forearm fractures. Compared to closed treatment methods, healing is slower after open reduction and internal fixation,[15] no matter what type of implant is used.[65] Crossed Kirschner wire (K-wire) fixation techniques that often are used successfully in the distal radius are technically difficult in the shaft region of the radius and ulna. In rare situations, external fixation has been used for pediatric forearm fixation, usually reserved for fractures with associated severe soft tissue injuries.

Preoperative planning is essential regardless of which surgical technique is chosen. Assessment of the fracture, including rotation and the presence or absence of comminution, is important. Bone-plate mismatch (because of narrow bones and wide plates) and extensive soft tissue dissection are risks when adult-sized plates are applied to pediatric bones. There fortunately are many size options of plates available if sufficient advanced planning is performed. Before intramedullary nailing of fractures, the forearm intramedullary canal diameter should be measured, especially at the narrowest canal dimension; typically this is the central portion of the radius[204] and the distal portion of the ulna near the junction of its middle and distal thirds. Precise canal measurement can be difficult, and the consequences of a nail or pin that is too large are probably worse than those of a nail or pin that is too small.[170,194] Modern digital radiography systems have made these measurements easier.[175]

Flexible Nail, Kirschner Wire, Rush Rod, and Steinmann Pin Intramedullary Fixation

Currently, intramedullary fixation is the preferred method for internal fixation of forearm fractures in children.[4,31,128,135,139,182,183] Intramedullary fixation of children's forearm fractures dates back at least to Fleischer's 1975 report in the German literature in which he called it "marrow wiring."[64] Closed intramedullary nailing (also known as indirect reduction and internal fixation) of diaphyseal forearm fractures in adolescents was later reported in the English literature by Ligier et al.,[137] Amit et al.,[4] and others.[18,132] A variety of implants have been used for forearm intramedullary nailing, including K-wires, Rush rods, and Steinmann pins. Continued favorable reports from around the world (e.g., England, Germany, New Zealand, Turkey, and the United States) have established intramedullary fixation as the surgical treatment of choice.[36,77,108,135,185]

Intramedullary fixation has several advantages over plate fixation, including improved aesthetics because of smaller incisions and less deep tissue dissection, potentially leading to a lower risk of stiffness.[46,128] Contoured pins are used in the radius to preserve its natural anatomic bow[4,46,182,185]; contoured pins are not necessary for the ulna.[4] Although the rotational stability of pediatric forearm fractures treated with intramedullary fixation has been questioned, Blasier and Salamon[18] suggested that the strong periosteum in children resists torsional stresses. In a cadaver study of the rotational stability of fractures of the ulna and radius treated with Rush rods, Ono et al.[174] found that intramedullary fixation of both bones reduced fracture rotation to one-eighth of that in unfixed fractures.

Elastic Stable Intramedullary Nailing

In the early 1980s, Metaizeau et al.[157] described elastic stable intramedullary nailing (ESIN) of pediatric forearm fractures with small-diameter (1.5–2.5 mm) contoured implants.[137] No effort was made to fill the medullary canal as with other intramedullary nailing techniques, and the "summit of the curve must be calculated preoperatively to lie at the level of the fracture."[132] The prebent flexible rods (known as Nancy nails) were reported to maintain satisfactory fracture alignment while encouraging development of normal physiologic fracture callus.[137,157] Biomechanically, these implants have been shown to act as internal splints provided the nails extend three or more diameters beyond the fracture site.[105] Good results with this technique have been reported by numerous authors (Fig. 10-22).[166,198,213]

Because the ESIN technique emphasizes the interdependence of the radius and ulna, if both bones are fractured, both bones are internally fixed.[132] It is also dependent on anchorage of the nails in the upper and lower metaphyseal portions of the bone to produce an internal three-point fixation construct.[132] Technique principles include fixing the radius first (if both bones need stabilization), using physeal-sparing entry points, and using small nails varying in diameter from 1.5 to 2.5 mm.[132] A nail that is too large may lead to nail incarceration and distraction at the fracture site, especially in the ulna.[170] Large nails may also increase the fixation rigidity, which may decrease the amount of callus formation, leading to delayed union and nonunion. Contouring of both nails is recommended, with particular attention to restoration of the appropriate radial bow (Fig. 10-23). Initially, nails were removed by about the fourth postoperative month, but several refractures led the originators of the technique to delay nail removal until 1 full year after surgery.[132] Pin ends should be cut short and buried to maintain prolonged fixation.

Immediate motion has been recommended by some authors after ESIN of pediatric forearm fractures,[15,132] whereas others have recommended immobilization for variable periods of time.[31] Early refracture with nails in place has been reported. Bellemans and Lamoureux[15] considered displaced oblique or comminuted midshaft forearm fractures in children older than 7 years of age to be an indication for ESIN. They considered bayonet apposition (overriding) to be unacceptable at any age because of concerns about rotational malalignment and frequent narrowing of the interosseous space.[15] Their fixation technique

Figure 10-22. A 10-year-old male whose both-bone complete forearm fracture near the junction of the middle and distal thirds was treated with elastic stable intramedullary nailing (ESIN). **A:** Injury radiographs demonstrating completely displaced radial and ulnar shaft fractures. **B:** Postreduction radiographs reveal unsatisfactory angular alignment as well as significant loss of radial bow. **C:** Anatomic appearance following ESIN. **D:** One-and-a-half-year follow-up radiographs. Nails were removed 6 months postoperatively. **E:** Clinical appearance with extended elbows and forearm midposition. **F:** Clinical appearance with extended elbows and pronated forearms. **G:** Clinical appearance with extended elbows and supinated forearms.

Figure 10-22. (*Continued*) **H:** Symmetrical pronation. **I:** Symmetrical supination.

involved passage of the intramedullary nails, followed by rotation of each nail until the greatest distance between the two bones was achieved in full supination.[15]

The two largest contemporary published series of ESIN-treated pediatric forearm shaft fracture patients come from Bochum, Germany and Nashville, Tennessee.[127,148] Together these studies comprise over 400 cases and thus offer insight into the application of this technique as well as complications. The average age of the patients in each of these two studies was 9.7 years of age, with a range of a bit less than 2 years of age to 16 years of age. Fourteen percent of the forearm shaft fractures were open fractures. Refracture rate and infection rate were both 3% for the combined cohort. Malunion, EPL injury, significant stiffness, and nerve injury were all less than 1%.

Single-bone fixation techniques for both-bone fractures have been reported. This involves fixation of a more unstable fracture, which is typically the radius, and closed treatment of the ulnar fracture. Based on previous data showing less risk of loss of forearm motion with ulnar shaft malunion, clinically acceptable results can be obtained using this technique. When performed, the first bone, which is usually the radius, is fixed using a flexible nail. The surgeon then checks the alignment of the ulnar fracture and assesses stability in both the frontal and lateral planes. If this bone is stable and amenable to immobilization, the surgery is completed. If there is instability, the surgeon can also perform fixation of the ulna. When compared to both-bone fixation, single-bone fixation has been shown to decrease operating room (OR) time and decrease costs associated with surgery, with similar radiographic and functional results.[122,238] Similarly, ulna-only fixation is possible as long as the radius remains stable after reduction of the angular and rotational deformity of the radius. In essence, single fixation converts a

Note 180-degree rotation
of radial Nancy nail

Figure 10-23. Metaizeau ESIN technique. The radial rod is twisted 180 degrees in step 4 to reestablish the radial bow.

both-bone complete fracture to an incomplete fracture equivalent of the bone not treated with fixation and allows the unfixed bone to be treated closed.[68] However, the authors advise caution with this approach, as malunion of the radius with ulna-only fixation (or ulna malunion with radius-only fixation) is possible if the nonfixed bone fracture reduction is unstable. In OR testing of stability under fluoroscopy is required, along with close follow-up to prevent a malunion that could lead to impairing loss of motion.

Plate Fixation

Open reduction and internal fixation of pediatric forearm shaft fractures with plates and screws is a well-documented procedure in both pediatric series[218] and adult series that include patients as young as 13 and even 7 years of age. In one of the early series of pediatric forearm fractures fixed with plates,[52] dynamic compression plates and one-third tubular plates applied with standard arbeitsgemeinshaft für osteosynthesefragen (AO) or Association for the Study of Internal Fixation (ASIF) technique (six cortices above and below the fracture site) obtained good results. Four-cortex fixation on either side of the fracture site has been shown to be equally effective in pediatric forearm fractures.[235]

Plate fixation uses the standard adult approach and technique except that smaller plates (2.7-mm compression and stacked one-third tubular), fewer screws, and single-bone fixation often are acceptable.[235] Plate fixation may allow more anatomic and stable correction of rotational and angular abnormalities and restoration of the radial bow than with noncontoured intramedullary rods; however, the larger incisions and extensive surgical exposures required for plate fixation have raised concerns regarding unsightly scars[218] and muscle fibrosis with consequent motion loss.[235] Although the aesthetic concerns seem valid, ultimate forearm motion is similar with the two techniques, with only minor losses reported in the literature after both plating and intramedullary nailing.[46] Fernandez et al.[61] recently documented these precise issues very nicely in that they found no significant differences in functional outcome in their plate fixation versus intramedullary nailing patients, but they noted the longer OR time and inferior appearance of the plated patients' scars.

Open reduction and internal fixation with plates and screws may be appropriate in the management of fractures with delayed presentation or fractures that angulate late in the course of cast care,[235] when significant fracture callus makes closed reduction and percutaneous passage of intramedullary nails difficult or impossible. Other indications for plate fixation include shaft fractures with significant comminution[65] and impending or established malunion[216] or nonunion.[89,136,170] Several authors have reported good results with plate fixation of the radius only[68] or the ulna only (Fig. 10-24).[16] Bhaskar and Roberts[16] compared 20 children with both-bone plate fixation to 12 with ulna-only fixation and found significantly more complications in the dual plating group, although motion was equal at 1-year follow-up. Single-bone fixation requires satisfactory reduction of both bones. Stabilization of one bone, usually the ulna, allows rotation reduction of the other bone with intact periosteum acting as a tension band to maintain reduction. Flynn and Waters[68]

stated that they usually performed intramedullary fixation of the ulna and manipulative reduction of the radius. However, when the radius is not reducible, it is usually due to interposed extensor muscle. In these less common cases, they preferentially plated the radius only when the fracture. Two patients in Bhaskar and Roberts'[16] study required open reduction and internal fixation of the radius when it was not adequately reduced after plate fixation of the ulna.

MANAGEMENT OF OPEN FRACTURES OF DIAPHYSEAL RADIUS AND ULNA FRACTURES

In one large epidemiologic study, open fractures of the shafts of the radius and ulna and open tibial shaft fractures occurred with equal frequency, making them the most common open fractures in children.[39] Although the infection rate is extremely low for open fractures, even grade I open forearm fractures in children have been associated with serious complications such as gas gangrene. Early irrigation and debridement[202] are indicated for open forearm fractures, and care should be taken to inspect and properly clean the bone ends. Both of the bone ends should be routinely inspected for the presence of intramedullary foreign material (Fig. 10-25). Once debrided, open forearm fractures can be stabilized by any of the available internal fixation methods without undue risk of infection (Fig. 10-26).[88,140] Open fractures tend to be more unstable than closed fractures (because of soft tissue stripping and comminution) and more commonly require internal fixation. Internal fixation also may facilitate soft tissue management and healing.[235] Lim et al.[138] from the KK Children's Hospital in Singapore recently reminded us that internal fixation is not an absolute prerequisite and many children with such open fractures may still be successfully managed with casting alone.

The amount of periosteal stripping and possible foreign body reaction associated with open forearm fractures may produce an unusual radiographic appearance: the "ruffled border sign" (Fig. 10-27). Usually, this seems to represent a normal healing response in growing children, but occasionally it is an early sign of osteomyelitis. The infection rate ranges from 0% to 33% for open fractures in children.[46,88,140,169,181,235] Even grade I open forearm fractures in children can be complicated by gas gangrene or osteomyelitis, and therapeutic amputation has been reported.[50] Open fracture grade does not appear to correlate with the infection rate in childhood forearm fractures, with most of the serious forearm infections reported in the literature occurring after grade I fractures.

Some centers in the United States have evaluated emergency department–based treatment of grade I open fractures of the forearm, wrist, and tibia in children and concluded that there was no significant difference in infection rates.[80] We would strike a strong note of caution regarding this treatment approach for two main reasons. First, existing studies appear to be at high risk of being underpowered (one infection occurred in the Godfrey et al. study and it was in the emergency department treatment group). Second, there is a dramatic difference in the nature of the two treatment approaches in that one involves formal surgical exposure and comprehensive visualization and

Figure 10-24. Single-bone plate fixation (radius only). **A:** A 12-year-old female with both-bone forearm fracture (AP and lateral). **B:** Immediate postoperative images. **C:** Two-year follow-up images. (Courtesy of Tom Welle, DO.)

Figure 10-25. Intramedullary organic soil contamination from open forearm fracture with benign-appearing skin laceration.

A   **B**

Figure 10-26. A 13-year-old girl with open forearm fracture. **A:** AP and lateral radiographs; note extrusion of ulna on lateral view. **B:** After irrigation and debridement and flexible nail internal fixation. Note the Penrose drain in the ulnar wound.

Figure 10-27. Ruffled border sign at the site of previous open fracture of ulna.

cleansing of the bone ends, while the other might be characterized as rinsing the skin. The risk to the child of a limb- or life-threatening infection is juxtaposed to unnecessary resource utilization.

Fracture Reduction/Conscious Sedation Protocol

Significantly displaced forearm shaft fractures are usually manipulated in the emergency department using a conscious sedation (also known as deep sedation) protocol. After obtaining informed consent for conscious sedation and fracture manipulation, an IV line is started, and the child's blood pressure, pulse, respirations, electrocardiogram, and peripheral oxygen level are monitored during the procedure and for about 30 minutes after the procedure. We use ketamine/atropine or fentanyl/midazolam administered intravenously in divided doses. Although many children moan or cry briefly during the manipulation, very few recall pain. Two recent reports have drawn attention to ketamine-related concerns. Perez-Garcia et al. reported the disturbing complication of severe hypertension in a 12 year old who had undiagnosed coarctation of the aorta, and Kinder et al. found that children with a high body mass index were at greater risk for nausea and vomiting.[123,176] Reductions are done under mini–C-arm (fluoroscopy) control. The initial position of forearm rotation is based on the level of the fracture, and the final position is based on the best reduction under fluoroscopy. Small portable fluoroscopy units improve the quality of the reduction, decrease the radiation exposure to the patient, and decrease the need for repeat fracture reduction and save time.[69] The level of experience of the physician correlates to the level of radiation exposure risk to the patient and health professionals involved in reduction. Finger-trap traction with 10 to 15 lb of counterweight frequently is used for completely displaced both-bone forearm shaft fractures (especially those with shortening). We do not complete greenstick fractures because the partial bone continuity adds stability.

Because of concerns about soft tissue swelling, we place nonmanipulated and manipulated fractures into a plaster sugar-tong splint (incorporating the elbow). We avoid the circumferential wrapping of the arm with cast padding by using a "sandwich splint" technique. Before manipulation, the sugar-tong splint is prepared by laying out 7 to 10 layers of appropriate-length 3-inch plaster casting material on top of a work surface. A four-layer matched length of cotton cast padding also is laid out and will form the inner padding (skin side) of the splint. A final single layer of cast padding is laid out and will form the outer layer of the splint to prevent elastic wrap adherence to the plaster. Once manipulation is completed, the plaster is dipped, wrung out, smoothed, and then sandwiched between the dry four- and one-ply cotton padding. This splint is then placed with the four-ply cotton side against the skin and secured with an elastic bandage (ace wrap). We prefer to avoid the circumferential application of cotton padding because it may limit splint expansion during follow-up swelling. If necessary, parents also can unwrap and loosen the elastic bandage at home to relieve pressure if swelling makes the splint bandage too tight. Patients are advised to use recommended nonsteroidal antiinflammatory drugs (NSAIDs) and acetaminophen and are rarely given a prescription for mild narcotic analgesics. Discharge instructions should be included to call back or return to the emergency room for pain not relieved by the pain medicine. With the continuing opioid abuse epidemic, there is a current trend to decrease opioid prescriptions after fracture treatment in the emergency room[124,231,234] and after operative fracture care.[82,115,231] Most children are prescribed more opioid doses than they use after fracture treatment. Decreasing or eliminating postfracture opioids does not cause an increase in discomfort or with return to the provider for opioid medications. Discharge prescription or over-the-counter NSAIDs and acetaminophen seem to be as effective as opioids after fracture reduction and immobilization. A disturbing study showed that adolescents who were legally prescribed opioids had had a 33% increased risk of nonlegal opioid abuse in the years right after high school as compared to adolescents who were never exposed to legal opioids.[158]

Patients usually return to the office within a week for repeat radiographs and clinical assessment. Provided that satisfactory alignment has been maintained, we remove the elastic wrap but leave the plaster sugar-tong splint in place. Nonmanipulated fractures can be converted to a conventional or waterproof cast on the first visit if it is more than 48 hours after the injury, but manipulated fractures that maintain good position are usually overwrapped with fiberglass for at least a week before converting to the definitive cast. The splint is "boxed

in" by applying cotton cast padding over the splint and the exposed upper arm, and by wrapping with fiberglass to convert the splint into an above-elbow cast. Follow-up radiographs are taken of manipulated fractures at about 1-week intervals for the next 2 weeks. Fractures that are losing position but are still in acceptable alignment usually require removal and remolding of a new cast to prevent further position deterioration in the upcoming week. Fractures that show increasing displacement at the initial follow-up visits can continue to angulate up until 4 to 5 weeks postinjury. Minor remanipulations can be done in the office after appropriate administration of oral analgesics and anxiolytics. Major remanipulations are best done with general anesthesia. The decision regarding the need for remanipulation may be tipped by viewing the arm position by the parents and physician after all splint and cast materials are removed. Aside from remanipulation and continued closed treatment, some fractures with loss of reduction into an unacceptable alignment will benefit from conversion to operative fixation.

Conversion from an above-elbow to a below-elbow cast at 3 to 4 weeks postinjury is not common in adults. This step may be omitted in younger children because of their faster healing and their minimal inconvenience from temporary elbow immobilization.[117] Patients who are converted to a short arm cast can return to sports as long as the cast is padded during play and league rules allow protected casts. Patients usually are required to have a physician's note allowing sports participation with a cast. This decision is made with the patient's and parents' understanding of potential increase in refracture risk and/or loss of acceptable alignment with sports play. The cast is removed at about 6 to 8 weeks after treatment, provided there is adequate callus formation. Most patients are given a Velcro brace or a customized thermoplastic forearm gauntlet brace to wear during daytime activity and sports if indicated until there is complete radiographic fracture healing (4/4 cortices completely healed and no transverse shaft lucency). Unfortunately, slow union may necessitate bracing for several months and even for a year, even for high-risk activities. Older children are given home elastic band strengthening exercises and allowed to participate in normal activities but formal physical therapy rarely is required. This fracture protocol is aimed at minimizing refracture risk.

Acceptable Limits of Angulation

Based on available evidence in the literature, we accept approximately 20 degrees of angulation in distal-third shaft fractures of the radius and ulna, 15 degrees at the midshaft level, and 10 degrees in the proximal third (for girls <8 years old and boys <10 years old). We accept 100% translation if shortening is less than 1 cm. Although other authors recommend accepting up to 45 degrees of rotation, we find this extremely difficult to measure accurately using the bicipital tuberosity and radial styloid as landmarks because of the lack of anatomic distinction in younger children. Plastic deformation fractures seem to have less remodeling potential than other fractures, and radiographically or aesthetically unacceptable angulation

Figure 10-28. Ulnar sag on serial radiographs. Note the prominent ulna fracture callus.

may require gradual, forceful manipulation under sedation or general anesthesia. Children approaching skeletal maturity (<2 years of remaining growth) should be treated using adult criteria because of their reduced remodeling potential. Parents should be cautioned that even mild angulation of the ulna, especially posterior sag, will produce an obvious deformity after cast removal because of the subcutaneous location of the bone (Fig. 10-28). This aesthetic deformity is exacerbated by abundant callus formation, but it will ultimately remodel if it falls within acceptable angulation criteria. Ulnar sag may be countered by remanipulation and placing the child in an extended elbow cast or with intramedullary fixation. Mild to moderate angulation of the radius usually produces much less aesthetic deformity but may limit motion more (Fig. 10-29). Even under the best care, some fractures will inadvertently lose position and show an early healing with unacceptable angulation. In this situation, the surgeon must decide if early osteotomy is indicated. If the child has greater than 2 years of growth remaining, watchful waiting is an option, with a delayed osteotomy if substantial loss of motion or unsightly angulation persists after a year. Proximal fracture malunions with apex ulnar deformity are more concerning for needing earlier intervention.

SURGICAL REPAIR OF DIAPHYSEAL RADIUS AND ULNA FRACTURES

Most forearm shaft fractures continue to be successfully treated with closed methods at our institution. Our top two indications

Figure 10-29. A 7-year-old girl with left both–bone complete forearm fracture. **A:** AP and lateral injury radiographs. **B:** Two-month follow-up radiographs.

Figure 10-29. (*Continued*) **C:** Two-year follow-up radiograph shows mild residual deformity. **D:** Pronation.
E: Supination. **F:** Five-year follow-up radiographs of left forearm with mild loss of radial bow.

(*continues*)

Figure 10-29. (*Continued*) **G:** Axial alignment at 2-year follow-up. **H:** Comparison radiographs of right forearm. **I:** Pronation. **J:** Supination. **K:** Axial alignment at 5-year follow-up.

for surgical treatment of these injuries are open shaft fractures and shaft fractures that exceed our stated reduction limits. If surgical treatment is deemed necessary, intramedullary fixation is preferred over plate fixation because of reduced soft tissue disruption. We occasionally fix one bone when both bones are fractured if overall forearm alignment is acceptable and stable after single-bone fixation.

Intramedullary Nailing

Preoperative Planning

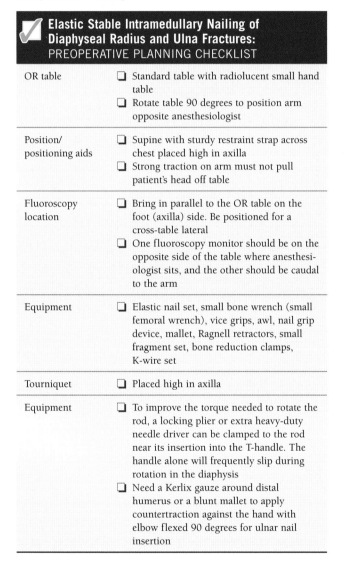

Elastic Stable Intramedullary Nailing of Diaphyseal Radius and Ulna Fractures:
PREOPERATIVE PLANNING CHECKLIST

OR table	❑ Standard table with radiolucent small hand table
	❑ Rotate table 90 degrees to position arm opposite anesthesiologist
Position/ positioning aids	❑ Supine with sturdy restraint strap across chest placed high in axilla
	❑ Strong traction on arm must not pull patient's head off table
Fluoroscopy location	❑ Bring in parallel to the OR table on the foot (axilla) side. Be positioned for a cross-table lateral
	❑ One fluoroscopy monitor should be on the opposite side of the table where anesthesiologist sits, and the other should be caudal to the arm
Equipment	❑ Elastic nail set, small bone wrench (small femoral wrench), vice grips, awl, nail grip device, mallet, Ragnell retractors, small fragment set, bone reduction clamps, K-wire set
Tourniquet	❑ Placed high in axilla
Equipment	❑ To improve the torque needed to rotate the rod, a locking plier or extra heavy-duty needle driver can be clamped to the rod near its insertion into the T-handle. The handle alone will frequently slip during rotation in the diaphysis
	❑ Need a Kerlix gauze around distal humerus or a blunt mallet to apply countertraction against the hand with elbow flexed 90 degrees for ulnar nail insertion

Positioning

The patient is positioned supine with the arm abducted 90 degrees on a hand table. A wide sturdy strap is placed in the axilla to allow traction without pulling the patient off the table. Traction helps to gain length of overriding fracture ends and allows the bones to seek their normal rotation.

Technique

Intramedullary Nailing of Diaphyseal Radius and Ulna Fractures:
KEY SURGICAL STEPS

- Expose the radius first with a 1–2-cm incision, just proximal to the Lister tubercle between the second and third tendon compartments. Alternatively, perform a styloid approach through the first dorsal compartment just proximal to the physis.
- Avoid major branches of the superficial radial nerve and retract the tendons to expose bone surface to avoid damage.
- Use an awl to create a start window between the APL/EPB and ECRL/B tendons for styloid approach (we feel this is superior to and safer than motorized drill techniques).
- Forcibly tighten the T-handle on the rod and insert the rod by hand with an oscillating twist motion.
- Pull traction on arm against the axillary strap.
- Use mallet to advance nail to fracture site if not possible by hand maneuvers. If rod fails to advance, the tip could be stuck in a rut. Tap the rod 5 mm backward; rotate the tip, then advance down the shaft again to the fracture.
- Pull heavy traction on the hand, manipulate the fracture, and use the small bone wrench to align the bone ends. If you miss, pull the nail back, rotate the rod 90 degrees, reattempt to pass, and repeat.
- If the fracture ends remain 100% translated despite manipulation, try the "shoehorn" K-wire technique before opening.
- If you have to open, make a 3–4-cm incision, grip the bone ends with small reduction clamps, and hold reduced while assistant passes nail. Use the volar (Henry) approach to open, carefully avoiding the PIN.
- Only advance the radius nail 1 cm past the fracture so it is just "perched." Full insertion will make it nearly impossible to reduce the ulna fracture next.
- Start the ulna about 3 cm distal to the olecranon tip about 4 mm lateral to the posterior crest. Palpate the radial head and stay clear of it. The starting incision can be 3–4 mm long and made percutaneously.
- Advance the nail with an oscillating twist technique to the fracture. With the radius rod just perched across the fracture by 1 cm, the ulna can be freely manipulated to ease nail passage across the ulna fracture.
- Insert nail about 1 cm short of the distal ulna physis to leave room for final impaction.
- Remove the T-handle, put about a 45-degree bend in the rod just as it enters the bone. Do not lever the rod against the bone because it will plough or fracture through the metaphyseal bone.
- Cut the nail as close to the bone as possible, then finally impact the nail so only 3-mm sticks out of the bone for purchase during removal.
- Rotate the radial rod so that the bow in the nail follows the natural bow of the radius. Leave 1 cm short of the end of the bone to allow for final impaction after cutting the rod similar to the ulna.

Our preferred intramedullary ulnar entry site is 2.5 cm distal to the olecranon tip (we prefer not to enter through the apophysis although many surgeons do), through the anconeus fossa just anterior to the subcutaneous crest of the proximal ulna on its lateral side. Care is taken not to enter the ulna more than 5 mm anterior to its subcutaneous crest to avoid encroachment into the region of the PRUJ. Pins placed directly through the tip of the olecranon apophysis can cause bursitis and pain until removal if left subcutaneous (that is why apophyseal entry surgeons usually leave the rods exterior and remove them soon after fracture healing). We prefer to open the cortex with an awl because it tends to wander less than motorized drills and it allows ulnar entry with little or no formal dissection through the thin anconeus muscle. The awl technique also simplifies OR setup in that no powered instrument hookups are necessary.

If dual-bone fixation is elected, the radius is almost always fixed first as it is usually more difficult to reduce, and it is also more difficult to approach with an open reduction than the ulna. If the ulna is fixed first, it will limit forearm mobility and make it more difficult to manipulate the radius and pass the nail, which forces a riskier, more complex open reduction on the radius deeply enveloped in muscle and critical neurovascular structures. Optimizing the closed rodding of the radius by fixing it first makes the ulna reduction a little more difficult, but open reduction of the ulna is often simpler than an open reduction of the radius fracture at any fracture level. We recommend the distal radial entry site in the lateral radial styloid be done through a physeal-sparing direct lateral approach through the floor of the first dorsal compartment. The tendons should be visualized, retracted, and the bone surface clearly exposed to avoid harpooning a tendon with the starting awl. This approach harbors less complications than the approach just proximal to Lister tubercle, which puts the EPL tendon at risk of rupture.[164] However, this risk can be lessened by careful surgical technique, ensuring the nail is placed in the bare area just proximal to the Lister tubercle, and keeping the nail tip bent 90 degrees from the shaft and cut off above the fascia, but below skin level. EPL ruptures, if they occur, can be treated with grafting or EIP tendon transfer. Radial sensory nerve complications from a first compartment approach are difficult to fully resolve. To protect against this risk, we insert the radial nail through a 1- to 2-cm incision, protecting the superficial radial nerve and the dorsal tendons with small blunt retractors. An awl is used to gain intramedullary access to the radius. We typically use small intramedullary nails (2–2.5 mm in diameter) to maintain some flexibility at the fracture site and stimulate appropriate callus formation. Larger nails may become incarcerated in either the narrow central canal of the radius or the distal third of the ulna and their rigidity may promote delayed or nonunion. Unbending the tip of the elastic nail minimizes the diameter of the implant and will ease its intramedullary passage. If the rod gets stuck, the hooked tip often needs to be backslapped out of a cortical rut and rotated slightly before proceeding forward (Fig. 10-30). False passage out of the cortex is to be avoided.

Backing the rod up 5 mm and rotating it away from the rut will ease passage down the shaft isthmus. If the nail fails to engage the shaft on the other side of the fracture, tap it back to the fracture, rotate it 90 to 180 degrees, and then retry. A "shoehorn" technique can be used to percutaneously align the fracture. A 2-mm K-wire is placed into the fracture between the

Figure 10-30. This illustrates the "rod rut" incurred during a femur Nancy nail insertion. This can happen in any IM rodding including radius and ulna. In the **left** figure, the tip of the rod has dug a rut in the cortex and is stuck. It was backed up 5 mm, leaving behind a visible rut. The rod was twisted 90 degrees and then passed up the shaft freely.

two ends of the translated bone. It is then levered to allow the bone ends to translate into alignment. With the K-wire lever in place, pass the nail across the fracture (Fig. 10-31).

Failure to pass the intramedullary nail across the fracture site after several attempts may necessitate a limited open reduction with at least a 2-cm incision to directly pass the rod across the fracture site (Fig. 10-32). Because of the thick soft tissue envelope, an open approach to the radius may need to be twice this long. Placing bone clamps on both sides of the fracture allows bone alignment control than trying to push the bone ends into place with a finger. Persistence in attempting to achieve closed reduction and rodding has been associated with compartment syndrome.[241] We are sensitive to both time and attempts during ESIN of forearm shaft fractures in our pediatric patients and recommend surgeons abandon prolonged attempts at reduction and fixation closed, and recommend relatively rapid conversion to a small open reduction if needed.

If single-bone fixation is contemplated, the more displaced bone is usually treated first. If the other bone remains minimally displaced and is grossly stable to manipulation, then single bone fixation may work. Weekly follow-up is recommended for the unfixed bone after single-bone fixation due to the higher risk of position loss than with both-bone fixation. Plating is preferred to intramedullary nailing when early malunion is present and callus formation is noted radiographically. Plating allows open osteoclasis and reduction. The plating technique is similar to that used in adults, except that smaller plates (2.7 mm vs. 3.5 mm) can be used and fewer cortices such as only four cortices above and below the fracture are required for adequate fixation. In children with both-bone forearm fractures, plating of a single bone may be adequate and reduce the morbidity associated with dual-bone plating.[16] This is more often with the radius fracture due to muscle interposition preventing anatomic reduction. Significant comminution of both bones also may be an indication for plate fixation.

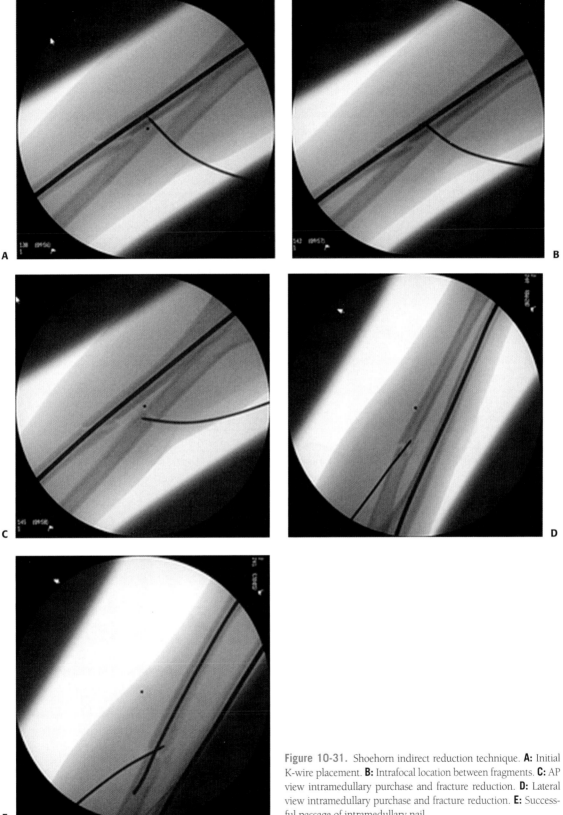

Figure 10-31. Shoehorn indirect reduction technique. **A:** Initial K-wire placement. **B:** Intrafocal location between fragments. **C:** AP view intramedullary purchase and fracture reduction. **D:** Lateral view intramedullary purchase and fracture reduction. **E:** Successful passage of intramedullary nail.

A

Figure 10-32. A 12-year-old girl with midshaft both bone complete forearm fracture. **A:** AP and lateral injury radiographs. **B:** Two-month follow-up radiographs. **C:** Six-month follow-up radiographs (ulnar nail removed). **D:** Pronation. **E:** Supination. **F:** Axial alignment.

B   C

D, E   F

Potential Pitfalls and Preventive Measures

Intramedullary Nailing of Diaphyseal Radius and Ulna Fractures:
KEY SURGICAL STEPS

Pitfall	Prevention
Refracture	• Keep elastic nails in place for nearly a year if there are no hardware irritation problems. Splint or cast for at least 6–8 weeks after elastic nailing to avoid early refracture. Splint during activity until achieving complete cortical healing and the disappearance of any transverse lucency
Delayed union	• Use the smallest nail that will pass to allow callus formation (1.75–2.5 mm) • Use a plate instead of a nail after skeletal maturity
Infection	• Wash out all open fractures, especially if they occur on organic surface (soccer field, fall from tree, dirt bike). Beware of the "lawn biopsy" in which a dirt clod can get stuck in the intramedullary canal in even a small grade 1 open fracture on an organic surface. Deliver, inspect, and curette the penetrating end of open organic surface fractures. A bloody dirt core is usually camouflaged as intramedullary bone marrow and can be deceptively easy to miss
Nail incarceration in canal	• Back up out of rut, rotate nail, then advance down canal. Keep rotating the nail as you advance the nail in the shaft. Change to a smaller nail if needed
Difficult nail passage across fracture	• Use a percutaneous K-wire to lever the ends of the fracture into alignment. Use a small radiolucent bone wrench to manipulate fracture during rod passage
Muscle/tendon entrapment or rupture	• Make sure that elastic nail does not rub on or impale EPL tendon. Open fracture sites that are not reducible
Neurapraxia	• Most will resolve spontaneously if noted prereduction. Fix radius first to minimize need to open which could injure PIN. Identify or avoid PIN during open reduction. Be certain ulnar nerve is not entrapped
Compartment syndrome	• During elastic nailing, perform an open reduction if nail does not pass after multiple attempts (20–30 minutes). Perform fasciotomy in any patient who has increasing anxiety, analgesia requirements, and apprehension postoperative. Prophylactic fasciotomies at time of nailing are often performed to lessen risk
Complex regional pain syndrome	• Early recognition and referral to physical therapy or pain service for treatment. Be certain there is not a nerve entrapment as underlying cause
Prominent/ penetrating rod end	• After full insertion, back out rod about 1 cm, cut rod, then final tamp into place to leave rod about 3 mm outside bone surface

MANAGEMENT OF EXPECTED ADVERSE OUTCOMES AND UNEXPECTED COMPLICATIONS IN DIAPHYSEAL RADIUS AND ULNA FRACTURES

Diaphyseal Radius and Ulna Fractures:
COMMON ADVERSE OUTCOMES AND COMPLICATIONS

• Malunion
• Delayed union or nonunion
• Stiffness
• Refracture
• Nail prominence with irritation/skin penetration
• Compartment syndrome

REDISPLACEMENT/MALALIGNMENT IN DIAPHYSEAL RADIUS AND ULNA FRACTURES

The most common short-term complication of forearm shaft fracture treatment is loss of satisfactory reduction in a previously well-reduced and well-aligned fracture, a complication that occurs in 10%[50,107,222] to 25% of patients.[50] Initial follow-up radiographs are a screening test aimed at identifying redisplacement. Kramhøft and Solgaard[125] recommended that children with displaced diaphyseal forearm fractures have screening radiography at 1 and 2 weeks after reduction. Voto also pointed out that most fractures that redisplace do so within the first 2 weeks after injury. However, if there is even slight change of position between successive weekly visits, angulation can increase for up to 4 weeks postinjury.[26] During early forearm fracture follow-up, it is important to look at the sequence of all postinjury alignment images, and not just the current images, to detect small changes in position that forebode unacceptable position loss. Inability to properly control fracture alignment with closed methods is the most commonly reported indication for operative intervention.[135,182,241]

The most common explanations for loss of fracture reduction are cast related (poor casting technique, no evidence of three-point molding).[40,222] The more experienced the surgeon, the greater the likelihood of successful reduction. Other factors that have been found to be associated with forearm fracture redisplacement are quality of initial reduction,[240] missed follow-up appointments,[43] proximal third fractures,[45,223,230] and failure of the doctor to respond to early warning signs such as slight loss of reduction at 1-week follow-up. Strategies for dealing with redisplacement include allowing the deformity to remodel,[96] cast wedging,[11] rereduction and recasting,[50,222] indirect reduction and internal fixation,[4] and open reduction and internal fixation.[235] Reports in the literature suggest that most forearm shaft fractures that redisplace can be successfully managed with repeat closed reduction and casting.[50,222] In addition, acute fracture displacement with injury has been shown to be predictive of fracture instability and difficulty with closed treatment.[230]

FOREARM STIFFNESS IN DIAPHYSEAL RADIUS AND ULNA FRACTURES

The forearm is a predominantly nonsynovial joint with high-amplitude motion as its main function. Sardelli et al.[192] have shown that common ADLs require nearly 75 degrees of pronation and 90 degrees of supination. The needs for forearm motion in ADLs may be changing with ever-increasing keyboard and cellphone usage. The most common long-term complication of forearm shaft fracture treatment is significant forearm stiffness,[96] with pronation loss occurring almost twice as frequently as supination loss.[97] Loss of pronation or supination motion sometimes occurs despite perfectly normal-appearing radiographs.[181] Abnormal bony alignment of the forearm bones can lead to motion deficits.[112] However, stiffness can exceed that expected from bony malalignment alone[112] and stiffness can occur with normal radiographs and both situations may be indicative of fibrosis of the interosseous membrane and/or contracture of the interosseous ligament.[181]

With focused testing of forearm motion, between 18%[33] and 72%[97] of patients show at least some minor deficits after nonsurgical treatment. Most minor deficits are not even noticed by patients and rarely are associated with functional limitations.[33] More severe losses of forearm rotation have far greater impact.[160] In their series of malunited forearm fractures (thus strongly weighted to demonstrate forearm stiffness), Price et al.[181] reported a 15% (6/39) rate of mild stiffness (up to 25-degree loss) and an 8% (3/39) rate of severe forearm stiffness (loss of 45 degrees or more of either pronation or supination). Holdsworth's series of malunited pediatric forearm fractures had a similar rate (6%) of severe forearm stiffness. Holdsworth[97] told the classic story of a female whose inability to properly pronate caused her to elbow her neighbors when eating at the table. It is possible to compensate for pronation losses with shoulder abduction, but no similar compensation mechanism exists for supination losses. Such severe motion loss is a very undesirable outcome.

Bhaskar and Roberts[16] published one of the only studies of plated pediatric forearm fractures to report goniometric pronation and supination data. Both their single-bone (ulna) and both-bone plated patients showed mild forearm motion losses (maximal 18% loss of pronation).[16] Variable rates of mild forearm range-of-motion losses have been reported after intramedullary fixation. Amit et al.[4] reported a 40% rate of mild stiffness (5–10 degrees) in 20 pediatric patients after Rush rod fixation of forearm fractures. Combined data from five series of the flexible intramedullary nailing (K-wires, Steinmann pins, Nancy nails) revealed a 1.6% rate (2/128) of mild forearm stiffness (up to a 20-degree loss) and a 0% (0/128) rate of severe motion loss (40 degrees or more loss of either pronation or supination).[4,15,128,242]

REFRACTURE IN DIAPHYSEAL RADIUS AND ULNA FRACTURES

Refracture occurs more often after forearm shaft fractures in children than after any other fracture.[129] Tredwell et al.[215] found that forearm refractures occurred at an average of 6 months after

original injury and were more common in males (3:1) and in older children (approximately 12 years old). Baitner and his San Diego colleagues suggested that middle- and proximal-third forearm shaft fractures created a higher risk of refracture for pediatric patients.[10] Refracture rates of 4% to 8%[207,214] have been reported in pediatric diaphyseal forearm fractures. Bould and Bannister[25] reported that diaphyseal forearm fractures were eight times more likely to refracture than metaphyseal fractures. Schwarz et al.[195] found that 84% (21/28) of the forearm refractures in their series had initially presented as greenstick fractures. Based on the stage of bony healing, refractures may occur through the original fracture site, through both the original site and partially through intact bone or completely through intact bone, but most seem to occur through the original fracture site.

Several authors have suggested that internal fixation is necessary after refracture,[179] but Schwarz et al.[195] reported good results with repeat closed reduction and casting in 14 of 17 patients with refractures. Closed reduction of the fracture and the bent rods has been shown to be effective for forearm refractures that occur with flexible nails in place (Fig. 10-33).[163] The best treatment of refracture is prevention, and patients should be splint protected (removable forearm splint or thermoplastic gauntlet) for up to 6 months depending on the activity after initial bone healing.[169,181,109] Refracture is rare during splint wear. However, two recent articles have challenged the effectiveness of prolonged post–forearm fracture bracing.[13,207] Parents must be cautioned about the risk of refracture for up to 12 months postinjury despite apparently adequate bone healing on radiographs.

Refracture after plate removal has been discussed frequently in the literature[65] and appears to be associated with decreased bone density beneath the plate.[120] This has led many authors to question the routine use of plate fixation for pediatric forearm fractures.[18,43] Refractures also have been reported after removal of intramedullary forearm fixation in children.[46,132] The main strategies aimed at decreasing the risk of refractures after implant removal are documentation of adequate bony healing before implant removal, delaying implant removal until a year postinjury, and an additional period of splint protection after implant removal.

MALUNION IN DIAPHYSEAL RADIUS AND ULNA FRACTURES

Evaluation of pediatric forearm fracture malunion must take into account established malreduction limits and expected pediatric remodeling potential. Thus, a malunion of 30 degrees may become less than 10 degrees during the course of follow-up. The level of the malunited fracture also must be considered, because the consequences of malreduction vary according to level.[193] More deformity in the predominant plane of motion is acceptable in fractures near physes of long bones than in diaphyseal fractures. Normal motion can be preserved despite persistent radiographic abnormality (Fig. 10-34).

Malunion of radial and ulnar shaft fractures can lead to an aesthetic deformity and loss of motion; however, significant loss of function occurs in a small percentage of patients.[33] Some

Figure 10-33. A 14-year-old ESIN patient who suffered refracture with the nails in place. **A:** Injury AP radiograph. **B:** Injury lateral radiograph. Skateboard mechanism. **C:** Early postoperative radiograph status post ESIN. **D:** Two-month postoperative AP radiograph. **E:** Two-month postoperative lateral radiograph. **F:** Refracture at 2.5 months postoperatively.

(continues)

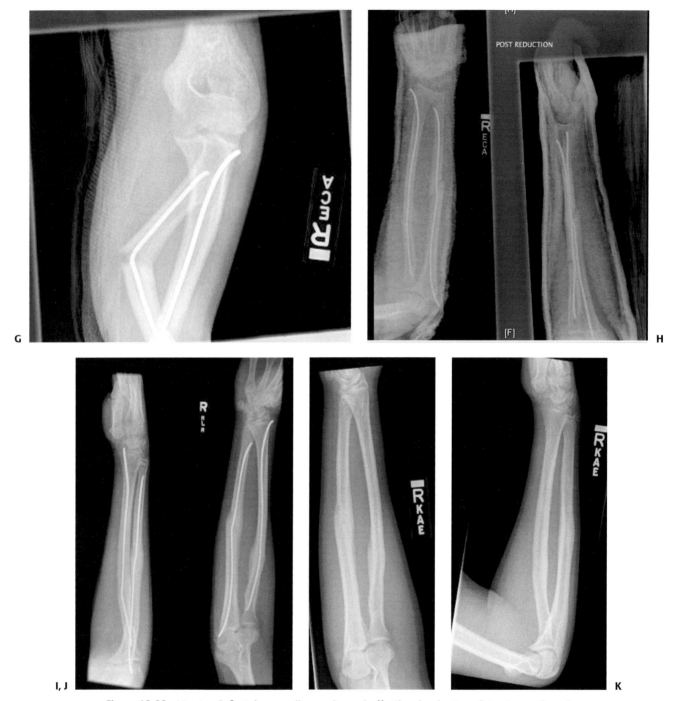

Figure 10-33. (*Continued*) **G:** Refracture elbow radiograph. **H:** Closed reduction of titanium nails and angulated radius and ulna fractures. **I:** Five months after refracture. **J:** AP radiograph 1 year after refracture. **K:** Lateral radiograph 1 year after refracture.

authors have recommended more aggressive efforts at correction of forearm fracture malunions.[155,180] Early malunions (up to 4 or 5 weeks after injury) can be treated with closed osteoclasis under anesthesia. If closed osteoclasis fails to adequately mobilize the fracture, a minimally invasive drill osteoclasis can be done. A small-diameter drill (or K-wire) is used to make multiple holes in the region of the malunion before forcefully

manipulating the bone back into alignment. Internal fixation is rarely needed if osteoclasis is performed in a timely fashion.

Once significant callus is present, indirect reduction and internal fixation with flexible intramedullary nails can be difficult or impossible because the intramedullary fracture site is now blocked with callus. Thus, established or impending malunions that cannot be adequately reduced closed and controlled

L, M   N

O   P

Figure 10-33. (*Continued*) **L:** Clinical appearance with extended elbows and forearm midposition. **M:** Clinical appearance with extended elbows and pronated forearms. **N:** Clinical appearance with extended elbows and supinated forearms. Note mild supination loss on right. **O:** Symmetrical pronation. **P:** Asymmetrical supination. Approximately 15-degree loss on right.

A   B

Figure 10-34. An 11-year-old with midshaft both-bone complete forearm fracture. **A:** AP and lateral injury radiographs. **B:** One-month follow-up radiographs.

(*continues*)

Figure 10-34. (*Continued*) **C:** Two-year follow-up radiographs. **D:** Pronation. **E:** Supination. **F:** Axial alignment. **G:** Six-year follow-up radiographs with substantial remodeling of radius and ulna fractures.

with a cast may require formal open reduction and plate fixation (Figs. 10-35 and 10-36). Many fractures that heal with angulation or rotation of more than the established criteria regain full motion and have an excellent cosmetic outcome. Fractures may require corrective osteotomy if they fail to remodel after an adequate period of observation or if adequate motion fails to return.[155,216] Such corrective osteotomies have been done long after injury (up to 27 years) and additional motion has still been regained.[216] There is a minor subset of malunions that does not remodel, that has functional limits (especially when there is limited supination deformity), and is therefore a candidate for osteotomy. Aside from planning traditional angular and rotational correction osteotomies, three-dimensional fracture

modeling can be used for patients with more complex deformity, where correction of both bones, or correction in more than one plane or multiple sites after refracture deformity, is required. Commercially available cutting guides and templates can be individually created for each patient's unique deformity, with good radiographic and clinical success noted.[12]

DELAYED UNION/NONUNION IN DIAPHYSEAL RADIUS AND ULNA FRACTURES

The diagnosis of delayed union is based on documentation of slower-than-normal progression toward union.[136] Daruwalla stated that normal healing of closed pediatric forearm shaft

Figure 10-35. An 8-year-old boy who underwent corrective osteotomy for forearm shaft malunion. **A:** Radiographs demonstrating significant angular malunion. **B:** Preoperative clinical appearance (dorsal view). **C:** Preoperative clinical appearance (volar view). **D:** Preoperative demonstration of full passive supination. **E:** Preoperative demonstration of marked limitation in passive pronation.

(continues)

F

G

H

J

I

K

Figure 10-35. (*Continued*) **F:** Early postoperative radiographs following corrective osteotomies (note intraosseous Kirschner wire tip from provisional fixation). **G:** Clinical appearance with extended elbows and forearm midposition. **H:** Clinical appearance with extended elbows and pronated forearms. **I:** Clinical appearance with extended elbows and supinated forearms. **J:** Symmetrical pronation. **K:** Symmetrical supination.

Figure 10-35. (*Continued*) **L:** AP radiograph 18 months after osteotomies (plates and screws have been removed). **M:** Lateral radiograph at 18-month follow-up. **N:** AP radiograph uninjured left forearm. **O:** Lateral radiograph uninjured left forearm.

Figure 10-36. A 16-year-old boy who underwent corrective osteotomy for forearm shaft malunion. **A:** AP radiograph at time of presentation. **B:** Lateral radiograph at time of presentation. Note rotational malunion of radius in addition to angular abnormalities of both bones. **C:** Clinical deformity (bump). **D:** Relatively symmetrical pronation noted preoperatively. **E:** Dramatic lack of supination on the right noted preoperatively. **F:** One-year postoperative radiographs following osteotomies. Note improved rotational alignment of radius. **G:** Uninjured left forearm radiographs.

Figure 10-36. (*Continued*) **H:** Clinical appearance with extended elbows and forearm midposition. **I:** Clinical appearance with extended elbows and pronated forearms. **J:** Clinical appearance with extended elbows and supinated forearms. **K:** Symmetrical pronation. **L:** Symmetrical supination.

fractures occurs at an average of 5.5 weeks (range 2–8 weeks). Delayed union can be practically defined as a failure to demonstrate complete healing (four cortices) on sequential radiographs by 12 weeks after injury, which exceeds the upper limit of normal healing by about 1 month. Nonunion can be defined as the absence of complete bony union by 6 months after injury, which exceeds the upper limit of normal healing by about 4 months.

Delayed unions and nonunions are rare after closed forearm shaft fractures in children.[62,136,206] In six large series of pediatric diaphyseal forearm fractures treated by closed methods, a less than 0.5% rate (1/263) of delayed union and no nonunions were reported.[33,97,125,181] Delayed unions and nonunions are more common after open reduction and internal fixation and open fractures. Particular concern has been raised about the potential of antegrade ulnar nailing (olecranon starting point) to distract the fracture site.[170] Combined data from four series of plated pediatric forearm fractures indicated a 3% (3/89) nonunion rate[16,218,235]; 24% (21/89) of these were open fractures and at least one[235] of the three nonunions occurred after a grade III open fracture.[218] Large series of open pediatric forearm fractures (treated by a variety of internal fixation methods) reported comparable numbers: 5% (8/173) delayed union rate and 1% (2/173) nonunion rate.[49,88] In a series of 30 nonunions in children, only 6 were in the forearm, and half of these were after open fractures.[136]

Because of the overall rarity of nonunions in children, the possibility of unusual diagnoses such as neurofibromatosis must be considered.[44] After open injury or surgical intervention for other reasons, the possibility of septic nonunion must be ruled out. In the absence of such extraneous factors, nonunion of pediatric forearm fractures seems to be related to surgical treatment.[44,206] Nonunions have been divided into atrophic and hypertrophic types. Atrophic nonunions probably are best treated with bone grafting and compression plating. Compression plating or other stable internal fixation without grafting usually is sufficient for hypertrophic nonunions.

CROSS-UNION/SYNOSTOSIS IN DIAPHYSEAL RADIUS AND ULNA FRACTURES

Posttraumatic radioulnar synostosis results in complete loss of forearm rotation. Most cross-unions that form after pediatric forearm shaft fractures are type II lesions (diaphyseal cross-unions), as described by Vince and Miller (Fig. 10-37).[220] Although some series of adult forearm fractures have reported concerning rates of posttraumatic synostosis, radioulnar synostosis is a rare complication of pediatric forearm shaft fractures.[220] In children, it is usually associated with high-energy injuries,[220] radial neck fractures, and surgically treated forearm fractures.[46,171] There may be a familial predisposition to this complication. Postoperative synostosis after forearm fractures in children is more often associated with plate fixation. The risk of cross-union is increased when open reduction and internal fixation of both-bone fractures are done through one incision.[43]

Both osseous and nonosseous cross-unions may form in the forearm,[5] but the more common type is osseous. After a synostosis matures (6–12 months), it can be excised along with any soft tissue interposition. The results of synostosis resection may be better in adults than children,[220] perhaps because of the more biologically active periosteum in children.[220] Complete synostoses have limited outcomes as compared to those with some lucency still present on CT scan between the two bones. Interposition of inert materials (such as Gore-Tex [W. L. Gore & Associates, Inc., Elkton, MD] or bone wax, local muscle (anconeus in proximal synostosis), and vascularized flaps has

A, B

C

Figure 10-37. Radioulnar synostosis following closed injury. **A:** Injury radiographs. **B:** Plain radiographs showing synostosis. **C:** CT scan showing synostosis. (Courtesy of Alan Aner, MD.)

been used to decrease the chances of recurrent synostosis.[5,171,220] NSAIDs and radiation treatment have been reported after synostosis excision in adults, but their use in children remains undefined. An alternative treatment is corrective osteotomy if the patient is synostosed from a position of either extreme pronation or supination to neutral. If the patient is stuck in a neutral position after posttraumatic synostosis, surgical intervention is usually not recommended.

INFECTION IN DIAPHYSEAL RADIUS AND ULNA FRACTURES

Infection occurs only in surgically treated forearm shaft fractures and open fractures. Appropriately timed preoperative antibiotic prophylaxis is believed to diminish the risk of infection. Children with open forearm fractures are considered to be at high risk for infection, and early (usually <24 hours)[202] irrigation and debridement in the OR is indicated. Whether in the backyard, the barnyard, the soccer field, or the dirtbike track, open forearm fractures that occur in organic settings are best treated with early irrigation and debridement with inspection of the intramedullary canal of both bone ends, where soil contamination tends to occur during injury (see Fig. 10-25). Soil contamination has been reported to lead to gas gangrene and subsequent upper extremity amputation in children with grade I open forearm fractures. Emergency room irrigation and debridement is not recommended and is considered inadequate with increased risk of serious infection.

In four published series of plated pediatric forearm fractures (25% open fractures), deep infection (osteomyelitis) occurred in 5% (4/83).[160,218,235] Such deep infections usually require extensive additional surgical treatment to eradicate them. Combined data from 12 series of similar pediatric forearm fractures (15% open fractures) treated with intramedullary K-wires, Steinmann pins, or Rush rods revealed a deep infection rate of 0.46% (2/437)[4,31,46,128,139,182,183,242] and a superficial infection rate of 2.5% (11/437). Six studies of ESIN fixation reported a 0.2% (1/370) deep infection rate and a 3% (12/370) superficial infection rate.[31,132,144] Superficial infections may require oral antibiotics, pin removal, or both.

Open forearm fractures clearly are at increased risk for infection. Most (96%) open forearm fractures in children are Gustilo and Anderson grade I or II.[88,140] It is often not possible to know if a fracture is grade I versus grade II open until more extensive exposure of deep tissues including the bone ends. Two studies specifically investigated the relationship between the time from injury until irrigation and debridement and the risk of later infection. Luhmann et al.[140] reported on 65 fractures (52 type I, 12 type II, 1 type III) that were irrigated and debrided an average of 5.6 hours (range 1.5–24 hours) after injury, and Greenbaum et al.[88] reported 62 fractures (58 type I, 4 type II) that were irrigated and debrided an average of 14.6 hours (range 1.7–37.8 hours) after injury. No statistically significant association was found in either of these studies; however, most (87%) of these fractures were grade I injuries. Pooled data revealed an overall 1.2% rate (2/173) of deep infection and a 0.6% rate (1/173) of superficial infection after current open fracture treatment protocols.[88,140]

NEURAPRAXIA IN DIAPHYSEAL RADIUS AND ULNA FRACTURES

The median nerve is the most commonly injured nerve with forearm shaft fractures (whether closed or open injuries),[50,88,140] but any peripheral nerve and at times multiple nerves may be involved.[46] In forearm fractures, the median nerve is injured by the radius and the ulnar nerve is injured by the ulna, including in cases where the nerve is entrapped in the fracture during closed reduction techniques.[9] Most of these injuries are simple neurapraxias that occur at the time of injury and resolve spontaneously over weeks to months.[50] Actual nerve entrapment within or perforation by the bony fragments has been reported, most often with long oblique greenstick fractures. Constricting fracture callus and fibrous tissue also have been known to cause nerve palsies. In patients who fail to recover normal nerve function within a satisfactory time period, nerve exploration, decompression, and possible nerve repair or reconstruction should be considered. If signs of progressive nerve recovery (e.g., advancing Tinel sign, needle-like paresthesias, return of function) are not present by the end of the third month after injury, or at a level where recovery should be seen, given that nerves recover at a rate of 1 mm/day or ~ 1 inch/month, further diagnostic workup (electromyography with nerve conduction studies) is indicated. Prolonged waiting can be harmful to long-term outcome as there is a limited window for nerve recovery to happen and earlier nerve decompression or reconstruction can lead to improved clinical outcomes.

Nerve injury after internal fixation is always a concern. Operative treatment of pediatric forearm fractures by either indirect reduction and internal fixation techniques or classic open reduction and internal fixation techniques requires fracture manipulation and soft tissue retraction, which have the potential to worsen existing subclinical nerve injury or to create a new injury. Such injuries are rare and may be underreported. Nerve injury after pediatric forearm plate fixation has been alluded to but not discussed extensively.[128] Luhmann et al.[139] reported an 8% (2/25) iatrogenic nerve injury rate after fixation with intramedullary K-wires or Rush rods: Both were ulnar nerve injuries that resolved in 2 to 3 weeks. Cullen et al.[46] reported one ulnar nerve injury that took 3 months to resolve in a group of 20 patients treated with K-wires or Rush rods.

Certain sensory nerves also are at risk for iatrogenic damage during surgical forearm fracture treatment, especially the superficial branch of the radial nerve.[31,139] Pooled data from six series that included 370 ESIN procedures revealed a 2% (7/370) rate of injury to the superficial branch of the radial nerve.[31,132,144] The branching pattern of this sensory nerve is complex, and efforts must be taken to protect it during careful insertion of intramedullary nails through an open incision at distal radial entry points.[1]

MUSCLE OR TENDON ENTRAPMENT/TENDON RUPTURE IN DIAPHYSEAL RADIUS AND ULNA FRACTURES

Severely displaced forearm fractures may trap portions of muscle between the fracture fragments.[99,182] Often, interposed tissue can

Figure 10-38. Muscle/tendon incarceration. **A:** Injury radiograph showing mild apex-volar fracture angulation. **B:** Flexor digitorum profundus entrapment in the ulna fracture site required surgical extirpation.

be effectively removed during standard fracture reduction, but the muscle may become an obstacle to successful closed reduction. Much of the volar aspects of the shafts of the radius and ulna are covered by the flexor pollicis longus and flexor digitorum profundus, respectively. Many displaced forearm shaft fractures also have apex-volar angulation.[169] As a result, portions of these muscles (or their tendons) are particularly prone to fracture site incarceration (Fig. 10-38). The pronator quadratus also is vulnerable to fracture site entrapment in the distal third of the radius and ulna, and it can block reduction of distal third forearm fractures.[99]

Flexor digitorum profundus entrapment within ulnar[93] and radial[226] shaft fractures has been reported. Entrapment of the flexor digitorum profundus typically restricts full extension of the involved finger (usually index, long, or ring fingers alone or in combination).[93] Isolated ring finger flexor digitorum profundus entrapment has also recently been reported.[205] Even if identified early, this complication rarely responds to occupational or physical therapy. Surgical intervention is the preferred treatment and requires only a small incision (usually over the ulna) through which the adherent tissue is elevated with a blunt instrument from the bone at the site of the fracture. Excellent restoration of finger motion can be achieved, even when the release is done up to 2 years after the fracture.

Extensor tendon injury has been reported after intramedullary nailing of pediatric forearm shaft fractures.[132,182] The extensor pollicis longus appears to be at particular risk for this injury if a dorsal entry point is utilized near the second and third dorsal compartments.[126,208,164] Primary tendon disruption may be caused by direct trauma during either nail insertion or extraction. Delayed tendon disruption is caused by slow erosion of the tendon as it glides past a sharp nail edge. The possibility of this complication can be minimized by using

surgical incisions large enough to allow insertion of small blunt retractors to protect adjacent tendons during nail insertion and extraction. Avoidance of tendon erosion requires nonsharp ends and pin lengths that extend beyond the tendon level into either the subcutaneous tissues[46] or through the skin (external pins).[182] Conceivably, the pins could be buried completely within the bone, but this would require either accepting them as permanent implants (something not commonly practiced at this time) or significantly increasing the level of difficulty of nail removal. The extensor pollicis longus is more at risk near the Lister tubercle and may require a late tendon reconstruction with extensor indicis proprius transfer if ruptured.

COMPARTMENT SYNDROME IN DIAPHYSEAL RADIUS AND ULNA FRACTURES

Compartment syndrome is rare after closed forearm fractures in children, but its consequences can be devastating. Yuan et al.[241] found no compartment syndromes in 205 closed forearm injuries, and Jones and Weiner[107] reported no compartment syndromes in their series of 730 closed forearm injuries. A single compartment syndrome that developed during cast treatment of a 12-year-old female with a closed both-bone forearm fracture was reported by Cullen et al.[46] Because the diagnosis of compartment syndrome can be difficult in children, the index of suspicion must be high.

Compartment syndrome should be suspected in any child who is not reasonably comfortable 3 to 4 hours after adequate reduction and immobilization of a forearm fracture. The risk of compartment syndrome is higher with open fractures[241] and fractures that are difficult to reduce and require extended operative efforts.[241] Yuan et al.[241] voiced concern that the 10% (3/30) rate of compartment syndrome in their patients with closed fractures might be caused by multiple passes or "misses" with intramedullary devices during efforts at indirect reduction and internal fixation. Compartment syndrome was reported by Haasbeek and Cole in 5 (11%) of 46 open forearm fractures in their series. The so-called floating elbow injury has been associated with a rate of compartment syndrome as high as 33%.[241] In children, the three As of increasing analgesia, anxiety, and agitation are the most reliable clinical signs of a pending compartment syndrome. Compartment pressure measurement is difficult in pediatric patients and is best used when the patient is brought to the OR for compartment release to document pre- and postoperative compartment pressures. Forearm compartment syndrome is best treated with fasciotomy, releasing both the superficial and deep volar compartments and the mobile wad. Both the lacertus fibrosus and the carpal tunnel should be released as part of the procedure.

COMPLEX REGIONAL PAIN SYNDROMES IN DIAPHYSEAL RADIUS AND ULNA FRACTURES

Complex regional pain syndromes such as reflex sympathetic dystrophy are uncommon complications after pediatric forearm shaft fractures.[218] Paradoxically, relatively minor injuries seem to place patients at greatest risk. The most reliable sign in children is true allodynia: significant reproducible pain with light touch on the skin. Swelling and other vasomotor changes often are accompanying signs.[134] The diagnosis in children is made based almost exclusively on the history and physical examination, with little reliance on studies such as bone scans. These pain syndromes are best treated initially with physical therapy aimed at range of motion and desensitization. Failure to respond to physical therapy may warrant a referral to a qualified pediatric pain specialist.[118,134]

Authors' Preferred Treatment for Diaphyseal Radius and Ulna Fractures (Algorithm 10-1)

We agree with Jones and Weiner that "closed reduction still remains the gold standard for closed isolated pediatric forearm fractures."[107] Most nondisplaced and minimally displaced radial and ulnar shaft fractures can be splinted in the emergency department and referred for orthopaedic follow-up within 1 week. Radiographs are repeated at the first orthopaedic visit, and a cast is applied. During warmer weather, when fracture incidence peaks, we tend to use waterproof cast liners. We avoid flexing the elbow past 80 to 90 degrees in waterproof casts because the soft tissue crease that forms in the

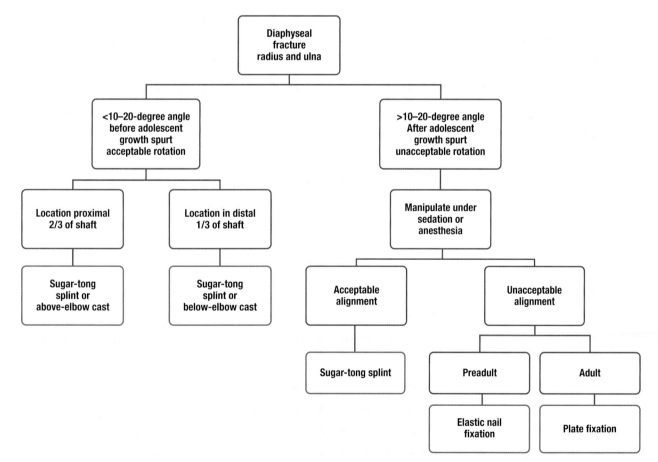

Algorithm 10-1. Authors' preferred treatment for diaphyseal radius and ulna fractures.

antecubital fossa tends to trap moisture. Because waterproof cast lining alone does not shield the skin from cast-saw cuts and burns as well as traditional padding does, specialized tape material may be added along the anticipated course of the cast saw to protect the skin during cast removal.

We prefer an above-elbow cast for all forearm fractures in children under the age of 4 years, because young children tend to lose or remove a below-elbow cast because of soft tissue differences (baby fat) common to the age group.[54] Most older children with forearm shaft fractures also are treated with above-elbow casting, except for those with distal third fractures. Good forearm casting technique should focus on the principles outlined earlier in this chapter. Patients with nondisplaced fractures usually are reevaluated radiographically in 1 to 2 weeks after initial immobilization to check for fracture displacement. Forearm shaft fractures heal more slowly than metaphyseal and physeal fractures of the distal radius and ulna.[50] The cast is removed in 6 to 8 weeks if adequate healing is present on radiographs. Because of the significant refracture rate after forearm shaft fractures, we brace these fractures for several weeks or even several months until all transverse lucency of the original fracture disappears and all four cortices are healed. It is extremely helpful to warn patients and their parents about the high rate of refracture with forearm shaft fracture throughout their treatment. Fractures that heal in bayonet apposition (complete translation and some shortening) can take longer to heal than those with end-to-end apposition and may require prolonged bracing to prevent refracture.[54]

SUMMARY, CONTROVERSIES, AND FUTURE DIRECTIONS RELATED TO DIAPHYSEAL RADIUS AND ULNA FRACTURES

FRACTURE RISK/FRACTURE PREVENTION

Over the past three decades, the rate of forearm fractures has increased dramatically in the United States: 33% higher for males and 56% higher for females.[121] Certain risk-taking behaviors demonstrated by children, as well as increased use of roller blades, hoverboards, skateboards, scooters, trampolines, wheeled shoes, bicycle ramping, snowboarding, and motorized vehicles such as all-terrain vehicles, may be at least partly to blame.[30,142] Electric bicycles have been shown to increase the rate of orthopaedic injuries in children as compared to nonelectric bicycles,[8,23] and this trend can probably be extrapolated to electric scooters and electric skateboards. Increased general physical activity patterns and decreased calcium intake also have been suggested as explanations,[121] but gaps persist in our epidemiologic understanding. Preventing these injuries remains an admirable but elusive goal. Two main avenues of research have been explored: optimizing safety during activities known to be associated with forearm fractures and investigating biologic mechanisms related to fracture risk.

The relationship between in-line skating (rollerblading) and pediatric forearm fractures has been shown, with one in eight children sustaining a fracture on their first skating attempt.[159] Prevention efforts have focused largely on protective gear. Wrist guards have been shown to decrease distal forearm bone strain and injury rates. Similar protective effects of wrist guards in snowboarders have been shown.[173] Trampolines are another target of injury prevention efforts aimed at a specific play activity.[58] Dramatic increases in trampoline-related injuries were reported during the 1990s, with rates doubling[204] or even tripling.[72] Safety recommendations have ranged from constant adult supervision and one-child-at-a-time use[131] to outright bans on public trampoline use.[72,204]

A variety of biologic risk factors have been studied relative to forearm fractures. Children who avoid drinking milk have been shown to have increased fracture risk,[86] as well as those who prefer to drink fruit juice and soda.[177] Several studies have shown an increased risk of fractures in females aged 3 to 15 years with low bone density.[83,85] Diet, nutrition, and exercise are being explored as causative factors, but the precise reason for the low bone density has not been confirmed. Too little physical activity (as measured by television, computer, and video viewing) has been associated with increased fracture risk, presumably because of decreased bone mineral density.[141] Caution also must be exercised when obtaining dual-energy x-ray absorptiometry data in children, as up to 88% of scans may be misinterpreted.[74] Childhood obesity is a growing problem in our society.[76,102] Increased body weight and decreased cross-sectional dimensions of the forearm bones also have been found in females who fracture their forearms.[203] Other researchers have found an increased risk of forearm fracture in obese children.[84,106]

PARENTAL PRESENCE DURING FRACTURE REDUCTION IN DIAPHYSEAL RADIUS AND ULNA FRACTURES

Parental presence is becoming increasingly popular for pediatric emergency department procedures. Several studies on chest tubes, IV cannulation, lumbar puncture, and urethral catheterization have shown increased parental satisfaction when parents are allowed to stay for these procedures.[90] Parental presence during induction of anesthesia also has been shown to have favorable effects on children older than 4 years of age.[110] To the best of our knowledge, there are no published studies on parental presence during orthopaedic procedures performed in the emergency department setting. There are also no parental presence studies on any emergency department procedures performed on children who are under sedation, when the child is probably not aware of the parent's presence.

Certain relationships between perceived procedural invasiveness and parental presence have been borne out in the literature. Four hundred parents from the Indiana area were surveyed, and with increasing invasiveness, the parents' desire to be present decreased.[20] A survey of academic emergency medicine attendings, residents, and nurses from across the country also showed that there is an inverse relationship between increasing invasiveness and support for parental presence.[14] Boudreaux et al. published their critical review of the parental presence literature and concluded that "randomized controlled trials are mixed regarding whether family presence actually helps the patient."[24]

Extrapolation of information from the previously mentioned studies to pediatric orthopaedic settings should be done with caution. We typically allow parents to be present for the induction of sedation, and once the patient is sedated, the parents are asked to wait in a designated area. If parents are allowed to be present, we strongly recommend a dedicated employee to attend to the parent or parents (a "spotter"). Several parents (typically fathers) have fainted during such orthopaedic procedures and injured themselves. Parents who stay for a reduction also should be counseled that the patient may moan or cry during reduction but will not remember it, and that the fracture manipulation may appear shockingly brutal. Parents who are not present during reduction should be asked to wait far enough away from the procedure room so that they cannot hear the child.

ACKNOWLEDGMENTS

The authors wish to acknowledge the priceless teaching and constructive feedback afforded us by our senior partner, Alvin H. Crawford, MD, FACS and previous author Charles T. Mehlman, DO, MPH.

Annotated References

Reference	Annotation
Abrams RA, Brown RA, Botte MJ. The superficial branch of the radial nerve: an anatomic study with surgical implications. *J Hand Surg Am.* 1992;17:1037–1041.	These two adult cadaver dissection papers give us important anatomic information that relates to distal radial entry sites for flexible nailing of forearm shaft fractures. Multiple branches of the terminal superficial radial nerve must be respected. Abrams et al. showed that in addition to branches "in" the first dorsal compartment, there may be a branch as close as 5 mm to Lister tubercle.
Auerbach DM, Collins ED, Kunkle KL, Monsanto EH. The radial sensory nerve: an anatomic study. *Clin Orthop Relat Res.* 1994;308:241–249.	Auerbach et al. showed an average of nearly six branches distally and 60% of specimens had branches overlying the so-called 3–4 wrist arthroscopy portal.
Bowman EN, Mehlman CT, Lindsell CJ, Tamai J. Nonoperative treatment of both-bone forearm shaft fractures in children: predictors of early radiographic failure. *J Pediatr Orthop.* 2011;31:23–32.	This study retrospectively analyzed a cohort of 282 children with displaced complete both-bone forearm shaft fractures who underwent closed reduction. Over the course of up to 4 weeks of radiographic follow-up, age-dependent criteria were used to assess radiographic failure rates: 20/15/10 degrees (distal third, middle third, proximal third) for girls less than 8 years old and boys less than 10 years old, and greater than 10 degrees for girls greater than 8 years old and boys greater than 10 years old. Overall, there was a 51% failure rate with age greater than 10 for either sex having three times higher odds of failure and proximal-third fractures nearly seven times higher.
Evans EM. Fractures of the radius and ulna. *J Bone Joint Surg Br.* 1951;33-B:548–561.	Evans also emphasized important management differences between greenstick and complete fractures.
Fee NF, Dobranski A, Bisla RS. Gas gangrene complicating open forearm fractures. Report of five cases. *J Bone Joint Surg Am.* 1977;59:135–138.	Four of the five patients presented in this paper were pediatric patients. All had outdoor injuries resulting in small grade 1 open forearm fractures. All had local wound care (rinsing the skin) and fracture reduction. Antibiotics were not routinely administered; an 8-year-old male, a 10-year-old female, and an 11-year-old male, all underwent upper extremity amputation while one 12-year-old male did not.
Lascombes P, Prevot J, Ligier JN, et al. Elastic stable intramedullary nailing in forearm shaft fractures in children: 85 cases. *J Pediatr Orthop.* 1990;10:167–171.	This is the classic paper produced by our French colleagues that effectively introduced this technique to the rest of the world. Eighty children with complete forearm shaft fractures (no greenstick fractures) were treated via their technique. Ninety-three percent were middle-third fractures, 8% were open fractures, and 6% required open reduction. They used distal lateral radial and proximal ulnar "anconeus" entry points (both respectful of adjacent growth areas). Contoured stainless steel and titanium flexible nails (1.5–2.5 mm) were implanted. They recommended no postoperative casting and encouragement of immediate motion. Nail removal by 10 to 12 months was recommended. They reported 92% excellent results at an average of 3½-year follow-up. There was an 8% rate of significant pronation/supination loss (>20 degrees) and a 16% rate of hypesthesia of superficial branch radial nerve.

Annotated References

Reference	Annotation
Matthews LS, Kaufer H, Garver DF, Sonstegard DA. The effect on supination-pronation of angular malalignment of fractures of both bones of the forearm. *J Bone Joint Surg Am.* 1982;64:14–17.	Classic adult cadaver study where they created midshaft forearm malunions with steel fixation plates angulated 10 and 20 degrees. A 10-degree angulation of either single bone resulted in little measurable loss, while 10-degree angulation of both bones led to approximately 20 degrees of motion loss and 20-degree angulation of both bones created motion losses of 40 degrees or more for both pronation and supination.
Murphy HA, Jain VV, Parikh SN, et al. Extensor tendon injury associated with dorsal entry flexible nailing of radial shaft fractures in children: a report of 5 new cases and review of the literature. *J Pediatr Orthop.* 2019;39(4):163–168.	This paper summarizes 33 reported cases of EPL tendon injury and how every single one of them is associated with the so-called dorsal radial entry point.
Price CT, Knapp DR. Osteotomy for malunited forearm shaft fractures in children. *J Pediatr Orthop.* 2006;26:193–196.	This is a 10-patient forearm shaft malunion report that emphasizes a commonsense surgical technique for corrective osteotomy. Rotate the bones under fluoro to find the plane of maximum deformity and then do a closing wedge osteotomy with internal fixation to correct it. Rotation is also accounted for via anatomic landmarks.
Price CT, Scott DS, Kurzner ME, Flynn JC. Malunited forearm fractures in children. *J Pediatr Orthop.* 1990;10:705–712.	This is a study of 39 patients with forearm shaft malunions. Fifty-six percent (22/39) had angular malunion exceeding 10 degrees (range 12–20 degrees) and/or rotational malunion (range 45–90 degrees). Twenty-three percent (5/22) of this subgroup lost either pronation or supination ranging from 25 to 60 degrees.
Sardelli M, Tashjian RZ, MacWilliams BA. Functional elbow range of motion for contemporary tasks. *J Bone Joint Surg Am.* 2011;93:471–477.	This paper amounts to a sophisticated update (30 years later) to the classic Morrey and Askew paper from 1981 that produced numbers that any orthopaedic resident worth their salt can recite: 30 of 130 and 50 of 50. It raises the stakes on what we should consider functional range of motion, pushing it as high as 20 to 155 degrees of elbow motion and nearly 75 degrees pronation and 90 degrees supination!!!
Trousdale RT, Linscheid RL. Operative treatment of malunited fractures of the forearm. *J Bone Joint Surg Am.* 1995;77:894–902.	Classic forearm shaft corrective osteotomy series (27 total patients) that is filled with patients whose injuries occurred while they were children)! Nearly 75% were less than 14 years old at the time of their initial injury and about 30% were actually less than 10 years old.
Younger AS, Tredwell SJ, Mackenzie WG, et al. Accurate prediction of outcome after pediatric forearm fracture. *J Pediatr Orthop.* 1994;14:200–206.	150 children (average age 8 years) with both-bone forearm shaft fractures were studied at an average of 4 years following injury. In conjunction with a concept they called axis deviation, they suggested cutoffs of 10 degrees in the midshaft, 12.5 degrees at the junction of middle and distal thirds, and 20 degrees in the distal third.

REFERENCES

1. Abrams RA, Brown RA, Botte MJ. The superficial branch of the radial nerve: an anatomic study with surgical implications. *J Hand Surg Am.* 1992;17:1037–1041.
2. Abrams RA, Ziets RJ, Lieber RL, Botte MJ. Anatomy of the radial nerve motor branches in the forearm. *J Hand Surg Am.* 1997;22:232–237.
3. Aktas S, Saridogan K, Moralar U, Ture M. Patterns of single segment non-physeal extremity fractures in children. *Int Orthop.* 1999;23:345–347.
4. Amit Y, Salai M, Chechik A, et al. Closing intramedullary nailing for the treatment of diaphyseal forearm fractures in adolescence: a preliminary report. *J Pediatr Orthop.* 1985;5:143–146.
5. Aner A, Singer M, Feldbrin Z, et al. Surgical treatment of posttraumatic radioulnar synostosis in children. *J Pediatr Orthop.* 2002;22:598–600.
6. Archibong AE, Onuba O. Fractures in children in south eastern Nigeria. *Cent Afr J Med.* 1996;42:340–343.
7. Assaf E, Mohs E, Dally FJ, et al. Vitamin D level and low-energy fracture risk in children and adolescents: a population-based case-control study of 45 cases. *J Pediatr Orthop B.* 2023. doi: 10.1097/BPB.0000000000001061
8. Avrahamov-Kraft E, Yulevich A, Sweed Y. Pediatric electrical bicycle road accidents. *Eur J Pediatr Surg.* 2022;32(1):120–126.
9. Aziz KA, Benfield C, Cornwall R, Little KJ. Characteristics and clinical outcomes of intraosseous nerve entrapment in closed pediatric upper extremity fractures. *American Society for Peripheral Nerve Annual Meeting,* Miami, FL. January 21, 2023.
10. Baitner AC, Perry A, Lalonde FD, et al. The healing forearm fracture: a matched comparison of forearm refractures. *J Pediatr Orthop.* 2007;27:743–747.
11. Bartl V, Gál P, Skotáková J, Kmosták P. Treatment of redislocated fragments of long bones using plaster cast wedging. *Rozhl Chir.* 2002;81:415–420.
12. Bauer AS, Storelli DAR, Sibbel SE, et al. Preoperative computer simulation and patient-specific guides are safe and effective to correct forearm deformity in children. *J Pediatr Orthop.* 2017;37(7):504–510.
13. Bauer MR, Albanese SA. Prescribing braces after forearm fractures does not decrease refracture rate. *J Pediatr Orthop B.* 2023;32(2):152–156.
14. Beckman AW, Sloan BK, Moore GP, et al; P50 (Parental Presence during Painful Pediatric Procedures) Research Group. Should parents be present during emergency department procedures on children and who should make the decision? A survey of emergency physician and nurse attitudes. *Acad Emerg Med.* 2002;9:154–158.
15. Bellemans M, Lamoureux J. Indications for immediate percutaneous intramedullary nailing of complete diaphyseal forearm shaft fractures in children. *Acta Orthop Belg.* 1995;61(Suppl I):169–172.
16. Bhaskar AR, Roberts JA. Treatment of unstable fractures of the forearm in children: is plating of a single bone adequate? *J Bone Joint Surg Br.* 2001;83:253–258.
17. Black GB, Amadeo R. Orthopedic injuries associated with backyard trampoline use in children. *Can J Surg.* 2003;46:199–201.
18. Blaisier RD, Salamon PB. Closed intramedullary rodding of pediatric adolescent forearm fractures. *Oper Tech Orthop.* 1993;3:128–133.
19. Blakemore LC, Cooperman DR, Thompson GH, et al. Compartment syndrome in ipsilateral humerus and forearm fractures in children. *Clin Orthop Relat Res.* 2000;376:32–38.
20. Boie ET, Moore GP, Brummett C, Nelson DR. Do parents want to be present during invasive procedures performed on their children in the emergency department? A survey of 400 parents. *Ann Emerg Med.* 1999;34:70–74.
21. Boone DC, Azen SP. Normal range of motion of joints in male subjects. *J Bone Joint Surg Am.* 1979;61:756–759.

22. Bot AGJ, Doornberg JN, Lindenhovius ALC, et al. Long-term outcomes of fractures of both bones of the forearm. *J Bone Joint Surg Am.* 2011;93(6):527–532.

23. Botton IN, Takagi D, Shlez A, et al. Road accidents in children involving light electric vehicles cause more severe injuries than other similar vehicles. *Eur J Pediatr.* 2021;180(11):3255–3263.

24. Boudreaux ED, Francis JL, Loyacano T. Family presence during invasive procedures and resuscitations in the emergency department: a critical review and suggestions for future research. *Ann Emerg Med.* 2002;40:193–205.

25. Bould M, Bannister GC. Refractures of the radius and ulna in children. *Injury.* 1999;30:583–586.

26. Bowman EN, Mehlman CT, Lindsell CJ, Tamai J. Nonoperative treatment of both-bone forearm shaft fractures in children: predictors of early radiographic failure. *J Pediatr Orthop.* 2011;31:23–32.

27. Boyer BA, Overton B, Schraeder W, et al. Position of immobilization for pediatric forearm fractures. *J Pediatr Orthop.* 2002;22:185–187.

28. Branovacki G, Hanson M, Cash R, Gonzalez M. The innervation of the radial nerve at the elbow and in the forearm. *J Hand Surg Br.* 1998;23:167–169.

29. Bratt HD, Eyres RL, Cole WG. Randomized double-blind trial of low-and moderate-dose lidocaine regional anesthesia for forearm fractures in childhood. *J Pediatr Orthop.* 1996;16:660–663.

30. Brown RL, Koepplinger ME, Mehlman CT, et al. All-terrain vehicle and bicycle crashes in children: epidemiology and comparison of injury severity. *J Pediatr Surg.* 2002;37:375–380.

31. Calder PR, Achan P, Barry M. Diaphyseal forearm fractures in children treated with intramedullary fixation: outcome of K-wires versus elastic stable intramedullary nail. *Injury.* 2003;34:278–282.

32. Cameron ML, Sponseller PD, Rossberg MI. Pediatric analgesia and sedation for the management of orthopedic conditions. *Am J Orthop (Belle Mead NJ).* 2000;29:665–672.

33. Carey PJ, Alburger PD, Betz RR, et al. Both-bone forearm fractures in children. *Orthopedics.* 1992;15:1015–1019.

34. Carsi B, Abril JC, Epeldegui T. Longitudinal growth after nonphyseal forearm fractures. *J Pediatr Orthop.* 2003;23:203–207.

35. Casey PJ, Moed BR. Greenstick fractures of the radius in adults: a report of two cases. *J Orthop Trauma.* 1996;10:209–212.

36. Celebi L, Muratli HH, Dogan O, et al. The results of intramedullary nailing in children who developed redisplacement during cast treatment of both-bone forearm fractures. *Acta Orthop Traumatol Turc.* 2007;41:175–182.

37. Ceroni D, Martin X, Delhumeau-Cartier C, et al. Is bone mineral mass truly decreased in teenagers with a first episode of forearm fracture? A prospective longitudinal study. *J Pediatr Orthop.* 2012;32:579–586.

38. Charnley J. *The Closed Treatment of Common Fractures.* Livingstone; 1957.

39. Cheng JC, Ng BK, Ying SY, Lam PK. A 10-year study of the changes in the pattern and treatment of 6,493 fractures. *J Pediatr Orthop.* 1999;19:344–350.

40. Chess DG, Hyndman JC, Leahey JL, et al. Short arm plaster cast for distal pediatric forearm fractures. *J Pediatr Orthop.* 1994;14:211–213.

41. Chung KC, Spilson SV. The frequency and epidemiology of hand and forearm fractures in the United States. *J Hand Surg Am.* 2001;26:908–915.

42. Committee on Drugs, American Academy of Pediatrics. Guidelines for monitoring and management of pediatric patients during and after sedation for diagnostic and therapeutic procedures: addendum. *Pediatrics.* 2002;110(4):836–838.

43. Crawford AH. Pitfalls and complications of fractures of the distal radius and ulna in childhood. *Hand Clin.* 1988;4:403–413.

44. Crawford AH, Schorry EK. Neurofibromatosis in children: the role of the orthopaedist. *J Am Acad Orthop Surg.* 1999;7:217–230.

45. Creasman C, Zaleske DJ, Ehrlich MG. Analyzing forearm fractures in children. The more subtle signs of impending problems. *Clin Orthop Relat Res.* 1984;188:40–53.

46. Cullen MC, Roy DR, Giza E, Crawford AH. Complications of intramedullary fixation of pediatric forearm fractures. *J Pediatr Orthop.* 1998;18:14–21.

47. Davids JR, Frick SL, Skewes E, Blackhurst DW. Skin surface pressure beneath an above-the-knee cast: plaster casts compared with fiberglass casts. *J Bone Joint Surg Am.* 1997;79:565–569.

48. Davidson AJ, Eyres RL, Cole WG. A comparison of prilocaine and lidocaine for intravenous regional anaesthesia for forearm fracture reduction in children. *Paediatr Anaesth.* 2002;12:146–150.

49. Davidson AW. Rock-paper-scissors. *Injury.* 2003;34:61–63.

50. Davis DR, Green DP. Forearm fractures in children: pitfalls and complications. *Clin Orthop Relat Res.* 1976;120:172–183.

51. DeFrate LE, Li G, Zayontz SJ, Herndon JH. A minimally invasive method for the determination of force in the interosseous ligament. *Clin Biomech (Bristol, Avon).* 2001;16:895–900.

52. Deluca PA, Lindsey RW, Ruwe PA. Refracture of bones of the forearm after the removal of compression plates. *J Bone Joint Surg Am.* 1988;70:1372–1376.

53. Dilberti T, Botte MJ, Abrams RA. Anatomical considerations regarding the posterior interosseous nerve during posterolateral approaches to the proximal part of the radius. *J Bone Joint Surg Am.* 2000;82:809–813.

54. Do TT, Strub WM, Foad SL, et al. Reduction versus remodeling in pediatric distal forearm fractures: a preliminary cost analysis. *J Pediatr Orthop B.* 2003;12:109–115.

55. Droll KP, Perna P, Potter J, et al. Outcomes following plate fixation of fractures of both bones of the forearm in adults. *J Bone Joint Surg Am.* 2007;89(12):2619–2624.

56. Dumont CE, Thalmann R, Macy JC. The effect of rotational malunion of the radius and ulna on supination and pronation. *J Bone Joint Surg Br.* 2002;84:1070–1074.

57. Duncan J, Weiner D. Unstable pediatric forearm fractures: use of "pins and plaster." *Orthopedics.* 2004;27:267–269.

58. Esposito PW. Trampoline injuries. *Clin Orthop Relat Res.* 2003;409:43–52.

59. Evans EM. Rotational deformity in the treatment of fractures of both bones of the forearm. *J Bone Joint Surg.* 1945;27:373–379.

60. Evans JK, Buckley SL, Alexander AH, Gilpin AT. Analgesia for the reduction of fractures in children: a comparison of nitrous oxide with intramuscular sedation. *J Pediatr Orthop.* 1995;15:73–77.

61. Fernandez FF, Egenolf M, Carsten C, et al. Unstable diaphyseal fractures of both bones of the forearm in children: plate versus intramedullary nailing. *Injury.* 2005;36:1210–1216.

62. Fike EA, Bartal E. Delayed union of the distal ulna in a child after both-bone forearm fracture. *J South Orthop Assoc.* 1998;7:113–116.

63. Firl M, Wünsch L. Measurement of bowing of the radius. *J Bone Joint Surg Br.* 2004;86:1047–1049.

64. Fleischer H. Marrow wiring in lower-arm fractures of children. *Dtsch Med Wochenschr.* 1975;100:1278–1279.

65. Flynn JM. Pediatric forearm fractures: decision making, surgical techniques, and complications. *Instr Course Lect.* 2002;51:355–360.

66. Flynn JM, Jones KJ, Garner MR, Goebel J. Eleven years experience in the operative management of pediatric forearm fractures. *J Pediatr Orthop.* 2010;30:313–319.

67. Flynn JM, Sarwark JF, Waters PM, et al. The surgical management of pediatric fractures of the upper extremity. *Instr Course Lect.* 2003;52:635–645.

68. Flynn JM, Waters PM. Single-bone fixation of both-bone forearm fractures. *J Pediatr Orthop.* 1996;16:655–659.

69. Fracture and dislocation compendium: Orthopaedic Trauma Association Committee for Coding and Classification. *J Orthop Trauma.* 1996;10:1–153.

70. Franklin CC, Robinson J, Noonan K, Flynn JM. Evidence-based medicine: management of pediatric forearm fractures. *J Pediatr Orthop.* 2012;32(Suppl 2):S131–S134.

71. Furia JP, Alioto RJ, Marquardt JD. The efficacy and safety of the hematoma block for fracture reduction in closed, isolated fractures. *Orthopedics.* 1997;20:423–426.

72. Furnival RA, Street KA, Schunk JE. Too many pediatric trampoline injuries. *Pediatrics.* 1999;103:e57.

73. Gabriel MT, Pfaeffle HJ, Stabile KJ, et al. Passive strain distribution in the interosseous ligament of the forearm: implications for injury reconstruction. *J Hand Surg Am.* 2004;29:293–298.

74. Gafni RI, Baron J. Overdiagnosis of osteoporosis in children due to misinterpretation of dual-energy x-ray absorptiometry (DEXA). *J Pediatr.* 2004;144:253–257.

75. Galpin RD, Webb GR, Armstrong DG, et al. *A comparison of short and long-arm plaster casts for displaced distal-third pediatric forearm fractures: a prospective randomized trial. Paper presented at Annual Meeting of the Pediatric Orthopaedic Society of North America;* April 27–May 1, 2004; St. Louis, MO.

76. Garcia VF, Langford L, Inge TH. Application of laparoscopy for bariatric surgery. *Curr Opin Pediatr.* 2003;15:248–255.

77. Garg NK, Ballal MS, Malek IA, et al. Use of elastic stable intramedullary nailing for treating unstable forearm fractures in children. *J Trauma.* 2008;65:109–115.

78. Giebel GD, Meyer C, Koebke J, Giebel G. Arterial supply of forearm bones and its importance for the operative treatment of fractures. *Surg Radiol Anat.* 1997;19:149–153.

79. Godambe SA, Elliot V, Matheny D, Pershad J. Comparison of propofol/fentanyl versus ketamine/midazolam for brief procedural sedation in a pediatric emergency department. *Pediatrics.* 2003;112:116–123.

80. Godfrey J, Choi PD, Shabtai L, et al. Management of pediatric type 1 open fractures in the emergency department or operating room: a multicenter perspective. *J Pediatr Orthop.* 2019;39(7):372–376.

81. Gonzalez MH, Lotfi P, Bendre A, et al. The ulnar nerve at the elbow and its local branching: an anatomic study. *J Hand Surg Br.* 2001;26:142–144.

82. Goodloe JB, Bailey EP, Luce LT, et al. A standardized order-set improves variability in opioid discharge prescribing patterns after surgical fixation of pediatric supracondylar humerus fractures. *J Surg Educ.* 2021;78(5):1660–1665.

83. Goulding A, Cannan R, Williams SM, et al. Bone mineral density in girls with forearm fractures. *J Bone Miner Res.* 1998;13:143–148.

84. Goulding A, Jones IE, Taylor RW, et al. Bone mineral density and body composition in boys with distal forearm fractures: a dual-energy x-ray absorptiometry study. *J Pediatr.* 2001;139:509–515.

85. Goulding A, Jones IE, Taylor RW, et al. More broken bones: a 4-year double cohort study of young girls with and without distal forearm fractures. *J Bone Miner Res.* 2000;15:2011–2018.

86. Goulding A, Rockell JEP, Black RE, et al. Children who avoid drinking cow's milk are at increased risk for prepubertal bone fractures. *J Am Diet Assoc.* 2004;104:250–253.

87. Gray H. *Gray's Anatomy: The Classic Collector's Edition.* Bounty; 1977:152–157.

88. Greenbaum B, Zionts LE, Ebramzadeh E. Open fractures of the forearm in children. *J Orthop Trauma.* 2001;15:111–118.

89. Hahn MP, Richter D, Muhr G, Ostermann PA. Pediatric forearm fractures: diagnosis, therapy, and possible complications. *Unfallchirurg.* 1997;100:760–769.

90. Haimi-Cohen Y, Amir J, Harel L, et al. Parental presence during lumbar puncture: anxiety and attitude toward the procedure. *Clin Pediatr (Phila).* 1996;35:2–4.

91. Harrington P, Sharif I, Fogarty EE, et al. Management of the floating elbow injury in children. Simultaneous ipsilateral fractures of the elbow and forearm. *Arch Orthop Trauma Surg.* 2000;120:205–208.

92. Helenius I, Lamberg TS, Kääriäinen S, et al. Operative treatment of fractures in children is increasing: a population-based study from Finland. *J Bone Joint Surg Am.* 2009;91:2612–2616.

93. Hendel D, Aner A. Entrapment of the flexor digitorum profundus of the ring finger at the site of an ulnar fracture: a case report. *Ital J Orthop Traumatol.* 1992;18:417–419.

94. Hennrikus WL, Shin AY, Klingelberger CE. Self-administered nitrous oxide and a hematoma block for analgesia in the outpatient reduction of fractures in children. *J Bone Joint Surg Am.* 1995;77:335–339.

95. Hoffman GM, Nowakowski R, Troshynski TJ, et al. Risk reduction in pediatric procedural sedation by application of an American Academy of Pediatrics/American Society of Anesthesiologists process model. *Pediatrics.* 2002;109:236–243.

96. Högström H, Nilsson BE, Willner S. Correction with growth following diaphyseal forearm fracture. *Acta Orthop Scand.* 1976;47:299–303.

97. Holdsworth BJ, Sloan JP. Proximal forearm fractures in children: residual disability. *Injury.* 1982;14:174–179.

98. Hollister AM, Gellman H, Waters RL. The relationship of the interosseous membrane to the axis of rotation of the forearm. *Clin Orthop Relat Res.* 1994;298:272–276.

99. Holmes JR, Louis DS. Entrapment of pronator quadratus in pediatric distal radius fractures: recognition and treatment. *J Pediatr Orthop.* 1994;14:498–500.

100. Hotchkiss RN, An KN, Sowa DT, et al. An anatomic and mechanical study of the interosseous membrane of the forearm: pathomechanics of proximal migration of the radius. *J Hand Surg Am.* 1989;14:256–261.

101. Hsu ES, Patwardhan AG, Meade KP, et al. Cross-sectional geometrical properties and bone mineral content of the human radius and ulna. *J Biomech.* 1993;26:1307–1318.

102. Inge TH, Krebs NF, Garcia VF, et al. Bariatric surgery for severely overweight adolescents: concerns and recommendations. *Pediatrics.* 2004;114:217–223.

103. Jacobsen FS. Periosteum: its relation to pediatric fractures. *J Pediatr Orthop B.* 1997;6:84–90.

104. Johari AN, Sinha M. Remodeling of forearm fractures in children. *J Pediatr Orthop B.* 1999;8:84–87.

105. Johnson CW, Carmichael KD, Morris RP, Gilmer B. Biomechanical study of flexible intramedullary nails. *J Pediatr Orthop.* 2009;29:44–48.

106. Jones IE, Williams SM, Goulding A. Associations of birth weight and length, childhood size, and smoking with bone fractures during growth: evidence from a birth cohort study. *Am J Epidemiol.* 2004;159:343–350.

107. Jones K, Weiner DS. The management of forearm fractures in children: a plea for conservatism. *J Pediatr Orthop.* 1999;19:811–815.

108. Jubel A, Andermahr J, Isenberg J, et al. Outcomes and complications of elastic stable intramedullary nailing of forearm fractures in children. *J Pediatr Orthop B.* 2005;14:375–380.

109. Kailis V, Hariga H, Docquier PL. Prevention of re-fractures of both bones of the forearm in children. *Acta Orthop Belg.* 2016;82(4):872–875.

110. Kain ZN, Mayes LC, Caramico LA, et al. Parental presence during induction of anesthesia: a randomized controlled trial. *Anesthesiology.* 1996;84:1060–1067.

111. Kang SN, Mangwani J, Ramachandran M, et al. Elastic intramedullary nailing of paediatric fractures of the forearm: a decade of experience in a teaching hospital in the United Kingdom. *J Bone Joint Surg Br.* 2011;93(2):262–265.

112. Kasten P, Krefft M, Hesselbach J, Weinberg AM. Computer simulation of forearm rotation in angular deformities: a new therapeutic approach. *Injury.* 2002;33:807–813.

113. Kasten P, Krefft M, Hesselbach J, Weinberg AM. How does torsional deformity of the radial shaft influence the rotation of the forearm? A biomechanical study. *J Orthop Trauma.* 2003;17:57–60.

114. Keenan WNW, Clegg J. Intraoperative wedging of casts: correction of residual angulation after manipulation. *J Pediatr Orthop.* 1995;15:826–829.

115. Keil LG, Sullivan MH, Dadoo S, et al. How much opioid do kids actually need? A prospective study of analgesic prescribing and postdischarge opioid use among pediatric patients with operative fractures. *J Pediatr Orthop.* 2021;41(10):e871–e876.

116. Kelly AM, Powell CV, Williams A. Parent visual analogue scale ratings of children's pain do not reliably reflect pain reported by child. *Pediatr Emerg Care.* 2002;18:159–162.

117. Kelly JP, Zionts LE. Economic considerations in the treatment of distal forearm fractures in children. *Paper presented at: Annual Meeting of the American Academy of Orthopaedic Surgeons;* February 28–March 4, 2001; San Francisco, CA.

118. Kemper KJ, Sarah R, Silver-Highfield E, et al. On pins and needles? Pediatric pain patients' experience with acupuncture. *Pediatrics.* 2000;105:941–947.

119. Kennedy RM, Porter FL, Miller JP, Jaffe DM. Comparison of fentanyl/midazolam with ketamine/midazolam for pediatric orthopedic emergencies. *Pediatrics.* 1998;102:956–963.

120. Kettunen J, Kröger H, Bowditch M, et al. Bone mineral density after removal of rigid plates from forearm fractures: preliminary report. *J Orthop Sci.* 2003;8:772–776.

121. Khosla S, Melton LJ III, Dekutoski MB, et al. Incidence of childhood distal forearm fractures over 30 years: a population-based study. *JAMA.* 2003;290:1479–1485.

122. Kim CY, Gentry M, Sala D, Chu A. Single-bone intramedullary nailing of pediatric both-bone forearm fractures a systematic review. *Bull Hosp Jt Dis (2013).* 2017;75(4):227–233.

123. Kinder KL, Lehman-Huskamp KL, Gerard JM. Do children with high body mass indices have a higher incidence of emesis when undergoing ketamine sedation? *Pediatr Emerg Care.* 2012;28:1203–1205.

124. Krakow AR, Talwar D, Mehta NN, et al. Getting the message: the declining trend in opioid prescribing for minor orthopaedic injuries in children and adolescents. *J Bone Joint Surg Am.* 2022;104(13):1166–1171.

125. Kramhøft M, Solgaard S. Displaced diaphyseal forearm fractures in children: classification and evaluation of the early radiographic prognosis. *J Pediatr Orthop.* 1989;9:586–589.

126. Kravel T, Sher-Lurie N, Ganel A. Extensor pollicis longus rupture after fixation of radius and ulna fracture with titanium elastic nail (TEN) in a child: a case report. *J Trauma.* 2007;63:1169–1170.

127. Kruppa C, Bunge P, Schildhauer TA, Dudda M. Low complication rate of elastic stable intramedullary nailing (ESIN) of pediatric forearm fractures: a retrospective study of 202 cases. *Medicine (Baltimore).* 2017;96(16):e6669.

128. Kucukkaya M, Kabukcuoglu Y, Tezer M, et al. The application of open intramedullary fixation in the treatment of pediatric radial and ulnar shaft fractures. *J Orthop Trauma.* 2002;16:340–344.

129. Landin LA. Epidemiology of children's fractures. *J Pediatr Orthop B.* 1997;6:79–83.

130. Larsen E, Vittas D, Torp-Pedersen S. Remodeling of angulated distal forearm fractures in children. *Clin Orthop Relat Res.* 1988;237:190–195.

131. Larson BJ, Davis JW. Trampoline-related injuries. *J Bone Joint Surg Am.* 1995;77:1174–1178.

132. Lascombes P, Prevot J, Ligier JN, et al. Elastic stable intramedullary nailing in forearm shaft fractures in children: 85 cases. *J Pediatr Orthop.* 1990;10:167–171.

133. Lautman S, Bergerault F, Saidani N, Bonnard C. Roentgenographic measurement of angle between shaft and distal epiphyseal growth plate of radius. *J Pediatr Orthop.* 2002;22:751–753.

134. Lee BH, Scharff L, Sethna NF, et al. Physical therapy and cognitive-behavioral treatment for complex regional pain syndromes. *J Pediatr.* 2002;141:135–140.

135. Lee S, Nicol RO, Stott NS. Intramedullary fixation for pediatric unstable fractures. *Clin Orthop Relat Res.* 2002;402:245–250.

136. Lewallen RP, Peterson HA. Nonunion of long bone fractures in children: a review of 30 cases. *J Pediatr Orthop.* 1985;5:135–142.

137. Ligier JN, Metaizeau JP, Prévot J, Lascombes P. Elastic stable intramedullary pinning of long bone shaft fractures in children. *Z Kinderchir.* 1985;40:209–212.

138. Lim YJ, Lam KS, Lee EH. Open Gustilo 1 and 2 midshaft fractures of the radius and ulna in children: is there a role for cast immobilization after wound debridement? *J Pediatr Orthop.* 2007;27:540–546.

139. Luhmann SJ, Gordon JE, Schoenecker PL. Intramedullary fixation of unstable bothbone forearm fractures in children. *J Pediatr Orthop.* 1998;18:451–456.

140. Luhmann SJ, Schootman M, Schoenecker PL, et al. Complications and outcomes of open pediatric forearm fractures. *J Pediatr Orthop.* 2004;24:1–6.

141. Ma D, Jones G. Television, computer, and video viewing; physical activity; and upper limb fracture risk in children: a population-based case control study. *J Bone Miner Res.* 2003;18:1970–1977.

142. Ma D, Morley R, Jones G. Risk-taking coordination and upper limb fractures in children: population-based case-control study. *Osteoporos Int.* 2004;15:633–638.

143. Mabrey JD, Fitch RD. Plastic deformation in pediatric fractures: mechanism and treatment. *J Pediatr Orthop.* 1989;9:310–314.

144. Mann DC, Schnabel M, Baacke M, Gotzen L. Results of elastic stable intramedullary nailing (ESIN) in forearm fractures in childhood. *Unfallchirurg.* 2003;106:102–109.

145. Manson TT, Pfaeffle HJ, Herdon JH, et al. Forearm rotation alters interosseous ligament strain distribution. *J Hand Surg Am.* 2000;25:1058–1063.

146. Markolf KL, Lamey D, Yang S, et al. Radioulnar load-sharing in the forearm: a study in cadavers. *J Bone Joint Surg Am.* 1998;80:879–888.

147. Martin J, Marsh JL, Nepola JV, et al. Radiographic fracture assessments: which ones can we reliably make? *J Orthop Trauma.* 2000;14:379–385.

148. Martus JE, Preston RK, Schoenecker JG, et al. Complications and outcomes of diaphyseal forearm fracture intramedullary nailing: a comparison of pediatric and adolescent age groups. *J Pediatr Orthop.* 2013;33:598–607.

149. Matthews LS, Kaufer H, Garver DF, Sonstegard DA. The effect on supination-pronation of angular malalignment of fractures of both bones of the forearm. *J Bone Joint Surg Am.* 1982;64:14–17.

150. McGinley JC, Hopgood BC, Gaughan JP, et al. Forearm and elbow injury: the influence of rotational position. *J Bone Joint Surg Am.* 2003;85:2403–2409.

151. McGinley JC, Kozin SH. Interosseous membrane anatomy and functional mechanics. *Clin Orthop Relat Res.* 2001;383:108–122.

152. McHenry TP, Pierce WA, Lais RL, Schacherer TG. Effect of displacement of ulna-shaft fractures on forearm rotation: a cadaveric model. *Am J Orthop.* 2002;31:420–424.

153. Mehlman CT. Clinical epidemiology. In: Koval KJ, ed. *Orthopaedic Knowledge Update.* 7th ed. AAOS; 2002:82.

154. Mehlman CT. Forearm, wrist, and hand trauma: pediatrics. In: Fischgrund JS, ed. *Orthopaedic Knowledge Update 9.* American Academy of Orthopaedic Surgeons; 2008:669–680.

155. Meier R, Prommersberger KJ, Lanz U. Surgical correction of malunited fractures of the forearm in children. *Z Orthop Ihre Grenzgeb.* 2003;141:328–335.

156. Mekhail AO, Ebraheim NA, Jackson WT, Yeasting RA. Vulnerability of the posterior interosseous nerve during proximal radius exposures. *Clin Orthop Relat Res.* 1995;315:199–208.

157. Metaizeau JP, Ligier JN. Surgical treatment of fractures of the long bones in children. Interference between osteosynthesis and the physiological processes of consolidation. Therapeutic indications. *J Chir (Paris).* 1984;121:527–537.

158. Miech R, Johnston L, O'Malley PM, et al. Prescription opioids in adolescence and future opioid misuse. *Pediatrics.* 2015;136(5):e1169–e1177.

159. Mitts KG, Hennrikus WL. In-line skating fractures in children. *J Pediatr Orthop.* 1996;16:640–643.

160. Morrey BF, Askew LJ, Chao EY. A biomechanical study of normal functional elbow motion. *J Bone Joint Surg Am.* 1981;63:872–877.

161. Moseley CF. Obituary: Mercer Rang, FRCSC (1933–2003). *J Pediatr Orthop.* 2004;24:446–447.

162. Mubarak SJ, Carroll NC. Volkmann's contracture in children: aetiology and prevention. *J Bone Joint Surg Br.* 1979;61:285–293.

163. Muensterer OJ, Regauer MP. Closed reduction of forearm refractures with flexible intramedullary nails in situ. *J Bone Joint Surg Am.* 2003;85:2152–2155.

164. Murphy HA, Jain VV, Parikh SN, et al. Extensor tendon injury associated with dorsal entry flexible nailing of radial shaft fractures in children: a report of 5 new cases and review of the literature. *J Pediatr Orthop.* 2019;39(4):163–168.

165. Murray WM, Delp SL, Buchanan TS. Variation of muscle moment arms with elbow and forearm position. *J Biomech.* 1995;28:513–525.

166. Myers GJ, Gibbons PJ, Glithero PR. Nancy nailing of diaphyseal forearm fractures: single bone fixation for fractures of both bones. *J Bone Joint Surg Br.* 2004;86:581–584.

167. Nakamura T, Yabe Y, Horiuchi Y. In vivo MR studies of dynamic changes in the interosseous membrane of the forearm during rotation. *J Hand Surg Br.* 1999;24:245–248.

168. Noonan KJ. Compartment syndrome in the pediatric patient. *J Pediatr Orthop.* 2010;30(Suppl 2):96–101.

169. Noonan KJ, Price CT. Forearm and distal radius fractures in children. *J Am Acad Orthop Surg.* 1998;6:146–156.

170. Ogonda L, Wong-Chung J, Wray R, Canavan B. Delayed union and nonunion of the ulna following intramedullary nailing in children. *J Pediatr Orthop B.* 2004;13:330–333.

171. Oğün TC, Sarlak A, Arazi M, Kapicioğlu MIS. Posttraumatic distal radioulnar synostosis and distal radial epiphyseal arrest. *Ulus Travma Derg.* 2002;8:59–61.
172. OlaOlorun DA, Oladiran IO, Adeniran A. Complications of fracture treatment by traditional bonesetters in southwest Nigeria. *Fam Pract.* 2001;18:635–637.
173. O'Neil DF. Wrist injuries in guarded versus unguarded first-time snowboarders. *Clin Orthop Relat Res.* 2003;409:91–95.
174. Ono M, Bechtold JE, Merkow RL, et al. Rotational stability of diaphyseal fractures of the radius and ulna fixed with Rush pins and/or fracture bracing. *Clin Orthop Relat Res.* 1989;240:236–243.
175. Parikh SN, Brody AS, Crawford AH. Use of a picture archiving and communication system (PACS) and computed plain radiography in preoperative planning. *Am J Orthop (Belle Mead NJ).* 2004;33:62–64.
176. Perez-Garcia MJ, Jiménez-Garcia R, Siles-Sanchez-Manjavacas A. Unexpected diagnosis of severe coarctation of the aorta after ketamine procedural sedation. *Pediatr Emerg Care.* 2012;28:1232–1233.
177. Petridou E, Karpathios T, Dessypris N, et al. The role of dairy products and non-alcoholic beverages in bone fractures among school-age children. *Scand J Soc Med.* 1997;25:119–125.
178. Pfaeffle HJ, Kischer KJ, Manson TT, et al. Role of the forearm interosseous ligament: is it more than just longitudinal load transfer? *J Hand Surg Am.* 2000;25:683–688.
179. Prevot J, Lascombes P, Guichet JM. Elastic stable intramedullary nailing for forearm fractures in children and adolescents. *Orthop Trans.* 1996;20:305.
180. Price CT, Knapp DR. Osteotomy for malunited forearm shaft fractures in children. *J Pediatr Orthop.* 2006;26:193–196.
181. Price CT, Scott DS, Kurzner ME, Flynn JC. Malunited forearm fractures in children. *J Pediatr Orthop.* 1990;10:705–712.
182. Pugh DM, Galpin RD, Carey TP. Intramedullary Steinmann pin fixation of forearm fractures in children: long-term results. *Clin Orthop Relat Res.* 2000;376:39–48.
183. Qidwai SA. Treatment of diaphyseal forearm fractures in children by intramedullary Kirschner wires. *J Trauma.* 2001;50:303–307.
184. Raiss P, Rettig O, Wolf S, et al. Range of motion of shoulder and elbow in activities of daily life in 3D motion analysis. *Z Orthop Unfall.* 2007;145:493–498.
185. Reinhardt KR, Feldman DS, Green DW, et al. Comparison of intramedullary nailing to plating for both-bone forearm fractures in older children. *J Pediatr Orthop.* 2008;28:403–409.
186. Rickert M, Bürger A, Günther CM, Schulz CU. Forearm rotation in healthy adults of all ages and both sexes. *J Shoulder Elbow Surg.* 2008;17:271–275.
187. Ring D, Waters PM, Hotchkiss RN, Kasser JR. Pediatric floating elbow. *J Pediatr Orthop.* 2001;21:456–459.
188. Roposch A, Reis M, Molina M, et al. Supracondylar fractures of the humerus associated with ipsilateral fractures in children: a report of forty-seven cases. *J Pediatr Orthop.* 2001;21:307–312.
189. Ryan LM, Teach SJ, Singer SA, et al. Bone mineral density and vitamin D status among African American children with forearm fractures. *Pediatrics.* 2012;130:e553–e560.
190. Salonen A, Salonen H, Pajulo O. A critical analysis of postoperative complications of antebrachium TEN-nailing in 35 children. *Scand J Surg.* 2012;101:216–221.
191. Sanders WE, Heckman JD. Traumatic plastic deformation of the radius and ulna: a closed method of correction of deformity. *Clin Orthop Relat Res.* 1984;188:58–67.
192. Sardelli M, Tashjian RZ, MacWilliams BA. Functional elbow range of motion for contemporary tasks. *J Bone Joint Surg Am.* 2011;93:471–477.
193. Sarmiento A, Ebramzadeh E, Brys D, Tarr R. Angular deformities and forearm function. *J Orthop Res.* 1992;10:121–133.
194. Schmittenbecker PP, Fitze G, Gödeke J, et al. Delayed healing of forearm shaft fractures in children after intramedullary nailing. *J Pediatr Orthop.* 2008;28:303–306.
195. Schwarz N, Pienaar S, Schwarz AF, et al. Refracture of the forearm in children. *J Bone Joint Surg Br.* 1996;78:740–744.
196. Segal D, Ziv A, Meisman A, et al. Relationship between hypovitaminosis d and fractures among adolescents with overweight or obesity. *Clin Pediatr (Phila).* 2023;62(2):107–114.
197. Shaer JA, Smith B, Turco VJ. Midthird forearm fractures in children: an unorthodox treatment. *Am J Orthop (Belle Mead NJ).* 1999;28:60–63.
198. Shah MH, Heffernan G, McGuinness AJ. Early experiences with titanium elastic nails in a trauma unit. *Ir Med J.* 2003;96:213–214.
199. Singer AJ, Gulla J, Thode HC Jr. Parents and practitioners are poor judges of young children's pain severity. *Acad Emerg Med.* 2002;9:609–612.
200. Sinikumpu JJ, Lautamo A, Pokka T, Serlo W. Complications and radiographic outcomes of children's both-bone diaphyseal forearm fractures after invasive and non-invasive treatment. *Injury.* 2013;44(4):431–436.
201. Sinikumpu JJ, Lautamo A, Pokka T, Serlo W. The increasing incidence of paediatric diaphyseal both-bone forearm fractures and their internal fixation during the last decade. *Injury.* 2012;43:362–366.
202. Skaggs DL, Kautz SM, Kay RM, Tolo VT. Effect of delay of surgical treatment on rate of infection in open fractures in children. *J Pediatr Orthop.* 2000;20:19–22.
203. Skaggs DL, Loro ML, Pitukcheewanont P, et al. Increased body weight and decreased radial cross-sectional dimensions in girls with forearm fractures. *J Bone Miner Res.* 2001;16:1337–1342.
204. Smith GA. Injuries to children in the United States related to trampolines, 1990–1995: a national epidemic. *Pediatrics.* 1998;101:406–412.
205. Song DJ, Kennebrew GJ Jr, Jex JW. Isolated ring finger flexor digitorum profundus entrapment after closed reduction and intramedullary fixation of both-bone forearm fracture. *Orthopedics.* 2012;35:e1283–e1285.
206. Song KS, Kim HKW. Nonunion as a complication of an open reduction of a distal radial fracture in a healthy child: a case report. *J Orthop Trauma.* 2003;17:231–233.
207. Soumekh L, Sylvanus T, Karlen A, et al. Refracture rate of both bone forearm fractures: a retrospective comparison of casting alone versus casting and extended functional bracing. *J Pediatr Orthop.* 2021;41(5):267–272.
208. Stahl S, Calif E, Eidelman M. Delayed rupture of the extensor pollicis longus tendon following intramedullary nailing of a radial fracture in a child. *J Hand Surg Eur Vol.* 2007;32:67–68.
209. Tabak AY, Celebi L, Murath HH, et al. Closed reduction and percutaneous fixation of supracondylar fracture of the humerus and ipsilateral fracture of the forearm in children. *J Bone Joint Surg Br.* 2003;85:1169–1172.
210. Tachakra S, Doherty S. The accuracy of length and angle measurement in videoconferencing teleradiology. *J Telemed Telecare.* 2002;8(Suppl 2):85–87.
211. Tarr RR, Garfinkel AI, Sarmiento A. The effects of angular and rotational deformities of both bones of the forearm: an in vitro study. *J Bone Joint Surg Am.* 1984;66:65–70.
212. Thomas EM, Tuson KW, Browne PS. Fractures of the radius and ulna in children. *Injury.* 1975;7:120–124.
213. Till H, Hüttl B, Knorr P, Dietz HG. Elastic stable intramedullary nailing (ESIN) provides good long-term results in pediatric long-bone fractures. *Eur J Pediatr Surg.* 2000;10:319–322.
214. Tisosky AJ, Werger MM, McPartland TG, Bowe JA. The factors influencing the refracture of pediatric forearms. *J Pediatr Orthop.* 2015;35(7):677–681.
215. Tredwell SJ, Van Peteghem K, Clough M. Pattern of forearm fractures in children. *J Pediatr Orthop.* 1984;4:604–608.
216. Trousdale RT, Linscheid RL. Operative treatment of malunited fractures of the forearm. *J Bone Joint Surg Am.* 1995;77:894–902.
217. Tynan MC, Fornalski S, McMahon PJ, et al. The effects of ulnar axial malalignment on supination and pronation. *J Bone Joint Surg Am.* 2000;82:1726–1731.
218. Van der Reis WL, Otsuka NY, Moroz P, Mah J. Intramedullary nailing versus plate fixation for unstable forearm fractures in children. *J Pediatr Orthop.* 1998;18:9–13.
219. VanderBeek BL, Mehlman CT, Foad SL, et al. The use of conscious sedation for forearm fracture reduction in children: does race matter? *J Pediatr Orthop.* 2006;26:53–57.
220. Vince KG, Miller JE. Cross-union complicating fracture of the forearm. Part II: children. *J Bone Joint Surg Am.* 1987;69:654–661.
221. Vorlat P, De Boeck H. Bowing fractures of the forearm in children: a long-term followup. *Clin Orthop Relat Res.* 2003;413:233–237.
222. Voto SJ, Weiner DS, Leighley B. Use of pins and plaster in the treatment of unstable pediatric forearm fractures. *J Pediatr Orthop.* 1990;10:85–89.
223. Wacker EM, Denning JR, Mehlman CT. Pediatric proximal radial shaft fractures treated nonoperatively fail to maintain acceptable reduction up to 70% of the time. *J Orthop Trauma.* 2019;33(10):e378–e384.
224. Walker JL, Rang M. Forearm fractures in children: cast treatment with the elbow extended. *J Bone Joint Surg Br.* 1991;73:299–301.
225. Waltzman ML, Shannon M, Bowen AP, Bailey MC. Monkeybar injuries: complications of play. *Pediatrics.* 1999;103:e58.
226. Watson PA, Blair W. Entrapment of the index flexor digitorum profundus tendon after fracture of both forearm bones in a child. *Iowa Orthop J.* 1999;19:127–128.
227. Weinberg DS, Park PJ, Boden KA, et al. Anatomic investigation of commonly used landmarks for evaluation rotation during forearm fracture reduction. *J Bone Joint Surg Am.* 2016;98(13):1103–1112.
228. Weiss JM, Mencio GA. Forearm shaft fractures: does fixation improve outcomes? *J Pediatr Orthop.* 2012;32(Suppl 1):S22–S24.
229. Wilkins KE. Operative management of children's fractures: is it a sign of impetuousness or do the children really benefit? *J Pediatr Orthop.* 1998;18:1–3.
230. Williams K, Whyte N, Carl JR, et al. Predictors for operative treatment in pediatric proximal third both-bone diaphyseal forearm fractures in children include age and translation, but not initial angulation. *J Child Orthop.* 2023;17(2):156–163.
231. Winslow L, Holstine J, Samora JB. Reducing the use of opioids for pediatric patients with supracondylar humerus fractures. *Jt Comm J Qual Patient Saf.* 2020;46(10):581–587.
232. Worlock P, Stower M. Fracture patterns in Nottingham children. *J Pediatr Orthop.* 1986;6:656–660.
233. Wright PB, Crepeau AE, Herrera-Soto JA, Price CT. Radius crossover sign: an indication of malreduced radius shaft greenstick fractures. *J Pediatr Orthop.* 2012;32:e15–e19.
234. Wynia EH, Lowing DM, Pan EJ, Schrock JW. Shifting practice in pediatric prescription opioid use in the emergency department for fractures. *Am J Emerg Med.* 2022;59:141–145.
235. Wyrsch B, Mencio GA, Green NE. Open reduction and internal fixation of pediatric forearm fractures. *J Pediatr Orthop.* 1996;16:644–650.
236. Yasin MN, Talwalkar SC, Henderson JJ, Hodgson SP. Segmental radius and ulna fractures with scaphocapitate fractures and bilateral multiple epiphyseal fractures. *Am J Orthop (Belle Mead NJ).* 2008;37:214–217.
237. Yasutomi T, Nakatsuchi Y, Koike H, Uchiyama S. Mechanism of limitation of pronation/supination of the forearm in geometric models of deformities of the forearm bones. *Clin Biomech (Bristol, Avon).* 2002;17:456–463.
238. Yong B, Yuan Z, Li J, et al. Single bone fixation versus both bone fixation for pediatric unstable forearm fractures: a systematic review and metaanalysis. *Indian J Orthop.* 2018;52(5):529–535.
239. Younger AS, Tredwell SJ, Mackenzie WG, et al. Accurate prediction of outcome after pediatric forearm fracture. *J Pediatr Orthop.* 1994;14:200–206.
240. Younger AS, Tredwell SJ, Mackenzie WG. Factors affecting fracture position at cast removal after pediatric forearm fracture. *J Pediatr Orthop.* 1997;17:332–336.
241. Yuan PS, Pring ME, Gaynor TP, et al. Compartment syndrome following intramedullary fixation of pediatric forearm fractures. *J Pediatr Orthop.* 2004;24:370–375.
242. Yung PSH, Lam CY, Ng BKW, et al. Percutaneous transphyseal intramedullary Kirschner wire pinning: a safe and effective procedure for treatment of displaced forearm fracture in children. *J Pediatr Orthop.* 2004;24:7–12.
243. Zionts LE, Zalavras CG, Gerhardt MB. Closed treatment of displaced both-bone forearm fractures in older children and adolescents. *J Pediatr Orthop.* 2005;25:507–512.

11

Radial Neck and Olecranon Fractures

Sumeet Garg, Mark A. Erickson, and Sarah E. Sibbel

INTRODUCTION TO FRACTURES OF THE PROXIMAL RADIUS AND ULNA

Fractures of the proximal radius in skeletally immature patients usually involve the metaphysis and/or physis. True isolated radial head fractures are less common. In the proximal ulna, the olecranon, which biomechanically is a metaphysis, often fails with a greenstick pattern. Fractures in this area also may involve the apophysis. Fractures of the olecranon associated with radial head dislocation are considered part of the Monteggia fracture pattern and are discussed in Chapter 12.

Fractures of the radial neck account for 1% to 3% of all children's fractures.[35] Radial neck fractures make up approximately 5% to 10% of elbow fractures in children. Radial head fractures are uncommon but concerning if there is articular displacement, and when they occur usually are Salter–Harris type IV injuries. The skeletally mature adolescent can have an adult-like intra-articular radial head fracture. Weight-bearing athletes such as gymnasts can develop a stress fracture of the radial head that can lead to a displaced nonunion. The median age at injury is 9 to 10 years in the pediatric population.[14,35,45,65] There is little difference in the occurrence rates between males and females[14,45]; however, this injury seems to occur on an average approximately 2 years earlier in girls than in boys.[58] Thorough assessment of radiographs is important due to the risk of associated fractures. Some reports suggest that 30% to 50% of patients will have additional fractures around the elbow, primarily medial epicondyle, elbow dislocations, and/or olecranon fractures.[3,59,79]

Fractures of the proximal ulna in skeletally immature children present in three different patterns: fractures involving the proximal apophysis, metaphyseal fractures of the olecranon, and fractures of the coronoid process.

Few fractures of the ulnar apophysis are described in the English literature, most recently by Carney.[5] In addition to acute injuries in children, some have been described in young adults with open physes.[68] Stress fracture nonunions can occur in throwing athletes. Most reports of apophyseal olecranon fractures occur in children with osteogenesis imperfecta (OI), who seem predisposed to this injury and are often treated using tension-band wiring.[52]

Isolated metaphyseal fractures of the olecranon are less common. It is important to assess the elbow for associated fractures or dislocations, such as a Monteggia variant of injury (Table 11-1; see Chapter 12). In the combined series of 4,684 elbow fractures reviewed, 230 were olecranon fractures, for an incidence of 4.9%. This agrees with the incidence of 4% to 6% in the major series reported.[18,49] Only 10% to 20% of the total fractures reported in these series required an operation. Six reports totaling 302 patients with fractures of the olecranon in children are in the English literature.[21,45] Considering all age groups, 25% of olecranon fractures in these reports occurred in the first decade and another 25% in the second decade.[35] During the first decade, the peak age for olecranon fracture was between age 5 and 10 years.[25] Approximately 20% of patients had an associated fracture or dislocation of the elbow, most involving the proximal radius.

TABLE 11-1. Incidence of Metaphyseal Fractures of the Olecranon
Age distribution: first decade, 25%; second decade, 25%; third decade, 50%
Peak age: 5–10 years
Extremity predominance: left (55%)
Sex predominance: male (65%)
Associated elbow injuries: 20%
Requiring surgical intervention: 19%

The incidence of fracture of the coronoid varies from less than 1% to 2% of elbow fractures; these fractures are often associated with elbow dislocations.

Fractures of the Proximal Radius

ASSESSMENT OF FRACTURES OF THE PROXIMAL RADIUS

MECHANISMS OF INJURY FOR FRACTURES OF THE PROXIMAL RADIUS

Most fractures of the proximal radius occur at the neck. Fractures of the proximal radius typically occur after a fall on an outstretched arm with the elbow extended and valgus stress.[23,45] The immature radial head is primarily cartilaginous with its primary blood supply coming from the metaphysis. This may predispose radial head fractures to avascular necrosis and nonunion. This can also occur with repetitive microtrauma, such as gymnastics.

In radial neck fractures, the cartilaginous radial head absorbs the loading force and transmits it to the weaker physis or metaphysis of the neck. These fractures characteristically produce an angular deformity of the head with the neck (Fig. 11-1). The direction of angulation depends on whether the forearm is in a supinated, neutral, or pronated position at the time of the fall. Vostal showed that in neutral forearm rotation, the pressure is concentrated on the lateral portion of the head and neck. In supination, the pressure is concentrated anteriorly, and in pronation, it is concentrated posteriorly.

Proximal radial fractures also may occur in association with an elbow dislocation. The fracture will usually occur during the dislocation event, typically displaced anteriorly. Alternatively, the fracture may occur during spontaneous reduction of the distal humerus, driving the displacement of the proximal radius posteriorly (Fig. 11-2).

INJURIES ASSOCIATED WITH FRACTURES OF THE PROXIMAL RADIUS

Proximal radius fractures can occur concomitantly with distal humerus, ulnar and/or radial shaft, or distal radius fractures.[23,65]

Figure 11-1. The most common mechanism of radial neck fractures involves a fall on the outstretched arm. This produces an angular deformity of the neck (**A**). Further valgus forces can produce a greenstick fracture of the olecranon (**B**) or an avulsion of the medial epicondylar apophysis (**C**). (Reproduced and redrawn with permission of The British Editorial Society of Bone & Joint Surgery. Jeffery CC. Fractures of the head of the radius in children. *J Bone Joint Surg Br.* 1950;32-B(3):314–324, permission conveyed through Copyright Clearance Center, Inc.)

Proximal radius fractures in combination with ulnar fractures often are part of the Monteggia fracture pattern, detailed in Chapter 12. The presence of associated fractures portends a poor prognosis for patients with proximal radius fractures with higher rates of persistent stiffness and pain compared to those with isolated proximal radius fractures.[67] As detailed further in Chapter 16, proximal radius fractures can also occur during traumatic elbow dislocations. The posterior interosseous nerve (PIN) wraps around the proximal radius and occasionally can be injured in association with proximal radius fractures. More typically, however, the PIN nerve is at risk during percutaneous manipulation or open reduction of proximal radius fractures.

SIGNS AND SYMPTOMS OF FRACTURES OF THE PROXIMAL RADIUS

Following a fracture, palpation over the radial head or neck is painful. If the patient moves or allows you to move the injured area, the pain is usually increased with forearm rotation more so than with elbow flexion and extension. Displaced fractures frequently result in visible bruising on the lateral aspect of the elbow with soft tissue swelling. Neurologic examination should include all neurovascular structures of the wrist and hand, but the PIN should get special attention (test for wrist, digital MCP, thumb IP, and MCP extension). Occasionally in a young child, the primary complaint may be wrist pain, and pressure over the proximal radius may accentuate this referred wrist pain. The wrist pain may be secondary to radial shortening and subsequent distal radioulnar joint dysfunction. This reinforces the principle of obtaining radiographs of both ends of a fractured long bone and complete examination of the entire affected extremity.

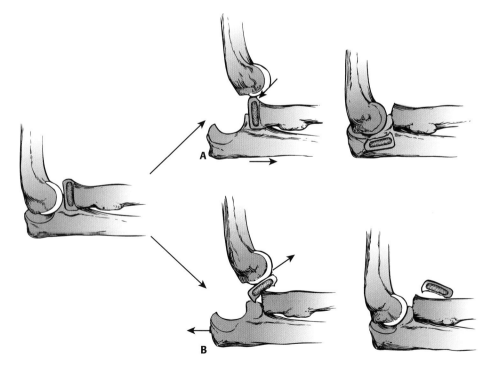

Figure 11-2. Dislocation fracture patterns. **A:** Type D: The radial neck is fractured during the process of reduction by the capitellum pressing against the distal lip of the radial head. **B:** Type E: The radial neck is fractured during the process of dislocation by the capitellum pressing against the proximal lip of the radial head.

Figure 11-2. (*Continued*) **C:** Radiographs of a radial head that was fractured during the reduction of the dislocation (type D). The radial head (*solid arrow*) lies posterior to the distal humerus, and the distal portion of the neck (*open arrow*) is anterior. **D:** Radiograph of the dislocated elbow in which the fracture of the radial neck occurred during the process of dislocation (type E). (**A, B: C:** Courtesy of Richard E. King, MD.)

IMAGING AND OTHER DIAGNOSTIC STUDIES FOR FRACTURES OF THE PROXIMAL RADIUS

Displaced proximal radius fractures are usually easy to identify on standard anteroposterior (AP) and lateral radiographs. Some ossification variants can resemble a fracture, so comparison views of the contralateral elbow can be a helpful tool to evaluate for a fracture.

If the elbow cannot be extended because of pain, special views are necessary to see the AP alignment of the proximal forearm and distal humerus. A regular AP view with the elbow flexed may not show the fracture because of obliquity of the beam and overlap of proximal forearm and distal humerus bones. One view is taken with the beam perpendicular to the distal humerus, and the other with the beam perpendicular to the proximal radius. The perpendicular views show the proximal radial physis in clear profile.

Figure 11-3. A: Radiocapitellar view. **B:** Angular stress deformity: Anterior angulation of the radial head and neck in a 12-year-old baseball pitcher. There is evidence of some disruption of the normal growth of the anterior portion of the physis (*black arrow*). The capitellum also shows radiographic signs of osteochondritis dissecans (*white arrow*). (Courtesy of Kenneth P. Butters, MD.)

Figure 11-4. The radiocapitellar view. **A:** Radiographs of an 11-year-old female who sustained a radial neck fracture associated with an elbow dislocation. There is ectopic bone formation (*arrows*). In this view, it is difficult to tell the exact location of the ectopic bone. **B:** The radiocapitellar view separates the radial head from the coronoid process and shows that the ectopic bone is from the coronoid process (*arrows*) and not the radial neck.

With a minimally displaced fracture, the fracture line may be difficult to see because it is superimposed on the proximal ulna, and oblique views of the proximal radius may be helpful. One oblique view that is especially helpful is the radiocapitellar view suggested by Greenspan et al.[26] and Hall-Craggs et al.[27] This view projects the radial head anterior to the coronoid process (Fig. 11-3) and is especially helpful if full supination and pronation views are difficult to obtain because of acute injury (Fig. 11-4).

The diagnosis of a partially or completely displaced fracture of the radial neck may be difficult in children whose radial head remains unossified.[40] The only clue may be irregularity in the smoothness of the proximal metaphyseal margin (Fig. 11-5). In the preossification stage, on the AP radiograph, the edge of the metaphysis of the proximal radius slopes distally on its lateral border. This angulation is normal and not a fracture. In the AP view, the lateral angulation varies from 0 to 15 degrees, with the average being 12.5 degrees. In the lateral view, the angulation can vary

from 10 degrees anterior to 5 degrees posterior, with the average being 3.5 degrees anterior.

The full extent of proximal radius injuries may be better evaluated with magnetic resonance imaging (MRI). Displacement of the supinator fat pad may also indicate fracture of the proximal radius; however, this fat pad and the distal humeral anterior and posterior fat pads are not always displaced with occult fractures of the radial neck or physis.[29] Arthrogram, ultrasound, and MRI are helpful to assess the extent of the displacement and the accuracy of reduction in children with an unossified radial epiphysis (Fig. 11-6).[9] Examination under anesthesia offers the best ability to optimize the radiographic view to assess maximal displacement of the fracture. An arthrogram can also easily be performed for additional diagnostic information. An added benefit is ability to assess range of motion of the elbow and forearm to help determine whether manipulation will offer benefit to the patient.

Posterior radiocapitellar subluxation following what appeared to be innocuous radial head fractures have been attributed to undiagnosed ligamentous injury (typically of the lateral ulnar collateral ligamentous complex) associated with the fracture. Waters and Kasser include these injuries among lesions described by the acronym "TRASH" for "*the radiographic appearance seemed harmless.*"[76] MRI provides excellent anatomic detail of the elbow joint and should be considered when evaluating displaced radial head fractures, particularly if change in position is noted on serial radiographs.

CLASSIFICATION OF FRACTURES OF THE PROXIMAL RADIUS

Chambers' Classification of Proximal Radial Fractures

Group	Description
\multicolumn{2}{|l|}{**Chambers' Classification of Fractures Involving the Proximal Radius[7]**}

Group	Description
I	**Primary displacement of the radial head (most common)**
	Valgus fractures
IA	Salter–Harris type I and II injuries of the proximal radial physis
IB	Salter–Harris type IV injuries of the proximal radial physis
IC	Fractures involving only the proximal radial metaphysis
	Fractures associated with elbow dislocation
ID	Reduction injuries
IE	Dislocation injuries
II	**Primary displacement of the radial neck**
IIA	Angular injuries (Monteggia type III variant)
IIB	Torsional injuries
III	**Stress injuries**
IIIA	Osteochondritis dissecans or osteochondrosis of the radial head
IIIB	Physeal injuries with neck angulation

Figure 11-5. Preosseous fracture. The only clue to the presence of a fracture of the radial neck with displacement of the radial head was loss of smoothness of the metaphyseal margin (*arrow*).

Head-Displaced Fractures (Group I)

With valgus elbow injuries, the fracture pattern of the radial head and neck can be one of three types (A, B, or C) (Fig. 11-7). In the first two types, the fracture line involves the physis. Type A represents either a Salter–Harris type I or II physeal injury. In a Salter–Harris type II injury, the metaphyseal fragment is triangular and lies on the compression side. In type B fractures, the fracture line courses vertically through the metaphysis, physis, and epiphysis to produce a Salter–Harris type IV fracture pattern. This is the only fracture type that involves the articular surface of the radial head in a skeletally immature child. In type C fractures, the fracture line lies completely within the metaphysis (Fig. 11-8), and the fracture can be transverse or oblique. Type B fractures, intra-articular radial head fractures, are rare. These can have poor long-term results if posterior radiocapitellar subluxation develops (Fig. 11-9).[73,76] The incidences of types A and C fractures are approximately equal.[65]

Figure 11-6. A, B: AP and lateral radiographs demonstrating a radial neck fracture in a patient with a non-ossified proximal radial epiphysis. **C:** Arthrogram prior to reduction demonstrating location/displacement of nonossified proximal radial epiphysis. **D–F:** Arthrogram/radiographs after reduction with intramedullary technique. (Reprinted with permission from Javed A, Guichet JM. Arthrography for reduction of a fracture of the radial neck in a child with a nonossified radial epiphysis. *J Bone Joint Surg Br.* 2001;83-B:542–543; permission conveyed through Copyright Clearance Center, Inc.)

Figure 11-7. Valgus (type B) injury. **A:** Three weeks after the initial injury, there was evidence of distal migration of this Salter–Harris type IV fracture fragment. Periosteal new bone formation has already developed along the distal metaphyseal fragment (*arrow*). **B:** Six months after the initial injury, there was evidence of an osseous bridge formation between the metaphysis and the epiphysis. Subsequently, the patient had secondary degenerative arthritis with loss of elbow motion and forearm rotation.

In two rare types of fractures of the radial neck fractures associated with elbow dislocation, the head fragment is typically totally displaced from the neck.[45] Fractures occurring during spontaneous reduction of elbow dislocation generally drive the radial head posterior as the capitellum applies a posteriorly directed force to the radial neck during reduction dislocation (type D) (see Fig. 11-2A). Fractures occurring during the dislocation event generally drive the radial head anteriorly as the capitellum applies an anteriorly direct force during the process of dislocating (type E) (see Fig. 11-2B).[45] Even with spontaneous or manipulative elbow reduction, the radial head fragment will usually remain anterior to the radial shaft with the fractured radial neck articulating with the capitellum.

Regardless of the type of fracture pattern, displacement can vary from minimal angulation to complete separation of the

Figure 11-8. Valgus type C injury. The fracture line is totally metaphyseal and oblique (*arrows*).

radial head from the neck (Fig. 11-10). With minimal angulation, the congruity of the proximal radio-ulnar joint (PRUJ) is usually retained. If the radial head is displaced in relation to the radial neck, the congruity of the PRUJ is lost. Completely displaced fractures are often associated with more severe injuries.

Neck-Displaced Fractures (Group II)

Rarely, angular or torsional forces cause a primary disruption or deformity of the radial neck while the head remains congruous within the PRUJ. Treatment of these fractures is manipulation of the distal neck fragment to align it with the head. For neck-displaced fractures, there are two subgroups: angular and torsional.

An angular fracture of the radial neck may be associated with a proximal ulnar fracture. This association is recognized as a Monteggia variant. A Monteggia type III fracture pattern is created when a varus force is applied across the extended elbow, resulting in a greenstick fracture of the olecranon or proximal ulna and a lateral dislocation of the radial head. Occasionally, however, the failure occurs at the radial neck (Monteggia III equivalent) and the radial neck displaces laterally, leaving the radial head and proximal neck fragment in anatomic position under the annular ligament (Fig. 11-11).[47]

Rotational forces may fracture the radial neck in young children before ossification of the proximal radial epiphysis. This has been described only in case reports with a supination force.[23] Reduction was achieved by pronation of the forearm. Diagnosis of these injuries is difficult and may require MRI, arthrography, ultrasound, and/or an examination under general anesthesia. This injury should be differentiated from the more common subluxation of the radial head ("nursemaid's elbow"), in which the forearm usually is held in pronation with resistance to supination.

Stress Injuries (Group III)

A final mechanism of injury is chronic repetitive stress, both longitudinal and rotational, on either the head or the proximal

Figure 11-9. **A:** Acute injury films revealing small displacement of radial head fracture on the flexed elbow anteroposterior (AP) view and subtle posterior subluxation not originally appreciated on the lateral view. **B:** Follow-up radiographs at 1 week noted more difficulty interpreting the AP view in cast, and more radiocapitellar posterior displacement on the lateral view. An MRI scan (**C**) was ordered urgently and revealed a marked effusion and intra-articular displacement of radial head fracture and posterior radiocapitellar subluxation. **D:** Open reduction internal fixation was performed to anatomically align the radial head fracture and reduce the joint. (Reprinted with permission from Waters PM, et al. Elbow "TRASH" [The Radiographic Appearance Seemed Harmless]. *J Pediatr Orthop.* 2010;30:S77–S81.)

Figure 11-10. Displacement patterns. The radial head can be angulated (**A**), translated (**B**), or completely displaced (**C**).

radial physis. These injuries are usually the result of athletic activity in which the upper extremity is required to perform repetitive motions or loading. Repetitive stresses disrupt growth of either the radial neck or the head with eventual deformity. A true stress fracture can occur with gymnastics.

In the United States, the popularity of organized sports has produced a number of unique injuries in children related to repetitive stress applied to growth centers. Many elbow stress injuries are related to throwing sports such as baseball. Most of this "Little League" pathology involves tension injuries on the medial epicondyle. In some athletes, however, the lateral side is involved as well because of the repetitive compressive forces applied to the capitellum and radial head and neck. Athletes

Figure 11-11. Angular forces. This 8 year old sustained a type III Monteggia equivalent in which the radial neck fractured (*arrow*), leaving the radial head reduced proximally. (Courtesy of Ruben D. Pechero, MD.)

Figure 11-12. Osteochondritis dissecans. Radiograph of this 11-year-old Little League pitcher's elbow shows fragmentation of the subchondral surfaces of the radial head. These changes and the accelerated bone age are evidence of overuse.

involved in sports requiring upper extremity weight bearing, such as gymnastics or wrestling, are also at risk. In the radial head, lytic lesions similar to osteochondritis dissecans may occur (Figs. 11-12 and 11-13).[69] Chronic compressive loading may cause an osteochondrosis of the proximal radial epiphysis, with radiographic signs of decreased size of the ossified epiphysis, increased radiographic opacity, and later fragmentation. If the stress forces are transmitted to the radial neck, the anterior portion of the physis may be injured, producing an angular deformity of the radial neck (see Fig. 11-3). The more complex aspect of this injury spectrum is loss of anterior radial head height, joint instability and malalignment, and at times, nonunion and avascular necrosis of the radial head stress fracture.

Judet and O'Brien Classifications of Radial Neck Fractures

Judet Classification of Radial Neck Fractures[30]	
Type	Description
I	Nondisplaced
II	<30 degrees of angulation
III	30–60 degrees of angulation
IVA	60–80 degrees of angulation
IVB	>80 degrees of angulation

Radial neck fractures, the most common type of proximal radius fracture (groups 1A and 1C per the chambers classification), have also been classified based on angulation by Judet.[30] Increasing grade has generally been associated with poorer

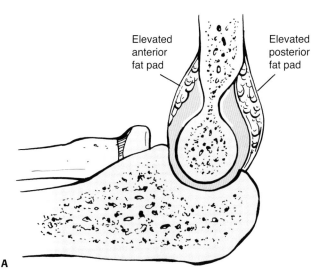

Elevated anterior fat pad   Elevated posterior fat pad

A

B

Figure 11-13. A: Elevated anterior and posterior fat pads. **B:** Radiographic appearance of posterior (*white arrow*) and anterior (*black arrow*) fat pad signs. (**A:** Adapted with permission from Skaggs DL, Mirzayan R. The posterior fat pad sign in association with occult fracture of the elbow in children. *J Bone Joint Surg Am.* 1999;81(10):1429–1433.)

TABLE 11-2. The Mayo Clinic Performance Index for the Elbow	
Function	**Point Score[a]**
Pain (45 points)	
None	45
Mild	30
Moderate	15
Severe	0
Motion (20 points)	
Arc 100 degrees	20
Arc 50–100 degrees	15
Arc 2 degrees	5
Stability[b] (10 points)	
Stable	10
Moderate instability	
Gross instability	0
Daily Function (25 points)	
Combing hair	5
Feeding oneself	5
Hygiene	5
Putting on shirt	5
Putting on shoes	5
Maximum possible total	**100**

[a]90 points or more, excellent; 75–89 points, good; 60–74 points, fair; and <60 points, poor.
[b]Stable, no apparent varus-valgus laxity clinically; moderate instability, <10 degrees of varus-valgus laxity; and gross instability, 10 degrees or more of varus-valgus laxity.
Reprinted with permission from Mayo Elbow Performance Score. *J Orthop Trauma.* 2006;20(8):S127.

outcomes with both nonoperative and operative care. O'Brien described a similar classification of radial neck fractures specifically for pediatric patients with slightly different grading[46]:

O'Brien Classification of Radial Neck Fractures in Children[46]	
Type	**Description**
I	<30 degrees of angulation
II	30–60 degrees of angulation
III	>60 degrees of angulation

OUTCOME MEASURES FOR FRACTURES OF THE PROXIMAL RADIUS

Most previously published literature on the outcomes of pediatric proximal radius fractures has used nonvalidated functional outcome measures. Various iterations of "excellent," "good," "fair," and "poor" with individualized descriptions have been utilized. The growing emphasis in orthopaedics on critical functional assessments following injury or surgery should improve the quality of future evidence on this topic. It is hoped that validated functional measures for upper extremity function and global pediatric and adolescent function be utilized in future research efforts in this area. The Mayo Elbow Performance Score is also used as a more objective functional measure (Table 11-2). More recently, the Patient Reported Outcomes Measurement Information System (PROMIS) has gained popularity in assessing patient-reported outcomes for a variety of conditions, including demonstrated use in pediatric orthopaedics.[16]

Range of motion following treatment of proximal radius fractures is a critical component of outcome. Usually, assessments have been done manually using a goniometer but have poor reliability within and between observers. Digital motion capture technology may provide more accurate measures of range of motion following extremity trauma in future studies but is not widely utilized.

A, B

C

Figure 11-14. Ossification pattern. **A:** At 5 years, ossification begins as a small oval nucleus. **B:** As the head matures, the center widens but remains flat. **C:** Double ossification centers in developing proximal radial epiphysis. (Reprinted with permission from Silberstein MJ, et al. Some vagaries of the radial head and neck. *J Bone Joint Surgery Am.* 1982;64(8):1153–1157.)

PATHOANATOMY AND APPLIED ANATOMY RELATING TO FRACTURES OF THE PROXIMAL RADIUS

In the embryo, the proximal radius is well defined by 9 weeks of gestation. By 4 years of age, the radial head and neck have the same contours as in an adult. Ossification of the proximal radius epiphysis begins at approximately 5 years of age as a small, flat nucleus (Fig. 11-14). This ossific nucleus can originate as a small sphere or it can be bipartite, which is a normal variation and should not be misinterpreted as a fracture.[38]

No ligaments attach directly to the radial neck or head. The radial collateral ligaments attach to the annular ligament, which originates from the radial side of the ulna. The articular capsule attaches to the proximal third of the neck. Distally, the capsule protrudes from under the annular ligament to form a pouch (recessus sacciformis). Thus, only a small portion of the neck lies within the articular capsule. Because much of the neck is extracapsular, fractures involving only the neck may not produce an intra-articular effusion, and the fat pad sign may be negative with fracture of the radial neck.[38]

The PRUJ has a precise congruence. The axis of rotation of the proximal radius is a line through the center of the radial head and neck. When a displaced fracture disrupts the alignment of the radial head on the center of the radial neck, the arc of rotation changes. Instead of rotating smoothly in a pure circle, the radial head rotates with a "cam" effect. This disruption of the congruity of the PRUJ (as occurs with displaced fractures of the proximal radius) may result in a loss of the range of motion in supination and pronation (Fig. 11-15).[77]

Table 11-3 lists the proposed mechanisms for fractures of the radial head and neck in children.

TREATMENT OPTIONS FOR FRACTURES OF THE PROXIMAL RADIUS

NONOPERATIVE TREATMENT OF FRACTURES OF THE PROXIMAL RADIUS

Indications/Contraindications

Nonoperative Treatment of Proximal Radius Fractures:
INDICATIONS AND CONTRAINDICATIONS

Indications

- <2-mm displacement of the radial head or neck
- <30- to 45-degree angulation of the radial neck (<30 degrees if age >10, <45 degrees if age <10) (relative indication depending on arc of motion; and if radial head is still aligned with capitellum)
- Full forearm pronation and supination

Relative Contraindications

- Open fracture
- Incongruent radiocapitellar or PRUJ joint(s)

Nonoperative treatment is indicated for most proximal radius fractures. Remodeling of the proximal radius can be expected in skeletally immature children as long as the joints are aligned. Based on multiple retrospective case series, radial neck angulation of up to 45 degrees can remodel if the radial head is not dislocated and conservative treatment will lead to good results.[11,14,44,45,65,78] It is critical to assess forearm rotation, and if a block to full rotation is appreciated, an attempt at reduction should be considered. Intra-articular aspiration of hematoma and injection of local anesthetic can assist with pain relief and

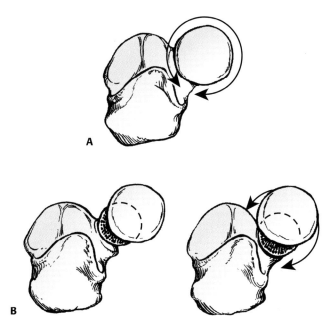

Figure 11-15. A: Normal rotation of the forearm causes the radial head to circumscribe an exact circle within the proximal radioulnar joint. **B:** Any translocation of the radial head limits rotation because of the "cam" effect described by Wedge and Robertson.[77]

assessment of range of motion. Examination under conscious sedation or anesthesia may also be indicated to properly assess range of motion and degree of displacement if adequate analgesia cannot be achieved with the patient awake.

In the case of nondisplaced radial head fractures (Salter–Harris IV, Group IB in the Chambers' classification), close follow-up with serial radiographs is warranted to monitor radiocapitellar alignment. If subluxation is suspected, advanced imaging with ultrasound or MRI, along with consideration of operative treatment, should be considered.

Closed reduction techniques should be attempted if there is displacement or unacceptable angulation at the fracture site, especially with a malaligned joint. The goal should be to restore acceptable alignment with full forearm rotation. Internal fixation is usually not necessary if successful, stable closed reduction can be accomplished.

TABLE 11-3. Proposed Mechanisms of Fractures of the Radial Head and Neck in Children

Primary Displacement of the Head (Incongruous)

Valgus injuries

Associated with dislocation of the elbow

• During reduction

• During dislocation

Primary Displacement of the Neck

Angular forces

Rotational forces

Chronic stress forces

Patients not requiring closed reduction should be immobilized for a short period of time to allow for comfort and soft tissue healing. This is generally 1 to 3 weeks based on extent of injury and age. After fracture pain has subsided, patients should work on progressively increasing range of motion and resumption of activities as symptoms allow. Short-term immobilization can be accomplished with a sling, posterior arm splint, elbow-hinged brace, or long-arm cast based on surgeon and patient preference.

Closed Reduction Techniques

Several closed reduction techniques for proximal radius fractures have been described in the literature, all with generally good results. The surgeon should be familiar with multiple techniques and apply them as needed because closed treatment of proximal radius fractures has been shown to have improved results compared to open treatment. No single closed technique has demonstrated to have superiority over another. Techniques are variations on either manipulating the proximal fragment to the fixed radial shaft or manipulating the radial shaft to the fixed proximal fragment; or both.

Patterson[50] described a reduction technique for the radial neck in 1934. Conscious sedation or general anesthesia is recommended in children to allow for adequate relaxation during the procedure. The annular ligament should be intact to stabilize the proximal radial head fragment.[45] An assistant grasps the arm proximal to the elbow joint with one hand (Fig. 11-16) and places the other hand medially over the distal humerus to provide a medial fulcrum for the varus stress

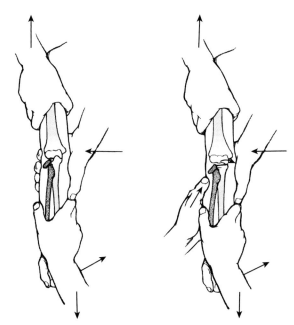

Figure 11-16. The Patterson manipulation technique.[49] **Left:** An assistant grabs the arm proximally with one hand placed medially against the distal humerus. The surgeon applies distal traction with the forearm supinated and pulls the forearm into varus. **Right:** Digital pressure applied directly over the tilted radial head completes the reduction. *Arrows* indicate direction of force applied by the manipulating hands.

Figure 11-17. Fluoroscopic view demonstrating maximal angulation of radial head. This is obtained by visualizing fracture radiographically with various degrees of forearm rotation until maximal angulation of the radial head is appreciated.

Figure 11-18. Neher and Torch reduction technique. (Reprinted with permission from Neher CG, Torch MA. New reduction technique for severely displaced pediatric radial neck fractures. *J Pediatr Orthop.* 2003;23(5):626–628.)

applied across the elbow. The surgeon applies distal traction with the forearm supinated to relax the supinator and biceps. A varus force is then placed on the elbow with added direct lateral pressure on the radial head to reduce the fracture. Kaufman et al.[31] proposed another technique in which the elbow is manipulated in the flexed position. The surgeon presses their thumb against the anterior surface of the radial head with the forearm in pronation.

Although forearm supination relaxes the supinator muscle, supination may not be the best position for manipulation of the head fragment. The tilt of the radial head depends on the position of the forearm at the time of injury. The direction of maximal tilt can be confirmed by radiographs and is also when fracture deformity will be most palpable clinically. The best position for reduction is the degree of rotation that places the radial head most prominent laterally (Fig. 11-17). With a varus force applied across the extended elbow, the maximal tilt directed laterally, and the elbow in varus, the radial head can be reduced with the pressure of a finger (see Fig. 11-16, right). An alternative technique with the elbow in extension was described by Neher and Torch.[43] An assistant uses both thumbs to place a laterally directed force on the proximal radial shaft while the surgeon applies a varus stress to the elbow. Simultaneously, the surgeon uses their other thumb to apply a reduction force directly to the radial head (Fig. 11-18).[41]

The Israeli technique involves stabilization of the proximal fragment with the thumb anteriorly while rotating the forearm into full pronation to reduce the shaft to the proximal fragment.[31] The elbow should be flexed to 90 degrees for the manipulation (Figs. 11-19 and 11-20). Another technique emphasizing reduction of the shaft to the proximal fragment was recently described by Monson. After adequate sedation or anesthesia,

the elbow is flexed to 90 degrees and forearm fully supinated. The proximal radial fragment should be stabilized in place by the annular ligament. A direct force is applied to the radial shaft to reduce the shaft to the head (Figs. 11-21 and 11-22).

Finally, use of an Esmarch bandage wrap, as is done for limb exsanguination prior to tourniquet use in extremity surgery, has been described to serendipitously promote fracture reduction (Fig. 11-23).[7] This can be used as an easy adjunct in nearly all the described closed reduction techniques.

Regardless of the technique chosen, alignment should be assessed by fluoroscopy. Radial neck angulation should be reduced to less than 45 degrees in children under 10 years of age, and less than 30 degrees in children greater than 10 years of age. Most importantly, the radiocapitellar joint needs to be congruent. The elbow joint must be stable to stress and range of motion of the forearm in pronation and supination restored. Immobilization for a short duration is recommended for pain control and soft tissue healing. Early range of motion should be encouraged once the acute pain has resolved, generally within 1 to 3 weeks.

A   B

Figure 11-19. Flexion-pronation (Israeli) reduction technique. **A:** Radiograph of the best reduction obtained by the Patterson method.[49] **B:** Position of the radial head after the flexion-pronation method. (Courtesy of Gerald R. Williams, MD.)

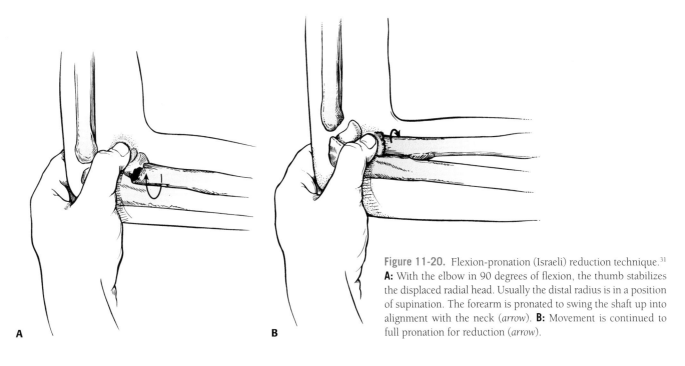

A   **B**

Figure 11-20. Flexion-pronation (Israeli) reduction technique.[31] **A:** With the elbow in 90 degrees of flexion, the thumb stabilizes the displaced radial head. Usually the distal radius is in a position of supination. The forearm is pronated to swing the shaft up into alignment with the neck (*arrow*). **B:** Movement is continued to full pronation for reduction (*arrow*).

OPERATIVE TREATMENT OF FRACTURES OF THE PROXIMAL RADIUS

Indications/Contraindications

Figure 11-21. As the fracture is usually displaced laterally, placing the forearm in supination results in the apex being anterior. The radial head is relatively stable and locked by the annular ligament. Pressure on the proximal radial shaft (*solid arrows*) with the arm in supination reduces the shaft to the radial head. (Reprinted with permission from Monson R, et al. A new closed reduction technique for the treatment of radial neck fractures in children. *J Pediatr Orthop.* 2009;29(3):243–247.)

Operative Treatment of Fractures of the Proximal Radius:
INDICATIONS AND CONTRAINDICATIONS

Indications

- Displacement remains over 2 mm following closed alignment
- Angulation is greater than 45 degrees (age <10)
- Angulation is greater than 30 degrees (age >10)
- Restricted range of motion of the elbow and/or forearm
- Incongruent radiocapitellar and/or PRUJ

Contraindications

- Acceptable alignment can be achieved with closed means
- No persistent elbow instability or incongruency
- Unrestricted range of motion after closed treatment

Figure 11-22. A: Preoperative anteroposterior and lateral radiographs of left elbow of a 9-year-old girl showing 34 degrees of angulation and 50% displacement.

(continues)   **A**

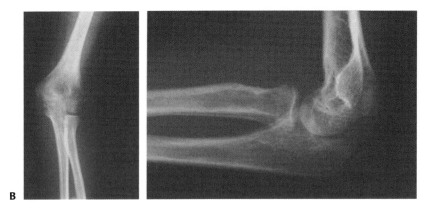

Figure 11-22. (*Continued*) **B:** Anteroposterior and lateral radiographs of the fracture 5 months postreduction showing maintenance of reduction with good callus formation. (Reprinted with permission from Monson R, et al. A new closed reduction technique for the treatment of radial neck fractures in children. *J Pediatr Orthop.* 2009;29(3):243–247.)

Figure 11-23. Elastic bandage wrap reduction. **A:** The final position achieved after manipulation by the Patterson[49] method. **B:** Position of the radial head after applying an elastic bandage to exsanguinate the extremity.

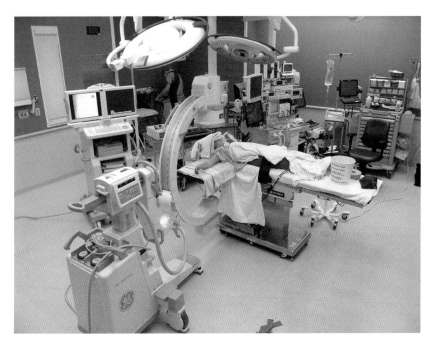

Figure 11-24. Preferred positioning and operative room setup for operative treatment of proximal radius and ulna fractures.

Surgical treatment is indicated when acceptable alignment cannot be achieved with closed means, or if there is persistent elbow instability or restricted range of motion after closed treatment. Most fractures of the proximal radius present to the surgeon with minimal deformity and do not require treatment other than a short period of immobilization. Operative treatment is considered when displacement remains over 2 mm, angulation is greater than 45 degrees (age <10) or greater than 30 degrees (age <10)—most importantly with persistent joint incongruity, and for open injuries. Nerve palsy is generally not an indication for surgery because most will recover function over time.

Instrument-Assisted Closed Reduction

Preoperative Planning

Instrument-Assisted Closed Reduction of Proximal Radius Fractures:
PREOPERATIVE PLANNING CHECKLIST

OR table	☐ Standard with radiolucent hand table
Position/ positioning aids	☐ Turn table 90 degrees, bring patient to edge of table toward hand table. Secure head with blanket/towel and tape. Safety strap over torso
Fluoroscopy location	☐ In line with affected extremity, perpendicular to OR table
Equipment	☐ Smooth K-wires
Tourniquet	☐ Nonsterile
Other	☐ Esmarch bandage

Positioning

The patient should be positioned supine on the operating table with a radiolucent hand table attached to the operating bed. The affected extremity should be placed directly in the middle of the hand table. The entire operating table should be rotated 90 degrees from standard position to place the injured extremity opposite the anesthesiologist. Fluoroscopy will be brought in directly in line with the injured extremity with surgeon and assistant on either side of the hand table (Fig. 11-24). The patient should be brought to the lateral edge of the bed and head secured to the operating room table. We suggest a towel or blanket draped over the head, surrounded by strong tape from one edge of the table to the other (Fig. 11-25). This is especially important for small patients, to allow for the fluoroscopy unit to be able to image the area of interest and not be blocked by the table. The torso should be secured to the table with a safety strap. A nonsterile tourniquet should be applied to the upper humerus. Surgeons may be standing or seated per their preference.

Surgical Approach

Percutaneous direct lateral approach is utilized as described in the technique below to minimize risk of injury to the PIN.

Technique

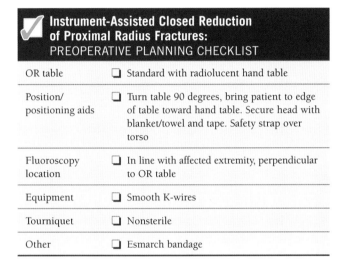

Instrument-Assisted Closed Reduction of Proximal Radius Fractures:
KEY SURGICAL STEPS

☐ Attempt closed reduction
☐ Percutaneous insertion of blunt end K-wire lateral forearm
☐ Reduce fracture by pushing on proximal fragment
☐ Assess stability and range of motion
  • If stable: Immobilize in long-arm cast
  • If unstable: Antegrade K-wire fixation
☐ Alternatively—use leverage technique described in text

Simple stainless steel smooth Kirschner wires (K-wires) generally are appropriate to assist with closed reduction. Size will range from 2 to 2.7 mm based on the size of the child. Other instruments utilized include Steinmann pins, periosteal elevators, freer elevator, or a double-pointed bident.[20] Fluoroscopy is used to localize the fracture site and intended entry site of the wire. This should be along the direct lateral cortex of the radial shaft to decrease risk of injury to the PIN. Pronating the forearm further moves the PIN away from the surgical field. The skin is incised with a small stab wound and a small curved clamp is utilized to bluntly dissect through the muscle to the radial cortex. The sharp end of the wire is cut for surgeon safety and the blunt end is inserted down to the radial cortex. Fluoroscopic guidance is used to localize the fracture site, and the blunt end of the wire can be used to push the distal fracture fragment back into an appropriate position (Fig. 11-26). Arthrography can be helpful to assess congruency of the elbow joint in the young.[8] Once the fracture is reduced to within appropriate guidelines, the pin is removed, and stability and range of motion are assessed. If the fracture remains stable through a normal arc of motion, no internal fixation is needed.[45,77] If instability is noted, then internal fixation can be placed. Small antegrade K-wires can be placed percutaneously to transfix the fracture (Fig. 11-27).

Figure 11-25. Detailed view of showing recommended method of securing head safely to the operative table while allowing for appropriate elbow positioning on the hand table for intraoperative fluoroscopy.

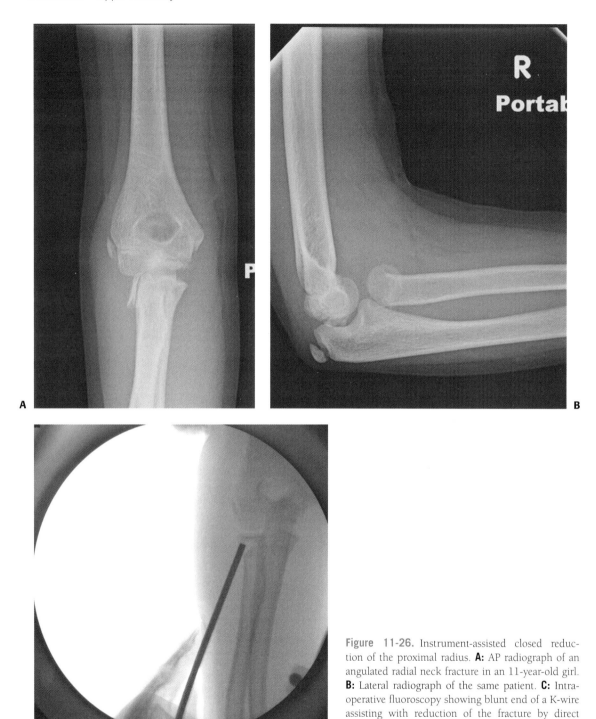

Figure 11-26. Instrument-assisted closed reduction of the proximal radius. **A:** AP radiograph of an angulated radial neck fracture in an 11-year-old girl. **B:** Lateral radiograph of the same patient. **C:** Intraoperative fluoroscopy showing blunt end of a K-wire assisting with reduction of the fracture by direct manipulation of the proximal fragment.

Intramedullary fixation can also be considered and is described in the next section. Pins should stay lateral to minimize injury to the PIN. Pins traversing the capitellum into the proximal radius should be avoided because they have a high rate of migration and/or pin breakage.[45,77] Various iterations of this technique have been described in the literature.[4,53,64]

Alternatively, the sharp end of the wire can be introduced into the fracture site and the wire used as a lever to correct angulation.[6,8,62,78] Similarly, if stable after pin removal, then further

fixation is not necessary. However, if unstable, the pin can be driven from proximal to distal across the radial cortex and serve as a buttress against recurrent angulation of the distal fragment. In this instance, the wire is introduced through the skin closer to the fracture site than in the prior described technique, to prevent soft tissue from blocking appropriate leverage of the distal fracture fragment. The pin is cut short but left out of the skin and underneath postoperative immobilization. It may be removed in a few weeks when the surgeon is comfortable and the level of the bicipital tuberosity of the proximal radius is marked. A 1-cm dorsal skin incision is made at that level just lateral to the subcutaneous border of the ulna. A periosteal elevator is gently inserted between the ulna and the radius, with care not to disrupt the periosteum of the radius or the ulna. The radial shaft is usually much more ulnarly displaced than expected, and the radial nerve is lateral to the radius at this level. While counterpressure is applied against the radial head, the distal fragment of the radius is levered away from the ulna. An assistant can aid in this maneuver by gently applying traction and rotating the forearm back and forth to disengage the fracture fragments. The proximal radial fragment can be reduced either manually with thumb pressure or assisted by a percutaneous instrument as described (Figs. 11-29 and 11-30).

Intramedullary Nail Reduction/Fixation

Preoperative Planning

Intramedullary Nail Reduction/Fixation of Proximal Radius Fractures: PREOPERATIVE PLANNING CHECKLIST	
OR table	☐ Standard with radiolucent hand table
Position/positioning aids	☐ Turn table 90 degrees, bring patient to edge of table toward hand table. Secure head with blanket/towel and tape. Safety strap over torso
Fluoroscopy location	☐ In line with affected extremity, perpendicular to OR table
Equipment	☐ Smooth K-wires
Tourniquet	☐ Nonsterile
Other	☐ Esmarch bandage

Implant size should be estimated prior to surgery by either measuring the intramedullary canal on preoperative radiographs or comparing the size of the implant to the intramedullary canal using intraoperative fluoroscopy. The intramedullary technique was initially described using K-wires, which are readily available and inexpensive. Some prefer using titanium flexible nails, but these are more costly. The isthmus of the radius should be measured on both AP and lateral views and implant size should be chosen to easily pass. In general, an implant 60% to 70% of the width of the isthmus will pass without too much difficulty. In adolescents, this will usually be 2- or 2.4-mm K-wires. It is advised to have one size larger and smaller than planned available if needed.

Positioning

Same as for instrument-assisted closed reduction.

Surgical Approaches

The implant is inserted at the distal radius via a radial entry. The distal radial physis should be localized with fluoroscopy. A direct lateral incision of 1 to 2 cm is made just proximal to

Figure 11-27. Oblique pin. **A:** Displaced fracture of the radial neck in an 11 year old. **B:** A closed reduction was performed, and to stabilize the head fragment, two pins were placed percutaneously and obliquely across the fracture site from proximal to distal. If open reduction and pinning are done, the preferred alignment is obliquely across the fracture site from distal to proximal. (Reproduced with permission from Wilkins KE, ed: *Operative Management of Upper Extremity Fractures in Children.* American Academy of Orthopaedic Surgeons; 1994.)

allowing range of motion at the elbow (Fig. 11-28). A slight variation of this technique was described in which the pin was temporarily inserted into the proximal fracture fragment instead of the fracture site. Similar leverage technique is used to reduce the fracture followed by intramedullary fixation with a separate wire as described in the next section, followed by removal of the temporary wire in the proximal fragment.[75]

A modification described by Wallace utilizes an instrument to provide counterforce on the radial shaft. Fluoroscopy in an AP projection is used to determine the forearm rotation that exposes the maximum amount of deformity of the fracture,

Figure 11-28. Leverage technique of instrument-assisted closed reduction of the proximal radius. **A:** Intra-operative AP fluoroscopy image demonstrating angulated radial neck fracture. **B:** K-wire inserted at fracture site and levering proximal fragment into a reduced position. **C:** AP view of elbow following pin removal in clinic showing anatomic alignment of proximal radius fracture. **D:** Same wire driven through the opposite cortex to hold reduced position of the proximal fragment.

the physis of the distal radius. Careful scissor dissection to the lateral radial cortex is made with care taken not to injure the superficial radial nerve. It is not required to search for the nerve; however, if encountered, it should be gently retracted. Extensor tendons from the first dorsal compartment may also be encountered and should be retracted.

Alternatively, the implant may be inserted via a direct dorsal approach over Lister tubercle of the radius. Either longitudinal or transverse incisions may be utilized. Extensor tendons, especially extensor pollicis longus, will be encountered and should be protected during opening of the radial cortex at the dorsal tubercle.

Figure 11-29. Wallace radial head reduction technique. **A:** A periosteal elevator is used to lever the distal fragment laterally while the thumb pushes the proximal fragment medially. **B:** K-wires are used to assist the reduction if necessary. *Arrows* indicate direction of movement of bone and instruments. **C:** The position of the reduction can be fixed with an oblique Kirschner wire.

Figure 11-30. A: Radial neck fracture angulated 45 degrees in a 14-year-old girl. **B:** Radiograph after closed reduction using thumb pressure on the radial head. **C:** Final reduction after manipulation of the distal fragment with an elevator using the Wallace technique. **D:** Lateral view of the elbow after reduction.

Technique

> ### ✓ Intramedullary Nail Reduction/Fixation of Proximal Radius Fractures:
> #### KEY SURGICAL STEPS
>
> ❏ Prebend implant at distal end
> ❏ Open distal radial cortex via radial or dorsal approach
> ❏ Advance implant to the fracture site
> ❏ Closed manipulation of fracture to allow implant to enter distal fragment
> ❏ Advance implant into distal fragment
> ❏ Rotate implant as needed to reduce fracture
> ❏ Assess stability and range of motion
> ❏ Cut implant distally under the skin
>   • Recheck to be certain there is no radial sensory nerve or extensor tendon impingement or risk of injury
> ❏ Close surgical wound
> ❏ Immobilize to allow for soft tissue healing

After selection of an appropriate-sized implant (K-wire or titanium flexible nail), the distal 3 to 4 mm of the implant should be bent sharply to about 40 degrees. The wire is advanced through the radial canal to the fracture site. If necessary, closed maneuvers should be used to improve alignment at the fracture site to allow for successful passage of the distal tip of the implant into the proximal fragment. The implant should be impacted into the epiphysis to achieve maximal fixation prior to reduction attempts with the implant. Once advanced appropriately, the nail should be rotated as needed to reduce the proximal fragment to the radial shaft. The forearm should be held by the assistant to prevent the radial shaft from rotating with the implant

(Fig. 11-31). Stability at the elbow joint and range of motion are assessed. The implant should be cut distally, balancing need for ease of recovery during implant removal with soft tissue irritation from implant prominence at the distal radius and to the extensor tendons. Rigid immobilization is not necessary with use of an intramedullary implant; however, most surgeons will immobilize the extremity in a long-arm splint or cast for at least 7 to 10 days for pain relief and to allow for soft tissue healing. Early range of motion is encouraged to minimize postoperative stiffness.

Open Reduction Internal Fixation

Preoperative Planning

> ### ✓ ORIF of Proximal Radius Fractures:
> #### PREOPERATIVE PLANNING CHECKLIST

OR table	❏ Standard with radiolucent hand table
Position/ positioning aids	❏ Turn table 90 degrees, bring patient to edge of table toward hand table. Secure head with blanket/ towel and tape. Safety strap over torso
Fluoroscopy location	❏ In line with affected extremity, perpendicular to OR table
Equipment	❏ 2- to 2.7-mm screws; mini-fragment plates versus fracture-specific plates (radial neck, radial head)
Tourniquet	❏ Nonsterile
Other	❏ Esmarch bandage

Figure 11-31. Intramedullary pin reduction. **A:** The insertion point for the curved flexible pin is in the metaphysis. **B:** The curved end of the rod passes in the shaft and engages the proximal fragment. **C:** Manipulation of the rod disimpacts the fracture. **D, E:** Once disimpacted, the head fragment is rotated into position with the intramedullary rod. (Reprinted with permission from Metaizeau JP, et al. Reduction and fixation of displaced radial neck fractures by closed intramedullary pinning. *J Pediatr Orthop.* 1993;13(3):355–360.)

Appropriate implants should be available if rigid internal fixation is planned. These may include mini-fragment screws, headless compression screws, mini- or modular-fragment plates, or specialty proximal radius plates. Small fragment screws and plates are often too large for fixation of the proximal radius. Specialty plates are produced by numerous manufacturers but are designed for adult patients. Many will be too large for children and young adolescents; however, they may fit appropriately in the older adolescent. Modular hand plates often are size appropriate for the young. Bioabsorbable rods and pins (poly-L-lactic acid) have been reported in small case series for fixation of radial head and neck fractures in children.[19,66]

Positioning

Same as for instrument-assisted closed reduction.

Surgical Approach

A lateral approach to the proximal radius should be used for open reduction of proximal radius fractures. Either the lateral Kocher or Kaplan approach provides appropriate exposure. In the Kocher approach, dissection is between the anconeus and extensor carpi ulnaris. Usually, the interval is easier to identify distally and can be traced back proximally. The muscle fibers will be seen to run in divergent directions distally, which assist with location of the interval. The Kaplan approach is more anterior and is ligament sparing. Often the annular ligament and joint capsule will be traumatically disrupted. Care should be taken to stay superior to the lateral collateral ligament of the elbow to prevent adding iatrogenic instability. The supinator may be released distally, if needed, for plate application.

When exposing the proximal radius, the forearm should be kept in a pronated position to move the PIN further away from the surgical field. Vigorous retraction should be avoided anteriorly to limit traction on the PIN.

Technique

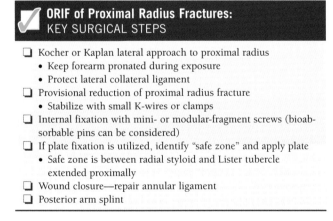

✓ **ORIF of Proximal Radius Fractures:**
KEY SURGICAL STEPS

- ❏ Kocher or Kaplan lateral approach to proximal radius
  - • Keep forearm pronated during exposure
  - • Protect lateral collateral ligament
- ❏ Provisional reduction of proximal radius fracture
  - • Stabilize with small K-wires or clamps
- ❏ Internal fixation with mini- or modular-fragment screws (bioabsorbable pins can be considered)
- ❏ If plate fixation is utilized, identify "safe zone" and apply plate
  - • Safe zone is between radial styloid and Lister tubercle extended proximally
- ❏ Wound closure—repair annular ligament
- ❏ Posterior arm splint

After adequate exposure of the fracture site, the anatomy of the fracture should be evaluated. Radial neck fractures are more common and can be reduced using manual pressure or instrumented manipulation. Often, a dental pick is useful to hold a

reduced position after manual reduction. The fracture can be either definitively or provisionally fixed at this point with small K-wires. Radial head fractures are usually more complex and may have multiple fragments. Attempts should be made to reduce the radial head in children and adolescents with use of small pins or bone clamps to hold provisional reduction. Radial head excision is a salvage operation and should be considered as a primary treatment only if there is extensive comminution prohibiting reconstruction. Results have been uniformly poor after excision with high incidence of cubitus valgus, radial deviation at the wrist, and relative ulnar-positive deformity. Radial head replacement has not been described for children or adolescents but is increasingly used for adults.

When proceeding with open reduction, most surgeons elect to place more rigid fixation to allow for early range of motion. Screw fixation with mini-fragment screws or headless compression screws provide stable fixation of radial head and neck fractures (Figs. 11-32 and 11-33).[60] Plates have been utilized for fixation of radial neck fractures requiring open reduction (Fig. 11-34). They should be placed in the "safe zone" of the proximal radius. This is an area of about 100 to 110 degrees of the circumference of the proximal radius that does not articulate with the proximal ulna during forearm rotation. With the forearm in 10 degrees of supination, the "safe zone" is directly lateral.[61,63] It is also found in the interval between the radial styloid and Lister tubercle. Screws should be kept unicortical to prevent perforation into the PRUJ. Plate application requires more extensive dissection than isolated screw fixation and has led some authors to strongly advocate for multiple screw fixation alone for radial head and neck fractures. An oblique headless screw can often provide adequate fixation. There is no good quality evidence supporting one form of internal fixation over another in the treatment of fractures of the proximal radius.

During closure, the annular ligament and joint capsule should be repaired if injured during the trauma or surgical dissection. The arm should be immobilized in a posterior splint for 1 to 2 weeks to allow for soft tissue healing before initiating range of motion. A regional anesthetic block prior to surgery or after surgery can provide improved patient comfort postoperatively. A detailed neurologic examination should be conducted preoperatively prior to regional nerve block and postoperatively after surgical exposure.

Outcomes

The severity of initial displacement and angulation are the best predictors of results of radial head and neck fractures after treatment. A higher incidence of good outcomes is found in patients with minimal fracture angulation and displacement, who do not require manipulation (closed or open).[13,46] For patients undergoing operative treatment, closed methods generally lead to improved results compared to open treatments. This is again largely because of increased severity of fractures requiring open reduction. All closed and percutaneous methods should be exhausted before proceeding to open management of proximal radius fractures.

The overall incidence of poor results in large series varies from 15% to 33%.[3,11,17,65,79] Considering only severely displaced fractures, the incidence of poor results was as high as 50%.[65] A

Authors' Preferred Treatment for Fractures of the Proximal Radius (Algorithm 11-1)

Algorithm 11-1. Authors' preferred treatment for fractures of the proximal radius.

Nonoperative management is our preferred treatment for most proximal radius fractures that are aligned and reduced in the joint. Operative treatment should aim to reduce displacement of the radial head/neck to less than 2 mm, restore angulation of radial neck fractures to less than 30 to 45 degrees (based on child's age), and reduce the joint while also confirming normal arc of forearm rotation. Open approaches are avoided if these goals can be achieved closed. Necessity for internal fixation should be evaluated on an individual basis and avoided, if possible. We have become more aggressive with operative treatment of radial head fractures because of the increased reports of adverse outcomes with progressive posterior radiocapitellar subluxation, articular incongruity, and joint malalignment. Low-profile internal fixation with mini-fragment or headless compression screws and, if needed, a mini-fragment plate is utilized for stable fixation to allow for early range of motion. MRI is utilized more frequently preoperatively in the evaluation of radial head fractures because of its improved ability to assess for articular congruity, radiocapitellar alignment, and for other associated soft tissue or cartilaginous injuries in skeletally immature patients.

Postoperative Care

Immobilization should only be for symptomatic relief from surgical trauma and soft tissue healing. In general, 1 to 2 weeks is sufficient in patients with open reduction internal fixation (ORIF) or intramedullary fixation. Longer immobilization times of 2 to 3 weeks may be required for some patients treated without open reduction and internal fixation to achieve enough symptom relief before mobilization. A collar and cuff, posterior splint, or long-arm cast are all appropriate methods of immobilization. Range of motion should be allowed and encouraged when acute fracture pain has resolved and the surgical scar has healed, to lessen risk of permanent stiffness.

Potential Pitfalls and Preventative Measures

Proximal Radius Fractures: POTENTIAL PITFALLS AND PREVENTIONS

Pitfall	Prevention
PIN injury	• Pronate forearm when using lateral-based open approaches to the proximal radius • Avoid vigorous retraction during open reduction • Insert percutaneous implants for reduction assistance directly lateral
Radiocapitellar subluxation	• Consider preoperative ultrasound or MRI for intra-articular radial head fractures, displaced extra-articular fractures • Close radiographic surveillance out of cast/splint for patients with radial head fracture
Failure to engage proximal fragment with intramedullary implant	• Choose appropriate-sized implant based on preoperative templating • Ensure distal end of implant has an appropriate bend to capture proximal fragment
Mechanical block to forearm rotation	• Ensure any plate fixation of the proximal radius is in the "safe zone" • Screws aiming toward the PRUJ should be unicortical

Iatrogenic PIN injury can occur during both percutaneous and open approaches to the proximal radius. Pronation of the forearm during a laterally based open exposure or during percutaneous K-wire insertion helps move the PIN away from the surgical field and reduces the risk of nerve injury. Vigorous anterior retraction during open exposures should also be avoided.

Knowledge of the anatomy of the PIN is required to safely place instrumentation and expose the proximal radius.

Radiocapitellar subluxation is an extremely poor prognostic factor for outcomes of proximal radius fractures. Close vigilance is warranted in fracture patterns predisposed to this complication, especially intra-articular radial head fractures or malaligned radial neck fractures with residual joint incongruity. In children with intra-articular fractures or those with an unossified proximal radial epiphysis, strong consideration should be made for ultrasound, MRI, or arthrogram to determine the anatomic extent of injury before surgery. Surgical treatment with in-depth understanding of the pathoanatomy can prevent this dangerous pitfall in appropriate cases.

The intramedullary technique has demonstrated good results in experienced hands. Surgeons with less experience may struggle with adequate engagement of the proximal fragment and loss of fixation with attempted rotation of the implant (Fig. 11-36). To decrease this adverse event, the implant should be bent sharply to 30 to 40 degrees at its distal end to promote engagement of the proximal fragment. The fragment should also be fixed all the way to the epiphysis, crossing the growth plate, to maximize purchase and decrease risk of implant failure with the corrective force during rotation of the implant. Percutaneous techniques to reduce displacement and angulation can also assist with engagement of the proximal fragment when using the intramedullary technique for fixation for highly angulated or displaced fractures.

Restricted range of motion after open reduction and internal fixation of proximal radius fractures is common. To minimize additional restriction because of implant placement, the surgeon should take care to apply plate fixation only to the "safe zone" of the proximal radius, and screws aiming toward the proximal radioulnar articulation should be unicortical.

Figure 11-36. Failure of fixation with intramedullary technique for proximal radius fracture. **A:** AP view showing loss of fixation of the proximal fragment. **B:** Lateral view showing loss of fixation of the proximal fragment.

Proximal Radius Fractures:
COMMON ADVERSE OUTCOMES AND COMPLICATIONS

- Loss of range of motion
- Radial head overgrowth
- Avascular necrosis of the radial head
- Nonunion
- Malunion
- Proximal radioulnar synostosis
- Cubitus valgus
- PIN injury

LOSS OF RANGE OF MOTION

Loss of motion is secondary to a combination of loss of joint congruity and posttraumatic or postoperative soft tissue scarring. Loss of pronation is more common than loss of supination. Flexion and extension are rarely significantly limited. Very little improvement in motion occurs after 6 months. Steinberg et al.[63] found that range of motion in their patients at 6 months was almost equal to that when the patients were examined years later. Patients should be encouraged to start range of motion early with both nonoperative and operative treatment to minimize loss of motion from posttraumatic stiffness. Both static and dynamic splinting can be useful along with aggressive therapy in the treatment of posttraumatic or postoperative elbow and forearm stiffness.

RADIAL HEAD OVERGROWTH

Next to loss of range of motion of the elbow and forearm, radial head overgrowth is probably the most common sequela (20%–40%).[70] The increased vascularity following the injury may stimulate epiphyseal growth, but the mechanisms of overgrowth following fractures are poorly understood. Radial head overgrowth usually does not compromise functional results, but it may produce some crepitus or clicking with forearm rotation.[14]

Premature Physeal Closure

Many series report premature physeal closure[22,45,46,65,77] after fractures of the radial head and neck. This complication did not appear to affect the overall results significantly, except in one patient, who had a severe cubitus valgus. Newman[45] found that shortening of the radius was never more than 5 mm compared with the opposite uninjured side.

Osteonecrosis

The incidence of osteonecrosis is probably higher than recognized. D'Souza et al.[14] reported the frequency to be 10% to 20% in their patients, 70% of whom had open reductions. In patients with open reduction, the overall rate of osteonecrosis was 25%. Other authors found that patients with osteonecrosis had poor functional

Figure 11-37. Osteonecrosis with nonunion in a radial head 1 year after open reduction. Both nonunion and osteonecrosis of the radial neck and head are present. Severe degenerative arthritis developed subsequently. (Courtesy of Richard E. King, MD.)

results.[45] It has been our experience, however, that revascularization can occur without any significant functional loss. Only in those with collapse and in whom a residual functional deficit occurs is osteonecrosis considered a problem (Fig. 11-37).

Malunion

Failure to reduce a displaced and angulated proximal radial fracture in a young child often results in an angulated radial neck with subsequent incongruity of both the PRUJ and the radiocapitellar joint (Fig. 11-38). Partial physeal arrest can also create this angulation (see Fig. 11-3). In our experience, this malunion, because of the incongruity of the radiocapitellar joint, often results in erosion of the articular surface of the capitellum, with subsequent osteochondral pain, loose bodies, and eventually degenerative joint disease.

Nonunion

Nonunion of the radial neck is rare; union may occur even after prolonged treatment (Fig. 11-39). Waters and Stewart[76] reported nine patients with radial neck nonunions, all of whom were treated with open reduction after failed attempts at closed reduction. They recommended observation of patients with radial neck nonunions who have limited symptoms and a functional range of motion. They suggested open reduction for displaced nonunions, patients

Figure 11-38. Angulation. **A:** Injury film showing 30 degrees of angulation and 30% lateral translocation of a radial neck fracture in an 11-year-old. **B:** Radiograph appearance of the proximal radius taken about 5 months later, showing lateral angulation of the neck. **C:** Lateral view showing the anterior relationship of the radial neck with proximal migration. At this point, the patient had full supination and pronation but a clicking sensation with forearm rotation in the area of the radial head. **D:** Three-dimensional reconstruction showing the incongruity of the proximal radiocapitellar joint. (Courtesy of Vincent Mosca, MD.)

Figure 11-39. Nonunion. **A:** Eight months after radial neck fracture in an 8.5-year-old girl. Patient had mild aching pain, but no loss of motion. There was some suggestion of proximal subluxation of the distal radioulnar joint. **B:** Three months later, the fracture is united after long-arm cast immobilization and external electromagnetic stimulation. (Courtesy of Charles T. Price, MD.)

Figure 11-40. Nonunion of intra-articular radial head fracture. This 15-year-old girl presented 1 year after elbow injury because of persistent pain. **A:** AP radiograph demonstrating nonunion of the radial head fracture. **B:** Lateral radiograph after open reduction and internal fixation. **C:** AP radiograph after open reduction and internal fixation. **D:** Lateral radiograph of the same patient.

with limited range of motion, and patients with restricting pain. Nonunion of intra-articular radial head fractures can also occur and should be treated with ORIF if symptomatic and radiocapitellar joint has remained congruent (Fig. 11-40). In many cases, nonunion of these fractures leads to progressive radiocapitellar subluxation and cartilage destruction as previously described. If seen earlier enough, radial head reconstruction with bone grafting and internal fixation can be successful.[32]

Changes in Carrying Angle (Cubitus Valgus)

In patients who have fractures of the radial neck, the carrying angle often is 10 degrees more (increased cubitus valgus)

than on the uninjured side.[14] The increase in the carrying angle appears to produce no functional deficit and no significant deformity.

Nerve Injuries

Partial ulnar nerve injury and PIN injury may occur as a direct result of the fracture, but most injuries to the PIN are caused by surgical exploration[14] or percutaneous pin reduction.[4] These PIN injuries usually are transient and exploration is not generally warranted. However, if there is failure of recovery in a timely manner (usually 3–4 months), then electrodiagnostics and surgical exposure are indicated.

A, B   C

Figure 11-41. Radioulnar synostosis. **A:** Surgical intervention with wire fixation was necessary for a satisfactory reduction in this patient who had a totally displaced radial neck fracture. **B:** Six weeks after surgery, there was evidence of a proximal radioulnar synostosis. **C:** Radiograph taken 6 months after reduction shows a solid synostosis with anterior displacement of the proximal radius. (Courtesy of R.E. King, MD.)

Radioulnar Synostosis

Proximal radioulnar synostosis can occur following treatment of proximal radius fractures (Fig. 11-41). It occurs most often after open reduction of severely displaced fractures[22,45,64] but has been reported to occur after closed reduction. Case reports argue that delayed treatment increases the likelihood of this complication. Treatment is based on functional limitation and disability.

Myositis Ossificans

Myositis ossificans is relatively common but usually does not impair function. Vahvanen[72] noted that some myositis ossificans occurred in 32% of his patients. In most, it was limited to the supinator muscle. If ossification was more extensive and was associated with a synostosis, the results were poor.

Fractures of the Proximal Ulna

ASSESSMENT OF FRACTURES OF THE PROXIMAL ULNA

MECHANISMS OF INJURY FOR FRACTURES OF THE PROXIMAL ULNA

Fractures Involving the Proximal Apophysis

The location of the triceps expansive insertion on the ulnar metaphysis, distal to the apophysis, probably accounts for the rarity of fractures along the apophyseal line. Only a few reports mention the mechanism of these apophyseal injuries. In our experience, this fracture is usually caused by avulsion forces across the apophysis with the elbow flexed, like the more common flexion metaphyseal injuries. Children with OI seem especially predisposed to this injury.[12]

Stress fractures of the olecranon apophysis can occur in athletes (especially throwing athletes) who place considerable recurrent tension forces on the olecranon.[20] Stress injuries also have been reported in surfers, elite gymnasts, and tennis players. If the recurring activity persists, a symptomatic nonunion can develop.[68,70] Paci et al.[48] described use of cannulated screw fixation of an olecranon stress fracture leading to union and return to play in an overhead throwing athlete.

Metaphyseal Fractures of the Olecranon

Three main mechanisms produce metaphyseal olecranon fractures. First, in injuries occurring with the elbow flexed, posterior tension forces play an important role. Second, in injuries where the fracture occurs with the elbow extended, the varus or valgus bending stress across the olecranon is responsible for the typical fracture pattern. Third, a less common mechanism involves a direct blow to the elbow that produces an anterior bending or shear force across the olecranon. In this type, the tension forces are concentrated on the anterior portion of the olecranon.

Flexion Injuries

A fall with the elbow in flexion places considerable tension forces across the posterior aspect of the olecranon process. Proximally, the triceps applies a force to the tip of the olecranon process. Distally, there is some proximal pull by the insertion of the brachialis muscle. Thus, the posterior cortex is placed

Figure 11-42. Mechanism of flexion injuries. **Center:** In the flexed elbow, a tension force develops on the posterior aspect of the olecranon (*small double arrow*). **Right:** Failure occurs on the tension side, which is posterior as a result of the muscle pull or a direct blow to the prestressed posterior olecranon. *Arrows* represent pull of brachialis (*left arrow*) and triceps (*right arrow*).

in tension. This tension force alone, if applied rapidly enough and with sufficient force, may cause the olecranon to fail at its midportion (Fig. 11-42). A direct blow applied to the posterior aspect of the stressed olecranon makes it more vulnerable to failure. With this type of mechanism, the fracture line is usually transverse and perpendicular to the long axis of the olecranon (Fig. 11-43). Because the fracture extends into the articular surface of the semilunar notch, it is classified as intra-articular.

The degree of separation of the fracture fragments depends on the magnitude of the forces applied and the integrity of the soft tissues. The low incidence of displaced olecranon fractures indicates that the soft tissues are quite resistant to these avulsion forces. In flexion injuries, there are relatively few associated soft tissue injuries or other fractures.

Figure 11-43. Radiograph of flexion injury showing greater displacement on the posterior surface.

Extension Injuries

Because children tend to have more ligamentous laxity, the elbow tends to hyperextend when a child breaks a fall with the outstretched upper extremity. In this situation, the olecranon may become locked into the olecranon fossa. If the elbow goes into extreme hyperextension, usually the supracondylar region of the distal humerus fails. If, however, the major direction of the force across the elbow is varus or valgus, a bending moment stresses the olecranon. Most of this force concentrates in the distal portion of the olecranon. Because the olecranon is metaphyseal bone, the force produces greenstick-type longitudinal fracture lines (Fig. 11-44). Most of these fracture lines are linear and remain extra-articular. In addition, because the fulcrum of the bending force is more distal, many of the fracture lines may extend distal to the coronoid process and into the proximal ulnar shaft regions. The major deformity of the olecranon with this type of fracture is usually an angulated greenstick type of pattern.

Many of these fractures are associated with other injuries in the elbow region, which depend on whether the bending force is directed toward varus or valgus. If a child falls with the forearm in supination, the carrying angle tends to place a valgus stress across the elbow. The result may be a greenstick fracture of the ulna with an associated fracture of the radial neck or avulsion of the medial epicondylar apophysis (Fig. 11-45). If the fracture involves the radial neck, it can be classified as an equivalent of the type I Monteggia injury.

Shear Injuries

Anterior tension failure is a rare injury that can occur when a direct blow to the proximal ulna causes it to fail with an anterior tension force; the PRUJ maintains its integrity. The most common type of shear injury is caused by a force applied directly to the posterior aspect of the olecranon, with the distal fragment displacing anteriorly (Figs. 11-46 and 11-47). The intact PRUJ displaces with the distal fragment. In this type of injury, the elbow may be either flexed or extended when the direct

Figure 11-44. A: Anteroposterior view of a linear greenstick fracture line (*arrow*) in the medial aspect of the olecranon. **B:** Lateral view showing the posterior location of the fracture line (*arrow*).

shear force impacts the posterior aspect of the olecranon. These fractures are caused by a failure in tension, with the force concentrated along the anterior cortex. This is opposite to the tension failure occurring on the posterior aspect of the cortex in the more common flexion injuries. In the shear-type injury, the fracture line may be transverse or oblique. The differentiating feature from the more common flexion injury is that the thick posterior periosteum usually remains intact. The distal

fragment is displaced anteriorly by the pull of the brachialis and biceps muscles.

Fractures of the Coronoid Process

Isolated coronoid fractures are theoretically caused by avulsion stress from the brachialis or secondary to an elbow dislocation. When associated with elbow dislocations, there is typically a

Figure 11-45. Valgus pattern of an extension fracture. **A:** A fall with the elbow extended places a valgus stress on the forearm. **B:** With increased valgus, a greenstick fracture of the olecranon can occur with or without a fracture of the radial neck or avulsion of the medial epicondylar apophysis (*arrows* denote direction of fracture displacement). **C:** Radiograph of a valgus extension fracture of the olecranon with an associated fracture of the radial neck.

Figure 11-46. Flexion shear injuries. **A, B:** Fracture with the elbow flexed. The direct blow to the distal portion of the posterior olecranon causes the fracture to fail in tension of the anterior surface. The intact proximal radioulnar joint displaces anteriorly. **C:** Radiograph of a flexion shear injury showing the distal fragments displaced anteriorly as a unit.

Figure 11-47. Extension shear injuries. **A, B:** Fracture with the elbow extended. If the elbow is extended when the direct blow to the posterior aspect of the elbow occurs, the olecranon fails in tension but with an oblique or transverse fracture line (*arrows*). **C:** With the elbow extended, the initial failure is in the anterior articular surface (*arrows*).

Figure 11-48. Lateral radiograph of an 11-year-old boy who injured his left elbow. Displaced anterior and posterior fat pads, plus a small fracture of the coronoid (*arrow*), indicate a probable partially dislocated elbow as the primary injury.

hemarthrosis and a small avulsion of the tip of the olecranon process (Fig. 11-48).

INJURIES ASSOCIATED WITH FRACTURES OF THE PROXIMAL ULNA

Metaphyseal Fractures of the Olecranon and the Proximal Apophysis

Associated injuries occur in 48% to 77% of patients with olecranon fractures,[25,49] especially varus and valgus greenstick extension fractures, in which the radial head and neck most commonly fracture (see Fig. 11-44). Other associated injuries include fractures of the ipsilateral radial shaft, Monteggia type I lesions with fractures of both the ulnar shaft and olecranon,[47] and fractures of the lateral condyle (Fig. 11-49).[36]

Fractures of the Coronoid Process

Although most coronoid fractures are associated with elbow dislocations, fractures of the olecranon, medial epicondyle, and lateral condyle can also occur.[45] The fracture of the coronoid may be part of a greenstick olecranon fracture (i.e., the extension-type metaphyseal fracture; Fig. 11-50).

SIGNS AND SYMPTOMS OF FRACTURES OF THE PROXIMAL ULNA

Metaphyseal Fractures of the Olecranon and the Proximal Apophysis

Flexion injuries cause soft tissue swelling and tenderness over the olecranon fracture. The abrasion or contusion associated with a direct blow to the posterior aspect of the elbow provides a clue as to the mechanism of injury. If there is wide separation, a defect can be palpated between the fragments. In addition, there may be weakness or even lack of active extension of the elbow, which is difficult to evaluate in an anxious young child with a swollen elbow. Associated proximal radius fractures may be noted clinically by swelling and tenderness laterally with palpation in this region.

Fractures of the Coronoid Process

Because of the common association of these fractures with elbow dislocations, a high index of suspicion is necessary when evaluating these injuries. Significant soft tissue swelling about

Figure 11-49. A: Undisplaced fracture of the lateral condyle (*arrows*) associated with a varus greenstick fracture of the olecranon. **B:** Lateral view showing greenstick fractures in the olecranon (*solid arrows*) and a nondisplaced fracture of the lateral condyle (*open arrows*).

Figure 11-50. Fracture of the coronoid (*solid arrows*) as part of an extension valgus olecranon fracture pattern. There was an associated fracture of the radial neck. Both the neck fracture and the distal portion of the coronoid process show periosteal new bone formation (*open arrows*).

the elbow is a consistent finding. The patient may also recall the "clunking" sensation of dislocation and spontaneous relocation with specific inquiry.

IMAGING AND OTHER DIAGNOSTIC STUDIES FOR FRACTURES OF THE PROXIMAL ULNA

Metaphyseal Fractures of the Olecranon and the Proximal Apophysis

The radiographic diagnosis may be difficult before ossification of the olecranon apophysis. The only clue may be a displacement of the small ossified metaphyseal fragment (Fig. 11-51), and the diagnosis may be based only on the clinical sign of tenderness over the epiphyseal fragment. If there is significant swelling, your index of suspicion for a more severe injury should be heightened. If there is any doubt about the degree of displacement, injection of radiopaque material into the joint (arthrogram) may delineate the true nature of the fracture. Alternatively, an MRI may be useful if uncertainty remains. Ultrasound is also being used more frequently to evaluate for olecranon fractures.

Fractures of the Coronoid Process

The radiographic diagnosis of this fracture is often difficult because on the lateral view, the radial head is superimposed over the coronoid process. Evaluation of a minimally displaced fracture may require oblique views (Fig. 11-52).[65] The radiocapitellar view (see Fig. 11-4) shows the profile of the coronoid process.

CLASSIFICATION OF FRACTURES OF THE PROXIMAL ULNA

Fractures Involving the Proximal Apophysis

Apophyseal Injuries of the Olecranon: CLASSIFICATION	
Type	**Description**
I	Apophysitis
II	Incomplete stress fracture
III	Complete fracture
IIIA	Pure apophyseal avulsion
IIIB	Apophyseal–metaphyseal combination

Injuries to the apophysis of the olecranon can be classified as one of three types. Type I is a simple apophysitis in which there is irregularity in the secondary ossification center (Fig. 11-53A).

Figure 11-51. Apophysitis. **A:** Chronic stimulation with irregular ossification of the articular apophyseal center (*arrows*) in a basketball player who practiced dribbling 3 hours per day. **B:** Normal side for comparison.

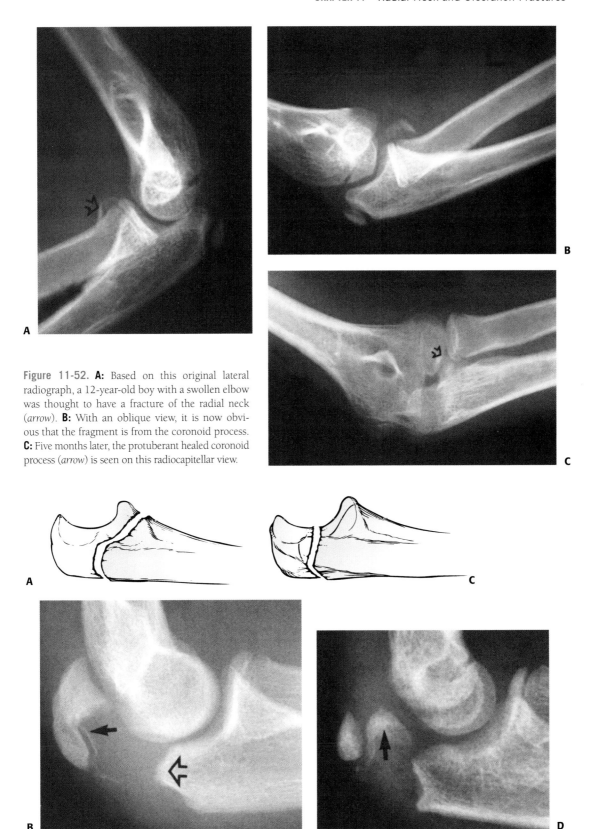

Figure 11-52. **A:** Based on this original lateral radiograph, a 12-year-old boy with a swollen elbow was thought to have a fracture of the radial neck (*arrow*). **B:** With an oblique view, it is now obvious that the fragment is from the coronoid process. **C:** Five months later, the protuberant healed coronoid process (*arrow*) is seen on this radiocapitellar view.

Figure 11-53. Apophyseal avulsions. Pure apophyseal avulsions. **A:** The fracture follows the contour of the apophyseal line. **B:** The distal fracture line is in the shape of the apophyseal line (*open arrow*) with a small metaphyseal flake attached to the apophysis (*solid arrow*). Apophyseal–metaphyseal combination. **C:** The fracture line follows the line of tension stress. **D:** A large portion of the metaphysis (*arrow*) is often with the proximal metaphyseal fragment.

The apophyseal line may widen. Type II is an incomplete stress fracture that involves primarily the apophyseal line, with widening and irregularity (Fig. 11-53B). A small adjacent cyst may form, but usually the architecture of the secondary ossification center is normal. These injuries occur primarily in sports requiring repetitive extension of the elbow, such as baseball pitching, tennis, or gymnastics. Type III injuries involve complete avulsion of the apophysis. True apophyseal avulsions (type IIIA) occur in younger children as a fracture through the apophyseal plate (Fig. 11-53A,B). In some of his amputation specimens in the 19th century, Poland found that the proximal apophyseal fragment included the distal tongue, which extended up to the coronoid process. Apophyseal–metaphyseal combination fractures (type IIIB), in which metaphyseal fragments are attached to the apophysis (Fig. 11-53C,D), usually occur in older children. These have been likened to Salter–Harris type II physeal injuries. Proximal displacement of the fragment is the only clue seen on a radiograph that a type IIIB fracture has occurred.

Metaphyseal Fractures of the Olecranon

Metaphyseal Fractures of the Olecranon: CLASSIFICATION	
Group	**Description**
A	Flexion injuries
B	Extension injuries
B1	Valgus pattern
B2	Varus pattern
C	Shear injuries

The classification is based on the mechanism of injury: flexion, extension, or shear. It is useful in guiding treatment options.

Fractures of the Coronoid Process

Fractures of the Coronoid Process: CLASSIFICATION[49]	
Type	**Description**
I	Involves only tip of coronoid
II	A single or comminuted fragment involving <50% of the coronoid process
III	A single or comminuted fragment involving >50% of the coronoid process

Regan and Morrey[49] classified coronoid fractures into three types based on the amount of the coronoid process involved. This classification is useful in predicting the outcome and in determining the treatment. Type I fractures involve only the tip of the process (see Fig. 11-48); type II fractures involve more than just the tip but less than 50% of the process (see Fig. 11-52); and type III fractures involve more than 50% of

the process. In addition, Mellema et al.[39] identified several relationships between specific injury patterns and their ability to predict the type of fracture as well as the distribution of subsequent fracture lines, which are also helpful for diagnosis and treatment planning.

OUTCOME MEASURES FOR FRACTURES OF THE PROXIMAL ULNA

The current literature is deficient in functional outcome instruments for fractures of the proximal ulna. The previously published studies on the outcomes of these fractures have used descriptive assessments that are currently nonvalidated techniques. Elbow range of motion after these injuries continues to be a driver of functional outcomes. As such, there is a definite need for both accurate methods of measuring range of motion as well as validated techniques for reporting the results. A recent systematic review by De Maio et al.[10] concluded that, in general, displaced olecranon fractures in children have good outcomes so long as an anatomic reduction is obtained.

PATHOANATOMY AND APPLIED ANATOMY RELATING TO FRACTURES OF THE PROXIMAL ULNA

At birth, the ossification of the metaphysis of the proximal ulna extends only to the midportion of the semilunar notch. At this age, the leading edge of the metaphysis is usually perpendicular to the long axis of the olecranon (Fig. 11-54A,B). As ossification progresses, the proximal border of the metaphysis becomes more oblique. The anterior margin extends proximally and to three-fourths of the width of the semilunar notch by 6 years of age. At this age, the physis extends distally to include the coronoid process (Fig. 11-54C). A secondary center of ossification occurs in the coronoid process. Just before the development of the secondary center of ossification in the olecranon, the leading edge of the metaphysis develops a well-defined sclerotic margin. Ossification of the olecranon occurs in the area of the triceps insertion at approximately 9 years of age (Fig. 11-54D). Ossification of the coronoid process is completed about the time that the olecranon ossification center appears.

The secondary ossification center of the olecranon may be bipartite (Fig. 11-54E). The major center within the tip of the olecranon is enveloped by the triceps insertion. This has been referred to as a traction center. The second and smaller center, an articular center, lies under the proximal fourth of the articular surface of the semilunar notch.

Fusion of the olecranon epiphysis with the metaphysis, which progresses from anterior to posterior, occurs at approximately 14 years of age. The sclerotic margin that defines the edge of the metaphysis may be mistaken for a fracture (Fig. 11-54F). Rarely, the physeal line persists into adulthood.[68] If this does occur, it is usually in athletes who have used the extremity in repetitive throwing activities.[70] The chronic tension forces applied across the apophysis theoretically prevent its normal closure.

Figure 11-54. Olecranon ossification. **A:** Limits of the border of ossification at birth, 8 years, and 12 years. **B:** Lateral view of olecranon at 6 months of age. The proximal margin is perpendicular to the long axis of the ulna. **C:** Lateral view of the olecranon at 6 years of age. The proximal margin is oblique. **D:** Secondary ossification center developing in the olecranon in an 11-year-old. A sclerotic border has developed on the proximal metaphyseal margin. **E:** Bipartite secondary ossification center. The larger center is the traction center (*open arrow*). The smaller, more proximal center is the articular center (*white arrow*). **F:** Before complete fusion, a partial line remains (*arrow*), bordered by a sclerotic margin.

Occasionally, a separate ossification center called a patella cubiti develops in the triceps tendon at its insertion on the tip of the olecranon. This ossicle is separate and can articulate with the trochlea. It is usually unilateral, unlike other persistent secondary ossification centers, which are more likely to be bilateral and familial. It has been posited that the patella cubiti was a traumatic ossicle rather than a developmental variation.

Metaphyseal Fractures of the Olecranon

Because the olecranon is a metaphyseal area, the cortex is relatively thin, allowing for the development of greenstick-type fracture deformities. The periosteum in children is immature and thick, which may prevent the degree of separation seen in adults. Likewise, the larger amount of epiphyseal cartilage in children may serve as a cushion to lessen the effects of a direct blow to the olecranon. In the production of supracondylar fractures, ligamentous laxity in this age group tends to force the elbow into hyperextension when the child falls on the outstretched upper extremity. This puts a compressive force across the olecranon and locks it into the fossa in the distal humerus, where it is protected. An older person, whose elbow does not go into hyperextension, is more likely to fall with the elbow partially flexed. The slightly flexed position, particularly with valgus or varus stress, puts the olecranon at increased risk for fracture. The unique biomechanical characteristics of the child's olecranon predisposes it to different fracture patterns than those in adults.

Fractures of the Coronoid Process

Up to age 6 years, the coronoid process consists of epiphyseal cartilage and physeal cartilage at the distal end of a tongue extending from the apophysis of the olecranon. The coronoid process does not develop a secondary center of ossification, but instead ossifies along with the advancing edge of the metaphysis (see Fig. 11-54).

TREATMENT OPTIONS FOR FRACTURES OF THE PROXIMAL ULNA

NONOPERATIVE TREATMENT OF FRACTURES INVOLVING THE PROXIMAL APOPHYSIS OF THE ULNA

Indications/Contraindications

Nonoperative Treatment of Fractures Involving the Proximal Apophysis of the Ulna:
INDICATIONS AND CONTRAINDICATIONS

Indications

- Nondisplaced fractures
- Apophysitis

Relative Contraindications

- Displaced fractures
- Open fractures

For apophysitis and nondisplaced stress fractures, we ask the patient to cease the offending activity, with or without a short course of immobilization. During this period of rest, the patient should maintain upper extremity strength with a selective muscle exercise program as well as maintain cardiovascular conditioning.

In a recently published series by Rath et al.,[55] isolated epiphyseal fractures of the olecranon were met with good long-term outcomes after nonoperative management with up to 2 mm of displacement.

Techniques

With minimal displacement (2–4 mm) of the fracture, satisfactory closed reduction can be obtained with the elbow extended. The elbow can then be immobilized in extension with a long-arm cast.

Outcomes

In general, these injuries recover well and the patient returns to full activities quickly. The highest-risk group for failure of nonoperative management are the stress injuries.

NONOPERATIVE TREATMENT OF METAPHYSEAL FRACTURES OF THE OLECRANON OF THE PROXIMAL ULNA

Indications/Contraindications

Nonoperative Treatment of Metaphyseal Fractures of the Olecranon of the Proximal Ulna:
INDICATIONS AND CONTRAINDICATIONS

Indications

- Nondisplaced fractures
- Fractures reducible to anatomic alignment by closed methods

Relative Contraindications

- Nonreducible fractures
- Open fractures

Flexion injuries are the most common type of olecranon fractures. In those with minimal displacement, nonoperative treatment is the preferred option. Nonoperative management is contraindicated in displaced olecranon fractures.

Treatment of extension injuries requires both adequate realignment of the angulation of the olecranon and treatment of the secondary injuries. Indications for nonoperative treatment in these injuries include the ability to restore anatomic alignment.

Zimmerman[79] reported that the original angulation tends to redevelop in some fractures. If a varus force produced the fracture, the proximal ulna or olecranon may drift back into varus, which can cause a painful subluxation of the radial head. A secondary osteotomy of the proximal ulna or olecranon may be necessary if the angulation is significant after a healed malunion.

Techniques

Flexion Injuries

Most displace minimally and require immobilization with the elbow in no more than 75 to 80 degrees of flexion (Fig. 11-55). Even if the fracture displaces significantly, immobilization in full or partial extension usually affords satisfactory healing and alignment.[18]

Extension Injuries

Often in varus injuries, correction of the alignment of the olecranon also reduces the radial head. The olecranon angulation corrects with the elbow in extension. This locks the proximal olecranon into the olecranon fossa of the humerus so that the distal angulation can be corrected at the fracture site with a valgus force applied to the forearm. Occasionally, in extension fractures, complete separation of the fragments requires open reduction and internal fixation (Fig. 11-56).

Shear Injuries

Some of these fractures are reduced better in flexion, and the posterior periosteum serves as a compressive force to maintain the reduction. This fracture has been treated using an overhead sling to apply a posteriorly directed force against the proximal portion of the distal fragment. The weight of the arm and forearm helps supplement the tension-band effect of the posterior periosteum.

Outcomes

Most nondisplaced or minimally displaced (<2 mm) proximal ulna fractures can be treated successfully with nonoperative methods. However, these injuries need to be followed closely to ensure maintenance of alignment. Any loss of reduction/alignment should be recognized and lead to surgical management.

Figure 11-55. Simple immobilization of a flexion injury. **A:** Injury film, lateral view, showing minimal displacement. **B:** Three weeks later, the fracture has displaced further. Periosteal new bone is along the posterior border of the olecranon (*arrow*). Healing was complete with a normal range of motion. (Courtesy of Jesse C. DeLee, MD.)

For anterior shear fractures, the key to management is recognition that the distal fragment is displaced anteriorly and the posterior periosteum remains intact. The intact posterior periosteum can serve as an internal tension band to facilitate reduction.

Figure 11-56. Open reduction of a valgus extension injury. **A:** Anteroposterior injury film shows complete displacement of the radial head. **B:** Lateral view also shows the degree of displacement of the olecranon fracture. This patient required surgical intervention with internal fixation to achieve a satisfactory reduction.

NONOPERATIVE TREATMENT OF FRACTURES OF THE CORONOID PROCESS OF THE PROXIMAL ULNA

Indications/Contraindications

Nonoperative Treatment of Fractures of the Coronoid Process of the Proximal Ulna:
INDICATIONS AND CONTRAINDICATIONS

Indications

- Elbow stability
- Mild displacement (types I and II)

Relative Contraindications

- Elbow instability
- Type III fractures

The degree of displacement or the presence of elbow instability guides the treatment. The associated injuries are also a factor in treatment. Regan and Morrey[56,57] treated type I and II fractures with early motion if there were no contradicting associated injuries.

Techniques

For initial immobilization, if the fracture is associated with an elbow dislocation, the elbow is placed in approximately 100 degrees of flexion, with the forearm in full supination.[42] Occasionally, in partial avulsion fractures, the fracture reduces more easily with the elbow in extension. In these rare cases, the brachialis muscle may be an aid in reducing the fragment in extension.

Outcomes

Regan and Morrey[56] found that the elbow often was unstable in type III fractures, and they secured these fractures with internal fixation. They had satisfactory results with type I and II fractures, but in only 20% of type III fractures were the results satisfactory with nonoperative treatment.

OPERATIVE TREATMENT OF FRACTURES INVOLVING THE PROXIMAL APOPHYSIS AND OLECRANON METAPHYSIS OF THE ULNA

Indications/Contraindications

Operative Treatment of Fractures Involving the Proximal Apophysis and Olecranon Metaphysis of the Ulna:
INDICATIONS AND CONTRAINDICATIONS

Indications

- Significant displacement
- Acceptable alignment cannot be achieved with closed methods
- Fractures with >4-mm displacement
- Fractures with incongruent intra-articular surface

Contraindications

- Acceptable alignment achieved with closed methods
- Fractures with ≤4-mm displacement
- Fractures with congruent intra-articular surface
- Percutaneous pinning allows stabilization of closed reduction

Apophyseal Fractures

There is no standard method of treatment of fractures of the apophysis because few such fractures have been described. Surgical treatment is indicated in situations where acceptable alignment cannot be achieved with closed methods. A recently published manuscript determined that fractures with more than 4 mm of displacement or with a noncongruent intra-articular surface should be treated surgically to achieve a better reduction and surgical outcome.[54] With mild to moderately displaced fractures, if a satisfactory closed reduction can be obtained, percutaneous pinning will stabilize the reduction. This can allow for casting in flexion, which is often better tolerated. For fractures with significant displacement (>4-mm malangulation), treatment is usually open reduction with internal fixation using a combination of axial pins and tension-band wiring (Fig. 11-57). Gortzak et al.[24] and Kim et al.[33] described techniques of open reduction using percutaneously placed K-wires and absorbable sutures instead of wires for the tension band. The percutaneously placed wires are subsequently removed 4 to 5 weeks postoperatively, eliminating the need for implant removal. More recently, a study by Perkins et al. compared outcomes by fixation type including tension band wire (TBW) versus tension band suturing (TBS). In their article, the outcomes were similar and good in both groups, with the exception being patients weighing more than 50 kg. In those patients, TBS constructs had a significantly higher rate of failure requiring revision surgery. Therefore, TBS should be avoided in patients weighing more than 50 kg.[51] Most stress injuries respond to simple rest from the offending activity. However, a chronic stress fracture can result in a symptomatic nonunion. Use of a compressive screw alone across the nonunion often is sufficient, but supplemental bone grafting may be necessary to achieve union if there is a fracture gap.

Metaphyseal Olecranon Fractures

Flexion Injuries

If the fracture is significantly displaced or comminuted, open reduction with internal fixation is usually required. Recommended fixation devices vary from absorbable or nonabsorbable suture to an axial screw through tension-band wiring with axial pins to a plate. Internal fixation allows early motion.

Extension Injuries

Treatment of extension injuries requires both adequate realignment of the angulation of the olecranon and treatment of the secondary injuries. Occasionally, in extension fractures, complete separation of the fragments requires open reduction and internal fixation (see Fig. 11-56).

Shear Injuries

For anterior shear fractures, the key to management is recognition that the distal fragment is displaced anteriorly, and the posterior periosteum remains intact. The intact posterior periosteum can serve as an internal tension band to facilitate reduction. If the periosteum is torn or early motion is desirable, internal fixation of the two fragments with an oblique screw perpendicular to the fracture line has also been recommended (Fig. 11-58).

Figure 11-57. Operative treatment of an apophyseal fracture. **A:** Postoperative radiograph of apophyseal fracture, which was stabilized with small Steinmann pins alone. **B:** Five months later, growth has continued in the traction center and the articular center is ossified (*arrow*). **C:** One year after injury, the apophysis was partially avulsed a second time. The two secondary ossification centers are now fused. **D:** Three months after the second fracture, the fracture gap has filled in, producing a normal olecranon.

Figure 11-58. Operative treatment of extension shear fractures. **A:** If the periosteum is insufficient to hold the fragments apposed, an interfragmentary screw can be used. **B:** An extension shear type of fracture secured with two oblique interfragmentary screws.

Closed Reduction and Percutaneous Pinning

Preoperative Planning

Closed Reduction and Percutaneous Pinning of Fractures Involving the Proximal Apophysis and Olecranon Metaphysis of the Ulna: PREOPERATIVE PLANNING CHECKLIST	
OR table	❏ Standard with radiolucent hand table
Position/ positioning aids	❏ Turn table 90 degrees, bring patient to edge of table toward hand table. Secure head with blanket/towel and tape. Safety strap over torso
Fluoroscopy location	❏ In line with affected extremity, perpendicular to OR table
Equipment	❏ Smooth K-wires; power drill; tension-band equipment available
Tourniquet	❏ Nonsterile

To adequately prepare for this technique, we must carefully assess the fracture pattern and determine that an attempt at closed reduction is feasible. It is good practice to also prepare for the possibility that this technique may need to be abandoned and transitioned to an open procedure if an adequate closed reduction is not attainable. Accordingly, the patient, family, and operating room team should all be informed of these possibilities. The OR table, positioning of the patient, and equipment necessary for both closed and open procedures should be identified and available before beginning the surgery. Equipment needed for a potential open procedure can be left unopened in the sterile packaging but should be visually accounted for and immediately available.

Positioning

Same as for instrument-assisted closed reduction of proximal radius fractures. Some surgeons prefer lateral or prone positioning. Take care to adequately protect the axilla and down arm in the lateral position; protect the face and keep the abdomen free from pressure in the prone position.

Surgical Approach(es)

A percutaneous approach is used, starting at the subcutaneous border of the tip of the olecranon.

Technique

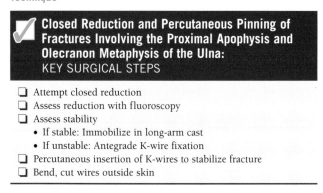

Closed Reduction and Percutaneous Pinning of Fractures Involving the Proximal Apophysis and Olecranon Metaphysis of the Ulna: KEY SURGICAL STEPS
❏ Attempt closed reduction
❏ Assess reduction with fluoroscopy
❏ Assess stability
• If stable: Immobilize in long-arm cast
• If unstable: Antegrade K-wire fixation
❏ Percutaneous insertion of K-wires to stabilize fracture
❏ Bend, cut wires outside skin

Simple stainless steel K-wires are appropriate to use for this technique. Size will range from 2 to 2.7 mm, based on the size of the child. Fluoroscopy is used to localize the fracture site and intended entry site of the wire. The fracture is then reduced with simultaneous elbow extension and thumb pressure over the olecranon. Once the fracture reduction is achieved, percutaneous K-wires are driven from the tip of the olecranon across the fracture site and exit the far cortex. Fracture stability and pin configuration are then assessed with fluoroscopy. The pins are then cut and bent outside of the skin. We prefer placing a sterile felt pad between the cut pins and the skin, followed by a long-arm cast for immobilization. The pins are then removed in the office after the fracture has healed, typically 3 to 4 weeks.

Open Reduction and Tension-Band Fixation

Preoperative Planning

Open Reduction and Tension-Band Fixation of Fractures Involving the Proximal Apophysis and Olecranon Metaphysis of the Ulna: PREOPERATIVE PLANNING CHECKLIST	
OR table	❏ Standard with radiolucent hand table
Position/positioning aids	❏ Turn table 90 degrees, bring patient to edge of table toward hand table. Secure head with blanket/towel and tape. Safety strap over torso
Fluoroscopy location	❏ In line with affected extremity, perpendicular to OR table
Equipment	❏ Smooth K-wires; tension-band equipment available
Tourniquet	❏ Nonsterile

Once it has been determined that a satisfactory reduction is not achievable by closed methods, an open reduction is indicated. The preparation for this procedure includes ensuring proper OR table, fluoroscopy, patient positioning, and necessary equipment.

Positioning

The positioning for this procedure is the same as for the closed reduction and percutaneous pinning technique described above. Some surgeons prefer lateral or prone positioning. Take care to adequately protect the axilla and down arm in the lateral position; protect the face and keep the abdomen free from pressure in the prone position.

Surgical Approaches

A standard posterior approach to the proximal ulna is used, with the incision spanning from 1 to 2 fingerbreadths proximal to the tip of the olecranon to 2 to 3 cm distal to the fracture site. The subcutaneous location of the ulna in this location allows for quick access to the fracture site. However, particularly close attention needs to be paid to delicate handling of the soft tissue envelope as there is commonly a fair amount of soft tissue trauma locally from the injury. It is recommended to shape the incision in a curvilinear fashion proximally to avoid placing the scar directly over the bony prominence of the olecranon.

Technique

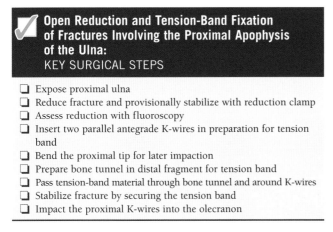

✓ **Open Reduction and Tension-Band Fixation of Fractures Involving the Proximal Apophysis of the Ulna:**
KEY SURGICAL STEPS

- ❏ Expose proximal ulna
- ❏ Reduce fracture and provisionally stabilize with reduction clamp
- ❏ Assess reduction with fluoroscopy
- ❏ Insert two parallel antegrade K-wires in preparation for tension band
- ❏ Bend the proximal tip for later impaction
- ❏ Prepare bone tunnel in distal fragment for tension band
- ❏ Pass tension-band material through bone tunnel and around K-wires
- ❏ Stabilize fracture by securing the tension band
- ❏ Impact the proximal K-wires into the olecranon

Once the fracture is exposed, a reduction can be performed with bone reduction forceps. The reduction maneuver can be facilitated by first placing a small unicortical drill hole distal to the fracture site along the diaphysis of the ulna. Then with one tine of the forceps in the drill hole and the other tine at the tip of the olecranon, applying gentle compression with the forceps will help reduce and stabilize the fracture.

With the fracture now reduced, two K-wires are driven in an antegrade fashion, parallel to each other, starting near the tip of the olecranon and coursing obliquely to cross the fracture site and exit the cortex of the anterior ulna. The fracture reduction and K-wire position are then assessed with fluoroscopy. The K-wires are then bent and cut in preparation for capture of the tension band. The wires are pulled back 3 to 4 mm at this point so that when fully impacted later, they will not protrude too far beyond the anterior ulnar cortex.

In preparation for tension-band application, a transverse tunnel is created in the ulnar diaphysis 1 to 2 cm distal to the fracture site. It is critical to leave an intact cortical bridge of bone along the posterior aspect of the ulna superficial to the tunnel. A drill is used to perforate the medial and lateral cortex of the ulna at the desired level of tunnel creation. A towel clip can then be inserted into these two pilot drill holes to finish creating the ulnar bone tunnel.

The tension-band material is then selected, either 18- to 20-gauge wire or large absorbable or nonabsorbable suture. We frequently utilize no. 2 polyethylene core braided polyester suture (Fiber Wire, Arthrex, Naples, FL) or no. 1 polydioxanone suture (PDS) instead of wire. As recently noted by Perkins et al., TBS technique should only be used in patients less than 50 kg.[51] The tension band is then passed through the ulnar bone tunnel and around the previously placed K-wires. Twisting the wires or tying the sutures tightens the tension band. At this point, the reduction clamp is removed and fracture stability assessed with elbow flexion/extension and fluoroscopy. The previously cut and bent K-wires are then impacted into the olecranon, finalizing the capture of the tension band.

Open Reduction and Compression Screw Fixation

Preoperative Planning

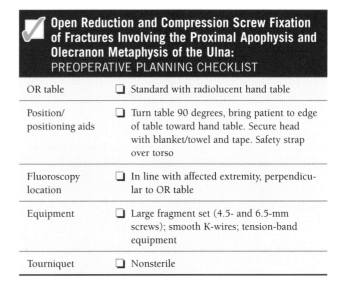

✓ **Open Reduction and Compression Screw Fixation of Fractures Involving the Proximal Apophysis and Olecranon Metaphysis of the Ulna:**
PREOPERATIVE PLANNING CHECKLIST

OR table	❏ Standard with radiolucent hand table
Position/ positioning aids	❏ Turn table 90 degrees, bring patient to edge of table toward hand table. Secure head with blanket/towel and tape. Safety strap over torso
Fluoroscopy location	❏ In line with affected extremity, perpendicular to OR table
Equipment	❏ Large fragment set (4.5- and 6.5-mm screws); smooth K-wires; tension-band equipment
Tourniquet	❏ Nonsterile

The preparation for this procedure is the same as for the above tension-band technique except for equipment/implant differences.

Positioning

The positioning for this procedure is the same as for the closed reduction and percutaneous pinning technique described above. Some surgeons prefer lateral or prone positioning. Take care to adequately protect the axilla and down arm in the lateral position; protect the face and keep the abdomen free from pressure in the prone position.

Surgical Approach

The approach for this procedure is the same as for the tension-band technique described above.

Technique

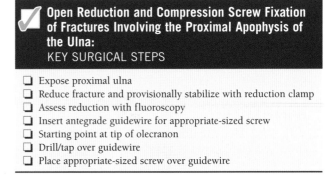

✓ **Open Reduction and Compression Screw Fixation of Fractures Involving the Proximal Apophysis of the Ulna:**
KEY SURGICAL STEPS

- ❏ Expose proximal ulna
- ❏ Reduce fracture and provisionally stabilize with reduction clamp
- ❏ Assess reduction with fluoroscopy
- ❏ Insert antegrade guidewire for appropriate-sized screw
- ❏ Starting point at tip of olecranon
- ❏ Drill/tap over guidewire
- ❏ Place appropriate-sized screw over guidewire

Once the fracture is exposed, a reduction can be performed with bone reduction forceps. The reduction maneuver can be facilitated by first placing a small unicortical drill hole distal to the fracture site along the diaphysis of the ulna. Then with one tine of the forceps in the drill hole and the other tine at the tip of the olecranon, applying gentle compression with the forceps will help reduce and stabilize the fracture.

With the fracture now reduced, the guide pin from the cannulated screw system can be placed in an antegrade fashion starting near the tip of the olecranon, across the fracture site, and into the intramedullary canal of the ulna. Most commonly a 6.5-mm cancellous bone screw is selected. The screw tract is then drilled and tapped over the guidewire, followed by placement of the appropriate-sized screw. The alignment and stability are then assessed with elbow flexion/extension and fluoroscopy.

Authors' Preferred Treatment for Fractures of the Proximal Ulna (Algorithm 11-2)

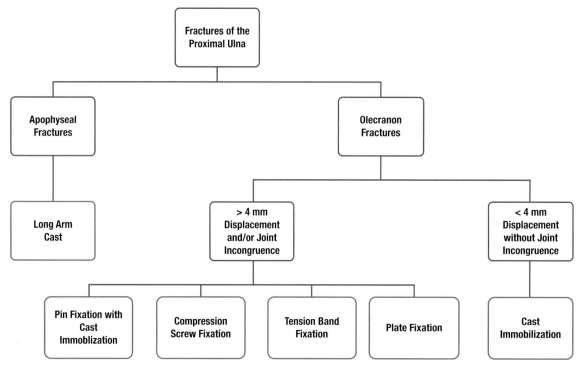

Algorithm 11-2. Authors' preferred treatment for fractures of the proximal ulna.

Apophyseal Fractures and Nondisplaced Fractures

For apophysitis and nondisplaced stress fractures, we ask the patient to cease the offending activity. During this period of rest, the patient should maintain upper extremity strength with a selective muscle exercise program as well as maintain cardiovascular conditioning. When a persistent nonunion of the olecranon in an adolescent does not demonstrate healing after a reasonable period of simple rest, we place a cannulated compression screw across the apophysis to stimulate healing.

Displaced Fractures

With minimal displacement of the fracture, satisfactory closed reduction can be obtained with the elbow extended. We usually immobilize the elbow in a long-arm cast in extension. Percutaneous pinning will stabilize the reduction if there is any concern about loss of reduction. Completely displaced fractures are treated operatively using a tension-band technique. In young children, we use small Steinmann or Kirschner pins. Patients with large ossification centers are treated with a compression screw like those with metaphyseal fractures. A recent publication reviewed the compression screw technique against TBW technique in patients with OI and displaced olecranon fractures. The compression screw technique was fraught with a significantly increased failure rate in this population, leading to the conclusion of TBW technique as the optimal choice for these injuries in patients with OI.[52]

Metaphyseal Olecranon Fractures

We use a classification based on the mechanism of injury in choosing the method of treatment.

Flexion Injuries

We immobilize most nondisplaced flexion injuries with the elbow in 5 to 10 degrees of flexion for approximately 3 weeks. It is important to obtain radiographs of these fractures after approximately 5 to 7 days in the cast to ensure that there has not been any significant displacement of the fragment.

Figure 11-59. Internal tension-band techniques. **A:** Standard AO technique with stainless steel wire. The wire can be prominent in the subcutaneous tissues. **B:** Axial wires plus polydioxanone sutures (PDSs) 6 weeks after surgery. **C:** A displaced flexion-type injury in an 11-year-old boy. There is complete separation of the fracture fragments. **D:** A cancellous lag screw plus PDS. The screw engages the anterior cortex of the coronoid process. The PDS passes through a separate drill hole in the olecranon (*open arrow*) and crosses in a figure-of-eight manner over the fracture site and around the neck of the screw.

To determine which injuries need internal fixation, we palpate the fracture for a defect and flex the elbow to determine the integrity of the posterior periosteum. If the fragments separate with either of these maneuvers, they are unstable and are fixed internally so that active motion can be started as soon as possible.

We prefer a modification of the tension-band technique. Originally, we used the standard AO technique with axial K-wires or Steinmann pins and figure-of-eight stainless steel as the tension band (Fig. 11-59A). Because removal of the wire often required reopening the entire incision, we now often use an absorbable suture for the figure-of-eight tension band. No. 1 PDS suture, which is slowly absorbed over a few months, is ideal so long as the patient is less than 50 kg (Fig. 11-59B).[51] When rigid internal fixation is applied, rapid healing at the fracture site produces internal stability before the PDS absorbs. We prefer K-wires in patients who

are very young and have very little ossification of the olecranon apophysis (see Fig. 11-57). If the axial wires become a problem, we remove them through a small incision. Most recently, we have used a combination of an oblique cortical screw with PDS as the tension band (Fig. 11-59C,D), and are pleased with the results. In the past, we had to remove almost all the axial wires; very few of the screws cause enough symptoms to require removal. Occasionally, we use the tension-band wire technique with 16- or 18-gauge wire in a heavier patient.

Extension Injuries

For extension injuries, we anesthetize the patient to allow forceful manipulation of the olecranon while it is locked in its fossa in extension. Because this is a greenstick fracture, we slightly overcorrect to prevent the recurrence of angular deformity. These fractures may require further manipulation in 1 to 2 weeks if the original angulation recurs. Associated fractures are treated simultaneously.

Shear Injuries

Most shear fractures can be treated nonoperatively. We usually immobilize them in enough flexion to hold the fragments together, if the posterior periosteum is intact (Fig. 11-60). If the periosteum is torn, an oblique screw is an excellent way to secure the fracture (see Fig. 11-58). If considerable swelling prevents the elbow from being hyperflexed enough to use the posterior periosteum as a tension band, an oblique screw is a good choice.

Figure 11-60. Shear injuries. **A:** Flexion pattern: Radiograph of the patient in Figure 11-46A after the elbow was flexed. The intact posterior periosteum acted as a tension band and held the fracture reduced. **B:** Radiograph taken 4 weeks after surgery shows new bone formation under the intact periosteum (*arrows*) on the dorsal surface of the olecranon. **C:** Extension pattern: Radiograph of patient with an extension shear injury showing an increase in the fracture gap (*arrows*). **D:** Because the dorsal periosteum and cortex were intact, the fracture gap (*arrows*) closed with flexion of the elbow.

Postoperative Care

A critical advantage of surgical management is the ability to allow and encourage early motion. Accordingly, with stable fixation, a brief period of immobilization postoperatively is in order. Typically, this would entail 10 to 14 days of immobilization to allow for wound healing, followed by active measures geared toward resumption of elbow/forearm range of motion.

Potential Pitfalls and Preventive Measures

Proximal Ulna Apophyseal and Metaphyseal Olecranon Fractures: POTENTIAL PITFALLS AND PREVENTIONS	
Pitfall	**Prevention**
Prominent implants	Attention to detail
	Plan for implant impaction
	Incision planning
	Consider use of suture instead of wire for tension band
Nonunion	Consider bone grafting
	Compression techniques
Loss of reduction in extension type	Reduce in extension, "over" reduce
	Pin if stability questionable

Murphy et al.[42] compared the failure of various fixation devices under rapid loading: (a) figure-of-eight wire alone, (b) cancellous screw alone, (c) AO tension band, and (d) cancellous screw with a figure-of-eight wire combination. The cancellous screw alone and figure-of-eight wire alone were by far the weakest. The greatest resistance to failure was found in the combination of a screw plus figure-of-eight wire, followed closely by the AO tension-band fixation. In their clinical evaluation of patients, comparing the AO tension band and combination of screw and figure-of-eight wire, they found more clinical problems associated with the AO technique. The main problem with the AO technique is the subcutaneous prominence of the axial wires.[49] To prevent proximal migration of these wires, Montgomery[41] devised a method of making eyelets in the proximal end of the wires through which he passed the figure-of-eight fixation wire.

Zimmerman[79] reported that the original angulation tends to redevelop in some extension-type olecranon fractures. If a varus force produced the fracture, the proximal ulna or olecranon may drift back into varus, which can cause a problematic subluxation of the radial head. A secondary osteotomy of the proximal ulna or olecranon may be necessary if the angulation is significant.

Outcomes

There are limited validated outcome measures on this population in the current literature. In general, the limited studies available report good-to-excellent outcomes with the techniques described above. Two recent systematic reviews confirmed that proper treatment of these injuries results in universally good outcomes.[10,28]

OPERATIVE TREATMENT OF FRACTURES OF THE CORONOID PROCESS OF THE PROXIMAL ULNA

Indications/Contraindications

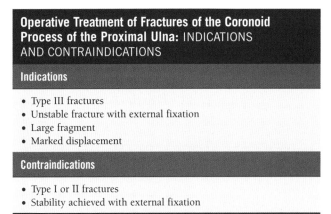

Operative Treatment of Fractures of the Coronoid Process of the Proximal Ulna: INDICATIONS AND CONTRAINDICATIONS
Indications
• Type III fractures
• Unstable fracture with external fixation
• Large fragment
• Marked displacement
Contraindications
• Type I or II fractures
• Stability achieved with external fixation

Regan and Morrey[55] found that the elbow often was unstable in type III fractures, and they secured these fractures with internal fixation. They had satisfactory results with type I and II fractures, but in only 20% of type III fractures were the results satisfactory that were treated nonoperatively. These indications were further supported by Aksu et al.,[2] who recommend surgical management for all type III injuries.

The presence of a coronoid fracture alerts us to be especially thorough in looking for other injuries. In children, surgery is rarely necessary. If there is a large fragment and marked displacement, open reduction is indicated.

ORIF of Coronoid Fractures

Preoperative Planning

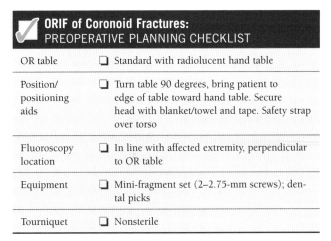

✓ ORIF of Coronoid Fractures: PREOPERATIVE PLANNING CHECKLIST	
OR table	❏ Standard with radiolucent hand table
Position/ positioning aids	❏ Turn table 90 degrees, bring patient to edge of table toward hand table. Secure head with blanket/towel and tape. Safety strap over torso
Fluoroscopy location	❏ In line with affected extremity, perpendicular to OR table
Equipment	❏ Mini-fragment set (2–2.75-mm screws); dental picks
Tourniquet	❏ Nonsterile

The preparation for ORIF of the coronoid process starts with ensuring familiarity with the local anatomy and anterior approach to this region. In addition, the surgeon needs to prepare for dealing with a relatively small-sized fracture fragment that will require significant precision for reduction and screw placement.

Positioning

The positioning for this technique is typically supine, with a hand table attachment.

Surgical Approach

This procedure is performed through either a medial or Henry anterior approach to the elbow. The anatomic plane of the anterior deep dissection lies between the brachioradialis and brachialis. The radial nerve lies within this interval and needs to be protected. In the medial approach, the ulnar nerve must be identified and protected. Either way, the brachial artery and median nerve are anteromedial in location. The fracture fragment will likely have at least partial attachment of the brachialis.

Technique

> ### ✓ ORIF of Coronoid Fractures:
> ### KEY SURGICAL STEPS
> ❑ Expose proximal ulna via either a medial or anterior Henry approach
> ❑ Protect the ulnar or radial nerve, depending upon approach used
> ❑ Reduce fracture fragment using dental picks
> ❑ Fix fracture with appropriate-sized mini-fragment screw

Because of the confined space anatomically in this location, the use of fracture reduction forceps will be challenging if not impossible. Accordingly, dental picks are very useful in obtaining reduction of this fracture. Once reduced, the fragment is fixed with a mini-fragment screw or sewn in place through two drill holes in the posterior aspect of the ulna. If there is significant comminution or the fragment is small, the pull-through suture technique is superior.

Authors' Preferred Treatment for Fractures of the Coronoid Process (Algorithm 11-3)

Algorithm 11-3. Authors' preferred treatment for fractures of the coronoid process.

We usually treat coronoid fractures with early motion, much as we do elbow dislocations. The presence of a coronoid fracture alerts us to be especially thorough in looking for other injuries. In children, surgery is rarely necessary. If there is a large fragment and marked displacement, open reduction is performed. The fragment is fixed with a mini-fragment screw or sewn in place through two drill holes in the posterior aspect of the ulna.

Postoperative Care

A short period of immobilization, 10 to 14 days, followed by active range of motion is preferred. However, tenuous fixation may be encountered when treating these injuries. Intraoperative assessment of fixation and stability is warranted, and depending on the assessment, the postoperative care may need to be adjusted accordingly.

POTENTIAL PITFALLS AND PREVENTIVE MEASURES

Coronoid Fractures: POTENTIAL PITFALLS AND PREVENTIONS	
Pitfall	**Prevention**
Loss of fixation	• Assess intraoperatively • Cast longer if fixation tenuous
Elbow instability	• Treat type III injuries operatively
Fragment comminution	• Be prepared for pull-through suture technique

Outcomes

As noted previously, Regan and Morrey[57] found that the elbow often was unstable in type III fractures, and they secured these fractures with internal fixation. They had satisfactory results with type I and II fractures, but in only 20% of type III fractures were the results satisfactory that were treated nonoperatively.

MANAGEMENT OF EXPECTED ADVERSE OUTCOMES AND UNEXPECTED COMPLICATIONS IN FRACTURES OF THE PROXIMAL ULNA

Fractures of the Proximal Ulna: COMMON ADVERSE OUTCOMES AND COMPLICATIONS
Fractures of the Proximal Apophysis and Olecranon Metaphysis of the Ulna
• Spur formation • Nonunion • Apophyseal arrest • Loss of reduction • Olecranon elongation • Prominent implants
Coronoid Fractures
• Elbow stiffness • Recurrent elbow instability

FRACTURES OF THE PROXIMAL APOPHYSIS AND OLECRANON METAPHYSIS OF THE ULNA

Spur Formation

Overgrowth of the epiphysis proximally may produce a bony spur. These can block extension. Symptomatic spurs can be treated with surgical excision.

Nonunion

Nonunion is a rare event in these fractures, most likely occurring in apophysitis/overuse injuries. Bone grafting the nonunion and ensuring stable fixation with compression is the

Figure 11-61. Congenital pseudarthrosis of the olecranon in a 9-year-old girl who had limited elbow extension and no antecedent trauma. The edges of the bone were separated by thick fibrous tissue. (Courtesy of Michael J. Rogal, MD.)

most efficacious method of treatment. More distal nonunion is unusual and should not be confused with congenital pseudarthrosis of the ulna, which is rare (Fig. 11-61). In the latter condition, there is no antecedent trauma.

Apophyseal Arrest

Apophyseal arrest appears to have no significant effect on elbow function (Fig. 11-62). There has been concern that applying compressive forces across the apophysis might cause premature growth arrest. In our experience, fusion of the apophysis to the metaphysis is accelerated. Apophyseal fractures usually occur when the physis is near natural closure. The growth proximally is appositional rather than longitudinal across the apophyseal plate. Thus, we have not found any functional shortening of the olecranon because of the early fusion of the apophysis to the metaphysis (see Fig. 11-57D). In practice, the use of a compression screw across an ossified olecranon fracture causes no loss of ulnar length. Children who sustain injuries before the development of the secondary ossification center may develop a deformity that is visible on radiographs (see Fig. 11-62). Although there may be shortening of the olecranon, it does not appear to produce functional problems. There are no reports of the effects of this injury in very young children or infants.

Irreducibility

An and Loder reported inability to reduce the fracture in one of their patients because the proximal fragment was entrapped in the joint.

Figure 11-62. Preosseous apophyseal arrest. **A:** Comminuted fracture of the proximal olecranon from a direct blow to the elbow in an 8-year-old boy. This fracture was treated nonoperatively. **B:** Radiograph 18 months later shows cessation of the proximal migration of the metaphyseal margin and a lack of development of a secondary ossification center. Despite this arrest of the apophysis, the patient had a full range of elbow motion.

Delayed Union

Delayed radiographic union usually is asymptomatic. In series,[37] one fracture treated with suture fixation ultimately progressed to a nonunion. Despite this, the patient had only a 11-degree extension lag and grade 4 triceps strength. An accessory ossicle, such as a patella cubiti, is not a nonunion.

Compartment Syndrome

Mathews[37] described one patient with Volkmann ischemic contracture after a nondisplaced linear fracture in the olecranon.

Nerve Injuries

Zimmerman[79] reported ulnar nerve neurapraxia from the development of a pseudarthrosis of the olecranon where inadequate fixation was used.

Elongation

Elongation of the tip of the olecranon may complicate healing of a fracture. Figure 11-63 illustrates a delayed union in which the apophysis became elongated to the point that it limited extension. This proximal overgrowth of the tip of the apophysis has

Figure 11-63. A: Injury film showing partial avulsion of the tip of the olecranon apophysis (*arrow*). **B:** Radiograph taken 4 years later shows a marked elongation and irregular ossification of the apophysis. (Courtesy of Joel Goldman, MD.)

A, B   **C**

Figure 11-64. Loss of reduction. **A:** Lateral radiograph of what appeared to be a simple undisplaced fracture (*arrow*) of the olecranon in an 11-year-old girl. **B:** On the anteroposterior film, the fracture also appears undisplaced. The mild lateral subluxation of the radial head was not recognized. **C:** Radiographs taken 5 months later showed further lateral subluxation with resultant incongruity of the elbow joint. (Courtesy of Richard W. Williamson, MD.)

occurred in olecranon fractures after routine open reduction and internal fixation.[49]

Loss of Reduction

Apparently, stable fractures treated with external immobilization may lose reduction, which results in a significant loss of elbow function (Fig. 11-64).

FRACTURES OF THE CORONOID PROCESS

Because of the high association of these coronoid fractures with elbow dislocations, postinjury stiffness is a concern. Accordingly, treatment modalities are selected to allow for early range of motion when possible. Complications are rare. In fractures with a large fragment (type III), the elbow may be unstable and prone to recurrent dislocations. Nonunion with the production of a free fragment in the joint occurs rarely in children.[48]

SUMMARY, CONTROVERSIES, AND FUTURE DIRECTIONS RELATED TO FRACTURES OF THE PROXIMAL RADIUS AND ULNA

A large portion of proximal radius and ulna fractures in children can be treated successfully by nonoperative methods. The surgical techniques described in this chapter are effective in achieving fracture union and good clinical results. However, the current literature is deficient in functional outcome instruments for fractures of the proximal ulna and radius in children. The previously published studies on the outcomes of these fractures have used descriptive assessments that are currently nonvalidated techniques. Elbow range of motion after these injuries continues to be a driver of functional outcomes. As such, there is a definite need for both accurate methods of measuring range of motion as well as validated techniques for reporting the results.

Annotated References

Reference	Annotation
Furushima K, Itoh Y, Iwabu S, et al. Classification of olecranon stress fractures in baseball players. *Am J Sports Med.* 2014;42(6):1343–1351.	Classification system for olecranon stress fractures to help guide treatment
Gortzak Y, Mercado E, Atar D, Weisel Y. Pediatric olecranon fractures: open reduction and internal fixation with removable K-wires wires and absorbable sutures. *J Pediatr Orthop.* 2006;26:39–42.	Surgical technique for tension-band fixation utilizing suture instead of wire to minimize need for secondary implant removal following surgical fixation
Greenspan A, Norman A. The radial head-capitellum view: useful technique in elbow trauma. *AJR Am J Roentgenol.* 1982;138:1186–1188.	Radiographic technique to assist in evaluation of radial head fractures
Metaizeau JP, Lascombes P, Lemelle JL, et al. Reduction and fixation of displaced radial neck fractures by closed intramedullary pinning. *J Pediatr Orthop.* 1993;13:355–360.	Surgical technique and results for closed intramedullary fixation of displaced radial neck fractures

Annotated References

Reference	Annotation
Regan W, Morrey BF. Classification and treatment of coronoid process fractures. *Orthopedics.* 1992;15:845–848.	Classification system for coronoid process fractures to help guide treatment
Smith GR, Hotchkiss RN. Radial head and neck fractures: anatomic guidelines for proper placement of internal fixation. *J Shoulder Elbow Surg.* 1996;5(2 Pt 1):113–117.	Anatomic study describing safe surgical exposure and implant placement for radial head and neck fractures
Van Zeeland NL, Bae DS, Goldfarb CA. Intra-articular radial head fracture in the skeletally immature patient: progressive radial head subluxation and rapid radiocapitellar degeneration. *J Pediatr Orthop.* 2011;31:124–129.	Case series describing high morbidity of untreated intra-articular radial head fractures in children
Waters PM, Beaty J, Kasser J. Elbow "TRASH" (the radiographic appearance seemed harmless) lesions. *J Pediatr Orthop.* 2010;30:S77–S81.	Overview of fracture patterns with high morbidity that appear harmless on initial review of radiographs
Zimmerman RM, Kalish LA, Hresko MT, et al. Surgical management of pediatric radial neck fractures. *J Bone Joint Surg Am.* 2013;95(20):1825–1832.	Large case series describing treatment of radial neck fractures in 151 children. Thirty-one percent overall poor results. Risk of poor result higher with age greater than 10 years, higher initial displacement, and need for open surgical procedures.

REFERENCES

1. Ackerson R, Nguyen A, Carry PM, et al. Intra-articular radial head fractures in the skeletally immature patient: complications and management. *J Pediatr Orthop.* 2015;35(5):443–448.
2. Aksu N, Korkmaz MF, Göğüş A, et al. [Surgical treatment of elbow dislocations accompanied by coronoid fractures]. *Acta Orthop Traumatol Turc.* 2008;42(4):258–264.
3. Basmajian HG, Choi PD, Huh K, et al. Radial neck fractures in children: experience from two level-1 trauma centers. *J Pediatr Orthop B.* 2014;23(4):369–374.
4. Bernstein SM, McKeever P, Bernstein L. Percutaneous pinning for radial neck fractures. *J Pediatr Orthop.* 1993;13:84–88.
5. Carney JR, Fox D, Mazurek MT. Displaced apophyseal olecranon fracture in a healthy child. *Mil Med.* 2007;172(12):1225–1227.
6. Cha SM, Shin HD, Kim KC, Han SC. Percutaneous reduction and leverage fixation using K-wires in paediatric angulated radial neck fractures. *Int Orthop.* 2012;36(4):803–809.
7. Chambers HG. Fractures of the proximal radius and ulna. In: Kasser JR, Beaty JH, eds. *Rockwood and Wilkins' Fractures in Children.* 5th ed. Lippincott Williams & Wilkins; 2001:483–528.
8. Cossio A, Cazzaniga C, Gridavilla G, et al. Paediatric radial neck fractures: one-step percutaneous reduction and fixation. *Injury.* 2014;45(Suppl 6):S80–S84.
9. Davidson RS, Markowitz RI, Dormans J, Drummond DS. Ultrasonographic evaluation of the elbow in infants and young children after suspected trauma. *J Bone Joint Surg Am.* 1994;76(12):1804–1813.
10. De Maio F, Gorgolini G, Caterini A, et al. Treatment of olecranon fractures in childhood: a systematic review. *Front Pediatr.* 2022;10:1046243.
11. De Mattos CB, Ramski DE, Kushare IV, et al. Radial neck fractures in children and adolescents: an examination of operative and nonoperative treatment and outcomes. *J Pediatr Orthop.* 2016;36(1):6–12.
12. DiCesare PE, Sew-Hoy A, Krom W. Bilateral isolated olecranon fractures in an infant as presentation of osteogenesis imperfecta. *Orthopedics.* 1992;15:741–743.
13. Dietzel M, Scherer S, Esser M, et al. Fractures of the proximal radius in children: management and results of 100 consecutive cases. *Arch Orthop Trauma Surg.* 2022 Aug;142(8):1903–1910.
14. D'Souza S, Vaishya R, Klenerman L. Management of radial neck fractures in children. a retrospective analysis of one hundred patients. *J Pediatr Orthop.* 1993;13:232–238.
15. Eberl R, Singer J, Fruhmann A, et al. Intramedullary nailing for the treatment of dislocated pediatric radial neck fractures. *Eur J Pediatr Surg.* 2010;4:250–252.
16. Eisenberg MT, Block AM, Ganapathy AK, et al. PROMIS utilization in pediatric orthopaedics: a scoping review. *J Pediatr Orthop.* 2022;42(9):521–531.
17. Falciglia F, Giordano M, Aulisa AG, et al. Radial neck fractures in children: results when open reduction is indicated. *J Pediatr Orthop.* 2014;34(8):756–762.
18. Fogarty EE, Blake NS, Regan BF. Fracture of the radial neck with medial displacement of the shaft of the radius. *Br J Radiol.* 1983;56:486–487.
19. Fuller CB, Guillen PT, Wongworawat MD, Riedel BB. Bioabsorbable pin fixation in late presenting pediatric radial neck fractures. *J Pediatr Orthop.* 2016;36(8):793–796.
20. Furushima K, Itoh Y, Iwabu S, et al. Classification of olecranon stress fractures in baseball players. *Am J Sports Med.* 2014;42(6):1343–1351.
21. Gaddy BC, Strecker WB, Schoenecker PL. Surgical treatment of displaced olecranon fractures in children. *J Pediatr Orthop.* 1997;17:321–324.
22. Gaston SR, Smith FM, Baab OD. Epiphyseal injuries of the radial head and neck. *Am J Surg.* 1953;85:266–276.
23. Gille P, Mourot M, Aubert F, et al. Fracture of the neck of the radius. *Rev Chir Orthop Reparatrice Appar Mot.* 1978;64:247–248.
24. Gortzak Y, Mercado E, Atar D, Weisel Y. Pediatric olecranon fractures: open reduction and internal fixation with removable Kirschner wires and absorbable sutures. *J Pediatr Orthop.* 2006;26:39–42.
25. Graves SC, Canale ST. Fractures of the olecranon in children: long-term follow-up. *J Pediatr Orthop.* 1993;13:239–241.
26. Greenspan A, Norman A, Rosen H. Radial head-capitellum view in elbow trauma: clinical application and radiographic-anatomic correlation. *AJR Am J Roentgenol.* 1984;143:355–359.
27. Hall-Craggs MA, Shorvon PJ, Chapman M. Assessment of the radial head-capitellum view and the dorsal fat-pad sign in acute elbow trauma. *AJR Am J Roentgenol.* 1985;145:607–609.
28. Holme TJ, Karbowiak M, Arnander M, Gelfer Y. Paediatric olecranon fractures: a systematic review. *EFORT Open Rev.* 2020;5(5):280–288.
29. Irshad F, Shaw NJ, Gregory RJ. Reliability of fat-pad sign in radial head/neck fractures of the elbow. *Injury.* 1997;28:433–435.
30. JudetH, Judet J. *Fractures et orthopédie de l'enfant. Indications et Techniques.* Maloine SA; 1974.
31. Kaufman B, Rinott MG, Tanzman M. Closed reduction of fractures of the proximal radius in children. *J Bone Joint Surg Br.* 1989;71:66–67.
32. Kim AE, Beatty EW, Bae D S. "Radial head stress fracture nonunion in adolescent overhead athletes: A Case Series: Original Research". *Journal of the Pediatric Orthopaedic Society of North America,* Vol. 4, No. 4, Nov. 2022, doi:10.55275/JPOSNA-2022-440.
33. Kim JY, Lee YH, Gong HS, et al. Use of Kirschner wires with eyelets for tension band wiring of olecranon fractures. *J Hand Surg Am.* 2013;38(9):1762–1767.
34. Klitscher D, Richter S, Bodenschatz K, et al. Evaluation of severely displaced radial neck fractures in children treated with elastic stable intramedullary nailing. *J Pediatr Orthop.* 2009;29(7):698–703.
35. Landin LA, Danielsson LG. Elbow fractures in children: an epidemiological analysis of 589 cases. *Acta Orthop Scand.* 1986;57:309–312.
36. Look N, Erickson M, Sibbel SE. Presentation and management of displaced lateral condylar mass fractures with ipsilateral displaced olecranon fractures in two pediatric cases. *Trauma Case Rep.* 2020;25:100278.
37. Mathews JG. Fractures of the olecranon in children. *Injury.* 1981;12:207–212.
38. McCarthy SM, Ogden JA. Radiology of postnatal skeletal development. VI. Elbow joint, proximal radius, and ulna. *Skeletal Radiol.* 1982;9:17–26.
39. Mellema JJ, Doornberg JN, Dyer GSM, Ring D. Distribution of coronoid fracture lines by specific patterns of traumatic elbow instability. *J Hand Surg Am.* 2014;39(10):2041–2046.
40. Merchan ECR. Percutaneous reduction of displaced radial neck fractures in children. *J Trauma.* 1994;37:812–814.
41. Montgomery RJ. A secure method of olecranon fixation: a modification of tension band wiring technique. *J R Coll Surg Edinb.* 1986;31:179–182.
42. Murphy DF, Greene WB, Gilbert JA, Dameron TB Jr. Displaced olecranon fractures in adults. Biomechanical analysis of fixation methods. *Clin Orthop Relat Res.* 1987;224:210–214.
43. Neher CG, Torch MA. New reduction technique for severely displaced pediatric radial neck fractures. *J Pediatr Orthop.* 2003;23:626–628.
44. Nenopoulos SP, Beslikas TA, Gigis JP. Long-term follow-up of combined fractures of proximal radius and ulna in childhood. *J Pediatr Orthop B.* 2009;18:252–260.
45. Newman JH. Displaced radial neck fractures in children. *Injury.* 1977;9:114–121.
46. O'Brien PI. Injuries involving the proximal radial epiphysis. *Clin Orthop Relat Res.* 1965;41:51–58.
47. Olney BW, Menelaus MB. Monteggia and equivalent lesions in childhood. *J Pediatr Orthop.* 1989;9:219–223.

48. Paci JM, Dugas JR, Guy JA, et al. Cannulated screw fixation of refractory olecranon stress fractures with and without associated injuries allows a return to baseball. *Am J Sports Med.* 2013;41(2):306–312.

49. Papavasiliou VA, Beslikas TA, Nenopoulos S. Isolated fractures of the olecranon in children. *Injury.* 1987;18:100–102.

50. Patterson RF. Treatment of displaced transverse fractures of the neck of the radius in children. *J Bone Joint Surg.* 1934;16:695–698.

51. Perkins CA, Busch MT, Christino MA, et al. Olecranon fractures in children and adolescents: outcomes based on fracture fixation. *J Child Orthop* 2018;12:497–501.

52. Persiani P, Ranaldi FM, Graci J, et al. Isolated olecranon fractures in children affected by osteogenesis imperfecta type I treated with single screw or tension band wiring system: outcomes and pitfalls in relation to bone mineral density. *Medicine (Baltimore).* 2017;96(20):e6766.

53. Pesudo JV, Aracil J, Barcelo M. Leverage method in displaced fractures of the radial neck in children. *Clin Orthop Relat Res.* 1982;169:215–218.

54. Prathapkumar KR, Garg NK, Bruce CE. Elastic stable intramedullary nail fixation for severely displaced fractures of the neck of the radius in children. *J Bone Joint Surg Br.* 2006;88(3):358–361.

55. Rath NK, Carpenter EC, Thomas DP. Traumatic pediatric olecranon injury: a report of suture fixation and review of the literature. *Pediatr Emerg Care.* 2011;27(12):1167–1169.

56. Regan W, Morrey BF. Classification and treatment of coronoid process fractures. *Orthopedics.* 1992;15:845–848.

57. Regan W, Morrey BF. Fractures of the coronoid process of the ulna. *J Bone Joint Surg Am.* 1989;71:1348–1354.

58. Roe SC. Tension band wiring of olecranon fractures: a modification of the AO technique. *Clin Orthop Relat Res.* 1994;308:284–286.

59. Schmittenbecher PP, Haevernick B, Herold A, et al. Treatment decision, method of osteosynthesis, and outcome in radial neck fractures in children: a multicenter study. *J Pediatr Orthop.* 2005;25(1):45–50.

60. Smith AM, Morrey BF, Steinmann SP. Low profile fixation of radial head and neck fractures: surgical technique and clinical experience. *J Orthop Trauma.* 2007;21(10):718–724.

61. Smith GR, Hotchkiss RN. Radial head and neck fractures: anatomic guidelines for proper placement of internal fixation. *J Shoulder Elbow Surg.* 1996;5(2 Pt 1):113–117.

62. Song KS, Kim BS, Lee SW. Percutaneous leverage reduction for severely displaced radial neck fractures in children. *J Pediatr Orthop.* 2015;35(4):e26–e30.

63. Soyer AD, Nowotarski PJ, Kelso TB, Mighell MA. Optimal position for plate fixation of complex fractures of the proximal radius: a cadaver study. *J Orthop Trauma.* 1998;12(4):291–293.

64. Steele JA, Graham HK. Angulated radial neck fractures in children: a prospective study of percutaneous reduction. *J Bone Joint Surg Br.* 1992;74:760–764.

65. Steinberg EL, Golomb D, Salama R, Wientroub S. Radial head and neck fractures in children. *J Pediatr Orthop.* 1988;8:35–40.

66. Su Y, Xie Y, Qin J, et al. Internal fixation with absorbable rods for the treatment of displaced radial neck fractures in children. *J Pediatr Orthop.* 2016;36(8):797–802.

67. Tan BHM, Mahadev A. Radial neck fractures in children. *J Orthop Surg (Hong Kong).* 2011;19:209–212.

68. Torg JS, Moyer R. Non-union of a stress fracture through the olecranon epiphyseal plate observed in an adolescent baseball pitcher. A case report. *J Bone Joint Surg Am.* 1977;59:264–265.

69. Tullos HS, King JW. Lesions of the pitching arm in adolescents. *JAMA.* 1972;220:264–271.

70. Turtel AH, Andrews JR, Schob CJ, et al. Fractures of unfused olecranon physis: a re-evaluation of this injury in three athletes. *Orthopedics.* 1995;18:390–394.

71. Ugutmen E, Ozkan K, Ozkan FU, et al. Reduction and fixation of radius neck fractures in children with intramedullary pin. *J Pediatr Orthop B.* 2010;19(4):289–293.

72. Vahvanen V, Gripenberg L. Fracture of the radial neck in children. A long-term follow-up study of 43 cases. *Acta Orthop Scand.* 1978;49:32–38.

73. Van Zeeland NL, Bae DS, Goldfarb CA. Intra-articular radial head fracture in the skeletally immature patient: progressive radial head subluxation and rapid radiocapitellar degeneration. *J Pediatr Orthop.* 2011;31:124–129.

74. Vocke AK, Von Laer L. Displaced fractures of the radial neck in children: long-term results and prognosis of conservative treatment. *J Pediatr Orthop B.* 1998;7:217–222.

75. Wang J, Chen W, Guo M, et al. Percutaneous reduction and intramedullary fixation technique for displaced pediatric radial neck fractures. *J Pediatr Orthop B.* 2013;22(2):127–132.

76. Waters PM, Beaty J, Kasser J. Elbow "TRASH" (the radiographic appearance seemed harmless) lesions. *J Pediatr Orthop.* 2010;30:S77–S81.

77. Wedge JH. Displaced fractures of the neck of the radius. *J Bone Joint Surg Br.* 1982;64:256.

78. Zhang FY, Wang XD, Zhen YF, et al. Treatment of severely displaced radial neck fractures in children with percutaneous K-wire leverage and closed intramedullary pinning. *Medicine (Baltimore).* 2016;95(1):e2346.

79. Zimmerman RM, Kalish LA, Hresko MT, et al. Surgical management of pediatric radial neck fractures. *J Bone Joint Surg Am.* 2013;95(20):1825–1832.

12

Monteggia Fracture-Dislocation in Children

Peter M. Waters and Kenneth J. Noonan

INTRODUCTION TO MONTEGGIA FRACTURE-DISLOCATIONS

Monteggia fracture-dislocations are a rare but complex injury usually involving a fracture of the ulna associated with proximal radioulnar joint dissociation and radiocapitellar dislocation. These injuries comprise less than 1% of all pediatric forearm fractures and typically affect patients between 4 and 10 years of age.[65,133] Unfortunately, this rare injury can have very serious consequences if not treated appropriately. The annual incidence of Monteggia fracture-dislocations in children is less than 1 in 100,000.[65] In 1814, Giovanni Battista Monteggia, a surgical pathologist and public health official in Milan, Italy, first described a variation of the injury that now bears his name as "a traumatic lesion distinguished by a fracture of the proximal third of the ulna and an anterior dislocation of the proximal epiphysis of the radius."[82,102] In 1967, José Luis Bado, while director of National Institute of Orthopaedics and Traumatology in Montevideo, Uruguay, published his classic monograph on the classification of Monteggia lesions.[8,10] He described a Monteggia lesion as a radial head fracture or dislocation in association with a fracture of the middle or proximal ulna. Over the last century, numerous authors have made significant contributions to pathoanatomy, classification, diagnosis, treatment, and complications.[7,20,26,28,30,31,45,54,58,71,79,80,90,104,107]

Despite the increased understanding of Monteggia lesions, the injury continues to represent a challenge for the orthopaedic surgeon. In 1943, Sir Watson-Jones wrote that "no fracture presents so many problems; no injury is beset with greater difficulty; no treatment is characterized by more general failure."[135] Even when fully diagnosed and treated appropriately, patients can still have compromised outcomes as a result of compartment syndrome, elbow stiffness, decreased forearm rotation, and even proximal radial and ulnar synostosis. Unfortunately, despite the increased awareness and understanding of the problematic nature of Monteggia lesions, full diagnosis of the entire injury is still missed by qualified radiologists, emergency department physicians, and orthopaedic surgeons among others.[17,34,35,49,107,109,128,138] In addition, less than optimal treatment of recognized but unstable injuries has also resulted in chronic Monteggia lesions.[28,31,46,51,58,104,106,107,137] A chronic Monteggia lesion is classically characterized by late diagnosis of a displaced radial head, can result in substantial morbidity, and is far more complex in terms of surgical decision making and management than treatment of an acute injury.[17,27,35,49,55,109,113]

ASSESSMENT OF MONTEGGIA FRACTURE-DISLOCATIONS

CLASSIFICATION OF MONTEGGIA FRACTURE-DISLOCATIONS

Bado Classification

Bado's original classification[8,10] has stood the test of time with minimal modifications except for the addition of various equivalent lesions (Fig. 12-1). The classification system is based on the direction of the radial head dislocation and the apex of the associated ulna fracture. Bado's[8,10] four true Monteggia types are as follows:

Bado Type I

A Bado type I lesion is an anterior dislocation of the radial head associated with an apex anterior ulnar diaphyseal fracture at any level. This is the most common Monteggia lesion in children and represents approximately 70% to 75% of all injuries.[31,43,107,133]

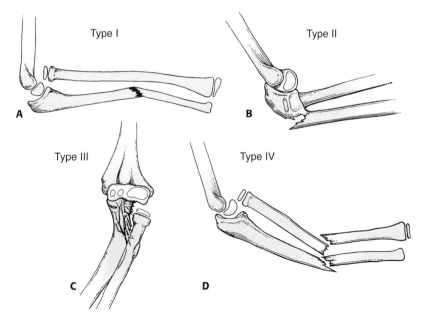

Figure 12-1. Bado classification. **A:** Type I (anterior dislocation): The radial head is dislocated anteriorly and the ulna has a short oblique or greenstick fracture in the diaphyseal or proximal metaphyseal area. **B:** Type II (posterior dislocation): The radial head is posteriorly or posterolaterally dislocated; the ulna is usually fractured in the metaphysis in children. **C:** Type III (lateral dislocation): There is lateral dislocation of the radial head with a greenstick metaphyseal fracture of the ulna. **D:** Type IV (anterior dislocation with radial shaft fracture): The pattern of injury is the same as with a type I injury, with the inclusion of a radial shaft fracture distal to the level of the ulnar fracture.

Figure 12-2. Type I equivalents. **A:** Isolated anterior radial head dislocation. **B:** Ulnar fracture with fracture of the radial neck. **C:** Isolated radial neck fractures. **D:** Elbow (ulnohumeral) dislocation with or without fracture of the proximal radius.

Bado Type II

A Bado type II lesion is a posterior or posterolateral dislocation of the radial head associated with an apex posterior ulnar diaphyseal or metaphyseal fracture. This pattern is the most common Monteggia lesion in adults but is relatively rare in children.[95,107] Type II lesions account for 6% of Monteggia lesions in children[65] and are usually found in older patients[95] who have sustained significant trauma.[33,104]

Bado Type III

A Bado type III lesion is a lateral dislocation of the radial head associated with a varus (apex lateral) fracture of the proximal ulna. This is the second most common pediatric Monteggia lesion.[89] When an injury is characterized by an olecranon fracture and a lateral or anterolateral radiocapitellar dislocation but no radioulnar dissociation, the injury is not a true Monteggia lesion.[52,106]

Bado Type IV

A Bado type IV lesion is an anterior dislocation of the radial head associated with fractures of both the ulna and the radius. The original description was of a radial fracture at the same level or distal to the ulna fracture. Type IV lesions are relatively rare in children.

EXPANSION OF THE BADO CLASSIFICATION: MONTEGGIA-EQUIVALENT LESIONS

Bado[8,10] classified certain injuries as equivalents to true Monteggia lesions because of their similar mechanisms of injury, radiographic appearance, or treatment methods. Since his original publication, the list of equivalent lesions has expanded case report by case report.

Type I Equivalent Fractures

Bado type I equivalents (Fig. 12-2) include isolated anterior dislocations of the radial head without ulnar fracture. This subclassification includes a "pulled elbow" or "nursemaid's elbow" because the mechanism of longitudinal traction, pronation, and hyperextension is similar to a true type I lesion. In nursemaid's elbow cases, the radiographs are normal. It is debatable if a "nursemaid's elbow" is really a part of the Monteggia spectrum but we will include it in this chapter for completeness. In type I equivalent lesions, the radial head is malaligned in its relationship to the capitellum and proximal ulna. However, the ulnar bow sign (Fig. 12-3) is normal as opposed to subtle plastic deformation of the ulna, which will have a concave ulnar bow and can be misdiagnosed as a type I equivalent when the injury is really a true Bado I lesion with plastic deformation fracture of the ulna. This distinction can be critical in terms of operative decision making in that the type I equivalent lesion requires an open reduction or repair of the displaced annular ligament while the Bado type I lesion with plastic deformation requires correction of the ulnar deformity with or without open reduction or repair of annular ligament depending on timing of intervention. Other type I equivalents (see Fig. 12-2) include (1) anterior dislocation of the radial head with ulnar metaphyseal or diaphyseal fracture and radial neck fracture; (2) anterior dislocation of the radial head with radial diaphyseal fracture more proximal to ulnar diaphyseal fracture; (3) anterior radial head dislocation with ulnotrochlear dislocation (Fig. 12-4)[107]; and (4) anterior dislocation of the radial head with a segmental ulna fracture.[2,43,97,112] More case reports will probably expand this subclassification over time. The type I equivalents have been shown to have poorer outcomes and require more frequent operative intervention than true Monteggia lesions.[43,89] Poor outcomes may relate to intra-articular injury, coronoid fracture, comminution of the ulna fracture, and comminution of the radial head fracture.[114]

Type II Equivalents

Bado[8,10] described type II equivalents to include posterior radial head dislocations associated with fractures of the proximal radial epiphysis or radial neck.

Type III and Type IV Equivalents

Bado[8,10] did not have equivalent lesions for the true type III and type IV lesions. Because mechanism of injury allows for this subclassification, case reports have emerged over time to include fractures of the distal humerus (supracondylar, lateral condylar) in association with proximal forearm fractures (Fig. 12-5).[5,15,16,29,37,43,44,78,86,97,103,108,112,116]

Figure 12-3. The ulnar bow line. This line, drawn between the distal ulna and the olecranon, defines the ulnar bow. The ulnar bow sign is a deviation of the ulnar border from the reference line by more than 1 mm.

Figure 12-4. Type I equivalent that includes elbow subluxation in addition to the radioulnar dislocation.

Monteggia equivalents

Type III equivalent   Type IV equivalent

Figure 12-5. Type III equivalent described by Ravessoud.[103] An oblique fracture of the ulna with varus alignment and a displaced lateral condylar fracture. Type IV equivalent described by Arazi[5]: fractures of the distal humerus, ulnar diaphysis, and radial neck.

Letts Classification

Letts et al.[69] have described an alternate classification schedule for pediatric Monteggia fracture-dislocations based both on direction of radial head dislocation and the type of ulnar fracture (Fig. 12-6). Letts types A, B, and C are analogous to Bado type I lesion with subclassifications as they are characterized by

anterior dislocation of the radial head with an associated ulnar fracture. In a type A lesion, there is plastic deformation of the ulna; in a type B lesion, there is an incomplete or greenstick ulnar fracture; and in a type C lesion, there is a complete ulnar fracture. The A, B, and C aspects of the Letts classification are useful for aiding in treatment decisions (see Ring, Jupiter, and Waters classification). Letts type D lesions are equivalent to

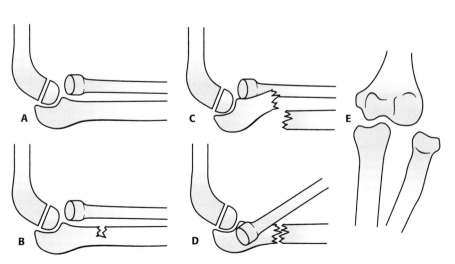

Figure 12-6. Pediatric Monteggia fracture-dislocation classification by Letts et al.[69] **A:** Anterior dislocation of the radial head with plastic deformation of the ulna. **B:** Anterior dislocation of the radial head with greenstick fracture of the ulna. **C:** Anterior dislocation of the radial head with complete fracture of the ulna. **D:** Posterior dislocation of the radial head with fracture of the ulnar metaphysis. **E:** Lateral dislocation of the radial head and metaphyseal greenstick fracture of the ulna.

Bado type II injuries and are characterized by posterior radial head dislocation. Letts type E lesions are equivalent to Bado type III injuries and are characterized by lateral radial head dislocation.

Authors' Preferred Classification

Monteggia Fracture-Dislocations: AUTHORS' PREFERRED CLASSIFICATION

Type	Radial Head Dislocation	Associated Fractures
True Lesions		
I	Anterior	Ulna metaphysis-diaphysis
II	Posterior	Ulna metaphysis-diaphysis
III	Lateral	Ulna metaphysis
IV	Anterior	Radial diaphysis, ulnar diaphysis
Hybrid lesion	Anterior, posterior, or lateral	Ulna metaphysis or olecranon

Type	Description
Equivalent Lesions	
I	Isolated dislocation of radial head
	Radial neck fracture (isolated)
	Radial neck fracture in combination with a fracture of the ulnar diaphysis
	Radial and ulnar fractures with the radial fracture above the junction of the middle and proximal thirds
	Fracture of ulnar diaphysis with anterior dislocation of radial head and an olecranon fracture
II	Posterior dislocation of the elbow
III	Ulnar fracture with displaced fracture of the lateral condyle
IV	None described

Ring, Jupiter, and Waters[106,107] defined a Monteggia lesion as a proximal radioulnar joint dislocation in association with a forearm fracture. In this classification system, it is the character of the ulnar fracture, more so than the direction of the radial head dislocation, that is most useful in determining the optimal treatment of Monteggia fracture-dislocations in both adults and children. Stable anatomic reduction of the ulnar fracture almost always results in anatomic, stable reduction of the radial head, proximal radioulnar joint, and radiocapitellar joint in the acute setting. The ulnar fracture is defined similarly to all pediatric forearm fractures: plastic deformation, incomplete or greenstick fractures, and complete fractures. Complete fractures are further subdivided into transverse, short oblique, long oblique, and comminuted fractures. Treatment directly relates to the fracture type: closed reduction for plastic deformation and greenstick fractures; intramedullary fixation for transverse and short oblique fractures; and open reduction and internal

fixation with plate and screws for long oblique and comminuted fractures. This fracture classification guides the surgeon to proper treatment that restores ulnar length and stability, which almost always results in a stable reduction of the radial head if treated acutely.

MECHANISMS OF INJURY FOR MONTEGGIA FRACTURE-DISLOCATIONS

Understanding mechanisms of injuries for each fracture-dislocation type provides knowledge on how the mechanical forces of injury at various ages impact normal anatomy and create the expected pathoanatomy of each Monteggia fracture-dislocation. We use this knowledge to "reverse engineer" the fracture and dislocation reduction maneuvers and stabilization techniques. This is especially true for closed reduction techniques.

Type I Mechanism of Injury

Three separate mechanisms of type I lesions have been described: direct trauma, hyperpronation, and hyperextension.[10,104,128]

Direct Blow Theory

The first theory proposed in English literature was the direct blow mechanism described by Speed and Boyd[118] and endorsed by Smith (Fig. 12-7). This theory was actually proposed by Monteggia,[82] who noted that the fracture occurs when a direct blow on the posterior aspect of the forearm first produces a fracture through the ulna. Then, either by continued deformation or direct pressure, the radial head is forced anteriorly with respect to the capitellum, causing the radial head to dislocate. Monteggia[82] explained that these injuries sometimes resulted from a blow by a "staff or cudgel" on the forearm raised to protect the head.

The "parry fracture," another term for the Monteggia fracture-dislocation, has been mentioned in the literature. During the American Civil War, Monteggia fractures were frequent because of direct blows on the forearm received while attempting to parry the butt of a rifle during hand-to-hand combat. The major

Figure 12-7. Mechanism of injury for type I Monteggia lesions: direct blow theory. The fracture-dislocation is sustained by direct contact on the posterior aspect of the forearm, either by falling onto an object or by an object striking the forearm. The continued motion of the object forward dislocates the radial head after fracturing the ulna.

Figure 12-8. Mechanism of injury for type I Monteggia lesions: hyperpronation theory.[34] Rotation of the body externally forces the forearm into pronation. The ulnar shaft fractures with further rotation, forcibly dislocating the radial head.

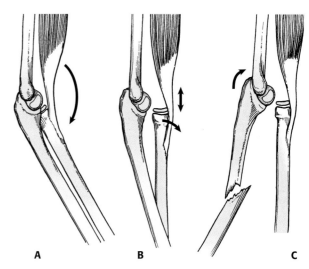

Figure 12-9. Mechanism of injury for type I Monteggia lesions: hyperextension theory.[128] **A:** Forward momentum caused by a fall on an outstretched hand forces the elbow into hyperextension. **B:** The biceps contracts, forcibly dislocating the radial head. **C:** Continued forward momentum causes the ulna to fracture because of tension on the anterior surface.

argument against this theory as the mechanism is that in the usual clinical situation, there rarely is evidence of a direct blow to the posterior aspect of the forearm, such as a contusion or laceration.[34,128]

Hyperpronation Theory

In 1949, Evans[34] published his observations regarding anterior Monteggia fracture-dislocations. Previous investigators had based their direct blow theory on hypothesis and clinical observation, but Evans used cadaveric investigation to support his hyperpronation theory. He demonstrated that hyperpronation of the forearm produced a fracture of the ulna with a subsequent dislocation of the radial head. He postulated that during a fall, the outstretched hand, initially in pronation, is forced into further pronation as the body twists above the planted hand and forearm (Fig. 12-8). This hyperpronation forcibly rotates the radius over the middle of the ulna, resulting in either anterior dislocation of the radial head or fracture of the proximal third of the radius, along with fracture of the ulna. In actual patients reported on by Evans, the ulnar fractures demonstrated a pattern consistent with anterior tension and shear or longitudinal compression. His cadaveric investigation, however, showed the ulnar fracture pattern to be consistent with a spiral or rotational force. The hyperpronation theory was also supported by Bado.[9]

Two arguments have been used to dispute the hyperpronation mechanism.[128] First, the ulnar fracture rarely presents clinically in a spiral pattern; it is often oblique, indicating an initial force in tension with propagation in shear rather than rotational. Second, the Evans experiments, which were performed

on totally dissected forearms,[34] did not take into consideration the dynamic muscle forces at play during a fall on an outstretched hand.

Hyperextension Theory

In 1971, Tompkins[128] analyzed both theories and presented good clinical evidence that type I Monteggia fracture-dislocations were caused by a combination of dynamic and static forces. His study postulated three steps in the fracture mechanism: hyperextension, radial head dislocation, and ulnar fracture (Fig. 12-9). The patient falls on an outstretched arm with forward momentum, forcing the elbow joint into hyperextension. The radius is first dislocated anteriorly by the violent reflexive contracture of the biceps, forcing the radius away from the capitellum. Once the proximal radius dislocates, the weight of the body is transferred to the ulna. Because the radius is usually the main load-bearing bone in the forearm, the ulna cannot handle the transmitted longitudinal force and, subsequently, fails in tension. This tension force produces an oblique fracture line or a greenstick fracture in the ulnar diaphysis or at the diaphyseal–metaphyseal junction. In addition to the momentum of the injury, the anterior angulation of the ulna results from the pull of the intact interosseous membrane on the distal fragment, causing it to follow the radius. The brachialis muscle causes the proximal ulnar fragment to flex.

Summary of Type I Mechanism of Injury

The type I lesion can probably be caused by any of the three proposed mechanisms, but the most common mechanism is a fall on an outstretched hand that forces the elbow into complete extension, locking the olecranon into the humerus. The forearm is in a rotational position of neutral to midpronation. As the proximal ulna locks into the distal humerus, the bending force stresses the proximal radioulnar joint. Because of the relatively pronated position of the joint, the ligamentous restraints are lax, providing only tenuous stability for the radial head. The anterior bending force, combined with a reflexive contraction of the biceps, violently dislocates the radial head anteriorly. The radioulnar joint and its ligamentous complex are at risk because of the ligamentous laxity and the decreased contact area between the proximal radius and ulna created by the rotation of the forearm. At midrotation, the short axis of the elliptical radial head is perpendicular to the ulna, causing the annular ligament and the dense anterior portion of the quadrate ligament to be relaxed. The contact area of the proximal radioulnar joint, because of the shape of the radial head, is also decreased, further reducing the stability of the joint. The ulna, now the main weight-bearing structure of the forearm, is loaded by a continued bending moment, causing tension on the anterior cortex and producing failure. The force at the site of failure is propagated in shear at approximately 45 degrees to the long axis of the ulna. This mechanism may produce plastic deformation with an anterior bow, a greenstick fracture, or an oblique fracture pattern, all of which are observed clinically. As the anterior bending movement continues, the vector of the biceps changes and acts as a tether and resists any further advance of the proximal radius. The distal fragment of the ulna continues to advance, acting as a fulcrum against the radial shaft. The anteriorly directed force of the distal ulnar fragment, combined with the retrograde resistance of the biceps, may create a fracture of the radius, or a type IV lesion.

Type II Mechanism of Injury

The cause of the type II Monteggia lesion is subject to debate. Bado[10] thought the lesion was caused by direct force and sudden supination. Penrose[96] analyzed seven fractures in adults and noted that a proximal ulnar fracture was the typical pattern. He postulated that the injury occurred by longitudinal loading rather than by direct trauma.[118] Olney and Menelaus[89] reported four type II lesions in their series of pediatric Monteggia fractures. Three of these patients had proximal ulnar fractures and one had an oblique midshaft fracture, suggesting two different mechanisms of injury.

The mechanism proposed and experimentally demonstrated by Penrose[96] was that type II lesions occur when the forearm is suddenly loaded in a longitudinal direction with the elbow in approximately 60 degrees of flexion. This investigation demonstrated that a type II lesion occurred consistently if the ulna fractured; otherwise, a posterior elbow dislocation was produced (Fig. 12-10). The difference in bone strength of the ulna, including its periosteum in the young, may explain the reason for the high incidence of type II Monteggia lesions in older adults and their rarity in children. Penrose[96] further noted that the rotational position of the forearm did not seem to affect the type of fracture produced.

Haddad et al.[47] described type II injuries caused by low-velocity injuries in six adults, five of whom were on long-term corticosteroid therapy. They suggested that this supports the

Figure 12-10. Mechanism of injury for type II Monteggia lesions. **A:** With the elbow flexed approximately 60 degrees, a longitudinal force is applied parallel to the long axis of the forearm. **B:** This force may result in a posterior elbow dislocation. **C:** If the integrity of the anterior cortex of the ulna is compromised, a type II fracture-dislocation occurs.

theory that the type II Monteggia injury is a variant of posterior elbow dislocation, in that it occurs when the ulna is weaker than the ligaments surrounding the elbow joint, resulting in an ulnar fracture before the ligament disruption required for dislocation. In essence, a fragility fracture.

Type III Mechanism of Injury

Wright[138] studied fractures of the proximal ulna with lateral and anterolateral dislocations of the radial head and concluded that the mechanism of injury was varus stress at the level of the elbow, in combination with an outstretched hand planted firmly against a fixed surface (Fig. 12-11). This usually produces a greenstick ulnar fracture with tension failure radially and compression medially. The radial head dislocates laterally, rupturing or displacing the annular ligament. Hume[52] suggested that type III lesions may be the result of hyperextension of the elbow combined with pronation of the forearm. Other

Figure 12-11. Mechanism of injury for type III Monteggia lesions. A forced varus stress causes a greenstick fracture of the proximal ulna and a true lateral or anterolateral radial head dislocation.

authors confirmed the mechanism of varus force at the elbow as the cause of type III injuries.[10,31,84] The direction of the radial head dislocation is probably determined by the rotational and angular force applied simultaneously to the varus moment at the elbow.[84]

Type IV Mechanism of Injury

Bado[8] proposed that a type IV lesion is caused by hyperpronation. Of the case reports discussing the mechanism of injury, both hyperpronation[40] and a direct blow[108] have been postulated. Olney and Menelaus[89] reported a single type IV lesion in their series but did not discuss the mechanism. Type IV lesions appear to be caused by the mechanism described for type I lesions.

INJURIES ASSOCIATED WITH MONTEGGIA FRACTURE-DISLOCATIONS

Monteggia lesions have been associated with fractures of the wrist and the distal forearm,[10] including distal radial and ulnar metaphyseal and diaphyseal fractures.[10,53,55,108] Galeazzi fractures may also occur with Monteggia lesions.[10,24,68] Radial head and neck fractures are commonly associated with type II fractures[10,65] but may occur with other types.[1,41,122] With a type II lesion, the radial head fracture is usually at the anterior rim.[33,95] Strong et al.[121] reported two type I equivalent lesions consisting of a fractured radial neck and midshaft ulnar fracture. This injury pattern is notable because of significant medial displacement of the distal radial fragment. Obtaining and maintaining reduction of the radius proved difficult with a closed technique.

Fractures of the distal humerus lateral condyle have also been associated with Monteggia fractures.[25] Ravessoud[103] reported an ipsilateral ulnar shaft lesion and a lateral condylar fracture without loss of the radiocapitellar relation, suggesting a type II equivalent (see Fig. 12-5). Kloen et al.[60] reported a bilateral Monteggia fracture-dislocation and described the operative technique for its treatment. Despite surgical and rehabilitative challenges, excellent results were obtained in both elbows. In essence, any fracture about the elbow and

forearm should be inspected for an associated Monteggia lesion. One should keep in mind the patterns of injury described above in order to avoid missing injuries as a result of "satisfaction of search." A valgus force applied to the elbow can result in a radial neck fracture, olecranon fracture, a medial epicondyle fracture, or even all three.

SIGNS AND SYMPTOMS OF MONTEGGIA FRACTURE-DISLOCATIONS

Type I Clinical Findings

Bado,[8,10] in his original description, provided an accurate clinical picture of Monteggia fracture-dislocations. In general, there is fusiform swelling about the elbow. The child has significant pain and has limitations in elbow flexion and extension as well as forearm pronation and supination. Usually, an angular change in the forearm itself is evident, with the apex shifted anteriorly and mild valgus apparent. There may be tenting of the skin or an area of ecchymosis on the volar aspect of the forearm. It is imperative to check for an open fracture wound. With displaced fracture dislocations, the child may not be able to extend the fingers at the metacarpophalangeal joints or retropulse the thumb secondary to a posterior interosseous nerve (PIN) branch of the radial nerve palsy. Later, as the swelling subsides, anterior fullness may remain palpable in the cubital fossa for the typical type I lesion radial head dislocation. However, this finding may be subtle because children will usually have an elbow flexion posture following injury. If the injury is seen late, there will be a loss of full flexion at the elbow and a palpable anterior dislocation of the radial head. The radial head–distal humerus impingement that occurs may be a source of pain with activities for a child with a chronic type I Monteggia fracture dislocation and a healed ulna fracture malunion. There can also be loss of forearm rotation with late presentation, although surprisingly children with chronic Monteggia lesions can remain relatively asymptomatic for a long time. Progressive valgus may occur if the anterior radial head dislocation worsens. With plastic deformation injuries, the clinical findings may be even more subtle, leading to late presentation or difficult radiographic diagnosis.

Type II Clinical Findings

Similar to type I lesions, the elbow region is swollen but exhibits posterior angulation of the proximal forearm and a marked prominence in the area posterolateral to the normal location of the radial head. The entire upper extremity should be examined because of the frequency of associated injuries.[63,95]

Type III Clinical Findings

Lateral swelling, varus deformity of the elbow, and significant limitation of motion (especially supination) are the hallmarks of type III Monteggia fracture-dislocations. Again, these signs can be subtle and missed by harried clinicians. Injuries to the radial nerve, particularly the posterior interosseous branch, occur more frequently with type III lesions than other Monteggia fracture-dislocations.[107]

Figure 12-12. Two examples of a Bado type I Monteggia fracture with anterior dislocation of the radial head. **A:** Proximal ulna fracture in the metadiaphyseal region. **B:** Midshaft diaphyseal ulna fracture. Note the disruption of the radiocapitellar line in both.

Type IV Clinical Findings

The appearance of the limb with a type IV lesion is similar to that of a type I lesion. However, more swelling and pain can be present because of the magnitude of force required to create this complex injury. Particular attention should be given to the neurovascular status of the limb, anticipating the possible increased risk for a compartment syndrome.

Clinical Findings in Monteggia Equivalents and Associated Injuries

In a Monteggia-equivalent injury, clinical findings are similar to those for the corresponding Bado lesion, with the common triad of pain, swelling, and deformity. Given the frequency of associated skeletal injuries, a careful examination of the entire upper extremity should be performed. This involves careful inspection of the skin and palpation of the distal humerus lateral condyle, the distal radius, and the distal radioulnar joint. Given the high frequency of radial nerve injuries with Monteggia fracture-dislocations,[13,107] a careful examination of neurologic examination should be performed. Because the posterior interosseous branch is most commonly injured, the clinician should routinely examine motor function of the extensor digitorum communis and the extensor pollicis longus. Failure to extend the fingers at the metacarpophalangeal joints or retropulse the thumb is indicative of a PIN palsy.

IMAGING AND OTHER DIAGNOSTIC STUDIES FOR MONTEGGIA FRACTURE-DISLOCATIONS

The standard evaluation of a Monteggia fracture-dislocation includes anteroposterior (AP) and lateral radiographs of the forearm and elbow. Any disruption of the ulna, including subtle changes in ulnar bowing, should alert the clinician to look for disruption of the proximal radioulnar joint.[26,56,58,71] Unfortunately, the dislocated radial head is all too often missed in the acute setting. It must be stressed that every forearm and elbow injury requires close scrutiny of the radial head–capitellar relationship. In cases where plain radiographs are concerning but equivocal, fluoroscopic imaging or cross-sectional imaging such as magnetic resonance imaging (MRI) in the young, computed tomography (CT) in older patients, or ultrasound scan in the hands of skilled technicians should be strongly considered. The goal for every radiologist, orthopaedist, and emergency department physician should be to never miss a Monteggia lesion in the acute setting.

Type I Radiographic Evaluation

The radiographic alignment of the radial head and capitellum is particularly important and is best defined by a true lateral view of the elbow (Fig. 12-12). In a type I Monteggia fracture-dislocation, the radiocapitellar relationship may appear normal or difficult to interpret on an AP radiograph despite

Figure 12-13. Radiocapitellar line. A composite drawing with the elbow in various degrees of flexion. A line drawn down the long axis of the radius bisects the capitellum of the humerus regardless of the degree of flexion or extension of the elbow.

obvious disruption on the lateral view. If there is any doubt regarding the radiocapitellar alignment, further radiographic evaluation must be obtained. A line drawn through the center of the radial neck and head should extend directly through the center of the capitellum. This alignment should remain intact regardless of the degree of flexion or extension of the elbow (Fig. 12-13). In some instances, there is disruption of the radiocapitellar line in a normal elbow. Miles and Finlay[81] pointed out that the radiocapitellar line passes through the center of the capitellum only on a true lateral projection. They reported five patients in whom the elbow was clinically normal but the radiocapitellar line appeared disrupted. In analyzing the radiographs, they found that the radiographic projection of the elbow was usually an oblique view or that the forearm was pronated in the radiograph. If this disruption appears on radiographs in a child with an acute injury, however, it is the treating surgeon's responsibility to ensure that it is an insignificant finding. This means further imaging until there is clarity of diagnosis.

It is still too frequent an occurrence that a highly qualified, distraught, orthopaedic surgeon will call for referral of a chronic Monteggia lesion that was missed acutely (Fig. 12-14). With late presentation of a chronic Monteggia injury, an MRI scan may be useful to determine the feasibility of a congruent radial head–capitellar reduction. If the radial head is no longer centrally concave or the capitellum is no longer symmetrically convex, surgical reduction may fail, with recurrent subluxation, persistent pain, and limited motion.

Type II Radiographic Evaluation

Standard AP and lateral radiographs of the forearm demonstrate the pertinent features for classifying type II Monteggia fracture-dislocations. The typical findings include a proximal metaphyseal fracture of the ulna, with possible extension into the olecranon (Fig. 12-15).[89,126] Oblique diaphyseal ulnar fractures can also result in a type II Monteggia lesion.[8,89] The radial head is dislocated posteriorly or posterolaterally[10] and should be carefully examined for other injuries. Accompanying fractures of the anterior margin of the radial head have been noted.[33,95] Initially, these rim fractures are subtle in children as they may be mostly cartilaginous with small bony fragment (see the radiographic appearance seemed harmless [TRASH] lesions) but can lead to progressive subluxation and make late reconstruction difficult. Cross-sectional imaging, such as an MRI or ultrasound scan, should be obtained if further characterization of the injury pattern is deemed warranted. Accurate diagnosis acutely is important.

Type III Radiographic Evaluation

In type III lesions, the radial head is displaced laterally or anterolaterally,[94] which is best visualized on the AP radiograph (Fig. 12-16). The ulnar fracture often is in the metaphyseal region,[10,57,107,138] but it can also occur more distally.[10,38] Varus deformity is common to all ulna fractures, regardless of the level. Radiographs of the entire forearm should be obtained because of the association of distal radial and ulnar fractures with this complex elbow injury.[126] As with all Monteggia injuries, the acute lesion can be missed if proper radiographs are not obtained and careful evaluation of the studies is not performed. Again, if in doubt, pursue further imaging acutely for accurate diagnosis.

Type IV Radiographic Evaluation

In a type IV Monteggia fracture-dislocation, the anterior radial head dislocation is similar to a type I lesion (Fig. 12-17). The radial and ulnar fractures generally are in the middle third of the shaft, with the radial fracture typically distal to the ulnar fracture. The fractures may be incomplete or complete. Although this injury pattern is uncommon in adults and rare in children, the radiocapitellar joint should always be examined in all midshaft forearm fractures to avoid missing the proximal radioulnar joint disruption (Fig. 12-18). Failure to recognize the radial head dislocation is the major complication of this fracture.[12]

Radiographic Evaluation of Monteggia Equivalents

As with the true Bado types, careful radiographic study should be made with at least two orthogonal views of the elbow in addition to standard views of the forearm. This is especially helpful for adequate views of both proximal forearm and distal humerus in the acute setting due to fracture deformity and patient and technician's restricted ability to ideally position the limb due to pain. Special views such as obliques should be obtained to clearly delineate the associated injuries (e.g., radial head or neck fracture, distal humerus lateral condyle fracture) and allow adequate pretreatment planning. Cross-sectional imaging, such as

Figure 12-14. A: Acute injury with anterior dislocation radial head on lateral view with reverse bow sign ulna. **B:** Lateral view of attempted closed reduction reveals persistent anterior dislocation radial head. The elbow joint was opened through a posterolateral incision and the entrapped annular ligament was extracted, reduced, and repaired over the radial neck. In the OR, closed reduction of plastic deformation ulna was not successful in reducing the radial head. **C:** Wire localization of planned olecranon osteotomy. **D:** Opening wedge acute osteotomy and internal fixation with intramedullary smooth K-wire. **E:** Healed osteotomy, radial head anatomically reduced to capitellum. Wire was removed.

an MRI, CT, or ultrasound scan, should be obtained as needed if further characterization of the injury is required.

Radiographic Determination of *Traumatic* Versus *Congenital* Dislocation

Distinguishing between chronic traumatic (see Fig. 12-14) and congenital radial head dislocations (Fig. 12-19) can be challenging. When radiocapitellar alignment is disrupted radiographically, evaluation of the shape of the radial head and capitellum can help determine the cause of the disruption, especially if there is no history of trauma or the significance of the trauma

is questioned. The presence of a hypoplastic capitellum and a convex deformed, dislocated radial head suggests a congenital etiology (see Fig. 12-19). True congenital radial head dislocations are usually (but not always) posterior, may be bilateral, and can be associated with various syndromes such as Ehlers–Danlos and nail–patella.[3,71] To avoid missing the diagnosis of an acute Monteggia fracture-dislocation, all anterior radial head dislocations should be at least suspected of having a traumatic origin.[3,73] MRI imaging can be very helpful when uncertain to avoid operating on a congenital dislocation that you misdiagnosis as posttraumatic and missing a traumatic dislocation that you interpret as congenital.

Figure 12-15. Bado type II lesion, with posterolateral dislocation of the radial head (**A**) with apex posterior ulna fracture (**B**).

OUTCOME MEASURES FOR MONTEGGIA FRACTURE-DISLOCATIONS

To assess recovery and patient outcome following closed or open treatment of Monteggia lesions, the clinician should carefully measure union rate, time to union, pain, patient satisfaction, elbow flexion and extension, and forearm rotation. Common treatment complications must be accurately recorded, especially because acute Monteggia injuries continue to be missed or inadequately treated, resulting in the development of chronic Monteggia lesions. An improved understanding of return to sports and functional outcomes is critical. The disabilities of the arm, shoulder, and hand (DASH) score can be used to measure the disability following Monteggia fracture-dislocations but has not been validated in children. Joint-specific outcome measures have been developed for the elbow, but many of these measures would benefit from further research into their validity, reliability, and applicability in children.[115] For pediatric patients, the pediatric outcomes data collection instrument (PODCI) offers a validated tool, but its upper limb disability measurement

Figure 12-16. AP (**A**) and lateral (**B**) radiographs of a Bado type III fracture pattern, with lateral dislocation of the radius and apex lateral fracture of the proximal ulna.

A
B

Figure 12-17. Bado type IV lesion with anterior dislocation of the radial head associated with a both-bone forearm fracture. Type IV lesion. There is an anterior dislocation of the radial head. The radial and ulnar fractures are usually in the middle third of the shaft, with the radial fracture distal to the ulnar fracture.

is broad and not joint or disease specific. The development and validation of pediatric upper limb outcome measures are needed and recent work with patient-reported outcome measurement instrument system (PROMIS) is encouraging.

PATHOANATOMY AND APPLIED ANATOMY RELATING TO MONTEGGIA FRACTURE-DISLOCATIONS

Understanding the anatomy of the proximal radioulnar joint, radiocapitellar joint, and proximal forearm is critical to understanding the treatment of acute and chronic Monteggia lesions. The bony architecture, joint contour, and periarticular ligaments provide stability to the proximal forearm and elbow. The muscle insertions and origins affect stability and determine surgical exposure along with the neighboring neurovascular structures.

LIGAMENTS

Annular Ligament

The annular (or orbicular) ligament (Fig. 12-20) is one of the prime stabilizers of the proximal radioulnar joint during forearm rotation. The annular ligament encircles the radial neck from its origin and insertion on the proximal ulna. Because of the shape of the radial head, the annular ligament tightens in supination. The annular ligament is confluent with the remainder of the lateral collateral ligamentous complex, which provides stability to the radiocapitellar and proximal radioulnar joints and resists varus stress. Displacement of the annular ligament occurs in a Monteggia lesion, often pulling off the ulna with a periosteal sleeve and eventually displacing over the head of the radius into the joint between the radial head and the capitellum.[124]

A, B
C

Figure 12-18. A: Forearm radiograph of a both-bone fracture, which does not adequately visualize the elbow. AP (**B**) and lateral (**C**) radiographs of the elbow clearly demonstrate the disrupted radiocapitellar line.

Figure 12-19. Congenital radial head versus traumatic dislocation. AP (**A**) and lateral (**B**) elbow radiographs and 3D CT scan (**C**) demonstrating a dysplastic radial head, posterior dislocation, and hypoplastic capitellum. All these findings are consistent with congenital radial head dislocation. AP (**D**) and lateral (**E**) elbow radiographs of a child with congenital radioulnar synostosis and posterior radial head dislocation. This is a case of congenital radioulnar synostosis.

Quadrate Ligament

The quadrate ligament[130] is just distal to the annular ligament and connects the proximal radius and ulna (see Fig. 12-20). It has a dense anterior portion, thinner posterior portion, and even thinner central portion. The quadrate ligament also provides stability to the proximal radioulnar joint during forearm rotation. The anterior and posterior borders become taut at the extremes of supination and pronation, respectively.

Oblique Cord

The oblique cord (Fig. 12-21), also known as the Weitbrecht ligament, extends at a 45-degree angle from the ulna proximally to the radius distally and is present in approximately 53% of forearms.[129] The oblique cord originates just distal to the radial

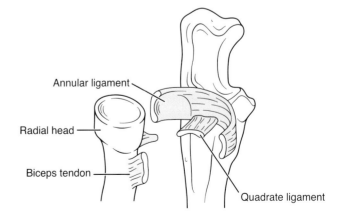

Figure 12-20. Ligamentous anatomy of the proximal radioulnar joint.

Figure 12-21. Ligaments of the forearm. In supination, the annular ligament, quadrate ligament, Weitbrecht ligament (oblique cord), and interosseous membrane are taut, providing increased stability to the proximal radioulnar joint.

Figure 12-22. The radial head is an elliptical structure secured by the annular ligament, which allows movement while providing stability. Because of the shape of the radial head, the stability provided by the annular ligament is maximized in supination.

notch of the ulna and inserts just distal to the bicipital tuberosity of the radius. With supination, the oblique cord tightens and may provide a marginal increase in stability to the proximal radioulnar joint. The clinical relevance of this structure is uncertain.

Interosseous Ligament

The interosseous ligament (see Fig. 12-21) is distal to the oblique ligament with its primary fibers running in the opposite direction (from radius proximally to ulna distally) to the oblique cord. However, similar to the oblique cord, it tightens in supination and provides further stability to the proximal radioulnar joint. The central band of the interosseous ligament is the stiffest stabilizing structure of the forearm.[136]

BONY ARCHITECTURE

The bony architecture of the elbow creates a relatively constrained hinge. The concave surface of the radial head matches the convex surface of the capitellum and provides stability to the radiocapitellar joint. In contrast, the bony geometry of the proximal radioulnar joint provides minimal inherent stability.

Radius

The shape of the radial head is generally elliptical in cross-section (Fig. 12-22).[23] In supination, the long axis of the ellipse is perpendicular to the proximal ulna, causing the annular ligament and the anterior portion of the quadrate ligament to tighten and stabilize the proximal radioulnar joint. In addition, the contact area between the radius and the radial notch of the ulna increases in supination because of the broadened surface of the elliptical radial head proximal to distal in that position. This may provide some additional stability.

The radius "radiates" around the ulna. For this reason, the radius must have an anatomic bow to achieve full forearm rotation while maintaining stability at the proximal and distal radioulnar joints (see Fig. 12-22). With the radius in supination, the bow tightens the oblique cord and interosseous ligament, thereby increasing stability of the proximal radioulnar joint.

MUSCULATURE

Biceps Brachii

The biceps brachii inserts into the bicipital tuberosity of the radius and acts as both flexor of the elbow and supinator of the forearm. The biceps acts as a deforming force in anterior Monteggia fracture-dislocations, pulling the radius anteriorly as the elbow is forcibly extended (see Fig. 12-9).[128] During treatment of type I and IV lesions, care is taken to maintain the elbow in flexion to prevent recurrent anterior subluxation of the radial head while the soft tissues heal. In chronic anterior Monteggia lesions, the biceps may foreshorten over time and resist anatomic reduction of the radial head.

Anconeus

The anconeus may act as a dynamic stabilizer of the elbow joint by providing a valgus moment at the joint during extension

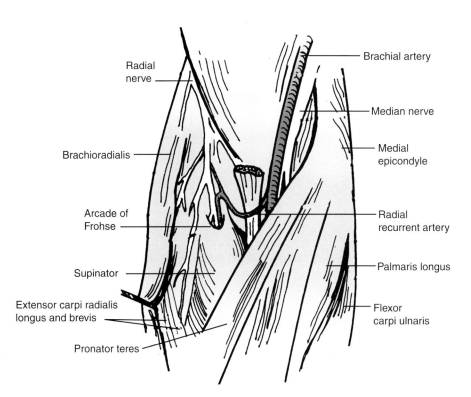

Figure 12-23. Dissection of the anterior elbow. Note the course of the radial nerve, which emerges from the biceps-brachioradialis interval and then divides into the superficial radial sensory branch and the posterior interosseous branch. The posterior interosseous nerve then passes under the Arcade of Frohse.

and pronation.[128] It may also act as a deforming force, along with the forearm flexors, on complete fractures of the ulna in a Monteggia lesion. Surgical exposure of the proximal radioulnar and radiocapitellar joints is usually performed through the anconeus–extensor carpi ulnaris interval.

NERVES

Posterior Interosseous Branch of the Radial Nerve

The radial nerve (Fig. 12-23) passes the distal humerus in the brachialis–brachioradialis interval. As the nerve descends into the forearm, it divides into the superficial radial sensory branch and the posterior interosseous motor branch. The PIN passes under the arcade of Frohse and between the two heads of the supinator, when present, or beneath the supinator when there is only one head. The nerve's close proximity to the radial head and neck makes it susceptible to injury with Monteggia fracture-dislocations.[58] Injuries to the PIN occur more frequently with type III lesions than other types of Monteggia fracture-dislocations.[107] Walton et al.[132] propose radiographic parameters that can possibly predict PIN palsy. In chronic Monteggia lesions, the PIN can be adherent to the dislocated radial head–neck or, less commonly, entrapped in the radiocapitellar joint.[109] Usually when the radial nerve is entrapped in the joint, there is complete motor palsy. Care must be taken to avoid injury to the radial nerve in surgical reconstructions of the chronic anterior dislocation.

Ulnar Nerve

The ulnar nerve passes posterior to the medial intermuscular septum of the upper arm, through the cubital tunnel behind the medial epicondyle of the distal humerus, and then between both heads of the flexor carpi ulnaris into the forearm. The ulnar nerve is at risk for injury with type II Monteggia lesions because of the stretch associated with varus deformity; and, also with ulnar lengthening in chronic Monteggia reconstructions.

GENERAL TREATMENT PRINCIPLES FOR MONTEGGIA FRACTURE-DISLOCATIONS

Although most treatment algorithms for Monteggia fracture-dislocations are based on the Bado classification, Ring and Waters[107] recommended that treatment choices be based on the type of ulnar fracture rather than on the Bado type. They recommended plastic deformation of the ulna be treated with closed reduction of the ulnar bow to obtain stable reduction of the radiocapitellar joint. Incomplete (greenstick or buckle) fractures of the ulna are similarly treated with closed reduction and casting. Closed treatment methods in the plastic deformation and incomplete ulna fracture types can restore ulnar length, alignment, and stability due to the periosteum. In children, most type I Monteggia injuries with plastic deformation of the ulna or incomplete ulnar fractures are stable when immobilized in 100 to 110 degrees of elbow flexion and full forearm supination to maintain radial head reduction.

However, any Monteggia lesion with a complete fracture of the ulna can be unstable after closed reduction. There are times where closed treatment will be successful, but the risk of failed closed treatment increases with complete fractures. Therefore, with complete transverse or short oblique ulnar fractures, intramedullary fixation of the ulna is recommended. Long oblique or comminuted ulnar fractures, which can develop shortening and malalignment even with intramedullary fixation, are best stabilized with plate and screw fixation. Monteggia lesions associated with a radial fracture (type IV lesions), can be treated with intramedullary or plate fixation. Using this treatment protocol, Ring and Waters[107] reported excellent results in all 28 patients treated within 24 hours of injury. A follow-up study by Ramski et al.[101] of 112 fractures confirmed the reliability of this ulnar-based treatment strategy. The only failures occurred when surgeons nonoperatively treated fractures that met operative treatment criteria by protocol.

As noted, successful treatment is dependent on three goals: (1) anatomical correction of the ulnar deformity; (2) achieving a stable congruent reduction of the radiocapitellar joint; and (3) maintenance of ulnar length and fracture stability (see Algorithm 12-1). For plastic deformation and incomplete fractures, these goals can usually be achieved with closed reduction and cast immobilization provided the treating professionals accurately diagnose the lesion in the acute setting. For complete fractures, fracture instability after closed reduction may lead to loss of anatomic ulnar length and redislocation of the radial head. These injuries are generally treated with internal fixation, usually IM rodding,[74] to lessen the risk of loss of reduction and development of a chronic Monteggia lesion.

Of note, open compared to closed pediatric Monteggia lesions have been noted to have a longer time of healing, higher complication rate, and worse long-term patient-reported outcome (QuickDASH) scores.[111]

TREATMENT OPTIONS FOR TYPE I MONTEGGIA FRACTURE-DISLOCATIONS

NONOPERATIVE TREATMENT OF TYPE I MONTEGGIA FRACTURE-DISLOCATIONS

Indications/Contraindications

Nonoperative Treatment of Type I Monteggia Fracture-Dislocations:
INDICATIONS AND CONTRAINDICATIONS

Indications

- Plastic deformation of the ulna
- Incomplete (greenstick or buckle) ulnar fracture

Relative Contraindications

- Open fracture
- Unstable ulnar fracture pattern
- Transverse or short oblique ulnar fracture
- Long oblique or comminuted ulnar fracture
- Residual or recurrent loss of congruency at radiocapitellar joint
- Late presentation

Closed reduction and cast immobilization is recommended as an initial treatment strategy for all type I Monteggia fracture-dislocations in which the ulna is plastically deformed or there is an incomplete fracture (greenstick or buckle). Operative intervention

Type I

Angulation correction

Longitudinal traction (Supination)

Flexion 90–100°

Immobilization/flexion 100–110° supination

Figure 12-24. Reduction technique for a type I Monteggia fracture-dislocation.

is recommended if there is a failure to obtain and maintain ulnar fracture reduction or a failure to obtain and maintain a congruent reduction of the proximal radioulnar and radiocapitellar joints. In patients with complete transverse or oblique fractures of the ulna, closed reduction alone can be successful but risks loss of reduction in a cast and development of a chronic Monteggia lesion if not followed closely with prompt change of treatment if fracture and radial head displacement occurs in the cast. In complete fractures, operative intervention is recommended to facilitate maintenance of ulnar alignment and the radiocapitellar reduction, especially if close patient follow-up is problematic.

Closed Reduction and Immobilization

Reduction of the Ulnar Fracture

The first step of the closed reduction is to reestablish the length of the ulna by longitudinal traction and manual correction of any angular deformity. The forearm is held in relaxed supination as longitudinal traction is applied with manual pressure directed over the apex of the deformity until the angulation is corrected clinically and radiographically (Figs. 12-24 and 12-25). With plastic deformation fractures, this may necessitate application of significant force that requires conscious sedation and often general anesthesia. With incomplete fractures, the correction of the ulnar deformity and radial head reduction can often be achieved with conscious sedation in the emergency room. Some papers have cited successful treatment of acute Monteggia lesions (defined as maintenance of the radiocapitellar reduction) with nonanatomic alignment of the ulnar fracture (Fig. 12-26).[40,98]

Figure 12-25. Closed reduction for type I lesion. **A:** Typical type I lesion in a 6 year old. Plastic deformation of the ulna must be corrected to prevent recurrence of the angular deformity, which allows reduction of the radial head and prevents its late subluxation. The deformity of the ulna is corrected first (**B**), but the radial head is still anteriorly subluxed because the ulna still has some anterior plastic deformation (**C**). **D:** By hyperflexing the elbow, the radiocapitellar line is restored.

However, anatomic reduction and healing of the ulna fracture are strongly advocated.

Reduction of the Radial Head

Once ulnar length and alignment have been reestablished, the radial head can be relocated. This is often accomplished by simply flexing the elbow to 90 degrees or more, thus producing spontaneous reduction (Fig. 12-27). Occasionally, posteriorly directed pressure over the anterior aspect of the radial head is necessary for reduction of the radial head. Flexion of the elbow to 110 to 120 degrees stabilizes the reduction. Once the radial head position is established, it should be scrutinized radiographically in numerous views to ensure a concentric reduction.

Figure 12-26. Nonanatomic alignment of the ulna fracture, with a residual posterior bow, but anatomic reduction of the radiocapitellar joint.

Figure 12-27. Schematic reduction maneuvers for type I lesion. Flexing the elbow spontaneously reduces the radial head. Occasionally, manual pressure is required in combination with flexion.

With a type I lesion, the optimal radiographic view is a true lateral of the elbow with the forearm held in supination. The longitudinal axis of the radius should pass directly through the center of the capitellum (see Fig. 12-27). There are rare occasions where the radial head will not reduce in the acute setting. This necessitates further investigation and care. Causes include undercorrected plastic deformation of the ulna; entrapment of the annular ligament in the joint despite reduction of the ulna fracture; and, less commonly, appreciated plastic deformation of the radius.

Radiographic Evaluation and Immobilization

Once the concentric reduction of the radial head is confirmed, the elbow should be placed in approximately 110 to 120 degrees of flexion to alleviate the potential deforming force of the biceps, which could redislocate the radial head. The forearm is placed in a position of midsupination to neutral rotation to alleviate the forces of the biceps, supinator muscle and the anconeus, as well as the forearm flexors, which tend to produce radial angulation of the ulna. After the fracture is reduced and the position of stability is established, a molded long-arm splint or cast is applied to hold the elbow joint in the appropriate amount of flexion, usually 110 to 120 degrees. Once the casting is completed, careful radiographic assessment should establish the concentric reduction of the radial head with respect to the capitellum, as well as satisfactory alignment of the ulna (Fig. 12-28).

Postreduction Care

The patient is followed at 1- to 2-week intervals to confirm continued satisfactory reduction by radiography. At 4 to 6 weeks after the initial reduction, if there is radiographic evidence of consolidation of the ulnar fracture and stability of the radial

A   B

Figure 12-28. Once the closed reduction is complete, radiographs should be analyzed for reestablishment of the radiocapitellar line (*arrows*) and ulnar alignment on both the lateral (**A**) and Jones (**B**) views.

head, the long-arm cast or splint can be removed with progressive guarded restoration of full motion and then return to full activity. A final set of radiographs should be obtained when the patient has achieved full motion to be certain the radiocapitellar and proximal radioulnar joints remain anatomically aligned.

Outcomes

In all series,[4,10,20,31,104,107] type I Monteggia lesions in children have uniformly good results when treated by manipulative closed reduction, if the radial head is properly aligned and the ulnar fracture is reduced with length preserved. These results most clearly apply to plastic deformation and incomplete fractures, which make up the majority of type I Monteggia lesions. Successful results can include complete fractures that do not lose reduction in the cast, but there is a risk. Similarly, if loss of reduction occurs in a patient treated closed and monitored closely, repeat reduction can achieve realignment.[48] You just cannot miss the loss of reduction by either poor radiographs, inaccurate review of the radiographs, or patients who do not follow up in a timely manner. No deterioration of results appears to occur at long term if healed anatomically.[67,92]

OPERATIVE TREATMENT OF TYPE I MONTEGGIA FRACTURE-DISLOCATIONS

Indications/Contraindications

Operative Treatment of Type I Monteggia Fracture-Dislocations:
INDICATIONS AND CONTRAINDICATIONS

Indications

- Open fracture
- Unstable ulnar fracture pattern
- Inability to obtain (or maintain) good alignment of the ulna and radiocapitellar joint in plastic deformation or incomplete fractures
- Transverse or short oblique ulnar fracture
- Long oblique or comminuted ulnar fracture

Relative Contraindications

- Plastic deformation of the ulna
- Incomplete (greenstick or buckle) ulnar fracture
- Good alignment with closed reduction and casting

There are two principal indications for operative treatment of type I fracture-dislocations: failure to obtain and maintain ulnar fracture reduction and a failure to obtain and maintain a congruent reduction of the radiocapitellar joint. The fractures most at risk for loss of reduction with nonoperative management are complete ulnar fractures. In these fractures, operative fixation of the ulna is recommended to facilitate maintenance of ulnar alignment and radiocapitellar reduction. In some cases, closed reduction of the radiocapitellar joint cannot be achieved, even after restoration of ulnar length and stabilization by intramedullary or plate fixation of the ulna. It is important not to accept a nonanatomic reduction as an imperfect reduction, which can

result in further joint malalignment and the development of a chronic Monteggia lesion. In these cases, the annular ligament is almost always avulsed or entrapped.[124] There is a high likelihood that annular ligament and/or periosteal interposition is preventing congruent reduction of the radiocapitellar joint. In these situations, an open reduction of the radiocapitellar joint should be performed with restoration of the annular ligament to its normal position around the proximal radius.[124,128]

Other reasons for failure include (1) failure to achieve anatomic reduction of a plastic deformation ulna fracture, which indicates a need for an acute incomplete osteotomy and fixation of the ulna with or without open reduction annular ligament; and (2) concomitant plastic deformation of the radius that requires closed or open reduction.

Preoperative Planning

Operative Treatment of Monteggia Fracture-Dislocations:
PREOPERATIVE PLANNING CHECKLIST

OR table	❏ Standard OR table with radiolucent arm board, table turned 90 degrees with operative limb pointing away from anesthesia team
Position/positioning aids	❏ Patient supine with adequate padding of heels and other bony prominences and neurovascular structures
Fluoroscopy location	❏ Generally from below arm (medial to lateral) ❏ Easy viewing of monitors for the entire OR team
Equipment	❏ Standard operating instruments, drill, Kirschner (K) wire or flexible titanium nail set, small or mini-fragment set, nonabsorbable 2-0 and 3-0 suture, splinting or casting supplies
Tourniquet	❏ Nonsterile tourniquet generally sufficient
[Other]	

Routine preoperative planning is required before embarking on any of the operative treatment pathways described below.

Intramedullary Fixation of Transverse or Short Oblique Ulnar Fractures

In patients with complete transverse or short oblique fractures, closed reduction alone can achieve alignment of radial head and ulna fracture but risks loss of reduction in a cast.[105] In these cases, closed reduction and intramedullary fixation of the ulna is recommended to facilitate maintenance of ulnar alignment and length along with reduction of the radiocapitellar joint. The quality of the ulnar reduction affects the ability to reduce the radial head, which is of primary importance.

Figure 12-29. AP (**A**) and lateral (**B**) type I fracture pattern. Entry site is via the olecranon apophysis. A smooth Steinmann pin (**C**) or a titanium elastic nail can be utilized.

If an ulnar fracture can be reduced but not maintained because of the obliquity of the fracture, internal fixation is also indicated.[40,89] Intramedullary fixation is standard in most series of Monteggia fracture-dislocations in children (Fig. 12-29).[8,10,31,38,66,77,99,107,110] Percutaneous intramedullary fixation reliably maintains alignment and preserves length without the additional concerns of open surgery or implant retention. This method of fixation can be accomplished using image intensification and with Steinmann pins, K-wires, or flexible titanium nails (Synthes, West Chester, PA). Entry can be through the olecranon apophysis (requires early removal) or proximal metaphysis (can be left in longer under the local muscle but then requires removal in OR). Steinmann pins and K-wires have the advantage of being universally available and inexpensive. Their stainless steel composition and smooth tip also permit easy removal in the office without need for additional anesthesia. Note that K-wires may not be of sufficient length for use in older children with longer, stronger forearms. Titanium rods usually have to be removed in the day surgery unit under anesthesia.

Technique

> **☑ Intramedullary Fixation of Transverse or Short Oblique Ulnar Fractures:**
> **KEY SURGICAL STEPS**

- ❑ Cortical entry through the apophysis or proximal metaphysis of the ulna
- ❑ Introduce appropriately sized intramedullary device (K-wire, Steinmann pin, or flexible titanium nail)
- ❑ Perform closed reduction based on mechanism of injury
  - Intramedullary device can be used in the proximal fragment to joystick the reduction
- ❑ Stabilize fracture with the intramedullary device, utilize fluoroscopy to confirm appropriate ulnar and radiocapitellar reduction, as well as proper placement of the intramedullary device
- ❑ Bend and cut intramedullary K-wire outside of skin for apophyseal entry to facilitate subsequent removal in the office; titanium nails or buried metaphyseal entry wires need to be removed in day surgery unit
- ❑ Apply long-arm splint, cast, or bivalved cast in a position of elbow flexion and supination appropriate for the specific Bado type

Entry can be through the apophysis or proximal metaphysis of the ulna depending on the level of the fracture and surgeon's preference. For type I lesions, a closed reduction maneuver is performed as described above. At times, an intramedullary device in the proximal fragment can be used to joystick the reduction. Intraoperative fluoroscopy is utilized to confirm appropriate ulnar and radiocapitellar reduction, as well as proper interosseous placement of the intramedullary device. Because ulnar fractures heal rapidly in children, the intramedullary device can generally be bent and cut outside of the skin to facilitate subsequent office removal. Some surgeons prefer to leave the intramedullary rod in a long time and therefore bury it beneath the skin. This is usually less problematic with metaphyseal entry and burying the device under the local muscle. Lightdale-Miric et al.[70] reviewed 59 acute Monteggia lesions. Some 75% were treated with exposed intramedullary (IM) fixation and 25% with buried fixation. There was no difference in clinical outcome including complications.

Only 4% of exposed IM fixation had to have OR removal while all of the buried wires did require OR removal under anesthesia. Of note, comparing IM rodding fixation to plate-screw construct fixation for oblique fractures revealed equivalent excellent results with less blood loss and operative time with IM fixation. A long-arm splint, cast (if minimal manipulation needed), or bivalved cast is then applied with the elbow in 90 to 110 degrees of flexion and forearm supination, which provides additional stability to the radiocapitellar joint.

Open Reduction and Plate Fixation of Long Oblique or Comminuted Ulnar Fractures

Although intramedullary fixation is preferred for transverse and short oblique fractures, long oblique and comminuted fractures may redisplace even with intramedullary fixation.[107] Plate and screw fixation (Fig. 12-30) is preferred with these rarer fractures.[66,94,107]

Figure 12-30. ORIF of type I Monteggia lesion in a 10-year-old male associated with a comminuted ulna fracture. Injury AP (**A**) and lateral (**B**) radiographs demonstrating the dislocated radial head and ulnar fracture pattern. Intraoperative AP (**C**) and lateral (**D**) images demonstrating plate and screw fixation.

Technique

Open Reduction and Plate Fixation of Long Oblique or Comminuted Ulnar Fractures:
KEY SURGICAL STEPS

- ❑ Longitudinal incision over subcutaneous border of the ulna
- ❑ Develop interval between extensor carpi ulnaris and flexor carpi ulnaris
- ❑ Carefully incise periosteum at fracture site and preserve for subsequent repair
- ❑ Perform open reduction
- ❑ Apply double-stacked one-third tubular plate or 2.7- or 3.5-mm dynamic compression plate depending on age and size of patient
  - • Four to six cortices of fixation both proximal and distal to the fracture
- ❑ Use fluoroscopy to confirm appropriate ulnar and radiocapitellar reduction, as well as proper placement of the plate and screws
- ❑ Repair periosteum over the fracture site and implant
- ❑ Layered wound closure
  - • If concerned about excessive swelling and compartment syndrome risk, prophylactically release forearm fascia after periosteal repair before superficial layer closure.
- ❑ Apply long-arm splint, cast, or bivalved cast in a position of elbow flexion and supination appropriate for the specific Bado type

A longitudinal incision, centered at the apex of the fracture, is made along the subcutaneous border of the ulna, at the extensor carpi ulnaris–flexor carpi ulnaris interval. An open reduction is performed, and a double-stacked one-third tubular plate or 2.7/3.5-mm dynamic compression plate (Synthes, West Chester, PA) is applied depending on age and size of patient utilizing standard Association of Osteosynthesis (AO) techniques. Four to six cortices of fixation are generally required both proximal and distal to the fracture. Intraoperative fluoroscopy is used to confirm appropriate ulnar and radiocapitellar reduction. The periosteum is repaired over the fracture site and implant. If concerned about excessive swelling and compartment syndrome risk, prophylactically release forearm fascia after periosteal repair before superficial layer closure. Again, a long-arm splint, cast, or bivalved cast is then applied with the elbow in 90 to 110 degrees of flexion and forearm supination, which provides additional stability to the radiocapitellar joint.

Open Reduction of the Annular Ligament

On occasion, a congruent closed reduction of the radiocapitellar joint cannot be achieved, even after intramedullary fixation or plate fixation of the ulna. In these situations, the position of the radial head may be improved, but the reduction remains imperfect. The surgeon may not feel a definitive clunk associated with an anatomic reduction but instead may feel a soft or rubbery resistance during manipulation. This suggests soft tissue interposition of either the annular ligament and/or periosteum.[128] First be certain the deformity of the ulna fracture is completely corrected. Also, assess the radius for plastic deformation fracture and correct if present. An open reduction of the radiocapitellar joint with restoration of the annular ligament to its normal position is recommended if fracture length and

alignment has been achieved. Soft tissue interposition more commonly occurs in type III lesions, but can also occur in type I lesions. Interposed cartilaginous or osteochondral fractures in the radiocapitellar joint or proximal radioulnar joint may also prevent complete reduction of the radial head.[128] Morris[83] described a patient in whom reduction of the radial head was obstructed by radial nerve entrapment between the radial head and ulna. When radial nerve entrapment occurs, it is usually with a complete PIN palsy. Care must be taken during exposure not to lacerate the nerve.

Technique

Open Reduction of the Annular Ligament:
KEY SURGICAL STEPS

- ❑ Posterolateral (Kocher) approach to the elbow under tourniquet control
- ❑ Develop interval between extensor carpi ulnaris and anconeus, maintain forearm in pronation to protect radial nerve from iatrogenic injury
- ❑ Perform elbow capsulotomy
- ❑ Identify annular ligament
  - • Ligament typically in continuity, usually torn off the ulna with a periosteal sleeve (generally not torn midsubstance)
- ❑ Reduce annular ligament over the radius, often with gentle manipulation inside ligament opening with freer elevator or small retractor.
  - • Repair the ligament back to the ulna with 2-0 and/or 3-0 nonabsorbable suture
  - • If necessary, perform olecranon open wedge osteotomy and use internal fixation
- ❑ Layered wound closure
- ❑ Apply long-arm splint, cast, or bivalved cast in a position of elbow flexion and supination appropriate for the specific Bado type

The most direct approach to the radiocapitellar joint is from the posterolateral aspect of the elbow. The interval between the anconeus and the extensor carpi ulnaris, using the distal portion of a Kocher incision, provides sufficient exposure of the radial head and the interposed structures. This approach protects the PIN when the forearm is pronated. A more extensile approach was described by Boyd and Boals (Fig. 12-31).[19] This exposure is begun by making an incision following the lateral border of the triceps posteriorly to the lateral condyle and extending it along the radial side of the ulna. The incision is carried under the anconeus and extensor carpi ulnaris in an extraperiosteal manner, elevating the fibers of the supinator from the ulna. This carries the approach down to the interosseous membrane, allowing exposure of the radiocapitellar joint, excellent visualization of the annular ligament, access to the proximal fourth of the entire radius, and approach to the ulnar fracture all through the same incision.[19,20] In addition, elevation of the extensor–supinator mass from the lateral epicondyle allows more proximal exposure of the dislocated radial head if entrapped behind the displaced capsule and annular ligament.

After obtaining adequate surgical exposure through either approach, a capsulotomy is performed, and the elbow joint is inspected. Careful exploration is required to identify the

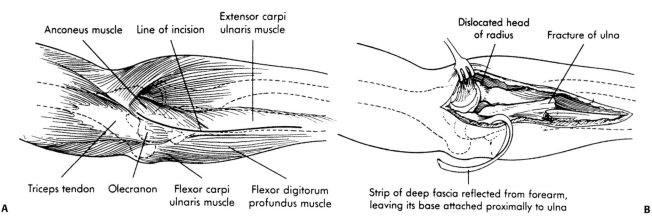

Figure 12-31. Boyd approach. **A:** The incision is carried under the anconeus and extensor carpi ulnaris to expose the radial head and annular ligament. **B:** The incision can be extended distally to allow exposure of the ulnar fracture and proximally to facilitate harvesting of a fascial strip for annular ligament reconstruction, if necessary.

annular ligament. The ligament is not typically torn in its midsubstance, but rather remains in continuity and tears of the ulna with a periosteal sleeve. The displaced in-continuity ligament usually slips off the radial neck over the radial head into the joint. Once the opening in the annular ligament is identified, a Freer elevator, forceps, soft tissue probe, or a small curette is used to reduce the annular ligament over the radial head. If a repair is required, 2-0 or 3-0 nonabsorbable sutures can be used. The congruency of the radiocapitellar and proximal radioulnar joint reductions should be confirmed under direct visualization (Fig. 12-32). Stability can then be confirmed by rotating the forearm under careful fluoroscopic imaging. If the radial head is still unstable, look for missed plastic deformation of the ulna or radius. If present, closed reduction of the ulna, or at times opening wedge osteotomy of the ulna, is required to anatomically and stably reduce the radial head. The same is true for the radius if there is plastic deformation and loss of normal radial bow. A layered wound closure is performed, followed by application of a long-arm splint or bivalved cast with the forearm in supination.

Authors' Preferred Treatment for Type I Monteggia Fracture-Dislocations (Algorithm 12-1)

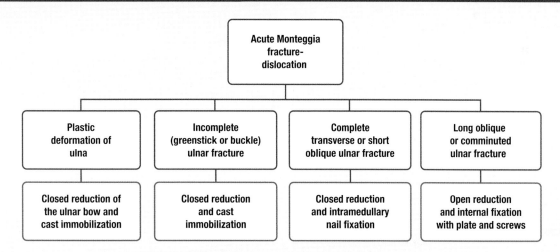

Algorithm 12-1. Authors' preferred treatment of all Monteggia fracture-dislocations.

An anatomic, stable reduction of the ulnar fracture almost always leads to a stable reduction of the radiocapitellar and proximal radioulnar joint. This in turn leads to an excellent long-term outcome. Failure to obtain and maintain ulnar fracture and radiocapitellar reduction will lead to a chronic Monteggia lesion, which is a complex clinical and surgical problem with risk of a suboptimum outcome. If a closed reduction can be achieved with a cast, close follow-up is warranted. If the reduction is lost at any point in the weekly follow-up evaluations, operative treatment is indicated. Although some authors have advocated conservative treatment,[39] it is not wrong to be very aggressive in treatment of acute

Monteggia fracture-dislocations and proceed directly to the operating room for stabilization. Overtreatment has been more successful than undertreatment in preventing a chronic Monteggia lesion.[101] Percutaneous intramedullary fixation of complete transverse and short oblique ulna fractures is standard. Open reduction and internal fixation with plate and screws for the less common long oblique and comminuted fracture is also standard.[101] Any irreducible or unstable radial head after fracture reduction and stabilization is approached surgically to define and correct the cause. This usually involves reducing an interposed annular ligament; further correction of the ulna deformity; or recognition and correction of associated radial deformity. This aggressive approach avoids late complications.[107]

POSTOPERATIVE CARE

After closed or open reduction of the ulna fracture and closed or open reduction of the radial head, a long-arm cast is used for 4 to 6 weeks with the forearm in slight supination and the elbow flexed 90 to 110 degrees depending on the degree of swelling. Radiographs are obtained every 1 to 2 weeks until fracture healing. Intramedullary hardware is removed with fracture healing. Plate and screw fixation may be removed after 6 to 12 months if there is any discomfort. Home rehabilitation is begun at 6 weeks and return to sports is dependent on restoration of motion and strength, usually around 8 to 12 weeks postoperatively.

Figure 12-32. **A, B:** Two views of diaphyseal ulna fracture with subluxed radial head that was unappreciated. **C, D:** Malunion ulna fracture with markedly displaced radial head noted on lateral radiographic views. **E:** Open reduction radiocapitellar joint with triceps fascia reconstruction annular ligament. **F, G:** Radiographs showing healed osteotomy radiographically with reduced radial head.

POTENTIAL PITFALLS AND PREVENTIVE MEASURES

Monteggia Fracture-Dislocations:
POTENTIAL PITFALLS AND PREVENTIONS

Pitfall	Prevention
Failure to identify radial head dislocation leading to chronic Monteggia lesion	• Always obtain dedicated elbow and forearm radiographs with forearm fractures to evaluate congruency of radiocapitellar reduction
Loss of radiocapitellar reduction leading to chronic Monteggia lesion	• Intramedullary fixation or plate fixation for unstable ulnar fractures • Regular postoperative radiographs every 1 to 2 weeks until fracture healing
Inadequate reduction of radial head leading to chronic Monteggia lesion	• Never accept an imperfect reduction of the radial head; make certain ulna fracture is completely reduced; any associated radius fracture is corrected; and perform an open reduction of radiocapitellar joint with restoration of the annular ligament to its normal position if complete, stable reduction does not occur after fracture realignment and stabilization
Radial nerve palsy	• During posterolateral approach to the elbow, pronate forearm to protect radial nerve from iatrogenic injury • During chronic Monteggia reconstructions, identify and protect radial nerve • Be careful during open reduction of an irreducible radial head dislocation if there is a complete PIN palsy
Compartment syndrome	• Monitor high-energy injuries in hospital with frequent neurovascular monitoring • Avoid hyperflexion in the cast or splint • Perform prophylactic volar and dorsal forearm fasciotomies during chronic Monteggia reconstructions • Consider bivalving postoperative casts or using splints

TREATMENT OPTIONS FOR TYPE II MONTEGGIA FRACTURE-DISLOCATIONS

The indications for nonoperative and operative treatment of type II lesions are similar to type I lesions as the ulnar fracture pattern dictates initial decision making. Following ulnar fracture reduction, any residual lack of congruency at the radiocapitellar joint should be treated surgically.

NONOPERATIVE TREATMENT OF TYPE II MONTEGGIA FRACTURE-DISLOCATIONS

As with type I injuries, incomplete type II fractures usually have a satisfactory result after closed reduction.[69,89] The ulnar

Figure 12-33. Schematic reduction maneuvers for type II lesion. Longitudinal traction and pronation of the forearm and immobilization in 60-degree flexion or complete extension.

fracture is reduced by longitudinal traction in line with the long axis of the forearm while the elbow is held at 60 degrees of flexion (Fig. 12-33). The radial head may reduce spontaneously or may require gentle, anteriorly directed pressure applied to its posterior aspect. The elbow is extended once the radial head is reduced and immobilized in that position to stabilize the radial head and allow molding posteriorly to maintain the ulnar reduction.[31,131] If the ulnar alignment cannot be maintained, an intramedullary Steinmann pin or K-wire should be used. Some surgeons prefer to fix the ulna fracture rather than cast in extension.

OPERATIVE TREATMENT OF TYPE II MONTEGGIA FRACTURE-DISLOCATIONS

Treatment goals are stable concentric reduction of the radial head and alignment of the ulnar fracture. When there is an unstable, complete ulnar fracture, percutaneous intramedullary fixation or open reduction and internal fixation with plate and screws are used similar to type I Monteggia fracture-dislocations.[94] The radial head should be reduced by open technique if there is interposed soft tissue or the Monteggia lesion is accompanied by a fractured capitellum or radial head.

Up to 10 degrees of ulnar angulation is acceptable in younger children, provided the radial head reduction is concentric and stable. Range-of-motion testing of stability is appropriate and necessary with reduced plastic deformation fractures because radiocapitellar alignment can be difficult to assess with AP radiographs in the cast. This is why testing reduction with motion assisted by fluoroscopy before cast application is important.

Reduction is maintained by the application of a long-arm splint, cast, or bivalved cast with a valgus mold and with the elbow in relative flexion. The degree of flexion varies depending on the direction of the radial head dislocation. When the radial head is dislocated in a straight lateral or anterolateral position, flexion to 100 to 110 degrees improves stability.[33,84] If there is a posterolateral component to the dislocation, flexion to 70 to 80 degrees has been recommended.[126] Forearm rotation in the cast is usually in supination, which tightens the annular ligament and interosseous membrane and further stabilizes the reduction.[10,31,84] Some have suggested positions of immobilization from pronation to slight supination.[126] Ramsey and Pedersen[100] recommended neutral as the best position of rotation to avoid loss of motion; their patients showed no loss of reduction using this position. It must be emphasized that the ulnar fracture and radial head reduction need to be truly stable for successful closed treatment because postreduction radiographs in cast are difficult to interpret accurately.

Postreduction Care

Cast immobilization is continued until fracture and soft tissue healing, usually by 6 weeks (see Fig. 12-36). Home rehabilitation is performed until restoration of motion and strength. A final set of radiographs is obtained when the patient has achieved full motion and strength to be certain that there is continued anatomic reduction of the proximal radioulnar and radiocapitellar joints.

OPERATIVE TREATMENT OF TYPE III MONTEGGIA FRACTURE-DISLOCATIONS

As noted earlier, the goals of surgical intervention are reduction and stabilization of both the ulnar fracture and the radial head. If there is an inability to obtain and maintain anatomic alignment of the ulnar fracture, proximal radioulnar joint, or radiocapitellar joint, then operative treatment is clearly indicated.

Ulnar Stabilization

Ulnar malalignment may prevent anatomic relocation of the radial head. The ulnar fracture can usually be reduced closed, but internal fixation may be necessary if the ulnar fracture is unstable to prevent recurrent lateral dislocation of the radial head. Persistent varus alignment, particularly with oblique ulnar fractures, can lead to recurrent subluxation of the radial head, radiocapitellar incongruence, and risk of a poor outcome.[40,89] Anatomic reduction of the ulna and fixation with plates and screws[40] or intramedullary wires[8] will yield excellent results.[101]

Open Reduction of the Annular Ligament

Failed closed reduction of the radial head with anatomic alignment of the ulna fracture implies interposition of soft tissue,

which is repaired through a Boyd approach (see Fig. 12-31).[19] This allows removal of the interposed tissues[128] and repair or reconstruction of the annular ligament and the periosteum of the ulna as necessary (Fig. 12-37).[13] The surgical technique is essentially the same as previously described for a type I Monteggia fracture-dislocation.

As with any Monteggia lesion, treatment is primarily aimed at obtaining and maintaining reduction of the radial head, either by an open or closed technique. This is usually performed by anatomic, stable closed reduction of the ulnar fracture, which in turn leads to a stable reduction of the proximal radioulnar and radiocapitellar joints. If there is any doubt about the stability of the fracture-dislocation reduction, operative fixation is indicated.

TREATMENT OPTIONS FOR TYPE IV MONTEGGIA FRACTURE-DISLOCATIONS

This complex lesion has been treated by both closed[89] and open[10] techniques. Percutaneous intramedullary fixation of the radial and ulnar fractures with flexible rods and closed reduction of the radial has also been described.[108] The goals of treatment for a type IV Monteggia lesion are similar to those of other Bado types. The presence of the free-floating proximal radial fragment hampers the ability to reduce the radial head. Stabilization of the radial fracture converts a type IV lesion to a type I lesion, making treatment simpler.

NONOPERATIVE TREATMENT OF TYPE IV MONTEGGIA FRACTURE-DISLOCATIONS

Closed reduction should be attempted initially, with the aim of transforming the type IV lesion to a type I lesion (see Fig. 12-37), especially if the radial and ulnar fractures have greenstick patterns. Use of the image intensifier allows immediate confirmation of reduction, especially of the radial head (Fig. 12-38). Closed treatment can occasionally be successful for type IV lesions (Fig. 12-39), but closed treatment without fixation of unstable ulnar lesions should not be attempted. If the initial fracture reduction cannot be obtained, an anatomic stable reduction with either intramedullary or plate fixation is performed.

OPERATIVE TREATMENT OF TYPE IV MONTEGGIA FRACTURE-DISLOCATIONS

Type IV fractures are usually unstable and the reduction of the radial head is easier to obtain and maintain after stable fixation of the radius. In young patients, this may be achieved by intramedullary fixation, usually from distal to proximal entry and passage. In children older than 12 years, plating of the radius

Figure 12-37. Irreducible type III lesion. **A:** Injury films showing typical greenstick olecranon fracture and lateral dislocation of a type III lesion. **B:** After manipulation and correction of the ulnar deformity, the radial head still remained dislocated. **C:** An open reduction was performed to extract the interposed torn annular ligament.

Type IV

Radial angulation correction

Traction longitudinal/supination transform to type I

Flexion 80–100°

Immobilization Flexion 100–110°/supination

Figure 12-38. Schematic reduction maneuvers for type IV lesion.

through a volar Henry extensile approach provides more rigid stabilization. Once stability is achieved, a closed reduction of the radial head is attempted. This is usually successful, but any intra-articular obstruction can be removed through a Boyd approach (see Fig. 12-31).

Authors' Preferred Treatment for Type IV Monteggia Fracture-Dislocations

As with any Monteggia lesion, treatment is primarily aimed at obtaining and maintaining reduction of the radial head, either by an open or closed technique. Percutaneous intramedullary fixation is frequently necessary because of inherent fracture instability (Fig. 12-40). At times, there can be both a proximal and distal radius fracture, which requires special consideration (Fig. 12-41). Following open treatment, the elbow is immobilized in a long-arm cast for 4 to 6 weeks in 110 to 120 degrees of flexion with the forearm in neutral rotation. A short-arm cast can be used thereafter if additional fracture protection is necessary. Home rehabilitation is performed until restoration of motion and strength. Final radiographs are obtained with full restoration of motion and strength to be certain there is anatomic reduction of the proximal radioulnar and radiocapitellar joints.

Figure 12-39. A, B: Type IV Monteggia fracture with radial neck fracture. **C, D:** Closed reduction and casting in the emergency department under conscious sedation. One-week follow-up AP (**E**) and lateral (**F**) radiographs demonstrating maintained alignment of the ulna fracture, radial neck fracture, and radio-capitellar line.

Figure 12-39. (*Continued*) Final follow-up AP (**G**) and lateral (**H**) images.

Figure 12-40. A, B: Injury radiographs of a type IV Monteggia fracture. **C–F:** Intraoperative images demonstrating intramedullary fixation of both bones.

(*continues*)

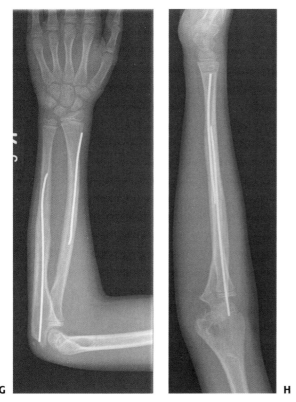

G   **H**

Figure 12-40. *(Continued)* **G, H:** Final follow-up radiographs.

TREATMENT METHODS FOR MONTEGGIA EQUIVALENT FRACTURE-DISLOCATIONS

Monteggia equivalent lesions vary in pattern and severity of injury; because of this, each particular injury has to be approached with a variety of different treatment options and strategies. They can be difficult to manage because the injuries of the radius and ulna can be in close proximity, the proximal radius can be broken and displaced and the proximal ulna may need to be stabilized in order to promote stable early motion and to decrease risk of cross-union.

NONOPERATIVE TREATMENT OF MONTEGGIA EQUIVALENT FRACTURE-DISLOCATIONS

Closed Reduction and Casting

Most Monteggia variants are usually not amenable to purely closed treatment as it can be difficult to align the fragments and maintain stability of the fractures while preventing malunion and allowing stable, full forearm motion.

OPERATIVE TREATMENT OF MONTEGGIA EQUIVALENT FRACTURE-DISLOCATIONS

As noted earlier, the goals of surgical intervention are reduction and stabilization of both the ulnar fracture and the proximal radius. If there is an inability to obtain and maintain anatomic alignment of the ulnar fracture, proximal radioulnar joint, or radiocapitellar joint, then operative treatment is clearly indicated.

Ulnar Reduction and Stabilization

Olecranon malalignment may prevent anatomic relocation of the radial head. The ulnar fracture can be reduced closed when the fracture is distal but it can be challenging to reduce when the fracture is proximal and internal fixation is usually necessary. In young patients, it can be difficult to fully appreciate the relationship of the radial head and the capitellum. In these cases, an arthrogram can be instructive after the reduction and stabilization. Using dye before the actual fracture fixation can make it challenging to assess the procedure as the dye can more easily leak out of the joint.

Reduction of the Proximal Radius Fractures

When the patient has a radial neck fracture as a component of their Variant pattern; it is best to approach these with a stepwise strategy as poor outcome (avascular necrosis [AVN], nonunion, stiffness)

A, B   **C**

Figure 12-41. A, B: Distal radius and radial neck fractures, in addition to disruption of the radiocapitellar alignment. **C, D:** Start with percutaneous pinning of the Salter–Harris 2 distal radius fracture with smooth pins.

Figure 12-41. *(Continued)* **E–G:** Then proceed to reduce the ulna, radial neck, and radiocapitellar joint. In this case, the ulna was opened to achieve appropriate reduction, but the radial neck fracture was close reduced. **H–I:** Intramedullary fixation of the ulna fracture maintained the alignment of the radiocapitellar joint.

A   B

Figure 12-42. Chronic Monteggia lesion with ulnar bow line. **A:** The injury radiograph of an 8-year-old girl who fell, spraining her arm. Note the anterior bow of the ulna (*black arrows*) and loss of the radiocapitellar relation (*open arrow*). The diagnosis of a Monteggia lesion was not established. **B:** Radiograph at time of late diagnosis. Note the persistent ulnar bow and overgrowth of radius.

is associated with open reductions of the proximal radius. As such, the surgeon should first try closed reduction techniques with direct pressure. This can be facilitated with a small incision and use of an awl to translate the proximal radius. Another method is to introduce a blunt hemostat or K-wire into the fracture site and leverage the radial head onto the radial shaft similar to the Kapandji method used for distal radius fractures. Another method to effectuate reduction is to use an intramedullary K-wire of a titanium nail to rotate the fracture fragment back into alignment (known as the "Metaizeau technique"). Caution is needed when the method is attempted in patients with a proximal radius fracture and a dislocated elbow as attempts to impact the wire into the radial head is thwarted when the fragment cannot be contained by the unstable elbow joint. Regardless of the technique used to reduce the proximal radius, an intramedullary implant is an excellent method to stabilize the fracture for 3 to 4 weeks, at which time gentle elbow and forearm motion can be instituted.

TREATMENT OPTIONS FOR CHRONIC MONTEGGIA FRACTURE-DISLOCATIONS

A late-presenting, previously undetected dislocation of the radial head is not as uncommon as orthopaedic surgeons would prefer.[26,28,31,35,62,91,93] The diagnosis of an acute Monteggia fracture-dislocation is often missed by skilled radiologists, emergency room physicians, pediatricians, and orthopaedic surgeons, particularly when the ulnar injury is subtle or in the form of plastic deformation. Ideally, a chronic Monteggia, especially from failure to accurately diagnose the lesion acutely, would be a *never event*. The shape of the ulna in patients with a seemingly isolated dislocation of the radial head usually indicates persistent plastic deformation or malunion of the ulna and a traumatic etiology to the radial head dislocation (see Figs. 12-3 and 12-42).[71,81] Isolated radial head dislocations with remote trauma have also been mistaken for congenital radial head dislocations. Elbow radiographs or MRI can help distinguish

a chronic Monteggia lesion from congenital dislocation of the radial head. As noted previously, the shape of the radial head is concave in most chronic Monteggia lesions but is convex in congenital radial head dislocation. In congenital radial head dislocation, the capitellum is often hypoplastic which can serve as another distinguishing radiographic feature.

Chronic Monteggia lesions have been diagnosed as early as several weeks after injury for a misdiagnosed, isolated ulnar fracture; or years later because of progressive pain, restriction of motion, or extremity malalignment. Even a few weeks after injury, treatment becomes much more complicated than acute recognition and intervention. Proper recognition and appropriate treatment of a dislocated radial head at the time of injury can prevent the difficult problem of a chronic Monteggia lesion. When a previously undetected proximal radioulnar and radiocapitellar dislocation is encountered (Fig. 12-43), there

Figure 12-43. Chronic Monteggia lesion with a persistent anterior radial head dislocation and ossification of the displaced annular ligament.

is controversy regarding subsequent care. At present, there are limited levels of evidence and conflicting retrospective literature on this problem. Some reports indicate that the natural history of the untreated lesion is not problematic.[87] Fahey[36] suggested that although persistent dislocations can do well in the short term, problems arise over time, resulting in substantial patient morbidity. In fact, the majority of reports support the view that the natural history of persistent dislocation is not benign and is associated with restricted motion, deformity, functional impairment, pain, potential degenerative arthritis, and late neuropathy.[1,6,14,17,43,53,55,71] Kalamchi[55] reported pain, progressive valgus deformity, and restricted motion, especially loss of forearm rotation and elbow flexion. Tardy ulnar, median, and PIN palsy have been reported secondary to cubitus valgus and radial head dislocation in the setting of chronic Monteggia lesions.[1,6,50,73] Unless there is concern regarding the morphology of the radial head or capitellum (convex radial head, flattening of capitellum) that will prevent congruency of reduction, we believe that relatively early asymptomatic, or later symptomatic, patients with chronic Monteggia lesions are candidates for surgical reconstruction.

In more long-standing lesions, MRI can be obtained to further delineate cartilage quality and potential radiocapitellar and proximal radioulnar joint congruity. Patients with radial head enlargement or deformity, flattening of the capitellum, or joint arthrosis are not candidates for reconstruction (see Fig. 12-14). In these patients, surgical decompression by radial head excision or ulnar lengthening can be considered if pain does not resolve with nonoperative treatment, but these interventions may place the patient at risk of developing wrist pain with either ulnar lengthening or radial head excision; or progressive cubitus valgus with radial head excision.

OPERATIVE TREATMENT OF CHRONIC MONTEGGIA FRACTURE-DISLOCATIONS

Descriptions of surgical reconstruction for pediatric chronic Monteggia lesions have been variable and include annular ligament repair or reconstruction alone,[46] ulnar osteotomy alone,[54,64] combined ulnar osteotomy with annular ligament repair or reconstruction,[28,51,85] and radial osteotomy.[27] The relative merit of each surgical technique has not been well defined and is likely to vary by patient and lesion. However, almost every expert advocates for an ulnar realignment osteotomy when reconstructing a chronic Monteggia lesion. The principal controversy revolves around whether an annular ligament reconstruction should be performed in addition to the ulnar osteotomy. The original technique for delayed open reduction of the radial head and annular ligament reconstruction for chronic Monteggia fracture-dislocations is attributed to Bell Tawse,[13] who used the surgical approach described by Boyd (see Fig. 12-31).[19] Other surgical approaches have been developed. Nakamura et al.[85] reported long-term clinical and radiographic outcomes in patients undergoing ulnar osteotomy with annular ligament reconstruction. At a mean follow-up of 7 years, they reported excellent results in 19 out of 22 patients. Of concern, the radial head remained subluxated in five patients at the time of latest

follow-up. Radiographic results did deteriorate when surgical reconstruction was performed more than 3 years after injury or in patients above 12 years of age. Zheng et al.[140] reviewed 52 patients with reconstruction of chronic Monteggia lesions. Seventy-five percent had sustained anatomic restoration of radiocapitellar joint and significant improvement in elbow and forearm motion, especially flexion and supination. Of the nine patients with early redislocation, six had successful early revision surgery with uncomplicated long-term outcome. Of note, those with annular ligament repair did better long term than those with reconstruction or not having surgery on the annular ligament. Similar to our ulnar osteotomy in conjunction with annular ligament repair presented here, Baydar et al.[11] presented on 14 patients with annular ligament repair and ulnar osteotomy. Twelve of 14 had excellent results. Systematic review and meta-analysis by Tan et al.[125] indicate most important factors in reconstruction were ulnar osteotomy and absence of a radiocapitellar pin.

Indications/Contraindications

Operative Treatment of Chronic Monteggia Fracture-Dislocations:
INDICATIONS/CONTRAINDICATIONS

Indications

- Symptomatic patients with a chronic Monteggia lesion (indication)
- Asymptomatic patients with a chronic Monteggia lesion (relative indication), especially if detected early

Contraindications

- Radial head enlargement and convex deformity
- Flattening of the capitellum joint arthrosis

Treatment indications have ranged from offering all patients with chronic Monteggia lesions surgical correction to limiting intervention to patients with pain, restricted motion, and functional disability. That wide spectrum of expert opinions makes individual case decisions difficult for patients, parents, and clinicians. Fowles et al.[40] suggested that reconstruction provides the best results in patients who have had a dislocation for 3 to 6 months or less. They also reported successful relocations up to 3 years after injury. Freedman et al.[42] advocated for surgical reconstruction up to 6 years after injury. Throughout the literature, the appropriate age for radial head reduction seems to be younger than 10 to 12 years.[120] Hirayama et al.[49] suggested that the reduction of a chronically dislocated radial head should be avoided if there is significant deformation of the radiocapitellar joint architecture including permanent irregularity of the radial head or flattening of the capitellum (see Fig. 12-14). Seel and Peterson[113] suggested that the age of the patient and the duration of the dislocation are unimportant. Their criteria for surgical repair were (1) normal concave radial head articular surface and (2) shape and contour of the ulna and radius deformity that is correctable by osteotomy. They treated seven patients ranging in age from 5 to 13 years for chronic dislocations that had been

Figure 12-44. Bell Tawse reconstruction. The central slip of the triceps is used to reconstruct an annular ligament in Bell Tawse reconstruction. The direction of stability is posterior (*thick arrow*).

present from 3 months to 7 years. All seven were fully active with no elbow pain or instability at an average of 4 years after surgery.

Zheng et al.[140] noted significant improvements in motion, function, and restoration of anatomic alignment in the majority of 52 pediatric patients with chronic Monteggia lesions treated surgically.

Although they recommended surgical treatment of chronic Monteggia lesions in children because of the long-term sequelae, Rodgers et al.[109] cautioned that the results of reconstructive procedures could be unpredictable and associated with a number of complications, including malunion of the ulnar shaft, recurrent radiocapitellar subluxation, and radial and ulnar neuropathy.

At present, most authors advocate surgical reconstruction of a chronic Monteggia (1) when the diagnosis is made early, (2) when there is preservation of the normal concave radial head and convex capitellum, (3) especially when there is progressive deformity (i.e., valgus), loss of motion and pain, and (4) when the patient and family are well aware of the concerns with operative reconstruction.

Annular Ligament Repair or Reconstruction

Most but not all authors advocate surgical repair or reconstruction of the annular ligament in conjunction with an ulnar osteotomy for a pediatric chronic Monteggia lesion.[28,51,85,109] Annular ligament repair or reconstruction without an osteotomy is very rarely indicated.[22] Kalamchi[55] restored stability after open reduction and osteotomy by utilizing the native annular ligament. The native ligament is generally present, even years later. The central opening can be dilated with a probe and/or surgical hemostat or by radial incisions. The annular ligament is then brought back over the radial head and down to its anatomic location on the neck before repair to the proximal ulna periosteum. Bell Tawse[13] used a strip of triceps tendon to reconstruct the annular ligament, as did Lloyd-Roberts[73] and Hurst and Dubrow.[53] Bell Tawse[13] used the central portion of the triceps tendon passed through a drill hole in the ulna and around the radial neck to stabilize the reduction and immobilized the elbow in a long-arm cast in extension (Fig. 12-44). Bucknill and Lloyd-Roberts[73] modified the Bell Tawse procedure by using the lateral portion of the triceps tendon, with a transcapitellar pin for stability. The elbow was immobilized in flexion. Hurst and Dubrow[53] used the central portion of the triceps tendon but carried the dissection of the periosteum

distally along the ulna to the level of the radial neck, which provided more stable fixation rather than stopping dissection at the olecranon as described by Bell Tawse.[13] They also used a periosteal tunnel rather than a drill hole for fixation of the tendinous strip to the ulna. Other authors have used other soft tissues for reconstruction, including the lacertus fibrosus, a strip of the forearm fascia (see Fig. 12-31),[117] palmaris longus free tendon graft,[134] and free fascia lata graft.[127]

Seel and Peterson[113] described the use of two holes drilled in the proximal ulna. The holes are placed at the original attachments of the annular ligament and allow repair of the annular ligament (frequently avulsed from one attachment and trapped within the joint) or reconstruction of the annular ligament with triceps tendon. This technique secures the radial head in its normal position from any dislocated position and allows osteotomy for correction of any accompanying deformity of the ulna and/or radius. Seel and Peterson[113] noted that the Bell Tawse procedure tends to pull the radius posterolaterally (Fig. 12-45A). A tight annular ligament reconstruction may constrict the neck of the radius, potentially limiting the growth of the radial neck ("notching") and reducing forearm rotation. Seel and Peterson[113] placed a single drill hole obliquely across the ulna to exit medially at the site of the medial attachment of the annular ligament on the coronoid process of the ulna (Fig. 12-45B). The tendon was routed through the tunnel, brought around the neck, and sutured to the lateral side of the ulna. With this construct, the direction of stability was posteromedial. The use of two drill holes to secure the annular ligament or other reconstructive

Figure 12-45. Schematic representation of annular ligament reconstruction techniques. **A:** The Bell Tawse reconstruction which results in a posteriorly directed force. **B:** The technique suggested by Seel and Peterson. In this technique, crossing drill holes are created at the anterior and posterior rim of the lesser sigmoid notch. The resulting reconstruction may improve stability of the radial head.

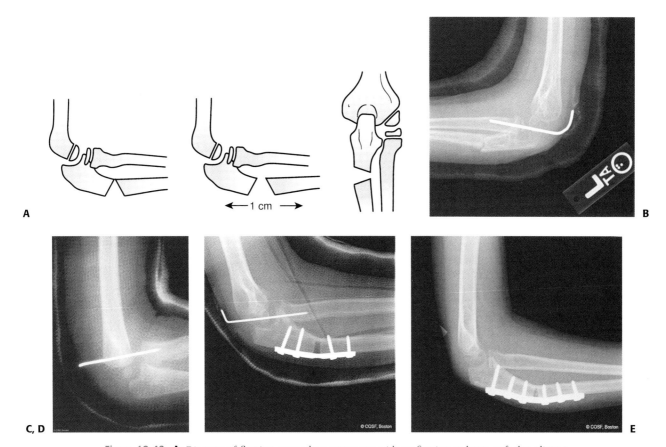

Figure 12-46. A: Diagram of floating open ulnar osteotomy without fixation or bone graft that aligns a reduced radial head. **B:** Similar ulnar osteotomy without fixation with radiocapitellar pin fixation in which the radial head is reduced. **C:** In a different case, however, the radial head was never reduced and the pin was placed without anatomic alignment. **D:** In this situation, a subsequent ulnar osteotomy was required including plate fixation without bone graft; annular ligament reconstruction and then protective radiocapitellar joint pinned anatomically for 4 weeks. **E:** Long-term follow-up with anatomic healing of the ulnar osteotomy and radial head reduction and ligament reconstruction.

graft at both normal attachments of the annular ligament on the ulna achieved a more normal posteromedial holding force on the neck of the radius. Alternatives to holes drilled in the bone are small-bone staples or bone-anchoring devices.

Ulnar Osteotomy

The majority of surgeons advocate an ulnar osteotomy, with or without ligament repair or reconstruction, for a chronic pediatric Monteggia lesion. Various types of osteotomies have been used to facilitate reduction of the radial head and prevent recurrent subluxation (Fig. 12-46). Kalamchi[55] reported using a "drill hole" ulnar osteotomy to obtain reduction of the radial head in two patients. Minimal periosteal stripping with this technique allowed the osteotomy to heal rapidly. Hirayama et al.[49] used a 1 cm distraction ulnar osteotomy approximately 5 cm distal to the tip of the olecranon with plate and screw fixation, but complications with loosening and plate breakage occurred. Mehta[79,80] used an osteotomy of the proximal ulna stabilized with bone graft. In neither series was annular ligament repair performed. Inoue and Shionoya[54] compared the results of simple corrective ulnar osteotomy in six patients with those of posterior angular (overcorrected) osteotomy in six others and found that better clinical outcomes were obtained with the overcorrected, angular osteotomy. Tajima and Yoshizu,[123] in a series of 23 neglected Monteggia fractures, found that the best results were obtained by opening wedge osteotomy of the proximal ulna without ligament reconstruction. Exner[35] reported that in patients with chronic dislocation of the radial head after missed type I Monteggia lesions, reduction was successfully obtained with ulnar corticotomy and gradual lengthening and angulation of the ulna using an external fixator. Liu et al.[72] compared gradual distraction lengthening and angulation correction of the ulnar deformity with reduction of the radial head over time; with acute correction and reduction. Ninety-two percent of the gradual correction and reduction patients had an excellent outcome compared with 50% with acute reduction by their techniques. Another option for chronic type IV Monteggia lesion is a shortening osteotomy of the radius, usually indicated for angulation of the radius without angulation of the ulna. Other surgeons have advocated performing corrective ulnar osteotomies stabilized by external fixation.[18,75]

Ulnar Osteotomy and Open Reduction of the Radial Capitellar and Radioulnar Joints With Annular Ligament Reconstruction

In patients younger than 10 to 12 years of age with delayed diagnosis of a Monteggia lesion, reduction and stabilization of the radial head to its anatomic relationship with the capitellum is indicated if the radial head remains concave. Even though the child may do well in the short term without reduction of the radial head, problems usually develop in adolescence or adulthood when progressive instability, pain, weakness of the forearm, and restriction of motion are likely. Appropriate discussion with the patient and family regarding the risks and complications of surgery is performed. This is not an operation for the inexperienced surgeon or uninformed patient and family. We perform an ulnar osteotomy and open reduction of the radiocapitellar and proximal radioulnar joints with annular ligament repair (preferred) or reconstruction (as needed).

Technique

> **✓ Ulnar Osteotomy and Open Reduction of the Radial Capitellar and Radioulnar Joints With Annular Ligament Reconstruction:**
> KEY SURGICAL STEPS

- ❏ An extensile curvilinear posterolateral incision is planned and used in the more complex and chronic lesions
- ❏ The midportion of the incision allows access to the radiocapitellar joint at the Kocher interval (between the anconeus and extensor carpi ulnaris)
- ❏ Incision extended proximally for identification of the radial nerve between the brachialis and brachioradialis if the radial head dislocation is markedly displaced or there is a PIN palsy; and for harvesting of the triceps fascia if required for annular ligament reconstruction
- ❏ Incision extended distally to allow access to the ulna for osteotomy between the extensor carpi ulnaris and the flexor carpi ulnaris
- ❏ Interval between the anconeus and extensor carpi ulnaris developed, the extensor–supinator mass can be elevated off of the anterior lateral epicondyle and lateral supracondylar if needed for visualization of the displaced annular ligament and radial head
- ❏ The elbow capsule incised anterior to the lateral ulnar collateral ligament in order to preserve the integrity of lateral ligamentous complex and ulnohumeral stability
- ❏ Pulvinar and synovitis are carefully debrided from the radiocapitellar joint to permit visualization of the radial head, annular ligament, and capitellum
- ❏ The lesser sigmoid notch should also be thoroughly debrided in order to permit reduction of the proximal radioulnar joint
- ❏ The annular ligament can generally be identified in an anterior, proximal position. Careful dissection and dilation of its aperture allows reconstitution of its typical ring shape. Rarely further dilation performed by making small radial incisions extending from the center toward the periphery but care must be taken not to overloosen the ligament
- ❏ At this stage, the surgeon must decide whether the native annular ligament can be reduced over the neck to provide desired soft tissue stability. Using the native annular ligament is preferred

- ❏ If the annular ligament can be salvaged, reduction over the radial head is performed
- ❏ If the ligament cannot be reduced over the radial head, the ligament may be incised along its posterior insertion (at or adjacent to the posterior rim of the lesser sigmoid notch) and repaired following reduction of the radial head. Or the native ligament needs to be excised and a local graft used
- ❏ If the annular ligament can be salvaged, the reduction of the radial head is evaluated with fluoroscopy and with direct inspection
- ❏ If there is anatomic restoration of radiocapitellar alignment with stability through full pronation and supination, then annular ligament repair alone may be sufficient (this is very unusual, typically ulnar osteotomy is required)
- ❏ If the annular ligament cannot be salvaged, its remnant is sharply excised in preparation for subsequent annular ligament reconstruction
- ❏ Annular ligament repair or reconstruction alone does not usually result in a congruent, stable radiocapitellar reduction due to the deforming force created by concomitant ulnar malunion and at times, biceps tendon foreshortening
- ❏ Opening wedge osteotomy of the ulna is normally required
- ❏ Opening wedge osteotomy of the ulna is usually performed at the apex of the malunion
- ❏ When the ulnar injury is characterized by plastic deformation, the osteotomy should be made proximal to the apex (closer to the elbow) in order to more effectively correct of radiocapitellar malalignment
- ❏ Temporary pinning of the radiocapitellar joint can help determine the size of the opening wedge osteotomy
- ❏ The radiocapitellar and proximal radioulnar joints are anatomically reduced and a K-wire is temporarily inserted across the radiocapitellar joint to stabilize the reduction
- ❏ Anatomic reduction of the radial head allows the ulnar osteotomy to open the necessary amount to maintain the reduction
- ❏ The osteotomy is then stabilized with appropriately contoured plate and screw fixation
- ❏ We prefer double-stacked one-third tubular plates in younger patients or a 2.7/3.5-mm dynamic compression plate dependent on the age and size of patient (Synthes, West Chester, PA)
- ❏ The radiocapitellar wire is then removed and fluoroscopy should be used to confirm stable reduction of the radial head
  - The annular ligament is repaired to the periosteum of the ulna or through drill holes in the ulna as needed
- ❏ If the annular ligament was not salvageable, a reconstruction should be performed with triceps fascia
- ❏ The extensor–supinator fascia may be used as an alternative
- ❏ Limited prophylactic fasciotomies of the volar and dorsal forearm compartments are performed to minimize risk of postoperative compartment syndrome
- ❏ Final orthogonal fluoroscopy imaging should be obtained to confirm stable reduction of the radiocapitellar and proximal radioulnar joints

The surgical approach may need to be extensile (Fig. 12-47B). The posterolateral skin incision is curvilinear in outline to allow for proximal triceps tendon harvesting, if necessary; radial nerve identification and decompression if indicated; and distally for an ulnar opening wedge osteotomy. Initially, only the midportion is opened.

The Kocher interval (between the anconeus and extensor carpi ulnaris) interval is used to expose the radiocapitellar joint. The joint exposure is carried proximal with elevation of the

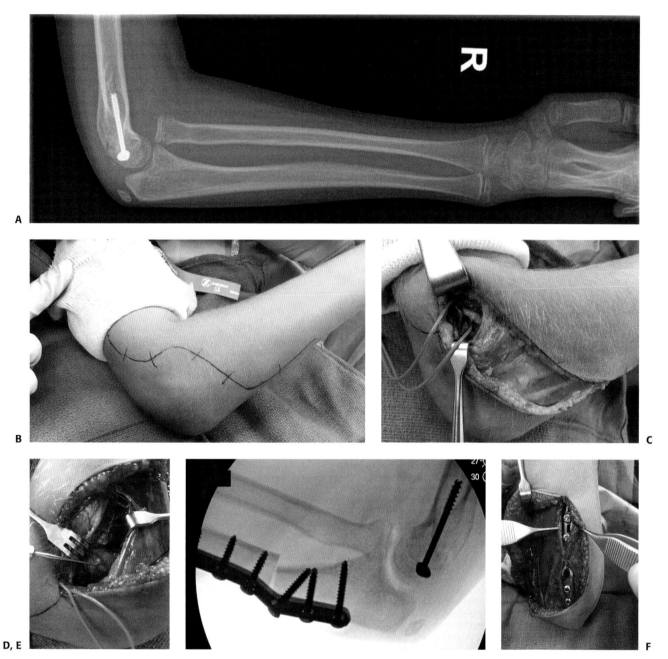

Figure 12-47. Authors' preferred technique for chronic Monteggia reconstruction. **A:** Lateral forearm radiograph in an 8-year-old girl with a chronic Bado type I Monteggia lesion, a prior history of ipsilateral medial epicondyle fracture that underwent open reduction and internal fixation. Note the positive ulnar bow sign with associated anterior dislocation of the radial head. **B:** Extensile incision for annular ligament reconstruction and ulnar osteotomy. **C:** Radial nerve identified and tagged in the interval between the brachialis and the brachioradialis. **D:** The annular ligament was identified and was dilated to allow delivery of the radial head through the aperture of the ligament. A nerve hook was used to reduce the annular ligament into its native position. Ulnar opening wedge osteotomy is performed proximal to the apex of the deformity, which is recommended in cases of plastic deformation to best facilitate reduction of the radial head. **E:** Fixation is achieved with contoured double-stacked one-third tubular plates. **F:** Limited prophylactic forearm fasciotomies are performed to minimize potential for compartment syndrome and to facilitate closure of the periosteum and fascia over the hardware.

extensor–supinator mass and capsule as a single tissue plane off the anterior aspect of the lateral epicondyle and the lateral supracondylar ridge. This improves visualization of the elbow joint. The radial head is usually dislocated anteriorly and superiorly with a wall of interposed capsule and displaced annular ligament blocking reduction. Pulvinar and synovitis are thoroughly debrided from the elbow joint. Particular attention is paid to a thorough debridement of the proximal radioulnar joint to allow the radial head to fit anatomically into place once reduced. At this stage, a decision needs to be made if the native annular ligament can be salvaged (see Fig. 12-47D). It almost always can and is preferred. There is a central perforation in the capsular and ligamentous wall that separates the dislocated radial head from the joint. This perforation indicates the site of the opening of the annular ligament. Dilation with curved elevators or small retractors is used to enlarge this opening. This usually enables the native annular ligament to be reduced over the radial neck with a tight fit. Rarely small radial incisions extending from the center outward are made to enable reduction. Again, you want the annular ligament to fit tightly around the neck, as it does in its uninjured state, so be careful not to make radial incisions too broadly and lessen the tension. Capsular adhesions are removed from the radial head to assist in reduction of the radial head and neck back into the joint. There will be some eccentricity and enlargement to the radial head due to its chronic dislocation. The native ligament usually detaches from the ulna with a large periosteal sleeve (the site of ossification on the radiographs of a chronic Monteggia lesion (see Fig. 12-43), and this is the desired site for suture reattachment to the ulna of the repaired ligament. If the native ligament cannot be used, and most of the time it can, then it is thoroughly debrided in preparation for harvesting of triceps fascia for ligament reconstruction.

In situations where the radial head is dislocated very anteriorly in a long-standing chronic state, or there is a PIN palsy, the incision is carried more proximal for identification and protection of the nerve. The radial nerve is identified proximally between the brachialis and brachioradialis (see Fig. 12-47C). Distal dissection of the nerve is performed to its motor (PIN) and sensory branches (see Fig. 12-23). In general, the PIN is adherent to the dislocated radial head. The nerves are mobilized and protected throughout the remainder of the reconstruction.

A radial head reduction is then attempted. The reduction is scrutinized for congruity between the radial head and the capitellum. If this is satisfactory, ligamentous repair or reconstruction alone can be done. This is exceedingly unusual. Most often the annular ligament repair comes after the ulnar osteotomy. If the radius cannot be reduced, or stay stable throughout pronation and supination, then an ulnar osteotomy is made either at the site of maximal deformity, or proximal at the metaphyseal–diaphyseal junction. A too-distal osteotomy may be insufficient for correction and stability (Fig. 12-48). When the ulnar injury is characterized by plastic deformation, the osteotomy can be made proximal to the apex of the deformity and closer to the

elbow to more effectively correct of radiocapitellar malalignment. Subperiosteal dissection of the ulna is performed at the planned osteotomy site. An opening wedge osteotomy is made with a laminar spreader to allow the radial head to align itself with the capitellum without pressure (see Fig. 12-46). Partial overcorrection of the ulnar alignment is the goal. A clever way to do this is to anatomically pin the radiocapitellar joint and allow the ulnar osteotomy to open the necessary amount for this reduction (Fig. 12-49). When reduced anatomically, the ulnar osteotomy is then fixed partially proximally and distally with contoured plate(s) and screws. The plate can be extraperiosteal proximal and distal to the osteotomy to maximize stability and promote healing without bone grafting. Further testing of a complete stable arc of rotation of the radial head is performed to ensure that the correct level and degree of osteotomy were obtained to maintain radiocapitellar and radioulnar alignment. If a temporary radiocapitellar pin was used, it is removed for this testing. If correct, the fixation is completed. No bone graft is used, and the periosteum is repaired. We prefer fixation with either 2.7 compression or 3.5 double-stacked one-third tubular plates in small children; and 3.5 dynamic compression plates in larger children (Synthes, West Chester, PA). Other standard fixation systems can be used depending on your preference and facility. Matching patient size and age to the implant choice is important regardless of which device is used. External fixation can also be used if that is your preference (see Fig. 12-48). Regardless of strategy and techniques, correction of the ulnar deformity and stable reduction of the radial head must be achieved for a successful outcome.

At this stage, the annular ligament repair or reconstruction is completed. Some authors have demonstrated repositioning of the annular ligament as an option.[76] If the native ligament is used, and it usually is in situations that are 2 years or less out from injury, then nonabsorbable braided sutures are placed in the annular ligament and the ligament is repaired through ulnar periosteal tunnels. None of the annular ligament sutures are tightened until all are placed. If reconstruction is necessary, an 8- to 10-cm strip of triceps fascia is developed from proximal to distal, carefully elevating the periosteum from the proximal ulna down to the level of the radial neck. Over the olecranon apophysis, this dissection will be delicate so as not to inadvertently amputate the fascia. The strip of tendon is then passed through the periosteum, around the radial neck, and then brought back and sutured to itself and the ulnar periosteum. The passage and securing in the periosteum are similar in design to the drill holes advocated by Seel and Peterson.[113] At this stage, the radial head and capitellum alignment should be anatomic throughout full rotation. Final closure involves repair of the capsule and extensor–supinator origin back to the lateral epicondylar region of the humerus. Final radiographs and fluoroscopic testing of a stable arc of motion in both flexion–extension and pronation–supination planes are gently tested before completion of closure. Prophylactic volar and dorsal forearm fasciotomies are carefully

Figure 12-48. A: Intraoperative photograph after open reduction and repair of annular ligament. The radiocapitellar joint is still subluxed. **B:** Next step is ulnar osteotomy to anatomically reduce radiocapitellar joint. **C:** External fixation used for maintaining alignment of ulnar osteotomy and radial head reduction.

Figure 12-49. A: After completion of the ulnar osteotomy, the radial head can be anatomically reduced with the respect to the capitellum and the lesser sigmoid notch. As seen in this radiograph, the radiocapitellar joint can be temporarily pinned, which allows the ulnar osteotomy to open to the necessary amount to maintain the reduction. The ulnar osteotomy should then be stabilized with contoured plates and screws. The temporary wire is then removed so that fluoroscopy can be used to confirm stability of the reduction. Annular ligament reconstruction is performed in the same surgery. **B:** Radiographs of the elbow 6 months after ulnar osteotomy and annular ligament repair demonstrate a healed osteotomy and anatomic reduction of the radiocapitellar joint.

performed through the original incision with elevation of the skin and subcutaneous tissues and a long tenotomy scissors. Final inspection of the radial nerve is performed before skin closure.

Radiocapitellar or radioulnar pin fixation is rarely needed postoperatively if the osteotomy and soft tissue repair tension are correct. As mentioned, at times, pin fixation is used intraoperatively for temporary stability to get the corrective ulnar osteotomy correct; it is then removed to test the range of motion. If there is radial head deformity in very chronic reconstructions, pinning the joint is sometimes useful for 3 to 4 weeks postoperatively. In our experience, postoperative radiocapitellar or radioulnar pinning has been occasionally necessary in when chronic Monteggia reconstruction fails early and repeat surgery is performed; or when there is more than the usual radial head eccentric and enlarged deformity but reconstruction is attempted because the head is still concave. Then, the radiocapitellar joint is secured by passing a smooth, transcapitellar pin through the posterior aspect of the capitellum into the radial head and neck with the elbow at 90 degrees and the forearm in supination. A pin of sufficient size is mandatory to avoid pin failure[59]; a small pin may fatigue and break. An alternative technique to secure the reduction of the radius is transversely pinning the radius to the ulna.[69]

After wound closure, a bivalved long-arm cast is applied with the forearm in 60 to 90 degrees of supination, and the elbow is flexed 80 to 90 degrees. The cast is maintained for 4 to 6 weeks and is then changed to a removable bivalved cast to allow active motion, especially pronation and supination. Elbow flexion and extension return more rapidly than rotary motion of the forearm which may take up to 6 months to improve, with pronation possibly limited, though minimally, permanently.[108] The final desired result is not determined until radiographs are anatomic with full restoration of motion.

MANAGEMENT OF EXPECTED ADVERSE OUTCOMES AND UNEXPECTED COMPLICATIONS RELATED TO MONTEGGIA FRACTURE-DISLOCATIONS

Monteggia Fracture-Dislocations:
COMMON ADVERSE OUTCOMES AND COMPLICATIONS

- Chronic Monteggia lesion
- Acute radial nerve palsy or PIN palsy
- Tardy radial nerve palsy
- Acute ulnar nerve palsy
- Acute anterior interosseous nerve palsy
- Myositis ossificans
- Compartment syndrome

Chronic Monteggia Lesions

As discussed at length, the highest risk for poor outcome from a pediatric Monteggia lesion is either failure to recognize the fracture-dislocation in the acute setting; or,

undertreatment that fails to restore and maintain ulnar alignment along with stable radial head reduction. Both will result in a chronic Monteggia lesion. Ideally, these still present diagnostic failures someday will be never events, either by improved human or artificial intelligence reading of acute injury radiographs.

In addition, reconstruction of a chronic Monteggia lesion late carries with it risk of repeat subluxation or dislocation. This can occur up to 25% of the time. If it is an early operative failure, repeat surgery should be performed. Reasons for failure include foreshortened biceps tendon providing dislocating force; inadequate realignment of ulna by osteotomy; persistent soft tissue interposed in radiocapitellar and/or radioulnar joint(s); unrecognized plastic deformation of the radius; or a combination of factors. All of these are examples of the surgeon potentially not understanding the precise pathoanatomy of their patient with a chronic Monteggia. Three-dimensional imaging and modeling from CT scans and use of advanced MRI imaging may improve our understanding of each patient's deformity and identify those patients with a deformity that does not fit the expected.

NERVE INJURIES

Radial Nerve Injury

The literature reflects a 10% to 20% incidence of radial nerve injury, making it the most common complication associated with Monteggia fractures.[52] It is most commonly associated with type I and III injuries.[13,87] The PIN is most commonly injured because of its proximity to the radial head–neck and its intimate relation to the arcade of Frohse (see Fig. 12-23). The arcade may be thinner and therefore more pliable in children than in adults. In addition, the periosteum is much thicker in pediatric patients. This may account in part for the rapid resolution of the nerve injury in children. A radial nerve injury in a child is treated expectantly. Nerve function usually returns by 12 weeks after reduction, if not sooner.[119] A review of a series of pediatric Monteggia lesions[89] recommends waiting up to 6 months before intervention for a PIN injury. Most series report 100% resolution in both fractures treated promptly and those treated late.[1,6]

Two reports[83,117] of irreducible Monteggia fractures caused by interposition of the radial nerve posterior to the radial head documented return of function approximately 4 months after the nerve was replaced to its normal anatomic position and the radial head was reduced. Morris,[83] in cadaver studies, showed that significant anterior dislocation of the radial head and varus angulation of the elbow allowed the radial nerve to slide posterior to the radial head and, with subsequent reduction of the radial head, become entrapped. If a chronic reconstruction is undertaken in the presence of a persistent radial nerve lesion, it is highly recommended that radial nerve exploration and decompression be performed before joint debridement. Rodgers et al.[109] cited a partial nerve injury during similar circumstances that was then microscopically repaired with full recovery. Rang[102] acknowledged the same experience in an open educational forum.

Ulnar Nerve Injury

Bryan[21] reported one adult with an ulnar nerve lesion associated with a type II Monteggia lesion with spontaneous resolution. Stein et al.[119] reported three combined radial and ulnar nerve injuries, two of which underwent exploration and decompression for functional return of the nerve.

Median Nerve Injury

Median nerve injuries are uncommon with Monteggia fractures, but injury to the anterior interosseous nerve has been reported.[134] Stein et al.,[119] in their report specifically examining nerve injuries in Monteggia lesions, reported no median nerve deficits. Watson and Singer[134] reported entrapment of the main trunk of the median nerve in a greenstick ulnar fracture in a 6-year-old girl. Completion of the fracture was necessary for release of the nerve. At 6 months after surgery, there was full motor recovery but the sensation was slightly reduced in the tips of the index finger and thumb.

Tardy Radial Nerve Palsy

Tardy radial nerve palsy associated with radial head dislocation has been infrequently reported.[1,6,50,139] Although reported treatment has varied, excision of the radial head with exploration and neurolysis of the nerve generally produced good results,[1,6] whereas exploration of the nerve alone produced variable results.[50] Yamamoto et al.[139] combined radial head resection and nerve exploration with tendon transfers, producing good results in two patients.

Compartment Syndrome

Compartment syndrome has been noted to occur at a higher rate with Monteggia fracture-dislocations than even type III supracondylar humerus fractures cited by Kopriva et al.,[61] at 15% in their retrospective series of 59 patients. Those patients with preoperative deficits and those undergoing IM fixation of the radius in a Monteggia equivalent lesion had a higher rate of acute compartment syndrome.

PERIARTICULAR OSSIFICATION

Two patterns of ossification after Monteggia fracture-dislocations have been noted radiographically: ossification around the radial head and myositis ossificans. Ossification around the radial head and neck[13,52] appears as a thin ridge of bone in a caplike distribution and may be accompanied by other areas resembling sesamoid bones. This typically resorbs with time. Ossification may also occur in the area of the annular ligament,[32] including in a chronic Monteggia with a displaced annular ligament (see Fig. 12-43). Elbow function generally is not affected by the formation of these lesions[13,52] as long as the radial head and neck are anatomically reduced.

The other form of ossification is true myositis ossificans, reported to occur in approximately 3% of elbow injuries and 7% of Monteggia lesions in adults and children.[88]

Myositis ossificans has a good prognosis in patients younger than 15 years of age, appearing at 3 to 4 weeks after injury and resolving in 6 to 8 months. Its occurrence is related to the severity of the initial injury, association with a fractured radial head, the number of remanipulations during treatment, and passive motion of the elbow during the postoperative period.[88]

SUMMARY, CONTROVERSIES, AND FUTURE DIRECTIONS RELATED TO MONTEGGIA FRACTURE-DISLOCATIONS

Adherence to several fundamental principles helps ensure a good outcome after Monteggia fracture-dislocations in children:

- With a high index of suspicion and careful radiographic evaluation, acute Monteggia injuries can be accurately diagnosed. Evaluation of radiocapitellar alignment requires AP and true lateral views of the elbow. All forearm fractures require careful inspection of the proximal radioulnar joint and the radiocapitellar joint before treatment.
- The radiocapitellar line must be anatomic in all views.
- If the radial head is dislocated, always look for ulnar fracture or plastic deformation. Conversely, if the ulna is fractured or plastically deformed, always look for a radial head subluxation or dislocation.
- In addition, always look for a fracture or plastic deformation of the radius.
- Stability of the ulnar reduction is required to maintain reduction of the radial head. Stability may be inherent to the fracture pattern (plastic deformation or incomplete fractures) or achieved by internal fixation (intramedullary fixation for short oblique and transverse fractures; plate and screw fixation for long oblique and comminuted fractures).
- Radial head reduction as confirmed by an intact radiocapitellar line must be achieved by open or closed means. The reduction must be stable and this usually is the result of a restoration of ulnar length, alignment, and stability.
- If the radial head is irreducible or unstable, this is either due to an inadequate ulnar fracture reduction; failure to recognize and reduce a radius fracture; or interposed soft tissue in the joint. If the bones are aligned and reduced, removal of interposed soft tissue is required. An annular ligament repair or reconstruction may be required.
- Treatment of an acute Monteggia lesion is more straightforward and much more successful than reconstruction of a chronic Monteggia lesion.
- Reconstruction of a chronic Monteggia lesion is not an operation for the uninitiated. There is a high risk of recurrent or residual radial head subluxation. Use of three-dimensional imaging, models, and templated osteotomies and hardware is indicated for more complex deformities.
- Acute Monteggia lesions if recognized promptly and treated as outlined can heal without problems and prevent complex chronic Monteggia lesions that have a high risk for long-term problems.

Annotated References

Reference	Annotation
Bado JL. *The Monteggia Lesion.* Charles C Thomas; 1962.	The original classification system that has stood the test of time.
Boyd HB, Boals JC. The Monteggia lesion. A review of 159 cases. *Clin Orthop Relat Res.* 1969;66:94–100.	Large early case series of this fracture pattern.
Foran I, Upasani VV, Walace CD, et al. Acute pediatric Monteggia fractures: a conservative approach to stabilization. *J Pediatr Orthop.* 2017;37(6):e335–e341.	Multicenter study demonstrating safety of a trial of conservative treatment for Monteggia fractures.
Inoue G, Shionoya K. Corrective ulnar osteotomy for malunited anterior Monteggia lesions in children. 12 patients followed for 1–12 years. *Acta Orthop Scand.* 1998;69:73–76.	Comparison of simple corrective ulna osteotomy with posterior angular osteotomy for chronic Monteggia lesions; finding the patients with angular osteotomies had better outcomes.
Kopriva J, Awowale J, Whiting P, et al. Compartment syndrome in operatively managed pediatric Monteggia fractures and equivalents. *J Pediatr Orthop.* 2020;40(8):387–395.	Acute compartment syndrome risk is very high, at 15%, in pediatric Monteggia lesions, especially with preoperative neurovascular injuries.
Leonidou A, Pagkalos J, Lepetsos P, et al. Pediatric Monteggia fractures: a single-center study of the management of 40 patients. *J Pediatr Orthop.* 2012;32(4):352–356.	Large single-center retrospective study with outcomes reported using Bruce–Harvey–Wilson scoring system demonstrating excellent outcomes with a conservative approach.
Letts M, Locht R, Wiens J. Monteggia fracture-dislocations in children. *J Bone Joint Surg Br.* 1985;67:724–727.	Alternate classification system for Monteggia fractures based both on direction of radial head dislocation and the type of ulnar fracture.
Lightdale-Miric NR, Obana KK, Fan BB, et al. Exposed intramedullary fixation produces similar outcomes to buried fixation for acute pediatric Monteggia fractures. *J Pediatr Orthop.* 2023;43(3):129–134.	Comparison of outcomes from exposed versus buried IM rods for acute Monteggia care with similar functional outcomes, no difference in infection or wound complications, and markedly less OR for exposed rod removal.
Ramski DE, Hennrikus WP, Bae DS, et al. Pediatric Monteggia fractures: a multicenter examination of treatment strategy and early clinical and radiographic results. *J Pediatr Orthop.* 2015;35(2):115–120.	Retrospective study at two large institutions analyzing the following treatment protocol: closed reduction for greenstick fractures, intramedullary fixation for transverse/short oblique fractures, and ORIF for long oblique/comminuted fractures.
Ring D, Waters PM. Operative fixation of Monteggia fractures in children. *J Bone Joint Surg Br.* 1996;78:734–739.	Large case series describing the importance of the characteristics of the ulna fracture influencing the treatment choice.
Roper B, Parikh S, Haidar L, et al. Outcomes after operative treatment of pediatric Monteggia fracture-dislocations: comparison between open and closed injuries. *J Pediatr Orthop.* 2022;42(7):361–366.	Open fractures have higher rates of complications and worse patient-reported outcomes by QuickDASH.
Tawse AJB. The treatment of malunited anterior Monteggia fractures in children. *J Bone Joint Surg Br.* 1965;47:718–723.	
Zheng ET, Waters PM, Vuillermin CB, et al. Surgical reconstruction of missed Monteggia lesions in children. *J Pediatr Orthop.* 2020;40(10):e916–e921.	Large series of chronic Monteggia reconstructions by open annular ligament repair (preferred) or reconstruction (less positive outcomes compared to repair) and ulnar osteotomy. Results were excellent in 75% and half the immediate redislocations could be fixed by immediate second surgery.

REFERENCES

1. Adams JP, Rizzoli HV. Tardy radial and ulnar nerve palsy: a case report. *J Neurosurg.* 1959;16:342–344.
2. Agarwal A. Type IV Monteggia fracture in a child. *Can J Surg.* 2008;51(2):E44–E45.
3. Almquist EE, Gordon LH, Blue AI. Congenital dislocation of the head of the radius. *J Bone Joint Surg Am.* 1969;51:1118–1127.
4. Anderson HJ. Monteggia fractures. *Adv Orthop Surg.* 1989;4:201–204.
5. Arazi M, Oğün TC, Kapicioğlu MI. The Monteggia lesion and ipsilateral supracondylar humerus and distal radius fractures. *J Orthop Trauma.* 1999;13(1):60–63.
6. Austin R. Tardy palsy of the radial nerve from a Monteggia fracture. *Injury.* 1976;7(3):202–204.
7. Babb A, Carlson WO. Monteggia fractures: beware! *S D J Med.* 2005;58(7):283–285.
8. Bado JL. La lesion de Monteggia. *Intermedica Sarandi.* 1958;328.
9. Bado JL. *The Monteggia Lesion.* Charles C Thomas; 1962.
10. Bado JL. The Monteggia lesion. *Clin Orthop Relat Res.* 1967;50:71–86.
11. Baydar M, Öztürk K, Orman O, et al. Use of corrective ulnar osteotomy and radial head relocation into preserved annular ligament in the treatment of radiocapitellar instability secondary to pediatric chronic Monteggia fracture-dislocation. *J Hand Surg Am.* 2022;47(5):481.e1–481.e9.
12. Beaty JH. Fractures and dislocations about the elbow in children: section on Monteggia fractures. *AAOS Instr Course Lect.* 1991;40:373–384.
13. Bell Tawse AJ. The treatment of malunited anterior Monteggia fractures in children. *J Bone Joint Surg Br.* 1965;47:718–723.
14. Best TN. Management of old unreduced Monteggia fracture dislocations of the elbow in children. *J Pediatr Orthop* 1994;14:193–199.
15. Bhandari N, Jindal P. Monteggia lesion in a child: variant of a Bado type-IV lesion. A case report. *J Bone Joint Surg Am.* 1996;78(8):1252–1255.
16. Biyani A. Ipsilateral Monteggia equivalent injury and distal radial and ulnar fracture in a child. *J Orthop Trauma.* 1994;8(5):431–433.
17. Blasier D, Trussell A. Ipsilateral radial head dislocation and distal fractures of both forearm bones in a child. *Am J Orthop (Belle Mead NJ).* 1995;24:498–500.
18. Bor N, Rubin G, Rozen N, Herzenberg JE. Chronic anterior monteggia lesions in children: report of 4 cases treated with closed reduction by ulnar osteotomy and external fixation. *J Pediatr Orthop.* 2015;35:7–10.
19. Boyd HB. Surgical exposure of the ulna and proximal one third of the radius through one incision. *Surg Gynecol Obstet.* 1940;71:86–88.

20. Boyd HB, Boals JC. The Monteggia lesion. A review of 159 cases. *Clin Orthop Relat Res.* 1969;66:94–100.
21. Bryan RS. Monteggia fracture of the forearm. *J Trauma.* 1971;11:992–998.
22. Cappellino A, Wolfe SW, Marsh JS. Use of a modified Bell Tawse procedure for chronic acquired dislocation of the radial head. *J Pediatr Orthop.* 1998;18(3):410–414.
23. Captier G, Canovas F, Mercier N, et al. Biometry of the radial head: biomechanical implications in pronation and supination. *Surg Radiol Anat.* 2002;24(5):295–301.
24. Cheung EV, Yao J. Monteggia fracture-dislocation associated with proximal and distal radioulnar joint instability. A case report. *J Bone Joint Surg Am.* 2009;91(4):950–954.
25. Dattani R, Patnaik S, Kantak A, Lal M. Distal humerus lateral condyle fracture and Monteggia lesions in a 3-year old child: a case report. *Acta Orthop Belg.* 2008;74(4):542–545.
26. David-West KS, Wilson NIL, Sherlock DA, Bennet GC. Missed Monteggia injuries. *Injury.* 2005;36(10):1206–1209.
27. De Boeck H. Radial neck osteolysis after annular ligament reconstruction. A case report. *Clin Orthop Relat Res.* 1997;342:94–98.
28. Degreef I, De Smet L. Missed radial head dislocations in children associated with ulnar deformation: treatment by open reduction and ulnar osteotomy. *J Orthop Trauma.* 2004;18(6):375–378.
29. Deshpande S, O'Doherty D. Type I Monteggia fracture dislocation associated with ipsilateral distal radial epiphyseal injury. *J Orthop Trauma.* 2001;15(5):373–375.
30. Devnani AS. Missed Monteggia fracture dislocation in children. *Injury.* 1997;28(2):131–133.
31. Dormans JP, Rang M. The problem of Monteggia fracture-dislocations in children. *Orthop Clin North Am.* 1990;21:251–256.
32. Earwaker J. Posttraumatic calcification of the annular ligament of the radius. *Skeletal Radiol.* 1992;21:149–154.
33. Edwards EG. The posterior Monteggia fracture. *Am Surg.* 1952;18:323–337.
34. Evans EM. Pronation injuries of the forearm, with special reference to the anterior Monteggia fracture. *J Bone Joint Surg Br.* 1949;31B(4):578–588.
35. Exner GU. Missed chronic anterior Monteggia lesion. Closed reduction by gradual lengthening and angulation of the ulna. *J Bone Joint Surg Br.* 2001;83(4):547–550.
36. Fahey JJ. Fractures of the elbow in children. *Instr Course Lect.* 1960;17:13–46.
37. Faundez AA, Ceroni D, Kaelin A. An unusual Monteggia type-I equivalent fracture in a child. *J Bone Joint Surg Br.* 2003;85(4):584–586.
38. Fernandez FF, Egenolf M, Carsten C, et al. Unstable diaphyseal fractures of both bones of the forearm in children: plate fixation versus intramedullary nailing. *Injury.* 2005;36(10):1210–1216.
39. Foran I, Upasani VV, Walace CD, et al. Acute pediatric Monteggia fractures: a conservative approach to stabilization. *J Pediatr Orthop.* 2017;37(6):e335–e341.
40. Fowles JV, Sliman N, Kassab MT. The Monteggia lesion in children. Fracture of the ulna and dislocation of the radial head. *J Bone Joint Surg Am.* 1983;65:1276–1282.
41. Frazier JL, Buschmann WR, Insler HP. Monteggia type I equivalent lesion: diaphyseal ulna and proximal radius fracture with a posterior elbow dislocation in a child. *J Orthop Trauma.* 1991;5:373–375.
42. Freedman L, Luk K, Leong JC. Radial head reduction after a missed Monteggia fracture: brief report. *J Bone Joint Surg Br.* 1988;70:846–847.
43. Givon U, Pritsch M, Levy O, et al. Monteggia and equivalent lesions. A study of 41 cases. *Clin Orthop Relat Res.* 1997;(337):208–215.
44. Givon U, Pritsch M, Yosepovich A. Monteggia lesion in a child: variant of a Bado type-IV lesion. A case report. *J Bone Joint Surg Am.* 1997;79(11):1753–1754.
45. Gleeson AP, Beattie TF. Monteggia fracture-dislocation in children. *J Accid Emerg Med.* 1994;11(3):192–194.
46. Gyr BM, Stevens PM, Smith JT. Chronic Monteggia fractures in children: outcome after treatment with the Bell-Tawse procedure. *J Pediatr Orthop B.* 2004;13(6):402–406.
47. Haddad ES, Manktelow AR, Sarkar JS. The posterior Monteggia: a pathological lesion? *Injury.* 1996;27:101–102.
48. Hart CM, Alswang J, Bram J, et al. Operative versus nonoperative management of acute pediatric Monteggia injuries with complete ulna fractures. *J Pediatr Orthop.* 2021;41(7):412–416.
49. Hirayama T, Takemitsu Y, Yagihara K, Mikita A. Operation for chronic dislocation of the radial head in children. *J Bone Joint Surg Br.* 1987;69:639–642.
50. Holst-Nielson F, Jensen V. Tardy posterior interosseus nerve palsy as a result of an unreduced radial head dislocation in Monteggia fractures: a report of two cases. *J Hand Surg Am.* 1984;9:572–575.
51. Hui JHP, Sulaiman AR, Lee HC, et al. Open reduction and annular ligament reconstruction with fascia of the forearm in chronic Monteggia lesions in children. *J Pediatr Orthop.* 2005;25(4):501–506.
52. Hume AC. Anterior dislocation of the head of the radius associated with undisplaced fracture of olecranon in children. *J Bone Joint Surg Br.* 1957;39-B:508–512.
53. Hurst LC, Dubrow EN. Surgical treatment of symptomatic chronic radial head dislocation: a neglected Monteggia fracture. *J Pediatr Orthop.* 1983;3:227–230.
54. Inoue G, Shionoya K. Corrective ulnar osteotomy for malunited anterior Monteggia lesions in children. 12 patients followed for 1 to 12 years. *Acta Orthop Scand.* 1998;69:73–76.
55. Kalamchi A. Monteggia fracture-dislocation in children. Late treatment in two cases. *J Bone Joint Surg Am.* 1986;68:615–619.
56. Karachalios T, Smith EJ, Pearse MF. Monteggia equivalent injury in a very young patient. *Injury.* 1992;23:419–420.
57. Kay RM, Skaggs DL. The pediatric Monteggia fracture. *Am J Orthop (Belle Mead NJ).* 1998;27(9):606–609.
58. Kemnitz S, De Schrijver F, De Smet L. Radial head dislocation with plastic deformation of the ulna in children. A rare and frequently missed condition. *Acta Orthop Belg.* 2000;66(4):359–362.
59. King RE. Treating the persistent symptomatic anterior radial head dislocation. *J Pediatr Orthop.* 1983;3:623–624.
60. Kloen P, Rubel IF, Farley TD, et al. Bilateral Monteggia fractures. *Am J Orthop (Belle Mead NJ).* 2003;32(2):98–100.
61. Kopriva J, Awowale J, Whiting P, et al. Compartment syndrome in operatively managed pediatric Monteggia fractures and equivalents. *J Pediatr Orthop.* 2020;40(8):387–395.
62. Koslowsky TC, Mader K, Wulke AP, et al. Operative treatment of chronic Monteggia lesion in younger children: a report of three cases. *J Shoulder Elbow Surg.* 2006;15(1):119–121.
63. Kristiansen B, Eriksen AF. Simultaneous type II Monteggia lesion and fracture separation of the lower radial epiphysis. *Injury.* 1986;17:51–52.
64. Lädermann A, Ceroni D, Lefèvre Y, et al. Surgical treatment of missed Monteggia lesions in children. *J Child Orthop.* 2007;1(4):237–242.
65. Landin LA. Fracture patterns in children. *Acta Paediatr Scand Suppl.* 1983;54:192.
66. Lascombes P, Prevot J, Ligier JN, et al. Elastic stable intramedullary nailing in forearm shaft fractures in children: 85 cases. *J Pediatr Orthop.* 1990;10:167–171.
67. Leonidou A, Pagkalos J, Lepetsos P, et al. Pediatric Monteggia fractures: a single-center study of the management of 40 patients. *J Pediatr Orthop.* 2012;32(4):352–356.
68. Letta C, Schmied M, Haller A, Rindlisbacher A. Combined Monteggia and Galeazzi lesions of the forearm: a rare injury. *Unfallchirurg.* 2012;115(11):1034–1037.
69. Letts M, Locht R, Wiens J. Monteggia fracture-dislocations in children. *J Bone Joint Surg Br.* 1985;67:724–727.
70. Lightdale-Miric NR, Obana KK, Fan BB, et al. Exposed intramedullary fixation produces similar outcomes to buried fixation for acute pediatric Monteggia fractures. *J Pediatr Orthop.* 2023;43(3):129–134.
71. Lincoln TL, Mubarak SJ. "Isolated" traumatic radial-head dislocation. *J Pediatr Orthop.* 1994;14:454–457.
72. Liu Y, Shi W, Li Y, et al. Ulnar osteotomy and monolateral external fixator for the treatment of chronic Monteggia fractures in children: comparison between gradual and acute radial head reduction. *J Pediatr Orthop B.* 2023;32(6):583–592.
73. Lloyd-Roberts GC, Bucknill TM. Anterior dislocation of the radial head in children: aetiology, natural history, and management. *J Bone Joint Surg Br.* 1977;59-B:402–407.
74. Louahem D, Jeandel C, Aldugman T, et al. Closed reduction by trans-physealantegrade elastic stable intramedullary nailing in acute pediatric Monteggia fractures: a report of 22 cases. *J Pediatr Orthop B.* 2022;31(1):43–49.
75. Lu X, Kun Wang Y, Zhang J, et al. Management of missed Monteggia fractures with ulnar osteotomy, open reduction, and dual-socket external fixation. *J Pediatr Orthop.* 2013;33(4):398–402.
76. Lu X, Yan G, Wang Y, et al. Repositioning of the annular ligament in the management of missed Monteggia fracture. *J Pediatr Orthop.* 2017;37(1):20–22.
77. Luhmann SJ, Gordon JE, Schoenecker PL. Intramedullary fixation of unstable both-bone forearm fractures in children. *J Pediatr Orthop.* 1998;18(4):451–456.
78. Maeda H, Yoshida K, Doi R, Omori O. Combined Monteggia and Galeazzi fractures in a child: a case report and review of the literature. *J Orthop Trauma.* 2003;17(2):128–131.
79. Mehta SD. Flexion osteotomy of ulna for untreated Monteggia fracture in children. *Ind J Surg.* 1985;47:15–19.
80. Mehta SD. Missed Monteggia fracture. *J Bone Joint Surg Br.* 1993;75:337.
81. Miles KA, Finlay DB. Disruption of the radiocapitellar line in the normal elbow. *Injury.* 1989;20:365–367.
82. Monteggia GB. *Instituzioni Chirurgiche.* Maspero; 1814.
83. Morris AH. Irreducible Monteggia lesion with radial nerve entrapment. A case report. *J Bone Joint Surg Am.* 1974;56:1744–1746.
84. Mullick S. The lateral Monteggia fracture. *J Bone Joint Surg Am.* 1977;59:543–545.
85. Nakamura K, Hirachi K, Uchiyama S, et al. Long-term clinical and radiographic outcomes after open reduction for missed Monteggia fracture-dislocations in children. *J Bone Joint Surg Am.* 2009;91(6):1394–1404.
86. Nakashima H, Kondo K, Saka K. Type II Monteggia lesion with fracture-separation of the distal physis of the radius. *Am J Orthop (Belle Mead NJ).* 2000;29(9):717–719.
87. Naylor A. Monteggia fractures. *Br J Surg.* 1942;29:323.
88. Neviaser RJ, LeFevre GW. Irreducible isolated dislocation of the radial head: a case report. *Clin Orthop Relat Res.* 1971;80:72–74.
89. Olney BW, Menelaus MB. Monteggia and equivalent lesions in childhood. *J Pediatr Orthop.* 1989;9:219–223.
90. Oner FC, Diepstraten AF. Treatment of chronic posttraumatic dislocation of the radial head in children. *J Bone Joint Surg Br.* 1993;75:577–581.
91. Osamura N, Ikeda K, Hagiwara N, Tomita K. Posterior interosseous nerve injury complicating ulnar osteotomy for a missed Monteggia fracture. *Scand J Plast Reconstr Surg Hand Surg.* 2004;38(6):376–378.
92. Ovesen O, Brok KE, Arreskøv J, Bellstrøm T. Monteggia lesions in children and adults: an analysis of etiology and long-term results of treatment. *Orthopedics.* 1990;13(5):529–534.
93. Papandrea R, Waters PM. Posttraumatic reconstruction of the elbow in the pediatric patient. *Clin Orthop Relat Res.* 2000;(370):115–126.
94. Parsch K. Die Morote-Drahtung bei proximalen und mittleren Unterarm Schaft Frakturen des Kindes. *Operat Orthop Traumatol.* 1990;2:245–255.
95. Pavel A, Pitman JM, Lance EM, Wade PA. The posterior Monteggia fracture: a clinical study. *J Trauma.* 1965;5:185–199.
96. Penrose JH. The Monteggia fracture with posterior dislocation of the radial head. *J Bone Joint Surg Br.* 1951;33-B:65–73.
97. Powell RS, Bowe JA. Ipsilateral supracondylar humerus fracture and Monteggia lesion: a case report. *J Orthop Trauma.* 2002;16(10):737–740.
98. Price CT, Scott DS, Kurzner ME, Flynn JC. Malunited forearm fracture in children. *J Pediatr Orthop.* 1990;10:705–712.
99. Pugh DM, Galpin RD, Carey TP. Intramedullary Steinmann pin fixation of forearm fractures in children. Long-term results. *Clin Orthop Relat Res.* 2000;(376):39–48.

100. Ramsey RH, Pedersen HE. The Monteggia fracture-dislocation in children. Study of 15 cases of ulnar-shaft fracture with radial-head involvement. *JAMA*. 1962;82:1091–1093.
101. Ramski DE, Hennrikus WP, Bae DS, et al. Pediatric Monteggia fractures: a multicenter examination of treatment strategy and early clinical and radiographic results. *J Pediatrc Orthop*. 2015;35(2):115–120.
102. Rang M. *The Story of Orthopaedics*. Saunders; 2000.
103. Ravessoud FA. Lateral condyle fracture and ipsilateral ulnar shaft fracture: Monteggia equivalent lesions. *J Pediatr Orthop*. 1985;5:364–366.
104. Reckling FW. Unstable fracture-dislocations of the forearm (Monteggia and Galeazzi lesions). *J Bone Joint Surg Am*. 1982;64:857–863.
105. Riccio AI, Blumberg TJ, Baldwin KD, Schoenecker JG. Intramedullary ulnar fixation for the treatment of Monteggia fracture. *JBJS Essent Surg Tech*. 2021;11(2):e19.00076.
106. Ring D, Jupiter JB, Waters PM. Monteggia fractures in children and adults. *J Am Acad Orthop Surg*. 1998;6(4):215–224.
107. Ring D, Waters PM. Operative fixation of Monteggia fractures in children. *J Bone Joint Surg Br*. 1996;78:734–739.
108. Rodgers WB, Smith BG. A type IV Monteggia injury with a distal diaphyseal radius fracture in a child. *J Orthop Trauma*. 1993;7:84–86.
109. Rodgers WB, Waters PM, Hall JE. Chronic Monteggia lesions in children. Complications and results of reconstruction. *J Bone Joint Surg Am*. 1996;78:1322–1329.
110. Rodríguez-Merchán EC. Pediatric fractures of the forearm. *Clin Orthop Relat Res*. 2005;(432):65–72.
111. Roper B, Parikh S, Haidar L, et al. Outcomes after operative treatment of pediatric Monteggia fracture-dislocations: comparison between open and closed injuries. *J Pediatr Orthop*. 2022;42(7):361–366.
112. Ruchelsman DE, Klugman JA, Madan SS, Chorney GS. Anterior dislocation of the radial head with fractures of the olecranon and radial neck in a young child: a Monteggia equivalent fracture-dislocation variant. *J Orthop Trauma*. 2005;19(6):425–428.
113. Seel MJ, Peterson HA. Management of chronic posttraumatic radial head dislocation in children. *J Pediatr Orthop*. 1999;19:306–312.
114. Singh AP, Dhammi IK, Jain AK, et al. Monteggia fracture dislocation equivalents: analysis of eighteen cases treated by open reduction and internal fixation. *Chin J Traumatol*. 2011;14(4):221–226.
115. Smith MV, Calfee RP, Baumgarten KM, et al. Upper extremity-specific measures of disability and outcomes in orthopaedic surgery. *J Bone Joint Surg Am*. 2012;94(3):277–285.
116. Sood A, Khan O, Bagga T. Simultaneous Monteggia type I fracture equivalent with ipsilateral fracture of the distal radius and ulna in a child: a case report. *J Med Case Rep*. 2008;2:190.
117. Spar I. A neurologic complication following Monteggia fracture. *Clin Orthop Relat Res*. 1977;(122):207–209.
118. Speed JS, Boyd HB. Treatment of fractures of ulna with dislocation of head of radius: Monteggia fracture. *JAMA*. 1940;125:1699.
119. Stein F, Grabias SL, Deffer PA. Nerve injuries complicating Monteggia lesions. *J Bone Joint Surg Am*. 1971;53:1432–1436.
120. Stoll TM, Willis RB, Paterson DC. Treatment of the missed Monteggia fracture in the child. *J Bone Joint Surg Br*. 1992;74:436–440.
121. Strong ML, Kopp M, Gillespie R. Fracture of the radial neck and proximal ulna with medial displacement of the radial shaft. Report of two cases. *Orthopedics*. 1989;12:1577–1579.
122. Sur YJ, Park JB, Song SW. Pediatric posterior monteggia lesion: a greenstick fracture of the proximal ulnar metaphysis with radial neck fracture. A case report. *J Orthop Trauma*. 2010;24(2):e12–e16.
123. Tajima T, Yoshizu T. Treatment of long-standing dislocation of the radial head in neglected Monteggia fractures. *J Hand Surg Am*. 1995;20:S91–S94.
124. Tan JW, Mu MZ, Liao GJ, Li JM. Pathology of the annular ligament in paediatric Monteggia fractures. *Injury*. 2008;39(4):451–455.
125. Tan SHS, Low JY, Chen H, et al. Surgical management of missed pediatric Monteggia fractures: a systematic review and meta-analysis. *J Orthop Trauma*. 2022;36(2):65–73.
126. Theodorou SD, Ierodiaconou MD, Rousis N. Fracture of the upper end of the ulna associated with dislocation of the head of the radius in children. *Clin Orthop Relat Res*. 1988;(228):240–249.
127. Thompson JD, Lipscomb AB. Recurrent radial head subluxation treated with annular ligament reconstruction. A case report and follow-up study. *Clin Orthop Relat Res*. 1989;(246):131–135.
128. Tompkins DG. The anterior Monteggia fracture: observations on etiology and treatment. *J Bone Joint Surg Am*. 1971;53:1109–1114.
129. Tubbs RS, O'Neil JT Jr, Key CD, et al. The oblique cord of the forearm in man. *Clin Anat*. 2007;20(4):411–415.
130. Tubbs RS, Shoja MM, Khaki AA, et al. The morphology and function of the quadrate ligament. *Folia Morphol (Warsz)*. 2006;65(3):225–227.
131. Walker JL, Rang M. Forearm fractures in children. Cast treatment with the elbow extended. *J Bone Joint Surg Br*. 1991;73:299–301.
132. Walton RDM, Ormsby NM, Brookes-Fazakerley SD, et al. Stability-based assessment of Monteggia-type injuries predicts failure of treatment. *J Pediatr Orthop B*. 2017;26(1):27–31.
133. Waters PM, Bae DS. *Pediatric Hand and Upper Limb Surgery: A Practical Guide*. Lippincott Williams & Wilkins; 2012:351–365.
134. Watson JA, Singer GC. Irreducible Monteggia fracture: beware nerve entrapment. *Injury*. 1994;25:325–327.
135. Watson-Jones R. *Fractures and Joint Injuries*. 3rd ed. Lippincott Williams & Wilkins; 1943.
136. Werner FW, Taormina JL, Sutton LG, Harley BJ. Structural properties of 6 forearm ligaments. *J Hand Surg Am*. 2011;36(12):1981–1987.
137. Wilkins KE. Changes in the management of Monteggia fractures. *J Pediatr Orthop*. 2002;22(4):548–554.
138. Wright PR. Greenstick fracture of the upper end of the ulna with dislocation of the radio-humeral joint or displacement of the superior radial epiphysis. *J Bone Joint Surg Br*. 1963;45:727–731.
139. Yamamoto K, Yanase Y, Tomihara M. Posterior interosseous nerve palsy as a complication of Monteggia fractures. *Nippon Geka Hokan*. 1977;46:46–56.
140. Zheng ET, Waters PM, Vuillermin CB, et al. Surgical reconstruction of missed Monteggia lesions in children. *J Pediatr Orthop*. 2020;40(10):e916–e921.

13

Evaluation of the Injured Pediatric Elbow

Peter M. Waters

INTRODUCTION

To the uninitiated, pediatric elbow fractures can be difficult to properly diagnose. The absence of ossification in the young, the vagaries of secondary centers of ossification, and the limits of plain radiographs in the skeletally immature, all contribute to risk of misdiagnosis, improper management, and poor outcome in some patients. Since most of these children present with their injuries initially to urgent care and emergency care units that may not have experienced pediatric orthopaedic surgeons and radiologists on site, the risk magnifies. Modern teleconsultation imaging services and review of radiographs by off-site subspecialty radiologists can reduce this risk. Even for experienced caregivers, a select group of injuries, the correct diagnosis, and thus management can be elusive. At the end of the 19th century, Sir Robert Jones[25] echoed the opinion of that era about elbow injuries: "The difficulties experienced by surgeons in making an accurate diagnosis; the facility with which serious blunders can be made in prognosis and treatment; and the fear shared by so many of the subsequent limitations of function, serve to render injuries in the neighborhood of the elbow less attractive than they might otherwise have proved." These concerns are applicable even today. The importance of correct diagnosis was emphasized in a study of litigation against the National Health Service in England: Over half of the cases involved missed or incorrectly diagnosed injuries, most of which were fractures about the elbow.[4] The difficulty in correctly diagnosing elbow injuries in children was shown by Shrader et al., who found that emergency room physicians accurately diagnosed elbow fractures in children only 53% of the time.[54] On the other hand, diagnostic errors with overcalls (1.1%) and miss rate (1.6%) of 1,235 abnormal cases and 2,630 normal cases were reported by Bisset and Crowe when senior certificate of added qualification pediatric radiologists read the films.[8] Front-line caregivers in pediatric emergency rooms continue to find accurate diagnosis of pediatric elbow injuries a challenge.[42] In other bones and joints, good results can often be obtained with minimal treatment, but in the elbow, more aggressive diagnostic testing and surgical treatment are often required to avoid complications. This was emphasized by Waters et al. in their writing on TRASH (The Radiographic Appearance Seemed Harmless) lesions of the pediatric elbow.[63,64] An understanding of the basic anatomy and radiographic landmarks of the elbow is essential in choosing appropriate treatment. In addition, the importance of a physical examination in the acute setting cannot be overemphasized: If the radiographs appear relatively benign, but the child's elbow is markedly swollen, then further diagnostic imaging is warranted.

EPIDEMIOLOGY

Because children tend to protect themselves with their outstretched arms when they fall, upper extremity fractures account for 65% to 75% of all fractures in children. The most common area of the upper extremity injured is the distal forearm.[6,31] Only 10% to 12% of all pediatric fractures involve the elbow but the highest complication rate of upper extremity fractures involve the elbow.

The distal humerus accounts for approximately 86% of fractures in the elbow region. Supracondylar fractures are the most frequent elbow injuries in children, reported to occur in 55% to 75% of patients with elbow fractures. Lateral condylar and radial neck are the second most common fractures,[23] followed by medial epicondylar fractures. Fractures of the radial head, medial condyle, and T-condylar fractures are much less common. Olecranon fractures can be occult initially in the acute setting and seen more commonly on follow-up than original x-rays.[23]

Elbow injuries are much more common in children and adolescents than in adults.[10] Voth et al.[62] reported on 15,300 patients presenting to a level 1 trauma center for care of major and minor injuries. Of the 3,953 patients with a major injury, 76% were fractures and 3% were dislocations. The majority were in the upper limb (73%), with the most common (16%) being fractures about the elbow. The peak age for fractures of the distal humerus is between 5 and 10 years old. Houshian et al.[32] reported that the average age of 355 children with elbow fractures was 7.9 years (7.2 years in boys and 8.5 years in girls). Contrary to most reports, these investigators found elbow fractures more frequent in girls (54%) than in boys. In a study of 450 supracondylar humeral fractures, Cheng et al.[16] found a median age of 6 years (6.6 years in boys and 5 years in girls) and a predominance of injuries (63%) in boys. These fractures are occurring at a time when the distal humerus and proximal forearm is predominately cartilaginous, making fracture diagnosis more challenging. In a series of 1,297 consecutive supracondylar humeral fractures, including 873 type III fractures, Fletcher et al. found that 18% occurred in children older than 8 years; these children had more open fractures from high-energy mechanisms than younger children.[24] Stoneback et al. reported that elbow dislocations were most frequent in those aged 10 to 19 years; 44% were sustained in sports.[58]

Physeal injuries in most parts of the body occur in older children between the ages of 10 and 13; however, the peak age for injuries to the distal humeral physes is 4 to 5 years in girls and 5 to 8 years in boys. In most physeal injuries, the increased incidence with advanced age is believed to be due to weakening of the perichondrial ring as it matures (see Chapter 2). Thus, some different biomechanic forces and conditions must exist about the elbow to make the physis and intra-articular anatomy more vulnerable to injuries at an earlier age. (For more data on the relationship of fractures about the elbow to all types of fractures, see Chapter 1.)

Finally, patient- and age-specific alignment (such as carrying angle) and mobility (such as hyperextension with ligamentous laxity) can predispose to different fracture types with injury. Elbow alignment may influence the transmission of traumatic force with a fall on an outstretched arm; with varus alignment more commonly resulting in lateral condyle fractures and valgus alignment more commonly causing radial neck fractures. Hyperextension leads to the olecranon locking into its fossa with a fall, transmitting fracture force to the supracondylar region of the humerus.

ANATOMY

The elbow is a complex joint composed of three individual joints contained within a common articular cavity. Several anatomic concepts are unique to the growing elbow.

THE OSSIFICATION PROCESS

The process of differentiation and maturation of the primary center of ossification begins at the center of the long bones and progresses both proximally and distally. The ossification process begins in the diaphyses of the humerus, radius, and ulna at the same time. By term, ossification of the humerus has extended distally to the condyles. In the ulna, it extends to more than half the distance between the coronoid process and the tip of the olecranon. The radius is ossified proximally to the level of the neck. The bicipital tuberosity remains largely unossified (Table 13-1).[19] Brodeur et al.[13] compiled a complete atlas of ossification of the structures about the elbow, and their work is an excellent reference source for finer details of the ossification process about the elbow.

Distal Humerus

Ossification of the distal humerus secondary centers of ossification proceeds at a relatively predictable rate; there are vagaries of ossification that need to be accounted for in an individual patient. In general, the rate of ossification in girls exceeds that of boys.[18,19,22] In some areas, such as the olecranon and lateral epicondyle, the difference between boys and girls in ossification age may be as great as 2 years.[18] During the first 6 months, the ossification border of the distal humerus is symmetric (Fig. 13-1).

Lateral Condyle

On average, the ossification center of the lateral condyle (capitellum) appears just before 1 year of age but may be delayed as late as 18 to 24 months.[10] Because the capitellar ossification center appears early, it is a reliable landmark for assessing injury and alignment in children aged 2 years and older. When the nucleus

TABLE 13-1. Sequence and Timing of Ossification in the Elbow

	Girls (years)	Boys (years)
Capitellum	1.0	1.0
Radial head	5.0	6.0
Medial epicondyle	5.0	7.5
Olecranon	8.7	10.5
Trochlea	9.0	10.7
Lateral epicondyle	10.0	12.0

Data from Cheng JC, et al. A new look at the sequential development of elbow-ossification centers in children. J Pediatr Orthop. 1998;18:161–167.

Figure 13-1. During the first 6 months, the advancing ossifying border of the distal humerus is fairly symmetric. Later, the lateral column becomes more vertical compared to the relatively more horizontal medial column on AP views.

of the lateral condyle first appears, the distal humeral metaphyseal border becomes asymmetric. The lateral border slants and becomes straight to conform with the ossification center of the lateral condyle (Fig. 13-2). By the end of the second year, this border becomes well defined, possibly even slightly concave. The capitellar ossification center is usually spherical when it first appears. It becomes more hemispherical as the distal humerus

Figure 13-3. At 24 months, the oval-shaped secondary ossification center of the lateral condyle extends into the lateral crista of the trochlea. The lateral border of the neck (metaphysis) of the radius is normally angulated both anteriorly and laterally. The secondary center of ossification of the radial head is usually not yet present.

matures,[9] and the ossific nucleus extends into the lateral ridge of the trochlea (Fig. 13-3). On the lateral view, the physis of the capitellum is wider posteriorly. This is a normal variation and should not be confused with a fracture.[9]

Medial Epicondyle

At about 5 to 6 years of age, a small concavity develops on the medial aspect of the metaphyseal ossification border. In this area, a medial epicondyle begins to ossify (Fig. 13-4).

Figure 13-2. Ossification at 12 months. As the ossification center of the lateral condyle develops (*arrow*), the lateral border of the metaphysis becomes straighter. The initial ossification is usually elliptical and often appears fragmented, not to be confused with fracture.

Figure 13-4. At about 5 or 6 years of age, a secondary center develops in the medial epicondylar apophysis (*white arrows*). At this same time, the ossification center of the radial head also develops (*open arrow*). Note that the physis of the proximal radius is widened laterally (*curved arrow*). Again, none of these findings should be viewed as fracture related.

A   B

Figure 13-5. A: At about 9 years of age, the ossification of the medial crista of the trochlea may begin as two well-defined centers (*arrows*). These multiple centers can give the trochlea a fragmented appearance. This is not to be confused with avascular necrosis of the trochlea. Also, remember what the trochlea ossification center normally looks like so that an entrapped medial epicondyle (**B**) will not be mistaken for normal ossification. Anteroposterior radiographs after a closed reduction of a medial epicondylar fracture associated with an elbow dislocation. Note the entrapment of the medial epicondyle in the joint.

Trochlea

At about 9 to 10 years of age, the trochlea begins to ossify. Initially, it may be irregular with multiple centers (Fig. 13-5).

Lateral Epicondyle

The lateral epicondyle is last to ossify and is not always visible (Fig. 13-6). At about 10 years of age, it may begin as a small, separate oblong center, rapidly fusing with the lateral condyle.[9]

THE FUSION PROCESS OF THE DISTAL HUMERUS

Just before completion of growth, the capitellum, lateral epicondyle, and trochlea fuse to form one epiphyseal center. Metaphyseal bone separates the extra-articular medial epicondyle from this common humeral epiphyseal center (Fig. 13-7).

Figure 13-6. The apophysis of the lateral epicondyle ossifies as either an oblong or a triangular center (*arrows*). The wide separation of this center from the metaphyseal and epiphyseal borders of the lateral condyle is normal. Fractures in this region are exceedingly rare.

Figure 13-7. The secondary ossification centers of the lateral condyle, trochlea, and lateral epicondylar apophysis fuse to form one center (*white arrows*). This common distal humerus epiphyseal ossification center is separated from the medial epicondylar apophysis by advancing metaphyseal bone (*black arrows*).

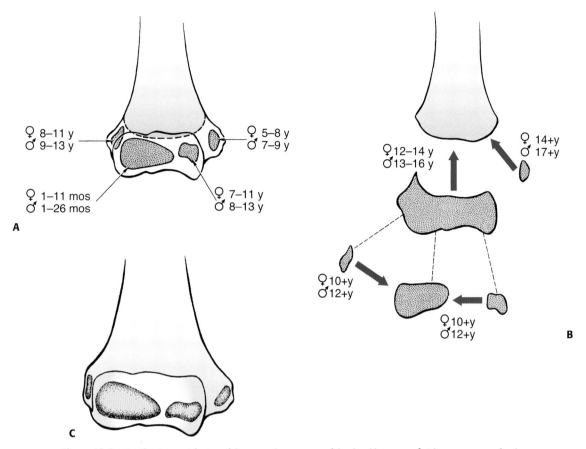

Figure 13-8. Ossification and fusion of the secondary centers of the distal humerus. **A:** The average ages for the onset of ossification of the various ossification centers are shown for both boys and girls. **B:** The ages at which these centers fuse with each other are shown for both boys and girls. **C:** The contribution of each secondary center to the overall architecture of the distal humerus is represented by the stippled areas. (**A, B:** Modified with permission of Medical Journals Sweden from Haraldsson S. On osteochondrosis deformans juvenilis capituli humeri including investigation of intraosseous vasculature in distal humerus. *Acta Orthop Scand Suppl.* 1959;38:1–232.)

The common epiphyseal center ultimately fuses with the distal humeral metaphysis. The medial epicondyle apophysis may not fuse with the metaphysis until the late teens. The ranges of onset of the ossification of various centers and their fusion to other centers or the metaphysis are summarized in Figure 13-8. Each center contributes to the overall architecture of the distal humerus (Fig. 13-8C).

Proximal Radius

The head of the radius begins to ossify before or even at about the same time as the medial epicondyles (see Fig. 13-4). The ossification center is present in at least 50% of girls by 3.8 years of age but may not be present in the same proportion of boys until around 4.5 years.[17] Initially, the ossification center is elliptical, and the physis is widened laterally due to the obliquity of the proximal metaphysis. The ossification center flattens as it matures. At about age 12, it develops an osseous concavity opposite the capitellum.[9]

Ossification of the radial head may be bipartite or may produce an irregularity of the second center. These secondary or irregular ossification centers should not be interpreted as

fracture fragments. However, an anterior compression fracture of the radial head epiphysis must not be interpreted as an aberrant or bipartite center of ossification. Clinical correlation and advanced imaging may be required to sort this out.

Olecranon

There is a gradual proximal progression of ossification to the proximal ulnar metaphysis. At birth, the ossification margin lies halfway between the coronoid process and the tip of the olecranon. By about 6 or 7 years of age, it appears to envelop about 66% to 75% of the capitellar surface. The final portion of the olecranon ossifies from a secondary ossification center that appears around 6.8 years of age in girls and 8.8 years in boys (Fig. 13-9A). Peterson[45] described two separate centers: one articular and the other traction type (Fig. 13-9B). This secondary ossification center of the olecranon may persist late into adult life.

Fusion of the Proximal Forearm Ossification Centers

Fusion of the proximal radial and olecranon epiphyseal centers with their respective metaphyses occurs at around the

Figure 13-9. Ossification of the olecranon. **A:** Secondary ossification begins as an oblique oblong center at about 6 to 8 years of age. **B:** It may progress as two separate ossification centers: articular (*open arrow*) and traction (*closed arrows*).

same time that the common distal humeral epiphysis fuses with its metaphysis (i.e., between 14 and 16 years of age).[41]

Noting that the pattern and ossification sequence of the six secondary ossification centers around the elbow were mainly derived from studies conducted more than 30 years ago, Cheng et al.[16] evaluated elbow radiographs of 1,577 Chinese children. They found that the sequence of ossification was the same in boys and girls—capitellum, radial head, medial epicondyle, olecranon, trochlea, and lateral epicondyle (mnemonic CRMTOL or CRITOE)—but ossification was delayed by about 2 years in boys in all ossification centers except the capitellum (see Table 13-1).

BLOOD SUPPLY

Extraosseous

There is a rich arterial network around the elbow (Fig. 13-10). The major arterial trunk, the brachial artery, lies anteriorly in the antecubital fossa crossing from the medial-anterior distal humerus into the forearm. Most of the intraosseous blood supply of the distal humerus comes from the anastomotic vessels that course posteriorly.

Three structural components govern the location of the entrance of the vessels into the developing epiphysis. First, there is no communication between the intraosseous metaphyseal vasculature and the ossification centers.[65] Second, vessels do not penetrate the articular surfaces. The lateral condyle is nonarticular only at the origin of the muscles and collateral ligaments. Third, the vessels do not penetrate the articular capsule except at the interface with the surface of the bone. Thus, only a small portion of the lateral condyle posteriorly is both nonarticular and extracapsular (Fig. 13-11).

Intraosseous

The most extensive study of the intraosseous blood supply of the developing distal humerus was conducted by Haraldsson (Fig. 13-12),[27,28] who demonstrated that there are two types of vessels in the developing lateral condyle. These vessels enter the posterior portion of the condyle just lateral to the origin of the capsule and proximal to the articular cartilage near the origin of the anconeus muscle. They penetrate the nonossified cartilage and traverse it to the developing ossific nucleus. In a young child, this is a relatively long course (Fig. 13-12A). These vessels communicate with one another within the ossific nucleus but do not communicate with vessels in either the metaphysis or nonossified chondroepiphysis. Thus, for practical purposes, they are end vessels.

The ossification center of the lateral condyle extends into the lateral portion of the trochlea. Thus, the lateral crista or ridge of the trochlea derives its blood supply from these condylar vessels. The medial ridge or crista remains unossified for a longer period of time. The trochlea is covered entirely by articular cartilage and lies totally within the confines of the articular capsule. The vessels that supply the nucleus of the ossific centers of the trochlea must therefore traverse the periphery of the physis to enter the epiphysis.

Haraldsson's[27,28] studies have shown two sources of blood supply to the ossific nucleus of the medial portion of the trochlea (Fig. 13-12B). The lateral vessel, on the posterior surface of the distal humeral metaphysis, penetrates the periphery of the physis and terminates in the trochlear nucleus. Because this vessel supplying the trochlea is an end vessel, it is especially vulnerable to injury by a fracture that courses through either the physis or the very distal portion of the humeral metaphysis. Injury to this vessel can markedly decrease the nourishment to the developing lateral ossific nucleus of the trochlea. A rare result of injury here is avascular necrosis of the distal humerus/trochlea. The medial

Profunda brachii artery

Radial collateral artery
Middle collateral branch
Profunda brachii artery

Radial recurrent artery

Posterior interosseous
recurrent artery

Radial artery

Brachial artery

Superior ulnar
collateral artery

Inferior ulnar
collateral artery

Supratrochlear artery

Ulnar recurrent artery
Anterior
Posterior

Common interosseous artery
Interosseous artery
Anterior
Posterior

Ulnar artery

Figure 13-10. The major arteries about the anterior elbow.

Figure 13-11. The vessels supplying the lateral condylar epiphysis enter the posterior aspect of the condyle, which is extra-articular.

Figure 13-12. Intraosseous blood supply of the distal humerus. **A:** The vessels supplying the lateral condylar epiphysis enter on the posterior aspect and course for a considerable distance before reaching the ossific nucleus. **B:** Two definite vessels supply the ossification center of the medial crista of the trochlea. The lateral vessel enters by crossing the physis. The medial one enters by way of the nonarticular edge of the medial crista.

Figure 13-13. The elbow fat pads. Some of the coronoid fat pad lies anterior to the shallow coronoid fossa. The olecranon fat pad lies totally within the deeper olecranon fossa. The clinical significance of a positive fat pad sign is discussed in detail in text.

vessel penetrates the nonarticulating portion of the medial crista of the trochlea. The multiple vascular sources may account for the development of multiple ossification centers in the maturing trochlea, giving it a fragmented appearance (see Fig. 13-5). When growth is complete, metaphyseal and epiphyseal vessels anastomose freely. The blood supply from the central nutrient vessel of the shaft reaches the epicondylar regions in the skeletally mature distal humerus.[27]

INTRA-ARTICULAR STRUCTURES

The articular surface lies within the confines of the capsule, but nonarticulating areas involving the coronoid and radial fossae anteriorly and the olecranon fossa posteriorly are also within the confines of the articular cavity. The capsule attaches just distal to the coronoid and olecranon processes. Thus, these processes are intra-articular. The entire radial head is intra-articular, with a recess or diverticulum of the elbow's articular cavity extending distally under the margin of the orbicular ligament. The medial and lateral epicondyles are extra-articular.

The elbow capsule is thickened anteriorly. These longitudinally directed fibers are very strong and become taut with the elbow in extension. In hyperextension, the tight anterior bands of the capsule force the ulna firmly into contact with the humerus. Thus, the fulcrum of rotation becomes transmitted proximally by the tip of the olecranon into the supracondylar area. This is an important factor in the etiology of supracondylar fractures.

FAT PADS

At the proximal portion of the capsule, between it and the synovial layer, are two large fat pads (Fig. 13-13). The posterior fat pad lies totally within the depths of the olecranon fossa when the elbow is flexed. The anterior fat pad extends anteriorly out of the margins of the coronoid fossa. The significance of these fat pads in the interpretation of radiographs of the injured elbow is discussed later.

LIGAMENTS

The pertinent ligamentous anatomy involving the orbicular and collateral ligaments is discussed in the sections on the specific injuries involving the radial neck, medial epicondyle, elbow dislocations, and Monteggia lesions (see Chapters 12, 14, and 19).

RADIOGRAPHIC FINDINGS

Because of the ever-changing ossification pattern, identification and delineation of fractures about the elbow in the immature skeleton may be subject to misinterpretation. The variables of ossification of the epiphyses should be well known to the orthopaedic surgeon who treats these injuries as well as the emergent care providers and radiologists. Even with that expertise, supplemental diagnostic use of contralateral radiographs, ultrasound, arthrograms, computed tomography (CT), and magnetic resonance imaging (MRI) scans may be appropriate and necessary.

Many studies have indicated that children with a normal range of elbow motion after elbow trauma do not require immediate radiographic evaluation.[29,48] Since cumulative radiation exposure is of concern in the pediatric population, and since there are increased unnecessary costs associated with unindicated radiographs, awareness of this body of literature is important for the treating physician in the acute setting. In a large multicenter prospective study, Appelboam et al.[3] found that of 780 children evaluated for elbow trauma, 289 were able to fully extend their elbow; among these, only 12 (4%) fractures were identified, all at their first evaluation. Among the 491 children who could not fully extend their injured elbow, 210 (43%) had confirmed fractures. These authors suggested that an elbow extension test can be used to rule out the need for radiographs, provided the physician is confident that an olecranon fracture is not present and that the patient can return for re-evaluation if symptoms have not resolved in 7 to 10 days. Lennon et al.[41] in a study involving 407 patients ranging in age from 2 to 96 years, proposed that patients aged no more than 16 years with a range of motion equal to the unaffected side do not require radiographic evaluation. Darracq et al.[18] found that limitation of active range of motion was 100% sensitive for fracture or effusion, while preservation of active range of motion was 97% specific for the absence of fracture. Other studies[15,30] have confirmed a high sensitivity (91%–97%) of an inability to extend the elbow as a predictor of elbow fracture in both children and adults. Vinson et al. noted that the four-way range of motion test (full elbow extension, 90 degrees elbow flexion, full pronation, and full supination) was 99% sensitive for radiographic elbow injuries and 100% sensitive for elbow injuries requiring surgical intervention in 251 patients seen prospectively in three emergency departments (EDs).[61] Instituting protocols for radiographs can reduce radiation exposure and imaging costs.[49] However, Baker and Borland[6] warned that in children with blunt trauma, a normal range of motion does not rule out significant injury and should not be used as a screening tool. In their 177 patients, an abnormal range of motion had a negative predictive value of only 77%.[6] In these circumstances, ultrasound is becoming increasingly a screening tool used in emergency care to assess for indications for formal radiographs.[21,47]

TABLE 13-2. Elbow TRASH Lesions

- Unossified medial condylar humeral fractures
- Unossified transphyseal distal humeral fractures
- Entrapped medial epicondylar fractures
- Complex osteochondral elbow fracture-dislocation in a child <10 years of age
- Osteochondral fractures with joint incongruity
- Radial head anterior compression fractures with progressive radiocapitellar subluxation
- Monteggia fracture-dislocations
- Lateral condylar avulsion shear fractures

Modified with permission from Waters PM, et al. Elbow "TRASH" (The Radiographic Appearance Seemed Harmless) lesions. *J Pediatr Orthop.* 2010;30(2 Suppl): S77–S81.

Waters et al.[63,64] described a subset of serious injuries to the pediatric elbow that they termed TRASH lesions (Table 13-2). These lesions represent predominantly intra-articular osteochondral injuries in children younger than 10 years of age who have sustained high-energy trauma; the lesions are often associated with unrecognized, spontaneously reduced elbow dislocations (Fig. 13-14). Similarly, transphyseal separations in the very young (<2 years of age) are rare but often misdiagnosed. Usually, the elbow is quite swollen and the range of motion is limited. Any elbow with marked swelling after injury in a child younger than 10 years of age should raise concern about a displaced, intra-articular osteochondral fracture, especially with a high-energy mechanism of injury and more swelling even when there is a seemingly benign radiograph. In children less than 2 years of age with a radiograph revealing posteromedial displacement of the radius and ulna relative to the distal humeral metaphysis and unossified epiphysis, a transphyseal injury should be suspected.[60] Ultrasound or MRI is diagnostic.[26,60] Since these young children are often victims of nonaccidental trauma and at risk not only for malunion but importantly more serious body harm, even permanent or fatal injuries, in the future, accurate diagnosis, treatment of the fracture, and evaluation of the human and social factors leading to injury are critical (see Chapter 7 for full details). Thus, a high index of suspicion and early additional imaging (ultrasound, arthrogram, or MRI) usually contribute to a more accurate diagnosis and best treatment of these injuries.[63,64]

When radiographs are indicated, a number of anatomic landmarks and angles should be evaluated and measured, including

Figure 13-14. A: Anteroposterior, lateral, and oblique views of an osteochondral fracture of the lateral condyle. If unrecognized, this can lead to painful nonunion and intra-articular incongruity. **B:** Magnetic resonance imaging scan documenting displacement and operative indications. **C:** Percutaneous reduction and screw fixation were done based on MRI findings. (Reprinted with permission from Waters PM, et al. Elbow "TRASH" (The Radiographic Appearance Seemed Harmless) lesions. *J Pediatr Orthop.* 2010;30(2 suppl):S77–S81.)

Figure 13-15. AP of the distal humerus (Jones axial radiographic view) that is important in acute trauma and follow-up care as an AP of the elbow will have overlapping radius and ulna and obscure injuries.

any displacement of the fat pads about the elbow. It is important to be familiar with these landmarks and angles and to be aware of the significance of any deviation from normal.

STANDARD VIEWS

The standard radiographs of the elbow include an anteroposterior (AP) view with the elbow fully extended and a lateral view with the elbow flexed to 90 degrees and the forearm neutral. As noted though, it is often difficult to obtain full elbow extension in the injured child. Thus, modification of imaging techniques is important.

AP OF THE DISTAL HUMERUS (JONES VIEW)

An axial view of the elbow, the Jones view, is very helpful when the patient cannot fully extend their, either in the acute injured state or postreduction, casting or pinning. (Fig. 13-15). The injured distal humerus is difficult to interpret due to the superimposed proximal radius and ulna when the elbow is flexed. In addition to AP and lateral views of the distal humerus, if there is a high index of suspicion for a fracture, but none is visible on routine AP and lateral radiographs, then internal and external oblique views may be helpful. This is especially true in identifying fractures of the radial head and coronoid process and judging displacement in lateral condylar, medial epicondylar, and supracondylar humerus fractures.

MEASUREMENT OF DISPLACEMENT: MEDIAL EPICONDYLAR FRACTURES

The determination of the amount of fracture displacement is critical to the choice of treatment of medial epicondylar fractures. The general consensus among pediatric orthopaedic surgeons seems to be that fractures with less than 2 mm of displacement can be treated nonoperatively, while those with more than

5 mm of displacement should be treated operatively. A difference of 1 or 2 mm in the measurement of displacement can change the management of these fractures. To determine the reliability of displacement measurements, Pappas et al.[44] had radiographs of 38 children with fractures of the medial humeral epicondyle evaluated by five reviewers with different levels of orthopaedic training. Pappas et al. found that the reviewers disagreed an average of 87% of the time about measurements on the lateral view, 64% of the time about measurements on the oblique view, and 54% about measurements on the AP view. The findings cast doubt on whether the amount of perceived displacement should be used as a criterion for choosing operative or nonoperative treatment of fractures of the medial epicondyle. Proposed methods for improving displacement measurement were (1) measuring displacement on AP views and (2) measuring displacement as the maximal distance between the fragment and the bone location from which it came in any view (Fig. 13-16). In contrast, Edmonds[22] suggested that internal

Figure 13-16. On anteroposterior radiograph of a left elbow with a medial epicondylar fracture, there are three different places where displacement could be measured. The *red line* represents 2 mm of displacement; the *green line*, 3 mm; and the *blue line*, 5 mm. (Reprinted with permission from Pappas N, et al. Intraobserver and interobserver agreement in the measurement of displaced humeral medial epicondyle fractures in children. *J Bone Joint Surg Am.* 2010;92(2):322–327.)

oblique views appear to best approximate the true anterior displacement. In addition, Edmonds et al. found that comparison of measurements of displacement on radiographs to those on three-dimensional CT scans demonstrated that fractures that appear to be minimally displaced or nondisplaced on radiographs, especially AP and lateral views, may have more than 1 cm of anterior displacement by CT scan. However, CT scans of all medial epicondylar fractures to assess accurate displacement would bring increased radiation exposure and risk to children and is not recommended. Klatt and Aoki[37] revealed that the center of the medial epicondyle throughout skeletal maturation consistently rests 0.5 mm (SD 2 mm) inferior to the olecranon line and 1.2 mm (SD 1.2 mm) anterior to the posterior humeral line.

Mini C-Arm and Ultrasound Assessment

Mini C-arm is increasingly used in the emergency setting for diagnosis and to assist and assess reduction of pediatric fractures. Conscious sedation reductions and casting with mini C-arm assessment is now commonplace in the pediatric emergent care setting (Chapter 3). While extremely convenient and accurate, caregivers need to be aware of the risks of radiation exposure to the injured children, hospital employees, and themselves if overutilized, especially by less experienced pediatric orthopaedic caregivers. Sumko et al. reported on increased exposure averaging 53 mrem with mini C-arm use in ED compared with 20 mrem with standard AP, lateral radiographs of the elbow in their institution.[59] For these reasons, in ED, ultrasound screening is increasingly used for children with suspected fractures. Expertise in these techniques is required to avoid misdiagnosis.[5] Ultrasound using standard plane of imaging has been shown to be useful for prompt diagnosis and appropriate treatment, potentially avoiding mismanagement of pediatric elbow injuries including TRASH lesions.[53]

ANTEROPOSTERIOR LANDMARKS

Baumann Angle

In the standard AP view, the major landmark is the angulation of the physeal line between the lateral condyle and the distal humeral metaphysis. The ossification center of the lateral condyle extends into the radial or lateral crista of the trochlea (see Fig. 13-9C). This physeal line forms an angle with the long axis of the humerus. The angle formed by the capitellar physeal line and the long axis of the humerus is the Baumann angle (Fig. 13-17A). The Baumann angle is not equal to the carrying angle of the elbow in older children.[8] It is a consistent angle when both sides are compared, and the x-ray beam is directed perpendicular to the long axis of the humerus. Acton and McNally[1] reviewed the descriptions of the Baumann angle in a number of commonly used textbooks and discovered three variations of measurement technique. They recommended that the angle should always be measured between the long axis of the humerus and the inclination of the capitellar physis, as Baumann described, and that it should be called the "shaft–physeal" angle to avoid confusion.

Caudad-to-cephalad angulation of the x-ray tube, or right or left angulation of the tube by as much as 30 degrees, changes the Baumann angle by less than 5 degrees. If, however, the tube becomes angulated in a cephalad-to-caudad direction by more than 20 degrees, the angle is changed significantly and the measurement is inaccurate. In their cadaver studies, Camp et al.[14] found that rotation of the distal fragment or the entire reduced humerus could also alter the projection of the Baumann angle. They found that to be accurate, the humerus must be parallel to the x-ray plate, with the beam directed perpendicular to the film as well. Thus, in the routine AP radiographs of the distal humerus, including the Jones view, the Baumann angle is a good measurement of any deviation of the angulation of the distal humerus.[55]

Other Angles

Two other angles measured on AP radiographs are commonly used to determine the proper alignment of the distal humerus or carrying angle. The humeral–ulnar angle is determined by lines longitudinally bisecting the shaft of the humerus with the shaft of the ulna on an AP view (Fig. 13-17B).[4] The metaphyseal–diaphyseal angle is determined by a line that longitudinally bisects the shaft of the humerus with a line that connects the widest points of the metaphysis of the distal humerus (Fig. 13-17C).[34] The humeral–ulnar angle is the most accurate in determining the true carrying angle of the elbow. The Baumann angle also has a good correlation with the clinical carrying angle, but it may be difficult to measure in adolescents in whom the ossification center of the lateral condyle is beginning to fuse with other centers. The metaphyseal–diaphyseal angle is the least accurate of the three.

LATERAL LANDMARKS

Teardrop

The lateral projection of the distal humerus presents a teardrop-like shadow above the capitellum.[41] The anterior dense line making up the teardrop represents the posterior margin of the coronoid fossa. The posterior dense line represents the anterior margin of the olecranon fossa. The inferior portion of the teardrop is the ossification center of the capitellum. On a true lateral projection, this teardrop should be well defined (Fig. 13-18A).

Shaft–Condylar Angle

On the lateral radiograph, there is an angulation of 40 degrees between the long axis of the humerus and the long axis of the lateral condyle/capitellar ossification center (see Fig. 13-18B). This can also be measured by the flexion angle of the distal humerus, which is calculated by measuring the angle of the lateral condylar physeal line with the long axis of the shaft of the humerus.[39]

Anterior Humeral Line

If a line is drawn along the anterior border of the distal humeral shaft, it should pass through the middle third of the ossification center of the capitellum. This is referred to as the anterior humeral line (see Fig. 13-18C). Passage of the anterior humeral

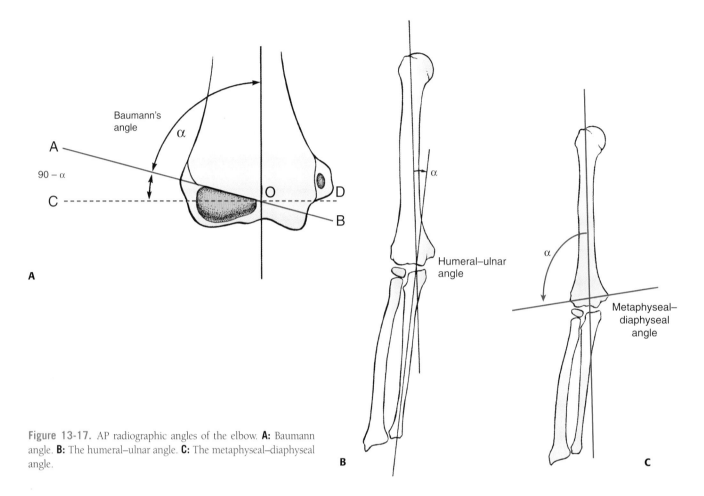

Figure 13-17. AP radiographic angles of the elbow. **A:** Baumann angle. **B:** The humeral–ulnar angle. **C:** The metaphyseal–diaphyseal angle.

line through the anterior portion of the lateral condylar ossification center or anterior to it indicates the presence of posterior angulation of the distal humerus. In a large study of minimally displaced supracondylar fractures, the anterior humeral line was the most reliable factor in detecting the presence or absence of occult fractures. Herman et al., however, found that the location of the anterior humeral line varied according to age: in almost half of children younger than 4 years of age, the line passed through the anterior third of the capitellum, while in older children, the anterior humeral line more consistently passed through the middle third.[31]

Coronoid Line

A line directed proximally along the anterior border of the coronoid process should barely touch the anterior portion of the lateral condyle (see Fig. 13-18D). Posterior displacement of the lateral condyle projects the ossification center posterior to this coronoid line.[41]

Figure 13-18. Lateral radiograph lines of the distal humerus. **A:** The teardrop of the distal humerus. **B:** The angulation of the lateral condyle with the shaft of the humerus. **C:** The anterior humeral line. **D:** The coronoid line. (Reprinted with permission from Shank CF, et al. The lateral capitellohumeral angle in normal children: mean, variation, and reliability in comparison to Baumann's angle. *J Pediatr Orthop.* 2011;31(3):266–271.)

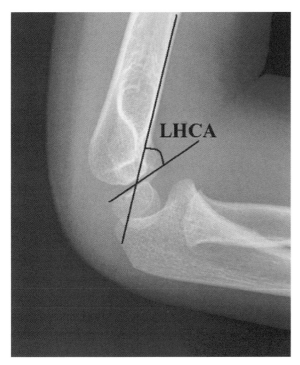

Figure 13-19. Lateral humerocapitellar angle (LHCA) on lateral radiograph of normal elbow. (From Shank CF, et al. The lateral capitellohumeral angle in normal children: mean, variation, and reliability in comparison to Baumann's angle. *J Pediatr Orthop.* 2011;31:266–271.)

Lateral Humerocapitellar Angle

Shank et al.[51] described measurement of the *lateral humerocapitellar angle (LHCA)* using digital measurement tools and digital radiographs (Fig. 13-19). This angle measures the angular relationship between the humeral shaft and the capitellum as seen on the lateral view. In normal elbows, the LHCA averaged 51 degrees and was not affected by age, sex, or side. Its reliability was found to be inferior to that of the Baumann angle but improved with increasing patient age. The correlation between the LHCA and clinical outcome is unclear, with some studies finding no correlation and others reporting a strong correlation between the LHCA and loss of flexion at skeletal maturity.[56] Although the exact relationship between the LHCA and clinical outcome is unclear, the authors suggested that an LHCA of more than three standard deviations from normal (absolute measurement of >69 degrees) should be accepted with reservation, especially in older patients, because some studies have suggested unpredictable remodeling of angular deformity.[56]

Radiocapitellar Line

Once ossified, the radial head should always align with the capitellum (see Chapter 12). Subtle changes in this alignment are missed and have long-term consequences (Fig. 13-20).

Pseudofracture

Some vagaries of the ossification process about the elbow may be interpreted as a fracture.[41] For example, the ossification of the trochlea may be irregular, producing a fragmented appearance (see Fig. 13-5). This fragmentation can be misinterpreted, especially if the distal humerus is slightly oblique or tilted. These secondary ossification centers may be mistaken for fracture fragments lying between the semilunar notch and lateral condyle (Fig. 13-21).

On the lateral view, the physeal line between the lateral condyle and the distal humeral metaphysis is wider posteriorly. This appearance may give a misinterpretation that the lateral condyle is fractured and tilted.[9]

On the AP view before the radial head ossifies, there is normally some lateral angulation to the radial border of the neck of the radius that may give the appearance of subluxation (see Fig. 13-3). The true position of the radial head can be confirmed by noting the relationship of the proximal radius to the ossification center of the lateral condyle on the lateral projection.[40]

A   B

Figure 13-20. A: Lateral radiograph of an injured elbow reveals the radial is subluxed anterior to the capitellum as noted by the incongruency of the narrow *arrow* up the proximal radius and the broader *arrow* through the capitellum. This can be very subtle and requires a high level of scrutiny. **B:** Contralateral lateral radiograph showing congruency of the radial head and capitellar lines.

Figure 13-21. Pseudofracture of the elbow. The trochlea with its multiple ossification centers may be misinterpreted as fracture fragments lying between the joint surfaces (*arrow*).

Fat Pad Signs of the Elbow

There are three areas in which fat pads overlie the major structures of the elbow. Displacement of any of the fat pads can indicate an occult fracture.[11] The first two areas are the fat pads that overlie the capsule in the coronoid fossa anteriorly and the olecranon fossa posteriorly. Displacement of either or both of these fat pads is usually referred to as the *classic elbow fat pad sign*. A third accumulation of fat overlies the supinator muscle as it wraps around the proximal radius.

Olecranon (Posterior) Fat Pad

Because the olecranon fossa is deep, the fat pad here is totally contained within the fossa. It is not visible on a normal lateral radiograph of the elbow flexed to 90 degrees.

Distension of the capsule with an effusion, as occurs with an occult intra-articular fracture, a spontaneously reduced dislocation, or even an infection, can cause the dorsal or olecranon fat pad to be visible.[44]

Coronoid (Anterior) Fat Pad

Likewise, the ventral or coronoid fat pad may be displaced anteriorly.[7] Because the coronoid fossa is shallow, the fat pad in this area projects anterior to the bony margins and can be seen normally as a triangular radiolucency anterior to the distal humerus (sail sign). Although displacement of the classic elbow fat pads is a reliable indication of an intra-articular effusion, there may be instances in which only one of the fat pads is displaced. Brodeur et al.[12] and Kohn[38] have shown that the coronoid fat pad is more sensitive to small effusions than the olecranon fat pad. The coronoid fat pad can be displaced without a coexistent displacement of the olecranon fat pad. Blumberg et al. analyzed the radiographs of 197 consecutive patients with elbow trauma and found that 113 (57%) had normal anterior fat pads; of these,

only two had fractures, giving a 98% negative predictive value to the presence of a normal anterior fat pad.[10]

Supinator Fat Pad

A layer of fat on the anterior aspect of the supinator muscle wraps around the proximal radius. This layer of fat or fat pad may normally bow anteriorly to some degree. Brodeur et al.[13] stated that displacement may indicate the presence of an occult fracture of the radial neck. Displacement of the fat line or supinator fat pad is often difficult to interpret; in a review of fractures involving the proximal radius, Schunk et al.[50] found it to be positive only 50% of the time.

Fat Pad Variations

For the fat pads to be displaced, the capsule must be intact. This can explain why there may be no displacement of the fat pads with an elbow dislocation that has spontaneously reduced due to capsule rupture. These elbows, however, will be more swollen clinically. Murphy and Siegel described other variations of classic fat pad displacement. If the elbow is extended, the fat pad is normally displaced from the olecranon fossa by the olecranon. Remember though, it is unusual to a significant acute elbow injury that maintains full elbow extension. Distal humeral fractures may cause subperiosteal bleeding and may lift the proximal portion of the olecranon fat pad without the presence of an effusion. These false-negative and false-positive determinations must be kept in mind when interpreting the presence or absence of a fat pad finding with an elbow injury.

Fat pad studies have drawn disparate conclusions. Corbett's[17] review of elbow injuries indicated that if a displacement of the posterior fat pad existed, a fracture was almost always present. Displacement of the anterior fat pad alone, however, could occur without a fracture. Corbett[17] also determined that the degree of displacement bore no relation to the extent of the fracture. Skaggs and Mirzayan[57] reported that 34 of 45 children (76%) with a history of elbow trauma and an elevated posterior fat pad had radiographic evidence of elbow fractures at an average of 3 weeks after injury, though AP, lateral, and oblique radiographs at the time of injury showed no other evidence of fracture. They recommended that a child with a history of elbow trauma and an elevated fat pad should be treated as if a nondisplaced elbow fracture were present. Donnelly et al.,[20] however, found evidence of fracture in only 9 of 54 children (17%) who had a history of trauma and elbow joint effusion but no identifiable fracture on initial radiographs. Donnelly et al. concluded that joint effusion without a visible fracture on initial radiographs does not correlate with the presence of occult fracture in most patients (83%). Persistent effusion did correlate with occult fracture: 78% of those with occult fractures had persistent effusions, whereas effusions were noted in only 16% of those without fractures. More recently, in a prospective MRI study of 26 children with positive fat pad signs, Al-Aubaidi and Torfing[2] concluded that the presence of a positive fat pad sign is not synonymous with an occult fracture. All 26 children had a positive fat pad sign on lateral radiographs, but MRI scans obtained an average of 7 days later found occult fractures in only 6 patients (23%), none of whom had a change in fracture treatment. Most (73%) had bone bruise by MRI. A meta-analysis of 10 papers, 250 patients, found 104 (45%) had an occult fracture with a positive fat pad sign. The most common fracture was supracondylar humerus (43%), followed by proximal ulna (19%), proximal radius (17%), and lateral condylar humerus (14%).[35]

COMPARISON RADIOGRAPHS

Although it is often tempting to order comparison radiographs in a child with an injured elbow due to the difficulty evaluating the irregularity of the ossification process, the indications for ordering comparison radiographs are rare.[33] Kissoon et al.[36] found that using routine comparison radiographs in children with injured elbows did not significantly increase the accuracy of diagnosis, regardless of the interpreter's training. Petit et al.[46] reviewed 3,128 radiographs of 2,470 children admitted to a pediatric ED for osteoarticular trauma and found that only 22% of the radiographs revealed abnormal findings; 33% of elbow radiographs revealed abnormalities. Fewer than half of clinically suspected fractures were confirmed by radiograph.

MAGNETIC RESONANCE IMAGING

Major and Crawford[43] used MRI to evaluate seven children who had radiographs that showed effusion but no fractures; four of the children had fractures identified by MRI. These investigators suggested that an occult fracture is usually present when effusion occurs, even if a fracture is not visible on radiograph. Griffith et al.[25] reviewed the radiographs and MRI scans of 50 children with elbow trauma. Radiographs identified effusions in 34% of the children and fractures in 52%; MRI identified effusions in 96% and fractures in 74%. Although MRI revealed a broad spectrum of bone and soft tissue injury beyond that shown on radiographs (bone bruising, muscle and ligament injuries, physeal injury, fracture), the additional information provided by MRI had little influence on patient treatment and no value in predicting clinical outcome. We have found MRI to be helpful in evaluating articular and osteochondral fractures to identify fracture pattern and extent, fragment position, and any interposed structure in the joint blocking reduction. MRI aids in proper level of care, including surgery for underappreciated injuries.

OTHER IMAGING MODALITIES

Sonography and arthrography can be useful in examining children with posttraumatic elbow effusions, but these can be painful (ultrasound with direct pressure) and invasive (arthrograms usually in operating rooms). The use of CT in the young can be limited by the need for sedation and lack of ossification of secondary centers. In adolescent T condylar humerus fractures, CT is extremely helpful for planning operative intervention. The development of multidetector CT (MDCT) technology allows examinations to be completed in seconds, eliminating the need for sedation in most cases. Studies using MDCT can also be reformatted and evaluated in multiple planes, reducing the manipulation necessary for a series of radiographs. Chapman et al.[15] reported that, in a series of 31 children with posttraumatic elbow effusion and normal radiographs, MDCT depicted occult injuries in 52%. Besides the minimal manipulation required, making it relatively easy and pain free, and the speed with which the image are obtained, they cited as additional advantages of MDCT the lower radiation dose than conventional radiographs and its sensitivity (92%), specificity (79%), and high negative predictive value (92%). A limitation of this method may be its high cost compared to standard radiographic examination.

Finally, there is progressive development in the use of artificial intelligence in orthopaedic surgery, including pediatric fracture assessment.[52] Deep learning algorithmic performance has been cited at 88% to 98% compared to human interpretation including pediatric elbows.

CONCLUSION

It is imperative to obtain an accurate diagnosis in the acute or short-term postacute setting of a pediatric elbow injury. Accurate diagnosis will prevent both over- and undertreatment, with undertreatment having the highest risk of a long-term poor outcome. Knowledge of the timing and sequence of secondary center of ossification appearance, and described vagaries of ossification, are important. This includes using these secondary centers, especially the capitellum, to accurately define fracture type, displacement, and treatment reductions. Use of additional imaging including ultrasound, arthrogram, and MRI studies, is warranted when in doubt; especially in young children with swollen elbow and painful, restricted range of motion.

Annotated References

Reference	Annotation
Cheng JC, Wing-Man K, Shen WY, et al. A new look at the sequential development of elbow-ossification centers in children. *J Pediatr Orthop.* 1998;18(2):161–167.	It is essential that professionals caring for skeletally immature children with elbow injuries know the normal sequence and vagaries of the appearance in timing and anticipated shape of the secondary centers of ossification.
Haraldsson S. On osteochondrosis deformans juvenilis capituli humeri including investigation of intraosseous vasculature in distal humerus. *Acta Orthop Scand Suppl.* 1959;38:1–232.	This study and the preliminary report in 1957 by lead author in same journal are important to understand the etiology of the rare but problematic posttraumatic avascular necrosis of the distal humerus in children.

Annotated References

Reference	Annotation
Kappelhof B, Roorda BL, Poppelaars MA, et al. Occult fractures in children with a radiographic fat pad sign of the elbow: a meta-analysis of 10 published studies. *JBJS Rev.* 2022;10(10).	Fat pad signs on radiographs are used in conjunction with physical examination, especially ability to extend the elbow, to determine diagnosis and treatments often. This study summarizes the best literature findings by meta-analysis,
Li W, Stimec J, Camp M, et al. Pediatric musculoskeletal radiographs: anatomy and fractures prone to diagnostic error among emergency physicians. *J Emerg Med.* 2022;62(4):524–533.	Accurate diagnosis of pediatric elbow injuries in the acute care setting is challenging for the evaluating physician. The study reviews the risk of errors of diagnosis and therefore treatment.
Rabiner JE, Khine H, Avner JR, et al. Accuracy of point of care ultrasonography for diagnosis of elbow fractures in children. Ann Emerg Med. 2013;61(1):9–17.	Ultrasound point of care imaging is now commonplace in many pediatric emergency rooms. This is one of many studies reviewing its accuracy in pediatric elbow trauma.
Shelmerdine SC, White RD, Liu H, et al. Artificial intelligence for radiological paediatric fracture assessment: a systematic review. *Insights Imaging.* 2022;13(1):94.	Artificial intelligence is advancing in many medical subspecialty fields, especially radiology. This systemic review is helpful to know the state of development when it was written in a rapidly changing field.
Shintani K, Hosomi R, Suzuki K, et al. Diagnostic imaging for elbow TRASH lesions in children and usefulness of ultrasonography using standard planes. *J Pediatr Orthop B.* 2023;32(6):557–564.	Discusses the utility of using ultrasound in skeletally immature pediatric elbow trauma to avoid missing a TRASH lesion, lessening the risk of a poor outcome.
Sumko MJ, Hennrikus W, Slough J, et al. Measurement of radiation exposure when using mini C-arm to reduce pediatric upper extremity fractures. *J Pediatr Orthop.* 2016;36(2):122–125.	Mini C-arm is frequently used in point of emergency care for pediatric elbow fractures. It is important to understand the occupational hazard risk to professionals and patients with single and repeated exposures and how to maximize safety.
Waters PM, Beaty J, Kasser J. Elbow "TRASH" (the radiographic appearance seemed harmless) lesions. *J Pediatr Orthop.* 2010;30(2 Suppl):S77–S81.	Review of injuries that are at high risk for poor outcome if the extent of osteochondral injury is underappreciated and untreated acutely in the skeletally immature pediatric elbow.

REFERENCES

1. Acton JD, McNally MA. Baumann's confusing legacy. *Injury.* 2001;32(1):41–43.
2. Al-Aubaidi Z, Torfing T. The role of the fat pad sign in diagnosing occult elbow fractures in the pediatric patient: a prospective magnetic resonance imaging study. *J Pediatr Orthop B.* 2012;21(6):514–519.
3. Appelboam A, Reuben AD, Benger JR, et al. Elbow extension test to rule out elbow fracture: multicentre, prospective validation, and observational study of diagnostic accuracy in adults and children. *BMJ.* 2008;337:a2428.
4. Atrey A, Nicolaou N, Katchburian M, Norman-Taylor F. A review of reported litigation against English health trusts for the treatment of children in orthopaedics: present trends and suggestions to reduce mistakes. *J Child Orthop.* 2010;4(5):471–476.
5. Averill LW, Kraft DB, Sabado JJ, et al. Ultrasonography of the pediatric elbow. *Pediatr Radiol.* 2023;53(8):1526–1538.
6. Baker M, Borland M. Range of elbow movement as a predictor of bony injury in children. *Emerg Med J.* 2011;28(8):666–669.
7. Beals RK. The normal carrying angle of the elbow. A radiographic study of 422 patients. *Clin Orthop Relat Res.* 1976;(119):194–196.
8. Bisset GS III, Crowe J. Diagnostic errors in interpretation of pediatric musculoskeletal radiographs at common injury sties. *Pediatr Radiol.* 2014;44(5):552–557.
9. Blount WP, Schulz I, Cassidy RH. Fractures of the elbow in children. *J Am Med Assoc.* 1951;146(8):699–704.
10. Blumberg SM, Kunkov S, Crain EF, Goldman HS. The predictive value of a normal radiographic fat pad sign following elbow trauma in children. *Pediatr Emerg Care.* 2011;27(7):596–600.
11. Bohrer SP. The fat pad sign following elbow trauma. Its usefulness and reliability in suspecting "invisible" fractures. *Clin Radiol.* 1970;21(1):90–94.
12. Brodeur AE, Silberstein MJ, Graviss ER. *Radiology of the Pediatric Elbow.* GK Hall; 1981.
13. Brodeur AE, Silberstein MJ, Graviss ER, Luisiri A. The basic tenets for appropriate evaluation of the elbow in pediatrics. *Curr Prob Diagn Radiol.* 1983;12(5):1–29.
14. Camp J, Ishizue K, Gomez M, et al. Alteration of Baumann's angle by humeral position: implications for treatment of supracondylar humerus fractures. *J Pediatr Orthop.* 1993;13(4):521–555.
15. Chapman V, Grottkau B, Albright M, et al. MDCT of the elbow in pediatric patients with posttraumatic elbow effusions. *AJR Am J Roentgenol.* 2006;187(3):812–817.
16. Cheng JC, Wing-Man K, Shen WY, et al. A new look at the sequential development of elbow-ossification centers in children. *J Pediatr Orthop.* 1998;18(2):161–167.
17. Corbett RH. Displaced fat pads in trauma to the elbow. *Injury.* 1978;9(4):297–298.
18. Darracq MA, Vinson DR, Panacek EA. Preservation of active range of motion after acute elbow trauma predicts absence of elbow fracture. *Am J Emerg Med.* 2008;26(7):779–782.
19. Docherty MA, Schwab RA, Ma OJ. Can elbow extension be used a test of clinically significant injury? *South Med J.* 2002;95(5):539–541.
20. Donnelly LF, Klostermeier TT, Klosterman LA. Traumatic elbow effusions in pediatric patients: are occult fractures the rule? *AJR Am J Roentgenol.* 1998;171(1):243–245.
21. Eckert K, Janssen N, Ackermann O, et al. Ultrasound diagnosis of supracondylar fractures in children. *Eur J Trauma Emerg Surg.* 2014;40(2):159–168.
22. Edmonds EW. How displaced are "nondisplaced" fractures of the medial humeral epicondyle in children? Results of a three-dimensional computed tomography analysis. *J Bone Joint Surg Am.* 2010;92(17):2785–2791.
23. Emery KH, Zingula SN, Anton CG, et al. Pediatric elbow fractures: a new angle on an old topic. *Pediatr Radiol.* 2016;46(1):61–66.
24. Fletcher ND, Schiller JR, Garg S, et al. Increased severity of type III supracondylar humerus fractures in the preteen population. *J Pediatr Orthop.* 2012;32(6):567–572.
25. Griffith JF, Roebuck DJ, Cheng JC, et al. Acute elbow trauma in children: spectrum of injury revealed by MR imaging not apparent on radiographs. *AJR Am J Roentgenol.* 2001;176(1):53–60.
26. Gufler H, Schulze CG, Wagner S, Baumbach L. MRI for occult physeal fracture detection in children and adolescents. *Acta Radiol.* 2013;54(4):467–472.
27. Haraldsson S. On osteochondrosis deformans juvenilis capituli humeri including investigation of intraosseous vasculature in distal humerus. *Acta Orthop Scand Suppl.* 1959;38:1–232.
28. Haraldsson S. The intra-osseous vasculature of the distal end of the humerus with special reference to capitulum; preliminary communication. *Acta Orthop Scand.* 1957;27(1):81–93.
29. Hawksworth CR, Freeland P. Inability to fully extend the injured elbow: an indicator of significant injury. *Arch Emerg Med.* 1991;8(4):253–256.
30. Henrikson B. Supracondylar fracture of the humerus in children. A late review of end-results with special reference to the cause of deformity, disability and complications. *Acta Chir Scand Suppl.* 1966;369:1–72.
31. Herman MJ, Boardman MJ, Hoover JR, Chafetz RS. Relationship of the anterior humeral line to the capitellar ossific nucleus: variability with age. *J Bone Joint Surg Am.* 2009;91(9):2188–2193.
32. Houshian S, Mehdi B, Larsen MS. The epidemiology of elbow fracture in children: analysis of 355 fractures, with special reference to supracondylar humerus fractures. *J Orthop Sci.* 2001;6(4):312–315.
33. Ippolito E, Caterini R, Scola E. Supracondylar fractures of the humerus in children. Analysis at maturity of 53 patients treated conservatively. *J Bone Joint Surg Am.* 1986;68(3):333–344.
34. Jenkins FA Jr. The functional anatomy and evolution of the mammalian humero-ulnar articulation. *Am J Anat.* 1973;137(3):281–297.

35. Kappelhof B, Roorda BL, Poppelaars MA, et al. Occult fractures in children with a radiographic fat pad sign of the elbow: a meta-analysis of 10 published studies. *JBJS Rev.* 2022;10(10).

36. Kissoon N, Galpin R, Gayle M, et al. Evaluation of the role of comparison radiographs in the diagnosis of traumatic elbow injuries. *J Pediatr Orthop.* 1995;15(4): 449–453.

37. Klatt JB, Aoki SK. The location of the medial humeral epicondyle in children: position based on common radiographic landmarks. *J Pediatr Orthop.* 2012;32(5): 477–482.

38. Kohn AM. Soft tissue alterations in elbow trauma. *Am J Roentgenol Radium Ther Nucl Med.* 1959;82:867–874.

39. Lamprakis A, Vlasis K, Siampou E, et al. Can elbow-extension test be used as an alternative to radiographs in primary care? *Eur J Gen Pract.* 2007;13(4): 221–224.

40. Landin LA, Danielsson LG. Elbow fractures in children: an epidemiological analysis of 589 cases. *Acta Orthop Scand.* 1986;57(4):309–312.

41. Lennon RI, Riyat MS, Hilliam R, et al. Can a normal range of elbow movement predict a normal elbow x-ray? *Emerg Med J.* 2007;24(2):86–88.

42. Li W, Stimec J, Camp M, et al. Pediatric musculoskeletal radiographs: anatomy and fractures prone to diagnostic error among emergency physicians. *J Emerg Med.* 2022; 62(4):524–533.

43. Major NM, Crawford ST. Elbow effusions in trauma in adults and children: is there an occult fracture? *AJR Am J Roentgenol.* 2002;178(2):413–418.

44. Pappas N, Lawrence JT, Donegan D, et al. Intraobserver and interobserver agreement in the measurement of displaced humeral medial epicondyle fractures in children. *J Bone Joint Surg Am.* 2010;92(2):322–327.

45. Peterson CA, Peterson HA. Analysis of the incidence of injuries to the epiphyseal growth plate. *J Trauma.* 1972;12(4):275–281.

46. Petit P, Sapin C, Henry G, et al. Rate of abnormal osteoarticular radiographic findings in pediatric patients. *AJR Am J Roentgenol.* 2001;176(4):987–990.

47. Rabiner JE, Khine H, Avner JR, et al. Accuracy of point of care ultrasonography for diagnosis of elbow fractures in children. *Ann Emerg Med.* 2013;61(1):9–17.

48. Sandegrad E. Fracture of the lower end of the humerus in children: treatment and end of the elbow in children. *J Bone Joint Surg Am.* 1999;81:1429–1433.

49. Schlacter JA, Roussos D, Masrouha K, et al. Effect of a protocol to reduce radiographic imaging in pediatric patients with suspected fractures. *J Pediatr Orthop.* 2023; 43(1):61–64.

50. Schunk K, Grossholz M, Schild H. Der supinatorfettkorper bei frakturen des ellbogengelenkes. *ROFO.* 1989;150(3):294–296.

51. Shank CF, Wiater BP, Pace JL, et al. The lateral capitellohumeral angle in normal children: mean, variation, and reliability in comparison to Baumann's angle. *J Pediatr Orthop.* 2011;31(3):266–271.

52. Shelmerdine SC, White RD, Liu H, et al. Artificial intelligence for radiological paediatric fracture assessment: a systematic review. *Insights Imaging.* 2022;13(1):94.

53. Shintani K, Hosomi R, Suzuki K, et al. Diagnostic imaging for elbow TRASH lesions in children and usefulness of ultrasonography using standard planes. *J Pediatr Orthop B.* 2023;32(6):557–564.

54. Shrader MW, Campbell MD, Jacofsky DJ. Accuracy of emergency room physicians' interpretation of elbow fractures in children. *Orthopedics.* 2008;31(12):1117–1119.

55. Silva M, Pandarinath R, Farng E, et al. Inter- and intra-observer reliability of the Baumann angle of the humerus in children with supracondylar humeral fractures. *Int Orthop.* 2010;34(4):553–557.

56. Simanovsky N, Lamdan R, Hiller N, Simanovsky N. The measurements and standardization of humerocondylar angle in children. *J Pediatr Orthop.* 2008;28(4): 463–465.

57. Skaggs DL, Mirzayan R. The posterior fat pad sign in association with occult fracture of the elbow in children. *J Bone Joint Surg Am.* 1999;81:1429–1433.

58. Stoneback JW, Owens BD, Sykes J, et al. Incidence of elbow dislocations in the United States population. *J Bone Joint Surg Am.* 2012;94(3):240–245.

59. Sumko MJ, Hennrikus W, Slough J, et al. Measurement of radiation exposure when using the mini C-arm to reduce pediatric upper extremity fractures. *J Pediatr Orthop.* 2016;36(2):122–125.

60. Supakul N, Hicks RA, Caltoum CB, Karmazyn B. Distal humeral epiphyseal separation in young children: an often-missed fracture-radiographic signs and ultrasound confirmatory diagnosis. *AJR Am J Roentgenol.* 2015;204(2):W192–W198.

61. Vinson DR, Kann GS, Gaona SD, Panacek EA. Performance of the 4-way range of motion test for radiographic injuries after blunt elbow trauma. *Am J Emerg Med.* 2016; 34(2):235–239.

62. Voth M, Lustenberger T, Auner B, et al. What injuries should we expect in the emergence room? *Injury.* 2017;48(10):2119–2124.

63. Waters PM, Bae DS. Elbow "TRASH" lesions. In: Waters PM, Bae DS, eds. *Pediatric Hand and Upper Extremity Surgery: A Practical Guide.* Lippincott Williams & Wilkins; 2012:379–390.

64. Waters PM, Beaty J, Kasser J. Elbow "TRASH" (the radiographic appearance seemed harmless) lesions. *J Pediatr Orthop.* 2010;30(2 Suppl):S77–S81.

65. Yang Z, Wang Y, Gilula LA, Yamaguchi K. Microcirculation of the distal humeral epiphyseal cartilage: implications for posttraumatic growth deformities. *J Hand Surg Am.* 1998;23(1):165–172.

Supracondylar Fractures of the Distal Humerus

Jonathan G. Schoenecker and Donald S. Bae

Supracondylar Fractures of the Distal Humerus

INTRODUCTION TO SUPRACONDYLAR FRACTURES OF THE DISTAL HUMERUS

Supracondylar humerus (SCH) fractures are the most common pediatric elbow fractures,[36] and the most common fracture requiring surgery in children. The peak age range at which most supracondylar fractures occur is 5 to 6 years.[26]

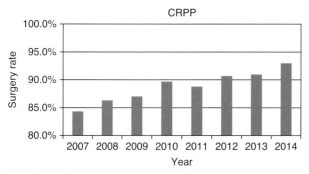

Figure 14-1. The percentage of patients who underwent CRPP for the treatment of a supracondylar humeral fracture. A significant increase in the rate of CRPP ($P < .0001$) was demonstrated.

The prevailing evidence and consensus advocate for the operative treatment of displaced SCH fractures with surgical reduction and fixation.[3,64,108,114] Advancements in the treatment methodologies for supracondylar fractures in pediatric patients have significantly reduced the incidence of malunion and compartment syndrome.[3,16,77,87,91,108,145] Over the past decade or so, more than 500 peer-reviewed articles have been published on supracondylar fractures, yet there still is no consensus in numerous treatment areas. A survey consisting of 88 questions was conducted among 35 pediatric orthopaedic surgeons, but agreement was only reached on 27% of the questions.[65]

A database search revealed that annually, over 10,000 pediatric supracondylar fractures are reported in emergency departments across the United States.[63] Out of these, 24% undergo surgical treatment, with 87% being closed reductions; the rate of surgical treatment has been rising over time (Fig. 14-1). The transfer rates for these fractures escalated from 5.6% in 2006 to 9.1% in 2011, typically from general or rural hospitals to urban or academic centers.

A study comparing the treatment outcomes of supracondylar fractures by pediatric orthopaedic fellowship–trained surgeons and general orthopaedic surgeons found no significant difference in the complication rates. However, patients treated by non–fellowship-trained surgeons were approximately four times more likely to experience insufficient fixation and 10 times more likely to undergo an open reduction.[37] There seems to be a trend toward a higher proportion of these injuries being treated by pediatric orthopaedic specialists, with one center reporting an increase of over 100% over a 10-year period.[160]

ASSESSMENT OF SUPRACONDYLAR FRACTURES OF THE DISTAL HUMERUS

In instances where a child experiences elbow pain or an inability to utilize the upper extremity postfall, an elbow or forearm fracture should be suspected. A comprehensive examination of the entire limb is crucial, with radiographs recommended for any areas exhibiting tenderness or swelling, as the co-occurrence of multiple fractures (e.g., SCH fracture combined with a radius/ulna fracture) is not uncommon (Fig. 14-2). For children presenting with acute elbow pain and nonuse of the upper extremity, the differential diagnosis includes fracture, nursemaid's elbow, inflammatory arthritis, and infection.

When dealing with a nondisplaced supracondylar fracture, one may observe tenderness around the distal humerus and movement restriction, particularly a lack of full elbow extension. The radiographs might not show any abnormalities except for a posterior fat pad sign. In contrast, completely displaced fractures are characterized by evident gross displacement of the elbow (Fig. 14-3).

An anterior "pucker sign" may be present if the proximal fracture fragment has pierced the brachialis and the anterior fascia of the elbow (Fig. 14-4). This sign, which involves skin puckering resulting from the proximal segment puncturing the brachialis muscle, engaging the deep dermis, and recoiling, indicates significant soft tissue damage. If there is any bleeding from a punctate wound, it should be treated as an open fracture.

All patients should undergo thorough motor, sensory, and vascular examinations. Although challenging in young children, these examinations should be comprehensively performed and accurately recorded. Sensory testing should be conducted in distinct areas of the radial nerve (dorsal first web space), median nerve (palmar index fingertip), and ulnar nerve (ulnar side little fingertip). If a child is uncooperative or has altered mental status, a wet cloth may be wrapped around the hand to assess for subsequent skin wrinkling, although in practice this is seldom done. In this test, areas where the skin does not wrinkle indicate a lack of sensory innervation.

The motor examination should assess finger, wrist, and thumb extension (radial nerve), index finger distal interphalangeal (DIP) flexion and thumb interphalangeal (IP) flexion (anterior interosseous nerve, or AIN), finger flexion strength (median), and interossei (ulnar nerve) muscle function. In young children, the intrinsic muscles may be tested by asking

Figure 14-2. Occult ipsilateral fracture. Type II supracondylar fracture (*open arrow*) with an occult distal radial fracture (*solid arrows*). (Reproduced with permission of Children's Orthopaedic Center, Los Angeles, CA.)

A

B

Figure 14-3. A: Clinical appearance of an extension-type supracondylar with diffuse swelling. **B:** The S-shaped configuration is created by the anterior prominence of the proximal fragment's spike and extension of the distal fragment. (**A:** Courtesy of Children's Orthopaedic Surgery Foundation.)

the child to pinch something with their thumb and first finger, while palpating the first dorsal interosseous and adductor pollicis for muscle contracture.

If not possible to accurately determine sensory and/or motor function preoperatively, it's crucial to document this in the medical record and communicate it to relevant caregivers.

Preoperative misinformation can complicate postoperative decision making when a nerve or vascular deficit is discovered.

The vascular examination should include determining the presence of palpable radial pulse, as well as warmth, capillary refill, and color of the hand. Assessment of the vascular status is essential, as series report up to 20% of displaced fractures

A

B

Figure 14-4. The pucker sign. This patient had penetration of the proximal fragment's spike into the subcutaneous tissue. **A:** Clinical photograph depicting the characteristic ecchymosis and anterior puckering of the skin. **B:** Laterally, there is puckering of the skin (*arrow*) in the area where the spike has penetrated into the subcutaneous tissue. (**A:** Courtesy of Children's Orthopaedic Surgery Foundation.)

present with vascular compromise.[28,137] The vascular status may be classified into one of three categories:

- Hand well perfused (warm and red), radial pulse present and palpable
- Hand well perfused (warm and red), radial pulse not palpable but Dopplerable
- Hand well perfused (warm and red), radial pulse not palpable and not Dopplerable
- Hand poorly perfused (cool and blue or blanched), radial pulse absent

During the physical examination, a high degree of suspicion is essential to avoid overlooking the development of a compartment syndrome and/or Volkmann ischemia. These conditions often occur in fractures associated with significant swelling and/or ecchymosis, anterior skin puckering, and/or an absent pulse. However, compartment syndrome may also occur in less severe-appearing fractures, so continual vigilance is necessary. The turgor or firmness of the volar compartment should be assessed, and excessive swelling around the elbow should be noted. Pain accompanying passive finger extension and flexion should be recorded. Studies suggest that escalating anxiety and an increased need for pain medication might be the earliest indicators of compartment syndrome. Pediatric patients with compartment syndromes often exhibit the three A's: anxiety, agitation, and an escalating need for analgesics.[12] Vital information can be overlooked when evaluating a child with pain after acute injury, coupled with high patient and parental anxiety. Therefore, a higher suspicion of compartment syndrome should be maintained, particularly in cases of delayed presentation or a dysvascular hand.

MECHANISMS OF INJURY OF SUPRACONDYLAR FRACTURES OF THE DISTAL HUMERUS

Supracondylar fractures can be categorized into extension and flexion types, based on the mechanism of injury that determines the direction of displacement of the distal fragment. Extension-type fractures, responsible for around 97% to 99% of supracondylar fractures,[92] are typically the result of a fall onto an outstretched hand with the elbow in full extension (often hyperextension in the young elbow) (Fig. 14-5). These fractures are mostly caused by falls, often from playground equipment.[144] Studies have shown that the overall safety of playground design can impact the likelihood of a supracondylar fracture. In particular, children who use the least safe playgrounds are nearly five times as likely to sustain an SCH fracture compared to those who use the safest playgrounds.[113]

Most of this chapter is on extension-type fractures, with flexion-type fractures being covered at the end of the chapter. The medial and lateral columns of the distal humerus are connected by a thin segment of bone between the olecranon fossa posteriorly and coronoid fossa anteriorly, resulting in a high risk of fracture to this area (Fig. 14-6).

During forced elbow hyperextension, the olecranon exerts substantial pressure into the olecranon fossa, acting as a fulcrum, while the anterior capsule concurrently applies a tensile force on the distal humerus at its insertion point. The resulting injury is

Figure 14-5. Mechanism of injury—elbow hyperextension. **A:** Most children attempt to break their falls with the arm extended, and the elbow then hyperextends. **B:** The linear applied force (*large arrow*) leads to an anterior tension force. Posteriorly, the olecranon is forced into the depths of the olecranon fossa (*small arrow*). **C:** As the bending force continues, the distal humerus fails anteriorly in the thin supracondylar area. **D:** When the fracture is complete, the proximal fragment can continue moving anteriorly and distally, potentially harming adjacent soft tissue structures such as the brachialis muscle, brachial artery, and median nerve.

Figure 14-6. Supracondylar fractures occur through the thinnest portion of the distal humerus in the AP plane. The thin bone makes the fracture unstable.

Figure 14-7. Relationship between fracture deformity to the adjacent neurovascular structures at risk, depending upon the pattern of displacement. **A:** In extension-type supracondylar humerus fractures with medial displacement of the epiphyseal fragment, the radial nerve is at risk. **B:** With posterior and lateral displacement, the brachial artery and median nerve are at risk. **C:** In flexion-type supracondylar fractures, the ulnar nerve is at greater risk.

an extension-type supracondylar fracture. It is hypothesized that ligamentous laxity leading to elbow hyperextension predisposes an individual to this fracture,[104] but this correlation remains unclear. Typically, medial displacement of the distal fragment is more prevalent than lateral displacement, occurring in roughly 75% of patients in most series. The direction of displacement—whether medial or lateral—is also crucial as it identifies the soft tissue structures at risk from the penetrating injury of the proximal metaphyseal fragment. Medial displacement of the distal fragment endangers the radial nerve, while lateral displacement poses a risk to the median nerve and brachial artery[90] (Fig. 14-7).

Generally, these injuries have been described as flexion or extension types with medial or lateral displacement of the epiphyseal segment, based on orthogonal radiographic imaging taken in the coronal and sagittal projections. However, rotational forces play an important role in the mechanism of injury in many cases. Understanding of the rotational component of SCH fractures will aid in evaluation of fracture stability and reduction maneuvers for displaced injuries. For example, the extension-type fractures with medial displacement of the distal segment often occur with obligate internal rotation, explaining the presence of internal rotation in patients with "varus" malunion and informing the use of internal rotation torque when assessing stability of pin fixation configurations.

IMAGING AND OTHER DIAGNOSTIC STUDIES OF SUPRACONDYLAR FRACTURES OF THE DISTAL HUMERUS

All patients with a history of falling onto an outstretched hand, accompanied by pain and an inability to use the extremity,

should undergo comprehensive radiologic evaluation. If physical examination does not localize the injury to the elbow alone, anteroposterior (AP) and lateral views of the entire upper extremity should be considered. While experienced providers rarely require comparison views, radiographs of the uninjured extremity may be useful for assessing the incompletely ossified epiphysis. The overall accuracy of an emergency room physician's interpretation of elbow fractures in children has been reported to be only 53%.[139]

Radiographic evaluation should commence with a true AP view of the distal humerus. (In contrast, an AP of an elbow in 90 degrees of flexion will provide approximately a 45-degree oblique view of the distal humerus and proximal radius and ulna.) A true AP view of the distal humerus facilitates a more precise evaluation of the distal humerus and reduces the error in determining Baumann angle. The lateral radiograph should be taken as a true lateral with the humerus held in the anatomic position and not externally rotated (Fig. 14-8). Oblique views of the distal humerus may occasionally be beneficial when a supracondylar fracture or occult condylar fracture is suspected but not visible on standard AP and lateral views; however, these need not be routinely ordered for evaluating a clear supracondylar fracture.

In patients with incomplete or nondisplaced fractures, initial radiographs may be negative except for a posterior fat pad sign; this is particularly true in very young patients, in whom much of epiphysis remains unossified (Fig. 14-9). A series of patients with traumatic elbow pain and a posterior fat pad sign but no visible fracture found that 53% (18/34) had a supracondylar fracture, 26% (9/34) a fracture of the proximal ulna, 12% (4/34) a fracture of the lateral condyle, and 9% (3/34) a fracture of

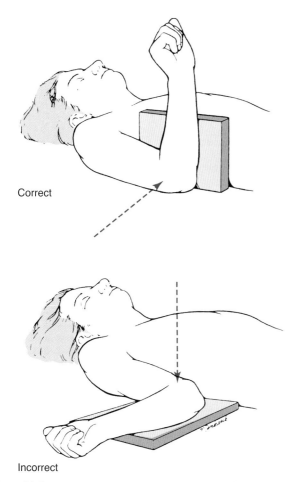

Correct

Incorrect

Figure 14-8. X-ray positioning. The correct method of taking a lateral view is with the upper extremity directed anteriorly rather than externally rotated.

the radial neck.[148] A more recent meta-analysis of 10 published papers noted that 43% of patients with a radiographic posterior fat pad sign had occult SCH fractures.[71]

The lateral radiograph, which is typically relied upon to identify fracture angulation and guide decision making, deserves special consideration. The anterior humeral line (AHL) should intersect the capitellum on a true lateral view of the elbow. Herman demonstrated that in a normal elbow, the AHL only passes through the middle third of the capitellum 52% of the time in children under 10 years of age. In children younger than 4 years old, the AHL is equally likely to pass through the anterior third of the capitellum as the middle third (Fig. 14-10).[57] Ryan et al.[127] found that in all children aged 5 years and above, the AHL should cross through the center of the capitellum. In an extension-type supracondylar fracture, the capitellum is positioned posterior to this line. Furthermore, it should be noted that on a true lateral view of a normal elbow, the "hourglass" shape of the coronoid and olecranon fossae should be tilted slightly anteriorly (see Fig. 14-9A); this radiographic feature can assist in diagnosing fractures with slight extension.

Baumann angle, also known as the humeral capitellar angle, is the angle subtended by lines drawn along the long axis of the humeral shaft and the capitellar physis (normal range is ~9–26 degrees) (Fig. 14-11). The interpretation of Baumann angle is subject to intra- and interobserver variability. In a prior report of five observers, differences of 7 degrees were seen in the measurement of Baumann angle.[142] As a general rule, a Baumann angle of at least 10 degrees is considered acceptable. A decrease in Baumann angle compared to the uninjured elbow indicates that a fracture is in varus malangulation.

If the AP and lateral views reveal a displaced supracondylar fracture but do not provide full details of the distal humeral fragment, further radiographic evaluation may aid in defining

Figure 14-9. A: Lateral radiograph demonstrating an elevated posterior fat pad (*white open arrow*) and a normal hourglass which is anteriorly tilted if there is not a displaced fracture. **B:** Another example of an elevated fat pad (*solid white arrows*). (Copyright © 2024 J. Schoenecker.)

A

B

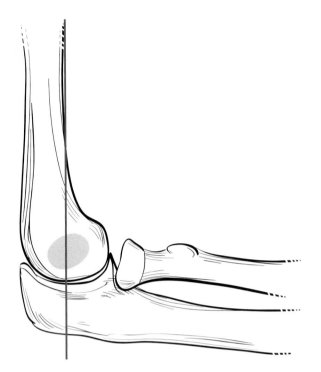

Figure 14-10. Anterior humeral line should cross the capitellum on a true lateral of the elbow, though not necessarily through the middle third of the capitellum as was previously believed. (From Tolo VT, Skaggs DL, eds. *Master Techniques in Orthopaedic Surgery: Pediatrics.* Lippincott Williams & Wilkins; 2007:1–15.)

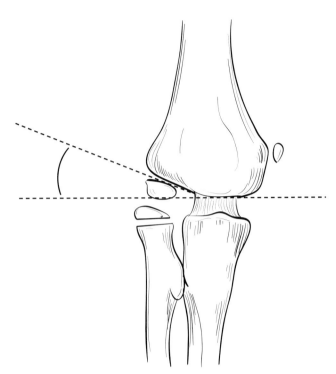

Figure 14-11. Baumann angle is between the line perpendicular to the long axis of the humeral shaft and the physeal line of the lateral condyle. A decrease in Baumann angle may indicate medial comminution. (From Tolo VT, Skaggs DL, eds. *Master Techniques in Orthopaedic Surgery: Pediatrics.* Lippincott Williams & Wilkins; 2007:1–15.)

fracture anatomy; this is done with a specific focus on impaction of the medial column, supracondylar comminution, and vertical split of the epiphyseal fragment. T-condylar fractures (Fig. 14-12) may be initially misdiagnosed as supracondylar fractures without intra-articular involvement. However,

T-condylar fractures usually occur in children over 10 years of age, a demographic where supracondylar fractures are less likely (see Chapter 15).

In very young children with primarily cartilaginous epiphyses, an epiphyseal separation can resemble an elbow dislocation.

Figure 14-12. Occult T-condylar fracture. **A:** Original x-rays appear to show a type II posteromedial supracondylar fracture. **B:** After manipulation, the vertical intercondylar fracture line (*arrows*) was visualized.

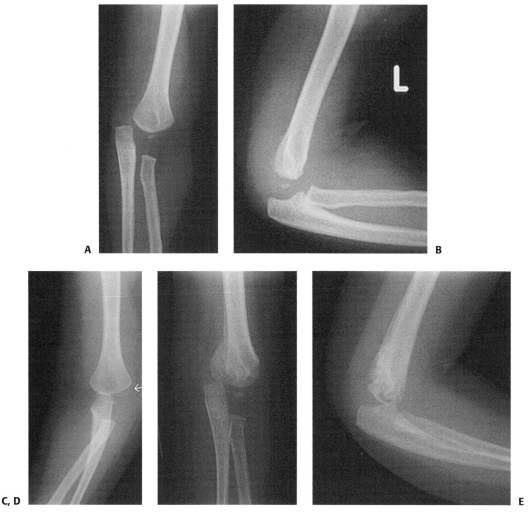

Figure 14-13. Twelve-month-old Salter II fracture resulting from child abuse. **A:** Note the radius points to the capitellum in all views, so this is not a dislocation. **B:** Lateral view. **C:** Oblique view shows the thin metaphyseal fragment, which defines this as a Salter II fracture. **D:** This fracture was not recognized at presentation to the emergency department. This AP view is 1 month old. **E:** Lateral view 1 month after injury. (Reproduced with permission of Children's Orthopaedic Center, Los Angeles, CA.)

In an epiphyseal separation, the fracture traverses the physis often without creating a metaphyseal fragment; therefore, no fracture line through ossified bone is seen. Furthermore, the ossified radius and ulna are malaligned in relationship with the humeral diaphysis. On physical examination, the patient presents with typical findings of a supracondylar fracture, including pronounced swelling around the elbow, malalignment, and significant discomfort. The key to diagnosing and differentiating an epiphyseal separation from an elbow dislocation radiographically lies in relationship between the proximal radius and the capitellar ossification center. In epiphyseal separations, the capitellum remains aligned with the radius.

In some cases, a thin metaphyseal fragment, which may give the impression of a lateral condyle fracture, may be seen, consistent with a Salter type II fracture pattern (Fig. 14-13). In such instances, additional data is necessary to diagnose and commence treatment. An arthrogram may prove useful (Fig. 14-14). In selected patients, magnetic resonance imaging or ultrasonography may also assist in evaluating the injury to the unossified epiphysis. This distinction is important because of the high risk of nonaccidental trauma in the young (age <3 years) with an epiphyseal separation with or without a metaphyseal fragment.

Of note, in one normal anatomical variant, the olecranon fossa may be absent (Fig. 14-15). Another normal anatomical variant is the supracondyloid process, which is present to some degree in approximately 1.5% of adult cadavers and should not be mistaken for fracture pathology. However, this anatomic variant can be the site of median nerve compression (Fig. 14-16).

CLASSIFICATION OF SUPRACONDYLAR FRACTURES OF THE DISTAL HUMERUS

Gartland Classification

A modified Gartland classification of supracondylar fractures is the most commonly accepted and used system.[3,108]

Figure 14-14. A: Salter II fracture in a 20-month-old is a bit easier to appreciate on arthrogram. **B:** Lateral view after reduction and pinning. (Reproduced with permission of Children's Orthopaedic Center, Los Angeles, CA.)

Figure 14-15. Normal anatomic variant in which there is no bone in the olecranon fossa. Note the minimally displaced radial neck fracture. (Reproduced with permission of Children's Orthopaedic Center, Los Angeles, CA.)

Supracondylar Fractures of the Distal Humerus:
MODIFIED GARTLAND CLASSIFICATION

Type	Description	Comments
I	<2-mm displacement	Periosteum torn and fat pad present acutely
II	Hinged posteriorly	Only sagittal plane displacement, AHL anterior to capitellum with greater angulation
III	Displaced	Sagittal and coronal plane displacement, variable amount of cortical continuity
IV	Multidirectional instability	Usually diagnosed with manipulation under fluoroscopic imaging
Medial comminution (not truly a separate type)	Collapse of medial column	Loss of Baumann angle, requires reduction

Type I

A Gartland type I fracture denotes a nondisplaced or minimally displaced (<2 mm) supracondylar fracture without change in the AHL. These fractures typically involve a tear of the anterior

Figure 14-16. **A:** AP radiograph of the distal humerus demonstrating a supracondylar process, a normal anatomic variant. **B:** Lateral radiograph demonstrating a supracondylar process. (Reproduced with permission of Children's Orthopaedic Center, Los Angeles, CA.)

periosteum with or without osseous injury; a posterior fat pad sign may be the only radiographic evidence of injury. There should be an intact olecranon fossa, no medial or lateral displacement, no medial column collapse, and a normal Baumann angle (Fig. 14-17).

Type II

A Gartland type II fracture involves a more significant tear of the anterior periosteum and at least a fracture of the anterior humeral cortex. These fractures typically lack a rotational or varus/valgus mechanism and are thus characterized by a pure sagittal plane deformity. It is displaced (>2 mm) with what is presumed to be an intact, yet hinged, posterior cortex. The AHL is usually located anterior to the capitellum on a true lateral view of the elbow (Fig. 14-18). However, in mildly angulated fractures, the AHL may intersect the capitellum (Fig. 14-19). If significant rotation in the coronal or transverse plane is present, it is classified as a type III fracture. The division of type II

Figure 14-17. Decision making using lateral x-rays. **A:** Typical type I fracture. The anterior humeral line (AHL) clearly goes through the capitellum. Cast with no more than 90 degrees of elbow flexion. **B:** Technically a type I fracture by definition as the AHL touches the capitellum. However, this fracture is at risk for displacement as the hourglass is not tilting forward, and the posterior cortex is broken as well. Initial treatment is casting at no more than 90 degrees of elbow flexion with the need for close follow-up stressed. **C:** Typical type II fracture, with the AHL missing the capitellum and the distal fragment hinged posteriorly. This is treated with closed reduction and pinning. **D:** As there is a hint of translation at the posterior cortex, this may be considered a type III fracture and should be reduced and pinned.

Figure 14-22. A: Intraoperative imaging demonstrates distal fragment falling into extension. **B:** As the elbow is flexed, the distal fragment falls into flexion, thus defining a Gartland type IV fracture. (Reprinted with permission from Leitch KK, et al. Treatment of multidirectionally unstable supracondylar humeral fractures in children: a modified Gartland type IV fracture. *J Bone Joint Surg Am.* 2006;88(5):980–985.)

The Special Case of Medial Column in Supracondylar Fractures of the Distal Humerus

A potential pitfall is failure to appreciate the malalignment of the medial column of the distal humerus, particularly in cases with medial column comminution and collapse (Fig. 14-23). With medial collapse, there is malrotation in the frontal plane, signifying that the injury is, at the very least, a Gartland type II

fracture. This collapse correlates with a decrease in Baumann angle and a varus malalignment, commonly known as cubitus varus. Most frequently, this is seen in type 3 valgus compression (comminution) or type 3 posterolateral (rotation) fractures. The lateral view, however, might display seemingly adequate alignment (Fig. 14-24). This can be misleading and lead to underestimation of fracture severity and instability, especially for those less familiar with the condition. Typically, these fracture patterns necessitate surgical reduction and pin fixation in order to avert late malunion.

Bahk et al.[14] reported that fractures with greater than 10 degrees of obliquity in the coronal plane or 20 degrees in the sagittal plane were more likely than fractures with less obliquity to result in malunion.

Figure 14-23. Medial (*arrow*) comminution is a subtle radiographic finding and indicates a more unstable variant that may collapse into the varus if not treated appropriately. (From Tolo VT, Skaggs DL. *Master Techniques in Orthopaedic Surgery: Pediatrics.* Lippincott; 2007:1–15.)

Figure 14-24. Note the lateral view does not show significant displacement. This view alone would suggest nonoperative treatment may be sufficient. (Reproduced with permission of Children's Orthopaedic Center, Los Angeles, CA.)

TABLE 14-1. Treatment Options for Subcondylar Fractures of the Distal Humerus

	Fracture Type			
Treatment	I	II	III	IV
Casting without reduction	Almost always			
Closed reduction and casting		Rarely indicated, do *not* flex elbow >90 degrees		
Closed reduction and pinning		Great majority of cases	Great majority of cases	Most cases
Open reduction and fixation		Uncommonly necessary	If closed reduction inadequate	If closed reduction inadequate

TREATMENT OPTIONS FOR SUPRACONDYLAR FRACTURES OF THE DISTAL HUMERUS

See Table 14-1 for treatment options for supracondylar fractures of the distal humerus based on fracture type.

INITIAL MANAGEMENT OF SUPRACONDYLAR FRACTURES OF THE DISTAL HUMERUS

Displaced supracondylar fractures requiring a reduction should be initially splinted with the elbow in a comfortable position, optimizing vascularity of the forearm/hand and minimizing soft tissue tension overlying the fracture fragment; this position is approximately 20 to 40 degrees of flexion. If the arm is pulseless, gentle traction and elbow flexion alone frequently restores a pulse. It can be helpful to palpate or doppler the radial pulse when determining the ideal position for immobilization, as it facilitates identification of the position that maximizes perfusion. Excessive flexion or extension may compromise the limb's vascularity and increase the risk of ischemia and/or compartment pressure.[17,95] The immobilized elbow and hand should then be gently elevated above the heart.

Urgency of Treatment

Several studies have concluded that delay of surgery of even over 24 hours had no deleterious effects on the outcomes of children with supracondylar fractures.[48,66,140,154,155] These studies were all retrospective and may have reported good results due to selection bias, as experienced pediatric orthopaedic surgeons move to more expedient treatment in select injuries, including those with neurovascular injuries.[48] A survey of 309 members of the Pediatric Orthopaedic Society of North America found that 81% of the respondents would treat a type III supracondylar humerus fracture (SCHF) presenting after normal work hours by splinting overnight and fixing the following morning, if there were no issues necessitating emergent fixation.[25]

Type II fractures may be a special case in this regard. Larson et al. reported on 399 consecutive cases in which it appears that timing for the operative treatment of type II fractures did

not affect outcome, with 52% of the fractures having surgery more than 24 hours after injury.[84] There were no compartment syndromes or vascular injuries in this group. Although there is little published data to support our opinion, we and others believe that if conditions such as poor perfusion, pulselessness, an associated displaced forearm fracture, firm compartments, skin puckering, antecubital ecchymosis, or very considerable swelling are present, operative treatment should not be unduly delayed.[3,102,114,121]

How Late Can Fractures Be Reduced?

Little has been written about how long after injury a fracture can still be closed reduced. Silva et al.[143] reported 42 type II SCH fractures treated 7 to 15 days after injury. They found that closed anatomic reduction was achieved in all fractures, with equal outcomes to fractures treated within 7 days of injury. We would caution that in very young children, reliable fracture reduction 2 weeks after injury with early callus formation is less likely. Two children closed reduced 8 days after injury developed avascular necrosis (AVN) of the trochlea.[143] Although these numbers are small, this phenomenon warrants further study. Lal and Bhan[90] reported that delayed open reduction (11–17 days after injury) did not increase the frequency of myositis ossificans. If a supracondylar fracture is unreduced or poorly reduced, delayed open reduction and pin fixation appear to be justified.

NONOPERATIVE MANAGEMENT OF SUPRACONDYLAR FRACTURES OF THE DISTAL HUMERUS

Closed Reduction and Casting

Closed reduction and casting of SCH fractures is not practiced in most modern centers. Most pediatric orthopaedic surgeons reserve cast immobilization for stable, nondisplaced fractures (type I) that do not require reduction.

Mildly displaced fractures can be reduced closed, using the intact posterior periosteum as a stabilizing force and then holding reduction by flexing the elbow greater than 120 degrees. Less flexion increases the risk of loss of reduction. The concern with closed reduction and flexion greater than 120 degrees is the risk of vascular compromise and/or compartment syndrome in the presence of anterior swelling and neurovascular compression. If closed reduction and casting are performed, the patients need to be monitored closely for neurovascular compromise and loss of reduction. Follow-up radiographs require AP views of the distal humerus to interpret with elbow flexion beyond 120 degrees. If necessary, rereduction or conversion to pinning needs to occur before full healing occurs, therefore, close radiographic follow-up is necessary for the first 3 weeks or less.

Traction

Traction as definitive treatment for supracondylar fractures in children is largely of historic interest. Indications for traction may include lack of anesthesia, medical conditions prohibiting anesthesia, lack of an experienced surgeon, or severe open wounds. Devnani[34] reported using traction in the gradual reduction of eight fractures with late presentation (mean of 5.6 days), though 18% of these children went on to a corrective osteotomy for malunion. Rates of cubitus varus from 9% to 33% have been reported in some traction-treated series, whereas others have reported excellent results.[47,62,171] Traction is difficult to justify economically due to the prolonged hospitalization necessary, given the excellent results with closed reduction and pinning, which usually requires no more than one-night hospitalization and is associated with a low rate of intraoperative complications.

OPERATIVE MANAGEMENT OF SUPRACONDYLAR FRACTURES OF THE DISTAL HUMERUS

Closed Reduction and Pinning

The most prevalent operative treatment for supracondylar fractures is closed reduction followed by percutaneous pin fixation.

For almost all displaced supracondylar fractures, barring those that are open, an initial attempt at closed reduction is advisable. Under general anesthesia and with the assistance of fluoroscopy, the frontal plane deformity is corrected, typically with longitudinal traction and medial or lateral translation of the distal fragment. The elbow is then flexed with anteriorly directed force on the olecranon, correcting the sagittal deformity and leading to fracture reduction. An appropriate reduction is determined by correction of Baumann angle (typically >10 degrees) on the AP fluoroscopic image, restoration of medial and lateral column alignment on oblique views, and confirmation that the AHL traverses the middle third of the capitellum on the lateral projection. Given the substantial compensatory rotation at the shoulder, slight rotational discrepancies at the fracture site are well tolerated. However, rotational malalignment may jeopardize fracture stability; if observed, one should exercise added caution in evaluating the postreduction stability.

The reduced fracture is typically secured with two to three Kirschner (K-) wires. Divergent pins may be placed via lateral insertion, or medial and lateral entry pins may be placed in a crossed configuration when lateral-only constructs do not achieve medial column stability. Depending on swelling and vascular conditions, the elbow is immobilized in flexion. Situations where a persistent fracture gap is seen fluoroscopically or a soft, "rubbery" sensation is felt during bony reduction raise concerns for soft tissue incarceration, including neurovascular bundle (NVB). In such instances, an open reduction should be considered (Fig. 14-25).

Crossed Pins Versus Lateral Entry Pins

Lateral entry pins are now being used more commonly than crossed pins for most supracondylar fractures.[1,5,18,25,79,93] A

Figure 14-25. Brachial artery and median nerve may be trapped at the fracture site. **A:** If a reduction feels rubbery and a gap at the fracture site is seen on imaging, entrapment is possible, especially in the setting of vascular compromise or median nerve or anterior interosseous nerve injury. **B:** Intraoperative photograph of a left elbow with the brachial artery (*red elastic loop*) and median nerve (*yellow elastic loop*) incarcerated at the fracture site during attempted closed reduction (*arrow*). (**A:** From Tolo VT, Skaggs DL, eds. *Master Techniques in Orthopaedic Surgery: Pediatrics.* Lippincott; 2007:1–15. **B:** Courtesy of Children's Orthopaedic Surgery Foundation.)

A

B

survey of 309 members of the Pediatric Orthopaedic Society of North America found that 70% of surgeon respondents prefer lateral pins.[25] Some series report that when a medial pin is used, there are more complications[168] or longer surgical time,[79] but other series find no difference.[48,170]

The decision regarding crossed versus lateral entry pin configurations is predicated on the balance between risks of iatrogenic injury to the ulnar nerve and loss for fracture reduction. Iatrogenic injury to the ulnar nerve with use of crossed pins has been reported to be as low as 0%, but large series of supracondylar fractures at major pediatric centers have shown the prevalence to be 5% to 6%.[1,33,122,147,172] Others have reported that these injuries occur more commonly.[166] A meta-analysis of 1,158 patients in seven randomized controlled trials (RCTs) and six prospective comparative cohorts found iatrogenic ulnar nerve injury was more than 10 times more likely when a medial pin was used, compared to lateral entry pins (4.1% [20/493] vs. 0.3% [2/666]) but no difference in loss of fixation between the two techniques.[33] Smaller series reported a 13% (5/39) risk of iatrogenic ulnar nerve injury when pediatric orthopaedic fellowship–trained surgeons used a medial pin,[37] and one series even reported a 21% (10/48) rate of iatrogenic ulnar nerve injury with a medial pin.[18]

Three meta-analyses have examined the issue of pin configuration and iatrogenic nerve injury. In 2010, Slobogean et al.[150] reported on 32 trials with 2,639 patients and found there was an iatrogenic ulnar nerve injury for every 28 patients treated with crossed pins compared to lateral pinning. In the same year, Babal et al.[8] reported on a systematic review of 35 articles discussing medial and lateral pinning versus lateral entry pinning and found that iatrogenic ulnar nerve injury occurred in 40 of 1,171 (3.4%) of crossed pins and 5 of 738 (0.7%) of lateral entry pins. The 2012 report by Woratanarat et al.[168] included 18 studies and 1,615 supracondylar fractures. They reported the risk of iatrogenic ulnar nerve injury to be 4.3 times higher in cross-pinning compared to lateral pinning. They found no difference in loss of fixation, late deformity, or Flynn criteria between the two types of pinning.

A prospective, surgeon-randomized study was performed on 104 children with type III supracondylar fractures, with surgeons using their preferred techniques of crossed pins or lateral entry pins. The authors found no statistical difference in the radiographic outcomes between lateral entry and crossed pin techniques, but two cases of iatrogenic injury to the ulnar nerve occurred with medially placed pins.[49]

Zaltz et al.[172] reported that in children less than 5 years of age, when the elbow is flexed more than 90 degrees, the ulnar nerve migrated over, or even anterior to, the medial epicondyle in 61% (32/52) of cases. Wind et al.[166] showed that the location of the ulnar nerve cannot be adequately determined by palpation to allow blind medial pinning. Unfortunately, making an incision over the medial epicondyle for medial pin placement does not ensure protection of the ulnar nerve.[147]

In a series of six cases of iatrogenic ulnar nerve injuries with early exploration, the nerve was directly penetrated by the pin in two cases (33.3%), with constriction of the cubital tunnel occurring in three cases (50%), and the nerve being fixed anterior to the medial epicondyle in one (16.7%) case.[122] Thus, even if direct penetration of the ulnar nerve is avoided, simply placing a medial epicondyle entry pin adjacent to the nerve can cause injury, presumably by constriction of the cubital tunnel or kinking of the nerve. Iatrogenic ulnar nerve injuries usually resolve spontaneously, but there have been several reports of permanent neurologic deficits.[120,122,147]

A series of 345 supracondylar fractures treated by percutaneous pinning showed that the use of a medial pin was associated with a 4% (6/149) risk of ulnar nerve injury when the medial pin was placed without hyperflexion and 15% (11/71) if the medial pin was placed with hyperflexion.[147] None of the 125 fractures treated with lateral entry pins alone resulted in iatrogenic injury. This is consistent with the findings of Zaltz et al.[172] of anterior subluxation of the ulnar nerve with elbow flexion beyond 90 degrees. Thus, the published literature supports the conclusion that if a medial pin is used, the lateral pins should be placed first, then the elbow extended and the medial pin placed without hyperflexion of the elbow.

The second issue with pin configuration is stability of fracture fixation. Biomechanical studies of stability of various pin configurations should be interpreted with care. Two studies evaluated the torsional strength of pin configurations and found crossed pins to be stronger than two lateral pins.[109,173] However, in these studies, the two lateral pins were placed immediately adjacent to each other and not separated at the fracture site as is recommended clinically for lateral entry pins.[56,116,131,145] In synthetic humeri study, Srikumaran et al.[153] found crossed pins to be stronger than two lateral entry pins, but did not test three lateral entry pins. Lee et al.[86] found that two divergent lateral pins separated at the fracture site were superior to crossed pins in extension loading and varus but were equivalent in valgus (Fig. 14-26). The greater

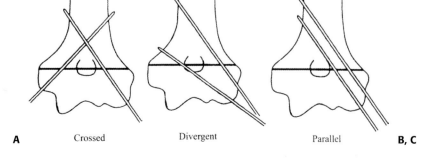

Figure 14-26. Three pinning techniques. **A:** Crossed: one medial and one lateral pin. **B:** Divergent: two divergent lateral pins. **C:** Parallel: two parallel lateral pins. (Reprinted with permission from Lee YH, et al. Three lateral divergent or parallel pin fixations for the treatment of displaced supracondylar humerus fractures in children. *J Pediatr Orthop.* 2008;28(4):417–422.)

A   Crossed   Divergent   Parallel   B, C strength was attributed to the location of the intersection of the two pins and greater divergence between the two pins, allowing for medial as well as lateral column fixation. Crossed pins are also more suitable to high medial oblique and other fracture patterns precluding adequate lateral pin fixation.[136]

Bloom et al.[20] reported that three lateral entry divergent pins were equivalent to cross-pinning and both were stronger than two lateral divergent pins. Another study with simulated medial comminution showed that three lateral divergent pins had equivalent torsional stability to standard medial and lateral crossed pinning.[85] Feng et al.[42] reported that two and three lateral entry pins had comparable construct stiffness to each other, and both were greater than crossed pins to all types of stress, except in valgus, in which crossed pins had greater stiffness. Thus, contemporary biomechanical studies mostly support clinical recommendations for lateral entry pins.[3,108,131,145]

Multiple biomechanical studies have reported that in addition to pin configuration, larger diameter pins provide more stability.[52,118,153]

A series of 124 consecutive fractures treated with lateral entry pins reported no malunions or loss of fixation.[145] From this successful series, combined with a failure analysis of eight fractures performed outside of this series, the authors concluded the important technical points for fixation with lateral entry pins as follows[145]:

- Maximize separation of the pins at the fracture site.[116]
- Engage the medial and lateral columns proximal to the fracture.
- Engage sufficient bone in both the proximal segment and the distal fragment.
- Maintain a low threshold for use of a third lateral entry pin if there is concern about fracture stability or the location of the first two pins.
- Use three pins for type III fractures.

In a study of eight cases of supracondylar fractures that lost reduction, Sankar et al. reported that loss of fixation in all cases was because of technical errors that were identifiable on the intraoperative fluoroscopic images and that could have been prevented with proper technique. They identified three types of pin fixation errors[131]: failure to engage both fragments with two or more pins, failure to achieve bicortical fixation with two pins or more, and failure to achieve adequate pin separation (>2 mm) at the fracture site. A systematic review of 35 articles reported loss of reduction in 0 out of 849 crossed pins and 4 out of 606 (0.7%) lateral entry pins.[22] Based on this study and the previous series by Skaggs et al.,[145] we recommend a minimum of two pins for a type II fracture and three pins for a type III fracture.

A study of 192 patients concluded that pin spread is an important factor associated with preventing loss of reduction, with the goal of pin spacing at least 13 mm or one-third the width of the humerus at the level of the fracture.[116]

Two prospective randomized clinical trials comparing lateral and cross-pinning techniques in the treatment of displaced SCH fractures showed no statistically significant difference between the two treatment groups in any radiographic or clinical outcome measures,[77,159] including nerve injury. It is interesting that

following the randomized clinical trial,[77] the same eight surgeons who used crossed pins in 59% of SCH fractures pretrial changed their practice to use crossed pins in only 15% of cases posttrial.[93]

An alternative technique using antegrade insertion of elastic intramedullary nailing has not been widely adopted, given that distal pinning of the fracture leads to reliably excellent results in most cases.

Open Reduction

Open reduction is indicated in cases of open fractures, failed closed reduction, a loss of pulse during fracture reduction, insufficient perfusion or nerve injury following fracture manipulation. Over time, the rate of open reductions in the United States has been steadily decreasing over time, with about 6% in the most recent year reported (Fig. 14-27).[63] Specialized pediatric trauma centers report even lower numbers, such as 0.7% (9/1,296) at Denver Children's Hospital,[48] and 2% (8/339) at Children's Hospital Los Angeles.[147] In the past, open reductions raised concerns of elbow stiffness, myositis ossificans, scarring, and iatrogenic neurovascular injury. However, several reports have demonstrated low rates of complications with open reduction, in the setting of more severe soft tissue and bony injuries. Ay et al.[7] found no loss of motion or clinical deformity in 61 patients treated with open reduction. In a prospective, randomized controlled study of 28 children, Kaewpornsawan[75] compared closed reduction and percutaneous pin fixation with open reduction (through a lateral approach); the patients treated with percutaneous pin fixation showed no differences with regard to cubitus varus, neurovascular injury, the range of motion (ROM), the infection rate, the union rate, or the criteria of Flynn et al.[45] In older children (8–14 years) with supracondylar fractures, Mollon et al.[98] reported a mean loss of 30 degrees of elbow flexion at final follow-up in patients treated with open reduction internal fixation compared with those treated with closed reduction percutaneous pinning. Twenty-two-year follow-up of 49 patients in Turkey showed 84% good functional outcomes, mean of 4 degrees varus/valgus difference from the contralateral side, mean of 5 degrees flexion deficit, and 4 degrees extension deficit.[54]

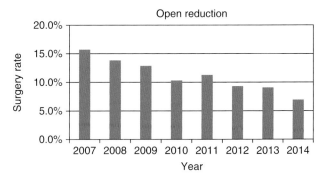

Figure 14-27. The percentage of patients who underwent open reduction for the treatment of a supracondylar humeral fracture. A significant decrease in the rate of open reduction (P < .0001) over time was demonstrated.

Figure 14-28. Intraosseous blood supply of the distal humerus. **A:** The vessels supplying the lateral condylar epiphysis enter on the posterior aspect and course for a considerable distance before reaching the ossific nucleus. **B:** Two definite vessels supply the ossification center of the medial crista of the trochlea. The lateral vessel enters by crossing the physis. The medial one enters by way of the nonarticular edge of the medial crista.

Surgical Approach

The direct anterior approach to the elbow is extremely useful for open reduction, particularly in cases of neurovascular compromise. The anterior approach has the advantage of allowing direct visualization of the brachial artery and median nerve as well as the fracture fragments. The exposure is through the torn periosteum and disrupted brachialis and therefore does not further destabilize the fracture with more soft tissue dissection. When performed through a relatively small (5–8 cm) transverse incision above or at the cubital fossa at the fracture site, the resulting scar is much more aesthetic than that of the lateral approach, and scar contracture limiting elbow extension is not an issue. A series of 26 patients treated with the anterior approach showed equivalent results to the traditional lateral or combined lateral and medial approach in terms of malunion, Flynn criteria,[45] and ROM.

The posterior approach for an extended supracondylar fracture risks a higher rate of loss of motion, further fracture instability with exposure through intact periosteum, and, most importantly, increased risk of AVN due to disruption of the posterior-end arterial supply to the trochlea of the humerus[5,80,97,167] (Fig. 14-28). This approach is not recommended.

OPERATIVE TREATMENT BY FRACTURE TYPE

Type I (Nondisplaced)

Simple immobilization with elbow flexion of 70 to 90 degrees, coupled with the forearm in a neutral rotation, is typically sufficient for type I fractures. In the absence of marked swelling around the elbow, a full cast can be applied; however, if swelling is pronounced, the cast should bivalved, or splints used for initial immobilization. Caregivers should be educated about the importance of elevation and signs and symptoms indicative of compartment syndrome. The elbow's flexion should generally not surpass 90 degrees. Through a Doppler study on the brachial artery postsupracondylar fractures, Mapes and Hennrikus observed reduced flow in the brachial artery during pronation and heightened flexion.[95] Prior to applying the splint, it's crucial to ensure a palpable pulse and to verify adequate perfusion in the position of intended elbow flexion. The immobilization should not be constrictive.

Radiographs may be taken 3 to 7 days after the fracture to evaluate for late displacement. If there is evidence of distal fragment extension, as assessed by the AHL not intersecting with the capitellum, the fracture ideally undergoes closed reduction followed by percutaneous pinning for optimal alignment and stabilization.

The desired alignment is characterized by the AHL intersecting the capitellum on the lateral x-ray, a Baumann angle exceeding 10 degrees or mirroring the opposite side, and an unblemished olecranon fossa. Regardless of fracture type, the immobilization period for supracondylar fractures is typically 3 to 4 weeks. Physical therapy is usually not beneficial or prescribed. Patients may be reevaluated at 4 to 6 weeks after the removal of immobilization to ensure recovery of elbow motion and strength, but more recently published information suggests these follow-up visits are not necessary.[4,115] Given that type I fractures predictably yield excellent outcomes when alignment is maintained, subsequent appointments may be decided upon based on medical circumstances and family preferences.

It is important to remember that the primary radiograph provides a static snapshot of the injury, which may involve soft tissue disruption greater than expected from the bony alignment. Pronounced swelling, disruptions in nerve function or vascularity, or excessive pain suggest a more severe injury than a type I fracture; concomitant periosteal disruption may contribute to fracture instability and late loss of reduction. Additionally, medial column comminution carries a risk of collapse into varus malalignment even during cast immobilization.

Type II Fracture (Hinged Posteriorly, With Posterior Cortex in Continuity)

The contemporary treatment of most type II fractures consists of closed reduction and percutaneous pin fixation. During this procedure, the fracture is reduced with elbow flexion, followed by verification of reduction on AP, lateral, and oblique fluoroscopy. Subsequently, two lateral pins are introduced[131,145,147] into the distal humeral segment, passed across the fracture, with engagement of the opposite cortex of the proximal fragment (see Figs. 14-4, 14-17C, D, and 14-29) (see Closed Reduction and Pinning section). The posterior cortex combined with the intact periosteum provides some intrinsic stability. Cross-pinning is rarely necessary for a type II fracture. Pins are left protruding through the skin to facilitate subsequent removal without the need for sedation or anesthesia, typically 3 weeks after fixation.

Figure 14-29. Properly placed divergent lateral entry pins. On the AP view, there should be maximal pin separation at the fracture site, the pins should engage both medial and lateral columns just proximal to the fracture site, and they should engage an adequate amount of bone proximal and distal to the fragments. On the lateral view, pins should incline slightly in the anterior to posterior direction in accordance with normal anatomy. (Reprinted with permission from Skaggs DL, et al. Lateral-entry pin fixation in the management of supracondylar fractures in children. *J Bone Joint Surg Am.* 2004;86(4):702–707.)

Casting Versus Closed Reduction and Percutaneous Pinning (CRPP) of Type II Supracondylar Fractures of the Distal Humerus

The distal humerus provides 20% of the longitudinal growth of the humerus and thus has little remodeling potential. The upper limb grows approximately 10 cm during the first year, 6 cm during the second year, 5 cm during the third year, 3.5 cm during the fourth year, and 3 cm during the fifth year of life.[36] In toddlers (<3 years of age) with greater growth remaining, some remodeling potential is present, so the surgeon may choose nonoperative treatment of a type II fracture in which the AHL abuts, but does not cross, the capitellum. In a child who is 8 to 10 years old, however, there is only 10% of growth of the distal humerus remaining, so adequate reduction and stabilization are essential to prevent malunion.

Recently, there has been a renewed enthusiasm for closed reduction and casting without pin fixation for some type II fractures. The interest in nonoperative treatment of type II fractures is based upon both subclassification of type II injuries and concerns regarding the risks and costs of surgical management. Wilkins previously distinguished between type IIA fractures, which have no rotational or translational displacement, and type IIB fractures, which do have rotation and translation. For type IIA fracture in which there is only extension deformity, closed reduction and casting may be sufficient. Sanders et al. published a prospective series of 99 type IIA patients, of which 45 were treated with closed reduction and casting.[130] Though 9% of casted patients converted to surgery, patient-reported outcomes at a mean of 2 years were equivalent in both treatment groups. McCartney et al.[96] reported their experience with 54 patients treated with closed reduction and casting of type IIA injuries. Sixteen (30%) of fractures converted to surgical treatment due to early displacement.

These series support the notion that a subset of type II injuries may be amenable to closed reduction alone but highlight the risks of late displacement and challenges in discerning instability based upon a single static set of radiographs. Along these lines, Hadlow et al.[55] noted that 23% (11/48) of type II patients in their series lost reduction following closed reduction and underwent delayed operative fixation. Fourteen percent (2/14) that were followed had a poor outcome by Flynn criteria.[45] Parikh et al.[112] similarly showed a 28% (7/25) loss of reduction, 20% (5/25) need for delayed surgery, and 2% (2/25) unsatisfactory outcome according to Flynn criteria in a smaller series of elbow treated with closed reduction.

Similarly, Fitzgibbons et al.[43] reported 20% lost reduction in the closed treatment of 61 type II fractures. They noted that failure was more likely to occur in more displaced fractures in which the AHL did not touch the capitellum, and in those children with wider upper arms. They concluded that "a reasonable protocol" would involve urgent pinning of fractures in which the capitellum extends beyond the AHL, whereas fractures that are less displaced could undergo reduction and casting and then be followed at 1-week intervals.[43] In a series of 155 type II SCH fractures treated nonoperatively, Camus et al.[24] reported that fractures were found to have radiographic evidence of sagittal plane (80% with abnormal AHL, decreased humerocapitellar angle), coronal plane (47% with abnormal Baumann angle), and rotational (44%) deformities. An additional consideration when treating SCH fractures nonsurgically is the likelihood of the child following up with an orthopaedic surgeon soon enough for a loss of reduction to be rereduced. Fletcher et al.[44] reported that children with supracondylar fractures seen at a large urban hospital in the United States were almost three times less likely to be seen back in clinic if they had public insurance or no insurance.

In contrast to the frequent loss of reduction seen with cast immobilization alone, closed reduction and percutaneous pin fixation have predictably good results. A consecutive series of 69 children with type II fractures treated with closed reduction and pinning reported no radiographic or clinical loss of reduction, no cubitus varus, no hyperextension, and no loss of motion. There were no iatrogenic nerve palsies, and no patient required additional surgery.[145] In another study of 189 consecutive type II fractures treated with CRPP, there were only four (2%) pin-tract infections, of which three were treated successfully with oral antibiotics and pin removal (1.5%) and one (0.5%) underwent operative irrigation and debridement for a wound infection not involving the joint. There were no nerve or vascular injuries, and no loss of reduction, delayed unions, or malunions. The authors concluded that pinning type II supracondylar fractures leads to a high probability of satisfactory outcome compared with previous studies of closed reduction without pinning.[149]

Another compelling rationale for pin fixation of type II fractures pertains to the amount of hyperflexion needed to maintain reduction in unpinned type II fractures, predisposing these patients to increased compartment pressures.[17] A study by Mapes and Hennrikus[95] showed that a pulse was lost to Doppler when type II fractures are flexed more than 110 degrees and type III fractures are flexed more than 70 degrees. Pronation also decreased flow in the brachial artery. To truly stabilize an extension fracture treated closed, greater than 120 degrees of flexion is required. Pinning these fractures obviates the need for immobilization with excessive elbow flexion. The basic tenet is that any fracture that requires greater than 90 degrees of elbow flexion to maintain bony alignment increases the risk of neurovascular compromise and/or compartment syndrome; therefore, the reduction should instead be held by pins, permitting immobilization of the elbow in less flexion (usually about 45–70 degrees).

Type III Fractures

For type III fractures, the standard of care in most contemporary centers is surgical reduction followed by pin fixation. Various studies have indicated that the outcomes of type III fractures managed with closed reduction and cast immobilization are inferior to those treated with pinning. Hadlow et al.[55] documented that a mere 61% of type III and 77% of type II fractures were effectively managed without the use of pins. It bears repeated emphasis that flexing the elbow with a type III supracondylar fracture beyond 90 degrees considerably increases the risk of compartment syndrome. Prolonged immobilization in hyperflexion should be seldom performed, particularly if modern operative facilities and a proficient surgeon are available. According to certain analyses,[107] type III fractures are more likely than type II injuries to lose reduction and require revision surgery.

Posteromedial Versus Posterolateral Displacement of Extension-Type Supracondylar Fractures of the Distal Humerus

The periosteum plays a key role with regard to treatment.[124] With extension-type injuries, the anterior periosteum is likely torn. The intact posterior periosteal hinge provides stability to the fracture and facilitates reduction with a flexion maneuver. Many authors have described adding forearm pronation to assist in reduction, but this need not be automatic. The direction of fracture displacement often indicates whether the medial or lateral periosteum remains intact. With a posteromedially displaced fracture, the mechanism of injury typically involves an external rotational moment initiating anterior and extending around the lateral column periosteum, leaving the medial periosteum intact. Elbow flexion and forearm pronation place the posterior periosteum and lateral soft tissues on tension, which corrects varus and extension malalignment and adds to stability of fracture reduction (Fig. 14-30). The anterior and medial periosteum, however, is often torn in a posterolaterally displaced fracture, occurring from an internal rotational moment, in which case pronation may be counterproductive.[119] Instead, in a posterolaterally displaced supracondylar fracture, forearm supination in addition to flexion, and external rotation, may be better because the lateral periosteum is usually intact (Table 14-2). If the posterior periosteal hinge is also disrupted, the fracture becomes unstable in both flexion and extension; this pattern has been described as a multidirectionally unstable, modified Gartland type IV fracture.[88]

The Special Case of Medial Column Comminution

Fractures with medial comminution may not have the dramatic displacement of most type III fractures but are best treated with operative reduction and pin fixation because collapse of the

Figure 14-30. Laterally torn periosteum in a posteromedially displaced supracondylar humerus fracture. (From Skaggs DL. Closed reduction and pinning of supracondylar humerus fractures. In: Tolo VT, Skaggs DL, eds. *Master Techniques in Orthopaedic Surgery: Pediatrics.* Lippincott Williams & Wilkins; 2007.)

medial column will lead to varus deformity (see Fig. 14-23). De Boeck et al.[32] recommended closed reduction with percutaneous pinning when a fracture had medial comminution even in otherwise minimally displaced fractures, to prevent cubitus varus. In this retrospective review, none of the six patients with medial comminution who underwent reduction and operative fixation had coronal plane deformity whereas four of seven (57%) patients who were treated nonoperatively developed cubitus varus.

The technique for reduction of a medial comminuted fracture is significant valgus force applied across a straight elbow. Often, so much force is required that one is fearful of creating a new fracture. Well-placed lateral entry pins are sufficient to hold the reduction.

Open Fractures

Open supracondylar fractures generally have an anterior puncture wound where the metaphyseal spike penetrates the skin (Fig. 14-31). Even if the wound is only a small puncture in the center of an anterior pucker, open irrigation and debridement are indicated. The open wound may be extended medially and laterally to provide a transverse incision for anterior approach.

TABLE 14-2. Forearm Rotation to Aid in Reduction as a Function of Direction of Fracture Displacement

Displacement	Periosteum Is Torn	Forearm Rotation to Aid in Reduction
Posterior medial	Lateral	Pronation
Posterior lateral	Medial	Supination

The NVB is usually directly under the skin and tented over the metaphyseal fragment, so care should be taken during the superficial surgical approach. The skin incision can be extended proximally along the medial aspect of the brachium (to follow the brachial artery and median nerve) and distally along the volar-lateral forearm if needed. Usually, only the transverse portion of the incision is required, which gives a better aesthetic result. The brachialis muscle is tethered distally by its insertion on the coronoid and is usually transected by the displaced proximal metaphyseal fragment. Blunt finger dissection is often sufficient to localize the fracture. After adequate exposure, the fracture surfaces are examined and washed, utilizing a curette to remove any foreign contaminant or entrapped soft tissue. Once the debridement and irrigation are complete, the fracture is reduced with elbow flexion, ensuring the periosteum does not become interposed in the fracture site. Stabilization is achieved with percutaneously placed K-wires. All patients with open fractures are also treated with intravenous antibiotics: generally, cefazolin for Gustilo type I, II, and IIIA injuries, with the addition of appropriate antibiotics to cover gram-negative organisms for type IIIB and C fractures.

OPERATIVE TECHNIQUES

Closed Reduction and Percutaneous Pinning

Preoperative Planning

Figure 14-31. Open supracondylar humerus fracture. The distal humerus metaphysis is completely protruding through the transverse open wound of the right elbow. (Courtesy of Children's Orthopaedic Surgery Foundation)

✓ Closed Reduction and Percutaneous Pinning: PREOPERATIVE PLANNING CHECKLIST

OR table	❑ Radiolucent arm board; alternatively may place affected limb on image intensifier of a fluoroscopy machine
Position	❑ Supine, with the fractured elbow on a short radiolucent arm board or image intensifier
Fluoroscopy location	❑ X-ray unit from head of bed, monitor opposite the surgeon
Equipment	❑ K-wires: most commonly, 0.062-inch smooth K-wires are used in patients less than 20 kg, and 5/64-inch K-wires in patients more than 20 kg, sterile coban, sterile felt, sterile foam

Technique

✓ Closed Reduction and Percutaneous Pinning: KEY SURGICAL STEPS

- ❑ Prep and drape
- ❑ Traction
- ❑ Fracture reduction
- ❑ Check reduction
- ❑ Tape or hold in reduced position
- ❑ Place K-wires
- ❑ Check reduction
- ❑ Bend and cut wires
- ❑ Apply felt, foam, and cast

Positioning

In the operating room, the patient receives a general anesthetic and prophylactic antibiotics. We prefer to have the fluoroscopy monitor opposite the surgeon for ease of viewing (Fig. 14-32).

The patient is positioned supine on the operating table, with the fractured elbow on a short radiolucent arm board.[145] Some surgeons use the wide end (image intensifier) of the fluoroscopy unit as the table, though this setup will limit rotation of the fluoroscopy unit to obtain lateral images of the elbow which is useful in very unstable fractures, such as type IV. Furthermore, recent information suggests that this alternative positioning may increase radiation exposure.[99] It is essential that the child's arm is far enough onto the arm board that the elbow can be well visualized with fluoroscopy. In very small children, this may necessitate placing the child's shoulder and head on the arm board (Fig. 14-33).

Figure 14-32. Positioning the fluoroscopy monitor on the opposite side of the bed allows the surgeon to easily see the images while operating. (From Tolo VT, Skaggs DL, eds. *Master Techniques in Orthopaedic Surgery: Pediatrics.* Lippincott Williams & Wilkins; 2007:1–15.)

Figure 14-33. In small children, imaging of the elbow may be difficult if the arm is not long enough to reach the center of the fluoroscopy unit. By placing the child's head in the crack between the operating room table and the arm board, the elbow is more easily imaged, and the child's head is unlikely to be inadvertently pulled off the side of the bed during the procedure. (From Tolo VT, Skaggs DL, eds. *Master Techniques in Orthopaedic Surgery: Pediatrics.* Lippincott Williams & Wilkins; 2007:1–15.)

Prep and drape the injured arm with an extremity drape. Apply traction with the elbow flexed approximately 20 degrees to minimize the risk of tethering neurovascular structures over an anteriorly displaced proximal fragment. For severely displaced fractures, hold significant traction for 60 seconds to allow soft tissue realignment, with the surgeon grasping the forearm with both hands, and the assistant providing countertraction in the axilla (Fig. 14-34). With the elbow almost straight, varus and valgus alignment in the coronal plane is corrected by movement of the forearm. Medial and lateral displacement of the distal fragment is corrected with direct translation of the distal fragment by the surgeon with image confirmation. The elbow is then slowly flexed while applying anteriorly directed pressure to the olecranon with the surgeon's thumb (Fig. 14-35). Pronate the forearm for posteromedially displaced fractures, and supinate for posterolaterally displaced fractures.

The reduction is then checked by fluoroscopic images in AP, lateral, and oblique planes. Verify four points to check for a good reduction: (1) the AHL intersects the capitellum (Fig. 14-36), (2) Baumann angle is greater than 10 degrees (Fig. 14-37), and (3 and 4) the medial *and* lateral columns are aligned on oblique views (Fig. 14-38). We will accept some translation of the distal fragment (up to 5 mm), as long as the above criteria are met. Once reduction is satisfactory, elastic tape or gauze may be placed around the elbow to hold the fracture in the reduced position while pinning (Fig. 14-39).

Figure 14-34. Reduction maneuver: Traction with elbow flexed 20 to 30 degrees. Assistant provides countertraction against patient's axilla (*white arrow*) to allow for significant traction to be applied. (From Tolo VT, Skaggs DL, eds. *Master Techniques in Orthopaedic Surgery: Pediatrics.* Lippincott Williams & Wilkins; 2007:1–15.)

Position elbow on a folded towel. Palpate the lateral humeral condyle. The K-wire is placed against the lateral condyle without piercing skin and checked under AP fluoroscopic guidance to assess the starting point. The K-wire may be held in the surgeon's hand at this point, not in the drill, to facilitate precise placement. If the starting point and trajectory are correct, the wire may be pushed through the skin and onto the cartilage

Figure 14-35. Reduction maneuver: Flex elbow while pushing anteriorly on olecranon with the thumb(s). (From Tolo VT, Skaggs DL, eds. *Master Techniques in Orthopaedic Surgery: Pediatrics.* Lippincott; 2007:1–15.)

Figure 14-36. Anterior humeral line should cross the capitellum on a true lateral of the elbow. (From Tolo VT, Skaggs DL, eds. *Master Techniques in Orthopaedic Surgery: Pediatrics.* Lippincott Williams & Wilkins; 2007:1–15.)

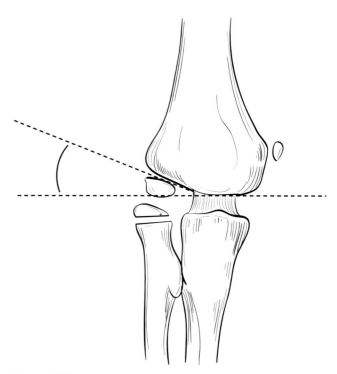

Figure 14-37. The Baumann angle is between the line perpendicular to the long axis of the humeral shaft and the physeal line of the lateral condyle. A decrease in the Baumann angle may indicate medial comminution. (From Tolo VT, Skaggs DL, eds. *Master Techniques in Orthopaedic Surgery: Pediatrics.* Lippincott Williams & Wilkins; 2007:1–15.)

of the distal lateral condyle; gentle force may allow the tip of the K-wire to engage the cartilage and maintain the appropriate starting point (Fig. 14-40). Place K-wires to maximally separate the pins at the fracture site to engage both the medial and lateral columns (see Fig. 14-29). In the sagittal plane, the reduced capitellum lies slightly anterior to the longitudinal axis of the

humerus, thus the pin may start a bit anterior to the plane of the fracture and angulate about 10 to 15 degrees posteriorly to maximize osseous purchase in the distal fragment. If imaging verifies correct pin placement, then advance each pin with a drill through the opposite cortex. After pin placement, the elbow is extended and the reduction is again checked under fluoroscopy

A   **B**

Figure 14-38. A: Oblique fluoroscopic view of the elbow demonstrating continuity of the medial column following adequate fracture reduction. **B:** Demonstration of lateral column continuity. (From Tolo VT, Skaggs DL, eds. *Master Techniques in Orthopaedic Surgery: Pediatrics.* Lippincott Williams & Wilkins; 2007:1–15.)

Figure 14-39. Fracture reduction is maintained by taping elbow in hyperflexed position. The wire may be pushed through the skin and into the cartilage using the cartilage of the distal lateral condyle as a pincushion that will hold the K-wire in place while carefully examining the AP and lateral images. (Reproduced with permission of Children's Orthopaedic Center, Los Angeles, CA.)

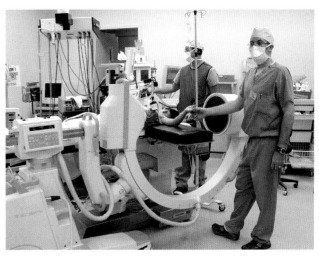

Figure 14-40. In very unstable fractures, rotation of the shoulder into external rotation to obtain a lateral image of the elbow may lead to a loss of reduction. In these rare instances, rotation of the C-arm, rather than the elbow, is a useful trick. (From Tolo VT, Skaggs DL, eds. *Master Techniques in Orthopaedic Surgery: Pediatrics.* Lippincott Williams & Wilkins; 2007:1–15.)

with lateral, oblique, and AP views (Fig. 14-41). Stress is applied in varus and valgus under fluoroscopy to ensure stable reduction. If there is any instability, you want to know about it now, rather than a week later. If there is instability, we will add a third lateral entry pin (Fig. 14-42). Vascular status is assessed. The wires are bent and cut. Take care to leave the wires at least 1 to 2 cm off the skin to prevent migration of the wires under the skin. A sterile felt square with a slit or drain sponge is then placed around the wires to protect the skin (Fig. 14-43). Foam may be loosely applied along the anterior and posterior aspects

of the elbow to allow for swelling[134] (Fig. 14-44). The cast is then applied in 45 to 70 degrees of elbow flexion, as flexion to 90 degrees may needlessly increase the risk of compartment syndrome (Fig. 14-45).

Medial Pin

In rare instances when three lateral pins do not stabilize the fracture, or there is an oblique fracture pattern preventing multiple lateral entry pins, a medial pin may be considered. The internal rotation stress test (IRST) may be utilized to ascertain the need

A, B   **C**

Figure 14-41. A: Assessment of sagittal alignment with lateral view. **B:** Both oblique views are checked to assess reduction of medial and lateral columns. **C:** If the lateral and oblique views show good reduction, the tape is removed and reduction and pin placement are checked in the AP view with elbow in relative elbow extension. (From Tolo VT, Skaggs DL, eds. *Master Techniques in Orthopaedic Surgery: Pediatrics.* Lippincott Williams & Wilkins; 2007:1–15.)

A, B

C

D

Figure 14-42. **A:** AP radiograph of a type III fracture in a 6-year-old boy. **B:** Lateral view. **C:** AP radiograph 3 weeks postoperative. **D:** Lateral view. (Reproduced with permission of Children's Orthopaedic Center, Los Angeles, CA.)

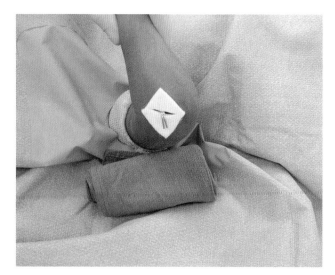

Figure 14-43. Skin is protected from pins with felt squares. (From Tolo VT, Skaggs DL, eds. *Master Techniques in Orthopaedic Surgery: Pediatrics.* Lippincott Williams & Wilkins; 2007:1–15.)

Figure 14-44. Sterile foam is placed directly on skin. If there is any circumferential dressing placed under the foam, it may be restricting. (From Tolo VT, Skaggs DL, eds. *Master Techniques in Orthopaedic Surgery: Pediatrics.* Lippincott Williams & Wilkins; 2007:1–15.)

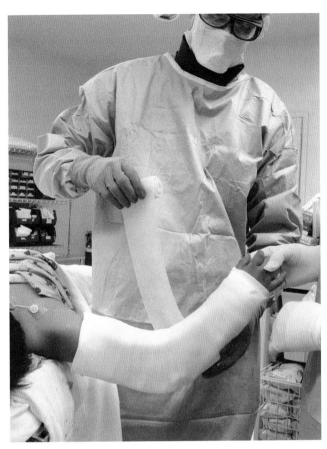

Figure 14-45. Cast with elbow flexion no more than 70 degrees and less flexion for very swollen elbows. (From Tolo VT, Skaggs DL, eds. *Master Techniques in Orthopaedic Surgery: Pediatrics.* Lippincott Williams & Wilkins; 2007:1–15.)

Figure 14-46. Algorithm for management of the pulseless supracondylar humerus fracture.

for crossed-pin configuration.[124] The elbow is extended to relax tension on the ulnar nerve and surrounding tissue, and the surgeon can palpate the medial epicondyle which is posterior to the center plane of the distal humerus. The entry site for medial pin placement is anterior on the medial epicondyle. A small incision is made to expose and protect the ulnar nerve. A drill guide is used to prevent binding of the perineural soft tissues that could kink the nerve. After desired pin placement is confirmed on fluoroscopy, the medial epicondyle and nerve are inspected to be certain there is no injury, impingement, or kinking of the nerve throughout flexion–extension arc of elbow motion.

Postreduction Perfusion

If there is any question of perfusion following fracture reduction in the operating room, the surgical prep (Betadine) is removed to evaluate the skin color. In addition, a Doppler is used to assess for the radial pulse at the wrist. In the case of a poorly perfused hand following reduction, open exploration and decompression or repair of the artery is required. In a case where the hand was well perfused prior to reduction and then poorly or not perfused after reduction and pinning, one must assume the artery is entrapped within the fracture site or compressed/kinked by adjacent soft tissue. Open exploration

of the artery is required. Either decompression of the intact artery or repair/reconstruction of an injured artery will be necessary; repeat open reduction and repinning of fracture may be necessary.

If there is no pulse postoperatively in an arm that had no pulse preoperatively, but the hand is warm and well perfused, Doppler examination provides helpful information. If a biphasic or triphasic signal is obtained at the wrist, our preference is careful observation of the child in hospital for 24 to 48 hours with the arm immobilized and mildly elevated[59] (Fig. 14-46). This is particularly true if there is associated preoperative median neuropathy, as the patient will not have the expected level of pain with a pending compartment syndrome. Any alteration in vascularity requires prompt operative intervention.

Open Reduction and Pinning

Technique

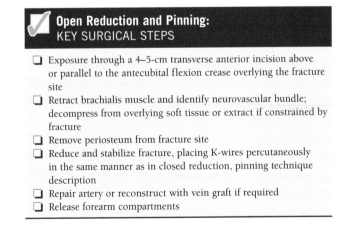

Open Reduction and Pinning:
KEY SURGICAL STEPS

- ❑ Exposure through a 4–5-cm transverse anterior incision above or parallel to the antecubital flexion crease overlying the fracture site
- ❑ Retract brachialis muscle and identify neurovascular bundle; decompress from overlying soft tissue or extract if constrained by fracture
- ❑ Remove periosteum from fracture site
- ❑ Reduce and stabilize fracture, placing K-wires percutaneously in the same manner as in closed reduction, pinning technique description
- ❑ Repair artery or reconstruct with vein graft if required
- ❑ Release forearm compartments

Make a 4- to 5-cm transverse anterior incision above and/or parallel to the antecubital flexion crease at the fracture site which allows access to the neurovascular structures and is aesthetic (see Fig. 14-42C). Retract the disrupted brachialis muscle and identify NVB proximal and distal to fracture site. Follow NVB to and across fracture site. If needed, untether or extract nerve and/or artery from fracture site. If more visualization is needed, this incision can be extended proximally along the medial aspect of the brachium or distally along the lateral volar forearm, based on fracture displacement. Liberate the periosteum, which is often entrapped in the fracture site. Open reduce and stabilize fracture. Place K-wires in the same manner as in closed reduction with percutaneous pinning. Just medial to the biceps tendon the brachial artery is noted, with the median nerve just medial to the artery. If the artery cannot be located in a patient presenting with a pulseless, poorly perfused hand, search for the lacerated ends of a torn artery, which may have retracted proximally and distally (Fig. 14-47). Repair artery or reconstruct with vein graft, if required. Release forearm compartments to prevent reperfusion compartment syndrome in cases of arterial reconstruction following prolonged periods of vascular insufficiency.

Figure 14-47. The brachial artery was lacerated by the proximal fragment. Bulldog clips have been placed on each end of the artery to control bleeding, and the median nerve is within the vessel loop. (Reproduced with permission from Children's Orthopaedic Center, Los Angeles, CA.)

Authors' Preferred Treatment for Supracondylar Fractures of the Distal Humerus

Algorithm 14-1. Authors' preferred treatment for type I to III supracondylar fractures of the distal humerus.

Type I to III Fractures (Algorithm 14-1)

Type I fractures are managed in a long-arm cast with approximately 80 to 90 degrees of elbow flexion for approximately 3 weeks. Follow-up x-rays at 1 week are recommended for assessment of fracture position.

We prefer closed reduction and pinning of type II supracondylar fractures. Two lateral pins are chosen as the initial postreduction fixation method in nearly all cases (see Fig. 14-17). If two lateral pins fail to provide acceptable fixation, we do not hesitate to place a third lateral pin. We

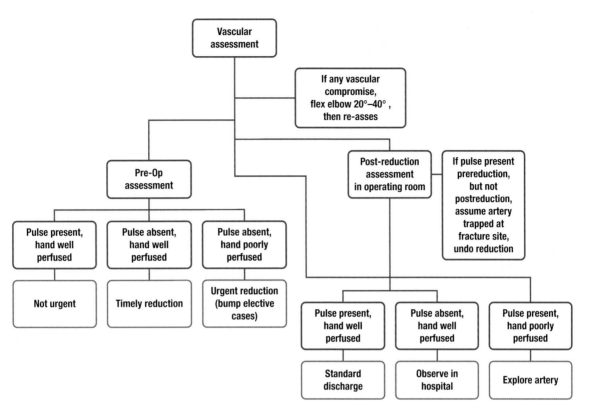

Algorithm 14-2. Authors' preferred treatment for type IV supracondylar fractures of the distal humerus.

believe it is safer to hold a type II fracture reduced with pins, rather than flex the elbow greater than 90 degrees.

For type III fractures, CRPP are attempted first. If closed reduction cannot be obtained, open reduction via an anterior approach and pinning is performed. A well-padded cast is applied, with x-rays and pin removal at week 3.

Type IV Fractures (Algorithm 14-2)

Although this extremely unstable fracture could be treated with open reduction, we follow the protocol recommended by Leitch et al.[88] First, place two K-wires into the distal fragment. Next, the fracture is reduced in the AP plane and verified by imaging. At this point, a lateral image may be obtained

by carefully rotating the limb through the shoulder, or by rotating the fluoroscopy unit into the lateral view (see Fig. 14-38B). The fracture is then reduced in the sagittal plane and the K-wires are driven across the fracture site. The reduction often is in midposition of flexion and extension (~60 degrees) and requires holding the reduction with distraction by the surgeon while the assistant places the first lateral entry stabilizing pin. In very unstable situations when distraction is insufficient, greater elbow flexion combined with longitudinal axial load through the forearm can be used to achieve the appropriate balance. Using these maneuvers, over 80% of type IV fractures can be closed reduced and pin stabilized with good results.[141]

Postoperative Care

Swanson et al.[156] reported that acetaminophen is as effective as narcotic analgesics for providing pain control after supracondylar fracture surgery in children, and Kay et al.[74] reported that perioperative ketorolac does not increase the risk of complications following operative fracture care. We use acetaminophen and a nonsteroidal anti-inflammatory drug (NSAID) as the first-line medications for pain relief, as narcotics are historically associated with more side effects.

A series of 618 patients found administration of postoperative antibiotics after CRPP of pediatric SCH fractures does not decrease the rate of surgical-site infection.[132]

Patients with minimal swelling felt to be at little risk for compartment syndrome may be discharged home with appropriate postoperative instructions, but otherwise, children are generally admitted overnight for elevation and observation. We recommend that the elbow is elevated over the heart for 48 hours postoperatively. Typically we do not have patients return for interval radiographic evaluation; however, in rare type IV fractures or cases with considerable comminution, imaging at 5 to 7 days postoperatively can be obtained.[117] In the unlikely event of loss of reduction, re-reduction is still feasible within the first week. The cast is generally removed 3 to 4 weeks postoperatively, at which time we have traditionally obtained radiographs out of the cast. A study of over 500 patients suggests that routine radiographs at 3 to 4 weeks are not necessary as they did not change treatment.[73] The authors suggested only taking radiographs at 3 to 4 weeks if clinically indicated by pain, deformity, or a severe fracture pattern. The pins are removed in the outpatient clinic at this time. ROM exercises are taught to the family, targeting gentle flexion and extension, to be started immediately after cast and pin removal. Families are counseled to return to clinic for follow-up evaluation if there is incomplete return of motion by 6 weeks postoperatively.

Potential Pitfalls and Preventions

Operative Treatment of Supracondylar Fractures of the Distal Humerus: POTENTIAL PITFALLS AND PREVENTIONS

Pitfall	Prevention
Closed Reduction and Percutaneous Pinning	
Nerve entrapment	If during the reduction maneuver, the fracture does not stay reduced and a "rubbery" feeling is encountered instead of the desired "bone-on-bone" feeling, the median nerve and/or brachial artery may be trapped within the fracture site (see Fig. 14-25). If this occurs, an open reduction is generally necessary to remove the neurovascular structures from the fracture site.
Proximal fragment has pierced the brachialis	"Milking maneuver"[118]: the biceps are forcibly "milked" in a proximal to distal direction past the proximal fragment, often culminating in a palpable release of the humerus posteriorly through the brachialis (Fig. 14-48).
Inability to obtain closed reduction	Milking maneuver; try pronation and/or supination to aid in rotational realignment and stability. If reduction is not acceptable, perform open reduction.
Loss of reduction	In general, plan on a minimum of two pins for type II fractures and three pins for type III fractures.
	If the first pin is in between where you really wanted two pins, just leave it and place one on either side of it for a total of three pins.
	Aim to separate the pins as far as possible at the fracture site—at least 13 mm or one-third the width of the humerus at the level of the fracture.
	Pin separation at the fracture line is more important than whether the pins are divergent or parallel.
	A key element to ensure stable fixation is to feel the pin go through the far proximal cortex. If this feeling is not clearly appreciated, careful fluoroscopic imaging with oblique views will often reveal the pin did not engage the second cortex of the proximal fragment.
	To optimize pin placement, think of the cartilaginous distal humerus as a "pincushion." With the K-wires in your fingers (not the drill), push them into the cartilage in the exact location and trajectory you want. Verify with imaging, then advance the pin with a drill.
	It is acceptable to cross the olecranon fossa, which adds two more cortices to improve fixation, but this means the elbow cannot be fully extended until the pins are removed.
	A small amount of translation or axial rotational malalignment may be accepted, but accept very little frontal or sagittal plane angular malalignment.
	Following reduction and fixation, stress the fracture under live imaging to the point where you are confident it will not displace postoperatively. The IRST (internal rotation stress test) is a helpful assessment tool to guide optimal pin placement.
	If there is difficulty maintaining fracture reduction when eternally rotating the shoulder for a lateral view of the elbow, move the C-arm instead of the patient's arm (see Fig. 14-40).
	The child's elbow should sufficiently flex so that the fingers touch the shoulder. If not, the fracture is likely not reduced and remains in too much extension (Fig. 14-49).
	In the rare instance when three lateral pins do not adequately stabilize the fracture, or there is an oblique fracture pattern preventing multiple lateral entry pins, a medial pin may be used.
Ulnar nerve damage	If you choose to place a medial pin, extend the elbow when placing the pin to keep the ulnar nerve posteriorly out of harm's way. If the nerve is out postoperatively, return to OR, explore nerve, decompress, and repeat pining as needed.
Decreased elbow flexion	We save the images in which the reduction looks the "worst," particularly if some translational or rotational malreduction is accepted, to have for comparison during postoperative visits to determine if movement of the fracture occurred. It has been noted that if the AHL is anterior to the capitellum following fracture healing, the child will go on to have less elbow flexion than if the AHL touches the capitellum; and, even the AHL crossing the anterior third of the capitellum is associated with less elbow flexion than crossing the middle or posterior third.[70]
Compartment syndrome	Cast the elbow in less than 90 degrees of flexion; the pins are holding; the reduction, not the cast.
	Be attentive to the three A's postoperatively: analgesia requirements increasing, anxiety, agitation.
	Measure compartment pressures and release compartments if there is index of suspicion of compartment syndrome to avoid Volkman ischemic contracture.
Postreduction perfusion	If any question of perfusion, remove Betadine to evaluate the skin color; undertake Doppler assessment for a triphasic radial pulse at the wrist.
	Open exploration and decompression or repair of the artery may be required.

Pitfall	Prevention
Open Reduction and Pinning	
Damage to the neurovascular structures	Care must be taken in dissection as the neurovascular bundle may be immediately superficial as it is pushed against the skin by the proximal fracture fragment.
	With an avascular or dysvascular hand, the brachial artery is usually tethered by soft tissues in fracture site and needs to be gently teased out of fracture without harm. Sometimes, the artery is in fracture site and requires atraumatic extraction. Rarely, it is completely lacerated and retracted away from fracture site proximally and distally. This requires repair or reconstruction of the artery with a vein graft.
Reduction difficulty	A Freer elevator can be used as a lever to extricate the periosteum from the fracture site to facilitate the reduction.
	Be certain to obtain anatomic alignment before pinning.
	Reconstruct the artery if needed once the fracture is anatomic and stable.
Compartment syndrome	Release the forearm compartments if revascularization is required to lessen risk of reperfusion compartment syndrome.

MANAGEMENT OF EXPECTED ADVERSE OUTCOMES AND UNEXPECTED COMPLICATIONS RELATED TO SUPRACONDYLAR FRACTURES OF THE DISTAL HUMERUS

VASCULAR INJURIES

Approximately 1% to 15% of patients with supracondylar fractures present with an absent pulse, though only a small minority of these patients sustain an anatomic injury requiring vascular repair.[11,28,48,53,137] While arterial lacerations or intimal injuries leading to thrombosis can occur, more commonly the diminution of distal pulses is due to traction, kinking, or extrinsic compression on the brachial artery in the zone of injury.[162] Indeed, even in patients with type III fractures and palpable radial pulses, Doppler ultrasonographic evaluation of the brachial artery will show stenosis and elevated peak systolic flow velocities.[61]

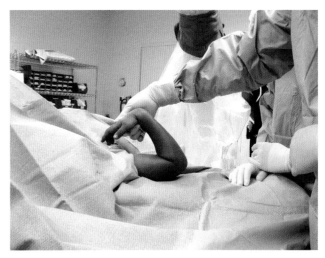

Figure 14-49. If fingers cannot touch shoulder, flexion deformity may not be reduced.

Figure 14-48. Brachialis muscle interposition is indicated on the left. The "milking maneuver" frees the brachialis muscle from its location in the fracture, allowing a closed reduction.

At the initial evaluation, the presence or absence of a pulse and perfusion of the hand should be determined. If there is no pulse, slight traction and gentle elbow flexion often restore the pulse and improve perfusion.[100] If there is not a palpable pulse, a Doppler may be used to assess the radial pulse at the wrist, which normally produces a triphasic signal. As one study found that every patient with a well-perfused yet pulseless hand had a Dopplerable pulse, a pulse that can be detected on Doppler may be an objective sign of good perfusion, but that has yet to be proven clinically.[48] Perfusion of the hand is estimated by color, warmth, pulp turgor, and arterial capillary refill, but there is no study yet with clear evidence of the reliability and validity of these standards. Capillary refill by itself can be deceiving. For example, after wrapping a rubber band around a finger, there is instant venous capillary refill but no artery inflow or venous outflow, so this must be differentiated from normal arterial capillary refill. Generally accepted normal perfusion criteria (viable hand) are capillary refill equivalent to the opposite side and less than 3 to 5 seconds, normal digital pulp turgor, and pink color. The clinician must distinguish between the nonviable and viable hand upon presentation and throughout care.

Hand perfusion, not presence or absence of a pulse, appears to be predictive of the need for arterial repair and risk of compartment syndrome. Choi et al.[28] reported on 25 pulseless patients whose hands were well perfused at presentation, and none (0%) required vascular repair or developed a compartment syndrome. In contrast, of eight patients who presented with poor distal perfusion, compartment syndrome developed in 25% and 38% underwent vascular repair. Garg et al.[48] reported 54 pulseless supracondylar fractures. Twenty-six of the patients (48%) had a return of palpable pulse following reduction. Twenty of these patients observed postreduction had a well-perfused hand with a pulse that could not be palpated but that could be detected on Doppler, one of which required vascular repair after loss of hand perfusion 9 hours after the operative reduction. All the other observed 19 patients had restoration of a palpable pulse by their first postoperative visit.

An absent radial pulse is not in itself an emergency, as collateral circulation may keep the limb well-perfused in the short term and potentially even long term. In the case of a pulseless, well-perfused hand, urgent reduction with pinning in the operating room is indicated.[108,128,137] In the presence of an associated median nerve injury, there is higher risk of a compartment syndrome and close observation with serial examinations until surgery is indicated.[101]

The pulseless arm with signs of poor perfusion (white color, decreased turgor, and/or slow capillary refill) constitutes a surgical emergency.[3] When a patient with a severely displaced supracondylar fracture presents to the emergency room and has compromised vascularity to the limb, the arm should be repositioned with the elbow in approximately 20 to 40 degrees of flexion which may improve vascular flow.[100,108] Regardless of return of pulse after repositioning of the elbow, the fracture should be reduced and pinned in a timely fashion.[100]

Fracture reduction should not be delayed by angiographic study or other advanced imaging modalities, as the location of the arterial lesion is known and fracture reduction usually restores the pulse.[3,27] Earlier studies support the notion that angiography is an unnecessary test that should not delay treatment.[100,137] Shaw et al.[137] reported on a series of 143 type III supracondylar fractures, 17 of which had vascular compromise. All underwent emergent reduction and percutaneous pinning without preoperative angiogram. In only 3 of the 17 (18%) patients, restored blood flow to the hand did not occur after reduction and required open exploration. In 14 of the 17 (82%) patients, restored blood flow to the hand occurred without complications. The authors concluded that prereduction angiography would add nothing to the management of these injuries. Choi et al.[27] reported that of 25 patients presenting with a pulseless but well-perfused hand, 100% did well clinically without arterial repair—52% (11) had a palpable pulse following surgery, and 48% (10) remained pulseless but well-perfused. Cheng et al.[26] in a series of 623 supracondylar fractures reported 9 cases presenting with an absent radial pulse (1.4%), of which only one required exploration. Garg et al.[48] reported 54 pulseless fractures, of which 9% (5/54) required vascular intervention.

Pulseless Hand

Prereduction White, Pulseless Hand

Standard treatment for a pulseless hand is CRPP. After closed reduction and stabilization, the pulse and perfusion of the hand should be reevaluated. Usually, hand perfusion is restored. Most extension-type supracondylar fractures are reduced and pinned with the elbow in hyperflexion. With more than 120 degrees of elbow flexion, the radial pulse generally is lost, and the hand becomes pale, even in patients with an initially intact pulse and a viable hand. Following pinning when the arm is extended, the pulse frequently does not return immediately. This is presumably secondary to arterial spasm, due to the original fracture displacement and aggravated by the adjacent soft tissue swelling and decreased peripheral perfusion in the anesthetized, somewhat cool intraoperative patient.

Because of this phenomenon, up to 10 to 15 minutes should be allowed for recovery of perfusion in the operating room before any decision is made regarding the need for exploring the brachial artery and restoring flow to the distal portion of the extremity. Because most patients without a palpable pulse regain and maintain adequate distal perfusion, the absence of a palpable pulse alone is not an indication for exploring a brachial artery. However, hand viability is imperative and all poorly perfused hands require exploration.

If there is a prolonged poor or absent pulse, and/or poor perfusion, there is a high risk of compartment syndrome and a low threshold for intraoperative compartment pressure measurements and documentation. In cases of poor limb perfusion for over 6 hours, prophylactic forearm compartment release should be considered.

Postreduction White (Poorly Perfused), Pulseless Hand

Following reduction and pinning, a poorly perfused pulseless hand requires urgent treatment.[3,108] If there was a pulse before fracture reduction, but not after reduction, one must assume the artery or surrounding tissue is trapped at the fracture site; the artery should be explored if the pulse does not return quickly. If there was not adequate perfusion before fracture reduction, and the hand remains poorly perfused after reduction, arterial exploration should be performed emergently.

Exploration through an anterior approach allows identification of the brachial artery. If the artery is obviously transected, vascular repair with or without interpositional vein graft is indicated.[6] If the vessel is in continuity, the artery is evaluated throughout the zone of injury for compression or kinking by adjacent soft tissues or incarceration between the fracture fragments. Once the artery is freely decompressed, associated arterial spasm may be relieved by application of lidocaine or papaverine, warming the operating room to promote peripheral vasodilation, and 10 to 15 minutes of observation. Following anatomic fracture reduction and decompression of the brachial artery, if the hand remains poorly perfused, vascular reconstruction is indicated by an appropriate specialist.

Postreduction Pink (Perfused), Pulseless Hand

If the pulse does not return, but the hand is well perfused following reduction, treatment is controversial.[100,126] At minimum, the patient should be admitted to the hospital with gentle arm elevation and carefully observed for at least 24 to 48 hours.[11] A vascular consult may be called, particularly if there is no pulse by Doppler. The patient should be observed for increasing narcotic requirements, increasing pain, and decreased passive finger motion (i.e., the three A's of a pending pediatric compartment syndrome: increasing anxiety, agitation, and analgesic requirement). Multiple authors report good results with observation of the postreduction pink pulseless hand.[3,27,53] However, a very low threshold for returning to the operating room for vascular exploration, decompression, and/or reconstruction along with forearm fasciotomies must be adhered to rather than assuming that perfusion from collaterals is sufficient. There are known disastrous cases of permanent impairment in this setting.

We have found intraoperative Doppler to be a helpful adjunct in cases of a well-reduced fracture, absent palpable pulse, but pink and perfused hand. Presence of a biphasic or triphasic signal at the wrist is reassuring and would prompt us to admit and observe for observation. One study found that every patient (20/20) with a well-perfused yet pulseless hand had a pulse that was detectable on Doppler, suggesting this may be an objective sign of good perfusion.[48] With absence of any Doppler signal at the wrist, or only a weakly monophasic signal, open exploration should be considered.

Vascular reconstruction may be performed on the pink pulseless hand with arterial injury. There has been some variance in results of reconstruction long term. Sabharwal et al.[128] have shown that early repair of the brachial artery has a high rate of symptomatic reocclusion or residual stenosis and recommended a period of close observation with frequent neurovascular checks before more invasive correction of this problem is contemplated. Many other studies report good results following vascular repair,[78,137] including an analysis of 19 studies with

a patency rate of 91% in 54 patients with surgically repaired arteries.[165] Repair by microscopic techniques appears to have better long-term results. Alves et al.[6] reported on 20 patients with brachial artery reconstruction with interposition vein grafting studied by duplex sonography, 19 of which had patent grafts with normal flow patterns and one had increased collateralization with reconstitution of normal flow distal to the elbow.

Lally et al.[83] reported on the long-term follow-up of 27 patients who had brachial artery ligation as a child for renal transplant. Decreased mean systolic pressure was noted in the affected limb in about 25% of patients and 67% had mildly decreased exercise tolerance. There was no significant difference in limb circumference or length.

VASCULAR STUDIES

There is currently no generally accepted evidence that further vascular studies beyond physical examination for perfusion and Doppler ultrasonography for radial pulse lead to improved outcomes, though this is an area of active research.[11] A review of articles subsequent to 1980 in the vascular surgical literature concludes, "Both angiography and color duplex ultrasound provide little benefit in the management of these patients. A child with a pink pulseless hand postfracture reduction can be managed expectantly unless additional signs of vascular compromise develop, in which exploration should be undertaken."[53] Similarly, some surgeons in the past have recommended pulse oximetry for evaluating postreduction circulation, but this has not been shown to discriminate the nonviable from the viable hand.

PULSELESS ARM WITH MEDIAN NERVE INJURY

If the arm is pulseless and has a median nerve deficit, special attention is warranted.[126] Injury to both the brachial artery and a nerve indicate significant soft tissue damage, which places the child at higher risk for a compartment syndrome. The pain of a compartment syndrome may be masked by the nerve injury, so very careful assessment and monitoring for a compartment syndrome are needed throughout the perioperative period, with a low threshold for vascular exploration and/or compartment release.[101] Mangat et al.[94] reported on seven patients who were pulseless with a median nerve injury, and all seven patients were found to have the brachial artery trapped or tethered at the fracture site. They recommend early exploration of the brachial artery in a Gartland type III supracondylar fracture in patients who present with an absent pulse and a coexisting anterior interosseous or median nerve palsy, as these appear to be strongly predictive of nerve and vessel entrapment. In contrast, they found only 20% of pulseless extremities without a nerve deficit had the artery trapped or tethered.

EXPLORATION OF THE BRACHIAL ARTERY

Often, during the open reduction of the fracture, release of a fascial band or an adventitial tether around the brachial artery resolves the problem of obstructed flow. In some patients, however, a formal vascular repair and/or vein grafting is required, at which time many orthopaedic surgeons will consult colleagues

Figure 14-50. Arterial pathology. **A:** The supratrochlear branch that arises from the anterior ulnar recurrent artery may bind the main trunk of the brachial artery against the sharp end of the proximal fragment. **B:** Intraoperative photograph of a right elbow after open decompression of the neurovascular bundle. The median nerve is retracted with a Ragnell retractor. The supratrochlear branch (*short arrow*) is seen arising from the main brachial artery (*long arrow*). (**A:** Reprinted from Rowell PJW. Arterial occlusion in juvenile humeral supracondylar fracture. *Injury.* 1974;6(3):254–256. Copyright © 1975 Elsevier Ltd. With permission. **B:** Courtesy of Children's Orthopaedic Surgery Foundation.)

with vascular expertise. The brachial artery is approached through an anteromedial transverse incision at the level of the fracture above the antecubital fossa. Often, this provides excellent exposure to the fracture site and neurovascular structures. Distal and proximal extension can be performed, as described in the authors' preferred method for open reduction (see Fig. 14-42C).

If the hand is still nonviable after reduction and pinning the fracture, care must be taken because the NVB may be difficult to identify when it is surrounded by hematoma or lies in a very superficial position. At the level of the fracture, the artery may seem to disappear into the fracture site, covered with shredded brachialis muscle. The artery is likely tethered by a fascial band or arterial adventitia attached to the proximal metaphyseal spike pulling the artery in the fracture site. Dissection is often best accomplished proximally to distally, along the brachial artery, identifying both the artery and the median nerve. Arterial injury is generally at the level of the supratrochlear artery (Fig. 14-50), which provides a tether, making the artery vulnerable at this location. Arterial transection or direct arterial injury can be identified at this level.

If arterial spasm is the cause of inadequate flow, and collateral flow is not sufficient to maintain the hand, attempts to relieve the spasm may be tried. Once the artery is no longer kinked or tethered, direct application of papaverine or local anesthetic to the artery has been found to be beneficial. Sympathetic block with a stellate ganglion block may prolong the vasodilatory effect. If these techniques do not relieve the spasm, and if collateral flow is insufficient to maintain a viable hand, there most likely is an intimal injury and occlusion. In these rare situations, the injured portion of the vessel is excised and a reverse vein graft of appropriate size is inserted, usually from the same extremity. Prophylactic release of forearm fascia is indicated in cases of prolonged ischemia to prevent a reperfusion compartment syndrome. When flow is restored, the wound is

closed, the patient is placed in a splint or foam and cast with the elbow in approximately 60 degrees of flexion, and the forearm is in neutral pronation and supination. Postoperative monitoring should include frequent examinations of perfusion and for signs of compartment syndrome or ischemia. Although injecting urokinase has been suggested to increase flow, we no longer advocate that technique because of systemic risks.

Compartment Syndrome

The prevalence of compartment syndrome in the setting of a supracondylar fracture is estimated to be 0.1% to 0.5%.[16,17] The classic five "P's" for the diagnosis of compartment syndrome—pain, pallor, pulselessness, paresthesias, and paralysis—are poor indicators of a compartment syndrome in children. Bae et al.[12] reported increasing analgesia requirement in combination with other clinical signs is a more sensitive and earlier indicator of compartment syndrome in children. They found that 10 children with access to patient-controlled or nurse-administered analgesia had increasing requirements for pain medication. Resistance to passive finger movement and dramatically increasing pain after fracture are clinical signs of compartment syndrome of the forearm. Special attention must be paid to supracondylar fractures with median nerve injuries, as the patient will not feel pain in the volar compartment.[101] A compartment syndrome of the forearm may occur with or without brachial artery injury and in the presence or absence of a radial pulse.

If the supracondylar fracture's mechanism of injury is high energy, as evidenced by crushing or associated fractures, there is an increased risk for compartment syndrome. A small series of patients suggested that an associated forearm fracture is associated with compartment syndrome, but Muchow reported a larger series of 1,288 patients that did not find an associated increased risk of compartment syndrome.[102] Similarly, a recent systematic review of 413 "floating elbow" patients across 11 published reports from 1999 and 2019 yielded only 8 cases (2%) of compartment syndrome.[13] Furthermore, retrospective studies are difficult to interpret, because those patients with forearm fractures may have been treated differently (more urgently, elevation, etc.). Ring et al.[125] found 6 of 10 pediatric floating elbows with pending or true compartment syndromes and recommend pinning of both forearm and SCH fractures. An arterial injury in association with multiple injuries or crush injury further diminishes blood flow to the forearm musculature and increases the probability of a compartment syndrome.

In a multicenter review, Ramachandran et al.[121] identified 11 cases in which children with supracondylar fractures developed compartment syndrome despite presenting with closed, low-energy injuries, and no associated fractures or vascular compromise. This series is disturbing as it demonstrates that compartment syndrome still occurs with modern treatment, even in children who may be thought to be at low risk. They found that in 10 of 11 patients' charts, excessive swelling was noted at time of presentation. The 10 cases with severe elbow swelling documented at presentation had a mean delay until surgery of 22 hours. This study suggests excessive swelling combined with delay in treatment is a risk factor for development of compartment syndrome. The authors also noted that even if distal pulse is found by palpation or Doppler examination, an evolving compartment syndrome may be present. In a similar series of 31 patients in whom volar forearm compartment pressures were measured pre- and postoperatively, Togac et al. found that delay to surgery and prolonged reduction with elbow flexion were associated with increased pressures.[158]

If there is concern that a compartment syndrome may be evolving, initial management includes removing all circumferential dressings. Battaglia et al.[16] documented the relationship between increasing elbow flexion above 90 degrees and increasing volar compartment pressure, so the elbow should be extended to a position well below 90 degrees. The volar compartment should be palpated, and again, the elbow should be extended. We believe that the fracture should be immediately stabilized with K-wires to allow proper management of the soft tissues.

Another factor that contributes to the development of compartment syndrome is warm ischemic time after injury. When blood flow is compromised and the hand is pale with no arterial flow, muscle ischemia is possible, depending on the duration of oxygen deprivation. After fracture reduction and flow restoration, the warm ischemic time should be noted. If this time is more than 6 hours, compartment syndrome secondary to ischemic muscle injury is likely. Prophylactic volar compartment fasciotomy can be performed at the time of arterial reconstruction. The exact indication for prophylactic fasciotomy in the absence of an operative revascularization is uncertain. Even when the diagnosis is delayed or if the compartment syndrome is chronic, fasciotomy and nerve decompression have been shown to be of some value.

Blakey et al.[19] reported on the experience of their specialized center over a 21-year period. At a mean of 3 months after sustaining an SCH fracture, 23 children with ischemic contractures

of the forearm were referred. The authors recommend that urgent exploration of the vessels and nerves in a child with a "pink pulseless hand" following fracture reduction with persistent and increasing pain suggests critical ischemia. No further conclusions regarding acute care of patients with a pink pulseless hand that does not have increasing pain suggestive of ischemia can be drawn from this retrospective study of established ischemic contractures.

Neurologic Deficit

A meta-analysis of 3,457 extension-type SCH fractures found an overall neurapraxia rate of 13%, with the AIN (5%) being the most common, followed by the radial nerve (4%).[8] A large single-center study of type III fractures reported 12% nerve injuries at presentation, with a rate of 19% of nerve injuries if there was an associated forearm fracture that required reduction.[48] A prospective study limited to surgical patients examined by pediatric fellowship-trained surgeons found a rate of 16% nerve injury: median 12% (12/100) (including 8 AIN injuries), radial 8% (8/100), ulnar 3% (3/100). A trend was seen between fracture severity and rate of a preoperative nerve injury: type II 7% (2/28), type III 19% (9/58), and type IV 36% (5/14) ($P = .058$).[69] A single-center study[138] of 244 nerve injuries associated with supracondylar fractures revealed 11% of extension fractures have a nerve injury: 86% were single nerve involvement (14% multiple nerves injured) and 29% had concurrent vascular injury. The most common nerve injured was also median nerve (62%). These observations have been further corroborated by recent retrospective series.[105]

AIN palsy presents as paralysis of the long flexors of the thumb (FPL) and index finger (FDP II) without sensory changes. Complete median nerve injury occurs from a more severe contusion, entrapment, or even rare transection of the nerve at the level of the fracture and presents with sensory loss in the median nerve distribution as well as motor loss of all muscles innervated by the median nerve (extrinsic and intrinsic). Nerve transections are rare and most commonly involve the radial nerve.

The direction of the fracture's displacement—and location of the associated ecchymosis—determines the nerve most likely to be injured.[133] If the distal fragment is displaced posteromedially, the radial nerve is more likely to be injured. Conversely, if the displacement of the distal fragment is posterolateral, the median nerve is stretched over the proximal fragment, injuring the complete median nerve or isolated AIN. In a flexion-type supracondylar fracture, which is rare, the ulnar nerve is the most likely nerve to be injured (see Fig. 14-7).[76]

Open reduction and exploration of the injured nerve are not necessarily indicated in cases of nerve injury in a closed fracture. Neural recovery, regardless of which nerve is injured, generally occurs with observation but may take 6 months or more.[138] In the large series of 244 displaced extension SCH fractures with nerve injuries out of Boston Children's Hospital, 60% of median nerve injuries had recovery at 3 months and 92% had complete recovery at follow-up, with median time to recovery of 2.3 months. Isolated median nerve injuries recovered faster

(70% by 3 months) than median nerve injuries associated with multiple nerve injuries, which took 54% longer to recovery. Radial nerve injuries took 30% longer to recover, with only 42% having recovered by 3 months.[138]

Culp et al.[31] reported identification of eight injured nerves in five patients in which spontaneous recovery did not occur by 5 months after injury. Neurolysis was successful in restoring nerve function in all but one patient. Shore et al.[138] noted five cases with poor recovery requiring surgery, none of which had decompression as part of open reduction internal fixation of fracture. None of the patients who had nerve decompression as part of operative treatment of the fracture and/or vascular injury had a long-term nerve deficit. Nerve grafting may be indicated for nerves not in continuity at the time of exploration. Release of tethering and entrapment with neurolysis for perineural fibrosis are generally successful in restoring nerve function if the nerve injury occurs in a timely fashion. There is no indication for early electromyographic analysis or treatment other than observation for nerve deficit until 3 to 6 months after fracture. Failure to observe an advancing Tinel sign and expected neural recovery as outlined above leads is an indication for exploration and treatment.

In the supracondylar area, nerve compression and perineural fibrosis appear to be the most common cause of prolonged nerve deficit. Although nerve injury is related to fracture displacement, a neural deficit can exist with even minimally displaced fractures. Sairyo et al.[129] reported one patient in whom radial nerve palsy occurred with a slightly angulated fracture that appeared to be a purely extension-type fracture on initial x-rays. However, the extent of fracture displacement and nerve trauma at the time of injury does not always correlate to the static x-ray in the emergency setting. Even in patients with mild injuries, a complete neurologic examination should be performed before treatment. An irreducible fracture with nerve deficit is an indication for open reduction of the fracture to ensure that there is no nerve entrapment. Chronic nerve entrapment in healed callus can give the appearance of a hole in the bone, the so-called Metev sign.[29]

Iatrogenic injury to the ulnar nerve with medial pinning has been reported to occur in 0.4% to 15% of patients with supracondylar fractures.[24,38,122,147] In the most recent, and largest, single-center study of the risk of ulnar nerve injury using a mini-open approach, the rate of iatrogenic injury was 0.4%, 10 times the previously reported rates.[123] In a large series of type III supracondylar fractures, the rate of iatrogenic injury to the radial nerve was less than 1%, but, in a meta-analysis, iatrogenic injury to the median and radial nerves from lateral pinning has been reported as high as 1.2%.[22] The course of the ulnar nerve through the cubital tunnel, between the medial epicondyle and the olecranon, makes it vulnerable during medial pin placement. Rasool[122] demonstrated with operative exploration that the pin usually did not impale the ulnar nerve, but more commonly constricted the nerve within the cubital tunnel by tethering adjacent soft tissue. These findings were later confirmed by an ultrasonographic study by Karakurt et al.[72] Zaltz et al.[172] reported that in children less than 5 years of age, when the elbow is flexed more than 90 degrees, the ulnar nerve

migrated over, or even anterior to, the medial epicondyle in 61% (32/52) of children. It has been suggested that placement of lateral entry pins first, followed by elbow extension to relax tension on the ulnar nerve and subsequent placement of a medial pin, could decrease the risk of iatrogenic nerve injury. Using this technique, Edmonds et al. reported a 1.1% (2/187) rate of iatrogenic ulnar nerve injury with medial pins.[38]

There is currently no consensus within the literature on the management of an iatrogenic ulnar nerve injury following medial pin placement. In the most recent, and largest, single-center study, two or three patients had spontaneous recovery of sensory or motor symptoms, while one had persistent mild weakness and paresthesias.[123] Lyons et al.[91] reported 17 patients with iatrogenic ulnar nerve injuries presumably due to a medial pin. All 17 patients had complete return of function, though many did not until 4 months. Only 4 of the 17 (24%) had the medial pins removed acutely. This study demonstrates that ulnar nerve function may eventually return without pin removal. Brown and Zinar[24] reported four ulnar nerve injuries associated with pinning of supracondylar fractures, all of which resolved spontaneously 2 to 4 months after pinning. Rasool[122] reported six patients with ulnar nerve injuries in whom early exploration was performed. In two patients, the nerve was penetrated, and in three, it was constricted by a retinaculum over the cubital tunnel, aggravated by the pin. In one patient, the nerve was subluxed and was fixed anterior to the cubital tunnel by the pin. Full recovery occurred in three patients, partial recovery in two, and no recovery in two. Spontaneous recovery of ulnar nerve function was reported in three patients. One nerve that was explored had direct penetration, and the pin was replaced in the proper position. Two patients had late-onset ulnar nerve palsies discovered during healing, and the medial pin was removed.

If an immediate postoperative neural injury is documented, we prefer to explore the ulnar nerve and replace the pin in the proper position or convert to an additional lateral pin construct. Common sense suggests that removal of the causative factor (the medial pin) earlier rather than later may lead to a quicker recovery of the nerve.[24,122,172]

Preventing ulnar nerve injury is obviously more desirable than treating ulnar neuropathy. Because of the frequency of ulnar nerve injury with crossed pinning, some surgeons prefer to use two or three lateral pins if possible and no medial pin. Successful maintenance of alignment of type III supracondylar fractures with lateral pins has been reported in many series.[77,145,147] However, in some circumstances, such as in flexion type and posterolateral type 3 supracondylar fractures, stabilization of the medial column is best achieved with a medial pin.[119,124] Further, one meta-analysis of 3,457 extension-type fractures reported an iatrogenic neurapraxia rate of 1.9% for laterally placed pins.[8] Thus, if stabilization of the medial column requires multiple pins, with multiple attempts, it may be more beneficial to place a medial pin through a safe technique.[123] Any nerve can be injured by any aberrant pin placement, and there are fracture patterns in which crossed pins provide more stable fixation.[68] When using medial pins, positioning the elbow in extension, creating small incisions, judiciously retracting adjacent soft tissues, and using a drill guide to protect the perineural tissue may help minimize the risk of ulnar nerve injury.[123]

Elbow Stiffness

Clinically significant loss of motion after extension-type supracondylar fractures is rare in children. In a study of 45 children with SCH fractures who did not undergo physical therapy, 90% of ROM returned at 30 days for extension and 39 days for flexion.[163] In another report of 63 patients with closed reduction percutaneous pinning of supracondylar fractures of the humerus stabilized with either two or three lateral entry pins, elbow ROM returned to 72% of contralateral elbow motion by 6 weeks after pinning and progressively increased to 86% by 12 weeks, 94% by 26 weeks, and 98% by 52 weeks.[174] Pins were removed by 3 to 4 weeks. No patient participated in formal physical therapy.

Although most children do not require formal physical therapy, we generally teach the parents ROM exercises to be performed at home following pin and cast removal at about 3 to 4 weeks postoperatively. We do not routinely schedule follow-up appointments, but instruct the families to contact us if ROM does not normalize in 6 to 8 weeks, at which time physical therapy may be initiated.

Aside from stiffness due to muscle atrophy, soft tissue scar, and prolonged immobilization, loss of elbow flexion can also be caused by a lack of anatomic fracture reduction: either posterior distal fragment angulation, posterior translation of the distal fragment with anterior impingement, or medial rotation of the distal fragment with a protruding medial metaphyseal spike proximally (Fig. 14-51). In young children with significant growth potential, there may be significant remodeling of anterior impingement, and any corrective surgery should be delayed for at least 1 year. Although anterior impingement can significantly remodel, there is risk of limited remodeling of persistent posterior angulation or hyperextension.

Pin-Tract Infections

The reported prevalence of pin-tract infections in SCH fractures ranges from less than 1% to 2.5% with closed reduction and standard pinning techniques[17,48,145] in most series; though one series reports a rate of 4.3% (21/490), noting that about half of the patients with infections did not receive preoperative antibiotics.[111] In a retrospective review of 622 operative treated patients, 1 patient developed a deep infection with septic arthritis and osteomyelitis (0.2%). Five additional patients had superficial skin infections and were treated with oral antibiotics for a total infection rate of 6 of 622 patients (1%).[16] Lateral entry pins can enter the elbow joint risk of deep-spaced infection, so expedient care of superficial infections is appropriate.[67]

Pin-tract infections generally resolve with pin removal and antibiotics. Fortunately, by the time a pin-tract infection develops, the fracture is usually stable enough to remove the pin without loss of reduction. However, an untreated pin-tract infection can result in a septic joint and should thus be treated as soon as is recognized or suspected. Interviews of patients 18 years after infected pin tracts show no long-term sequelae.[111]

Pin Migration

In one retrospective series of 622 patients,[16] the most common complication was pin migration, necessitating unexpected return to the operating room for pin removal in 11 patients (1.8%). In a more recent multicenter retrospective analysis of 7,862 patients, 15 children (0.2%) required return to the

Figure 14-51. Distal fragment rotation. **A:** Posterior angulation only of the distal fragment. **B:** Pure horizontal rotation without angulation. **C:** Pure posterior translocation without rotation or angulation. **D:** Horizontal rotation with coronal tilting, producing a cubitus varus deformity. There is a positive crescent sign.

Figure 14-52. Myositis ossificans. Ossification of the brachialis muscle developed in this 8-year-old who had undergone multiple attempts at reduction. (Courtesy of John Schaeffer, MD.)

operating room for pin migration.[89] Risk factors for pin migration include increased delay to pin removal and patient body mass index greater than 95%.[10] The pin migration complications can be minimized by both bending at least 1 cm of pin at a 90-degree angle, at least 1 cm from the skin, and protecting the skin with thick felt over the pin (see Fig. 14-42A) or using commercially available pin covers.

Myositis Ossificans

Myositis ossificans is a remarkably rare complication of supracondylar fractures, but it can occur (Fig. 14-52). This complication has been described after closed and open reductions due to disruption of the brachialis with injury, but vigorous postoperative manipulation or physical therapy is believed to be an associated factor.[124]

Postoperative myositis ossificans can be observed with the expectation of spontaneous resolution of both restricted motion and the myositis ossificans. There is no indication of early excision. O'Driscoll et al [106] reported a single case of myositis ossificans associated with sudden onset of pain posttrauma in which a 1-year-old lesion of myositis ossificans was fractured. With excision, the pain was relieved and full ROM returned.

Nonunion

The distal humeral metaphysis is a well-vascularized area with remarkably rapid healing, and nonunion of a supracondylar

fracture is rare. With infection, devascularization, and soft tissue loss, the risk of nonunion would presumably increase.

Avascular Necrosis

AVN of the trochlea after supracondylar fracture has been reported.[40] The blood supply of the trochlea's ossification center is limited, with two separate sources. One small artery is lateral and courses directly through the physis of the medial condyle. It provides blood to the medial crista of the trochlea. If the supracondylar fracture line is very distal, this artery can be injured, producing AVN of the ossification center and resulting in a classic fishtail deformity. Kim et al.[75] identified 18 children with trochlear abnormalities after elbow injuries, 5 of which were supracondylar fractures. MRI indicated low-signal intensity on T2 indicative of cartilage necrosis. Cubitus varus deformity developed in all cases.

Symptoms of AVN of the trochlea do not occur for months or years. Healing of the fracture is normal, but mild pain and occasional locking eventually may develop with characteristic radiologic findings and motion may be limited depending on the extent of AVN. Glotzbecker et al.[50] described 15 cases of symptomatic fishtail deformity presenting an average of 4.7 years after fracture, 80% of whom had mechanical symptoms of locking, catching, and painful limited motion. An important risk for AVN of the trochlea is following an open reduction of a supracondylar fracture through a posterior approach, which presumably disrupts the blood supply of the trochlea (Fig. 14-53). Treatment options at present are limited but distal

Figure 14-53. Avascular necrosis of the trochlea developed following open reduction through a posterior approach. The child had limited motion and symptoms of occasional catching. (Reproduced with permission from Children's Orthopaedic Center, Los Angeles, CA.)

humeral epiphyseodeses of the medial and lateral columns may halt deformity progression, and arthroscopic debridement and removal of osteochondral loose bodies have been reported to provide clinical improvement.

Loss of Reduction

Sankar et al.[131] in a series of 322 fractures reported 2.9% had postoperative loss of fixation. All eight were Gartland type III fractures treated with just two pins (seven lateral entry and one crossed pin). In all cases, loss of fixation was due to technical errors that were identifiable on the intraoperative fluoroscopic images and that could have been prevented with proper technique. They identified three types of pin fixation errors: (1) failure to engage both fragments with two pins or more, (2) failure to achieve bicortical fixation with two pins or more, and (3) failure to achieve adequate pin separation (>2 mm) at the fracture site (Fig. 14-54). As noted above, the IRST is helpful in the operating room to determine the stability of fixation and whether an additional lateral or medial pin is indicated.

Clinical experience of a series of 124 consecutive supracondylar fractures including completely unstable fractures has taught us that lateral entry pins, when properly placed, are usually strong enough to maintain reduction, while some fractures remain unstable using an intraoperative internal rotational stress of the medial column, and benefit from a medial pin.[124,145] Pennock et al.[116] reported that pins separated by at least 13 mm, or one-third the width of the humerus, at the level of the fracture on an AP view is an important factor in helping to prevent loss of reduction.

When loss of reduction is noted within the first 1 to 2 weeks, revision closed reduction and pin fixation are usually effective. A report of 21 supracondylar fractures that lost reduction underwent revision surgery at a mean of 7.6 days (range 3–18 days). Seventeen were treated with closed reduction and four required open reduction. Two cases resulted in cubitus varus, and three patients lacked 10 degrees of motion at final follow-up.[110] Other authors have proposed closed osteoclasis techniques to address late loss of reduction when fracture callus is already present.[169]

Cubitus Varus

Cubitus varus, also known as a "gunstock deformity," refers to the characteristic appearance of the malunited SCH fracture in the coronal plane (Fig. 14-55A). While the varus malalignment is most conspicuous, the typical supracondylar malunion also results in extension and internal rotation of the distal metaphyseal–epiphyseal segment, clinically manifesting as elbow hyperextension and decreased elbow flexion (Fig. 14-55B,C). The appearance of cubitus varus deformity is distinctive on plain radiographs. On the AP view, the angle of the physis of the lateral condyle (Baumann angle) is more horizontal than normal (Fig. 14-56A). On the lateral view, hyperextension of the distal fragment posterior to the AHL correlates with the clinical findings of increased extension and decreased flexion of the elbow (Fig. 14-56B).

It has been proposed that unequal growth in the distal humerus causes cubitus varus deformity, but this seems unlikely, as there is not enough growth in this area to cause cubitus varus within the time it is recognized. The most common reason for cubitus varus in patients with supracondylar fractures is likely malunion rather than growth arrest. Cubitus varus can be prevented by making certain Baumann angle is intact at the time of reduction and remains so during healing by achieving stable fixation. Pirone et al.[124] reported cubitus varus deformities in 8 of 101 (7.9%) patients treated with cast immobilization compared to 2 of 105 (1.9%) patients with pin fixation, with ages ranging from 1.5 to 14 years (mean of 6.4 years). A decrease in frequency of cubitus varus deformity after the use of percutaneous pin fixation has been reflected in other series.[45,124]

The distal humerus growth is 20% of that of its overall length. In a 5-year-old then, the amount of distal humeral growth in 1 year postfracture is approximately 2 mm, making it unlikely that growth asymmetry is a significant cause of varus deformity that occurs within the first 6 to 12 months after fracture. AVN of the trochlea or medial portion of the distal humeral fragment can result in progressive varus deformity. However, in a series of 36 varus deformities reported by Voss et al.,[161] only four patients had medial growth disturbance and distal humeral AVN as a cause of progressive varus deformity.

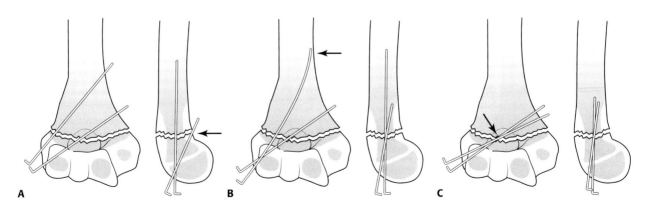

Figure 14-54. Illustrations depicting errors in pin-fixation technique. **A:** The *black arrow* demonstrates the anterior pin failing to transfix the proximal bone. **B:** The *black arrow* demonstrates one pin without bicortical purchase. **C:** The *black arrow* demonstrates pins too close together at the fracture site.

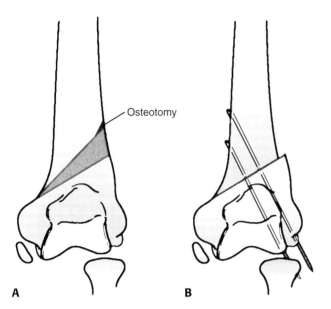

Figure 14-58. A: By moving the apex of the closing wedge distally, the osteotomy's center of rotation is moved closer to the deformity. **B:** Upon closing a distally based wedge osteotomy, there is less translational effect than in a more proximally based osteotomy.

in historic series have led to controversy about the value of a distal humeral corrective osteotomy for cubitus varus deformity. In a review of 41 patients undergoing distal humeral osteotomies for malunions following SCH fractures at two major pediatric centers, Weiss et al.[164] reported a complication rate of 53% with a 32% return to the operating room in surgeries performed between 1987 and 1997. However, in surgeries performed from 1998 to 2002, the complication rate was 14% with a 0% reoperation rate. When lateral entry pins were used to fix the osteotomy, there were significantly less complications.[164]

Because malunion is the cause of most cubitus varus deformities, the angular deformity usually occurs at the level of the fracture. Rotation and hypertension may contribute to the deformity, but varus is the most significant factor. Hyperextension can produce a severe deformity in some patients. During corrective osteotomy, an oblique bone cut (Fig. 14-58) places the osteotomy's center of rotation as close to the actual level of the deformity as possible. On an AP x-ray of the humerus with the forearm in full supination, the size of the lateral wedge and the angular correction needed are determined. An "incomplete" lateral closing wedge osteotomy may be performed, leaving a small medial hinge of bone intact. This protects the ulnar nerve and provides rotational stability to the osteotomy. The osteotomy usually is fixed with two or three K-wires placed laterally with appropriate spread and divergence. In the absence of an intact medial hinge, two lateral wires probably are not sufficient to secure this osteotomy.[161] Crossed wires may be useful in this situation. In general, an oblique lateral closing wedge osteotomy with a medial hinge will correct the varus deformity, with minor correction of hyperextension unless one of the two osteotomy cuts has slightly more anterior wedge removed at the time of lateral wedge excision.[161] A transverse lateral closing wedge

has more risk of a lateral bump with poor aesthetics. Residual rotational deformity was not found to be a significant problem in studies by Voss et al.,[161] which is logical given the amount of rotation available from the shoulder. More recent published series have corroborated the safety and efficacy of lateral closing wedge osteotomy for cubitus varus.[157]

Higaki and Ikuta[60] described a dome osteotomy in which a curved osteotomy is made in the supracondylar area. Proponents of this osteotomy suggest that multiplane correction is possible without inducing translation in the distal fragment and that rotation can be corrected. DeRosa and Graziano[39] described a step-cut osteotomy in which the distal fragment is slotted into the proximal fragment and the osteotomy is secured with a single screw. Most recently, Herzog et al. noted excellent clinical and radiographic results in a series of 18 patients treated via a posterior triceps-splitting approach, plate fixation, and early mobilization.[58] Overall, functional outcomes are generally good.

Alternatively, a Wiltse-type osteotomy, similar to that described by DeRosa and Graziano but with the complete transverse cut distal as possible, just superior to the olecranon fossa, to have the axis of rotation of the osteotomy as close as possible to the deformity (Fig. 14-59).[146]

Preoperative templating is performed to determine the angle of correction required for correction of the varus and, if

Figure 14-59. This osteotomy can address frontal and sagittal plane malalignment, and offer some inherent bony stability, while not producing a lateral bump which occurs with simple closing wedge osteotomies. *Open arrows* show triangles of bone that are removed, *solid arrow* shows rotation of fragment.

necessary, for correction of any extension deformity. Templating is based on AP of bilateral upper extremities centered on the elbow combined with clinical examination comparing one arm to the other in terms of frontal plane appearance and arc of motion. For example, if the affected arm has 20 degrees more extension and 20 degrees less flexion than the contralateral arm, a 20-degree wedge is planned in the sagittal plane.

Hyperextension deformity may remodel over time (see Fig. 14-56A), but correction is slow and inconsistent. In one series,[161] hyperextension deformities remodeled as much as 30 degrees in very young children, but in older children, there was no significant remodeling in the flexion/extension plane. If hyperextension appears to be a major problem, osteotomy should also be directed at this deformity rather than simple correction of the varus deformity; this situation requires a multiplane osteotomy.

Technique

A longitudinal incision measuring approximately 6 cm is made over the lateral distal humerus along the metaphysis. Dissection is carried out in the interval between the brachioradialis and triceps. Subperiosteal dissection is performed to expose the extra-articular distal humerus in the region of the planned osteotomy. Posterior dissection is continued toward, but not distal, to the olecranon fossa so as to prevent harming the blood supply to the trochlea. Hohmann or Chandler retractors are used for circumferential protection with special care medially near the ulnar nerve. An oblique closing wedge osteotomy is created just above the olecranon fossa from proximal-lateral to distal-medial. To facilitate precise correction, two K-wires may be passed along the intended path of the subsequent bony cuts, converging at a point just proximal to the medial epicondyle and just beyond the medial cortex. Intraoperative fluoroscopy may be used to assess the appropriate pin position, accounting for the angular correction desired.

At this point, K-wires are preplaced percutaneously into the lateral condyle, directed up the lateral column of the distal humerus. These pins are passed to a level just distal to the planned osteotomy, allowing for ease of fixation later in the procedure.

Following this, osteotomies are performed with a sagittal saw blade along the previously placed K-wires, preserving the medial cortex/periosteum if possible. The intercalary wedge of bone is removed, the osteotomy site is closed with manual pressure, using the medial cortex/periosteum as a fulcrum. Once the correction is achieved, the previously placed K-wires in the distal lateral condyle are passed across the osteotomy site, engaging the far proximal cortex. As in an SCH fracture, typically two or three pins are sufficient.

If there is excessive preoperative hyperextension deformity, the lateral closing wedge osteotomy cuts may also be inclined, taking more longitudinal bone anteriorly than posterior. This will allow for biplanar correction and improve the position of the AHL on the lateral fluoroscopy view.[124]

Stability is tested with stress under fluoroscopy. If necessary, an additional pin is added. The wound is irrigated, and a small amount of local bone graft from the excised wedge is packed around the osteotomy site but making certain bone graft is not in the olecranon fossa. The periosteum is reapproximated. A well-padded or bivalved long-arm cast is applied in 60 to 80 degrees of flexion with the arm at neutral in regard to supination

and pronation. The cast is removed when good callus is demonstrated on radiographs, usually approximately 4 weeks postoperatively, and the pins are removed in clinic at that time (Fig. 14-60).

Flexion-Type Supracondylar Fractures of the Distal Humerus

INTRODUCTION TO FLEXION-TYPE SUPRACONDYLAR FRACTURES OF THE DISTAL HUMERUS

Flexion-type supracondylar humeral fractures account for about 2% of humeral fractures.[92] Unlike the more common extension-type injuries, flexion-type supracondylar fractures have disruption of the posterior periosteum, resulting in greater fracture displacement and instability with elbow flexion. Radiographic differences may be subtle, and a flexion pattern of injury may not be recognized until reduction is attempted. A supracondylar fracture with apparent lateral displacement may actually be a flexion-type injury.

ASSESSMENT OF FLEXION-TYPE SUPRACONDYLAR FRACTURES OF THE DISTAL HUMERUS

Patients with flexion-type supracondylar fracture present with elbow pain, swelling, and limited ROM. Given the mechanism of injury and nature of periosteal disruption, there will often be a distinctive bruising posteromedially, imparted by the displaced proximal medial metaphysis; this is in contrast to the typically anteromedial or anterolateral ecchymosis of extension-type fractures.[133]

Vascular injury is rare in flexion-type injuries, though a comprehensive neurologic evaluation is warranted. A meta-analysis of 146 flexion-type SCH fractures found an overall neuropraxia rate of 15%, with the ulnar nerve injury as the most common nerve injured (91%),[8] as the flexed displaced fracture fragment places the nerve under tension. A more recent single-institution retrospective series identified ulnar neuropraxia in 26% of flexion-type supracondylar fractures.[76] Mahan et al.[92] and Flynn et al.[46] together noted a higher rate of open reduction for flexion-type supracondylar humeral fractures with an associated ulnar nerve injury.

MECHANISMS OF INJURY FOR FLEXION-TYPE SUPRACONDYLAR FRACTURES OF THE DISTAL HUMERUS

The mechanism of injury is generally believed to be a fall directly onto the elbow rather than a fall onto the outstretched hand with hyperextension of the elbow (Fig. 14-61). The distal fragment is displaced anteriorly and may migrate proximally in a totally displaced fracture. The ulnar nerve is vulnerable in this fracture pattern.[92] Rarely, it may be entrapped in the fracture or later in the healing callus.

Figure 14-60. Lateral closing wedge osteotomy for cubitus varus. **A:** Clinical photograph depicting cubitus varus of the left elbow. In addition to varus alignment in the coronal plane, there was extension and internal rotation. **B:** AP radiographic demonstrating cubitus varus with typical change in Bauman angle. **C:** Via a lateral approach, guide pins were placed in the trajectory of the planned osteotomy. Note the obliquity of the planned osteotomy to minimize the lateral bony prominence. **D:** A microsagittal saw used to create the osteotomy. Lateral pins have been placed laterally in preparation for subsequent stabilization of the osteotomy. **E:** The lateral wedge has been removed, preserving the medial periosteum and cortex. **F:** The osteotomy is reduced and pins passed, engaging the far proximal cortices. **G:** Postoperative elbow motion, demonstrating restoration of symmetric carrying angle. **H:** Postoperative elbow flexion. **I:** Postoperative elbow extension. (Courtesy of Children's Orthopaedic Surgery Foundation)

Figure 14-61. Flexion mechanism. Flexion-type fractures usually result from a blow to the posterior aspect of the elbow. The obliquity of the fracture line may be opposite that of an extension type. The large *white arrow* demonstrates the usual direction of fragment displacement.

IMAGING AND OTHER DIAGNOSTIC STUDIES FOR FLEXION-TYPE SUPRACONDYLAR FRACTURES OF THE DISTAL HUMERUS

Anterior displacement may be accompanied by medial or lateral translation. Associated fractures of the proximal humerus and radius can occur and any tenderness in these areas mandates a full x-ray evaluation of the upper extremity. Fracture classification is similar to extension-type supracondylar fractures[56]: type I, nondisplaced fracture; type II, flexion angulation only with anterior cortical contact; and type III, totally unstable displaced distal fracture fragment.

TREATMENT OPTIONS FOR FLEXION-TYPE SUPRACONDYLAR FRACTURES OF THE DISTAL HUMERUS

NONOPERATIVE TREATMENT OF FLEXION-TYPE SUPRACONDYLAR FRACTURES OF THE DISTAL HUMERUS

In general, stable, nondisplaced, flexion-type I fractures can simply be protected in a long-arm cast. If mild angulation, as in a type II fracture, requires some reduction in extension, the arm can be immobilized with the elbow fully extended; the addition of a thumb spica component and D-ring may provide additional support and prevent longitudinal slippage of the cast

distally. Radiographic evaluation with the elbow extended is easily obtained and accurate in determining the adequacy of reduction. Reduction is assessed by evaluating Baumann angle, the AHL intersecting the lateral condyle, and the integrity of the medial and lateral columns at the olecranon fossa.

If reduction cannot be obtained, as is often the case, or if malrotation persists, soft tissue interposition, possibly the ulnar nerve, should be suspected. De Boeck[36] studied 22 flexion-type supracondylar fractures. He found cast treatment to be satisfactory in nondisplaced cases. In the other 15 cases, CRPP were successful in most patients.

Type I and II fractures (Figs. 14-62 and 14-63) are generally reduced if any angular displacement is seen on fluoroscopic intraoperative evaluation. Type II fractures can be immobilized in an extension cast with the elbow fully extended. The cast is removed at 3 weeks. If closed reduction is performed without skeletal stabilization, follow-up x-rays usually are taken at 1 week and when the cast is removed at 3 weeks. True lateral x-rays in a fully extended cast are important and may require a few attempts or the use of live fluoroscopy.

OPERATIVE TREATMENT OF FLEXION-TYPE SUPRACONDYLAR FRACTURES OF THE DISTAL HUMERUS

Pinning of Unstable Flexion-Type Supracondylar Fractures

Pinning is generally required following the reduction of unstable type II and III flexion supracondylar fractures. The pinning

Figure 14-62. Type I flexion injury. A type I flexion supracondylar fracture pattern (*arrows*) in a 6-year-old below-the-elbow amputee. There is only about a 10-degree increase in the shaft condylar angle. The patient was treated with a simple posterior splint.

technique described for extension-type supracondylar fractures is not appropriate for flexion injuries fractures; greater elbow flexion will only exacerbate fracture displacement.

Because the posterior periosteum is torn in the flexion-type supracondylar fracture, reduction can be obtained in extension, which places tension across the intact anterior periosteum. In general, a slightly less than anatomic reduction can be accepted

as long as three conditions are met: there is no soft tissue interposition of tissue, Baumann angle is acceptable to the other side, and neither flexion nor extension is seen on the lateral view. Although rotating the arm is often possible for a lateral view of extension supracondylar fracture, the C-arm must be moved to obtain satisfactory x-ray results when pinning a flexion-type supracondylar fracture, because they are often rotationally unstable even when reduced (see Fig. 14-40).

Technique

> **Pinning of Flexion-Type Supracondylar Fractures:**
> **KEY SURGICAL STEPS**
>
> ❏ Place pin in distal fragment
> ❏ Check pin placement in both AP and lateral planes
> ❏ Place second parallel or divergent pin
> ❏ Reduce fracture in both planes
> ❏ Drive pins across fracture site
> ❏ Assess reduction and stability of reduction
> ❏ Cut and bend pins
> ❏ Apply cast

Place a lateral entry pin in the distal fragment. Check pin placement in the AP plane then the lateral plane by rotating the C-arm, not the elbow. Adjust pin placement as needed, then place a second parallel or divergent pin. Reduce fracture in the AP plane by correcting both medial-lateral translation and varus/valgus angulation. Rotate the C-arm and reduce fracture in the lateral plane, either by extension and flexion of the elbow, or using the "push–pull" technique[30] (Fig. 14-64). In addition to preplacing the pins in the distal fracture fragment, some have advocated placing a joystick pin in the proximal segment for assistance with closed reduction.[9]

Figure 14-63. Closed reduction, extension cast. **A:** A 5-year-old girl sustained a type II flexion pattern. **B:** She was manipulated into extension and found to be stable, and thus was maintained in a long-arm cast in extension.

Figure 14-64. The "push–pull" method. **A:** Prereduction with a rolled towel used as a fulcrum. **B:** Push with overreduction into extension. **C:** Pull back to align the anterior humeral line with the middle third of the capitellum. (Reprinted with permission from Chukwunyerenwa C, et al. Treatment of flexion-type supracondylar fractures in children: the 'push–pull' method for closed reduction and percutaneous K-wire fixation. *J Pediatr Orthop B.* 2016;25(5):412–416.)

Figure 14-65. Lateral view of a flexion-type supracondylar fracture. **A:** The capitellum in front of the anterior humeral line. **B:** AP view of fracture often underestimates the amount of displacement if an AP is taken of a bent elbow rather than a true AP of the distal humerus. **C:** Intraoperative view shows anatomy has been restored, with the anterior humeral line crossing the middle third of the capitellum. **D:** AP view demonstrates three well-placed lateral pins with maximal separation at fracture site, with all pins engaging solid bone.

Once the fracture is reduced, drive the pins across the fracture site and through the cortex of the proximal bone. Assess reduction with AP and lateral images; Baumann angle should be at least 10 degrees, and the AHL should go through the capitellum (Fig. 14-65). Assess stability of reduction with stress under live imaging.[124] If the fracture is not stable with lateral-only pins, the medial column can be stabilized with a medially placed pin. Cut and bend pins, protect skin with sterile bandage or felt, and cast to allow for swelling, with less than 90 degrees of elbow flexion.

Open Reduction of Flexion-Type Supracondylar Fractures

Open reduction is required for flexion-type supracondylar fractures in up to 31% of cases; and if the ulnar nerve is injured, the rates of open reduction increase to as high as 60% (6/10) in one series.[46,92] A medial or posterior surgical approach is used if closed reduction cannot be obtained. If a posterior approach is used, care is taken to avoid posterior soft tissue dissection of distal fragment to avoid injuring the blood supply to the trochlea. The ulnar nerve is identified and protected throughout the exposure and fracture stabilization.

Authors' Preferred Treatment for Flexion-Type Supracondylar Fractures of the Distal Humerus (Algorithm 14-3)

Algorithm 14-3. Authors' preferred treatment for flexion-type supracondylar fractures of the distal humerus.

In general, we treat type I flexion supracondylar fractures with a splint or cast with the elbow flexed for comfort. Minimally displaced type II fractures that reduce in extension are treated in an extension cast. Unstable type II and III fractures are surgically reduced and pinned. We have a low threshold for open reduction, particularly in patients with preoperative nerve palsy or difficult manipulative closed reduction. The medial approach is used, to avoid risks of excessive posterior soft tissue dissection in the very young.

Operative Treatment of Flexion-Type Supracondylar Humerus Fractures:
POTENTIAL PITFALLS AND PREVENTIONS

Pitfall	Prevention
Loss of fracture reduction	Pins spaced at least 13 mm or one-third the width of the humerus at the level of the fracture
	Use three pins in type III and IV fractures
Iatrogenic compartment syndrome	Do not flex humerus >70 degrees if elbow very swollen
Not recognizing compartment syndrome	Recognize promptly the three A's: analgesia requirements increasing, anxiety, agitation; and intervene.
Inability to reduce closed	Application of proximally directed axial load through the forearm may be used to reduce the metaphyseal–epiphyseal fragment posteriorly
	Placement of joystick pins in the distal and/or proximal fragment(s) may facilitate closed reduction
	Low threshold for open reduction via a medial approach, particularly in cases of preexisting ulnar nerve palsy

ACKNOWLEDGMENTS

With appreciation to David L. Skaggs and John M. Flynn, who prepared this chapter for the 9th edition and on which this revision is based.

Annotated References

Reference	Annotation
Bae DS, Kadiyala RK, Waters PM. Acute compartment syndrome in children: contemporary diagnosis, treatment, and outcome. *J Pediatr Orthop.* 2001;21(5):680–688.	Pain, pallor, paresthesia, paralysis, and pulselessness were relatively unreliable signs and symptoms of compartment syndrome in children. An increasing analgesia requirement in combination with other clinical signs such as anxiety and agitation were more sensitive indicators of compartment syndrome: All 10 patients with access to patient-controlled or nurse-administered analgesia demonstrated an increasing requirement for pain medication.
De Boeck H, De Smet P, Penders W, De Rydt D. Supracondylar elbow fractures with impaction of the medial condyle in children. *J Pediatr Orthop.* 1995;15(4):444–448.	In this retrospective review, none of six patients with medial comminution who underwent operative fixation had cubitus varus whereas four of seven (57%) patients who were treated nonoperatively developed cubitus varus. De Boeck et al. recommended closed reduction with percutaneous pinning when a fracture had medial comminution even in otherwise minimally displaced fractures, to prevent cubitus varus.
Leitch KK, Kay RM, Femino JD, et al. Treatment of multidirectionally unstable supracondylar humeral fractures in children: a modified Gartland type-IV fracture. *J Bone Joint Surg Am.* 2006;88(5):980–985.	Type IV fractures with multidirectional instability are described. These fractures are characterized by an incompetent periosteal hinge circumferentially and are defined by being unstable in both flexion and extension. This multidirectional instability is usually determined under anesthesia at the time of operation when on a lateral view the capitellum is anterior to the AHL with elbow flexion, and posterior to the AHL with elbow extension. This pattern of instability may result from the initial injury or may occur iatrogenically during a forceful attempted reduction. A specialized approach to closed reduction of this type of fracture is described in this chapter.

Annotated References	
Reference	Annotation
Mapes RC, Hennrikus WL. The effect of elbow position on the radial pulse measured by Doppler ultrasonography after surgical treatment of supracondylar elbow fractures in children. *J Pediatr Orthop.* 1998; 18(4):441–444.	Doppler is not able to detect pulse when type II fractures are flexed >110 degrees, and type III fractures are flexed >70 degrees. Supination also decreased flow in the brachial artery.
Pennock AT, Charles M, Moor M, et al. Potential causes of loss of reduction in supracondylar humerus fractures. *J Pediatr Orthop.* 2014;34(7):691–697.	Loss of reduction after percutaneous fixation of supracondylar fractures occurs at a rate of 4.2%. Pin spread is an important factor associated with preventing loss of reduction with a goal of pin spacing at least 13 mm or one-third the width of the humerus at the level of the fracture.
Rees AB, Schultz JD, Wollenman LC, et al. A mini-open approach to medial pinning in pediatric supracondylar humeral fractures may be safer than previously thought. *J Bone Joint Surg Am.* 2022;104(1):33–40.	The mini-open approach for medial pin insertion is safer than previous estimates. Here, in the largest single-center study of cross-pinning for SCHFs, the iatrogenic ulnar nerve injury rate of 0.43% was nearly 10 times lower than estimated rates from recent meta-analyses. Considering all nerves, the iatrogenic injury rate for this cross-pinning cohort was also lower than the estimated iatrogenic nerve injury rate for lateral pinning.
Ryan DD, Lightdale-Miric NR, Joiner ERA, et al. Variability of the anterior humeral line in normal pediatric elbows. *J Pediatr Orthop.* 2016;36(2):e14–e16.	In children 5 years and older, the AHL goes through the middle third of the capitellum in all patients, so if it does not, it is appropriate to look for pathology. However, with decreasing age, variability increases, with the AHL going through the anterior third of the capitellum in almost one-third of children under age 2 years.
Sanders JS, Ouillette RJ, Howard R, et al. Nonoperative versus operative treatment of type IIA supracondylar humerus fractures: a prospective evaluation of 99 patients. *J Pediatr Orthop.* 2023;43(1):e9–e16.	No clinical differences and equal patient-reported outcomes at mean 2 years were noted in patients treated with closed reduction and casting versus pinning for type IIA fractures. Nine percent of nonoperatively treated patients converted to surgical treatment at first clinical follow-up.
Skaggs DL, Cluck MW, Mostofi A, et al. Lateral-entry pin fixation in the management of supracondylar fractures in children. *J Bone Joint Surg Am.* 2004;86(4):702–707.	A series of 345 SCH fractures treated by percutaneous pinning showed that the use of a medial pin was associated with a 4% (6/149) risk of ulnar nerve injury when the medial pin was placed without hyperflexion and 15% (11/71) if the medial pin was placed with hyperflexion. None of the 125 fractures treated with lateral entry pins alone resulted in iatrogenic injury. Thus, one apparently undeniable conclusion is that if a medial pin is used, place the lateral pin(s) first, then extend the elbow and place the medial pin without hyperflexion of the elbow.
Skaggs DL, Sankar WN, Albrektson J, et al. How safe is the operative treatment of Gartland type 2 supracondylar humerus fractures in children? *J Pediatr Orthop.* 2008;28(2):139–141.	189 consecutive cases of type II fractures treated with closed reduction and percutaneous pinning were reviewed. There were 2% (4/189) pin-tract infections, of which three were treated successfully with oral antibiotics and pin removal 1.5% (3/191) and one (0.5% [1/191]) had operative irrigation and debridement for a wound infection not involving the joint. There were no nerve or vascular injuries, and no loss of reduction, delayed unions, or malunions. Pinning type II supracondylar fractures leads to a high probability of satisfactory outcome compared with previous studies of closed reduction without pinning.
Woratanarat P, Angsanuntsukh C, Rattanasiri S, et al. Meta-analysis of pinning in supracondylar fracture of the humerus in children. *J Orthop Trauma.* 2012;26(1):48–53.	Eighteen of 1,829 studies were included with 1,615 supracondylar fractures (837 and 778 children with cross and lateral pinning, respectively). The average age was 6.1 ± 0.9 years. The risk of iatrogenic ulnar nerve injury was 4.3 (95% CI, 2.1–9.1) times higher in cross-pinning compared with lateral pinning. There was no significant difference in loss of fixation, late deformity, or Flynn criteria between the two types of pinning. Conclusions: Lateral pinning is preferable to cross-pinning for fixation of pediatric supracondylar humerus fractures as a result of decreased risk of ulnar nerve injury.
Zaltz I, Waters PM, Kasser JR. Ulnar nerve instability in children. *J Pediatr Orthop.* 1996;16(5):567–569.	In children less than 5 years of age, when the elbow is flexed more than 90 degrees, the ulnar nerve migrated over, or even anterior to, the medial epicondyle in 61% (32/52) of children.

REFERENCES

1. Abbott MD, Buchler L, Loder RT, Caltoum CB. Gartland type III supracondylar humerus fractures: outcome and complications as related to operative timing and pin configuration. *J Child Orthop*. 2014;8(6):473–477.
2. Abe M, Ishizu T, Shirai H, et al. Tardy ulnar nerve palsy caused by cubitus varus deformity. *J Hand Surg Am*. 1995;20(1):5–9.
3. Abzug JM, Herman MJ. Management of supracondylar humerus fractures in children: current concepts. *J Am Acad Orthop Surg*. 2012;20(2):69–77.
4. Acosta AM, Li YJ, Bompadre V, et al. The utility of the early postoperative follow-up and radiographs after operative treatment of supracondylar humerus fractures in children. *J Pediatr Orthop*. 2020;40(5):218–222.
5. Aktekin CN, Toprak A, Ozturk AM, et al. Open reduction via posterior triceps sparing approach in comparison with closed treatment of posteromedial displaced Gartland type III supracondylar humerus fractures. *J Pediatr Orthop B*. 2018;17(4):171–178.
6. Alves K, Spencer H, Barnewolt CE, et al. Early outcomes of vein grafting for reconstruction of brachial artery injuries in children. *J Hand Surg Am*. 2018;43(3):287.e1–287.e7.
7. Ay S, Akinci M, Kamiloglu S, Ercetin O. Open reduction of displaced pediatric supracondylar humeral fractures through the anterior cubital approach. *J Pediatr Orthop*. 2005;25(2):149–153.
8. Babal JC, Mehlman CT, Klein G. Nerve injuries associated with pediatric supracondylar humeral fractures: a meta-analysis. *J Pediatr Orthop*. 2010;30(3):253–263.
9. Badawy M, Amin HED, Abdel-Ghani H, et al. Technique for facilitating closed reduction of difficult flexion type supracondylar humeral fracture in children. *J Pediatr Orthop B*. 2023;32(6):565–568.
10. Badin D, Boustany M, Lee RJ, et al. Incidence, risk factors, and consequences of radiographic pin migration after pinning of pediatric supracondylar humeral fractures. *J Pediatr Orthop B*. 2023;32(6):575–582.
11. Badkoobehi H, Choi PD, Bae DS, Skaggs DL. Management of the pulseless pediatric supracondylar humeral fracture. *J Bone Joint Surg*. 2015;97(11):937–943.
12. Bae DS, Kadiyala RK, Waters PM. Acute compartment syndrome in children: contemporary diagnosis, treatment, and outcome. *J Pediatr Orthop*. 2001;21(5):680–688.
13. Baghdadi S; CORTICES. Pediatric floating elbow injuries are not as problematic as they were once thought to be: a systematic review. *J Pediatr Orthop*. 2020;40(8):380–386.
14. Bahk MS, Srikumaran U, Ain MC, et al. Patterns of pediatric supracondylar humerus fractures. *J Pediatr Orthop*. 2008;28(5):493–499.
15. Barton KL, Kaminsky CK, Green DW, et al. Reliability of a modified Gartland classification of supracondylar humerus fractures. *J Pediatr Orthop*. 2001;21(1):27–30.
16. Bashyal RK, Chu JY, Schoenecker PL, et al. Complications after pinning of supracondylar distal humerus fractures. *J Pediatr Orthop*. 2009;29(7):704–708.
17. Battaglia TC, Armstrong DG, Schwend RM. Factors affecting forearm compartment pressures in children with supracondylar fractures of the humerus. *J Pediatr Orthop*. 2002;22(4):431–439.
18. Begovic N, Paunovic Z, Djuraskovic Z, et al. Lateral pinning versus others procedures in the treatment of supracondylar humerus fractures in children. *Acta Orthop Belg*. 2016;82(4):866–871.
19. Blakey CM, Biant LC, Birch R. Ischaemia and the pink, pulseless hand complicating supracondylar fractures of the humerus in childhood. *J Bone Joint Surg Br*. 2009;91(11):1487–1492.
20. Bloom T, Robertson C, Mahar A, Newton P. Biomechanical analysis of supracondylar humerus fracture pinning for slightly malreduced fractures. *J Pediatr Orthop*. 2008;28(7):766–772.
21. Boyd DW, Aronson DD. Supracondylar fractures of the humerus: a prospective study of percutaneous pinning. *J Pediatr Orthop*. 1992;12(6):789–794.
22. Brauer CA, Lee BM, Bae DS, et al. A systematic review of medial and lateral entry pinning versus lateral entry pinning for supracondylar fractures of the humerus. *J Pediatr Orthop*. 2007;27(2):181–186.
23. Bronfen CE, Geffard B, Mallet JF. Dissolution of the trochlea after supracondylar fracture of the humerus in childhood: an analysis of six cases. *J Pediatr Orthop*. 2007;27(5):547–550.
24. Camus T, MacLellan B, Cook PC, et al. Extension type II pediatric supracondylar humerus fractures: a radiographic outcomes study of closed reduction and cast immobilization. *J Pediatr Orthop*. 2011;31(4):366–371.
25. Carter CT, Bertrand SL, Cearley DM. Management of pediatric type III supracondylar humerus fractures in the United States: results of a national survey of pediatric orthopaedic surgeons. *J Pediatr Orthop*. 2013;33(7):750–754.
26. Cheng JC, Lam TP, Maffulli N. Epidemiological features of supracondylar fractures of the humerus in Chinese children. *J Pediatr Orthop B*. 2001;10(1):63–67.
27. Choi PD, Melikian R, Skaggs DL. Management of vascular injuries in pediatric supracondylar humeral fractures. San Francisco, CA: Presented at the Annual Meeting of American Academy of Pediatrics, Section of Orthopaedics; 2008.
28. Choi PD, Melikian R, Skaggs DL. Risk factors for vascular repair and compartment syndrome in the pulseless supracondylar humerus fracture in children. *J Pediatr Orthop*. 2010;30(1):50–56.
29. Choong J, Baldrighi C, Oestreich K, Jester A. Successful delayed neurolysis of the median nerve in a teenager 7 years after supracondylar fracture: a case report and review of the literature. *Ann Plast Surg*. 2021;87(4):e37–e39.
30. Chukwunyerenwa C, Orlik B, El-Hawary R, et al. Treatment of flexion-type supracondylar fractures in children: the 'push–pull' method for closed reduction and percutaneous K-wire fixation. *J Pediatr Orthop B*. 2016;25(5):412–416.
31. Culp RW, Osterman AL, Davidson RS, et al. Neural injuries associated with supracondylar fractures of the humerus in children. *J Bone Joint Surg Am*. 1990;72(8):1211–1215.
32. De Boeck H, De Smet P, Penders W, De Rydt D. Supracondylar elbow fractures with impaction of the medial condyle in children. *J Pediatr Orthop*. 1995;15(4):444–448.
33. Dekker A, Krijnen P, Schipper IB. Results of crossed versus lateral entry K-wire fixation of displaced pediatric supracondylar humeral fractures: a systematic review and meta-analysis. *Injury*. 2016;47(11):2391–2398.
34. Devnani AS. Late presentation of supracondylar fracture of the humerus in children. *Clin Orthop Relat Res*. 2005;(431):36–41.
35. Dietz HS, Schmittenbecher PP, Slongo T, et al. *AO Manual of Fracture Management: Elastic Stable Intramedullary Nailing in Children*. Thieme Medical Publishers; 2006.
36. Dimeglio A. Growth in pediatric orthopaedics. In: Morrissy RT, Weinstein SL, eds. *Lovell and Winters's Pediatric Orthopaedics*. 6th ed. Lippincott Williams & Wilkins; 2006:35–65.
37. Dodds SD, Grey MA, Bohl DD, et al. Clinical and radiographic outcomes of supracondylar humerus fractures treated surgically by pediatric and non-pediatric orthopedic surgeons. *J Child Orthop*. 2015;9(1):45–53.
38. Edmonds EW, Roocroft JH, Mubarak SJ. Treatment of displaced pediatric supracondylar humerus fracture patterns requiring medial fixation: a reliable and safer cross-pinning technique. *J Pediatr Orthop*. 2012;32(4):346–351.
39. Ernat J, Ho C, Wimberly RL, et al. Fracture classification does not predict functional outcomes in supracondylar humerus fractures: a prospective study. *J Pediatr Orthop*. 2017;37(4):e233–e237.
40. Etier BE Jr, Doyle JS, Gilbert SR. Avascular necrosis of trochlea after supracondylar humerus fractures in children. *Am J Orthop (Belle Mead NJ)*. 2015;44(10):E390–E393.
41. Fatemi MJ, Habibi M, Pooli AH, Mansoori MJ. Delayed radial nerve laceration by the sharp blade of a medially inserted Kirschner-wire pin: a rare complication of supracondylar humerus fracture. *Am J Orthop (Belle Mead NJ)*. 2009;38(2):E38–E40.
42. Feng C, Guo Y, Zhu Z, et al. Biomechanical analysis of supracondylar humerus fracture pinning for fractures with coronal lateral obliquity. *J Pediatr Orthop*. 2012;32(2):196–200.
43. Fitzgibbons PG, Bruce B, Got C, et al. Predictors of failure of nonoperative treatment for type-2 supracondylar humerus fractures. *J Pediatr Orthop*. 2011;31(4):372–376.
44. Fletcher ND, Sirmon BJ, Mansour AS, et al. Impact of insurance status on ability to return for outpatient management of pediatric supracondylar humerus fractures. *J Child Orthop*. 2016;10(5):421–427.
45. Flynn JC, Zink WP. Fractures and dislocations of the elbow. In: MacEwen GD, Kasser JR, Heinrich SD, eds. *Pediatric Fractures: A Practical Approach to Assessment and Treatment*. Lippincott Williams & Wilkins; 1993:133–164.
46. Flynn K, Shah AS, Brusalis CM, et al. Flexion-type supracondylar humeral fractures: ulnar nerve injury increases risk of open reduction. *J Bone Joint Surg*. 2017;99(17):1485–1487.
47. Gadgil A, Hayhurst C, Maffulli N, Dwyer JS. Elevated, straight-arm traction for supracondylar fractures of the humerus in children. *J Bone Joint Surg Br*. 2005;87(1):82–87.
48. Garg S, Weller A, Larson AN, et al. Clinical characteristics of severe supracondylar humerus fractures in children. *J Pediatr Orthop*. 2014;34(1):34–39.
49. Gaston RG, Cates TB, Devito D, et al. Medial and lateral pin versus lateral-entry pin fixation for type 3 supracondylar fractures in children: a prospective, surgeon-randomized study. *J Pediatr Orthop*. 2010;30(8):799–806.
50. Glotzbecker MP, Bae DS, Links AC, Waters PM. Fishtail deformity of the distal humerus: a report of 15 cases. *J Pediatr Orthop*. 2013;33:592–597.
51. Got C, Thakur N, Marcaccio EJ Jr, et al. Delayed presentation of a brachial artery pseudoaneurysm after a supracondylar humerus fracture in a 6-year-old boy: a case report. *J Pediatr Orthop*. 2010;30(1):57–59.
52. Gottschalk HP, Sagoo D, Glaser D, et al. Biomechanical analysis of pin placement for pediatric supracondylar humerus fractures: does starting point, pin size, and number matter? *J Pediatr Orthop*. 2012;32(5):445–451.
53. Griffin KJ, Walsh SR, Markar S, et al. The pink pulseless hand: a review of the literature regarding management of vascular complications of supracondylar humeral fractures in children. *Eur J Vasc Endovasc Surg*. 2008;36(6):697–702.
54. Guven MF, Kaynak G, Inan M, et al. Results of displaced supracondylar humerus fractures treated with open reduction and internal fixation after a mean 22.4 years of follow-up. *J Shoulder Elbow Surg*. 2015;24(4):640–646.
55. Hadlow AT, Devane P, Nicol RO. A selective treatment approach to supracondylar fracture of the humerus in children. *J Pediatr Orthop*. 1996;16(1):104–106.
56. Hamdi A, Poitras P, Louati H, et al. Biomechanical analysis of lateral pin placements for pediatric supracondylar humerus fractures. *J Pediatr Orthop*. 2010;30(2):135–139.
57. Herman MJ, Boardman MJ, Hoover JR, Chafetz RS. Relationship of the anterior humeral line to the capitellar ossific nucleus: variability with age. *J Bone Joint Surg Am*. 2009;91(9):2188–2193.
58. Herzog AN, Wirth T, Fernandez FF. Supracondylar dome osteotomy with a posterior triceps-splitting approach for acute correction of posttraumatic cubital axis deformities in adolescent patients. *J Pediatr Orthop*. 2023;43(1):e17–e24.
59. Heyer JH, Mitchell SL, Garcia S, et al. A modern day timeline for in-hospital monitoring in perfused, pulseless pediatric supracondylar humerus fractures. *J Pediatr Orthop*. 2022;42(10):589–594.
60. Higaki T, Ikuta Y. The new operation method of the domed osteotomy for 4 children with varus deformity of the elbow joint. *J Jpn Orthop*. 1982;31:300–335.
61. Ho CA, Podeszwa DA, Riccio AI, et al. Pathologic arterial changes in neurovascularly intact Gartland III supracondylar humerus fractures: a pilot study. *J Pediatr Orthop*. 2020;29(2):137–144.
62. Holden CE. The pathology and prevention of Volkmann's ischaemic contracture. *J Bone Joint Surg Br*. 1979;61-B(3):296–300.
63. Holt JB, Glass NA, Bedard NA, et al. Emerging U.S. national trends in the treatment of pediatric supracondylar humeral fractures. *J Bone Joint Surg*. 2017;99(8):681–687.

64. Howard A, Mulpuri K, Abel ML, et al. The treatment of pediatric supracondylar humerus fractures. *J Am Acad Orthop Surg.* 2012;20(5):320–327.
65. Iobst CA, Stillwagon M, Ryan D, et al. Assessing quality and safety in pediatric supracondylar humerus fracture care. *J Pediatr Orthop.* 2017;37(5):e303–e307.
66. Ismayl G, Kim WJ, Iqbal M, Sajid S. Early versus delayed treatment for Gartland type III supracondylar humeral fractures in children: a systematic review and meta-analysis. *Indian J Orthop.* 202;56(11):1871–1881.
67. Jardaly AH, LaCoste K, Gilbert SR, Conklin MJ. Late deep infections complicating percutaneous pinning of supracondylar humerus fractures. *Case Rep Orthop.* 2021;2021:7915516.
68. Jenkins SM, Mehlman CT, Denning JR. Unicolumnar pin fixation of type III supracondylar humeral fractures is associated with over 3 times higher odds of lost reduction. *J Orthop Trauma.* 2022;36(1):e30–e34.
69. Joiner ERA, Skaggs DL, Arkader A, et al. Iatrogenic nerve injuries in the treatment of supracondylar humerus fractures: are we really just missing nerve injuries on preoperative examination? *J Pediatr Orthop.* 2014;34(4):388–392.
70. Kao HK, Lee WC, Yang WE, Chang CH. Clinical significance of anterior humeral line in supracondylar humeral fractures in children. *Injury.* 2016;47(10):2252–2257.
71. Kappelhof B, Roorda BL, Poppelaars MA, et al. Occult fractures in children with a radiographic fat pad sign of the elbow: a meta-analysis of 10 published studies. *JBJS Rev.* 2022;10(10).
72. Karakurt L, Ozdemir H, Yilmaz E, et al. Morphology and dynamics of the ulnar nerve in the cubital tunnel after percutaneous cross-pinning of supracondylar fractures in children's elbows: an ultrasonographic study. *J Pediatr Orthop B.* 2005;14(3):189–193.
73. Karalius VP, Stanfield J, Ashley P, et al. The utility of routine postoperative radiographs after pinning of pediatric supracondylar humerus fractures. *J Pediatr Orthop.* 2017;37(5):e309–e312.
74. Kay RM, Directo MP, Leathers M, et al. Complications of ketorolac use in children undergoing operative fracture care. *J Pediatr Orthop.* 2010;30(7):655–658.
75. Kim HT, Song MB, Conjares JNV, Yoo CI. Trochlear deformity occurring after distal humeral fractures: magnetic resonance imaging and its natural progression. *J Pediatr Orthop.* 2002;22(2):188–193.
76. Kim KY, Conaway W, Schell R, Hennrikus WL. Prevalence of ulnar nerve palsy with flexion-type supracondylar fractures of the humerus. *J Pediatr Orthop B.* 2020;29(2):133–136.
77. Kocher MS, Kasser JR, Waters PM, et al. Lateral entry compared with medial and lateral entry pin fixation for completely displaced supracondylar humeral fractures in children: a randomized clinical trial. *J Bone Joint Surg Am.* 2007;89(4):706–712.
78. Konstantiniuk P, Fritz G, Ott T, et al. Long-term follow-up of vascular reconstructions after supracondylar humerus fracture with vascular lesion in childhood. *Eur J Vasc Endovasc Surg.* 2011;42(5):684–688.
79. Kwak-Lee J, Kim R, Ebramzadeh E, Silva M. Is medial pin use safe for treating pediatric supracondylar humerus fractures? *J Orthop Trauma.* 2014;28(4):216–221.
80. Kzlay YO, Aktekin CN, Özsoy MH, et al. Gartland type 3 supracondylar humeral fractures in children: which open reduction approach should be used after failed closed reduction? *J Orthop Trauma.* 2017;31(1):e18–e23.
81. Lacher M, Schaeffer K, Boehm R, Dietz HG. The treatment of supracondylar humeral fractures with elastic stable intramedullary nailing (ESIN) in children. *J Pediatr Orthop.* 2011;31(1):33–38.
82. Ladenhauf HN, Schaffert M, Bauer J. The displaced supracondylar humerus fracture: indications for surgery and surgical options: a 2014 update. *Curr Opin Pediatr.* 2014;26(1):64–69.
83. Lally KP, Foster CE III, Chwals WJ, et al. Long-term follow-up of brachial artery ligation in children. *Ann Surg.* 1990;212(2):194–196.
84. Larson AN, Garg S, Weller A, et al. Operative treatment of type II supracondylar humerus fractures: does time to surgery affect complications? *J Pediatr Orthop.* 2014;34(4):382–387.
85. Larson L, Firoozbakhsh K, Passarelli R, Bosch P. Biomechanical analysis of pinning techniques for pediatric supracondylar humerus fractures. 2006;26(5):573–578.
86. Lee SS, Mahar AT, Miesen D, Newton PO. Displaced pediatric supracondylar humerus fractures: biomechanical analysis of percutaneous pinning techniques. *J Pediatr Orthop.* 2002;22(4):440–443.
87. Lee YH, Lee SK, Kim BS, et al. Three lateral divergent or parallel pin fixations for the treatment of displaced supracondylar humerus fractures in children. *J Pediatr Orthop.* 2008;28(4):417–422.
88. Leitch KK, Kay RM, Femino JD, et al. Treatment of multidirectionally unstable supracondylar humeral fractures in children: a modified Gartland type-IV fracture. *J Bone Joint Surg Am.* 2006;88(5):980–985.
89. Lindsay SE, Crawford L, Holmes S, et al. Return to the operating room for unplanned pin removal after percutaneous pinning of supracondylar humerus fractures: a retrospective review. *J Pediatr Orthop.* 2023;43(7):e508–e512.
90. Louahem DM, Nebunescu A, Canavese F, Dimeglio A. Neurovascular complications and severe displacement in supracondylar humerus fractures in children: defensive or offensive strategy? *J Pediatr Orthop B.* 2006;15(1):51–57.
91. Lyons JP, Ashley E, Hoffer MM. Ulnar nerve palsies after percutaneous cross-pinning of supracondylar fractures in children's elbows. *J Pediatr Orthop.* 1998;18(1):43–45.
92. Mahan ST, May CD, Kocher MS. Operative management of displaced flexion supracondylar humerus fractures in children. *J Pediatr Orthop.* 2007;27(5):551–556.
93. Mahan ST, Osborn E, Bae DS, et al. Changing practice patterns: the impact of a randomized clinical trial on surgeons preference for treatment of type 3 supracondylar humerus fractures. *J Pediatr Orthop.* 2012;32(4):340–345.
94. Mangat KS, Martin AG, Bache CE. The 'pulseless pink' hand after supracondylar fracture of the humerus in children. *J Bone Joint Surg Br.* 2009;91(11):1521–1525.
95. Mapes RC, Hennrikus WL. The effect of elbow position on the radial pulse measured by Doppler ultrasonography after surgical treatment of supracondylar elbow fractures in children. *J Pediatr Orthop.* 1998;18(4):441–444.
96. McCartney CC, Thompson S, Waller G, et al. Gartland type IIa supracondylar humerus fractures: outcomes of attempted nonoperative management. *J Pediatr Orthop.* 2022;42(6):314–320.
97. Mehlman CT. Invited commentary related to: "Gartland type-3 supracondylar humeral fractures in children: which open reduction approach should be used after failed closed reduction?" *J Orthop Trauma.* 2017;31(1):e23–e24.
98. Mollon BG, McGuffin WS, Seabrook JA, et al. Supracondylar humerus fractures in older children: treatment modalities and outcomes. *J Bone Joint Surg Br.* 2011;93-B(Suppl III):284.
99. Montgomery BK, Cidambi EO, Birch CM, et al. Minimizing surgeon radiation exposure during operative treatment of pediatric supracondylar humerus fractures. *J Pediatr Orthop.* 2023;43(7):414–417.
100. Mooney JF III, Hosseinzadeh P, Oetgen M, Cappello T. AAOS appropriate use criteria: management of pediatric supracondylar humerus fractures with vascular injury. *J Am Acad Orthop Surg.* 2016;24(2):e24–e28.
101. Mubarak SJ, Carroll NC. Volkmann's contracture in children: aetiology and prevention. *J Bone Joint Surg Br.* 1979;61-B(3):285–293.
102. Muchow RD, Riccio AI, Garg S, et al. Neurological and vascular injury associated with supracondylar humerus fractures and ipsilateral forearm fractures in children. *J Pediatr Orthop.* 2015;35(2):121–125.
103. Mulpuri K, Dobbe A, Schaeffer E, et al. Management of displaced supracondylar fractures of the humerus using lateral versus cross K wires: a prospective randomised trial. *Bone Joint J.* 2016;98(Suppl 21):93–93.
104. Nork SE, Hennrikus WL, Loncarich DP, et al. Relationship between ligamentous laxity and the site of upper extremity fractures in children: extension supracondylar fracture versus distal forearm fracture. *J Pediatr Orthop B.* 1999;8(2):90–92.
105. Norrell KN, Muolo CE, Sherman AK, Sinclair MK. The frequency and outcomes of nerve palsies in operatively treated supracondylar humerus fractures. *J Pediatr Orthop.* 2022;42(8):408–412.
106. O'Driscoll SW, Spinner RJ, McKee MD, et al. Tardy posterolateral rotatory instability of the elbow due to cubitus varus. *J Bone Joint Surg Am.* 2001;83(9):1358–1369.
107. Oetgen ME, Mirick GE, Atwater L, Lovejoy JF. Complications and predictors of need for return to the operating room in the treatment of supracondylar humerus fractures in children. *Open Orthop J.* 2015;9:139–142.
108. Omid R, Choi PD, Skaggs DL. Supracondylar humeral fractures in children. *J Bone Joint Surg Am.* 2008;90(5):1121–1132.
109. Onwuanyi ON, Nwobi DG. Evaluation of the stability of pin configuration in K-wire fixation of displaced supracondylar fractures in children. *Int Surg.* 1998;83(3):271–274.
110. Or O, Weil Y, Simanovsky N, et al. The outcome of early revision of malaligned pediatric supracondylar humerus fractures. *Injury.* 2015;46(8):1585–1590.
111. Parikh SN, Lykissas MG, Roshdy M, et al. Pin tract infection of operatively treated supracondylar fractures in children: long-term functional outcomes and anatomical study. *J Child Orthop.* 2015;9(4):295–302.
112. Parikh SN, Wall EJ, Foad S, et al. Displaced type II extension supracondylar humerus fractures: do they all need pinning? *J Pediatr Orthop.* 2004;24(4):380–384.
113. Park MJ, Baldwin K, Weiss-Laxer N, et al. Composite playground safety measure to correlate the rate of supracondylar humerus fractures with safety: an ecologic study. *J Pediatr Orthop.* 2010;30(2):101–105.
114. Park MJ, Ho CA, Larson AN. AAOS appropriate use criteria: management of pediatric supracondylar humerus fractures. *J Am Acad Orthop Surg.* 2015;23(10):e52–e55.
115. Patel HA, Chaudhry S, Lee MC, Solomito M. Streamlining postoperative care after pediatric supracondylar humerus fractures: is follow-up after pin removal routinely needed? *J Pediatr Orthop.* 2021;41(6):e464–e469.
116. Pennock AT, Charles M, Moor M, et al. Potential causes of loss of reduction in supracondylar humerus fractures. *J Pediatr Orthop.* 2014;34(7):691–697.
117. Ponce BA, Hedequist DJ, Zurakowski D, et al. Complications and timing of follow-up after closed reduction percutaneous pinning supracondylar humerus fractures: follow-up after percutaneous pinning of supracondylar humerus fractures. *J Pediatr Orthop.* 2004;24:610–614.
118. Pradhan A, Hennrikus W, Pace G, et al. Increased pin diameter improves torsional stability in supracondylar humerus fractures: an experimental study. *J Child Orthop.* 2016;10(2):163–167.
119. Prusick VW, Gibian JT, Ross KE, et al. Surgical technique: closed reduction and percutaneous pinning of posterolaterally displaced supracondylar humerus fractures. *J Orthop Trauma.* 2021;35(3):e108–e115.
120. Ramachandran M, Birch R, Eastwood DM. Clinical outcome of nerve injuries associated with supracondylar fractures of the humerus in children: the experience of a specialist referral centre. *J Bone Joint Surg Br.* 2006;88(1):90–94.
121. Ramachandran M, Skaggs DL, Crawford HA, et al. Delaying treatment of supracondylar fractures in children: has the pendulum swung too far? *J Bone Joint Surg Br.* 2008;90:1228–1233.
122. Rasool MN. Ulnar nerve injury after K-wire fixation of supracondylar humerus fractures in children. *J Pediatr Orthop.* 1998;18(5):686–690.
123. Rees AB, Schultz JD, Wollenman LC, et al. A mini-open approach to medial pinning in pediatric supracondylar humeral fractures may be safer than previously thought. *J Bone Joint Surg Am.* 2022;104(1):33–40.
124. Rees AB, Schultz JD, Wollenman LC, et al. Internal rotation stress test reduces cross-pinning and improves outcomes in displaced pediatric supracondylar humeral fractures. *JB JS Open Access.* 2021;6(3):e21.0014.
125. Ring D, Waters PM, Hotchkiss RN, Kasser JR. Pediatric floating elbow. *J Pediatr Orthop.* 2001;4:456–459.

126. Robb JE. The pink, pulseless hand after supracondylar fracture of the humerus in children. *J Bone Joint Surg Br*. 2009;91(11):1410–1412.

127. Ryan DD, Lightdale-Miric NR, Joiner ERA, et al. Variability of the anterior humeral line in normal pediatric elbows. *J Pediatr Orthop*. 2016;36(2):e14–e16.

128. Sabharwal S, Tredwell SJ, Beauchamp RD, et al. Management of pulseless pink hand in pediatric supracondylar fractures of humerus. *J Pediatr Orthop*. 1997;17(3):303–310.

129. Sairyo K, Henmi T, Kanematsu Y, et al. Radial nerve palsy associated with slightly angulated pediatric supracondylar humerus fracture. *J Orthop Trauma*. 1997;11(3):227–229.

130. Sanders JS, Ouillette RJ, Howard R, et al. Nonoperative versus operative treatment of type IIa supracondylar humerus fractures: a prospective evaluation of 99 patients. *J Pediatr Orthop*. 2023;43(1):e9–e16.

131. Sankar WN, Hebela NM, Skaggs DL, Flynn JM. Loss of pin fixation in displaced supracondylar humeral fractures in children: causes and prevention. *J Bone Joint Surg Am*. 2007;89(4):713–717.

132. Schroeder NO, Seeley MA, Hariharan A, et al. Utility of postoperative antibiotics after percutaneous pinning of pediatric supracondylar humerus fractures. *J Pediatr Orthop*. 2017;37(6):363–367.

133. Schultz JD, Rees AB, Wollenman LC, et al. Bruise location in supracondylar humerus fractures predicts specific neurovascular injuries. *J Pediatr Orthop*. 2022;42(3):e250–e256.

134. Seehausen DA, Kay RM, Ryan DD, Skaggs DL. Foam padding in casts accommodates soft tissue swelling and provides circumferential strength after fixation of supracondylar humerus fractures. *J Pediatr Orthop*. 2015;35(1):24–27.

135. Shah AS, Waters PM, Bae DS. Treatment of the "pink pulseless hand" in pediatric supracondylar humerus fractures. *J Hand Surg Am*. 2013;38(7):1399–1403.

136. Shah M, Han JH, Park H, et al. Prevalence and treatment outcome of displaced high-long oblique supracondylar humeral fractures in children. *Front Pediatr*. 2021;9:739900.

137. Shaw BA, Kasser JR, Emans JB, Rand FF. Management of vascular injuries in displaced supracondylar humerus fractures without arteriography. *J Orthop Trauma*. 1990;4(1):25–29.

138. Shore BJ, Gillespie BT, Miller PE, et al. Recovery of motor nerve injuries associated with displaced, extension-type pediatric supracondylar humerus fractures. *J Pediatr Orthop*. 2019;39(9):e652–e656.

139. Shrader MW, Campbell MD, Jacofsky DJ. Accuracy of emergency room physicians' interpretation of elbow fractures in children. *Orthopedics*. 2008;31(12).

140. Sibinski M, Sharma H, Bennet GC. Early versus delayed treatment of extension type-3 supracondylar fractures of the humerus in children. *J Bone Joint Surg Br*. 2006;88(3):380–381.

141. Silva M, Cooper SD, Cha A. The outcome of surgical treatment of multidirectionally unstable (type IV) pediatric supracondylar humerus fractures. *J Pediatr Orthop*. 2015;35(6):600–605.

142. Silva M, Pandarinath R, Farng E, et al. Inter- and intra-observer reliability of the Baumann angle of the humerus in children with supracondylar humeral fractures. *Int Orthop*. 2010;34(4):553–557.

143. Silva M, Wong TC, Bernthal NM. Outcomes of reduction more than 7 days after injury in supracondylar humeral fractures in children. *J Pediatr Orthop*. 2011;31(7):751–756.

144. Siriwardhane M, Siriwardhane J, Lam L, et al. Supracondylar fracture of the humerus in children: mechanism of injury. *J Bone Joint Surg Br*. 2012;94B(Suppl 23):141.

145. Skaggs DL, Cluck MW, Mostofi A, et al. Lateral-entry pin fixation in the management of supracondylar fractures in children. *J Bone Joint Surg Am*. 2004;86(4):702–707.

146. Skaggs DL, Glassman D, Weiss JM, Kay RM. A new surgical technique for the treatment of supracondylar humerus fracture malunions in children. *J Child Orthop*. 2011;5(4):305–312.

147. Skaggs DL, Hale JM, Bassett J, et al. Operative treatment of supracondylar fractures of the humerus in children: the consequence of pin placement. *J Bone Joint Surg Am*. 2001;83(5):735–740.

148. Skaggs DL, Mirzayan R. The posterior fat pad sign in association with occult fracture of the elbow in children. *J Bone Joint Surg Am*. 1999;81(10):1429–1433.

149. Skaggs DL, Sankar WN, Albrektson J, et al. How safe is the operative treatment of Gartland type 2 supracondylar humerus fractures in children? *J Pediatr Orthop*. 2008;28(2):139–141.

150. Slobogean BL, Jackman H, Tennant S, et al. Iatrogenic ulnar nerve injury after the surgical treatment of displaced supracondylar fractures of the humerus: number needed to harm, a systematic review. *J Pediatr Orthop*. 2010;30(5):430–436.

151. Slongo T, Audigé L, Schlickewei W, et al. Development and validation of the AO pediatric comprehensive classification of long bone fractures by the Pediatric Expert Group of the AO Foundation in collaboration with AO clinical investigation and documentation and the International Association for Pediatric Traumatology. *J Pediatr Orthop*. 2006;26(1):43–49.

152. Soldado F, Diaz-Gallardo P, Cherqaoui A, et al. Unsuccessful mid-term results for distal humeral hemiepiphysiodesis to treat cubitus varus deformity in young children. *J Pediatr Orthop B*. 2022;31(5):431–433.

153. Srikumaran U, Tan EW, Belkoff SM, et al. Enhanced biomechanical stiffness with large pins in the operative treatment of pediatric supracondylar humerus fractures. *J Pediatr Orthop*. 2012;32(2):201–205.

154. Suganuma S, Tada K, Yasutake H, et al. Timing of surgery for pediatric supracondylar humerus fractures and early postoperative results. *J Hand Surg Asian Pac Vol*. 2020;25(2):226–231.

155. Sullivan MH, Wahlig BD, Broida SE, et al. Does shorter time to treatment of pediatric supracondylar humerus fractures impact clinical outcomes? *J Pediatr Orthop*. 2023;43(6):350–354.

156. Swanson CE, Chang K, Schleyer E, et al. Postoperative pain control after supracondylar humerus fracture fixation. *J Pediatr Orthop*. 2012;32(5):452–455.

157. Tarabishi MM, Almigdad AK, Ganger R, Farr S. Distal humeral corrective osteotomy for treatment of supracondylar fracture malunions in children. *J Child Orthop*. 2023;17(3):232–238.

158. Toğaç S, Eken G, Ermutlu C, Sarisözen B. Forearm compartment pressure change in children operated for supracondylar humerus fracture. *J Pediatr Orthop*. 2022;42(9):509–515.

159. Tripuraneni KR, Bosch PP, Schwend RM, Yaste JJ. Prospective, surgeon-randomized evaluation of crossed pins versus lateral pins for unstable supracondylar humerus fractures in children. *J Pediatr Orthop B*. 2009;18(2):93–98.

160. Tuason D, Hohl JB, Levicoff E, Ward WT. Urban pediatric orthopaedic surgical practice audit: implications for the future of this subspecialty. *J Bone Joint Surg Am*. 2009;91(12):2992–2998.

161. Voss FR, Kasser JR, Trepman E, et al. Uniplanar supracondylar humeral osteotomy with preset Kirschner wires for posttraumatic cubitus varus. *J Pediatr Orthop*. 1994;14(4):471–478.

162. Vu TN, Phung SHD, Vo LH, Nguyen UH. Diagnosis and treatment for pediatric supracondylar humerus fractures with brachial artery injuries. *Children (Basel)*. 2021;8(10):933.

163. Wang YL, Chang WN, Hsu CJ, et al. The recovery of elbow range of motion after treatment of supracondylar and lateral condylar fractures of the distal humerus in children. *J Orthop Trauma*. 2009;23(2):120–125.

164. Weiss JM, Kay RM, Waters P, et al. Distal humerus osteotomy for supracondylar fracture malunion in children: a study of perioperative complications. *Am J Orthop (Belle Mead NJ)*. 2010;39(1):22–25.

165. White L, Mehlman CT, Crawford AH. Perfused, pulseless, and puzzling: a systematic review of vascular injuries in pediatric supracondylar humerus fractures and results of a POSNA questionnaire. *J Pediatr Orthop*. 2010;30(4):328–335.

166. Wind WM, Schwend RM, Armstrong DG. Predicting ulnar nerve location in pinning of supracondylar humerus fractures. *J Pediatr Orthop*. 2002;22(4):444–447.

167. Wingfield JJ, Ho CA, Abzug JM, et al. Open reduction techniques for supracondylar humerus fractures in children. *J Am Acad Orthop Surg*. 2015;23(12):e72–e80.

168. Woratanarat P, Angsanuntsukh C, Rattanasiri S, et al. Meta-analysis of pinning in supracondylar fracture of the humerus in children. *J Orthop Trauma*. 2012;26(1):48–53.

169. Wu X, Lin R, Chen J, Chen S. Closed reduction with percutaneous Kirschner wire drill-and-pry for pediatric supracondylar humeral fractures with bony callus formation and delayed presentation. *Injury*. 2023;54(2):547–551.

170. Yang K, Willoughby R, Donald G. Radiological comparison of lateral entry compared with combined medial and lateral entry pin fixation for type IIIS supracondylar fractures in children with particular focus on rotational displacement. *J Bone Joint Surg Br*. 2012;94B(Suppl 23):142.

171. Young S, Fevang JM, Gullaksen G, et al. Deformity and functional outcome after treatment for supracondylar humerus fractures in children: a 5- to 10-year follow-up of 139 supracondylar humerus fractures treated by plaster cast, skeletal traction or crossed wire fixation. *J Child Orthop*. 2010;4(5):445–453.

172. Zaltz I, Waters PM, Kasser JR. Ulnar nerve instability in children. *J Pediatr Orthop*. 1996;16(5):567–569.

173. Zionts LE, McKellop HA, Hathaway R. Torsional strength of pin configurations used to fix supracondylar fractures of the humerus in children. *J Bone Joint Surg Am*. 1994;76(2):253–256.

174. Zionts LE, Woodson CJ, Manjra N, et al. Time of return of elbow motion after percutaneous pinning of pediatric supracondylar humerus fractures. *Clin Orthop Relat Res*. 2009;467(8):2007–2010.

15

T-Condylar Fractures of the Distal Humerus

Brian P. Scannell

INTRODUCTION TO T-CONDYLAR FRACTURES OF THE DISTAL HUMERUS

Distal humerus fractures in children are common but T-condylar fractures compose just some proportion of these fractures. Their treatment, however, is usually more invasive and extensive surgically. In T-condylar fractures, the fracture line most commonly originates in the central groove of the trochlea and courses proximal to the olecranon and coronoid fossae, where it divides and separates the medial and lateral bony columns of the distal humerus. If the proximal fracture lines are oblique, the fracture may be termed *Y-condylar.* T- and Y-condylar fractures are rare injuries in skeletally immature children and are often a transitional fracture seen in adolescents at the end of skeletal development.[6,25]

The early modern literature reflects only reports by Blount[9] and Zimmerman,[44] who each described a case of a T-condylar distal humerus fracture in an 11-year-old patient. The average age of pediatric patients reported in four major case series[20,23,33,36] was 12.8 years. Three studies have found that the nondominant arm is more likely to be injured 2.5 times greater than the dominant arm.[11,26,31,36] Thus, Maylahn and Fahey,[28] who reported six patients near skeletal maturity, were accurate when they said, "the fractures (T-condylar) take on the characteristics of an adult fracture and should be treated as such."

The actual incidence in younger children is certainly low, but it may be underdiagnosed because it is often confused with other fractures, such as those involving the isolated lateral condylar physis or total distal humeral physis. Special imaging studies such as elbow arthrograms or MRI scans may be necessary to demonstrate the intracondylar aspects in young children. The combination of an increased awareness of the possibility of this injury and a more aggressive diagnostic approach may result in more cases being recognized acutely and appropriately treated in this younger age group. The poorer outcomes from these relatively rare injuries are due to either failure to recognize the complex nature of the fracture or treat in a more comprehensive manner.

ASSESSMENT OF T-CONDYLAR FRACTURES OF THE DISTAL HUMERUS

MECHANISMS OF INJURY OF T-CONDYLAR FRACTURES OF THE DISTAL HUMERUS

The primary mechanism of this injury is most commonly an axial load onto an outstretched arm or a direct fall onto a flexed elbow. The position of the elbow results in either an extension- or flexion-type injury. This mechanism of injury results in a direct wedge effect of the articular surface of the olecranon on the distal end of the humerus. The sharp edge of the semilunar notch or coronoid process acts as a wedge to break the trochlea and split the condyles, which in turn separates the two columns of the distal humerus.

The most common mechanism producing a flexion injury is a direct blow to the posterior aspect of the elbow, usually when the child falls directly on the flexed elbow. This flexion mechanism in young children contributes to its rarity because most upper extremity injuries in children result from a fall on an outstretched hand and have a component of elbow hyperextension. In these flexion injuries, the wedge effect is produced at the apex of the trochlea by the central portion of the trochlear notch. The condylar fragments usually lie anterior to the shaft in these flexion injuries (Fig. 15-1A,B).

A T-condylar fracture may also be caused by a fall on the outstretched arm with the elbow in only slight flexion. This extension mechanism has been suggested by patients in their description of the dynamics of their fall; and indirectly by the posterior position of the distal fragments in relation to the diaphyses of the humerus (Fig. 15-1C,D). In the extension type of injury, the coronoid portion of the semilunar notch produces the wedge effect.

It has been suggested that the attachment of the forearm flexor and extensor muscles and their contraction during the injury may play a role in the displacement pattern of this

Figure 15-1. Mechanism patterns. **A, B:** The more common flexion pattern in which the condylar fragments are situated anterior to the distal shaft. **C, D:** An extensor pattern in which the condylar fragments are situated posterior to the distal shaft. The muscle origins on the respective condyles cause them to diverge in the coronal plane (*arrows*) and flex in the sagittal plane.

fracture. Because of their origins on the epicondyles, they accentuate both the separation in the coronal plane and the forward displacement in the sagittal plane. This displacement pattern is often evident on the injury films (see Fig. 15-1C,D), and consideration will aid later reduction maneuvers.

INJURIES ASSOCIATED WITH T-CONDYLAR FRACTURES DISTAL OF THE HUMERUS

Very little has been written on the type of associated injuries seen with T-condylar fractures of the distal humerus in children. In general, these are high-velocity injuries that are typically the result of high-energy mechanisms, such as motor vehicle collisions, high-speed sporting accidents, or falls from significant heights.[19] Open wounds, other ipsilateral upper limb injuries, and systemic injuries can occur because of the high-energy trauma that occurs. A recent series has documented that in adolescents with intra-articular distal humerus fractures, nearly 25% were open injuries.[11]

SIGNS AND SYMPTOMS OF T-CONDYLAR FRACTURES OF THE DISTAL HUMERUS

The history should focus on the mechanism, time of injury, and the identification of other sites of injury. It is important to recognize any prior elbow injury or upper extremity surgery. Focused examination of the injured extremity should include inspection for bruising, swelling, deformity, and evidence of any open injuries. A thorough circumferential inspection of the elbow is critical to avoid missing open wounds, which commonly occur on the posterior aspect.[26] Careful examination of distal vascular status is performed, inspecting the distal extremity for color, turgor, capillary refill, and palpating the radial and ulnar pulses. If there is a questionable pulse in the setting of gross malalignment of the arm, gentle longitudinal traction can be used to realign the limb and often restore the distal pulse. A detailed and accurate distal neurologic examination including motor function, hand sensibility, and two-point discrimination or sweating pattern in younger children (median and ulnar nerves) should be performed to identify injury to the median, ulnar, radial, anterior, and/or posterior interosseous nerves. Recognition and documentation of these associated injuries is very important as there is a high rate of associated nerve injuries, and failure to document preoperatively may lead to attribution of the deficit to the surgery rather than the injury. At the conclusion of the examination, the arm is splinted in 30 to 70 degrees of flexion at the elbow for comfort in a padded posterior, above-elbow splint.

IMAGING AND OTHER DIAGNOSTIC STUDIES FOR T-CONDYLAR FRACTURES OF THE DISTAL HUMERUS

Clinically, these fractures are most often confused with extension-type supracondylar fractures, especially in younger patients. The extended position of the elbow, along with the massive swelling, is almost identical to that of the displaced extension type of supracondylar fracture.

Plain radiographs are the cornerstone to the diagnosis. In older children, the differentiation must be made from that of a comminuted supracondylar fracture without intercondylar extension. Sometimes, the diagnosis is not obvious until the fragments have been partially reduced, which allows the vertical fracture lines splitting the trochlea to become more evident. In younger children, the diagnosis is much more difficult because the articular surface is cartilaginous and not visible on plain radiographs. In addition, because of its rarity, the possibility of a T-condylar fracture may not be considered in this age group.

The diagnosis must exclude common fracture patterns of either the isolated lateral or medial condyles and complete separation of the distal humeral physis. In these latter fractures, an important sign is the presence of a medial or lateral Thurstan Holland fragment in the metaphysis.[7] The key differential for the T-condylar fracture is the presence of a vertical fracture line extending down to the apex of the trochlea.

Although difficult to obtain in children secondary to pain, a traction view radiograph can help with better visualization of the articular fracture.[27] It may help avoid further axial imaging. This type of imaging can also be performed in the operating room prior to commencing surgery in order to obtain better visualization of the distal fracture fragments.

If the diagnosis is suspected after a careful evaluation of the static radiographs or traction radiographs, it can be confirmed with a preoperative CT scan for adolescent children or MRI in younger children.[7] CT scans can allow for proper surgical planning and fracture-specific fixation, particularly in the adolescent patient. MRI may be preferred in the younger patient if there is suspicion for intra-articular extension. Finally, the use of contrast medium in the form of an arthrogram intraoperatively can also be helpful to distinguish fracture lines and aid in the assessment of the quality of the articular reduction and fracture fixation.

CLASSIFICATION OF T-CONDYLAR FRACTURES OF THE DISTAL HUMERUS

Fracture Pattern

The fracture pattern in adolescents is similar to that in adults. The condylar fragments are often separated, with the articular surface completely disrupted. In addition to separation of the condylar fragments by the force of the original injury, the muscles that originate on these condylar fragments rotate them in both the coronal and sagittal planes (see Fig. 15-1C,D). In the sagittal plane, the position of the condylar fragments in relation to the humeral shaft and metaphysis can either be anterior (flexor mechanism; see Fig. 15-1B) or posterior (extension mechanism; see Fig. 15-1D).

In skeletally immature patients, the central portions of the condylar fragments are usually separated, but the articular surface may remain intact because of its large cartilage component (Fig. 15-2).[33] Thus, the disruption and displacement are primarily in the osseous supracondylar area. The elasticity of the cartilage of the distal end of the humerus often acts as

Figure 15-2. Intact articular surface. In this T-condylar fracture in a 7-year-old boy, the thick articular cartilage remains essentially intact, preventing separation of the condylar fragments. This fracture was secured with simple percutaneous pins.

an opening hinge but protects the articular surface from being completely disrupted. At times, this is not seen until the patient is in the operating room and an arthrogram is performed. It also can be seen on a preoperative MRI scan.

Classification Systems

Various classifications[20,38] for adult T-condylar fractures have been proposed, but there are problems with applying these classifications to children's injuries. For example, the number of young children with this fracture is so small that it limits the experience of any clinician in treating all types of fracture patterns. In addition, there is no useful classification for younger patients, in whom the unossified intact articular cartilage is not visible on plain radiographs. Toniolo and Wilkins[41] proposed a simple classification based on the degree of displacement and comminution of the fracture fragments for pediatric T-condylar fractures. Type I fractures are minimally displaced (Fig. 15-3). Type II fractures are displaced but do not have comminution of the metaphyseal fragments (Fig. 15-4). Type III fractures are displaced fractures with comminution of the metaphyseal fragments (Fig. 15-5A,B).

Figure 15-3. Examples of type I T-condylar fractures. **A:** Lateral view of type I undisplaced T-condylar fracture in a 6 year old. **B:** AP of the T-condylar fracture line (*open arrows*) was not appreciated until it healed. There are both medial and lateral Thurstan Holland fragments (*solid arrows*). (Courtesy of Ruben D. Pechero, MD.) **C:** Pre- and postoperative x-rays of minimally displaced intra-articular type I T-condylar fracture in a 16-year-old boy treated with closed reduction and percutaneous screw fixation.

Figure 15-4. Type II displaced T-condylar factures. **A, B:** Type II displaced T-condylar fracture with no metaphyseal comminution—AP (A) and lateral (B) injury radiographs. **C, D:** Postoperative images of displaced type II T-condylar fracture with significant displacement but no comminution, treated bicolumn rigid fixation to facilitate early range of motion.

Figure 15-5. Type III T-condylar fractures with significant displacement and comminution. **A, B:** Type III—two views of markedly comminuted T-condylar fracture with multiple displaced fragments (*arrows*) in a 12 year old. **C–F:** Pre-, intra-, postoperative, and final healed radiographs of a 12-year-old girl with displaced and severely comminuted distal humerus and ipsilateral distal radius fracture, treated with a combination of transarticular screw and cross-wire fixation. At 1 year, she has made a complete recovery with comparable range of motion to her contralateral elbow.

In adolescents aged 12 years or older, classification and treatment follow similar patterns to those for adults. In general, intra-articular humerus fractures are defined by column (medial, lateral, or both) and degree of comminution. The Arbeitsgemeinschaft für Osteosynthesefragen (AO) classification is used most often (Fig. 15-6). T-condylar fractures in the adolescent are usually AO C1 and C2 injuries.[36] Fortunately, C3 injuries with marked comminution are rare in the adolescent. Metaphyseal–diaphyseal fractures are separate entities and need to be recognized as such for proper treatment and fixation decisions.[14]

OUTCOME MEASURES FOR T-CONDYLAR FRACTURES OF THE DISTAL HUMERUS

Common clinical outcomes recorded in T-condylar fractures of the distal humerus include time to union, range of motion, and elbow strength as measured through standardized quantitative tools such as Cybex testing. Functional outcome scores for both operative and nonoperative treatments such as the Mayo Elbow Performance Score[30] and the Disability of the Arm, Shoulder, and Hand[12] (DASH) are frequently used to measure functional improvement after upper extremity surgery. Patient Reported

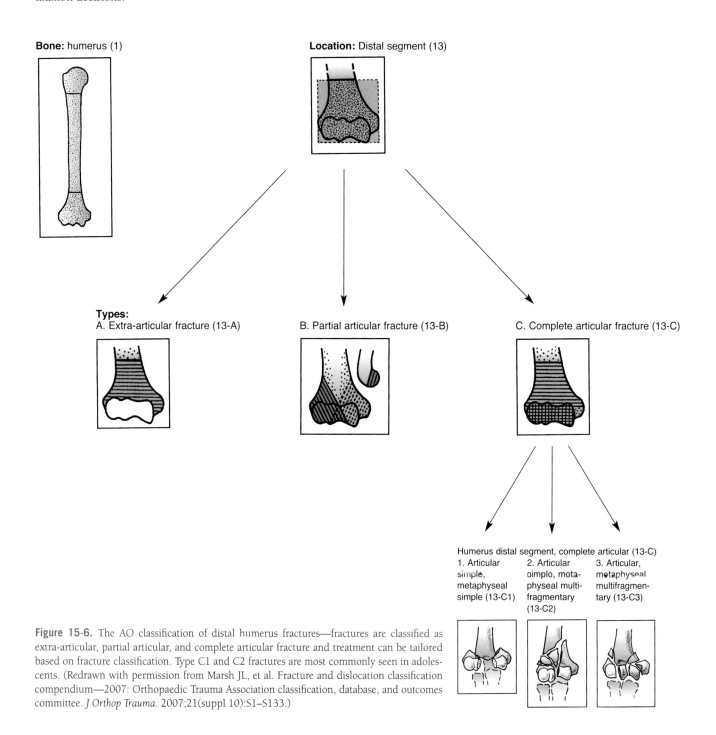

Figure 15-6. The AO classification of distal humerus fractures—fractures are classified as extra-articular, partial articular, and complete articular fracture and treatment can be tailored based on fracture classification. Type C1 and C2 fractures are most commonly seen in adolescents. (Redrawn with permission from Marsh JL, et al. Fracture and dislocation classification compendium—2007: Orthopaedic Trauma Association classification, database, and outcomes committee. *J Orthop Trauma.* 2007;21(suppl 10):S1–S133.)

Outcome Measurement scores are increasingly used in adult trauma and applied to pediatric trauma outcomes.

PATHOANATOMY AND APPLIED ANATOMY RELATING TO T-CONDYLAR FRACTURES OF THE DISTAL HUMERUS

The elbow is a complex joint composed of three individual joints contained within a common articular cavity. Ossification of the distal humerus proceeds in a predictable order. However, the rate of ossification in girls generally exceeds that of boys.[13,15,17,34] In some areas, such as the olecranon and lateral epicondyle, the difference between boys and girls in ossification age may be as great as 2 years.[15] Knowledge of the sequence and timing of ossification in the elbow will aid the treating physician in differentiating true intercondylar pathology from normal anatomic variant.

The bone of the distal humerus is triangular in shape. The medial and lateral columns of the distal humerus form the supracondylar region and are characterized by sharp and thin ridges of bone, respectively.[5] At the base of the triangle lies the trochlea, which represents the most distal portion of the humerus. It is important to realize that the lateral column of the distal humerus curves anteriorly along with the anteriorly translated articular surface of the distal humerus, but the medial column is straight in line with the humeral diaphysis. The spatial relationship among the medial column, lateral column, and trochlea is conceptually similar to a spool of thread being held between the thumb and index finger.[21] Failure to understand and appreciate the distal humerus anatomy may result in functional malunions.

The surgical approach for distal humerus fractures most widely accepted is an extensile posterior incision through which all aspects of the elbow can be exposed including the anterior structures.[35] The ulnar nerve is frequently a structure that needs to be identified and protected during open reduction and internal fixation. It passes through the cubital tunnel just posterior to the medial epicondyle and is held in close proximity to the distal humerus by Osborne fascia. Higher on the lateral side the radial nerve pierces the intermuscular septum where it is vulnerable to injury by a fracture or a surgical exposure extending proximally, as may be necessary in the uncommon fracture with metaphyseal with comminution.

TREATMENT OPTIONS FOR T-CONDYLAR FRACTURES OF THE DISTAL HUMERUS

Because of the rarity of this injury, treatment recommendations are based on isolated case or small retrospective case series and/or the application of adult treatment principles.[1,7,8,20,23,33,36,37,42] Regardless of the treatment method, certain basic principles must be considered in dealing with these fractures.

A treatment plan must be individualized for the specific fracture, patient age, and the surgeon's level of expertise and experience. The following principles must be considered in planning a treatment method:

- The T-condylar fracture is an articular fracture, so the first goal is to restore and stabilize the joint surface.
- Stability depends on the integrity of the lateral and medial supracondylar columns.
- Elbow articular mobility depends on articular congruity, correct alignment of the axis of motion, and debris- and bone-free fossae.
- Closed methods alone usually cannot produce an acceptable result because the muscle and collateral ligament forces applied to the fragments make the fracture unstable.
- Most patients are adolescents with minimal potential for bone remodeling and may need treatment with bicolumn open reduction and internal fixation similar to an adult. Stable internal fixation that allows for immediate postoperative movement is important in reducing the risk of contracture development postoperatively.

NONOPERATIVE TREATMENT OF T-CONDYLAR DISTAL HUMERUS FRACTURES

Indications/Contraindications

Nonoperative Treatment of T-Condylar Fractures of the Distal Humerus: INDICATIONS AND CONTRAINDICATIONS

Indications

Young children aged <8 years with intact periosteum
- Simple fractures without comminution, displacement, or angulation

Relative Contraindications

Fracture displacement >2 mm
Fracture comminution
- Ipsilateral arm injuries

Most T-condylar fractures of the distal humerus are best treated with some form of open reduction and internal fixation. However, there is a narrow range of fractures that are indicated for management of these injuries with closed treatment and casting. Children who are under 8 years of age with robust periosteum and essentially nondisplaced fractures may be candidates for closed treatment and casting. Preoperative advanced imaging may be necessary and close follow-up radiographically is required if closed treatment is used.

Closed Treatment

Nondisplaced and stable fractures can be immobilized until healing with close radiographic follow-up. An above-elbow cast is applied for at least 3 weeks with repeat x-rays on a weekly interval to detect interval displacement. Closed reduction and immobilization without fracture fixation is not recommended. If closed reduction is required for improved alignment, this is an unstable injury that requires fixation.

Outcomes

Most T-condylar fractures of the distal humerus are treated operatively, and therefore it is very difficult to tease out the results of nonoperative management of these fractures. In our review of several series, only 4 of 48 combined fractures were treated nonoperatively.[23,33,36] In these limited cases, all patients achieved a full arc of motion without complications from their fracture or treatment. These results can only be expected with very careful selection of nondisplaced and stable fractures.

OPERATIVE TREATMENT OF T-CONDYLAR DISTAL HUMERUS FRACTURES

Indications/Contraindications

Adolescents with T-condylar fractures of the distal humerus are usually treated with reduction and fixation: rarely closed reduction and percutaneous pin/screw fixation; or more commonly, bicolumn open reduction and internal fixation similar to an adult. Indications for open reduction and internal fixation include all displaced extra-articular fractures, displacement of the articular surface greater than 2 mm, comminution of the distal humerus with greater than two fracture fragments, and ipsilateral fracture(s) of the upper extremity. Open fractures, pending compartment syndromes, and avascular limbs are surgical emergencies. However, the majority of T-condylar fractures of the distal humerus can be treated electively within 72 hours from the initial injury. The fracture reduction and instrumentation is complex enough that having the best OR team available can be in everyone's best interest.

In adolescents, most T-condylar fractures of the distal humerus are C1 according to the AO classification (see Fig. 15-6). Therefore, choosing either a triceps-splitting or triceps-reflecting approach is sufficient to facilitate access for open reduction and internal fixation. In the rare circumstances of C2 or C3 fractures, especially in the setting of anterior comminution, an olecranon osteotomy is warranted to facilitate visualization and fixation of the articular surface.

Closed Reduction and Percutaneous Pin/Screw Fixation

In young children (<8 years) with robust periosteum, the T-condylar distal humerus fracture may represent isolated hinging of the periosteum with minimal displacement of the intercondylar fracture. Careful preoperative imaging will demonstrate merely hinging of the articular surface without significant displacement. In younger children with minimal displacement, it is not unreasonable to perform a fluoroscopic guided reduction and stabilization with multiple percutaneous pins. Generally smooth, appropriate-sized pins are used: one pin horizontally from the lateral to medial to stabilize the joint surface and multiple pins to stabilize the medial and lateral columns. These pins can either be divergent lateral-entry or both medial- and lateral-entry pins. An arthrogram can be used after fixation to confirm anatomic alignment of the articular surface.

In older children with minimal displacement, percutaneous reduction and cannulated column screw fixation is acceptable.

This, to some degree, violates standard adult principles of open reduction internal fixation; it relies on the adolescent periosteum and rapid healing potential. However, if anatomic articular alignment and stable internal fixation can be achieved percutaneously, then less invasive treatment is appropriate. It is critical to have superior fluoroscopic images intraoperatively to prevent the realization of persistent fracture fragment displacement and/or inadvertent screw malposition on follow-up radiographs. Again, an arthrogram can be very helpful to confirm reduction at the articular surface.

Preoperative Planning

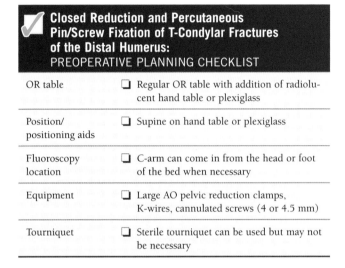

Closed Reduction and Percutaneous Pin/Screw Fixation of T-Condylar Fractures of the Distal Humerus:
PREOPERATIVE PLANNING CHECKLIST

OR table	❏ Regular OR table with addition of radiolucent hand table or plexiglass
Position/ positioning aids	❏ Supine on hand table or plexiglass
Fluoroscopy location	❏ C-arm can come in from the head or foot of the bed when necessary
Equipment	❏ Large AO pelvic reduction clamps, K-wires, cannulated screws (4 or 4.5 mm)
Tourniquet	❏ Sterile tourniquet can be used but may not be necessary

Surgical planning includes decisions on percutaneous pin versus screw fixation and patient positioning in the operative room. Careful scrutiny of preoperative radiographs and 3D imaging (usually CT scans) is imperative. Sometimes, intraoperative fluoroscopy images with traction realignment are essential in final decision making about surgical approach and fixation methods. These images should be performed prior to final positioning, prepping and draping as changing course intraoperative is difficult. Percutaneous treatment should only be chosen if anatomic reduction and stable fixation can be achieved with limited postoperative immobilization to lessen the risk of elbow contracture.

Similar principles for displaced adult distal humerus intra-articular fractures are employed, with reduction and stabilization of the articular surface first, followed by stabilization of the medial and lateral columns. If percutaneous reduction and fixation is performed, a large, external bone holding the reduction clamp is used to facilitate interfragmentary reduction and compression of the joint, prior to pin or screw fixation. Accurate placement of a transverse pin to hold the articular segments in an anatomic position is critical (Fig. 15-7). Depending on the degree of displacement and fracture fragment configuration, provisional or definitive fixation can be achieved with standard medial and lateral column pins as in a supracondylar humerus fracture. As noted above, in limited scenarios, these fractures can be treated definitively with closed reduction and percutaneous fixation using either smooth wires or cannulated screws.

Figure 15-7. Percutaneous fixation of a T-condylar fracture. **A:** This 8-year-old had a displaced intra-articular distal humerus. **B:** A reduction was successful with longitudinal traction and compression of the articular surface manually with a clamp. A lateral-to-medial pin was placed perpendicular to the fracture to stabilize the articular surface first. **C:** Pin fixation was then performed with lateral and medial column fixation. **D:** An arthrogram was completed following fixation demonstrating anatomic articular surface.

Positioning

Percutaneous fixation of T-condylar fractures of the distal humerus is usually performed in the supine position but can be facilitated also in the lateral or prone position. Most commonly, the patient is positioned supine with arm on a hand table. The arm is elevated on a stack of towels to facilitate easier pin/screw insertion. Bringing the shoulder into abduction and elbow into extension can improve the quality of visualization of the fracture with C-arm imaging. In general, the young have enough rotatory motion about the shoulder to allow for proper visualization in the supine position. Alternative positions are discussed further with open reduction and internal fixation.

Surgical Approach

In closed reduction and percutaneous pin/screw fixation, limited surgical exposure is performed. In some settings, small stab incisions are made to ensure that the large bone-reducing forceps can be placed directly on bone (medial and lateral epicondyles most commonly) to generate the desired compressive effect. In general, wires are placed percutaneously from the lateral column of the distal humerus. On the medial side, small 1- to 2-cm incisions can be made to prevent inadvertent injury to the ulnar nerve, there is a much higher incidence of ulnar nerve instability in children than adults. In addition, the arm is placed in a semiextended position when passing wires/screws from the medial to lateral, to decrease the risk of iatrogenic ulnar nerve injury.

Technique

Closed Reduction and Percutaneous Pin/Screw Fixation of T-Condylar Fractures of the Distal Humerus: KEY SURGICAL STEPS

- Begin with performance of accurate AP/lateral and oblique fluoroscopic images of the distal humerus. Longitudinal traction images may help with planning and can be performed prior to prep/drape.
- Make small stab incisions, to facilitate bone clamp application.
- Under dynamic fluoroscopy, verify that fracture reduction is being achieved with dynamic compression.
- Consider the use of an arthrogram. This can be performed before or after fixation based on surgeon preference.
- Reduce the fracture into an acceptable position.
- Place appropriate wires to achieve provisional stability. If planning to utilize cannulated screws, wires specific for these screws can be used for the provisional stability.
- Fix the articular fragment first.
- Address column stability second.
- Once the wires are in the correct position, confirm with live fluoroscopy to ensure adequate reduction and wire placement.
- If using cannulated screws:
- Measure screw lengths when appropriate and then overdrill guide wires.
- Place the screw across the articular fragment first and then stabilize the medial/lateral columns.
- Test stability with flexion and extension.

OPEN REDUCTION AND INTERNAL FIXATION

Preoperative Planning

ORIF of T-Condylar Fractures of the Distal Humerus: PREOPERATIVE PLANNING CHECKLIST

OR table	Regular OR table with addition of radiolucent hand table or plexiglass
Position/ positioning aids	Prone position on bolsters to decompress abdomen and protect neurovascular structures
Fluoroscopy location	C-arm can come in from the head or foot of the bed when necessary
Equipment	Large AO pelvic reduction clamps, K-wires, cannulated screws and precontoured distal humerus plates or pelvic reconstruction plates, Penrose drain, and vessel loop to isolate and protect the ulnar nerve
Tourniquet	Sterile tourniquet used but can be let down if necessary because of timing
Other	Monopolar and bipolar cautery to facilitate dissection of the ulnar nerve

The surgical treatment of T-condylar fractures of the distal humerus involves consideration of three critical components: (1) body positioning—prone, lateral decubitus, or supine; (2) surgical approach—triceps splitting, paratricipital, triceps reflecting, or olecranon osteotomy; and (3) type of fixation—single column, bicolumn orthogonal, or parallel plating.

Positioning

Fixation of distal humerus fractures can be facilitated in the supine, lateral, or prone positions with the choice determined primarily based on the anticipated exposure, presence of concomitant injuries, and surgeon experience.

In the setting of polytrauma, patients may be positioned in supine/sloppy lateral position with a large bump placed under the ipsilateral shoulder. Surgery can be performed with the arm across the chest, held in place by an assistant, a sterile weight off the hand, or a towel clamp. Bringing the arm into abduction and extension can aid with visualization of the fracture and improve the quality of C-arm imaging.

An alternative approach is to position the patient in the lateral position with an axillary roll to protect the brachial plexus on the nonoperative limb. In this position, a large bump is fashioned or a specialized arm holder is used to hold the arm in internally rotated position at the shoulder with 90 degrees of flexion at the elbow. The C-arm machine can obtain acceptable images coming from the head or feet parallel to the bed.

Finally, patients can be positioned in the prone position with the operative limb exposed on a separate small arm board/table. In this position, bolsters are used in standard fashion similar to a spinal procedure to decompress the abdomen and protect neurovascular structures. The arm is held similar to the lateral position, with internal rotation of the shoulder and 90 degrees

A, B   C

Figure 15-8. Paratricipital approach. The paratricipital approach is done through a longitudinal posterior skin incision. Medially (**A**) the ulnar nerve (*black arrow*) is identified. The medial intermuscular septum (forceps) is excised and the triceps muscle is elevated off the posterior aspect of the distal humerus (**B**). Laterally, the triceps muscle is elevated off the posterolateral aspect of the distal humerus, allowing exposure of the lateral column, olecranon fossa, and posterior aspect of the trochlea (**C**). L, lateral column; T, triceps. (Reprinted with permission from Bucholz RW, et al. *Rockwood and Green's Fractures in Adults.* 7th ed. Lippincott Williams & Wilkins; 2010.)

of flexion at the elbow with minimal tension. Again, C-arm imaging is accessible from the head or foot of the bed.

Surgical Approach

A universal skin approach is used for most surgical approaches associated with T-condylar fractures of the distal humerus. A long curvilinear posterior skin incision is used, with the distal extension lateral to the olecranon and then back to the midline onto the proximal ulna. Avoiding the tip of the olecranon prevents an irritating posterior scar. Skin and subcutaneous fasciocutaneous flaps are elevated extensively at the level of the fascia. The ulnar nerve requires careful attention, protection, mobilization, and decompression at this stage and throughout the remainder of the operation. An elastic loop is placed around the nerve, and the nerve is handled gently for the entire surgical procedure.

Triceps-Splitting Approach

- Achieved either via a direct posterior incision in the triceps fascia (Fig. 15-8).[29]
- Or using long oblique fascial incisions from the medial and lateral epicondyles, to a more proximal connecting point in the midline and reflect the resultant tongue of fascia from proximal to distal down to its insertion on the olecranon, separating the tendon from the muscle, while protecting the ulnar nerve on the medial side.[42]
- The triceps muscle is split in the midline and is retracted beyond the medial and lateral columns, respectively, with broad retractors.
- The radial and ulnar nerves are protected behind retractors during exposure, reduction, and fixation. The radial nerve proximally limits this approach in fractures with metaphyseal

comminution.Flexion of the elbow allows for visualization and fixation of the articular fragments.

- With this approach, the intra-articular fracture assessment is still made indirectly. However, with C1 and C2 fractures, this can be seen well with fluoroscopy.

Triceps-Reflecting Approach (Bryan and Morrey)

- The medial aspect of the triceps is elevated from the humerus along the intermuscular septum to the level of the posterior capsule. In children and adolescents, this can be achieved with subperiosteal elevation (Fig. 15-9).[10,37]
- The superficial fascia of the forearm is incised distally for about 6 cm to the periosteum of the medial aspect of the proximal ulna.
- The periosteum and fascia are carefully elevated as a single layer from the medial to lateral, distal to proximal. Care must be taken to maintain the continuity of the triceps, periosteum, and fascia. The medial aspect of the junction between the triceps insertion and the superficial fascia and periosteum of the ulna is the weakest portion of the reflected tissue. Elevation off the apophysis is also delicate as buttonholing can occur here which will limit the length and strength of the triceps fascial flap and risk destabilizing the triceps insertion into the olecranon.
- At the conclusion of skeletal fixation, the triceps insertion periosteal sleeve is repaired directly to the bone with transosseous sutures or suture anchors.
- This approach is contraindicated in open fractures, where a portion of the triceps may become avascular secondary to the initial trauma from the fracture and further dissection increases this risk.

A, B   **C**

Figure 15-9. Triceps split. A midline approach is made through the center of the triceps tendon and medial head (**A**). The approach can be extended distally by splitting the triceps insertion to the olecranon and raisin medial and lateral full-thickness fasciotendinous flaps (**B, C**). To gain further exposure of the posterior trochlea, the elbow is flexed and the olecranon tip may be excised. (Reprinted with permission from Bucholz RW, et al. *Rockwood and Green's Fractures in Adults.* 7th ed. Lippincott Williams & Wilkins; 2010.)

Triceps-Reflecting Anconeus Pedicle Flap

- The triceps-reflecting anconeus pedicle (TRAP) flap approach is similar to the Bryan–Morrey approach, with the triceps reflected off the olecranon in continuity with the anconeus. The difference is that in the TRAP approach, a V-shaped incision is made to reflect the triceps and anconeus completely off the triceps. The anconeus muscle is fully released from insertion on the proximal lateral ulna.[32]
- This approach allows adequate exposure of the articular surface with no significant difference from the transolecranon approach.

Olecranon Osteotomy

- The olecranon osteotomy has been described as a standard approach for adult T-condylar distal humerus fractures (Fig. 15-10).
- In our hands, we reserve this approach in children and adolescents for complex T-condylar fractures of the distal humerus with significant intra-articular comminution (AO C3 T-condylar fractures).
- Similar to the paratricipital approach, the triceps is mobilized from the medial and lateral septa and followed distally to the elbow joint.

A, B   **C, D**

Figure 15-10. Olecranon osteotomy. The olecranon osteotomy is approached via a longitudinal posterior skin incision (**A**). The ulnar nerve is exposed and may be prepared for anterior subcutaneous transposition (**B**). The subcutaneous border of the proximal ulnar is exposed and the nonarticular portion of the greater sigmoid notch between the olecranon articular facet and the coronoid articular facet is clearly defined. Medial and lateral retractors are then placed into the ulnohumeral joint and an apex distal chevron osteotomy entering into the bare area is marked on the subcutaneous border of the ulna. A microsagittal saw is used to complete two-thirds of the osteotomy (**C**) and two osteotomes, placed into each arm of the chevron, apply controlled leverage to fracture the remaining third (**D**). (Reprinted with permission from Bucholz RW, et al. *Rockwood and Green's Fractures in Adults.* 7th ed. Lippincott Williams & Wilkins; 2010.)

- A longitudinal cancellous screw is predrilled down the olecranon from the tip or apophysis.
- Careful planning of the screw size is important as too large of a screw may engage the ulnar diaphysis prior to fully seating the screw head. Too small of a screw size may result in poor fixation of the osteotomy and loss of reduction.
- This screw is removed, and a chevron-type osteotomy is performed at the deepest portion of the trochlear notch of the olecranon process and corresponding with the area devoid of articular cartilage (bare area).
- The chevron osteotomy points distally, and is initiated with a fine oscillating saw and completed with a thin osteotome.
- The triceps muscle and the osteotomized proximal half of the olecranon are then reflected superiorly.
- The osteotomy can alternatively be fixed with a precontoured olecranon plate or parallel K-wires and tension band technique.
- At the end of the reduction, the osteotomy is reduced and fixed with compression fixation with cancellous screw and washer fixation.

Technique

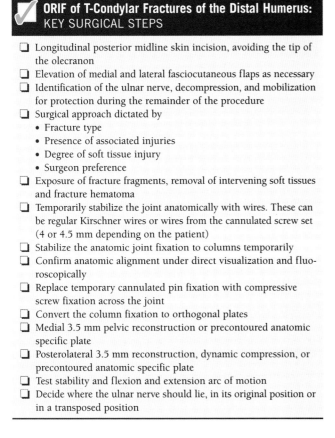

✓ ORIF of T-Condylar Fractures of the Distal Humerus:
KEY SURGICAL STEPS

☐ Longitudinal posterior midline skin incision, avoiding the tip of the olecranon
☐ Elevation of medial and lateral fasciocutaneous flaps as necessary
☐ Identification of the ulnar nerve, decompression, and mobilization for protection during the remainder of the procedure
☐ Surgical approach dictated by
  • Fracture type
  • Presence of associated injuries
  • Degree of soft tissue injury
  • Surgeon preference
☐ Exposure of fracture fragments, removal of intervening soft tissues and fracture hematoma
☐ Temporarily stabilize the joint anatomically with wires. These can be regular Kirschner wires or wires from the cannulated screw set (4 or 4.5 mm depending on the patient)
☐ Stabilize the anatomic joint fixation to columns temporarily
☐ Confirm anatomic alignment under direct visualization and fluoroscopically
☐ Replace temporary cannulated pin fixation with compressive screw fixation across the joint
☐ Convert the column fixation to orthogonal plates
☐ Medial 3.5 mm pelvic reconstruction or precontoured anatomic specific plate
☐ Posterolateral 3.5 mm reconstruction, dynamic compression, or precontoured anatomic specific plate
☐ Test stability and flexion and extension arc of motion
☐ Decide where the ulnar nerve should lie, in its original position or in a transposed position

Reconstruction of the Articular Surface

The first priority is to reestablish the integrity of the articular fragments—in other words, to convert it to a supracondylar fracture (Fig. 15-11). The olecranon and coronoid fossae must be cleared of bony fragments or debris to eliminate the chance

of bony impingement against their respective processes with motion. The best way to stabilize the condyles is with a screw passed transversely through the center of the axis of rotation in such a manner as to apply transverse compression. This stabilization method may require other temporary transverse pins to prevent rotation of the fragments as the guide hole is drilled or when the compression screw is being applied. These pins can be placed in a position that will not interfere with later plate placement.

In most adolescents, this is essentially an adult type of fracture pattern. Direct visualization of the reduction of all fracture fragments is mandatory. It is critical to get the joint surface anatomically and rigidly fixed. Regardless of surgical exposure (Bryan–Morey, triceps splitting, triceps-reflecting anconeus pedicle flap, olecranon osteotomy), it is imperative that the surgeon visualize the articular fracture reduction completely. This is best accomplished through direct visualization. In some C1-type fractures, however, indirect reduction can be performed but must be verified fluoroscopically or with an arthrogram. A single, short-threaded cancellous screw is most commonly used. A 3.5- to 4.5-mm diameter screw is placed from lateral to medial depending on the size of the bone and the available space between the articular surface and the olecranon fossa. Open physes further complicate the delicacy of exact screw placement in this region. The ulnar nerve is protected on the medial side. Once anatomic reduction and fixation of the articular surface are achieved, secure fixation of the columns is performed next. However, do not rush to column fixation unless the joint surface is reduced correctly. Fortunately, rarely do adolescent injuries have the same degree of extensive periarticular bony comminution like the more complex adult fracture-dislocations.

Stabilization of the Supracondylar Columns

Once the condylar and articular integrity has been reestablished, the distal fragments must be secured to the proximal fragment by stabilizing the supracondylar fragment columns. A factor in the column fixation decision is how important is it to initiate early motion. In a younger child with rapid bony healing, pin fixation is often satisfactory; the pins can be removed after 3 to 4 weeks to allow for protected motion. In an older adolescent nearer to skeletal maturity, we prefer rigid fixation—usually plates or less commonly, screws—that allows early motion (Fig. 15-12; see Fig. 15-4C,D). Before applying the plates, the supracondylar columns can be stabilized temporarily with pin fixation.

Principles of Plate Fixation

The plates must be strong; thin semitubular plates can be inadequate and may break.[43] However, double stacking semitubular plates can be used in younger or thinner teenagers. Proper rotational bending is harder in these plates. Usually the reinforced malleable reconstructive type of plates used for fixation of pelvic fractures can be anatomically contoured and provide very secure fixation of the distal humerus. Plating can be accomplished with orthogonal or parallel plating systems. Some studies have shown no difference in load to failure.[4,16] However, some recommend orthogonal plating (or plates 90 degrees to each other), which provides for a more stable construct.[18,24,39,40]

Figure 15-11. Sequence of distal humerus reconstruction. **A–C:** First, the articular portions are reassembled with provisional K-wire fixation, followed by screw fixation. **D:** K-wires can then also be used to provide temporary fixation of the distal humerus. **E:** A one-third tubular plate is attached to the medial side. **F:** A 3.5-mm pelvic reconstruction plate was attached to the posterolateral border.

Figure 15-12. T-condylar humeral fracture with plate and screw fixation. **A, B:** Injury films of a type II flexion pattern in a 16-year-old boy. **C, D:** Articular integrity was first restored with a transcondylar compression screw. The condyles were secured to the metaphysis and distal shaft using pelvic reconstruction plates placed at 90 degrees to each other.

Author's Preferred Treatment for T-Condylar Fractures of the Distal Humerus (Algorithm 15-1)

Algorithm 15-1. Author's preferred treatment of T-condylar fractures of the distal humerus according to age and displacement.

Because this fracture is rare in children, there are limited standard recommendations for treatment. The author suggestions are based on a combination of clinical experience and the experience of others in a few series.[8,14,20,23,33,36,37,42] The most imperative step in these fractures is to reestablish the integrity of the articular surface to maintain the congruity of the joint. Occasionally in the young, this can be achieved percutaneously and confirmed arthrographically. However, anatomic articular reduction may not be achieved adequately by closed methods, so we proceed with an open surgical technique. In the young child, we use the simple classification of Toniolo and Wilkins,[41] separating the fractures into three types based on the degree of displacement or comminution to be helpful in guiding the aggressiveness of our treatment. In adolescents, we guide our treatment according to the AO classification.

Type I (Undisplaced or Minimally Displaced)

In type I injuries, there is little displacement of the bony supracondylar columns. In children, the periosteum is often intact and can provide some intrinsic stability. In addition, the thicker articular and epiphyseal cartilage in skeletally immature children may still be intact, even if the bony epiphysis appears severed by a vertical fracture line. Because of this condition, we have found two methods to be successful for these types of fractures.

Closed Treatment
Cast Application

Truly nondisplaced fractures can be treated in a cast. Again, it is imperative to judge completely stable fractures from injuries

that can displace. Careful radiographic follow-up is necessary to avoid an articular malunion. Because of the rapid healing in these nondisplaced fractures, the cast can be removed in 4 weeks and a hinged elbow brace initiated to permit early protected motion if children are older (>8 years old).

Percutaneous Pin Fixation or Screw Fixation

The minimally displaced fractures in the young require manipulation under general anesthesia and radiographic control to reestablish the supracondylar columns and articular surface anatomy. If there is minor anterior or posterior rotation in the sagittal plane of the metaphyseal portion of the column, a pin placed into that column can be used as a "joystick" to manipulate the fragment into a satisfactory position. Once a satisfactory reduction is achieved, the pin can then be advanced across the fracture site for fixation. These fractures usually require multiple pins placed percutaneously, such as those used in comminuted supracondylar fractures (see Fig. 15-7). Because of the rapid healing, the pins can be removed at 3 to 4 weeks to allow early active motion.

In the setting of mild intra-articular displacement, we employ the use of a large bone-reducing forceps to help facilitate with our reduction. Often this can be applied percutaneously or through small stab incisions to ensure that the tines of the clamp are placed directly onto the bone (usually medial and lateral epicondyles) of the distal humerus without injury to the neighboring neurovascular structures. Once the articular diastasis is corrected, guide wires from the cannulated screw set are placed with bicortical fixation perpendicular to the fracture line. Appropriate-length screws with washers are placed over the guide wires. Compression is applied sequentially, alternating between screws to ensure optimal and balanced compression. This percutaneous technique can only be used when anatomic articular reduction is achieved.

Type II (Displaced Without Comminution)
Open Reduction and Internal Fixation

For some of these fractures with mild/moderate displacement, an attempt at a closed reduction of the articular surface can be performed as previously described (see Fig 15-7). In a supine position, longitudinal traction can be pulled on the arm. Without intra-articular comminution, it may be possible to reduce the articular surface and perform an arthrogram after pin or screw fixation.

However, if there is wide separation of the condylar fragments with marked disruption of the articular surface, stability and articular congruity can be established only with an open surgical procedure. We prefer a triceps-splitting approach for C1 distal humerus fractures and a triceps-sparing Bryan–Morrey approach for C2 distal humerus fractures. Olecranon osteotomy or triceps-reflecting aconeus pedicle (TRAP) exposure techniques are used for comminuted C3 articular fractures in adolescents. We place the patient supine in a "sloppy lateral" position to allow for easier lateral fluoroscopic imaging. A sterile tourniquet is used throughout the surgery.

Initial reconstruction is directed to restoration of the articular surface and then stable fixation of the articular block to the shaft.

Some of the plates specifically designed for distal humerus fracture fixation in the adult either do not fit anatomically or are too prominent for many pediatric patients. In these smaller patients, choosing an appropriate-sized plate that provides rigid fixation is necessary. In the larger, skeletally mature adolescent, use of adult distal humerus specific plates is appropriate. Later plate removal may be necessary though.

Type III (Displaced With Comminution)
Multiple Pin Fixation Treatment

In this time of extreme sports even in the young, there are instances of severely comminuted fractures in which the patient's bone will not allow for screw or plate fixation but the fracture is too displaced and/or comminuted to be successfully treated closed. In these instances, open reduction and pin fixation of each fracture fragment is a treatment option. There are times when even suture repair of fractures is required. The fixation does not allow for immediate motion but is started as soon as feasible (see Fig. 15-5 and Algorithm 15-1). The very distal comminuted injury, especially if there is an open physis, is amenable to this treatment and relies on the rapid healing biology of the younger patient.

Open Reduction and Internal Fixation

Often open reduction and internal fixation is necessary for the treatment of the type III fracture. The author uses the technique described in Figure 15-11 in a prone position. Approach is dictated by the fracture fragments.

Postoperative Care

In situations in which closed reduction and pin fixation is performed, a well-padded circumferential cast is applied for a total of about 4 weeks depending on the degree of healing appreciated on the postreduction radiographs. Patients are then transitioned into a hinged elbow brace and physical therapy is initiated until full range of motion is achieved. Wires are removed when appropriate healing is appreciated.

Children treated with closed reduction and percutaneous screw fixation are transitioned from their circumferential cast at 7 to 14 days and placed into a hinged elbow brace. Increasing motion is permitted over time and healing. Physical therapy is initiated at the first postoperative visit and protected therapy is continued until full range of motion is achieved. Return to sports is dependent on bony healing, restoration of strength, and maximum motion, usually at 3 months.

If plate fixation is used, we place the extremity in a well-padded soft dressing and hinged brace. Continuous passive motion (CPM) can be initiated in hospital followed by home CPM for complex T-condylar fractures treated with ORIF can aid in regaining elbow motion sooner. The active motion of postoperative therapy is performed in a hinged elbow brace with full motion allowed. A mild 10-degree extension contracture in these patients is anticipated in the best results.

Potential Pitfalls and Preventative Measures

T-Condylar Fractures of the Distal Humerus: POTENTIAL PITFALLS AND PREVENTIONS

Pitfall	Prevention
Articular malreduction	• Appropriate skin and soft tissue exposure, with visualization of critical articular components. • Begin with joint reduction and stabilization, convert from three- or four-part fracture to a two-part supracondylar-type fracture.
Inadequate stabilization to allow for early range of motion	• In most T-condylar fractures, rigid fixation is necessary to allow for early range of motion. • Use rigid plate fixation for both medial and lateral columns to facilitate early mobilization especially in adolescent patients.
Ulnar nerve irritation	• At the end of the case, examine the ulnar nerve with flexion and extension. Ensure that it is not irritated by contact with the plate. • Consider ulnar nerve transposition if there is evidence of tether or impingement of the nerve during an arc of motion.

Outcomes

The literature reflects good results with surgical management of displaced distal humerus articular fractures. Zimmerman[44] advocated establishing an anatomic reduction with internal fixation so that early motion could facilitate a more rapid rehabilitation. In the two young children described by Beghin et al.,[7] operative intervention was necessary to achieve a satisfactory reduction. A review of four series[20,23,33,36] supports surgical management: 44 of the 48 elbows in these combined series were treated operatively. The investigators of these series maintained that open reduction and internal fixation was the best way to restore the integrity of the articular surface and stabilize the fracture sufficiently to allow early mobilization. All but one of the patients treated surgically in this combined series had good or very good results at follow-up.

Kanellopoulos and Yiannakopoulos[22] described closed reduction of the intra-articular component, with fixation by partially threaded pins for interfragmentary compression. Two elastic titanium intramedullary nails were used for stabilizing the supracondylar component. The T-condylar fractures in two adolescents healed without complications after using this technique. Both patients returned to sports with full elbow range of motion at 6 weeks after surgery.

The triceps-splitting approach, as described by Campbell, was first advocated by Van Gorder.[42] Kasser et al.[23] have demonstrated in children that the triceps-splitting approach did not appear to cause significant muscle dysfunction according to Cybex testing and concluded that an olecranon osteotomy was unnecessary. The authors concluded that this approach gives adequate exposure of the fracture and the articular surface and does not seem to produce any loss of strength from splitting the triceps. Although one reported patient had radiographic evidence of osteonecrosis of the trochlea,[33] another had a nonunion,[23] and many had some loss of range of motion; none of these surgically treated patients demonstrated any significant loss of elbow function or discomfort. Anari et al.[3] found that younger children may benefit from a less invasive approach such as the triceps splitting when the fracture pattern allows.

Alonso-Llames[2] described a paratricipital approach for the treatment of supra- and intracondylar fractures in children. A recent series suggests caution using this approach due to less optimal outcome.[11] Bryan and Morrey[10] described a triceps-sparing approach in which the extensor mechanism is reflected laterally, exposing the whole distal humerus. Re et al.[36] found that both the Bryan–Morrey (triceps reflecting) and olecranon osteotomy approaches yielded improved extension compared to the triceps-splitting approach. Remia et al.[37] evaluated triceps function and elbow motion in nine patients with T-condylar fractures treated with open reduction through a Bryan and Morrey triceps-sparing approach and compared them to those reported after a triceps-splitting approach. No statistically significant differences were found in function or range of motion. Recent literature additions support the treatment algorithms outlined in this chapter and prior study findings. Bell[8] has published retrospectively a large series of adolescent distal humerus fractures with 37 of 81 being intra-articular fractures. They found that younger children were more likely to have fractures amenable to management by percutaneous reduction and older adolescents by open reduction. Open reduction was associated with higher complications. However, this may be a product of the original injury rather than the management. Regardless, families should be counseled accordingly. Cook[11] in a retrospective review of 31 type C distal humeral fractures found that C2 and C3 fractures had significantly less motion postoperatively.

The surgeon must choose the surgical approach that allows for the best exposure with the least risk. The priority is adequate visualization of all fracture fragments, especially the joint surface, to achieve rigid anatomic fixation. Early motion is desired to lessen the risk of postinjury contractures about the elbow.

MANAGEMENT OF EXPECTED ADVERSE OUTCOMES AND UNEXPECTED COMPLICATIONS RELATED TO T-CONDYLAR FRACTURES OF THE DISTAL HUMERUS

T-Condylar Fractures of the Distal Humerus: COMMON ADVERSE OUTCOMES AND COMPLICATIONS

- Postoperative elbow stiffness
- Fracture malunion
- Fracture nonunion and hardware failure
- Osteonecrosis of trochlea
- Hardware impingement and irritation
- Need for additional surgery
- Hardware removal
- Manipulation under anesthesia

It is important to emphasize to the parents initially that this is a serious fracture. Because of the considerable soft tissue injury and the involvement of the articular surface of the distal humerus, stiffness and loss of motion of the elbow can be expected regardless of the treatment mode.[20,28,33] In adolescents, failure to provide solid internal fixation that facilitates early motion (i.e., using only pin fixation) can result in a satisfactory radiographic appearance but considerable dysfunction because of residual loss of elbow motion. Ultimately, many of these patients may have a final healed fracture lacking terminal extension. Cook et al. demonstrated that patients on average lacked 10 degrees of terminal extension.[11]

Although neurovascular complications have not been mentioned in the few cases reported in the literature, the incidence is probably about equal to that of supracondylar fractures. A recent paper[11] has documented a 16% incidence of preoperative neurologic injuries with these fractures in adolescents. Nerve injuries are predominantly of the ulnar nerve but have also involved the radial and median nerves. Although nerve injuries may be associated with the injury or fracture, they have also been documented during surgical fixation.[11] The ulnar nerve is most at risk both during exposure of fracture fragments and with internal fixation. Postoperative incidence of ulnar nerve symptoms is 5% to 8%.[6,8] Ulnar nerve transposition should be considered when either nerve instability is noted with flexion–extension elbow motion or there is concern for hardware impingement on the nerve.

Because these fractures occur late in the growth process, partial or total growth arrest caused by the injury or internal fixation has not been a major complication. Likewise, because these are older children, little remodeling of a malunion can be expected. Nonunion,[23] osteonecrosis of the trochlea,[33] and failure of internal fixation have also been reported as complications.

Aside from stiffness, the biggest risk is fracture malunion caused by inadequate reduction and/or fixation. Extra-articular malunion may be tolerated if there is not a block to motion. Intra-articular malunion is clearly a real risk for pain, loss of motion and function, and eventually arthritis. Intra-articular malreduction should be avoided.

Hardware irritation and/or impingement can occur. Obviously, all smooth wires need to be removed after the fracture is healed. Hardware that contributes to impingement pain and/or loss of motion needs to be similarly removed. Secondary surgery for hardware removal or stiffness unfortunately is not uncommon following this injury and is reported to be as high as 24%.[8] It is paramount that this complication is discussed with families preoperatively.

ACKNOWLEDGMENTS

The authors thank Benjamin Shore, MD, Carley Vuillermin, MD, and Peter Waters, MD as previous coauthors of this chapter for contributions that have been carried forward to this edition.

Annotated References

Reference	Annotation
Bell P, Scannell BP, Loeffler BJ, et al. Adolescent distal humerus fractures: ORIF versus CRPP. *J Pediatr Orthop.* 2017;37(8):511–520.	A recent series of distal humeral fractures managed operatively contrasting the outcomes of extra- and intra-articular distal humerus fractures.
Bryan RS, Morrey BF. Extensive posterior exposure of the elbow. A triceps-sparing approach. *Clin Orthop Relat Res.* 1982;(166):188–192.	Seminal paper describing the triceps-sparing approach to the elbow.
Cheung EV, Steinmann SP. Surgical approaches to the elbow. *J Am Acad Orthop Surg.* 2009;17(5):325–333.	This article outlines contemporaneous approaches to the elbow joint. It provides a discussion of their uses and limitations.
Cook JB, Riccio AI, Anderson T, et al. Outcomes after surgical treatment of adolescent intra-articular distal humerus fractures. *J Pediatr Orthop.* 2016;36(8):773–779.	This article provides a comprehensive audit of a recent series of adolescent intra-articular distal humerus fractures, their associated injuries, and the expected outcomes.
Toniolo RM, Wilkins KE. *T-Condylar Fractures.* Lippincott-Raven; 1996.	Original description of the pediatric intra-articular distal humeral fracture types.

REFERENCES

1. Abraham E, Gordon A, Abdul-Hadi O. Management of supracondylar fractures of humerus with condylar involvement in children. *J Pediatr Orthop.* 2005;25(6):709–716.
2. Alonso-Llames M. Bilaterotricipital approach to the elbow: its application in the osteosynthesis of supracondylar fractures of the humerus in children. *Acta Orthop Scand.* 1972;43(6):479–490.
3. Anari JB, Neuwirth AL, Carducci NM, et al. Pediatric T-condylar humerus fractures: a systematic review. *J Pediatr Orthop.* 2017;37(1):36–40.
4. Atalar AC, Tunalı O, Erşen A, et al. Biomechanical comparison of orthogonal versus parallel double plating systems in intraarticular distal humerus fractures. *Acta Orthop Traumatol Turc.* 2017;51(1):23–28.
5. Bareri P, Hanel D. Fractures of the distal humerus. In: Wolfe SW, Hotchkiss Robert H, Pederson WC, et al., eds. *Green's Operative Hand Surgery.* 7th ed. Elsevier; 2017:697–733.
6. Beck NA, Ganley TJ, McKay S, et al. T-condylar fractures of the distal humerus in children: does early motion affect final range of motion? *J Child Orthop.* 2014;8(2):161–165.
7. Beghin JL, Bucholz RW, Wenger DR. Intercondylar fractures of the humerus in young children: a report of two cases. *J Bone Joint Surg Am.* 1982;64(7):1083–1087.
8. Bell P, Scannell BP, Loeffler BJ, et al. Adolescent distal humerus fractures: ORIF versus CRPP. *J Pediatr Orthop.* 2017;37(8):511–520.
9. Blount WP, Schulz I, Cassidy RH. Fractures of the elbow in children. *J Am Med Assoc.* 1951;146(8):699–704.
10. Bryan RS, Morrey BF. Extensive posterior exposure of the elbow. A triceps-sparing approach. *Clin Orthop Relat Res.* 1982;(166):188–192.
11. Cook JB, Riccio AI, Anderson T, et al. Outcomes after surgical treatment of adolescent intra-articular distal humerus fractures. *J Pediatr Orthop.* 2016;36(8):773–779.
12. Ek ETH, Goldwasser M, Bonomo AL. Functional outcome of complex intercondylar fractures of the distal humerus treated through a triceps-sparing approach. *J Shoulder Elbow Surg.* 2008;17(3):441–446.
13. Elgenmark O. Relationship between ossification and age. *Acta Paediatr Scand.* 1946;33(Suppl 1):31–52.
14. Fayssoux RS, Stankovits L, Domzalski ME, Guille JT. Fractures of the distal humeral metaphyseal-diaphyseal junction in children. *J Pediatr Orthop.* 2008;28(2):142–146.
15. Francis CC. The appearance of centers of ossification from 6–15 years. *Am J Phys Antropol.* 1940;27:127–138.
16. Got C, Shuck J, Biercevicz A, et al. Biomechanical comparison of parallel versus 90-90 plating of bicolumn distal humerus fractures with intra-articular comminution. *J Hand Surg Am.* 2012;37(12):2512–2518.
17. Haraldsson S. The intra-osseous vasculature of the distal end of the humerus with special reference to capitulum: preliminary communication. *Acta Orthop Scand.* 1957;27(2):81–93.
18. Helfet DL, Hotchkiss RN. Internal fixation of the distal humerus: a biomechanical comparison of methods. *J Orthop Trauma.* 1990;4(3):260–264.
19. Henley MB, Bone LB, Parker B. Operative management of intra-articular fractures of the distal humerus. *J Orthop Trauma.* 1987;1(1):24–35.
20. Jarvis JG, D'Astous JL. The pediatric T-supracondylar fracture. *J Pediatr Orthop.* 1984;4(6):697–699.
21. Jupiter JB, Mehne DK. Fractures of the distal humerus. *Orthopedics.* 1992;15(7):825–833.
22. Kanellopoulos AD, Yiannakopoulos CK. Closed reduction and percutaneous stabilization of pediatric T-condylar fractures of the humerus. *J Pediatr Orthop.* 2004;24(1):13–16.
23. Kasser JR, Richards K, Millis M. The triceps-dividing approach to open reduction of complex distal humeral fractures in adolescents: a Cybex evaluation of triceps function and motion. *J Pediatr Orthop.* 1990;10(1):93–96.
24. Kirk P, Goulet J, Freiberg A, et al. A biomechanical evaluation of fixation methods for fractures of the distal humerus. *Orthop Trans.* 1990;14:674.
25. Kraus R. The pediatric vs. the adolescent elbow. Some insight into age-specific treatment. *Eur J Trauma Emerg Surg.* 2014;40(1):15–22.

26. Landin LA, Danielsson LG. Elbow fractures in children: an epidemiological analysis of 589 cases. *Acta Orthop Scand.* 1986;57(4):309–312.

27. Lauder A, Richard MJ. Management of distal humerus fractures. *Eur J Orthop Surg Traumatol.* 2020;30(5):745–762.

28. Maylahn DJ, Fahey JJ. Fractures of the elbow in children: review of three hundred consecutive cases. *J Am Med Assoc.* 1958;166(3):220–228.

29. McKee MD, Wilson TL, Winston L, et al. Functional outcome following surgical treatment of intra-articular distal humeral fractures through a posterior approach. *J Bone Joint Surg Am.* 2000;82-A(12):1701–1707.

30. Morrey BF, An KN, Chao EYS. Functional evaluation of the elbow. In: Morrey BF, ed. *The Elbow and Its Disorders.* 2nd ed. WB Saunders Co; 1993:95.

31. Mortensson W, Thönell S. Left-side dominance of upper extremity fracture in children. *Acta Orthop Scand.* 1991;62(2):154–155.

32. O'Driscoll SW. The triceps-reflecting anconeus pedicle (TRAP) approach for distal humeral fractures and nonunions. *Orthop Clin North Am.* 2000;31(1):91–101.

33. Papavasiliou VA, Beslikas TA. T-condylar fractures of the distal humeral condyles during childhood: an analysis of six cases. *J Pediatr Orthop.* 1986;6(3):302–305.

34. Patel B, Reed M, Patel S. Gender-specific pattern differences of the ossification centers in the pediatric elbow. *Pediatr Radiol.* 2009;39(3):226–231.

35. Patterson SD, Bain GI, Mehta JA. Surgical approaches to the elbow. *Clin Orthop Relat Res.* 2000;370:19–33.

36. Re PR, Waters PM, Hresko T. T-condylar fractures of the distal humerus in children and adolescents. *J Pediatr Orthop.* 1999;19(3):313–318.

37. Remia LF, Richards K, Waters PM. The Bryan-Morrey triceps-sparing approach to open reduction of T-condylar humeral fractures in adolescents: cybex evaluation of triceps function and elbow motion. *J Pediatr Orthop.* 2004;24(26):615–619.

38. Riseborough EJ, Radin EL. Intercondylar T fractures of the humerus in the adult. A comparison of operative and non-operative treatment in twenty-nine cases. *J Bone Joint Surg Am.* 1969;51(1):130–141.

39. Sanders RA, Raney EM, Pipkin S. Operative treatment of bicondylar intraarticular fractures of the distal humerus. *Orthopedics.* 1992;15(2):159–163.

40. Schemitsch EH, Tencer AF, Henley MB. Biomechanical evaluation of methods of internal fixation of the distal humerus. *J Orthop Trauma.* 1994;8(6):468–475.

41. Toniolo RM, Wilkins KE. *T-Condylar Fractures.* Lippincott-Raven; 1996.

42. Van Gorder GW. Surgical approach in supracondylar "T" fractures of the humerus requiring open reduction. *J Bone Joint Surg.* 1940;22:278–292.

43. Wildburger R, Mähring M, Hofer HP. Supraintercondylar fractures of the distal humerus: results of internal fixation. *J Orthop Trauma.* 1991;5(3):301–307.

44. Zimmerman H. *Fractures of the Elbow.* Springer-Verlag; 1980.

16

Medial Epicondyle Fractures and Dislocations of the Elbow

Benjamin R. Wilson and Vishwas Talwalkar

Fractures of the Medial Epicondyle

MEDIAL EPICONDYLE FRACTURES

INTRODUCTION TO MEDIAL EPICONDYLE FRACTURES

It has long been recognized that the medial epicondyle fracture is often associated with elbow dislocation and that the apophyseal fragment could become entrapped within the joint. The reported incidence of medial epicondyle fracture associated with dislocation of the elbow in children and adolescents has varied from as low as 30% to as high as 60% in many of the reported series.[123] Two bilateral injuries associated with bilateral elbow dislocations have been reported,[48] both patients having sustained their injuries while participating in gymnastics. Fractures involving the medial epicondylar apophysis constitute approximately 14% of fractures involving the distal humerus and 11% of all fractures in the elbow region.[29] The youngest reported patient with this injury was 3.9 years old.[29] In the large series of fractures of the medial epicondylar apophysis, most occurred between ages 9 and 14, and the peak age incidence was 11 to 12 years.[75,89,122,134] Fractures of the epicondylar apophysis preferentially affect males by a ratio of almost 4 to 1 over females. In six large series in the literature, boys constituted 79% of the patients.[52,115,154]

Figure 16-1. Ossification of the medial epicondyle. **A:** The concentric oval nucleus of ossification of the medial epicondylar apophysis (*arrow*). **B:** As ossification progresses, parallel smooth sclerotic margins develop in each side of the physis. **C:** Because it is somewhat posterior, on a slightly oblique anteroposterior view the apophysis may be hidden behind the distal metaphysis. **D:** The posterior location of the apophysis (*arrow*) is appreciated on this slightly oblique lateral view. **E:** On the anteroposterior view, the line created by the overlapping of the metaphysis (*arrow*) can be misinterpreted as a fracture line (pseudofracture).

Incidence of Medial Epicondyle Fractures

Overall incidence: Fractures of the elbow region, 11.5%

Age: peak, 11 to 12 years

Sex: males, 79% (4:1, male:female)

Association with elbow dislocation: approximately 50% (15%–18% of these involve incarceration of the epicondylar apophysis)

The medial epicondyle represents a traction apophysis because the forces across its physis are in tension rather than the compressive forces present across the other condylar physis of the distal humerus. The medial epicondylar apophysis actually arises from the posterior surface of the medial distal humeral metaphysis. Ossification begins at about 4 to 6 years of age and fuses at about 15 years of age, making it the last secondary ossification center to fuse with the distal humeral metaphysis (Fig. 16-1). The ossification center starts as a small eccentric oval nucleus (see Fig. 16-1A). As it matures, parallel sclerotic margins develop along both sides of the physis (see Fig. 16-1B). There may be some irregularity of the ossification process, which gives the ossific nucleus a fragmented appearance. This fragmentation may be falsely interpreted as a fracture (see Fig. 16-1E).

Superficially, the flexor–pronator mass, which includes the origin of the flexor carpi radialis, flexor carpi ulnaris, flexor digitorum superficialis, palmaris longus, and part of the pronator teres, originates from the anterior aspect of the medial epicondylar apophysis (Fig. 16-2).[166] Part of the flexor carpi ulnaris also originates on the posterior aspect of the epicondyle. Deep to these muscular insertions, the medial ulnar collateral ligament originates from the medial epicondyle. In younger children, some of the capsule's origin extends up to the physeal line of the

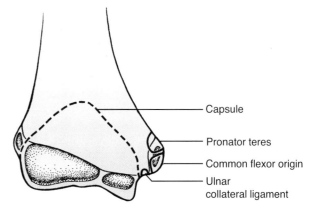

Figure 16-2. Soft tissue attachments. The AP view of the distal humerus demonstrates the relationship of the apophysis to the origins of the medial forearm muscles. The origin of the ulnar collateral ligament lies outside the elbow capsule. The margin of the capsule is outlined by the *dotted line*.

epicondyle. In older children and adolescents, as the epicondyle migrates more proximally, the capsule is attached only to the medial crista of the trochlea.[11] Thus, in older children, if there is a pure muscular avulsion force on the epicondyle, the capsule and part of the medial ligamentous complex may remain attached to the trochlea's outer border and relative elbow stability preserved. However, if the medial epicondyle is avulsed via the medial ulnar collateral ligament, given the importance of this ligament in elbow stability, relative elbow instability usually results.

ASSESSMENT OF MEDIAL EPICONDYLE FRACTURES

Mechanisms of Injury for Medial Epicondyle Fractures

Injuries to the medial epicondylar apophysis most commonly occur as acute injuries in which a distinct event produces a partial or a complete separation of the apophyseal fragment. Three theories have been proposed about the mechanism of acute medial epicondylar apophyseal injuries: a direct blow; avulsion mechanisms; or association with elbow dislocation.

Direct Blow

This type of injury may occur as a result of a direct blow on the posterior aspect of the epicondyle or be associated with a direct blow to the posterior medial aspect of the elbow. In rare patients in whom the fragment is produced by a direct blow to the medial aspect of the joint, the medial epicondylar fragment is often fragmented (Fig. 16-3). In these injuries, there may also be more superficial ecchymosis in the skin.

Avulsion Mechanisms

Various investigators have suggested that some of these injuries are due to a pure avulsion of the epicondyle by the flexor–pronator muscles of the forearm.[89,139] This muscle avulsion force can occur in combination with a valgus stress in which the elbow is locked in extension, or as a pure musculature contraction that may occur with the elbow partially flexed.

When a child falls on their outstretched upper extremity with the elbow in extension, the wrist and fingers are often hyperextended as well, placing an added tension force on the epicondyle by the forearm flexor muscles (Fig. 16-4). The normal valgus carrying angle tends to accentuate these avulsion forces when the elbow is in extension. Many proponents of this theory point to the other associated elbow fractures that have been seen with this injury as evidence to confirm that a valgus force is applied across the elbow at the time of the injury. These associated injuries include radial neck fractures with valgus angulation and greenstick valgus fractures of the olecranon.[89]

Isolated avulsion can also occur in adolescents with the simple act of throwing a ball. In this instance, the sudden contracture of the forearm flexor muscles may be sufficient to cause the epicondyle to fail[22,34] (Fig. 16-5). Cain et al.[22] reported on their experience with 29 overhead athletes who sustained medial epicondyle fractures of this mechanism, 97% of which were able to return to sports after completion of treatment. They recommend a low threshold for operative intervention with

Figure 16-3. Direct fragmentation. The fragmented appearance of the medial epicondyle (*arrows*) in a 13-year-old who sustained a direct blow to the medial aspect of the elbow. (From Wilkins KE. Fractures of the medial epicondyle in children. *Instr Course Lect.* 1991;40:1–8, with permission.)

Figure 16-4. Hyperextension forces. When a person falls on the outstretched upper extremity, the wrist and fingers are forced into hyperextension (*solid arrow*), which places tension on the forearm flexor muscles. This sudden tension along with the normal valgus carrying angle tends to place a strong avulsion force on the medial epicondyle (*open arrow*).

Figure 16-5. Muscle avulsion. Isolated avulsion of the medial epicondyle occurred suddenly in this 13-year-old football quarterback after throwing a deep pass.

these types of mechanisms due to the demand for elbow stability in higher-level athletics. The literature has also reflected a relatively high incidence of medial epicondylar apophyseal avulsions occurring with arm wrestling in patients near skeletal maturity.[107,129] The largest series, reported by Nyska et al.[129] from Israel, involved eight boys of 13 to 15 years of age, all of whom were treated nonoperatively with good results.

Medial Epicondyle Fractures Associated With Elbow Dislocation

Avulsion fractures of the medial epicondyle may also be associated with elbow dislocation in which the ulnar collateral ligament provides the avulsion force. If the patient presents with the elbow dislocated, there is no doubt that the dislocation is the major factor causing this fracture. If the patient presents with the elbow concentrically reduced, it is less clear as to whether the medial epicondyle fracture may have been caused by an occult or partial elbow dislocation that has reduced spontaneously. Thus in these cases, it is important to elicit a history from the patient of dislocation and subsequent spontaneous reduction. A marked degree of swelling often heralds a dislocation or subluxation that self-reduced. Some investigators have noted later calcification development in the lateral collateral ligaments and adjacent lateral periosteum after fracture. They believed this calcification was evidence that the ligament had been stretched during the process of elbow dislocation. Marion and Faysse[115] found that most elbow dislocations associated with medial epicondyle fractures were posterolateral, but some pure lateral, posterior, and posteromedial dislocations were also observed. A question has also arisen as to whether incarceration of the epicondylar fragment into the joint can occur without

a dislocation. Patrick[139] believed that when an extreme valgus stress was applied to the joint, a vacuum was created within the joint that "sucks in" the avulsed epicondylar fragment.

Signs and Symptoms of Medial Epicondyle Fractures

Medial epicondyle fractures associated with elbow dislocation are associated with gross deformity of the elbow, swelling, and distracting injuries so that the medial epicondyle fracture can be easily overlooked. A careful and focused evaluation looking specifically at the medial epicondyle is necessary to avoid missing this injury. If a fracture of the medial epicondyle has occurred, then tenderness to palpation will likely be present in this location. Due to its proximity to the zone of injury, ulnar nerve function must be carefully tested before initiating treatment and the status of the nerve documented in the medical record.

Because the anterior oblique band of the ulnar collateral ligament may be attached to the medial epicondylar apophysis, the elbow may exhibit some instability after injury. To evaluate the medial stability of the elbow, Woods and Tullos[180] and Schwab et al.[163] advocated a simple valgus stress test (gravity stress test). This test is performed with the patient supine and the arm abducted 90 degrees. The shoulder and arm are externally rotated 90 degrees. The elbow must be flexed at least 15 degrees to eliminate the stabilizing force of the olecranon. If the elbow is unstable, simple gravity forces will open the medial side. This subtle opening may be difficult to discern, especially in the acutely injured and guarding patient. For this reason, stress testing is no longer recommended in the awake patient.

Imaging and Other Diagnostic Studies of Medial Epicondyle Fractures

Good quality anteroposterior (AP) and lateral radiographs are essential. Alternative radiographs such as internal or external oblique as well as distal humerus axial are often helpful when the interpretation of initial images is not conclusive.[24,65] Widening or irregularity of the apophyseal line may be the only clue in fractures that are slightly displaced or nondisplaced. If the fragment is significantly displaced, the radiographic diagnosis is usually obvious. If the fragment is totally incarcerated in the joint, however, it may be hidden by the overlying proximal ulna or distal humerus. The clue here is the total absence of the epicondyle from its normal position just medial and posterior to the medial metaphysis. Knowledge of the order and approximate age of appearance of elbow ossification centers is necessary to appreciate the absence of the epicondyle when it should be present. Computed tomography (CT) scans can be diagnostic in confusing situations.

Potter[142] suggested that properly performed magnetic resonance imaging (MRI) might disclose acute or chronic injury to the medial epicondylar apophysis, recommending pulse sequences for evaluating the apophysis including fat-suppressed gradient-echo imaging. On MRI, increased signal intensity and abnormal widening of the medial epicondylar physis are seen, typically with surrounding soft tissue edema.

Fractures of the medial epicondyle, even if displaced, may not produce positive fat pad signs.[68,166] If the fracture is only minimally displaced and if it is the result of an avulsion injury, there may be no effusion because all the injured tissues remain extra-articular. In fractures associated with elbow dislocation, there is rupture of the capsule, so its ability to confine the hemarthrosis inside the joint is lost. In minimally displaced apparent fractures of the medial epicondyle in the young with significant hemarthrosis and soft tissue swelling, the evaluation must be especially thorough to ensure that an unrecognized fracture involving the medial condylar physis is not present.

The ability to accurately measure medial epicondyle fracture displacement has been questioned by several authors who have published work regarding this concern. In a study of medial epicondyle fracture radiographs in 38 patients, Pappas et al.[135] reported poor intra- and interobserver agreement with regard to fracture displacement measurement and questioned the value of perceived fracture displacement as a criterion for choosing surgical versus nonsurgical treatment. In a separate publication, a series of 11 patients judged to have nondisplaced or minimally displaced medial epicondyle fractures had their fractures imaged by both standard radiography and CT.[44] Medial and anterior displacement were then measured on standard radiographs and CT images and compared. Edmonds reported statistically significant differences between standard radiographs and CT images in all measurements with marked increased displacement appreciated on CT scan including six fractures with greater than 10 mm of displacement. To improve our ability to accurately measure fracture displacement on standard radiographs, Klatt and Aoki[92] performed a review of 171 normal AP and lateral elbow radiographs describing the relationship between the medial epicondyle center and reproducible local anatomic landmarks. On the AP radiographs, the medial epicondyle center was located 0.5 mm inferior to a line based on the inferior olecranon fossa, and on the lateral radiograph, the medial epicondyle center was located 1.2 mm anterior to the posterior humeral line.

Nondisplaced or Minimally Displaced Fractures

The apophyseal line remains intact in nondisplaced medial epicondyle fractures. The clinical manifestations usually consist only of swelling and local tenderness over the medial epicondyle. Crepitus and motion of the epicondyle are usually not present. On radiographs, the smoothness of the edge of the apophyseal line remains intact. Although there may be some loss of soft tissue planes medially on the radiograph, displacement of the elbow fat pads may not be present because the pathology is extra-articular.[68]

Fractures with displacement usually result from a stronger avulsion force, so there is often more soft tissue swelling. Palpating the fragment may elicit crepitus because the increased displacement allows unstable motion of the fragment. On radiographs, there is a loss of parallelism of the smooth sclerotic margins of the physis (Fig. 16-6).[166] The radiolucency in the area of the apophyseal line is usually increased in width.

Significantly Displaced Fractures

In significantly displaced fractures, the fragment may be palpable and freely movable. When displaced a considerable distance from the distal humerus, crepitus between the fragments

Figure 16-6. AP radiograph shows loss of normal smooth margins of the physis.

may not be present. Significantly displaced fractures may be associated with an elbow dislocation that reduced spontaneously and there may be no documentation of the original dislocation. On radiograph, the long axis of the epicondylar apophysis is typically rotated medially (Fig. 16-7). The displacement often exceeds 5 mm, but the fragment remains proximal to the true joint surface. These displaced medial epicondylar fractures can also present acutely with a yet unreduced elbow dislocation.

Figure 16-7. Displaced medial epicondylar fracture. Oblique view of an elbow in which the epicondyle (*arrow*) is significantly displaced both distally and medially. In addition, the fragment is rotated medially.

Figure 16-8. Dislocation with incarceration. **A:** AP view showing a posterolateral elbow dislocation. The presence of the medial epicondyle within the elbow joint (*arrow*) prevented a closed reduction. **B:** The lateral view of the same elbow demonstrates the fragment (*arrow*) between the humerus and olecranon.

Entrapment of the Epicondylar Fragment in the Joint

In some cases of severe displacement associated with an elbow dislocation, the fragment can lie within the joint and prevent reduction (Fig. 16-8). Recognition of this fragment as being within the joint before a manipulation should alert the physician to the possible need for open reduction. There should be adequate relaxation during the manipulative process. At times with closed reduction, the medial epicondylar fragment remains in the joint and prevents a congruent ulnar-trochlear reduction. There are instances when the elbow will spontaneously reduce prior to evaluation. In these cases, the fragment may still be entrapped even though the elbow appears reduced. The key clinical finding is a block to motion, especially extension. The epicondylar fragment is usually between the joint surfaces of the trochlea and the semilunar notch of the olecranon. On a radiograph, any time the fragment appears at the level of the joint, it must be considered to be totally or partially within the elbow joint until proven otherwise.[139] If the radiograph is examined carefully, the elbow is usually found to be incompletely reduced. Because of an impingement of the fragment within the joint, a good AP view may be difficult to obtain because of the inability to extend the elbow fully. If the fracture is old, the fragment may be fused to the coronoid process, and widening of the medial joint space may be the only clue that the fragment is lying in the joint. The epicondylar ossification center may become fragmented and mistaken for the fragmented appearance of the medial crista of the trochlea.[29,154] Absence of the apophyseal center on the radiograph may be further confirmatory evidence that the fragment is within the joint. Comparison radiographs of the opposite elbow may be necessary to delineate the true pathology.

Fractures Through the Epicondylar Apophysis

Fractures through the body of the epicondyle can result from either a direct blow or avulsion of only part of the apophysis. In either case, the fragments may or may not be displaced. The normal lucent line formed by the overlying metaphyseal border should not be confused with this injury. Although described by Silberstein et al.,[166] this intrafragment fracture is a rare presentation usually seen with throwing athletes.

Differential Diagnosis of Medial Epicondyle Fractures

The major injuries to differentiate from isolated medial epicondyle fractures are those fractures involving the medial condylar physis. This is especially true if secondary ossification centers are not present (see Chapter 18). If there is a significant hemarthrosis or a significant piece of metaphyseal bone accompanying the medial epicondylar fragment, arthrography or MRI may be indicated to determine if there is an intra-articular component to the fracture. Other elbow fractures that can be associated with this injury include fracture of the radial neck, olecranon, or coronoid process.

TREATMENT OPTIONS FOR MEDIAL EPICONDYLE FRACTURES

Better implants, improved surgical technique, greater appreciation of the importance of the ulnar collateral ligament inserting on the medial epicondyle, and increased understanding of the degree of displacement in fractures previously thought to be nondisplaced, all contribute to a general trend toward more frequent surgical treatment of medial epicondyle fractures.[59] In a 2012 article, Mehlman and Howard[120] acknowledged the dearth of high-level evidence in the published literature on this topic but reports that meta-analysis of clinical research with a particular focus on harm supports surgical treatment for most patients. Independent of whether a nonoperative or operative approach is chosen for the management of a particular medial epicondyle fracture, treatment goals remain to obtain fracture healing and to promote the return of full motion, strength, and stability to the elbow.[137,138]

Even though our ability to measure fracture displacement may be less accurate than we believed in the past, displacement remains an important fracture to consider when making treatment decisions. Additional factors to consider include intra-articular fragment entrapment, ulnar nerve symptoms, dominant arm, and patient-specific activity level.

Nonoperative Treatment of Medial Epicondyle Apophysis Fractures

Indications/Contraindications

Nonoperative Treatment of Medial Epicondyle Fractures: INDICATIONS AND CONTRAINDICATIONS	
Indications	**Relative Contraindications**
Displacement less than 2 mm	Displacement greater than 10 mm
Low-to-moderate activity demands	Displaced fracture involving the dominant arm in a throwing athlete; either arm in gymnast or wrestler
	Incarcerated fragment within joint

There appears to be consensus that fractures that are nondisplaced or minimally displaced less than 2 mm should be treated nonoperatively. Minimally displaced fractures may be treated using simple immobilization for comfort or cast immobilization for 2 to 3 weeks. Often, a hinged brace can be employed to allow for flexion and extension, but to prevent excessive valgus stress to the elbow. Early initiation of motion is recommended to prevent stiffness, which is the most common complication of this injury. Likewise, there is agreement that if the medial epicondyle fragment is irreducible and is incarcerated within the elbow joint, the accepted treatment is surgical extraction and stable internal fixation. However, controversy remains as to the optimal treatment method for patients with displacement more than 2 mm.

Outcomes

Josefsson and Danielsson[82] reported 35-year follow-up results in 56 isolated fractures treated nonoperatively. Although more than 60% of their patients demonstrated nonunion on radiograph, these investigators reported a high percentage of good and excellent results. Other reports in the literature[3,134] also demonstrated overall good results with nonoperative management. Knapik and co-authors performed a meta-analysis to compare nonoperative treatment of medial epicondyle fractures in patients with and without associated elbow dislocation.[93] While patients with associated elbow dislocation had a higher fracture nonunion rate, both groups had minimal clinical or functional limitations at final follow-up.

Operative Treatment of Medial Epicondyle Apophysis Fractures

Recent literature describes excellent results obtained with surgical treatment. Louahem et al.[105] from Montpellier, France, report excellent results in 130 and good results in 9 of 139 displaced medial epicondyle fractures treated surgically. Hines et al.,[75] whose practice was to surgically repair all fractures displaced more than 2 mm, found that 96% of their patients had good-to-excellent results. Poor results were attributed mainly to technical errors. Using contemporary outcome measures, Canavese and co-authors describe good and excellent results following surgical treatment of medial epicondyle fractures.[23]

Indications/Contraindications

Operative Treatment Indications for Medial Epicondyle Fractures
Absolute Indication
• Incarceration of the epicondylar fragment
Relative Indications
• Ulnar nerve dysfunction
• Presence of elbow instability
• Desire to avoid symptomatic nonunion

Indications for operative intervention in acute injuries are divided into two categories: absolute and relative. The single absolute indication is incarceration of the epicondylar fragment within the joint. The relative indications include ulnar nerve dysfunction, a need for elbow stability, and a desire to avoid symptomatic nonunion.

Incarceration of the Epicondylar Fragment

If the epicondylar fragment is found in the joint acutely, it must be removed. There are proponents of both nonsurgical and surgical techniques for extraction.

Various methods of extracting the fragment by nonoperative methods have been proposed. The success rate of extracting the fragment successfully from the joint by manipulation alone at best has been reported at approximately 40%.[139] All the nonoperative methods require either heavy sedation or light general anesthesia.

The manipulative technique most commonly used is the method popularized by Roberts.[47,152] It involves placing a valgus stress on the elbow while supinating the forearm and simultaneously dorsiflexing the wrist and fingers to place the forearm muscles on stretch; theoretically, this maneuver should extract the fragment from the joint. To be effective, this procedure should be carried out within the first 24 hours after injury.

Failure to extract the fragment by manipulative techniques is an indication to proceed with open surgical extraction.[177] Once open extraction and reduction have been performed, many methods have been advocated to stabilize the fragment, including screw fixation, smooth pins, or suture fixation in comminuted fractures. Excision of the bony fragment with soft tissue repair has also been advocated, especially if the fragment is too small for adequate fixation; or, is comminuted.

Ulnar Nerve Dysfunction

Ulnar nerve dysfunction, which occurs more frequently when the medial epicondyle is incarcerated within the joint,[41,177] is a relative indication for operative intervention. If there are mild-to-moderate ulnar nerve symptoms at the time of the injury, there is usually no need to explore the nerve, because most of these mild symptoms resolve spontaneously.[39] If the dysfunction is complete, then the ulnar nerve may be directly impinged upon by the fracture or entrapped within the fracture site and should be explored surgically.

There has been some question as to whether delayed ulnar nerve symptoms can occur after fractures of the epicondyle that are not associated with elbow dislocation. However, in a review of more than 100 patients with uncomplicated fractures involving the medial epicondylar apophysis, Patrick[139] could not find any instance in which a delayed ulnar neuritis developed.

Joint Stability

For some patients, even minor forms of valgus instability after elbow injuries involving the medial epicondylar apophysis can cause significant disability. This condition is especially true in athletes who must have a stable upper extremity, such as baseball pitchers, gymnasts, or wrestlers. In younger adolescents (younger than 14 years of age), the anterior band of the ulnar collateral ligament often displaces with the apophyseal fragment. In older individuals (15 years or older), large fragments may be avulsed without a ligamentous injury. Rather than depending on arbitrary measurements of fracture displacement, some authors believe that demonstration of a significant valgus instability was an indication for surgical intervention in patients who require a stable elbow for their athletic activities. Recent studies have suggested that a history of elbow dislocation with medial epicondyle fracture should be used as an indication for operative management, likely due to the more extensive soft tissue injury and the risk of residual instability after conservative treatment.[54,93,161,185]

Open Reduction and Internal Fixation of Medial Epicondyle Fractures

Preoperative Planning

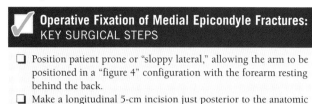

Operative Fixation of Medial Epicondyle Fractures:
PREOPERATIVE PLANNING CHECKLIST

OR table	❏ Spine table or flat radiolucent table ❏ Hand table extension
Position/ positioning aids	❏ Prone, "sloppy lateral," or supine position
Fluoroscopy location	❏ C-arm and monitor may be positioned on the same side or side opposite the surgeon
Equipment	❏ 4- or 4.5-mm diameter cannulated or solid screws
Tourniquet	❏ Nonsterile tourniquet high on the affected arm

Technique

✓ Operative Fixation of Medial Epicondyle Fractures:
KEY SURGICAL STEPS

- ❏ Position patient prone or "sloppy lateral," allowing the arm to be positioned in a "figure 4" configuration with the forearm resting behind the back.
- ❏ Make a longitudinal 5-cm incision just posterior to the anatomic location of the medial epicondyle.
- ❏ Expose the ulnar nerve and release the fascia.
- ❏ Anatomically reduce the medial epicondyle to the distal humeral metaphysis.
- ❏ Under fluoroscopic guidance, place a cannulated guide pin or solid drill through the center of the medial epicondyle fragment into the center of the medial column of bone in the distal humerus and confirm anatomic reduction of the fracture.
- ❏ Drill and tap (if needed) into the medial column of the distal humeral metaphysis.
- ❏ Place a single screw within the dense cancellous bone of the medial column.
- ❏ Confirm anatomic reduction and stability of the fracture and position of the implant with visual inspection and fluoroscopy before wound closure.

Our preferred operative technique involves positioning the patient prone on a radiolucent table (Fig. 16-9). The arm is placed in a "figure 4" position with the forearm resting across the patient's back. This position places a varus stress on the elbow, which facilitates fracture reduction while allowing a direct medial approach to the fracture site. Recent studies have found that the prone technique produces results similar to supine positioning. However, the ease with which the fracture can be reduced prone has led many surgeons to switch to prone positioning.[13,58,116]

A longitudinal 5-cm incision is made just posterior to the anatomic location of the medial epicondyle. The fragment is usually displaced distally and anteriorly. Interposed periosteum and soft tissue are removed from the fracture site, and clot is extracted by irrigation. Expose the ulnar nerve and ensure that it is not trapped within the fracture. If not already disrupted by the fracture, we typically release the cubital tunnel retinaculum, but a complete dissection of the nerve is usually unnecessary. Transposition of the nerve is not typically necessary in these cases. The fascia overlying the ulnar nerve as the nerve travels in its groove behind the medial epicondyle is then released, which allows for mobilization of the nerve and gentle retraction. Exposure of the ulnar nerve will also expose the fracture site.

Preserve soft tissue attachments to the medial epicondyle and elevate just enough soft tissue at the fracture site to allow adequate visualization to achieve an anatomic reduction. A small towel clip or clamp is used to grasp the fascia and tendinous origin of the flexor–pronator group, avoiding fragmentation of the medial epicondyle, and the fracture is reduced while the elbow is flexed and the forearm is pronated. A large suture may also be placed temporarily in the flexor–pronator tendon and used to apply traction to the fragment. A dental pick instrument also works well to manipulate and position the fracture fragment and fine-tune the reduction if needed.

Figure 16-9. The patient is positioned prone on a radiolucent table with the shoulder internally rotated. The arm can be positioned on a hand table (**A**) or the arm can be positioned on a radiolucent table with a radiolucent support placed beneath the elbow (**B**). **C:** When using a radiolucent table, fluoroscopy can be positioned on the opposite side of the table, allowing excellent visualization of the fracture and the fluoroscopy monitor. **D:** A cannulated guide pin maintains the medial epicondyle fracture reduction with the ulnar nerve in close proximity. **E, F:** A 4.5-mm cannulated screw with washer securely holds the medial epicondyle fragment. Bone wax is placed into the head of the cannulated screw to minimize intraosseous bleeding and postoperative swelling.

The medial epicondyle is reduced under direct vision to its anatomic position on the posterior aspect of the distal medial humerus. Temporarily stabilization with one or two small K-wires, or the guide pin for a cannulated screw, is performed under fluoroscopic guidance.

Final fixation is achieved using a partially threaded screw to compress the medial epicondyle fragment against the humeral metaphysis. In large male patients, a 4.5-mm diameter screw is used, but 3.5- or 4-mm diameter screws may be appropriate for smaller elbows. In fragments that are too small for screws, K-wire or suture anchor fixation can also be considered.[150] Fixation techniques must be strong enough to allow early motion, therefore every effort should be made to optimize its strength. Bicortical fixation has been used but injury to the radial nerve when penetrating the opposite cortex with a cannulated screw has been reported.[114] The dense cancellous bone of the medial column of the distal humerus provides excellent fixation and care should be taken to avoid using a longer screw with threads solely within the hollow central intramedullary canal proximal to the olecranon fossa where fixation is less secure (Fig. 16-10).

A washer may be added to increase fixation surface area and reduce the risk of fragmenting the medial epicondyle with compression but this does make the implant slightly more prominent, theoretically increasing the need for hardware removal after fracture healing.[133] After removal of the guide pin or K-wires, the elbow is assessed to ensure valgus stability and reestablishment of a full range of motion. After the surgical incision is closed, the extremity is placed in a well-padded posterior splint, which is removed 1 to 2 weeks postoperatively and replaced with a removable splint or hinged brace, allowing initiation of early active range-of-motion exercise.

If the epicondyle is fragmented and if there is a need to achieve elbow stability, a spiked washer can be used to secure the multiple pieces to the metaphysis. If internal fixation is impossible, simply excise the fragments and reattach the ligament to the bone and periosteum at the base of the epicondylar defect using suture anchors or transosseous sutures for fixation.

Figure 16-10. A 13-year-old boy was referred for treatment following posterolateral elbow dislocation. **A, B:** On the AP and lateral radiographs, a medial epicondyle fracture cannot be easily seen but the medial epicondyle ossification center is absent from its normal anatomic position at the distal medial posterior humerus. **C, D:** A prereduction CT scan was obtained at the outside facility clearly demonstrating the medial epicondyle fragment within the elbow joint. **E, F:** Four months following surgical removal of the incarcerated medial epicondyle fragment and internal fixation of the fracture, a follow-up CT scan demonstrates anatomic reduction and excellent position of the single screw (with washer) within the medial column of bone, engaging subcortical bone for maximum fixation. The fracture is completely healed, and the patient has returned to virtually all activities.

Authors' Preferred Treatment for Medial Epicondyle Fractures (Algorithm 16-1)

Algorithm 16-1. Authors' preferred treatment of medial epicondyle fractures.

Determining the appropriate treatment for each patient involves a process of shared decision making in which the benefits and risks of each treatment alternative are discussed with the family. We use the general treatment guidelines outlined in Algorithm 16-1 as a starting point for discussion with the patient and family. We strongly consider the expected activity of the patient and extremity in deciding with the patient and family on nonoperative or operative treatment.

For uncomplicated fractures of less than 2 mm of displacement, we recommend nonoperative treatment. The elbow is immobilized for 7 to 14 days and then range of motion is initiated. A removable splint is then used to protect the elbow at school and outside the home but is not worn indoors.

Redislocation or instability is rare but elbow stiffness is common, so early motion is important. Physical therapy can be used if voluntary active motion is difficult to obtain. The therapist should emphasize modalities designed to decrease swelling and pain and to reestablish strength. Range of motion should be achieved only by active means, not by passive stretching.

Our three primary indications for operative intervention are (1) reduction of any medial epicondyle fragment incarcerated within the elbow joint, (2) significant ulnar nerve deficit, and (3) stabilization of the elbow in patients anticipated to place significant stress on the medial epicondyle and its associated structures. We realize that it is difficult to predict the athletic potential of a young child but most parents do see great possibilities for their children. We are more likely to treat with internal fixation if the injury involves the dominant extremity of baseball pitchers, tennis players, or football quarterbacks. In wrestlers and gymnasts, the stability of the nondominant extremity also must be considered.

Potential Pitfalls and Preventive Measures

Medial Epicondyle Fractures:
POTENTIAL PITFALLS AND PREVENTIONS

Pitfalls	Prevention
Failure to recognize a medial epicondyle fragment entrapped within the joint following elbow dislocation	• All children older than age 5 years should have a medial epicondyle ossification center, which must be visualized in its normal anatomic location following elbow dislocation reduction.
Fragmentation of the medial epicondyle during ORIF	• Instead of grasping the medial epicondyle bone with a clamp, grasp the flexor–pronator fascia where it attaches to the medial epicondyle. • Avoid overtightening the screw that is fixing the medial epicondyle in place. • Consider using a washer to distribute pressure over greater surface area.
Injury to the radial nerve	• Do not obtain bicortical fixation in the lateral cortex of the distal humerus with the medial epicondyle screw.

OUTCOMES AND COMPLICATIONS RELATED TO MEDIAL EPICONDYLE FRACTURES

Fractures of the Medial Epicondyle:
ADVERSE OUTCOMES AND COMPLICATIONS

Major Complications

• Failure to recognize incarceration in the elbow
• Ulnar nerve dysfunction
• Symptomatic nonunion
• Valgus instability
• Radial nerve injury
• Marked elbow contracture

Minor Complications

• Mild loss of motion
• Myositis ossificans
• Calcification of the collateral ligaments
• Irritation from prominent implants
• Cosmetic appearance
• Nonunion in the high-performance athlete

Although much has been written about fractures involving the medial epicondylar apophysis, few complications are attributed to the fracture itself. The major complications that result in loss of function are failure to recognize incarceration in the joint and ulnar or median nerve dysfunction. Most of the other complications are minor and result in only minimal functional or cosmetic sequelae.

Major Complications

Failure to Recognize Fragment Incarceration

Failure to recognize incarceration of the epicondylar fragment into the joint can result in significant loss of elbow motion

and premature arthritis, especially if it remains incarcerated for any length of time. Fowles et al.[51] challenged the opinion that surgery is detrimental in patients with late incarceration, and the idea remains controversial. In their patients in whom the fragment was surgically extracted, an average of 14 weeks after injury, 80% more elbow motion was regained. In addition, the patients' preoperative pain was relieved and the ulnar nerve dysfunction resolved. Lopez et al.[104] described a case report of an incarcerated fragment treated 12 weeks following injury by excision of the fragment. Twelve months following surgery, the ulnar neuropathy had resolved, the patient had minimal symptoms and excellent motion.

The long-term outcome following intra-articular retention of the medial epicondyle fragment is unpredictable. Rosendahl[154] reported an 8-year follow-up of a fragment retained within the joint. The epicondyle had fused to the semilunar surface of the ulna, producing a large bony prominence clinically. There was only minor loss of elbow motion, with little functional disability. Potenza et al.[141] described a case report of a neglected intra-articular medial epicondyle fracture with 48-year follow-up resulting in minimal symptoms. Similar to the case reported by Rosendahl, the fragment had fused to the olecranon where it caused minimal problems.

Ulnar Nerve Dysfunction

The other major complication associated with this injury is the development of ulnar nerve dysfunction. The incidence of ulnar nerve dysfunction varies from 10% to 16%.[115] If the fragment is entrapped in the joint, the incidence of ulnar nerve dysfunction may be as high as 50%.[48] More profound ulnar nerve injury has been reported after manipulative procedures.[139] Thus, in patients with fragments incarcerated in the joint, closed manipulation may not be the procedure of choice if a primary ulnar nerve dysfunction is present. Patients in whom the fragment was left incarcerated in the joint for a significant time have experienced poor recovery of the primary ulnar nerve injury.[115] A consistent finding noted by surgeons when exploring the ulnar nerve and removing the incarcerated fragment from the joint has been a thick fascial band binding the ulnar nerve to the underlying muscle.[11,139] Constriction by this band has been noted to cause immediate or late dysfunction of the ulnar nerve.

Delayed ulnar nerve palsy has also been reported following surgical treatment. Anakwe et al.[8] described two cases in which open reduction of a medial epicondyle was performed. Patients presented at 1- and 2-week follow-up with complete ulnar nerve palsy despite normal neurologic examination immediately postoperatively. In both patients, on reexploration the ulnar nerve was found to be compressed by scar tissue between two heads of the flexor carpi ulnaris just distal to the medial epicondyle. Both patients experienced a complete recovery following ulnar nerve decompression.

Symptomatic Nonunion

Nonunion of the medial epicondyle fragment with the distal metaphysis occurs in up to 50% of fractures with significant displacement treated nonoperatively. Although the majority of the

Figure 16-11. Nonunion in an athlete. This 15-year-old baseball pitcher had an untreated medial epicondyle fracture 1 year before this radiograph. He developed a fibrous union, but the epicondyle was shifted distally (*arrow*). His elbow was unstable enough to prevent him from pitching.

nonunions cause minimal problems, symptomatic nonunions do occur (Fig. 16-11). Kulkarni and colleagues described 14 patients with symptomatic medial epicondyle nonunions experiencing symptoms including medial-sided elbow pain, ulnar nerve dysfunction, valgus instability, and limited motion.[98] Smith et al.[168] from Boston Children's Hospital reviewed 137 patients treated for medial epicondyle fracture at their institution. Of the 42 fractures who were treated nonoperatively, nonunion occurred in 19 fractures and 8 of those fracture nonunion patients experienced symptoms significant enough to warrant surgical treatment at a mean of 12 months following their initial injury. All patients were treated with open reduction and internal fixation of the nonunited fragment, three of whom underwent grafting of the nonunion site. Successful fracture union was achieved in seven of the eight fractures and all patients experienced significant symptomatic improvement. Shukla and Cohen[165] described the treatment results of five patients with chronic medial epicondyle nonunion using a tension band construct. At a mean follow-up of 31 months, all fractures were healed, patients reported being satisfied with their surgery, and measurable outcome measures were significantly improved.

Valgus Instability

Valgus instability following displaced medial epicondyle fracture nonunion is a very challenging problem and has been used as an argument for surgical treatment. Gilcrist and McKee[56] reported good and excellent treatment results following excision of the nonunited fragment and advancement of the medial collateral ligament complex with fixation to the distal humerus

with suture anchors in five patients with symptomatic valgus elbow instability. Mayo Elbow Performance Score improved from 66 preoperatively to 91 postoperatively, and all patients were satisfied with the result.

Radial Nerve Injury

When fixing a medial epicondyle fragment, the operating surgeon must decide whether to accept fixation within the cancellous bone of the medial column or achieve bicortical fixation by gaining purchase in the lateral cortex of the proximal humeral metaphysis. Unfortunately, the radial nerve travels on the surface of the humerus at the location where a bicortical screw penetrates the cortex. Marcu et al.[114] have reported two cases of radial nerve injury with cannulated screw fixation.

Minor Complications

Loss of Motion

The most common minor complication is loss of the final degrees of elbow extension. A loss of 5% to 10% can be expected to develop in about 20% of these fractures. Minimal functional deficit is attributed to this loss of elbow motion. Prolonged immobilization seems to be the key factor contributing to loss of elbow extension. It is important to discuss with parents before treatment is begun that loss of motion is common after this injury, regardless of the treatment method used. Sufficient fracture stability to allow for early motion is paramount to lessening the risk of functional loss of motion. Severe contractures are rare; more often associated with more complex fracture dislocations; and may require nonoperative management with therapy, serial casting, dynamic splinting, and at times, operative intervention.

Myositis Ossificans

Myositis ossificans is a rare occurrence following vigorous and repeated manipulation to extract the fragment from the joint. As with many other elbow injuries, myositis may be a result of the treatment rather than the injury itself. Myositis ossificans must be differentiated from ectopic calcification of the collateral ligaments, which involves only the ligamentous structures. This condition may occur after repeated injuries to the epicondyle and ligamentous structures (Fig. 16-12). Often, this calcified ligament is asymptomatic and does not seem to create functional disability. The esthetic effects are minimal. In some patients, an accentuation of the medial prominence of the epicondyle creates a false appearance of an increased carrying angle of the elbow.

Hardware Prominence

Finally, following open reduction and internal fixation, the implants are sometimes prominent and cause discomfort. Pace and Hennrikus found that using a washer with a screw was more likely to cause discomfort significant enough for patients to undergo implant removal, compared to patients who underwent medial epicondyle fixation with a screw alone.[133]

A   **B**

Figure 16-12. Heterotopic calcification. **A:** Injury to an 11-year-old who had moderate displacement of the medial epicondyle (*arrow*). **B:** One year later, they had considerable calcification of the ulnar collateral ligament (*arrows*). Other than mild instability with valgus stress, the patient had full range of motion and was asymptomatic. (Courtesy of Mark R. Christofersen, MD.)

Dislocations of the Elbow

INTRODUCTION TO ELBOW DISLOCATIONS

Disruptions of the elbow joint represent a spectrum of injuries involving three separate articulations: the radiocapitellar, the ulnohumeral, and the proximal radioulnar joints. Dislocations of the elbow joint in children are not common. Of all elbow injuries in skeletally immature patients, Henrikson[73] found that only about 3% of all were dislocations. The peak incidence of pediatric elbow dislocations typically occurs in the second decade of life, usually between 13 and 14 years of age when the physes begin to close.[73,87] Based on the National Electronic Injury Surveillance System database, the calculated incidence of elbow dislocations in adolescents aged 10 to 19 years was 6.87 dislocations per 100,000 person-years with an almost 2:1 ratio of injuries in males compared to females (incidence 8.91 vs. 4.72 per 100,000 person-years).[172] The largest proportion of elbow dislocations (44.5%) occur in conjunction with sports activities; football/rugby, wrestling, and basketball being the most common sports for males and gymnastics and skating being the most common sports for females.[172] A recent report of the epidemiology of elbow dislocations in athletes showed that elbow dislocations occurred in 0.38 per 100,000 athletic exposures.[40] Almost 60% of medial epicondyle fractures are associated with elbow dislocations in this age group.[97] As with all joint dislocations, the principles of treatment include promptly obtaining a concentric reduction of the elbow joint while identifying and treating all associated injuries. The ultimate goal

is allowing protected motion and rehabilitation with the goal of restoring full elbow motion and function without recurrent instability.

PATHOANATOMY AND APPLIED ANATOMY RELATING TO ELBOW DISLOCATIONS

Constraints about the elbow preventing dislocation can be considered as either dynamic or static. Dynamic elbow stabilizers consist of the elbow musculature, over which the patient has conscious control, which changes depending on the degree of muscular contraction. Unlike the shoulder, dynamic stabilizers play only a modest role in elbow stability.

Static constraints are of greater importance and can be divided into osseous and ligamentous restraints (Figs. 16-13 to 16-15). The bony geometry of the elbow creates a relatively constrained hinge. The coronoid and olecranon form a semicircle of approximately 180 degrees into which the trochlea of the humerus securely articulates. The concave surface of the radial head matches the convex capitellum and provides stability to the lateral aspect of the elbow joint. The bony configuration of the medial and lateral aspects of the elbow complements each other with the ulnohumeral articulation providing stability against mediolateral or longitudinal translation, whereas the radiocapitellar joint provides resistance to axial compression. The circular nature of the proximal radius allows for nearly 180 degrees of rotation through the full range of flexion and extension, allowing for maintenance of these relationships with forearm rotation.

Lateral ligamentous constraints include the annular ligament that is attached to proximal ulna and encircles the radial neck and the lateral collateral ligaments that originate from the lateral

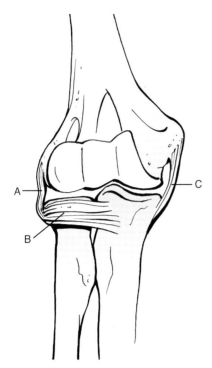

Figure 16-13. Anteroposterior view of the elbow illustrates the bone and ligamentous structures which contribute to elbow stability. (*A*, lateral collateral ligament; *B*, annular ligament; *C*, medial collateral ligament.)

epicondyle and insert into the annular ligament and the lateral aspect of the proximal ulna. The primary role of the annular ligament and the lateral collateral ligament complex is to provide stability to the radiocapitellar and proximal radioulnar joints by resisting varus stress.

The medial ulnar collateral ligament is the primary ligamentous restraint to valgus stress, resisting pathologic opening of the medial aspect of the elbow. Having its origin from the inferior

Figure 16-14. The annular ligament and lateral collateral ligament complex provides stability to the proximal radioulnar joint and radial capitellar articulation. (*A*, annular ligament; *B*, lateral collateral ligament insertion on annular ligament; *C*, lateral collateral ligament insertion on ulna.)

Figure 16-15. The medial elbow is stabilized by the hinge articulation between the proximal ulna and the humerus. Three components of the ulnar collateral ligament provide additional elbow stability. (*A*, coronoid process; *B*, olecranon process; *C*, anterior oblique medial collateral ligament; *D*, posterior oblique medial collateral ligament; *E*, transverse medial collateral ligament.)

aspect of the medial epicondyle, the medial collateral ligament has two primary components that contribute to elbow stability, the anterior and the posterior bands. The band's anterior portion is taut in extension and the posterior fibers are taut in flexion. There is also a fan-shaped posterior oblique ligament that inserts on the olecranon and functions mainly in flexion and a small transverse ligament runs from the olecranon to the coronoid that is thought to have little functional importance. Woods and Tullos[180] pointed out that the major stabilizing ligamentous structure in the elbow is the anterior band of the ulnar collateral ligament.

CLASSIFICATION OF ELBOW DISLOCATIONS

Because of the location of critical stabilizing factors and surrounding neurovascular structures, elbow dislocations should be considered based on the direction of dislocation and the associated fractures that may be present. As the mechanism of injury, the associated injuries, and imaging differ based on the nature of the injury, these factors should be considered for each dislocation pattern.

Elbow dislocations are described by the position of the proximal radioulnar joint relative to the distal humerus: posterior, anterior, medial, or lateral. Posterior dislocations are typically further subdivided into posterolateral and posteromedial injuries. Occasionally, the proximal radioulnar joint is disrupted. When this happens, the radius and ulna can diverge from each other. Rarely, the radius and ulna translocate, with the radius medial and the ulna lateral. Isolated traumatic dislocations of the radial head must be differentiated from congenital dislocations. Isolated dislocations of the proximal ulna are exceedingly rare and have not been reported in children. Included in this chapter is a discussion of the commonly occurring subluxation of the radial head, referred to as "pulled elbow" or "nursemaid's elbow." This is not a true subluxation but rather a partial entrapment of the annular ligament in the radiocapitellar joint. Monteggia fracture-dislocations are discussed in detail in Chapter 12.

POSTERIOR ELBOW DISLOCATIONS

ASSESSMENT OF POSTERIOR ELBOW DISLOCATIONS

Mechanisms of Injury for Posterior Elbow Dislocations

O'Driscoll et al.[131] have proposed that most posterior elbow dislocations begin with disruption of the lateral ligaments and proceed along the anterior capsular structures to the medial ligaments. Although this is likely the mechanism for the more rarely seen posteromedial elbow dislocation, for the more common posterior and posterolateral elbow dislocations, this notion has been challenged. Clinical and MRI-based studies noting that medial ulnar collateral ligament injuries occur more frequently than lateral ulnar collateral injuries[83,84,86,148] have led to the competing theory[148] that most posterior elbow dislocations initiate from a valgus force at the elbow leading to failure of the medial ulnar collateral ligament or the medial epicondyle apophysis, to which it is attached, creating a medial epicondyle fracture. As the proximal radius and ulna displace laterally, the coronoid disengages with the intact biceps tendon acting as the center of rotation for the displaced forearm (Fig. 16-16). Application of both an abduction and an extension force leads to forearm external rotation and, with anterior soft tissue disruption, the result is a posterior or posterolateral elbow dislocation.[131,148]

Injuries Associated With Posterior Elbow Dislocations

Fractures

Concomitant fractures occur in over one-half of posterior elbow dislocations.[102,109,127,153,156] Recent evaluations have found that number to be very high 78%.[181] The most common fractures involve the medial epicondyle (55%), with fractures also possibly involving the coronoid process, and the radial head and neck. Fractures involving the lateral epicondyle, lateral condyle, olecranon, capitellum, and trochlea occur less frequently.[28,109,123] Given the significant association among fractures of the medial epicondyle, the coronoid process, and the proximal radius (especially markedly displaced radial neck fractures) and posterior elbow dislocations, evaluating for elbow stability when these fractures are noted is important.

Soft Tissue Injuries

Posterior dislocations normally produce moderate soft tissue injury and can be associated with neurovascular injuries in addition to concomitant fractures (Fig. 16-17). The anterior

Figure 16-16. Mechanism of injury producing a posterior elbow dislocation. **A:** The elbow is forced into extension that ruptures the medial collateral ligaments. The normal valgus alignment of the elbow accentuates the valgus force at the elbow. **B:** The lateral slope of the medial crista of the trochlea forces the proximal ulna posterolaterally (*small arrow*). The biceps tendon serves as a fulcrum for rotation (*medium arrow*) leading to valgus hinging (*large arrow*) of the forearm. **C:** The proximal ulna and radius are then impacted posteriorly and held against the distal articular surface by the contraction of the biceps and triceps (*arrows*).

Figure 16-17. Injuries associated with elbow dislocation. (*1*) The radial head and olecranon are displaced posterolaterally. (*2*) The brachialis muscle is stretched across the articular surface of the distal humerus. (*3*) The origins of the medial forearm flexion muscles are either torn or avulsed with the medial epicondyle from the medial condyle. (*4*) The median nerve and brachial artery are stretched across the medial condyle and held firmly by the lacertus fibrosus. (*5*) The medial condyle lies in the subcutaneous tissue between the brachialis anteriorly and the pronator teres posteriorly. (*6*) The lateral (radial) collateral ligaments often avulse a piece of cartilage or bone from the lateral condyle.

capsule fails in tension, opening the joint cavity. Radial head displacement strips the capsule from the posterolateral aspect of the lateral condyle with the adjacent periosteum. Because of the large amount of cartilage on the posterolateral aspect of the lateral condyle, the posterior capsule may not reattach firmly with healing. This lack of a strong reattachment is believed to be a factor in the rare recurrent elbow dislocation.[132] In a series of 62 adults and adolescents with elbow dislocations requiring surgical treatment, McKee et al.[118] reported that disruption of the lateral collateral ligament complex occurred in all 62 elbows.

Medially, the ulnar collateral ligament complex is disrupted either by an avulsion of the medial epicondyle or a direct tear of the ligament.[163,171] Cromack[33] found that with medial epicondylar fractures, the origins of the ulnar collateral ligaments and the medial forearm flexor muscles remain as a unit, along with most of the pronator teres, which is stripped from its humeral origin proximal to the epicondyle. These structures are then displaced posterior to the medial aspect of the distal humerus. The ulnar collateral ligaments and the muscular origins of the common flexor muscles tear if the epicondyle remains attached to the humerus. With posterolateral displacement of the forearm, the medial aspect of the distal humerus most often passes into the intermuscular space between the pronator teres posteriorly and the brachialis anteriorly. The brachialis, because it has little distal tendon, is easily ruptured. The rent in the anterior capsule usually is in this same area.

The structure most commonly torn on the lateral aspect of the elbow is the annular ligament.[171] On occasion, the lateral collateral ligament either avulses a small osteochondral fragment from the lateral epicondyle or tears completely within its substance.

Neurovascular Injuries

When the elbow is dislocated, the medial aspect of the distal humerus typically protrudes between the pronator teres posteriorly and the brachialis anteriorly. The median nerve and brachial artery lie directly over the distal humerus in the subcutaneous tissues. In a cadaver and clinical study by Louis et al.,[106] there was a consistent pattern of disruption of the anastomosis between the inferior ulnar collateral artery and the anterior ulnar recurrent artery. If the main brachial arterial trunk also is compromised, the loss of this collateral system can result in the loss of circulation to the forearm and hand. An avascular hand can occur acutely; or a dysvascular hand with cold intolerance late if there is a brachial artery disruption. This is more common in adults with severe trauma.

The ulnar nerve is at risk in posterior elbow dislocation because of its position posterior to the medial epicondyle. In clinical cases, the ulnar nerve is the most common neurovascular injury.[123] The injury is usually a stretch neurapraxia that resolves but at times the ulnar can be tethered or entrapped by the medial epicondyle displaced fracture. The median nerve is at risk for entrapment in the elbow with hyperextension reduction techniques due to disruption of the anteromedial soft tissue structures.

Signs and Symptoms of Posterior Elbow Dislocations

Posterior elbow dislocations must be differentiated from extension-type supracondylar or physeal fractures of the distal humerus. With all these injuries, the elbow is held semiflexed and swelling may be considerable. Swelling initially is usually less with a dislocation than with a type III supracondylar humeral fracture. Crepitus is usually absent in children with a dislocation and the forearm appears shortened. The prominence produced by the distal humeral articular surface is more distal and is palpable as a blunt articular surface. The tip of the olecranon is displaced posteriorly and proximally so that its triangular relationship with the epicondyles is lost. The skin may have a dimpled appearance over the olecranon fossa. If the dislocation is posterolateral, the radial head also may be prominent and easily palpable in the subcutaneous tissues. In children less than age 2 years, a physeal fracture can occur, especially in the setting of nonaccidental trauma. The physeal fracture is usually posteromedially displaced compared to the more common posterolateral displacement with an elbow dislocation.

Imaging and Other Diagnostic Studies for Posterior Elbow Dislocations

AP and lateral x-rays usually are diagnostic of a posterior elbow dislocation. There is a greater superimposition of the distal humerus on the proximal radius and ulna in the AP view. The radial head may be proximally and laterally displaced, or it may be directly behind the middistal humerus, depending on whether the dislocation is posterolateral, posterior, or posteromedial (Fig. 16-18). The normal valgus angulation between the forearm and the arm usually is increased with the most common posterolateral dislocation. On the lateral view, the coronoid process lies posterior to the condyles. Pre- and postreduction x-rays must be examined closely for associated fractures. The medial epicondyle should be identified on the postreduction films. If it should be present based on the patient's age and elbow ossification pattern and it is not visible, the medial epicondyle is likely fractured and may be entrapped in the joint. Additional radiographs may be necessary to further evaluate an associated medial epicondyle fracture. In the young, contralateral elbow radiographs to confirm the presence or absence of the medial epicondyle on the normal elbow can assist in the radiographic evaluation for fractures. Postreduction radiographs should be carefully scrutinized for a congruent reduction and for subtle osteochondral fracture fragments that can become entrapped in the joint. If reduction is not anatomic or is noncongruent or if osteochondral fragments are visualized, further evaluation with CT tomography or MRI is utilized. MRI also may be used to further define the extent of soft tissue injury in complex injury patterns. Ultrasound has been used for further diagnostic accuracy in the emergency room setting.

TREATMENT OPTIONS FOR POSTERIOR ELBOW DISLOCATIONS

If untreated, elbow dislocation predictably results in dramatic loss of elbow function characterized by loss of motion and eventually pain. In comparison, reduction of the dislocated elbow usually achieves marked improvement of acute pain as well as restoration of long term function, especially in children and young adolescents.

Nonoperative Treatment of Posterior Elbow Dislocations

Indications/Contraindications

Nonoperative Treatment Following Successful Closed Reduction of Posterior Elbow Dislocation: INDICATIONS AND CONTRAINDICATIONS
Indication
• Stable concentric elbow reduction obtained following closed treatment
Relative Contraindications
• Unable to obtain a concentric and stable elbow reduction • Intra-articular entrapment of fracture fragments • Vascular injury • Change in neurologic status following reduction, especially median nerve, or other indication of nerve entrapment

Figure 16-18. Radiographic findings. **A:** Anteroposterior radiograph. The radial head is superimposed behind the distal humerus. There is increased cubitus valgus. The medial epicondyle has not been avulsed. **B:** Lateral radiograph demonstrating that the proximal radius and ulna are both displaced posteriorly to the distal humerus.

Expected progressive elbow swelling secondary to the soft tissue injury associated with an elbow dislocation makes it imperative that all acute elbow dislocations be promptly reduced under adequate sedation or anesthesia. Royle[156] found that dislocations reduced soon after the injury had better outcomes than those in which reduction was delayed. Immediately after reduction, the surgeon should determine and document the stability of the elbow by examination under anesthesia or sedation. Definitive nonoperative treatment following closed reduction should be considered if the elbow is stable through a functional range of motion; a concentric anatomic reduction can be obtained and maintained; and there is no evidence to suggest a vascular injury, nerve entrapment, or significant intra-articular osteochondral fragments.

Closed Reduction of Posterior Elbow Dislocations

Closed reduction of pediatric elbow dislocations should always be done with adequate analgesia, sedation, or anesthesia. In addition to making the experience much less frightening and traumatic for the child, adequate analgesia, sedation, or anesthesia will achieve sufficient muscle relaxation for the reduction to be obtained more effectively with less force, thereby reducing the risk of creating an iatrogenic fracture (such as fracture of the radial neck) during reduction.

A careful neurologic examination must be done before and after the reduction with special attention to the ulnar nerve prereduction, and to the median nerve postreduction in terms of entrapment. This same careful examination must be made at all follow-up evaluations. Ulnar neuropathy is not uncommon with these injuries and usually resolves spontaneously if reduction is anatomic. Persistent median nerve motor–sensory loss associated with severe pain and resistance with elbow flexion–extension arc of motion may be indicative of entrapment.

All methods of closed reduction must overcome the deforming muscle forces so that the coronoid process and the radial head can slip past the distal end of the humerus. Adequate sedation or anesthesia is necessary to permit muscle relaxation. If adequate sedation to achieve full muscular relaxation cannot be achieved in the emergency department (ED), the procedure should be performed in the operating room (OR) under general anesthesia. An assistant who can provide adequate stabilizing force is required. Before the primary reduction forces are applied, the forearm is hypersupinated to dislodge the coronoid process and radial head from their position behind the distal humerus and to reduce tension on the biceps tendon.[132] The reducing forces are applied in two major directions (Fig. 16-19). The first reducing force must be along the long axis of the humerus to overcome the contractions of the biceps and brachialis anteriorly and the triceps posteriorly.

Once these forces are neutralized, the proximal ulna and radius must be passed from posterior to anterior. The "pusher" technique of reduction of an elbow dislocation is preferred in children 9 years of age or younger. In this age group, the child often can be seated comfortably in the parent's lap (Fig. 16-20). Hanging the arm over the back of a well-padded

Figure 16-19. Forces required to reduce posterior elbow dislocations. **A:** The forearm is hypersupinated (*arrow 1*) to unlock the radial head. **B:** Simultaneous forces are applied to the proximal forearm along the axis of the humerus (*arrow 2*) and distally along the axis of the forearm (*arrow 3*). **C:** The elbow is then flexed (*arrow 4*) to stabilize the reduction once the coronoid is manipulated distal to the humerus.

Figure 16-20. Reduction by "pusher" techniques. **A:** Lavine method. The child is held by the parent while the elbow is draped over the edge of the chair. The olecranon is pushed distally past the humerus by the thumb of the physician while the other arm pulls distally along the axis of the forearm. **B:** Meyn technique with patient lying prone on the table. (**B.** Adapted with permission from Meyn MA, Quigley TB. Reduction of posterior dislocation of the elbow by traction on the dangling arm. *Clin Orthop.* 1974; 103:106–107.)

chair may provide some stabilization. For a child 10 years of age and older, the puller technique advocated by Parvin[136] is used (see Fig. 16-21). Combined pusher–puller techniques are also possible.[67]

Several authors[102] have strongly advised against initial hyperextension before reduction forces are applied to the elbow. Loomis[103] demonstrated that when the coronoid process is locked against the posterior aspect of the humerus and the elbow is extended, the force applied to the anterior muscles is multiplied by as much as five times because of the increased leverage. This places a marked strain on the injured structures in the antecubital fossa including the anterior capsule, the brachialis muscle, and the neurovascular structures. By contrast, when force is applied to the proximal forearm with the elbow flexed, the force exerted against the muscles across the elbow is equal to the distracting force. For patients with posterolateral dislocations, the lateral displacement of the proximal radius and ulna must first be corrected to prevent the median nerve from being entrapped or injured during reduction.[17,25] Hyperextension reduction puts the median nerve more at risk for entrapment.

Once successful reduction is accomplished, the range of stable elbow motion is assessed. Fluoroscopy can be helpful during and after the reduction to assess stability as well. Formal x-rays are obtained after the manipulation to assess the adequacy of the

Figure 16-21. Reduction by "puller" techniques in a supine position. **A:** With the elbow flexed to almost 90 degrees, a force is applied to the anterior portion of the forearm with one hand while the other hand pulls distally along the forearm. A counterforce is applied to offset the manipulating forces by direct stabilization of the patient by a second medical person. **B:** The counterforce is applied with a sheet around the chest in the ipsilateral axilla.

reduction, to be certain the joint is congruently reduced, and to assess for the presence of any intra-articular fragments. If the elbow is stable through a functional range of motion, the elbow is immobilized in a posterior splint, hinged brace, or a split cast with the elbow flexed 90 degrees. If there is a question of persistent relative instability, the forearm is held in full supination. If the elbow is absolutely stable following reduction, the forearm can be immobilized in midpronation to allow the patient to be more functional with early progressive motion.

Closed Reduction of an Elbow Dislocation Prereduction Planning

✓ **Closed Reduction of a Posterior Elbow Dislocation:**
PREPROCEDURE PLANNING CHECKLIST

Location	❏ ED if muscular relaxation can be obtained.
	❏ If not, under general anesthesia in the OR is preferred.
	❏ Most are performed in ED under conscious sedation.
OR table	❏ Any supportive stretcher or OR table will suffice.
Position/ positioning aids	❏ For puller technique, the patient is placed either supine with the shoulder abducted 90 degrees and the elbow over the edge of the bed, or prone with the shoulder abducted 90 degrees and the elbow draped over the side of the table.
	❏ For the Pusher technique, the patient is either held by the parent with the elbow draped over the edge of a well-padded chair or prone with the shoulder abducted 90 degrees and the elbow draped over the side of the table.
	❏ Proper padding of all peripheral pressure points is critical.
Fluoroscopy location	❏ The image intensifier is placed alongside the table on the side of elbow dislocation and arranged to assess a lateral x-ray once the elbow is reduced.
Equipment	❏ Postreduction immobilization supplies (cast or splint)

Closed Reduction of a Posterior Elbow Dislocation
by the "Puller" Technique

✓ **Closed Reduction of a Posterior Elbow Dislocation by the "Puller" Technique:**
KEY STEPS

❏ Ensure adequate sedation with near-complete muscular relaxation
❏ Have assistant to stabilize the body and the humerus
❏ Flex the elbow to about 90 degrees
❏ "Milk" the distal humerus out of anterior soft tissues
❏ Apply force on the anterior forearm in line with the humeral shaft
❏ Correct any medial or lateral displacement
❏ Apply a distally directed force in line with the forearm to reduce the elbow joint
❏ Check the elbow reduction with static and dynamic fluoroscopic evaluation
❏ Assess elbow stability
❏ Immobilize elbow in about 90 degrees of flexion

The puller technique can be performed in various positions including the supine position and the prone position.

The patient is placed on the table in the chosen position with the shoulder abducted 90 degrees and the elbow off the side of the table. An assistant is positioned on the opposite side of the patient to provide the counterforce. A sheet can be placed around the patient for stabilization purposes if desired. If this is done, an additional assistant may be required to stabilize the upper arm during the reduction.

With the elbow flexed to almost 90 degrees, a traction force is applied to the anterior portion of the forearm along the longitudinal axis of the humerus with one hand while the other hand pulls distally along the forearm. If any medial or lateral displacement is present, this should be corrected before the forearm is translated distally to release soft tissue structures from the distal humerus and prevent entrapment of tissue around the distal humerus. Gently "milking" the anterior soft tissue out from around the distal humerus, by gently pinching and pulling the tissues enveloping the distal humerus forward, as the reduction is performed can also help the reduction. During the procedure, a counterforce is applied by an assistant to offset the manipulating forces and stabilize the humerus. The physician performing the procedure usually appreciates a palpable clunk of the reduction. Using fluoroscopic evaluation, if available, the reduction is assessed in multiple projections.

Closed Reduction of a Posterior Elbow Dislocation
by the "Pusher" Technique

✓ **Closed Reduction of a Posterior Elbow Dislocation by the "Puller" Technique:**
KEY STEPS

❏ Ensure adequate sedation with near-complete muscular relaxation
❏ Have assistant to stabilize the body and the humerus over the edge of a fixed surface
❏ Flex the elbow to about 90 degrees
❏ "Milk" the distal humerus out of anterior soft tissues
❏ Using the thumb, apply force on the prominent olecranon, translating it distally in line with the humeral shaft
❏ Correct any medial or lateral displacement
❏ Apply a distally directed force in line with the forearm with the other hand to reduce the elbow joint
❏ Check the elbow reduction with static and dynamic fluoroscopic evaluation
❏ Assess elbow stability
❏ Immobilize elbow in about 90 degrees of flexion

Like the puller technique, the pusher technique can be performed in various positions. Again, adequate sedation is required and fluoroscopy can be helpful for postreduction evaluation. The patient is positioned with the distal humerus over a fixed surface, either the back of a chair or the edge of the bed.

With the elbow flexed to almost 90 degrees, the thumb is used to push the olecranon distally past the humerus. The other arm then pulls distally along the axis of the forearm affecting the reduction. Again, if any medial or lateral displacement is present, this should be corrected before the forearm is translated distally. Fluoroscopic evaluation, if available, can then be performed as with the puller technique.

Postreduction Care

Elbow stability should be assessed and the elbow then immobilized in a position of stability. In the postreduction examination, an estimation of the direction of instability should be performed: valgus, varus, or posterolateral rotatory instability. In these circumstances, evaluation with a postreduction MRI to assess the extent of the soft tissue injury may help direct treatment.

Some type of immobilization, usually a posterior splint or circumferential cast, is advocated by most investigators. A frequently recommended period of immobilization is 3 weeks,[102,103,136,164] although some have advocated earlier motion.[155,156,180] Murphy et al. evaluated 145 pediatric dislocations and found that immobilization greater than 2 weeks led to loss of extension. O'Driscoll et al.[131] suggested that if the elbow was stable in response to valgus stress with the forearm pronated, then the anterior portion of the medial collateral ligament was intact and the patient could begin early motion. Ninety degrees of elbow flexion appears to be the standard position of immobilization. Hinged elbow braces with adjustable blocks to motion are very useful for obtaining progressive, protected motion.

Outcomes

Closed reduction of posterior elbow dislocations is successful in most cases. In the combined series of 317 dislocations,[102,127,153,156] only two cases[102] could not be reduced by closed methods. In the Carlioz and Abols[28] series, two dislocations reduced spontaneously and closed reduction was successful in 50 cases, but failed in 6 cases (10%). Josefsson et al.[85] reported that all 25 dislocations without associated fractures were successfully reduced. In the largest reported series of pediatric elbow dislocations to date, Murphy et al. reported that only 1 of 145 cases required open treatment to obtain reduction.[123]

Potential Pitfalls and Preventive Measures

Reduction of Posterior Elbow Dislocation: POTENTIAL PITFALLS AND PREVENTIONS

Pitfall	Prevention
Stiffness	• Early mobilization
Inadequate analgesia	• Perform the reduction in the OR if adequate analgesia for muscular relaxation is not available in the emergency setting
Median nerve entrapment	• Correct lateral displacement before translating anteriorly • Avoid hyperextension reduction
Coronoid fracture during reduction	• Attempt reduction with the elbow in flexion

Operative Treatment of Posterior Elbow Dislocations

Indications/Contraindications

Operative Treatment of Posterior Elbow Dislocation: INDICATIONS AND CONTRAINDICATIONS

Indications
- Unable to obtain a concentric and stable elbow reduction
- Intra-articular entrapment of fracture fragments
- Vascular injury
- Open injuries
- Change in neurologic status following reduction or other indication of nerve entrapment

Contraindication
- Stable concentric elbow reduction obtained following closed treatment

Indications for primary open reduction include an inability to obtain or maintain a concentric closed reduction, an open dislocation, a displaced osteochondral fracture with entrapment in the joint, a vascular injury, or a neurologic injury for which there is any indication that there may be entrapment of the nerve.

Primary ligament repair is not routinely indicated. Adults with posterior elbow dislocations without concomitant fracture have no better function or stability following a primary ligamentous repair than those treated nonoperatively.[83,84] There was a recent report of more aggressive ligamentous repair if instability persisted following reduction with good clinical results.[101] However, this report is difficult to interpret as it did not have a control group where the ligaments were treated without repair. All fractures preventing concentric reduction need to be repaired with an open reduction of an elbow dislocation. Beware of elbow dislocations in children less than age 10 as they often have associated osteochondral fractures that can block reduction. More detailed examination and imaging may be required in the young.

Open Dislocations

Open dislocations have a high incidence of associated arterial injury.[71,102,106] Operative intervention is necessary in open posterior dislocations to irrigate and debride the open wound and elbow and to evaluate the brachial artery (Fig. 16-22). If there is vascular disruption, some authors advocate vascular repair or reconstruction with a vein graft even in the presence of adequate capillary refill. This may lessen the risk of late cold intolerance, dysesthesias, or dysvascularity.

Fractures

Children with an elbow dislocation usually have an associated fracture of the coronoid, lateral condyle, olecranon, radial neck, or medial epicondyle (see previous section). In the Murphy et al. series of 145 pediatric dislocations, 80% had an associated fracture, 60% of which involved the medial epicondyle.[123] Fractures of the anteromedial facet of the coronoid

Figure 16-22. A: A 13-year-old male presented to the emergency department following a rollover ATV injury with a contaminated, open posterior elbow dislocation. The brachial artery can be seen traversing the articular cartilage of the distal humerus. **B:** Following debridement and elbow reduction, the brachial artery and median nerve are seen in the traumatic wound. Intraoperative assessment revealed palpable radial pulse and Doppler ultrasound studies found no evidence of vascular injury. **C, D:** Three months following injury elbow range of motions is from −20 extension to 130 degrees flexion with no pain and minimal functional limitations. Periarticular calcification is present with worrisome joint space irregularity.

have been recognized as an important injury associated with elbow dislocations in adolescents and adults.[42,151] The presence of a concomitant displaced fracture is a common indication for surgical intervention.[28,178] Surgery for associated fractures produced better results than nonoperative treatment of fracture-dislocations in the series of Carlioz and Abols,[28] and similar results were reported by Wheeler and Linscheid.[178] Repair of an associated medial epicondylar fracture may also improve elbow stability in throwing athletes when the injury is in the dominant arm.[22,163,180] Entrapment of any fracture fragments within the joint is an absolute indication for surgical treatment. Displaced medial epicondyle fractures can be entrapped within the joint after reduction and are often overlooked on the radiographs. Because of the high association of this fracture with elbow dislocations, the location of the medial epicondyle should be confirmed in every case. Ultimately, the surgical treatment for fractures associated with an elbow dislocation is based on the circumstances surrounding each individual patient. Factors favoring operative treatment

include older patient age, instability of the elbow during examination under sedation at the time of reduction, the presence of a displaced intra-articular fracture, injury to multiple elbow stabilizers, injury to the patient's dominant arm, and anticipated high-demand sports, especially overhead sports or activities on the elbow. Murphy reported a high rate of fixation of the medial epicondyle fractures (79%) when associated with an elbow dislocation.[123] This may be a reflection of increased national trends in both operative fixation rates and youth sports participation. See the previous section for a more thorough discussion on the management of medial epicondyle fractures.

Vascular Injuries

With initial evidence of vascular compromise, treatment should consist of urgent reduction of the elbow dislocation that usually returns the displaced brachial vessels to their normal position[72,179] followed by reassessment of the vascular status. With prompt normalization of the vascular status, serial observation is still recommended to evaluate for evolving circulatory compromise. If there is evidence of persistent vascular compromise after reduction, vascular exploration followed by operative repair of those structures that are ruptured or severely damaged should be pursued emergently. Even though collateral vessels may provide adequate vascular flow to give a warm hand with good capillary refill if there has been a significant vascular injury, failure to repair the injury may predispose the patient to late ischemic changes such as claudication, cold sensitivity, or even late amputation.

Neurologic Injuries

As with vascular injuries, initial evidence of neurologic compromise should prompt urgent reduction. A significant negative change in the neurologic status following closed reduction may indicate intra-articular nerve entrapment and should prompt exploration. This is particularly true for median nerve injuries postreduction. If missed, this may have significant consequences for hand function if not addressed surgically.[18]

Open Reduction of an Irreducible Posterior Elbow Reduction

Preoperative Planning

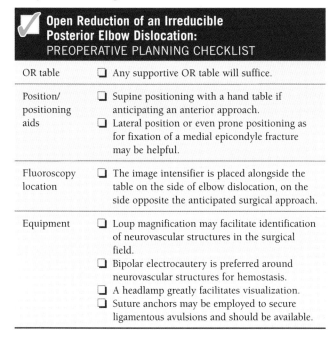

	Open Reduction of an Irreducible Posterior Elbow Dislocation: PREOPERATIVE PLANNING CHECKLIST	
OR table	❏ Any supportive OR table will suffice.
Position/ positioning aids	❏ Supine positioning with a hand table if anticipating an anterior approach. ❏ Lateral position or even prone positioning as for fixation of a medial epicondyle fracture may be helpful.
Fluoroscopy location	❏ The image intensifier is placed alongside the table on the side of elbow dislocation, on the side opposite the anticipated surgical approach.
Equipment	❏ Loup magnification may facilitate identification of neurovascular structures in the surgical field. ❏ Bipolar electrocautery is preferred around neurovascular structures for hemostasis. ❏ A headlamp greatly facilitates visualization. ❏ Suture anchors may be employed to secure ligamentous avulsions and should be available.

Positioning

Supine positioning with a hand table will usually suffice. With an associated medial epicondyle fracture, the lateral position or the prone position may be employed as well. (See section on medial epicondyle fractures.)

Approach

The surgical approach will be dictated by the goals of the procedure and based on an estimation of the structures that may be blocking the reduction. Loose osteochondral fracture fragments can block a congruent reduction and CT and/or MRI scanning may be required to visualize the fragments and determine operative approach. The most common structures preventing

reduction via closed means include the distal humerus being buttonholed through the brachialis musculature; the radial head being buttonholed through the capsule and lateral collateral ligament; and entrapment of fracture fragments, especially the medial epicondyle, with their attached ligamentous or muscular structures wedging them in place. If the distal humerus or the radial head is easily palpable in the subcutaneous tissues and not able to be milked out of these tissues through closed means, an operative approach to perform this will be necessary. A lateral approach is best if radial head is noted to be subcutaneous indicating possible block to reduction because of buttonholing through the lateral capsule and around the lateral collateral ligaments.[61,90] A medial approach is best if the distal humerus is noted to be subcutaneous indicating a block to reduction because of buttonholing through the brachialis or if an associated medial epicondyle fracture is present and surgical fixation is planned. With the lateral approach, the radial nerve needs to be protected; with the medial approach, the ulnar needs protection. The median nerve and brachial artery are of concern either way and are best visualized and protected with an anteromedial approach or extensile exposure.

Open Reduction

After making the appropriate approach based on the injury and planned surgical procedures, with gentle spreading of the subcutaneous tissues, the significant soft tissue trauma is evident. The buttonholed distal humerus, the median and ulnar nerves, and the brachial artery should be identified. Any intervening tissue or osteochondral fragments are removed from the interval between the joint surfaces. The joint is then reduced through a similar set of distraction and translational forces as described for the closed reduction techniques. Once reduced, joint stability is evaluated and a thorough assessment of the capsular and ligamentous structures is performed. Primary repair or reattachment of the medial collateral ligament complex with small suture anchors or transosseous drill holes may be performed to improve stability.

Entrapped intra-articular fragments should be removed before mobilizing the elbow. With the capsule disrupted and the joint full of blood clot, early arthroscopic removal of loose bodies is not recommended. Thus, it is preferable to perform loose body removal with an open arthrotomy in the early postreduction period. Given the extensive medial soft tissue disruption, a medial approach with visualization of the joint through the windows created by the injury allows for easy access to all aspects of the joint. Be certain to locate the ulnar nerve and medial antebrachial cutaneous nerves with operative exposure.

Persistent significant elbow instability should prompt a thorough investigation for associated fractures or incongruity of the reduction suggesting incarceration of soft tissue or chondral fragments in the joint.

Fractures associated with elbow dislocations may necessitate reduction and fixation as dictated by the guiding principles for the individual fracture. Failure to reduce and fix fractures associated with an elbow dislocation may lead to persistent instability. As is discussed at length in the first half of this chapter, we prefer to reduce and fix medial epicondyle fractures associated with elbow dislocations.

Open Reduction of an Irreducible Posterior Elbow Dislocation:
KEY SURGICAL STEPS

❏ Make a medially based incision just anterior to the humerus curving distally at the elbow (note that the neurovascular structures may be very subcutaneous because of the injury).
❏ Identify the median and ulnar nerves and the brachial artery. Protect medial antebrachial cutaneous nerves.
❏ Remove any tissue or any other intervening structures.
❏ Visually inspect the joint surfaces and remove any loose osteochondral fragments that are too small to be fixed back in place.
❏ Flex the elbow to about 90 degrees.
❏ Apply force on the forearm in line with the humerus, translating it distally in line with the humeral shaft and opening the joint surface.
❏ Correct any medial or lateral displacement.
❏ Apply a distally directed force in line with the forearm, or directly posteriorly translate the distal humerus to reduce the elbow joint.
❏ Check the elbow reduction with visual evaluation as well as dynamic fluoroscopic evaluation.
❏ Assess elbow stability through range of motion.
❏ Assess the extent of capsular and ligamentous damage and repair critical elements such as the medial ulnar collateral ligament and/or the medial epicondyle (see separate medial epicondyle section).
❏ Reassess elbow stability through range of motion if repairs are performed.
❏ Be certain there is no neurovascular impingement or entrapment.
❏ Immobilize elbow in about 90 degrees of flexion.

Postoperative Care

Immobilization after surgery depends on the procedure performed. After open reduction, management is similar to that after satisfactory closed reduction.

Because the major complication of elbow dislocations is stiffness, the initial full-time immobilization is removed after approximately 1 week and the patient transitioned to a removable splint or the hinged brace is unlocked for progressive motion. The patient begins intermittent protected active elbow motion out of the splint multiple times a day as limited by pain. In a reliable patient with minimal risk of additional trauma, the patient can usually dispense with the splint after 10 to 14 days and use a sling. If there are times at high risk for another fall, a removable splint or brace can be continued up till about 5 to 6 weeks postinjury during these times (i.e., during school) but should be removed at other times of the day when there is minimal risk (i.e., mealtime) to promote range of motion. The emphasis is on early active motion in a safe environment to prevent stiffness that often occurs after this injury. Before reduction, it is important to emphasize to the parents that there may be some loss of motion, especially extension, regardless of the treatment. This is usually less than 30 degrees and not of functional or aesthetic significance. If open reduction is required, mobilization is begun after wounds have healed (1–2 weeks) as described above.

Authors' Preferred Method of Treatment for Posterior Elbow Dislocations (Algorithm 16-2)

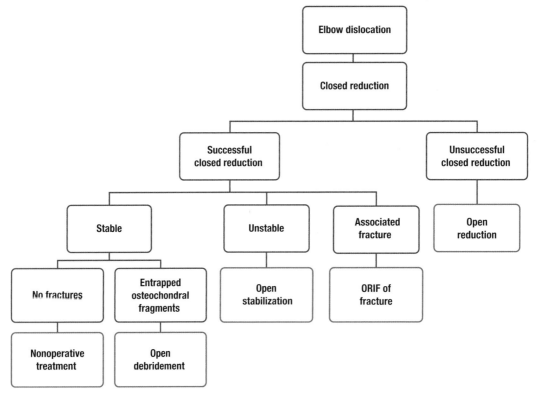

Algorithm 16-2. Authors' preferred treatment for posterior elbow dislocation.

OUTCOMES AND COMPLICATIONS RELATED TO POSTERIOR ELBOW DISLOCATIONS

Di Gennaro et al. evaluated elbow dislocations in children at an average of 15 years of follow-up and found that most patients had a good prognosis.[38] Murphy et al. noted less than excellent outcomes with dislocations associated with multiple fractures, need for operative intervention, and immobilization greater than 2 weeks.

Complications associated with posterior elbow dislocations can be divided into those occurring early and those occurring later. Early complications include neurologic and vascular injuries. Late complications include loss of motion, myositis ossificans, recurrent dislocations, radioulnar synostosis, and cubitus recurvatum. The special problems of chronic, unreduced dislocations are not considered complications of treatment.

Posterior Elbow Dislocations:
COMMON ADVERSE OUTCOMES AND COMPLICATIONS

Early Complications

- Neurologic injuries: Ulnar nerve is the most commonly injured nerve with elbow dislocations with high rate of spontaneous resolution. Median nerve is less common but has higher rate of entrapment requiring surgical intervention.
- Vascular injuries: Injury to the brachial artery can occur requiring surgical decompression and vascular repair if not resolved with closed reduction.

Late Complications

- Loss of elbow range of motion
- Heterotopic bone formation
- Recurrent posterior dislocations
- Radioulnar synostosis
- Cubitus recurvatum

Special Problem

- Unreduced posterior elbow dislocations

Early Complications

Neurologic Injuries

Median Nerve Lesions

The most serious neurologic injury involves the median nerve, which can be damaged directly by the dislocation or can be entrapped within the joint. Median nerve injuries occur most commonly in children 5 to 12 years of age. These injuries, either isolated median nerve (7/317 total dislocations) or combined median and ulnar nerve injuries (4/317 total dislocations), were present in only 3% of dislocations.[102,127,153,156] These injuries can present late[18] and can present after spontaneous elbow reduction.[167]

Fourrier et al.[49] in 1977 delineated three types of medial nerve entrapment (Fig. 16-23).

In type 1 entrapment, the child has an avulsion fracture of the medial epicondyle or has a rupture of the origin of the flexor–pronator muscle and ulnar collateral ligament (see Fig. 16-23A). This

allows the median nerve, with or without the brachial artery, to displace posteriorly, essentially wrapping posteriorly around the medial aspect of the humerus and then coursing distally around the articular surface of the distal humerus. In type 2 entrapment, the nerve is entrapped between the fracture surfaces of the medial epicondyle and the distal humerus (see Fig. 16-23B). Finally, in type 3 entrapment, the nerve is kinked and entrapped between the distal humerus and the olecranon (see Fig. 16-23C).

If median nerve dysfunction is present prior to reduction, it is often difficult to identify nerve entrapment postreduction. Certainly, any significant decrease in median nerve function following a closed reduction or incongruity in the reduction should prompt evaluation for this injury pattern. In some patients with an associated medial epicondyle fracture, the nerve can be so severely damaged after being entrapped that neuroma resection, nerve transposition, and direct repair or grafting is necessary.[17,60] Good recovery of nerve function has been reported after operative decompression and repair.

If the nerve has been entrapped for a considerable period, the Matev sign may be present on the x-rays. This represents a depression on the posterior surface of the medial epicondylar ridge where the nerve has been pressed against the bone.[12,35,60,66,143,145] This groove is seen on x-ray as two sclerotic lines parallel to the nerve. This sign disappears when the nerve has been decompressed.

The combination of an associated fracture of the medial epicondyle and significant median nerve dysfunction was cited by Rao and Crawford[145] as an absolute indication for surgical exploration of the nerve because of the frequency of median nerve entrapment with fractures of the medial epicondyle. This has been reviewed recently by Simon et al.,[167] who came to the same conclusion. MRI may be helpful in defining the course of the median nerve if entrapment is suspected.[2] Electromyography and nerve conduction studies have been utilized to assist in operative decision making. Painful dysesthesias with arc of motion is usually indicative of entrapment. Once the entrapped nerve is removed from the joint, neurologic function typically improves. Resection and repair or nerve grafting may be necessary.

Ulnar Nerve Lesions

In a combined series of 317 patients,[102,123,127,153,156] the most commonly injured nerve was the ulnar nerve. Of the 32 patients (10%) who had nerve symptoms after reduction, 21 had isolated ulnar nerve injuries, 7 had isolated median nerve injuries, and in 4 patients both the median and ulnar nerves were involved. During open reduction of elbow fracture dislocations, the ulnar nerve needs to be identified and protected.[102] Ulnar nerve transposition is recommended if there is concern about the nerve instability or impingement on the fixation screw.

Radial Nerve Lesions

Radial nerve injury with posterior elbow dislocation is very rare. Watson-Jones reported two radial nerve injuries associated with elbow dislocation; in both, the symptoms rapidly resolved after reduction. Rasool[146] reported a third case, which also resolved spontaneously within 4 weeks.

Figure 16-23. Median nerve entrapment. **A:** Type 1. Entrapment within the elbow joint with the median nerve coursing posterior to the distal humerus. **B:** Type 2. Entrapment of the nerve between the fracture surfaces of the medial epicondyle and the medial condyle. **C:** Type 3. Simple kinking of the nerve into the anterior portion of the elbow joint. (Redrawn from Hallett J. Entrapment of the median nerve after dislocation of the elbow. A case report. *J Bone Joint Surg Br.* 1981;63-B(3):408–412, with permission, permission conveyed through Copyright Clearance Center, Inc.)

Arterial Injuries

Arterial injuries are uncommon with posterior elbow dislocations in children and adolescents with only eight vascular injuries (3%) reported in the combined series of 317 patients.[102,127,153,156] However, Carlioz and Abols[28] reported four patients with diminished radial pulses that resolved after reduction. Arterial injuries have been associated with open dislocations in which collateral circulation is disrupted.[71,106,157] In these situations, usually, the brachial artery is ruptured,[63,71,76,106,157] but it can also be thrombosed[179] as well as entrapped in the elbow joint.[72,140,179] Pearce[140] reported an entrapped radial artery in which there was a high bifurcation of the brachial artery. When there is a complete rupture, there usually is evidence of ischemia distally. However, the presence of good capillary circulation to the hand or a Doppler pulse at the wrist does not always mean the artery is intact.[63,76] Arteriograms usually are not necessary because the arterial injury is at the site of the dislocation. If imaging is indicated to evaluate possible arterial injury, its minimal risk and invasiveness make vascular ultrasound an attractive initial imaging choice.

For surgical treatment of vascular injuries about the elbow, simple ligation of the ends has been done in the past with adults, especially if there was good capillary circulation distally.[71] However, this may predispose to late ischemic changes such as claudication, cold sensitivity, or even late amputation. Most investigators recommend direct arterial repair or a vein graft, but this subject remains controversial.[63,76,106,157]

Late Complications

Loss of Motion

Almost all patients with elbow dislocations lose some range of elbow motion.[28,83–85] This loss is less in children than in adults[85] and usually is no more than 10 degrees of extension. This rarely is of functional or aesthetic significance (Fig. 16-24). However, the potential for loss of motion must be explained to the parents before reduction and may be an indication for a supervised rehabilitation program. If there is a displaced medial epicondylar fracture, because of the loss of isometry in the medial ligaments, the loss of major range of motion can be severe and limiting. Similarly, an incongruent elbow joint will have marked limitations of motion. In situations where the loss of motion is greater than 45 to 60 degrees, late operative release, either arthroscopic or open, may be indicated for an elbow release. Successful release requires high level of patient cooperation with extensive therapy.

Myositis Ossificans Versus Heterotopic Calcification

True myositis ossificans should be differentiated from heterotopic calcification, which is a dystrophic process. Myositis ossificans involves ossification within the muscle sheath that can lead to a significant loss of range of motion of the elbow. Disruption of the brachialis muscle is believed to be a contributory factor.[103] Fortunately, myositis ossificans is rare in children.[85] Although heterotopic calcification in the ligaments and capsule of the elbow is common,[85,153] it rarely results in loss of elbow function.

Figure 16-24. Outcomes. **A, B:** AP and lateral radiographs of a posterolateral elbow dislocation in a 10-year-old gymnast. **C, D:** AP and lateral radiographs after elbow reduction and ORIF of the medial epicondyle with a single 4.0-mm cannulated screw. **E:** Clinical photograph taken 6 months postoperatively. The patient has returned to full activities and is satisfied with her function. Note the slight loss of motion in the right elbow, which can extend to 0 degrees, but is not able to hyperextend like her uninvolved left elbow.

In Neviaser and Wickstrom's[127] series of 115 patients, 10 had x-ray evidence of myositis ossificans; all, however, were asymptomatic. Roberts[153] differentiated true myositis ossificans from heterotopic calcification in his series of 60 elbow dislocations and noted that only three patients had true myositis ossificans. Linscheid and Wheeler[102] reported that the incidence of some type of heterotopic calcification was 28%, which was most common around the condyles. Only in five patients was it anterior to the capsule (which probably represented true myositis ossificans

in the brachialis muscle). Four of these patients had some decrease in elbow function. Josefsson et al.[85] reported that 61% of 28 children with posterior dislocations had periarticular calcification, but this did not appear to be functionally significant.

Radioulnar Synostosis

In dislocations with an associated fracture of the radial neck, the incidence of a secondary proximal radioulnar synostosis is

A, B   **C**

Figure 16-25. Radioulnar synostosis. An 11-year-old boy fell, injuring his nondominant left elbow. An elbow dislocation was reduced by emergency personnel prior to arrival at the hospital. **A:** Initial radiographs demonstrated a significantly displaced radial neck fracture. This was reduced using percutaneous techniques. **B:** Five months later radiographs and (**C**) a CT scan noted a complete radioulnar synostosis.

increased (Fig. 16-25). This can occur regardless of whether the radial neck fracture is treated operatively or nonoperatively[25,28,131] and likely occurs because of the extensive periosteal stripping that occurs along the anterior aspect of the forearm between the proximal radius and ulna. Carlioz and Abols[28] reported a synostosis in one of three patients with posterior elbow dislocations associated with radial neck fractures.

Cubitus Recurvatum

Occasionally, a severe elbow dislocation results in significant tearing of the anterior capsule. As a result, after reduction, when all the stiffness created by the dislocation has subsided, the patient may have some hyperextension (cubitus recurvatum) of the elbow. This is usually minimally symptomatic but if asymmetric, may be aesthetically disturbing to the parents and adolescent.

Posterolateral Rotatory Instability

O'Driscoll et al.[130] described posterolateral instability in five patients, including two children, in whom laxity of the ulnar part of the radial collateral ligament allowed a transitory rotary subluxation of the ulnohumeral joint and a secondary dislocation of the radiohumeral joint. This was confirmed with a report of another nine pediatric patients, most of whom had a history of posterior elbow dislocation.[99] Patients with posterolateral instability often complain of a feeling of apprehension with certain activities or describe a history of recurrent temporary dislocation of the elbow but, when examined, exhibit no unusual clinical findings. They also may present with contracture. The instability is diagnosed with a posterolateral rotary instability test, which is done by holding the patient's arm over

the head while applying proximal axial compression plus a valgus and supination force to the forearm (Fig. 16-26). As the elbow is slowly flexed from an extended position, the radial head, which is initially posteriorly subluxated, reduces producing the appreciation of a "clunk" or "shift." In some cases, the only positive finding is apprehension with the examination; in others, posterolateral rotary instability can be detected only with the patient completely relaxed under general anesthesia. The prone push-up test (performed with the forearms

Figure 16-26. Posterolateral rotary instability. Posterolateral rotational instability is best demonstrated with the upper extremity over the head with the patient supine. The radial head can be subluxated or dislocated by applying a valgus and supination force to the forearm at the same time proximal axial compression is applied along the forearm. (Reprinted with permission from O'Driscoll SW, et al. Posterolateral rotatory instability of the elbow. *J Bone Joint Surg Am.* 1991;73(3):440–446.)

Figure 16-27. Pathology associated with recurrent elbow dislocations. The three components that allow the elbow to dislocate: a lax ulnar collateral ligament, a "pocket" in the radial collateral ligament, and a defect in the lateral condyle. (Adapted from Osborne G, Cotterill P. Recurrent dislocation of the elbow. *J Bone Joint Surg Br.* 1966;48(2):340–346, permission conveyed through Copyright Clearance Center, Inc.)

maximally supinated) or the chair push-up test (also performed with the arms maximally supinated) can often reproduce the patient's symptoms of pain or a feeling of subluxation or apprehension in the office setting, and thus can often help establish the diagnosis. O'Driscoll et al.[130] reported that surgical repair of the lax ulnar portion of the radial collateral ligament eliminated the posterolateral rotary instability. In children and adolescents, the same instability can occur from cartilage nonunion of the origin of the radial collateral ligament.

Recurrent Posterior Dislocations

Recurrent posterior elbow dislocation is rare. In the combined series of dislocations, only 2 of 317 patients (0.6%) experienced recurrent dislocations.[102,127,153,156] Approximately 80% of recurrent dislocations are in males. Three investigators have reported bilateral cases.[88,147] The pathology of recurrent dislocation involves any or all of a combination of collateral ligament instability, capsular laxity, and bone and articular cartilage defects.

Contributing Pathology

Osborne and Cotterill[132] suggested that articular changes are secondary and that the primary defect is a failure of the posterolateral ligamentous and capsular structures to become reattached after reduction (Fig. 16-27). Osborne and Cotterill[132] proposed that the extensive articular cartilage covering the surface of the distal humerus leaves little surface area for soft tissue reattachment and the presence of synovial fluid further inhibits soft tissue healing. With recurrent dislocations, the radial head impinges against the posterolateral margin of the capitellum, creating an osteochondral defect. In addition to the defect in the capitellar articular surface, a similar defect develops in the anterior articular margin of the radial head. When these two defects oppose each other, recurrence of the dislocation is more likely. Subsequent studies have confirmed these findings in almost all recurrent dislocations, especially in children.[43,70,130] In addition to the osteochondral defects in the capitellum and radial head, bone defects may include a shallow semilunar notch resulting

from a coronoid fossa process fracture or multiple recurrent dislocations.

Treatment Options

There is only one report of successful nonsurgical management of recurrent elbow dislocations. Herring and Sullivan[74] used an orthosis that blocked the last 15 degrees of extension. After his patient wore this orthosis constantly for 2 years and with vigorous activities for another 6 months, there were no further dislocations, but the follow-up period was only 1 year. Beaty and Donati[14] emphasized that physical therapy and the use of an orthosis should be tried before surgery is considered.

Because nonsurgical management is so often unsuccessful, the treatment of recurrent posterior elbow dislocations is predominately surgical. Various surgical procedures have been described to correct bone and soft tissue abnormalities (Fig. 16-28).

Bony procedures are directed toward correcting dysplasia of the semilunar notch of the olecranon. Both boomerang-shaped bone blocks and simple bone blocks have been used (see Fig. 16-28A). Mantle[113] increased the slope of the semilunar notch in two patients with an opening wedge osteotomy of the coronoid process (see Fig. 16-28B).

Various soft tissue procedures have been described as well. Reichenheim[147] and King[91] transferred the biceps tendon just distal to the coronoid process to reinforce it (see Fig. 16-28C). Kapel[88] developed a cruciate ligament-type reconstruction in which distally based strips of the biceps and triceps tendon were passed through the distal humerus (see Fig. 16-28D). Beaty and Donati[14] modified this technique by transferring a central slip of the triceps through the humerus posterior to anterior and attaching it to the proximal ulna.

The most widely accepted technique is that described by Osborne and Cotterill,[132] in which the lateral capsule is reattached to the posterolateral aspect of the capitellum with sutures passing through holes drilled in the bone (see Fig. 16-28E). The joint should be inspected at surgery because osteocartilaginous loose bodies may be present.[70,112] Since Osborne and Cotterill's[132] initial report of eight patients, successful use of

Figure 16-28. Surgical procedures for recurrent dislocation. **A:** Simple coronoid bone block. **B:** Open wedge coronoid osteotomy. **C:** Biceps tendon transfer to coronoid process. **D:** Cruciate ligament reconstruction. **E:** Lateral capsular reattachment of Osborne and Cotterill. (**A, C, D,** and **E:** Adapted with permission from Osborne G, Cotterill P. Recurrent dislocation of the elbow. *J Bone Joint Surg Br.* 1966;48(2):340–346, permission conveyed through Copyright Clearance Center, Inc.)

this technique has been reported in numerous others.[43,70,112,130] Zeier[184] and O'Driscoll et al.[130] reinforced the lateral repair with strips of fascia lata, triceps fascia, or palmaris longus tendon.

Postoperative Care

Postoperatively, especially after the repair described by Osborne and Cotterill,[132] the arm is immobilized in a long arm cast with the elbow flexed 90 degrees for 4 to 6 weeks. Protected active range-of-motion exercises are performed for an additional 4 to 6 weeks. Strenuous activities are avoided for 12 weeks postoperative.

Complications

Major complications after correction of recurrent dislocations include loose osteocartilaginous fragments and destruction of the articular surface of the joint, elbow stiffness, or recurrent instability.

Unreduced Posterior Elbow Dislocations

Untreated posterior dislocations of the elbow in children are extremely rare in North America. Most reported series are from other countries.[50]

Children with untreated dislocations typically have pain and limited midrange of motion. Pathologically, there is usually subperiosteal new bone formation that produces a radiohumeral

horn, myositis ossificans of the brachialis muscle, capsular contractures, shortening of the triceps muscle, contractures of the medial and lateral collateral ligaments, and compression of the ulnar nerve.[49,50] These factors have to be considered when planning treatment.

Treatment Options

Closed reduction of dislocations recognized within 3 weeks of injury may be possible.[4,50] If this fails or if the dislocation is of longer duration, open reduction is necessary.

Open reduction through a posterior approach involves lengthening of the triceps muscle and decompression or transposition of the ulnar nerve.[50] Satisfactory results usually can be obtained if a stable concentric reduction is achieved within 3 months of the initial dislocation.[4] Results after surgical reconstruction decline thereafter but still may produce some improvement in function.[37,50,110,121,124] After reduction, stabilization of the elbow joint with transarticular pins, external fixation, or newer internal fixation devices may be considered.[5,50,124,170]

Mahaisavariya et al.[111] reported improved extension and better functional results 1 to 3 months after injury in 34 patients with chronic elbow dislocation reconstruction in whom the triceps tendon was not lengthened compared with 38 patients who had the triceps lengthened at surgery.

ANTERIOR ELBOW DISLOCATIONS

Anterior elbow dislocations are rare. Of the 317 elbows in the combined series,[102,127,153,156] only 5 were anterior, for an incidence of slightly over 1%. They are associated with an increased incidence of complications, such as brachial artery disruption and associated fractures, compared with posterior dislocations.

Assessment of Anterior Elbow Dislocations

Anterior elbow dislocations usually are caused by a direct blow to the posterior aspect of the flexed elbow.[79] Hyperextension of the elbow also has been implicated in one study.

The elbow is held in extension upon presentation. There is fullness in the antecubital fossa. Swelling usually is marked because of the soft tissue disruption associated with this type of dislocation. There is severe pain with attempted motion. A careful neurovascular examination is mandatory.

Routine AP and lateral x-rays are diagnostic. In most cases, the proximal radius and ulna dislocate in an anteromedial direction (Fig. 16-29). As with posterior dislocations, postreduction radiographs should be carefully scrutinized for a congruent reduction and for subtle osteochondral fracture fragments. Evaluation with CT or MRI can be used to further define the extent of soft tissue injury in complex injury patterns.

Associated fractures are common. In children, the triceps insertion may be avulsed from the olecranon with a small piece of cortical bone or even a displaced fracture through the olecranon itself.[64] Inoue and Horii[79] reported an 11-year-old girl with an anterior elbow dislocation with displaced fractures of the trochlea, capitellum, and lateral epicondyle. These were repaired with open reduction and internal fixation using Herbert bone screws. A recent report reviews three cases, all of which had

fractures.[21] Interestingly, the displaced olecranon fracture was not visualized in one of the cases because of the children's age, thus prompting a warning from the authors in children under age 10. Fixation options from these studies varied from tension band constructs and plate fixation for the olecranon fractures and cannulated screws for the medial epicondyle.

There appears to be an increased incidence of brachial artery rupture or thrombosis associated with anterior elbow dislocations. As discussed with posterior elbow dislocations, early and persistent vigilance for circulatory issues should be exercised. When compromised, as discussed above in more detail with posterior elbow dislocations, a prompt evaluation with consideration for arterial repair or reconstruction with vein grafting may be necessary.

Treatment of Anterior Elbow Dislocations

As with posterior elbow dislocations, because of the significant amount of soft tissue swelling and potential for neurovascular compromise, all anterior elbow dislocations should be reduced with adequate analgesia and relaxation as soon as possible. Consideration for nonoperative treatment following closed reduction should be considered if the elbow is stable through close to a functional range of motion, a concentric anatomic reduction can be obtained and maintained, and there is no evidence to suggest a vascular injury, nerve entrapment, or significant intra-articular osteochondral fragments.

Surgery usually is not required unless the dislocation is open, there is a brachial artery injury, or there is an associated fracture that does not realign satisfactorily after closed reduction. Open reduction and internal fixation of the fracture may then be necessary.[79]

Reduction usually is accomplished by flexing the elbow and pushing the forearm proximally and downward at the same time. As with posterior dislocations, a force must first be applied longitudinally along the axis of the humerus with the

Figure 16-29. Anterior dislocation of the elbow. **A:** Initial lateral radiograph. The olecranon lies anterior to the distal humerus. **B:** Initial anteroposterior radiograph. The proximal ulna and radial head lie anteromedial, and the elbow carrying angle is in varus. (Courtesy of Hilario Trevino, MD.)

Figure 16-30. Reduction of anterior dislocation. **A:** With the elbow semi-flexed, a longitudinal force is applied along the long axis of the humerus (*arrow 1*). Pulling distally on the forearm may be necessary to initially dislodge the olecranon. **B:** Once the olecranon is distal to the humerus, the distal humerus is pushed anteriorly (*arrow 2*) whereas a proximally directed force is applied along the long axis of the forearm (*arrow 3*). **C:** Finally, the elbow is immobilized in some extension (*arrow 4*).

elbow semiflexed to overcome the forces of the biceps and triceps. The longitudinal force along the axis of the forearm is directed toward the elbow (Fig. 16-30). To make reduction easier, the distal humerus can be forced in an anterior direction by pushing on the posterior aspect of the distal arm.

Because most anterior dislocations occur in flexion, the elbow should be immobilized in some extension for 1 to 3 weeks, followed by protected active range-of-motion exercises. Early motion after open reduction and internal fixation of an associated olecranon fracture usually can be allowed.[79]

MEDIAL AND LATERAL ELBOW DISLOCATIONS

Medial and lateral elbow dislocations are also rare types of dislocations. In the recent series of 145 pediatric elbow dislocations, Murphy reported 10 medial dislocations and no lateral dislocations.[123]

Assessment of Medial and Lateral Elbow Dislocations

In a complete lateral dislocation, the olecranon is displaced lateral to the capitellum. This gives the elbow a markedly widened appearance. In an incomplete lateral dislocation, the semilunar notch articulates with the capitulotrochlear groove, and the radial head appears more prominent laterally. There is often good flexion and extension of the elbow, increasing the likelihood that a lateral dislocation will be overlooked. Similarly, in a medial dislocation, the forearm appears translated medially relative to the humerus.

AP x-rays of the elbow usually are diagnostic. On the lateral view, the elbow may appear reduced (Fig. 16-31).

Treatment of Medial and Lateral Elbow Dislocations

These rare dislocations can be treated by closed reduction in virtually all patients.[182] A longitudinal force is applied along the axis of the humerus to distract the elbow, and then direct medial or lateral pressure (opposite the direction of the dislocation) is applied over the proximal forearm.

DIVERGENT ELBOW DISLOCATION

Divergent dislocation represents a posterior elbow dislocation with disruption of the interosseous membrane between the proximal radius and ulna with the radial head displaced laterally and the proximal ulna medially (Fig. 16-32). These dislocations are extremely rare.[9,26,36,55,77,78,117,125,164]

Assessment of Divergent Dislocations

Divergent dislocations are often caused by high-energy trauma. Associated fractures of the radial neck, proximal ulna, and coronoid process are common.[1,26,46] It has been speculated that, in addition to the hyperextension of the elbow that produces the dislocation, a strong proximally directed force is applied parallel to the long axis of the forearm, disrupting the annular ligament and interosseous membrane and allowing the divergence of the proximal radius and ulna. In a cadaveric study, Altuntas et al.[6] confirmed that only after release of all the ligamentous stabilizers of the elbow and release of the intraosseous membrane from the elbow to the distal third of the forearm could a divergent dislocation be replicated.

Treatment of Divergent Dislocations

Divergent dislocations are typically easily reduced using closed reduction under general anesthesia. Reduction is achieved by applying longitudinal traction with the elbow semiextended and at the same time compressing the proximal radius and ulna together.

Figure 16-31. A 12-year-old girl experienced a lateral elbow dislocation while playing basketball. **A, B:** AP and lateral radiographs demonstrate lateral translation of radius and ulna. Soft tissue shadows reflect visible clinical deformity in which forearm is laterally displaced relative to the arm. **C, D:** Images following attempted close reduction under general anesthesia confirm incarceration of the fractured medial epicondyle fragment within the elbow joint and incomplete reduction. **E, F:** Three months following open reduction and internal fixation of the medial epicondyle fragment, the elbow joint is concentrically reduced, and elbow range of motion is restricted from –20 degrees of extension to 125 degrees of flexion.

After successful closed reduction, the elbow is immobilized in 90 degrees of flexion and the forearm in neutral. Postreduction CT scan may be useful to confirm the anatomic relationships have been restored between the humerus, radius, and ulna, as well as to evaluate for possible fracture displacement.[181] Active range-of-motion exercises are then begun after approximately 2 to 3 weeks following the injury. Most patients regain full elbow motion, including forearm pronation and supination.

PROXIMAL RADIOULNAR TRANSLOCATIONS

Translocation of the proximal radius and ulna is another extremely rare injury with only case reports being described in the English literature.[10,26,27,31,45,57,69,80]

Assessment of Proximal Radioulnar Translocations

Radioulnar translocation is commonly missed on the AP x-ray unless the proximal radius and ulna are noted to be completely

A, B   **C**

Figure 16-32. Mediolateral divergent dislocation. **A:** Anteroposterior view demonstrating disruption of the proximal radioulnar joint with the radius lateral and the ulna medial. **B:** Lateral radiograph confirms that the radius and ulna are both posterior to the distal humerus. **C:** A radiograph taken 4 weeks after injury shows periosteal new bone formation (*arrows*), indicating where the soft tissues were extensively torn away from the proximal ulna.

reversed in relation to the distal humerus. Translocations are believed to be caused by a fall onto the pronated hand with the elbow in full or nearly full extension, producing an axial force on the proximal radius. The anterior radial head dislocation occurs first, followed by the posterior dislocation of the olecranon. Combourieu et al.[31] suggest that avulsion of the brachialis insertion is necessary for the radial head to translate medially. The radial head, depending on the degree of pronation, can be lodged in the coronoid fossa or dislocated posteriorly. As a consequence, fractures of the radial head, radial neck, or coronoid process may occur.[26,27,45] Harvey and Tchelebi[69] reported a case in which the cause of radioulnar translocation may have been iatrogenic: the result of inappropriate technique used to reduce a posterior elbow dislocation.

Swelling and pain may obscure the initial examination, and minimal deformity may be apparent. Once pain has been adequately managed with analgesics, the most consistent finding on clinical examination is limited elbow range of motion, especially in supination.

Radial neck fracture is the most common fracture associated with proximal radioulnar translocation.[77,45,80] Eklof et al[45] also reported one patient who sustained a fracture of the tip of the coronoid. Proposed soft tissue injuries include radial collateral ligament, medial collateral ligament, annular ligament, interosseous ligament, and avulsion of the brachialis.[31,45,80] Transient ulnar nerve paresthesia that resolved after reduction of the translocation has been reported in several patients.[31,80] Osteonecrosis of the radial head was noted in one patient after open

reduction of a proximal radioulnar translocation and premature closure of the proximal radial physis has been reported.[31,69]

Treatment of Proximal Radioulnar Translocations

Successful closed reduction of proximal radioulnar translocation has been reported.[31,80] The patient must be completely relaxed under general anesthesia, as sedation or regional anesthesia is unlikely to provide sufficient relaxation. With the elbow flexed approximately 90 degrees, longitudinal traction is applied to the elbow while the forearm is supinated (Fig. 16-33). If the radial head can be palpated, gentle anterior-directed pressure may help slide the radial head and neck over the coronoid process, allowing the proximal radius and ulna to resume their normal configuration. As always, just the right amount of force should be used; excessive force risks iatrogenic fracture to the proximal radius. Successful closed reduction should be confirmed on x-ray, and the elbow should be immobilized for approximately 3 to 4 weeks with the forearm supinated and the elbow flexed 90 to 100 degrees.

Radioulnar translocations may require open reduction.[26,27,45,57,69,80] A lateral approach provides adequate exposure to the translocation and radial neck fracture if present. At surgery, the radial head and neck are typically found trapped beneath the trochlea of the distal humerus. Elbow extension tightens the biceps tendon, making reduction more difficult. With the elbow flexed, a freer or joker elevator can be placed beneath the radial head and neck facilitating delivery over the coronoid process as

Figure 16-33. Proximal radioulnar translocation. **A:** Position of the proximal radius and ulna with a proximal radioulnar translocation. **B:** Closed reduction is rarely successful but may be attempted under general anesthesia using gentle longitudinal traction while supinating the forearm. (Redrawn with permission from Harvey S, Tchelebi H. Proximal radioulnar translocation. A case report. *J Bone Joint Surg Am.* 1979;61(3):447–449.)

the forearm is supinated. If present, a radial neck fracture may now be treated in standard fashion. Internal fixation also may be necessary for an unstable displaced fracture.

Harvey and Tchelebi[69] used an osteotomy of the proximal ulna to expose and reduce the radius that was complicated by a postoperative ulnar nerve paralysis that recovered completely over 2 months. Just like after successful closed reduction, following open reduction, the upper extremity is immobilized for approximately 3 to 4 weeks with the forearm supinated and the elbow flexed 90 to 100 degrees, followed by active elbow range-of-motion exercises.

PULLED ELBOW SYNDROME

INTRODUCTION TO PULLED ELBOW SYNDROME

Subluxation of the annular ligament, or pulled elbow syndrome, is a common elbow injury in young children.[7,30,78,81] The term "nursemaid's elbow" and other synonyms have been used to describe this condition. The demographics associated with subluxation of the radial head have been well described.[7,30,78,81] The mean age at injury is 2 to 3 years, with the youngest reported patient 2 months of age. It rarely occurs after 7 years of age; 60% to 65% of the children affected are girls, and the left elbow is involved in approximately 70%. It is difficult to determine the actual incidence because many subluxations are treated in

primary care physician's offices, by parents, or resolve spontaneously before being seen by a physician.

Mechanisms of Injury for Pulled Elbow Syndrome

Longitudinal traction on the extended elbow is the usual mechanism of injury (Fig. 16-34), although other mechanisms such as falls or direct blows have been described.[100] Cadaver studies have shown that longitudinal traction on the extended elbow can produce a partial slippage of the annular ligament over the head of the radius and into the radiocapitellar joint, sometimes tearing the subannular membrane.[121,159] Displacement of the annular ligament occurs most easily with the forearm in pronation. In this position, the lateral edge of the radial head, which opposes the main portion of the annular ligament, is narrow and round at its margin. In supination, the lateral edge of the radial head is wider and more square at its margin, thereby restricting slippage of the annular ligament. McRae and Freeman[119] demonstrated that forearm pronation maintained the displacement of the annular ligament.

After 5 years of age, the distal attachments of the subannular membrane and annular ligament to the neck of the radius have strengthened sufficiently to prevent its tearing and subsequent displacement.[159] Previously, the theory was proposed that the radial head diameter was less in children than in adults and this contributed to subluxation of the annular ligament. However, cadaver studies of infants, children, and adults have shown that the ratio of the head and neck diameters is essentially the same.[159] Griffin[62] suggested that the lack of ossification of the proximal radial epiphysis in children less than 5 years of age made it more pliable, thereby facilitating slippage of the annular ligament.

Amir et al.[7] performed a controlled study comparing 30 normal children with 100 who had pulled elbow syndrome. They found an increased frequency of hypermobility or ligamentous laxity among children with pulled elbows. Also, there was an increased frequency of hypermobility in one or both parents of the involved children compared with noninvolved children, suggesting that hypermobility could be a factor predisposing children to this condition.

Thus, the most widely accepted mechanism is that the injury occurs when the forearm is pronated, the elbow extended, and longitudinal traction is applied to the patient's wrist or hand (see Fig. 16-34).[119,162] Such an injury typically occurs when a young child is lifted or swung by the forearm or when the child suddenly steps down from a step or off a curb while one of the parents is holding the hand or wrist.

Newman[128] reported that five of six infants under 6 months of age with a pulled elbow sustained the injury when rolling over in bed with the extended elbow trapped under the body. It was believed that this maneuver, especially if the infant was given a quick push to turn over by an older sibling or a parent, provided enough longitudinal traction to displace the annular ligament proximally.

Signs and Symptoms of Pulled Elbow Syndrome

The history is usually that of an episode of a longitudinal pull on the elbow of the young child. The initial pain usually subsides

Figure 16-34. The injury most commonly occurs when a longitudinal pull is applied to the upper extremity. Usually, the forearm is pronated. There may be a partial tear in the subannular membrane, allowing the annular ligament to subluxate into the radiocapitellar joint.

rapidly, and the child does not appear to be in distress except that they are reluctant to use the involved extremity. The upper extremity is typically held at the side with the forearm pronated. A limited painless arc of flexion and extension may be present; however, any attempt to supinate the forearm produces pain and is met with resistance. Although there is no evidence of an elbow effusion, local tenderness may be present over the radial head and annular ligament. In some patients, the pain may be referred proximally to the shoulder and many complain of pain distally toward the wrist, usually on the dorsal forearm.[7,78]

Unfortunately, the classic history is not always present.[30,144,158,162] In some studies, 33% to 49% of patients had no clear history of longitudinal traction to the elbow.[158,162] In patients without a witnessed longitudinal traction injury, other causes, such as occult fracture or early septic arthritis, must be carefully ruled out.

Imaging and Other Diagnostic Studies for Pulled Elbow Syndrome

Radiography

If there is a reliable history of traction to the elbow, the child is 5 years of age or younger, and the clinical findings strongly support the diagnosis, x-rays are not necessary.[7,30,144,159,175] However, if there is an atypical history or clinical examination, x-rays should be obtained to be certain that there is not a fracture before manipulation is attempted.

AP and lateral x-rays usually are normal,[20,30,62,144,159,162,169] but subtle abnormalities may be present. Normally, the line down the center of the proximal radial shaft should pass through the center of the ossification center of the capitellum (radiocapitellar line).[53,169] Careful review of x-rays may demonstrate the radial capitellar line to be lateral to the center of the capitellum in

up to 25% of patients.[53,169] Determination of this subtle change requires a direct measurement on the x-ray. Interestingly, the pulled elbow can be reduced by the radiology technician because the elbow x-rays are usually taken with the forearm supinated. The subluxation is reduced inadvertently when the technician places the forearm into supination to position it for the x-ray. Bretland[19] suggested that if the best x-ray that can be obtained is an oblique view with the forearm in pronation, pulled elbow syndrome is the likely diagnosis.

Ultrasonography

When the diagnosis is not evident, ultrasonography may be helpful,[95] although not always reliable.[160] The diagnosis is made by demonstrating an increase in the echo-negative area between the articular surfaces of the capitellum and the radial head and increased radial capitellar distance. Kosuwon et al.[95] found that this distance is normally about 3.8 mm with forearm pronated. With a subluxated radial head, this measured 7.2 mm. A difference of 3 mm between the normal and affected sides, therefore, suggests radial head subluxation.

Magnetic Resonance Imaging

While MRI is rarely indicated, if the source of elbow pain and disability is in doubt, and diagnoses such as fracture or infection are being considered, MRI may be helpful. Richardson described such a case in which subluxation of the annular ligament was revealed on MRI, reduction of the annular ligament performed while the patient was sedated in the MRI scanner, and additional images were obtained to confirm restoration of the annular ligament to its anatomically correct position.[149]

TREATMENT OPTIONS FOR PULLED ELBOW SYNDROME

Nonoperative Treatment of Pulled Elbow Syndrome

Closed Reduction

Virtually all annular ligament subluxations are successfully treated by closed reduction. The traditional reduction maneuver has been to supinate the forearm.[30,62,78,144,162] Some authors have recommended that supination be done with the elbow flexed, and others have found that supination alone with the elbow extended can affect a reduction. In many patients, a snapping sensation can be both heard and palpated when the annular ligament reduces.

As an alternative, hyperpronation may also be used as a reduction maneuver.[15,16,96,108] Macias reported that reduction was successful in 40 of 41 patients (98%) in the hyperpronation group compared with 38 of 44 patients (86%) in the supination group. They concluded that the hyperpronation technique was more successful, required fewer attempts, and was often successful when supination failed.

Prereduction Planning

It is important to elicit a reliable history as to whether or not the child had a traction force applied across the extended elbow. The entire extremity is then carefully examined. Focal tenderness should be present directly over the radiocapitellar joint. If the history or physical examination is not entirely consistent with annular ligament subluxation, then x-rays of the upper extremity are obtained to assess for other injuries before manipulating the elbow.

Technique

Closed Reduction of Annular Ligament Subluxation:
KEY STEPS

- ☐ Obtain accurate history for evidence of appropriate injury mechanism.
- ☐ Examination should demonstrate the elbow to be held in extension with no visible deformity but with tenderness at radiocapitellar joint.
- ☐ Perform AP and lateral elbow radiographs if history or examination is not consistent with annular ligament subluxation.
- ☐ Perform initial reduction maneuver by supinating forearm with elbow in hyperflexion.
- ☐ After 10 minutes, if no resolution of symptoms, then perform alternative reduction maneuver with forearm extension and hyperpronation.

Once the diagnosis of annular ligament subluxation is clearly established, reduction is performed. It is first explained to the parents that there will be a brief episode of pain followed by relief of the symptoms. The patient usually is seated on the parent's lap. The patient's forearm is held with the elbow extended while the thumb of the surgeon's opposite hand is placed over the lateral aspect of the elbow (Fig. 16-35). The forearm is then supinated and brought into hyperflexion. Gentle side-to-side pronation–supination in this position may help the annular ligament slip back in place over the radial head. A palpable or audible "click" may be appreciated as the annular ligament reduces. If no improvement is noted after 10 minutes, perform the alternative hyperextension-extension reduction maneuver.

Figure 16-35. Supination reduction technique for nursemaid's elbow. **Left:** The forearm is first supinated. **Right:** The elbow is then hyperflexed. The surgeon's thumb is placed laterally over the radial head to feel the characteristic snapping as the ligament is reduced.

What should be done if a definite snap or pop is not felt or if the patient fails to use the extremity after manipulation? In a subgroup of patients, discomfort may persist despite successful annular ligament reduction. If the subluxation has occurred more than 12 to 24 hours before the child is seen, there often is a mild secondary synovitis, and recovery may not be immediate and dramatic. One must confirm that the initial diagnosis was correct. If not taken before the manipulation, x-rays should be obtained and the entire extremity carefully reexamined. If the x-ray results are normal and the elbow can be fully flexed with free supination and pronation, the physician can be assured that the subluxated annular ligament has been reduced. Reexamination clinically and by x-ray in 5 to 10 days may be appropriate.

Postreduction Care

The value of immobilizing the elbow following reduction has been debated. Taha[173] reported a decreased rate of recurrence during the 10 days following reduction if the elbow was splinted in a flexed supinated position for 2 days following reduction. Salter and Zaltz[159] recommended the use of a sling, mainly to prevent the elbow from being pulled a second time. Kohlhaas and Roeder[94] recommended a T-shirt technique for flexed elbow stabilization in very young children. This provides adequate immobilization without the use of a sling by pinning the sleeve of the long-sleeved T-shirt to the opposite chest. In general, after a successful closed reduction of a first-time annular ligament subluxation, immobilization of the extremity is not necessary if the child is comfortable and using the arm normally. After the reduction, it is important to explain to the parents the mechanism of injury and to emphasize the need to prevent longitudinal pulling on the upper extremities. Picking the child up under the axillae and avoiding games such as "ring around the rosie" involving longitudinal traction to the arm are stressed. However, recurrence rate is high even with the most diligent parents. Therefore, instruction in home reduction of the pulled elbow is useful and reduces the number of visits to the ED and primary care physician.

Operative Treatment of Pulled Elbow Syndrome

Even if untreated, most annular ligament subluxations eventually reduce spontaneously. There are no reported cases of negative long-term sequelae following untreated annular ligament subluxation. Therefore, open reduction is rarely, if ever, indicated for annular ligament subluxation. An indication for surgery might be the chronic, symptomatic, irreducible subluxation.[32,175] In such a circumstance, the annular ligament may need to be partially transected to achieve reduction.

OUTCOMES AND COMPLICATIONS RELATED TO PULLED ELBOW SYNDROME

There are no reports of long-term sequelae from unrecognized and unreduced subluxations. Almost all subluxations reduce spontaneously. The only problem seems to be discomfort to the patient until the annular ligament reduces.

Recurrent Subluxations

The reported incidence of recurrent subluxation has varied from 5% to 39%.[30,62,78,144,162,174] Children 2 years of age or younger appear to be at greatest risk for recurrence.[162,175] Recurrent subluxations usually respond to the same manipulative procedure as the initial injury. They eventually cease after 4 to 5 years when the annular ligament strengthens and ligament laxity lessens. Recurrences do not lead to any long-term sequelae. If recurrent annular ligament subluxation significantly impacts a patient's quality of life because of pain or limited activity, immobilization in an above-elbow cast with the forearm in supination or neutral position for 2 to 3 weeks is usually effective at preventing recurrence.

SUMMARY, CONTROVERSIES, AND FUTURE DIRECTIONS RELATED TO MEDIAL EPICONDYLE FRACTURES AND ELBOW DISLOCATIONS

Most dislocations of the elbow in children and adolescents can be successfully managed nonoperatively. Recurrent dislocation and instability appear to be very rare complications with stiffness being a much more common potential occurrence. Following elbow dislocation reduction, patients may be successfully managed in a well-padded posterior splint for 5 to 10 days at which time a removable splint may be applied and early elbow range of motion initiated. Medial epicondyle fractures commonly occur in association with elbow dislocation and the treating physician must have a high index of suspicion for this injury. Careful physical examination and thoughtful use of imaging studies will allow the treating physician to detect medial epicondyle fractures in all patients. The most common cause of a missed medial epicondyle fracture is that the treating physician did not think to specifically look for this injury. There is general agreement that medial epicondyle fractures displaced less than 2 mm can be effectively treated with immediate splint immobilization and initiation of active elbow range of motion 5 to 10 days following the injury. Medial epicondyle fractures entrapped within the elbow joint must be extracted, with open reduction and stable internal fixation allowing early elbow range of motion indicated in most patients. Controversy remains regarding treatment of medial epicondyle fractures displaced more than 2 mm. Shared decision making with patient and family, considering activity demands, dominant extremity, and displacement allow formulation of an optimal treatment strategy for each patient. Better implants, improved surgical technique, greater appreciation of the importance of the ulnar collateral ligament function, and increased understanding of the degree of displacement in fractures previously thought to be nondisplaced, all contribute to a general trend toward more frequent surgical treatment of medial epicondyle fractures.

ACKNOWLEDGMENTS

We thank James H. Beaty, James R. Kasser, Stephen D. Heinrich, Kaye Wilkins, George Thompson, Anthony Stans, and Todd Milbrandt for their contributions to this chapter. The information presented in this chapter is based on their efforts in previous editions.

Annotated References

Reference	Annotation
Di Gennaro GL, Spina M, Fosco M, et al. Dislocations of the elbow in children: long-term follow-up. *Musculoskel Surg*. 2013;97(Suppl 1):3–7.	Thirty-six nonoperative elbow dislocation patients were followed for an average of 15 years demonstrating no recurrent dislocation and good results overall.
Edmonds EW. How displaced are "nondisplaced" fractures of the medial humeral epicondyle in children? Results of a three-dimensional computed tomography analysis. *J Bone Joint Surg Am*. 2010;92(17):2785–2791.	A prospective study comparing CT and standard radiograph imaging which demonstrates that standard radiograph interpretation consistently underappreciates medial epicondyle fracture displacement.

Annotated References	
Reference	**Annotation**
Glotzbecker MP, Shore B, Matheney T, et al. Alternative technique for open reduction and fixation of displaced pediatric medial epicondyle fractures. *J Child Orthop*. 2012;6(2):105–109.	Nicely illustrated description of effective technique for open reduction and fixation of medial epicondyle fractures.
Linscheid RL, Wheeler DK. Elbow dislocations. *JAMA*. 1965;194(11): 1171–1176.	Seminal paper beginning the modern era of elbow dislocation diagnosis and treatment.
Murphy RF, Vuillermin C, Naqvi M, et al. Early outcomes of pediatric elbow dislocation: risk factors associated with morbidity. *J Pediatr Orthop*. 2017;37(7):440–446.	Analysis of this contemporary large series of pediatric elbow dislocation demonstrated a relatively high percentage of concomitant elbow fractures which may benefit from surgical treatment. Early mobilization was associated with improved elbow range of motion.
O'Driscoll SW, Bell DF, Morrey BF. Posterolateral rotatory instability of the elbow. *J Bone Joint Surg Am*. 1991;73:440–446.	O'Driscoll and co-authors introduced the concept of posterolateral elbow instability.

REFERENCES

1. Afshar A. Divergent dislocation of the elbow in an 11-year-old child. *Arch Iran Med*. 2007;10(3):413–416.
2. Akansel G, Dalbayrak S, Yilmaz M, et al. MRI demonstration of intra-articular median nerve entrapment after elbow dislocation. *Skeletal Radiol*. 2003;32(9): 537–541.
3. Albright JA, Jokl P, Shaw R, Albright JP. Clinical study of baseball pitchers: correlation of injury to the throwing arm with method of delivery. *Am J Sports Med*. 1978;6(1):15–21.
4. Allende G, Freytes M. Old dislocation of the elbow. *J Bone Joint Surg Am*. 1944; 26:692–706.
5. AlQahtani S, Aibinder WR, Parry JA, et al. Static and dynamic external fixation are equally effective for unstable elbow fracture-dislocations. *J Orthop Trauma*. 2021; 35(3):E82–E88.
6. Altuntas AO, Balakumar J, Howells RJ, Graham HK. Posterior divergent dislocation of the elbow in children and adolescents: a report of three cases and review of the literature. *J Pediatr Orthop*. 2005;25(3):317–321.
7. Amir D, Frankl U, Pogrund H. Pulled elbow and hypermobility of joints. *Clin Orthop Relat Res*. 1990;(257):94–99.
8. Anakwe RE, Watts AC, McEachan JE. Delayed ulnar nerve palsy after open reduction and internal fixation of medial epicondylar fractures. *J Pediatr Orthop B*. 2010; 19(3):239–241.
9. Andersen K, Mortensen AC, Gron P. Transverse divergent dislocation of the elbow. A report of two cases. *Acta Orthop Scand*. 1985;56(5):442–443.
10. Antonis K, Leonidou OA, Sbonias G, Fligger I. Convergent type proximal radioulnar translocation complicating posterior elbow dislocation: watch out for dual dislocations in children's elbows. *J Pediatr Orthop B*. 2011;20(3):138–141.
11. Ashurst APC. *An Anatomical and Surgical Study of Fractures of the Lower End of the Humerus*. Lea & Febiger; 1910.
12. Ayala H, De Pablos J, Gonzalez J, Martinez A. Entrapment of the median nerve after posterior dislocation of the elbow. *Microsurgery*. 1983;4(4):215–220.
13. Baghdadi S, Weltsch D, Arkader A, et al. Open reduction of medial epicondyle fractures in the pediatric population: supine versus prone position. *J Pediatr Orthop*. 2021;41(5):273–278.
14. Beaty JH, Donati NL. Recurrent dislocation of the elbow in a child: case report and review of the literature. *J Pediatr Orthop*. 1991;11(3):392–396.
15. Bek D, Yildiz C, Köse O, et al. Pronation versus supination maneuvers for the reduction of 'pulled elbow': a randomized clinical trial. *Eur J Emerg Med*. 2009;16(3): 135–138.
16. Bexkens R, Washburn FJ, Eygendaal D, et al. Effectiveness of reduction maneuvers in the treatment of nursemaid's elbow: a systematic review and meta-analysis. *Am J Emerg Med*. 2017;35(1):159–163.
17. Boe S, Holst-Nielsen F. Intra-articular entrapment of the median nerve after dislocation of the elbow. *J Hand Surg Br*. 1987;12(3):356–358.
18. Bono KT, Popp JE. Intraosseous median entrapment following pediatric posterior elbow dislocation. *Orthopedics*. 2012;35(4):e592–e594.
19. Bretland PM. Pulled elbow in childhood. *Br J Radiol*. 1994;67(804):1176–1185.
20. Broadhurst BW, Buhr AJ. The pulled elbow. *Br Med J*. 1959;1(5128):1018–1019.
21. Butler MA, Martus JE, Schoenecker JG. Pediatric variants of the transolecranon fracture dislocation: recognition and tension band fixation: report of 3 cases. *J Hand Surg Am*. 2012;37(5):999–1002.
22. Cain EL Jr, Liesman WG, Fleisig GS, et al. Clinical outcomes and return to play in youth overhead athletes after medial epicondyle fractures treated with open reduction and internal fixation. *Orthop J Sport Med*. 2021;9(2):2325967120976573.
23. Canavese FM, Marengo L, Tiris A, et al. Radiological, clinical and functional evaluation using the quick disabilities of the arm, shoulder and hand questionnaire of children with medial epicondyle fractures treated surgically. *Int Orthop*. 2017;41(7):1447–1452.

24. Cao J, Smetana BS, Carry P, et al. A pediatric medial epicondyle fracture cadaveric study comparing standard AP radiographic view with the distal humerus axial view. *J Pediatr Orthop*. 2019;39(3):E205–E209.
25. Capo SR, Tito AV, Cuesta FJG, et al. Median nerve paralysis following elbow fractures and dislocations. Apropos of a series of 12 cases [article in French]. *Ann Chir*. 1984;38:270–273.
26. Carey RP. Simultaneous dislocation of the elbow and the proximal radio-ulnar joint. *J Bone Joint Surg Br*. 1984;66(2):254–256.
27. Carl A, Prada S, Teixeira K. Proximal radioulnar transposition in an elbow dislocation. *J Orthop Trauma*. 1992;6(1):106–109.
28. Carlioz H, Abols Y. Posterior dislocation of the elbow in children. *J Pediatr Orthop*. 1984;4(1):8–12.
29. Chessare JW, Rogers LF, White H, Tachdjian MO. Injuries of the medial epicondylar ossification center of the humerus. *AJR Am J Roentgenol*. 1977;129(1):49–55.
30. Choung W, Heinrich SD. Acute annular ligament interposition into the radiocapitellar joint in children (nursemaid's elbow). *J Pediatr Orthop*. 1995;15(4):454–456.
31. Combourieu B, Thevenin-Lemoine C, Abelin-Genevois K, et al. Pediatric elbow dislocation associated with proximal radioulnar translocation: a report of three cases and a review of the literature. *J Bone Joint Surg Am*. 2010;92(8):1780–1785.
32. Corella F, Horna L, Villa A, et al. Irreducible 'pulled elbow' report of two cases and review of the literature. *J Pediatr Orthop B*. 2010;19(4):304–306.
33. Cromack PI. The mechanism and nature of the injury in dislocations of the elbow and a method of treatment. *Aust N Z J Surg*. 1961;30:212–216.
34. Cruz AI Jr, Steere JT, Lawrence JTR. Medial epicondyle fractures in the pediatric overhead athlete. *J Pediatr Orthop*. 2016;36(Suppl 1):S56–S62.
35. Danielsson LG. Median nerve entrapment in elbow dislocation. A case report. *Acta Orthop Scand*. 1986;57(5):450–452.
36. DeLee JC. Transverse divergent dislocation of the elbow in a child. Case report. *J Bone Joint Surg Am*. 1981;63(2):322–323.
37. Devnani AS. Outcome of longstanding dislocated elbows treated by open reduction and excision of collateral ligaments. *Singapore Med J*. 2004;45(1):14–19.
38. Di Gennaro GL, Spina M, Fosco M, et al. Dislocations of the elbow in children: long-term follow-up. *Musculoskel Surg*. 2013;97(Suppl 1):3–7.
39. Dias JJ, Johnson GV, Hoskinson J, Sulaiman K. Management of severely displaced medial epicondyle fractures. *J Orthop Trauma*. 1987;1(1):59–62.
40. Dizdarevic I, Low S, Currie DW, et al. Epidemiology of elbow dislocations in high school athletes. *Am J Sports Med*. 2016;44(1):202–208.
41. Dodd SD, Flanagin BA, Bohl DD, et al. Incarcerated medial epicondyle fracture following pediatric elbow dislocation: 11 cases. *J Hand Surg Am*. 2014;39(9): 1739–1745.
42. Doornberg JN, Ring D. Coronoid fracture patterns. *J Hand Surg Am*. 2006;31(1): 45–52.
43. Dürig M, Gauer EF, Muller W. [The operative treatment of recurrent and simple traumatic dislocations of the elbow by the method of Osborne and Cotterill (author's transl)]. *Arch Orthop Unfallchir*. 1976;86:141–156.
44. Edmonds EW. How displaced are "nondisplaced" fractures of the medial humeral epicondyle in children? Results of a three-dimensional computed tomography analysis. *J Bone Joint Surg Am*. 2010;92(17):2785–2791.
45. Eklöf O, Nybonde T, Karlsson G. Luxation of the elbow complicated by proximal radio-ulnar translocation. *Acta Radiol*. 1990;31(2):145–146.
46. El Bardouni A, Mahfoud M, Ouadghiri M, et al. [Divergent dislocation of the elbow. Apropos of a case]. *Rev Chir Orthop Reparatrice Appar Mot*. 1994;80(2):150–152.
47. Fahey JJ, O'Brien ET. Fracture-separation of the medial humeral condyle in a child confused with fracture of the medial epicondyle. *J Bone Joint Surg Am*. 1971; 53(6):1102–1104.
48. Fairbank HAT, Buxton SJD. Displacement of the internal epicondyle into the elbow joint. *Lancet*. 1934;2:218.
49. Fourrier P, Levai JP, Collin JP. [Median nerve entrapment in elbow dislocation]. *Rev Chir Orthop Reparatrice Appar Mot*. 1977;63(1):13–16.

50. Fowles JV, Kassab MT, Douik M. Untreated posterior dislocation of the elbow in children. *J Bone Joint Surg Am*. 1984;66(6):921–926.

51. Fowles JV, Kassab MT, Moula T. Untreated intra-articular entrapment of the medial humeral epicondyle. *J Bone Joint Surg Br*. 1984;66:562–565.

52. Frances R, Bunch T, Chandler B. Little league elbow: a decade later. *Phys Sportsmed*. 1978;6(4):88–94.

53. Frumkin K. Nursemaid's elbow: a radiographic demonstration. *Ann Emerg Med*. 1985;14(7):690–693.

54. García-Mata S, Arbeloa-Gutierrez L, Brun M, Sánchez-Guardamino D. Prospective study of pediatric medial humeral epicondyle fractures nonoperatively treated. Clinical, radiologic, and functional evaluation at long term. *J Pediatr Orthop B*. 2021;30(2):180–189.

55. George HL, Unnikrishnan PN, Bass A, et al. Transverse divergent dislocation of elbow in a child: a case report and review of current literature. *Pediatr Emerg Care*. 2011;27(5):411–413.

56. Gilcrist AD, McKee MD. Valgus instability of the elbow due to medial epicondyle nonunion: treatment by fragment excision and ligament repair—a report of five cases. *J Shoulder Elbow Surg*. 2002;11:493–497.

57. Gillingham BL, Wright JG. Convergent dislocation of the elbow. *Clin Orthop Relat Res*. 1997;(340):198–201.

58. Glotzbecker MP, Shore B, Matheney T, et al. Alternative technique for open reduction and fixation of displaced pediatric medial epicondyle fractures. *J Child Orthop*. 2012;6(2):105–109.

59. Gottschalk HP, Eisner J, Hosalkar HS. Medial epicondyle fractures in the pediatric population. *J Am Acad Orthop Surg*. 2012;20(4):223–232.

60. Green NE. Entrapment of the median nerve following elbow dislocation. *J Pediatr Orthop*. 1983;3(3):384–386.

61. Greiss M, Messias R. Irreducible posterolateral elbow dislocation. A case report. *Acta Orthop Scand*. 1987;58:421–422.

62. Griffin ME. Subluxation of the head of the radius in young children. *Pediatrics*. 1955;15(1):103–106.

63. Grimer RJ, Brooks S. Brachial artery damage accompanying closed posterior dislocation of the elbow. *J Bone Joint Surg Br*. 1985;67(3):378–381.

64. Guitton TG, Albers RGH, Ring D. Anterior olecranon fracture-dislocations of the elbow in children. A report of four cases. *J Bone Joint Surg Am*. 2009;91(6):1487–1490.

65. Guzek RH, Harwood K, Isaacs D, et al. A corresponding point measurement system provides reliable measurement of displacement for medial epicondyle fractures. *JB JS Open Access*. 2022;7(4):e22.00039.

66. Hallett J. Entrapment of the median nerve after dislocation of the elbow. A case report. *J Bone Joint Surg Br*. 1981;63-B(3):408–412.

67. Hankin FM. Posterior dislocation of the elbow. A simplified method of closed reduction. *Clin Orthop Relat Res*. 1984;(190):254–256.

68. Harrison RB, Keats TE, Frankel CJ, et al. Radiographic clues to fractures of the unossified medial humeral condyle in young children. *Skeletal Radiol*. 1984;11(3):209–212.

69. Harvey S, Tchélébi H. Proximal radio-ulnar translocation. A case report. *J Bone Joint Surg Am*. 1979;61(3):447–449.

70. Hassmann GC, Brunn F, Neer CS II. Recurrent dislocation of the elbow. *J Bone Joint Surg Am*. 1975;57(8):1080–1084.

71. Henderson RS, Roberston IM. Open dislocation of the elbow with rupture of the brachial artery. *J Bone Joint Surg Br*. 1952;34-B(4):636–637.

72. Hennig K, Franke D. Posterior displacement of brachial artery following closed elbow dislocation. *J Trauma*. 1980;20(1):96–98.

73. Henrikson B. Supracondylar fracture of the humerus in children. A late review of end-results with special reference to the cause of deformity, disability and complications. *Acta Chir Scand Suppl*. 1966;369:1–72.

74. Herring JA, Sullivan JA. Recurrent dislocation of the elbow. *J Pediatr Orthop*. 1989;9(4):483–484.

75. Hines RF, Herndon WA, Evans JP. Operative treatment of medial epicondyle fractures in children. *Clin Orthop Relat Res*. 1987;223:170–174.

76. Hofamann KE, Moneim MS III, Omer GE, Ball WS. Brachial artery disruption following closed posterior elbow dislocation in a child—assessment with intravenous digital angiography. A case report with review of the literature. *Clin Orthop Relat Res*. 1984;(184):145–149.

77. Holbrook JL, Green NE. Divergent pediatric elbow dislocation. A case report. *Clin Orthop Relat Res*. 1988;(234):72–74.

78. Illingsworth CM. Pulled elbow: a study of 100 patients. *Br Med J*. 1975;2:672–674.

79. Inoue G, Horii E. Combined shear fractures of the trochlea and capitellum associated with anterior fracture-dislocation of the elbow. *J Orthop Trauma*. 1992;6(3):373–375.

80. Isbister ES. Proximal radioulnar translocation in association with posterior dislocation of the elbow. *Injury*. 1991;22(6):479–482.

81. Jongschaap HC, Youngson GG, Beattie TF. The epidemiology of radial head subluxation ('pulled elbow') in the Aberdeen city area. *Health Bull (Edinb)*. 1990;48(2):58–61.

82. Josefsson PO, Danielsson LG. Epicondylar elbow fracture in children. 35 year follow-up of 56 unreduced cases. *Acta Orthop Scand*. 1986;57(4):313–315.

83. Josefsson PO, Gentz CF, Johnell O, Wendeberg B. Surgical versus non-surgical treatment of ligamentous injuries following dislocation of the elbow joint. A prospective randomized study. *J Bone Joint Surg Am*. 1987;69(4):605–608.

84. Josefsson PO, Gentz CF, Johnell O, Wendeberg B. Surgical versus nonsurgical treatment of ligamentous injuries following dislocations of the elbow joint. *Clin Orthop Relat Res*. 1987;(214):165–169.

85. Josefsson PO, Johnell O, Gentz CF. Long-term sequelae of simple dislocation of the elbow. *J Bone Joint Surg Am*. 1984;66(6):927–930.

86. Josefsson PO, Johnell O, Wendeberg B. Ligamentous injuries in dislocations of the elbow joint. *Clin Orthop Relat Res*. 1987;221:221–225.

87. Josefsson PO, Nilsson BE. Incidence of elbow dislocation. *Acta Orthop Scand*. 1986;57(6):537–538.

88. Kapel O. Operation for habitual dislocation of the elbow. *J Bone Joint Surg Am*. 1951;33-A(3):707–710.

89. Kilfoyle RM. Fractures of the medial condyle and epicondyle of the elbow in children. *Clin Orthop Relat Res*. 1965;41:43–50.

90. Kim SJ, Ji JH. Irreducible posteromedial elbow dislocation: a case report. *J Shoulder Elbow Surg*. 2007;16(6):e1–e5.

91. King T. Recurrent dislocation of the elbow. *J Bone Joint Surg Br*. 1953;35-B (1):50–54.

92. Klatt JB, Aoki SK. The location of the medial humeral epicondyle in children: position based on common radiographic landmarks. *J Pediatr Orthop*. 2012;32(5):477–482.

93. Knapik DM, Fausett CL, Gilmore A, Liu RW. Outcomes of nonoperative pediatric medial humeral epicondyle fractures with and without associated elbow dislocation. *J Pediatr Orthop*. 2017;37(4):e224–e228.

94. Kohlhaas AR, Roeder J. Tee shirt management of nursemaid's elbow. *Am J Orthop (Belle Mead NJ)*. 1995;24(1):74.

95. Kosuwon W, Mahaisavariya B, Saengnipanthkul S, et al. Ultrasonography of pulled elbow. *J Bone Joint Surg Br*. 1993;75(3):421–422.

96. Krul M, van der Wouden JC, Kruithof EJ, et al. Manipulative interventions for reducing pulled elbow in young children. *Cochrane Database Syst Rev*. 2017;7:CD007759.

97. Lee HH, Shen HC, Chang JH, et al. Operative treatment of displaced medial epicondyle fractures in children and adolescents. *J Shoulder Elbow Surg*. 2005;14(2):178–185.

98. Kulkarni VS, Arora N, Gehlot H, et al. Symptomatic medial humeral epicondylar fracture non-union- rare presentation of a relatively common injury. *Injury*. 2017;48(Suppl 2):S50–S53.

99. Lattanza LL, Goldfarb CA, Smucny M, Hutchinson DT. Clinical presentation of posterolateral rotatory instability of the elbow in children. *J Bone Joint Surg Am*. 2013;95(15):e105.

100. Li N, Khoo B, Brown L, Young T. Nonaxial traction mechanisms of nursemaid's elbow. *Pediatr Emerg Care*. 2021;37(6):E292–E294.

101. Lieber J, Zundel SM, Luithle T, et al. Acute traumatic posterior elbow dislocation in children. *J Pediatr Orthop B*. 2012;21(5):474–481.

102. Linscheid RL, Wheeler DK. Elbow dislocations. *JAMA*. 1965;194(11):1171–1176.

103. Loomis LK. Reeducation and after-treatment of posterior dislocation of the elbow. With special attention to the brachialis muscle and myositis ossificans. *Am J Surg*. 1944;63:56–60.

104. López JT, Vílches Fernández JM, Domínguez Amador JJD, Ruiz MAF. Chronic incarceration of the medial epicondyle: a case report. *J Shoulder Elbow Surg*. 2012;21(5):e12–e15.

105. Louahem DM, Bourelle S, Buscayret F, et al. Displaced medial epicondyle fractures of the humerus: surgical treatment and results. A report of 139 cases. *Arch Orthop Trauma Surg*. 2010;130(5):649–655.

106. Louis DS, Ricciardi JE, Spengler DM. Arterial injury: a complication of posterior elbow dislocation. A clinical and anatomical study. *J Bone Joint Surg Am*. 1974;56(8):1631–1636.

107. Low BY, Lim J. Fracture of humerus during armwrestling: report of 5 cases. *Singapore Med J*. 1991;32(1):47–49.

108. Macias CG, Bothner J, Wiebe R. A comparison of supination/flexion to hyperpronation in the reduction of radial head subluxations. *Pediatrics*. 1998;102(1):e10.

109. Magee LC, Baghdadi S, Gohel S, Sankar WN. Complex fracture-dislocations of the elbow in the pediatric population. *J Pediatr Orthop*. 2021;41(6):e470–e474.

110. Mahaisavariya B, Laupattarakasem W. Neglected dislocation of the elbow. *Clin Orthop Relat Res*. 2005;(431):21–25.

111. Mahaisavariya B, Laupattarakasem W, Supachutikul A, et al. Late reduction of dislocated elbow. Need triceps be lengthened? *J Bone Joint Surg Br*. 1993;75(3):426–428.

112. Malkawi H. Recurrent dislocation of the elbow accompanied by ulnar neuropathy: a case report and review of the literature. *Clin Orthop Relat Res*. 1981;(161):270–274.

113. Mantle JA. Recurrent posterior dislocation of the elbow. *J Bone Joint Surg Br*. 1966;4:85–90.

114. Marcu DM, Balts J, McCarthy JJ, et al. Iatrogenic radial nerve injury with cannulated fixation of medial epicondyle fractures in the pediatric humerus: a report of 2 cases. *J Pediatr Orthop*. 2011;31(2):e13–e16.

115. Marion J, Faysse R. Fractures de l'epitrochlee. *Rev Chir Orthop*. 1962;48:447–469.

116. May CJ, Shore BJ. Open reduction and internal fixation of pediatric medial epicondylar humeral fractures in the prone position. *JBJS Essent Surg Tech*. 2021;11(2):e19.00069.

117. McAuliffe TB, Williams D. Transverse divergent dislocation of the elbow. *Injury*. 1988;19(4):279–280.

118. McKee MD, Schemitsch EH, Sala MJ, O'driscoll SW. The pathoanatomy of lateral ligamentous disruption in complex elbow instability. *J Shoulder Elbow Surg*. 2003;12(4):391–396.

119. McRae R, Freeman PA. The lesion of pulled elbow. *J Bone Joint Surg Br*. 1965;47:808.

120. Mehlman CT, Howard AW. Medial epicondyle fractures in children: clinical decision making in the face of uncertainty. *J Pediatr Orthop*. 2012;32(Suppl 2):S135–S142.

121. Mehta S, Sud A, Tiwari A, Kapoor SK. Open reduction for late-presenting posterior dislocation of the elbow. *J Orthop Surg (Hong Kong)*. 2007;15(1):15–21.

122. Murakami Y, Komiyama Y. Hypoplasia of the trochlea and the medial epicondyle of the humerus associated with ulnar neuropathy. Report of two cases. *J Bone Joint Surg Br*. 1978;60-B(2):225–227.

123. Murphy RF, Vuillermin C, Naqvi M, et al. Early outcomes of pediatric elbow dislocation: risk factors associated with morbidity. *J Pediatr Orthop*. 2017;37:440–446.

124. Naidoo KS. Unreduced posterior dislocations of the elbow. *J Bone Joint Surg Br*. 1982;64(5):603–606.

125. Nakano A, Tanaka S, Hirofuji E, et al. Transverse divergent dislocation of the elbow in a six-year-old boy: case report. *J Trauma.* 1992;32(1):118–119.

126. Nanno M, Sawaizumi T, Ito H. Transverse divergent dislocation of the elbow with ipsilateral distal radius fracture in a child. *J Orthop Trauma.* 2007;21(2):145–149.

127. Neviaser JS, Wickstrom JK. Dislocation of the elbow: a retrospective study of 115 patients. *South Med J.* 1977;70(2):172–173.

128. Newman J. "Nursemaid's elbow" in infants six months and under. *J Emerg Med.* 1985;2(6):403–404.

129. Nyska M, Peiser J, Lukiec F, et al. Avulsion fracture of the medial epicondyle caused by arm wrestling. *Am J Sports Med.* 1992;20(3):347–350.

130. O'Driscoll SW, Bell DF, Morrey BF. Posterolateral rotatory instability of the elbow. *J Bone Joint Surg Am.* 1991;73:440–446.

131. O'Driscoll SW, Morrey BF, Korinek S, An KN. Elbow subluxation and dislocation. A spectrum of instability. *Clin Orthop Relat Res.* 1992;(280):186–197.

132. Osborne G, Cotterill P. Recurrent dislocation of the elbow. *J Bone Joint Surg Br.* 1966;48(2):340–346.

133. Pace GI, Hennrikus WL. Fixation of displaced medial epicondyle fractures in adolescents. *J Pediatr Orthop.* 2017;37(2):e80–e82.

134. Papavasilou VA. Fracture-separation of the medial epicondylar epiphysis of the elbow joint. *Clin Orthop Relat Res.* 1982;171:172–174.

135. Pappas N, Lawrence JT, Donegan D, et al. Intraobserver and interobserver agreement in the measurement of displaced humeral medial epicondyle fractures in children. *J Bone Joint Surg Am.* 2010;92(2):322–327.

136. Parvin RW. Closed reduction of common shoulder and elbow dislocations without anesthesia. *AMA Arch Surg.* 1957;75(6):972–975.

137. Patel NM, Ganley TJ. Medial epicondyle fractures of the humerus: how to evaluate and when to operate. *J Pediatr Orthop.* 2012;32(Suppl 1)S10–S13.

138. Patel RM, Tarkunde Y, Wall LB, et al. Long-term outcomes of operatively treated medial epicondyle fractures in pediatric and adolescent patients. *J Hand Surg Glob Online.* 2021;3(3):124–128.

139. Patrick J. Fracture of the medial epicondyle with displacement into the elbow joint. *J Bone Joint Surg Am.* 1946;28:143–147.

140. Pearce MS. Radial artery entrapment. A rare complication of posterior dislocation of the elbow. *Int Orthop.* 1993;17(2):127–128.

141. Potenza V, Farsetti P, Caterini R, et al. Neglected fracture of the medial humeral epicondyle that was entrapped into the elbow joint: a case report. *J Pediatr Orthop B.* 2010;19(6):542–544.

142. Potter HG. Imaging of posttraumatic and soft tissue dysfunction of the elbow. *Clin Orthop Relat Res.* 2000;(370):9–18.

143. Pritchett JW. Entrapment of the median nerve after dislocation of the elbow. *J Pediatr Orthop.* 1984;4(6):752–753.

144. Quan L, Marcuse EK. The epidemiology and treatment of radial head subluxation. *Am J Dis Child.* 1985;139(12):1194–1197.

145. Rao SB, Crawford AH. Median nerve entrapment after dislocation of the elbow in children. A report of 2 cases and review of literature. *Clin Orthop Relat Res.* 1995;(312):232–237.

146. Rasool MN. Dislocations of the elbow in children. *J Bone Joint Surg Br.* 2004;86(7):1050–1058.

147. Reichenheim PP. Transplantation of the biceps tendon as a treatment for recurrent dislocation of the elbow. *Br J Surg.* 1947;35(138):201–204.

148. Rhyou IH, Kim YS. New mechanism of the posterior elbow dislocation. *Knee Surg Sports Traumatol Arthrosc.* 2012;20(12):2535–2541.

149. Richardson M, Kuester VG, Hoover K. The usefulness of MRI in atypical pulled/nursemaid's elbow: a case report. *J Pediatr Orthop.* 2012;32(5):e20–e22.

150. Rickert KD, Sarrel KL, Sanders JS, et al. Medial epicondyle fractures: biomechanical evaluation and clinical comparison of 3 fixation methods used in pediatric patients. *J Pediatr Orthop.* 2020;40(9):474–480.

151. Ring DC, Doornberg JN. Fracture of the anteromedial facet of the coronoid process. Surgical technique. *J Bone Joint Surg Am.* 2007;89(Suppl 2)267–283.

152. Roberts NW. Displacement of the internal epicondyle into the elbow joint. *Lancet.* 1934;2:78–79.

153. Roberts PH. Dislocation of the elbow. *Br J Surg.* 1969;56(11):806–815.

154. Rosendahl B. Displacement of the medical epicondyle into the elbow joint: the final result in a case where the fragment has not been removed. *Acta Orthop Scand.* 1959;28(3):212–219.

155. Ross G, McDevitt ER, Chronister R, Ove PN. Treatment of simple elbow dislocation using an immediate motion protocol. *Am J Sports Med.* 1999;27(3):308–311.

156. Royle SG. Posterior dislocation of the elbow. *Clin Orthop Relat Res.* 1991;(269):201–204.

157. Rubens MK, Aulicino PL. Open elbow dislocation with brachial artery disruption: case report and review of the literature. *Orthopedics.* 1986;9(4):539–542.

158. Sacchetti A, Ramoska EE, Glascow C. Nonclassic history in children with radial head subluxations. *J Emerg Med.* 1990;8(2):151–153.

159. Salter RB, Zaltz C. Anatomic investigations of the mechanism of injury and pathologic anatomy of "pulled elbow" in young children. *Clin Orthop Relat Res.* 1971;77:134–143.

160. Scapinelli R, Borgo A. Pulled elbow in infancy: diagnostic role of imaging. *Radiol Med.* 2005;110(5–6):655–664.

161. Scherer S, Dietzel M, Jordan N, et al. Changes in the management of pediatric medial humeral epicondyle fractures with and without associated elbow dislocation. *Injury.* 2021;52(8):2257–2264.

162. Schunk JE. Radial head subluxation: epidemiology and treatment of 87 episodes. *Ann Emerg Med.* 1990;19(9):1019–1023.

163. Schwab GH, Bennett JB, Woods GW, Tullos HS. Biomechanics of elbow instability: the role of the medial collateral ligament. *Clin Orthop Relat Res.* 1980;(146):42–52.

164. Shankarappa YK. Transverse divergent dislocation of the elbow with ipsilateral distal radius epiphyseal injury in a seven year old. *Injury.* 1998;29(10):798–802.

165. Shukla SK, Cohen MS. Symptomatic medial epicondyle nonunion: treatment by open reduction and fixation with a tension band construct. *J Shoulder Elbow Surg.* 2011;20(3):455–460.

166. Silberstein MJ, Brodeur AE, Graviss ER, Luisiri A. Some vagaries of the medial epicondyle. *J Bone Joint Surg Am.* 1981;63(4):524–528.

167. Simon D, Masquijo JJ, Duncan MJ, Kontio K. Intra-articular median nerve incarceration after spontaneous reduction of a pediatric elbow dislocation: case report and review of the literature. *J Pediatr Orthop.* 2010;30(2):125–129.

168. Smith JT, McFeely ED, Bae DS, et al. Operative fixation of medial humeral epicondyle fracture nonunion in children. *J Pediatr Orthop.* 2010;30(7):644–648.

169. Snyder HS. Radiographic changes with radial head subluxation in children. *J Emerg Med.* 1990;8(3):265–269.

170. Sochol KM, Andelman SM, Koehler SM, Hausman MR. Treatment of traumatic elbow instability with an internal joint stabilizer. *J Hand Surg Am.* 2019;44(2):161. e1–161.e7.

171. Søjbjerg JO, Helmig P, Kjaersgaard-Andersen P. Dislocation of the elbow: an experimental study of the ligamentous injuries. *Orthopedics.* 1987;12:461–463.

172. Stoneback JW, Owens BD, Sykes J, et al. Incidence of elbow dislocations in the United States population. *J Bone Joint Surg Am.* 2012;94(3):240–245.

173. Taha AM. The treatment of pulled elbow: a prospective randomized study. *Arch Orthop Trauma Surg.* 2000;120(5–6):336–337.

174. Teach SJ, Schutzman SA. Prospective study of recurrent radial head subluxation. *Arch Pediatr Adolesc Med.* 1986;150:164–166.

175. Triantafyllou SJ, Wilson SC, Rychak JS. Irreducible "pulled elbow" in a child. A case report. *Clin Orthop Relat Res.* 1992;(284):153–155.

176. van Wagenberg JMF, van Huijstee PJ, Verhofstad MHJ. Pediatric complex divergent elbow dislocation. *J Orthop Trauma.* 2011;25(1):e5–e8.

177. Vuillermin C, Donohue KS, Miller P, et al. Incarcerated medial epicondyle fractures with elbow dislocation: risk factors associated with morbidity. *J Pediatr Orthop.* 2019;39(9):e647–e651.

178. Wheeler DK, Linscheid RL. Fracture-dislocations of the elbow. *Clin Orthop Relat Res.* 1967;50:95–106.

179. Wilmshurst AD, Millner PA, Batchelor AG. Brachial artery entrapment in closed elbow dislocation. *Injury.* 1989;20(4):240–241.

180. Woods GW, Tullos HS. Elbow instability and medial epicondyle fractures. *Am J Sports Med.* 1977;5(1):23–30.

181. Wu Y, Jiang H, Miao W. A case report of children's divergent dislocation of the elbow and review of literature. *Medicine (Baltimore).* 2016;95(44):e4772.

182. Zaraa M, Saied W, Bouchoucha S, Ben Ghachem M. [Purely lateral elbow dislocation in a child, case report and literature review]. *Chir Main.* 2012;31(1):38–40.

183. Zaricznyj B. Transverse divergent dislocation of the elbow. *Clin Orthop Relat Res.* 2000;373:146–152.

184. Zeier FG. Recurrent traumatic elbow dislocation. *Clin Orthop Relat Res.* 1982;(169):211–214.

185. Zhuang J, Hu X, Lou Y, Zheng P. Comparison of surgical treatment outcomes of pediatric medial epicondyle fractures with and without elbow dislocation. *J Hand Surg Am.* 2023;48(9):949.e.1–949.e6.

17

Lateral Condylar and Capitellar Fractures of the Distal Humerus

Benjamin W. Sheffer and Jeffrey R. Sawyer

Lateral Condylar Fractures

INTRODUCTION TO LATERAL CONDYLAR FRACTURES

All the physes of the distal humerus are vulnerable to injury, each with a distinct fracture pattern. The vulnerability of the various distal humeral physes to injury is altered by age and injury mechanism. Fractures traversing the entire distal humeral physis may occur in neonates or within the first 2 to 3 years of life.[12,48] Fractures involving the lateral condylar physis occur later, with the average age around 6 years.[21,30,35] Fractures of the medial condylar physis are rare and occur most often in children 8 to 12 years of age.[21,30,35] Obesity and a larger varus carrying angle have been cited as indicators of the likelihood of a lateral condylar fracture rather than a supracondylar fracture.[19,33]

Fractures of the lateral condylar physis, which are less common than supracondylar fractures, constitute 17% of distal humeral fractures. Fractures involving the lateral condyle in the immature skeleton can either cross the physis into the epiphysis or extend across the physis for a short distance before exiting the more medial trochlear cartilage.

Lateral condylar fractures usually are isolated skeletal injuries and rarely associated with skeletal injuries outside the elbow region.[24,28,44] Unlike supracondylar humeral fractures, fractures of the lateral condyle rarely are associated with neurovascular injuries. Within the elbow region, the associated injuries that do occur, though rarely, with this fracture include elbow dislocation, radial head fractures, and fractures of the olecranon, which are often greenstick fractures.[32] Although a rare cause of these injuries, nonaccidental trauma must always be considered in the differential diagnosis, especially in young children.[37] Acute fractures involving only the capitellum are uncommon but serious injuries in skeletally immature patients that need to be recognized and treated appropriately.

ASSESSMENT OF LATERAL CONDYLAR FRACTURES

MECHANISMS OF INJURY FOR LATERAL CONDYLAR FRACTURES

Two mechanisms have been suggested for lateral condylar fractures: "push-off" and "pull-off." The pull-off or avulsion theory has more advocates than the push-off mechanism.[31] In early studies, this injury was consistently produced in young cadavers by adducting the forearm with the elbow extended and the forearm supinated. The push-off mechanism has also been reproduced in cadavers by applying a sharp blow to the palm with the elbow flexed, causing the radial head to push off the lateral condyle. This push-off injury also can result from a direct blow to the olecranon.

It is likely that both mechanisms can produce this injury. The more common type of fracture, which extends to the apex of the trochlea, probably is a result of avulsion forces on the condyle, with the olecranon's sharp articular surface serving to direct the force along the physeal line into the trochlea. When a child falls forward on their palm with the elbow flexed, the radial head is forced against the capitellum and may cause the less common physeal fracture that courses through the ossific nucleus of the capitellum.

SIGNS AND SYMPTOMS OF LATERAL CONDYLAR FRACTURES

Compared with the marked distortion of the elbow that occurs with displaced supracondylar fractures, little distortion of the elbow, other than that produced by the fracture hematoma, may be present with lateral condylar fractures. The key to the clinical evaluation of this fracture is the soft tissue swelling and pain concentrated over the lateral aspect of the distal humerus.[42] Nondisplaced or minimally displaced fractures may produce only local tenderness at the condylar fracture site. The benign appearance of the elbow in some minimally displaced fractures may account for the delay in parents seeking treatment for a child with such injuries. With more displaced fractures, there often is hematoma present laterally, and attempted manipulation may result in local crepitus with motion of the lateral condylar fragment. This manipulation causes pain and should be avoided if there is clear radiographic evidence of a fracture.

IMAGING AND OTHER DIAGNOSTIC STUDIES FOR LATERAL CONDYLAR FRACTURES

The radiographic diagnosis of lateral condylar injury may be less obvious than that of a supracondylar fracture (Fig. 17-1), especially if the fracture is minimally displaced.

Figure 17-1. A: Injury film of a 7-year-old child with a nondisplaced fracture of the lateral condyle (*small arrows*). Attention was drawn to the location of the fracture because of extensive soft tissue swelling on the lateral aspect (*white arrows*). **B:** Because of the extensive soft tissue injury, there was little intrinsic stability, allowing the fracture to become displaced at 7 days (*arrow*).

A   B

Figure 17-2. Unossified lateral condyle. **A:** AP view. A small ossific nucleus can barely be seen (*arrow*) in the swollen lateral soft tissues. **B:** An arthrogram shows the defect left by the displaced lateral condyle (*closed arrow*). The displaced condyle is outlined in the soft tissues (*solid arrow*). Note the large cartilaginous fragment that is not visible on radiograph.

The radiographic appearance varies according to the fracture line's location and the severity of displacement. On standard anteroposterior (AP) and lateral radiographs, the metaphyseal fragment or "flake" may be small and seemingly minimally displaced. Internal oblique views are especially helpful in patients in whom displacement is suspected but not evident on AP and lateral views. To determine the importance of the internal oblique view in the radiographic evaluation of nondisplaced or minimally displaced lateral condylar fractures, Song et al.[73] compared the oblique view to standard AP views and found that the amount of displacement differed between the two views in 75% of children. The authors recommended routine use of an internal oblique view to make the diagnosis of lateral condylar fracture, evaluate the amount of fracture displacement, and assess fracture stability.

Arthrography, MRI, and more recently ultrasound evaluation[6] have been suggested to identify unstable fractures in the acute setting if it is unclear based on radiographs and to aid in preoperative planning for those with late displacement, delayed union, or malunion. Although not used with all fractures, MRI can be a very useful diagnostic aid to guiding treatment, especially with delayed unions, but often requires sedation in younger patients.

A major diagnostic difficulty lies in differentiating a lateral condylar fracture from a fracture of the entire distal humeral physis in a young child in whom the capitellar ossification center is unossified. In this scenario, an arthrogram or MRI may be helpful (Figs. 17-2 to 17-4).[10,24] Ultrasonography, which often can avoid MRI sedation issues, can be used to distinguish occult elbow fractures including lateral condyle from transphyseal separations in young patients.[9]

In fractures of the entire distal humeral physis, the proximal radius and ulna usually are displaced posteromedially (Fig. 17-5A). The relationship of the lateral condylar ossification center to the proximal radius remains intact. In true fractures involving only the lateral condylar physis, the relationship of the condylar ossification center to the proximal radius is disrupted (Fig. 17-5B). In addition, displacement of the proximal radius and ulna is more likely to be lateral because of the loss of stability provided by the lateral crista of the distal humerus.

Figure 17-3. Arthrogram of stage I fracture of the lateral condyle (*large arrows*). Articular surface is intact with no displacement (*small arrows*).

Figure 17-4. A: Radiograph of what appears to be a stable type II fracture of the lateral condyle in a 10-year-old child. **B:** Gradient-echo MRI clearly shows that this is a fracture of the entire distal humeral physis.

CLASSIFICATION OF LATERAL CONDYLAR FRACTURES

Lateral condylar fractures can be classified by either the fracture line's anatomic location or by the amount of displacement of the fracture.

Classification by Anatomic Location

The Milch classification is based on whether or not the fracture extends through (type I) or medially around (type II) the capitellar ossific nucleus. The Milch classification is used infrequently because of its poor reliability and predictive value[84] and is primarily of historical interest. Salter and Harris[61] classified lateral condylar injuries as a form of Salter–Harris type IV injuries. Because the fracture line starts in the metaphysis and then courses along the physeal cartilage, a lateral condylar humeral fracture has some of the characteristics of both type II and IV injuries. The

Salter–Harris classification is of little clinical use and is debatable as to the accuracy of terminology, because the fracture exits the joint in the not-yet-ossified cartilage of the trochlea.

Classification by Stage of Displacement

Lateral Condylar Fractures: JAKOB CLASSIFICATION BY STAGE OF FRACTURE DISPLACEMENT	
Stage	**Description**
I	Fracture relatively nondisplaced, articular surface intact
II	Articular surface disrupted; capitellum not rotated or significantly displaced
III	Fragment rotated and displaced

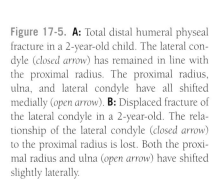

Figure 17-5. A: Total distal humeral physeal fracture in a 2-year-old child. The lateral condyle (*closed arrow*) has remained in line with the proximal radius. The proximal radius, ulna, and lateral condyle have all shifted medially (*open arrow*). **B:** Displaced fracture of the lateral condyle in a 2-year-old. The relationship of the lateral condyle (*closed arrow*) to the proximal radius is lost. Both the proximal radius and ulna (*open arrow*) have shifted slightly laterally.

The amount of fracture displacement (as measured at metaphyseal fracture gap) was described by Jakob et al.[31] in three stages (Fig. 17-6). In the first stage, the fracture is relatively nondisplaced, and the articular surface is intact (see Fig. 17-6A,B). In the second stage, the fracture extends completely through the articular surface (see Fig. 17-6C,D). In the third stage, the condylar fragment is rotated and displaced laterally and proximally, which allows translocation of both the olecranon and the radial head (see Fig. 17-6E,F).

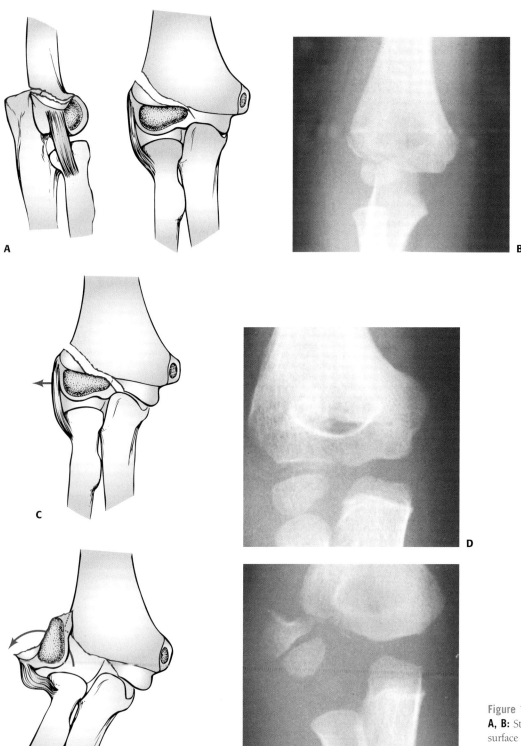

Figure 17-6. Stages of displacement. **A, B:** Stage I displacement—articular surface intact. **C, D:** Stage II displacement—articular surface disrupted. **E, F:** Stage III displacement—fragment rotated.

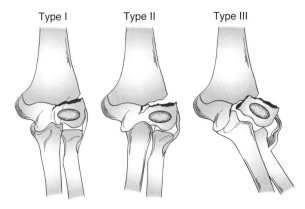

Type I   Type II   Type III

Figure 17-7. Classification of lateral humeral condylar fractures: type I, less than 2 mm of displacement; type II, 2 mm or more of displacement and congruity of the articular surface; type III, more than 2 mm of displacement and lack of articular congruity. (Reprinted with permission from Weiss JM, et al. A new classification system predictive of complications in surgically treated pediatric humeral lateral condyle fractures. *J Pediatr Orthop.* 2009;29[6]:602–605.)

Lateral Condylar Fractures:
WEISS CLASSIFICATION BY FRACTURE
DISPLACEMENT AND CARTILAGINOUS HINGE

Type	Description
I	<2 mm of displacement
II	>2 mm of displacement with intact cartilaginous hinge
III	>2 mm of displacement with nonintact cartilaginous hinge

Weiss et al.[84] modified the Jakob classification based on fracture displacement and disruption of the cartilaginous hinge (Fig. 17-7). Type I fractures are displaced less than 2 mm, type II fractures are displaced more than 2 mm but have an intact cartilaginous hinge, and type III fractures are displaced more than 2 mm and do not have an intact cartilaginous hinge. In

their series of 158 type II and III fractures, they found that all type II fractures had less than 4 mm of displacement on initial radiographs and all type III fractures had more than 4 mm of displacement. This classification was found to be predictive of complications, with type III fractures having a three times higher rate of complications than type II fractures.

Lateral Condylar Fractures:
SONG ET AL. CLASSIFICATION BY FRACTURE
DISPLACEMENT AND FRACTURE PATTERN[73]

Stage	Displacement (mm)	Fracture Pattern	Stability
1	≤2	Limited to metaphysis	Stable
2	≤2	Indefinable; extends to epiphyseal articular cartilage	Indeterminate
3	≤2	Medial and lateral displacement of distal fragment	Unstable
4	>2	No rotation of fragment	Unstable
5	>2	Rotation of fragment	Unstable

Finally, Song et al.[73] proposed a five-stage system based on fracture stability where stage 1 (≤2-mm displacement) is limited to the metaphysis and therefore inherently stable. Stage 2 (≤2-mm displacement), in which the fracture line is indefinable because of the cartilaginous nature of the epiphysis, extends to the epiphyseal articular cartilage and carries an indeterminate risk of displacement. Stage 3 (≤2-mm displacement) is unstable and at higher risk of displacement because of the medial and lateral displacement of the distal fragment. Stage 4 (>2-mm displacement) and stage 5 (>2 mm displaced and rotated) are unstable fractures, which by definition are displaced (Fig. 17-8). This classification helps refine surgical indications.

Stage I   Stage II   Stage III   Stage IV   Stage V

Figure 17-8. Stages of displacement of fractures of the lateral humeral condyle in children. Stage I, stable fracture with 2 mm or less of displacement and fracture line limited to within the metaphysis. Stage II, indefinable fracture with 2 mm or less of displacement and fracture line extending to the epiphyseal articular cartilage; there is a lateral gap. Stage III, unstable fracture with 2 mm or less of displacement and a gap that is wide laterally as medially. Stage IV, unstable fracture with displacement of more than 2 mm. Stage V, unstable fracture with displacement of more than 2 mm with rotation. (Reproduced with permission from Song KS, et al. Closed reduction and internal fixation of displaced unstable lateral condylar fractures of the humerus in children. *J Bone Joint Surg Am.* 2008;90(12):2673–2681.)

Displacement of the Fracture and Elbow Joint

The fracture line usually begins in the posterolateral metaphysis, with soft tissue disruption between the origins of the extensor carpi radialis longus and the brachioradialis muscle. The extensor carpi radialis longus and brevis muscles remain attached to the distal fragment, along with the lateral collateral ligaments of the elbow. If there is much displacement, both the anterior and posterior aspects of the elbow capsule are usually torn. This soft tissue injury, however, usually is localized to the lateral side and may help identify a minimally displaced fracture. More extensive soft tissue swelling at the fracture site may indicate more severe soft tissue injury[42,56] and predict that the fracture is unstable and prone to late displacement.

The degree of displacement varies according to the magnitude of the force applied and whether the cartilaginous hinge of the articular surface remains intact.[29] If the articular surface is intact, the condylar fragment may be either nondisplaced or tilted, hinging on the intact medial articular surface. If the fracture is complete, the fragment can be rotated and displaced in varying degrees; in the most severe fractures, rotation is almost 180 degrees so that the lateral condylar articular surface opposes the denuded metaphyseal fracture surface.

Because the usual fracture line disrupts the lateral crista of the trochlea, the elbow joint may be unstable, creating the possibility of posterolateral subluxation of the proximal radius and ulna. Thus, the forearm rotates along the coronal plane into valgus, and there may also be lateral translocation of the lateral condyle with the radius and ulna (Fig. 17-9). This concept of lateral translocation is important in understanding secondary deformities and planning late reconstruction of untreated fractures.

When the fracture line traverses the lateral condylar ossific nucleus, the elbow remains reasonably stable because the trochlea remains intact. Total coronal rotation of the condylar fragment can occur with this injury. The axial deformity that results is pure valgus without translocation.

This posterolateral elbow instability with the lateral condyle fracture has led to a mistaken concept that this injury is associated with a primary dislocation of the elbow, which is rarely the case. The posterolateral instability of the elbow is usually a result, not a cause, of the injury, as the displacement of the joint is through the fracture.[59]

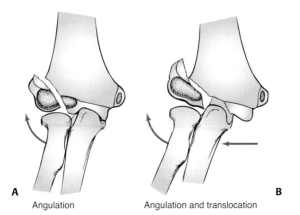

A   Angulation   B   Angulation and translocation

Figure 17-9. Angular deformities. **A:** Capitellar fracture. **B:** Fracture extending into the trochlea.

TREATMENT OPTIONS FOR LATERAL CONDYLAR FRACTURES

Fractures involving the lateral condylar physis can be treated with immobilization alone, closed reduction and percutaneous pinning, or open surgical reduction depending on the degree of fracture displacement and amount of fragment instability.[75]

NONOPERATIVE TREATMENT OF LATERAL CONDYLAR FRACTURES

Immobilization

Nonoperative Treatment of Lateral Condylar Fractures: INDICATIONS AND CONTRAINDICATIONS
Indication
• Stable articular reduction with <2 mm of displacement
Relative Contraindication
• Inability to obtain acceptable reduction

About 40% of lateral condylar fractures are nondisplaced, are at low risk for late displacement, and can be treated with immobilization alone. If the fracture line is barely perceptible on the original radiographs, including internal oblique views (stage I displacement), the chance for subsequent displacement is low. Minimally displaced fractures (<2 mm) may be stable and have intact soft tissue attachments that prevent displacement of the distal fragment. Immobilization of nondisplaced or minimally displaced (<2 mm) fractures in a posterior splint or cast is adequate.[4,6,74] Some authors advocate for casting in supination[63] while other authors advocate casting in neutral forearm position.[2] Radiographs are important during the first 3 weeks after injury to ensure that late displacement does not occur. Typically, radiographs are obtained within 7 to 10 days of the injury to ensure no further displacement and again at cast removal.

OPERATIVE TREATMENT OF LATERAL CONDYLAR FRACTURES

Closed Reduction and Percutaneous Pinning

Closed Reduction and Percutaneous Pinning of Lateral Condylar Fractures: INDICATIONS AND CONTRAINDICATIONS
Indications
• Anatomic reduction with closed reduction
• Arthrographic confirmation of articular congruity
Contraindications
• Inability to obtain adequate reduction
• Unstable fracture that cannot be maintained with percutaneous pins

When a lateral condylar fracture is displaced more than 2 mm, closed or open reduction is required to restore anatomic alignment of the joint and physis. Unfortunately, it is difficult to maintain reduction of a displaced lateral condylar fracture without supplemental fixation, so closed reduction alone is not recommended for treating displaced lateral condylar fractures. Several techniques have been described for initial closed reduction, with the recommended elbow position ranging from hyperflexion to full extension. However, clinical experience and some authors[63] indicate that closed reduction is best achieved with the forearm supinated and the elbow extended. Placing a varus stress on the extended elbow allows easier manipulation of the fragment. Fractures that are found to be stable with an intact cartilaginous hinge, either by stress maneuvers, arthrography, or other imaging modalities, can be percutaneously pinned with the elbow in flexion, similar to a supracondylar humeral fracture. Several studies, including that of Mintzer et al.,[45] have shown good results with percutaneous reduction and fixation for unstable, moderately displaced lateral condylar fractures, which can then be stabilized with Kirschner (K-) wires or a cannulated screw.[55,68,85] A percutaneous pin from the lateral column also can be used as a "joystick" to maneuver the distal fragment and aid in reduction. The smooth pins or cannulated screw is then advanced across the fracture site to the opposite cortex to obtain stability.[45]

A comparison study of displaced lateral condylar fractures (>2 mm) treated with percutaneous or open reduction found that patients treated with percutaneous fixation had shorter operating room (OR) times and fewer complications (13% vs. 26%) with equal healing times compared to patients treated with open reduction and internal fixation (ORIF).[34] Anatomic alignment of the joint and fracture stability are confirmed by stress testing and/or arthrography. If a satisfactory reduction cannot be obtained, then reduction can be achieved with open reduction and maintained by internal fixation.

Technique

> ☑️ **Closed Reduction and Percutaneous Pinning of Lateral Condylar Fractures:**
> KEY SURGICAL STEPS

- ❏ Always be prepared in terms of equipment, personnel, and setup to do an open reduction
- ❏ Consider general anesthesia with endotracheal tube and muscular paralysis
- ❏ Use C-arm receiver when open reduction is unlikely; use radiolucent table when the possibility of open reduction is unclear or likely
- ❏ Perform arthrogram/stress radiographs to assess stability
- ❏ Reduce the fracture with the elbow extended, forearm supinated, and wrist extended using thumb pressure and varus elbow stress
- ❏ Use smooth K-wire "joystick" to help reduction if necessary
- ❏ Pin with two or three smooth (0.062- or 5/64-inch) K-wires in divergent fashion depending on stability of fracture and size of the patient
- ❏ Consider 4.0- or 4.5-mm cannulated screw as alternative
- ❏ Assess reduction and stability with stress radiographs and arthrography
- ❏ Cut and bend pins outside skin. Repeat radiographs to ensure cutting/bending did not change pin position
- ❏ If stable, place patient in long-arm bivalved cast. If unstable or poor reduction, proceed with ORIF

Outcomes

Song et al.[73] reported good results in 46 (73%) of 63 unstable lateral condylar fractures, 53 of which were treated with closed reduction and percutaneous pinning. Closed reduction was attempted in all fractures, regardless of the amount of displacement. If closed reduction was successful (n = 53), then percutaneous fixation was used. If closed reduction failed to achieve less than 2 mm of displacement, ORIF was performed (n = 10). They listed three elements as essential to obtaining good results with percutaneous reduction and pinning treatment: (1) accurate interpretation of the amount and direction of fracture displacement (mainly posterolaterally), (2) routine intraoperative confirmation of the reduction on both AP and internal oblique radiographs, and (3) maintenance of the reduction with two percutaneous, smooth K-wires.

Open Reduction and Internal Fixation

> **ORIF of Lateral Condylar Fractures:**
> INDICATIONS AND CONTRAINDICATIONS
>
> **Indication**
> - Displaced, unstable fracture with articular malangulation and malrotation
>
> **Contraindication**
> - Able to obtain an adequate reduction and stabilize it with percutaneous reduction and pinning

Because of the risk of poor functional and esthetic results, open reduction has traditionally been the advocated treatment method for unstable fractures that are irreducible with closed manipulation.[46,53,64,74] About 60% of all fractures involving the lateral condylar physis have at least 2 mm of displacement and are potentially unstable.[31,84]

Preoperative Planning

> ☑️ **ORIF of Lateral Condylar Fractures:**
> PREOPERATIVE PLANNING CHECKLIST

OR table	❏ Radiolucent table, seated
Position/positioning aids	❏ Patient supine
Fluoroscopy location	❏ At the foot of the table to allow surgeon and assistant to work
Equipment	❏ Hohmann and metacarpal retractor, reduction clamp, K-wire, or 4.0- or 4.5-mm cannulated screws
Tourniquet	❏ Nonsterile if possible
Other	❏ In a patient with endotracheal tube and muscular paralysis, consider headlamp or other light sources such as lighted retractors

Surgical Approach

The standard lateral Kocher approach is most commonly used because it is familiar to most surgeons and allows direct joint visualization while protecting the posterior blood supply to the distal fragment. Often, a tear in the aponeurosis of the brachioradialis muscle laterally leads directly to the fracture site. Alternatively, a posterolateral approach has been proposed because of proposed advantages of excellent exposure with minimal dissection and improved cosmetic results because of more posterior placement of the surgical scar.[39] This posterolateral approach requires special care to avoid excessive dissection of the posterior soft tissue attachment and for this reason, it is less commonly used. Finally, some surgeons are now approaching displaced lateral condylar via an anterior incision, similar to open supracondylar fracture care. An anterior approach enters the joint and fracture site via the torn capsule and periosteum and protects the posterior blood supply to the fragment. The comparative benefit and risk of this approach have yet to be defined.

Technique

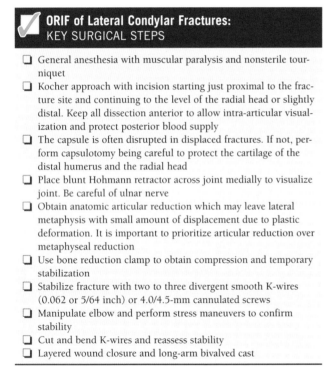

ORIF of Lateral Condylar Fractures:
KEY SURGICAL STEPS

- ☐ General anesthesia with muscular paralysis and nonsterile tourniquet
- ☐ Kocher approach with incision starting just proximal to the fracture site and continuing to the level of the radial head or slightly distal. Keep all dissection anterior to allow intra-articular visualization and protect posterior blood supply
- ☐ The capsule is often disrupted in displaced fractures. If not, perform capsulotomy being careful to protect the cartilage of the distal humerus and the radial head
- ☐ Place blunt Hohmann retractor across joint medially to visualize joint. Be careful of ulnar nerve
- ☐ Obtain anatomic articular reduction which may leave lateral metaphysis with small amount of displacement due to plastic deformation. It is important to prioritize articular reduction over metaphyseal reduction
- ☐ Use bone reduction clamp to obtain compression and temporary stabilization
- ☐ Stabilize fracture with two to three divergent smooth K-wires (0.062 or 5/64 inch) or 4.0/4.5-mm cannulated screws
- ☐ Manipulate elbow and perform stress maneuvers to confirm stability
- ☐ Cut and bend K-wires and reassess stability
- ☐ Layered wound closure and long-arm bivalved cast

The elbow is exposed through a 3- to 4-cm lateral approach, placing two-thirds of the incision proximal and one-third distal to the joint line (Fig. 17-10). In the interval between the brachioradialis and the triceps, the dissection is carried down to the lateral humeral condyle. In displaced fractures, much of the soft tissue is traumatically disrupted. If not, the joint's anterior surfaces are exposed by separating the fibers of the common extensor muscle mass. An arthrotomy, if not already present from the injury, is created slightly anteriorly, from the radiocapitellar joint to the distal humeral shaft. With severely displaced fractures, these soft tissues often are already stripped

Figure 17-10. Lateral approach for open reduction and internal fixation of a lateral humeral condylar fracture of the left elbow. The approach is made through the brachioradialis-triceps interval; an anterior retractor is used to expose the joint surface. Note the large unossified articular fragment.

and the surgeon can follow the fracture hematoma directly into the joint. Care must be taken to prevent injury to the distal humeral articular surface, which often is rotated into the wound immediately beneath the capsule. Retracting the antecubital soft tissues exposes the anterior joint surface. To protect the brachial artery and medial nerve, a small metacarpal or blunt Hohmann retractor can be passed across the joint to the opposite side, taking care to protect the ulnar nerve during its placement. The trochlea and fracture site are inspected. The joint is irrigated to remove blood clots and debris, the articular surface is reduced anatomically, and the reduction is confirmed by observing the articular surface, particularly at the trochlea. It may be hard to see far medially and distally around the trochlea, and a headlamp or lighted suction/retractors can aid visualization. It is important to assess the quality of the reduction on the articular surface and not the lateral humeral cortex, because often there is plastic deformation of the lateral cortex. Reducing the lateral cortex may lead to a nonanatomic articular reduction. In some cases, when mobilizing the distal fragment, the tourniquet may need to be deflated to detether the soft tissues, especially in young children. The reduction is provisionally held with a small tenaculum clamp, towel clip, or percutaneous pins as joysticks. Two smooth K-wires are inserted in a divergent configuration, entering the distal fragment, crossing the physis, and through the far medial humeral metaphysical cortex. Occasionally a third lateral-entry pin, more parallel to the joint surface, is used if greater stability is required. Smooth pins can be safely placed across the physis, particularly when there is only a small metaphysical fragment. Alternatively, instead of smooth K-wire fixation, a cannulated screw from the lateral metaphysis of the fracture fragment can be placed into the lateral column of the

A, B   **C**

Figure 17-11. A: Severe soft tissue infection after open reduction internal fixation of lateral condylar fracture with pins outside of skin in patient with a wet cast. **B:** T2-weighted MRI showing septic arthritis and osteomyelitis. **C:** Plain radiograph demonstrating healed fracture with extensive osteomyelitis.

distal humerus. This is done by advancing a K-wire that starts lateral to the articular surface and is placed up the lateral column of the distal humerus, lateral to the olecranon fossa. A 4.0- or 4.5-mm screw is then advanced up the lateral column giving compression at the fracture site.

The reduction and the position of the internal fixation are checked by direct observation as well as by AP, lateral, and oblique fluoroscopy images before wound closure. If used, the ends of the smooth wires are cut outside the skin to allow easy removal. There is evidence that pins left out of the skin have less complications than buried pins and have fewer returns to the OR.[10] The arm is placed in a posterior splint or bivalved long-arm cast with the elbow flexed 90 degrees.

The cast is worn for 4 to 6 weeks after surgery until the fracture is healed. The pins may be removed at 4 to 6 weeks postoperatively if bony union is progressing. Gentle active motion of the elbow is then resumed and continued until full range of motion (ROM) returns.

Outcomes

Generally good results with ORIF of lateral condylar fractures have been reported, with infrequent complications of delayed union or nonunion (1%) and osteonecrosis (1%).[8,40,55,69] Elbow stiffness is more common after open reduction than after closed treatment but resolves in most patients by 24 to 48 months after injury.[8]

While most authors advocate early surgical treatment of these injuries, Silva et al.[69] reported a series of 181 children (mean age 5 years, mean follow-up 38 weeks) who had either early (0–7 days) or late (8–14 days) fixation. There were no major neurovascular injuries in either group, and the complication rate, surgical time, ROM, and patient satisfaction were similar between the two groups. A small study of 16 patients treated at a mean of 7.4 weeks (3–15.6 weeks) after fracture found that

approximately half the patients developed a small partial fishtail deformity but none developed full osteonecrosis of the lateral condyle.[40] Yang et al.[86] described the use of an olecranon osteotomy to obtain anatomic reduction in 6 patients (mean age, 4.5 years) who had delayed treatment almost 4 months after injury. The optimal timing of surgery remains unknown given the heterogeneity of fracture presentation; a host of patient and fracture characteristics, including degree of concomitant soft tissue injury, influence timing to definitive treatment. Risk factors for delayed/nonunion include more than 1 mm of residual displacement after fixation and increased intraoperative fluoroscopy time.[9] Pin-related complications and infections are more common (1%–2%) but are decreasing because of the increased use of cannulated screw fixation. Surgery alone does not ensure a good result unless an anatomic reduction is obtained and the fixation is secure enough to maintain the reduction.

Smooth pins are the most frequently used method of fragment fixation.[18,25,31] The passage of a smooth wire through the physis does not result in any growth disturbance,[41] which may be due to the fact that the cross-sectional area of the pins is small relative to the surface area of the physis and because only 20% of humeral growth occurs through the distal humeral physis. The effects of a transphyseal screw are unknown, but the risk of growth arrest following screw fixation of these fractures is extremely low, most likely due to reasons stated above.

Several studies comparing pins left outside or below the skin found that, while exposed pins had a slightly higher or no different initial infection rate (Fig. 17-11), buried pins had higher rates of pin migration, symptomatic implants, and protrusion through the skin (up to 40%) causing late infection and increased treatment cost.[11,50]

Because of the issues related to pin fixation, as well as a biomechanical in vitro study showing increased rigidity of screw fixation compared to pin fixation,[62] there has been increased use of cannulated screws in this setting.[66,77] In a series of 62 patients,

Li and Xu[38] found lower rates of infection (0% vs. 17%), lateral prominence (13% vs. 37%), and loss of motion (6% vs. 30%) in patients treated with open reduction and fixation with cannulated screws compared to those treated with K-wires. Although the two groups were similar, the type of fixation was not randomized. Gilbert et al.[22] in a similar-sized series found a higher rate of union, shorter cast time, and greater postoperative ROM in patients treated with cannulated screws compared to wires; however, they did note that those with screw fixation did require a second surgical procedure to remove the screw.

Authors' Preferred Treatment for Lateral Condylar Fractures (Algorithm 17-1)

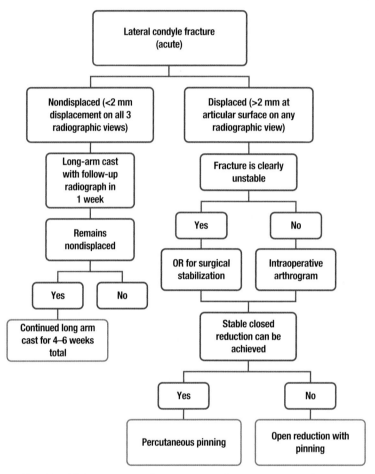

Algorithm 17-1. Authors' preferred treatment for lateral condylar fractures.

Immobilization

If the fracture is minimally displaced on all three radiographic views (i.e., the metaphyseal fragment is less than 2 mm from the proximal fragment on AP, lateral, and internal oblique views) and the clinical signs also indicate there is reasonable soft tissue integrity, the elbow is immobilized in a long-arm cast with the forearm in neutral rotation and the elbow flexed 80 to 90 degrees. Radiographs, including internal oblique views, are taken within the first week after the fracture with the cast removed and the elbow extended. If there is no displacement, the radiographs are repeated once again during the next 1 to 2 weeks. Immobilization is continued until fracture union is apparent, usually between 4 and 6 weeks after injury.

In some fractures with more than 2 mm of displacement (type II injury), the fracture pattern is such that the articular cartilage appears intact. If there is any question about the integrity of the cartilaginous articular surface and it is believed that the fracture may be stable and not require pinning, an MRI may be obtained. If the stability is questionable and it is believed that the fracture is likely to displace, or that the patient's family will not comply with close follow-up, the patient is examined under general anesthesia using arthrography and stress maneuvers to determine fracture stability.

Percutaneous Pinning

For fractures with stage II displacement (2–4 mm), closed reduction and percutaneous pin fixation are attempted because open reduction often is not necessary (Fig. 17-12). We use a lateral-entry pin to joystick the fracture into the correct alignment. The surgeon may also apply a gentle valgus force to the elbow, using the intact articular cartilage as a hinge to reduce the metaphysical fracture displacement. If there are concerns about reduction or stability after percutaneous pinning, varus stress radiography and elbow arthrography are performed to assess fracture displacement. Most commonly for these fractures, due to more stable soft tissue attachments, we use two to three smooth divergent K-wires left outside the skin to be removed in the office: We occasionally use a cannulated screw; however, this implant

Figure 17-12. A: Anteroposterior radiograph demonstrating Weiss type II lateral condylar fracture. **B:** Arthrogram demonstrating fracture line and lack of intra-articular step-off (*arrow*). **C:** Anteroposterior radiograph demonstrating metaphyseal healing 4 weeks after closed reduction and percutaneous pinning.

A, B   C

Figure 17-13. **A:** Lateral condylar fracture-dislocation in a 5-year-old boy. **B:** Intraoperative fluoroscopy showing placement of a cannulated screw. **C:** Radiographic union. Note lateral overgrowth (*arrow*).

choice does require a return to the OR for removal. If stress radiography and/or arthrography show residual or indeterminate malalignment, we proceed with ORIF to directly visualize the articular surface.

Open Reduction and Internal Fixation

If the fracture is completely displaced, malrotated, and/or grossly unstable (type III), ORIF is indicated. We prefer ORIF within a few days of injury if the soft tissues will allow for all fractures with type III displacement. We use a nonsterile tourniquet when possible and find a headlamp, illuminated suction tips, or illuminated retractors to be helpful, especially in obese or extremely swollen patients. In fractures with significant displacement and soft tissue injury, we prefer a single cannulated screw (Fig. 17-13) to K-wires, allowing for earlier mobilization and faster return of motion, especially in patients with higher-energy injuries such as fracture-dislocations. However, consideration must be given to the young child in whom a second surgical procedure will be necessary to remove the screw. Patients are placed in a bivalved long-arm cast which is then removed at approximately 4 to 6 weeks to start ROM.

Lateral Condylar Fractures:
PITFALLS AND PREVENTIONS

Pitfall	Prevention
Intraoperative	
Difficulty visualizing articular surface reduction	• Head lamp • Extend capsular incision to radio-capitellar joint
Difficulty mobilizing fragment	• Release tourniquet
Postoperative	
Difficulty maintaining reduction with pins	• Use cannulated screw • Use larger/additional pin(s)
Capitellar osteonecrosis	• Avoid all posterior dissection of displaced fragment
Elbow stiffness	• Use cannulated screw instead of pins for early ROM
Surgical pin complications	• Pins left outside the skin, removed in clinic

LATERAL CONDYLAR FRACTURE ADVERSE OUTCOMES AND COMPLICATIONS

If an adequate reduction is obtained promptly and maintained with stable fixation, results are uniformly good. With supracondylar fractures, an incomplete reduction may result in an esthetic deformity, but functional results are generally good. In contrast, with displaced fractures of the lateral condylar physis and joint surface, a marginal reduction can result in both esthetic deformities and functional loss of motion.[76] The complications that affect the outcome are numerous and can result from both biologic and technical problems. Biologic problems such as lateral spur formation, stiffness, physeal arrest, and fish-tail deformities may occur even when stable anatomic reduction is obtained. Osteonecrosis of the capitellar fragment, delayed neurologic injury, malunion, and nonunion are all more often related to technical problems, which may include failure to recognize a displaced fracture, immobilization treatment of an unstable fracture that displaces in a cast, internal fixation of a malreduced articular fracture fragment, and extensive posterior soft tissue dissection that results in osteonecrosis.

A   B

Figure 17-14. **A:** Five-year-old boy with type III lateral condylar fracture who underwent open reduction and pinning. **B:** Six-month follow-up radiographs demonstrating significant overgrowth and cosmetic deformity.

LATERAL SPUR FORMATION

Lateral condylar spur formation is one of the most common sequelae after a fracture involving the lateral condylar physis.[34,84] The spur occurs after both nonoperative and operative treatment. Rates of lateral spur formation are high, approximately 75%. More severe initial fragment displacement and the need for surgical intervention increase the risk of spur formation.[34,58]

After nonoperative treatment, lateral spurs result from the minimal displacement of the metaphyseal fragment and usually have a smooth outline. In patients with no real change in carrying angle, the lateral prominence of the spur may produce an appearance of mild cubitus varus (pseudovarus). The spur that occurs after operative treatment has a more irregular contour and is hypothesized to be the result of hypertrophic bone formation from ORIF (Fig. 17-14; see Fig. 17-13). During open reduction, care should be taken to limit the amount of dissection and to carefully replace the lateral periosteal flap overlying the metaphyseal fragment to lessen the size of lateral spur formation. Before treatment of lateral condylar fractures, the parents should be told that a lateral spur with pseudovarus may develop, regardless of the treatment method. This mild deformity usually is not of functional significance and may resolve over the subsequent 1 to 2 years.

ELBOW STIFFNESS

Elbow stiffness can occur after lateral condylar fractures, but most patients regain nearly full elbow ROM within 4 to 6 months after cast removal.[39,81] Older patients, those requiring

longer immobilization, patients presenting more than 3 weeks after injury,[67] and those requiring surgical treatment can be expected to have a greater loss of motion. Physiotherapy and dynamic splinting are both options for treating early persistent stiffness. Elbow release is rarely needed if fracture and joint alignment are anatomic in healing.

CUBITUS VARUS

Reviews of lateral condylar fractures show that a surprising number heals with some residual cubitus varus angulation (Fig. 17-15).[20,28,47,70,71,79] In some series, the incidence of cubitus varus is as high as 40%,[20,71] and the deformity seems to be as frequent after operative treatment as after nonoperative treatment.[71] The exact cause is not completely understood. Varus malalignment can be due to an inadequate reduction, growth stimulation of the lateral condylar physis from the fracture insult, or a combination of both (Fig. 17-16).[71] The cubitus varus deformity rarely is severe enough to cause concern or require further treatment, but, like lateral spur formation and stiffness, families should be warned of the risk of cubitus varus so that this common adverse outcome is not a surprise.

CUBITUS VALGUS

The most common sequela of nonunion with displacement is the development of a progressive cubitus valgus deformity. The fragment migrates both proximally and laterally, producing not only an angular deformity but also lateral translocation of the proximal radius and ulna (Fig. 17-17). Lateral translocation is

A

Figure 17-15. Cubitus varus. **A:** Follow-up radiograph of a boy whose lateral condylar fracture was treated nonoperatively and healed with a mild varus angulation. **B:** Clinical appearance of deformity.

B

A

B

Figure 17-16. True varus. **A:** Injury film demonstrating a minimally displaced fracture (*arrow*). This 6-year-old boy was treated with cast immobilization with complete fracture healing. **B:** Five years later, he presented with a clinically apparent, asymptomatic 10-degree cubitus varus deformity.

A   B

Figure 17-17. **A:** An 11-year-old girl with cubitus valgus resulting from a fracture of the lateral condylar physis with nonunion. **B:** Nonunion with cubitus valgus. Radiograph showing both angulation and translocation secondary to nonunion of the condylar fragment.

not as likely to develop in the more lateral type of these fractures because the lateral crista of the trochlea is intact (Fig. 17-18).

Cubitus valgus not associated with nonunion is much less common after united lateral condylar fractures than is cubitus varus. It has rarely been reported to result from premature arrest of the lateral condylar physis.[80] As with cubitus varus, cubitus valgus usually is minimal and rarely of clinical or functional significance. If cubitus valgus is symptomatic, it can be treated with a medial closing wedge or dome osteotomy and internal fixation or corrected gradually with osteotomy and distraction using an external fixator.[57] The more difficult type of cubitus valgus is associated with nonunions.

PHYSEAL ARREST

Physeal arrest resulting from premature fusion of the various secondary ossification centers may result in little or no deformity. Because only 20% of humeral growth occurs in the distal physis, complete physeal arrest seldom causes any clinically significant angular deformity or length discrepancy; however, partial physeal arrest may be the cause of cubitus valgus or fishtail deformity in some patients.

GROWTH DISTURBANCE: FISHTAIL DEFORMITY

Two types of "fishtail deformity" of the distal humerus may occur. The first is more common and radiographically manifests as a sharp-angled wedge (Fig. 17-19). It is believed that this type of malformation is caused by persistence of a gap between the lateral condylar physis ossification center and the medial ossification of the trochlea.[25,80] Because of this gap, the lateral

Figure 17-18. Nonunion without translocation. Despite nonunion, elbow stability was maintained because the lateral crista of the trochlea had remained intact (*arrow*). Valgus angulation also developed.

Figure 17-19. An angular "fishtail" deformity that persisted in this 14-year-old boy after operative treatment of a lateral condylar fracture, which occurred 6 years previously.

Figure 17-20. Radiographic appearance of capitellar fragment osteonecrosis 6 months after open reduction and internal fixation of a severely displaced lateral condylar fragment; extensive surgical dissection and multiple reduction attempts were the likely cause.

crista of the trochlea may be underdeveloped, which may represent a small "bony bar" in the distal humeral physis.[28] Thus, this type of fishtail deformity represents both an articular malunion and minor growth disturbance problem. Despite some reports of loss of elbow motion and functional pain with this type of fishtail deformity,[44,80] most investigators[4,13,20] have not found this type of radiographic deformity to cause major functional deficiencies. Arthroscopic debridement of the articular flap has been used in symptomatic individuals.[82] The second type of fishtail deformity manifests as a gentler, smoother concavity of the distal humerus. It is believed to be associated with osteonecrosis or larger growth arrest of the lateral part of the medial crista of the trochlea.[47]

OSTEONECROSIS

Osteonecrosis of the condylar fragment may be iatrogenic and is most commonly associated with loss of the posterior blood supply of the developing lateral condyle due to the initial traumatic injury or extensive dissection necessary to effect a late reduction.[31] Haraldsson et al. highlighted the fact that the primary blood supply to the lateral condyle consists of two vessels that enter the lateral condyle posteriorly and cross the lateral condylar ossification center before terminating in the medial trochlea.[27] Partial osteonecrosis, however, has been described in an essentially nondisplaced fracture of the lateral condylar physis that had a radiographic appearance and clinical course similar to those of osteochondritis dissecans.[25] Osteonecrosis is rare in fractures of the lateral condylar physis that receive little or no initial treatment and result in nonunion.[31,87]

Overly vigorous dissection of fresh fractures can result in osteonecrosis of either the lateral condylar ossification center[20,53]

(Fig. 17-20) or, rarely, the metaphyseal portion of the fragment, leading to nonunion (Fig. 17-21). Central osteonecrosis that is extensive can be quite problematic; the proximal forearm migrates into the defect resulting in bony impingement, osteochondral injury, loss of motion, and pain. There is no complete anatomic solution. Growth arrest of the lateral and medial columns of the distal humerus has been proposed to lessen deformity progression. Arthroscopic debridement of loose bodies has been used with positive short-term results.[23]

NEUROLOGIC COMPLICATIONS

Neurologic complications can be divided into two categories: acute nerve injury sustained at the time of the injury and/or treatment, which are very rare, and delayed neuropathy involving the ulnar nerve (the so-called tardy ulnar nerve palsy).

Tardy ulnar nerve palsy is a known late complication of fractures of the lateral condylar physis, especially after the development of cubitus valgus from malunion or nonunion. The symptoms usually are gradual in onset. Motor loss occurs first, with sensory changes developing somewhat later. The average interval from onset of symptoms has been reported as long as two decades from the time of injury. Various treatment methods have been advocated, ranging from anterior transposition of the ulnar nerve (originally the most commonly used procedure) to simple in situ decompression of the cubital tunnel. We prefer subcutaneous anterior transposition of the nerve. As noted in

A   B

Figure 17-21. Osteonecrosis and nonunion developed in this child after extensive dissection and difficulty in obtaining a primary open reduction. **A:** Injury film. **B:** Two years later, there was extensive bone loss in the metaphysis and a nonunion of the condyle.

the following nonunion section, there are times when ulnar nerve decompression and/or transposition is part of a more extensive reconstruction.

MALUNION

If not properly reduced and stabilized, the fragment can unite in an undesirable position. Cubitus valgus has been reported to occur as a result of malunion of the fracture fragments.[80] Malunion can result in the development of a bifid lateral condyle that may not be symptomatic if the malalignment is minor (Fig. 17-22). However, more severe articular malunion is problematic short and long term. Late three-dimensional corrective osteotomy is challenging but can provide symptomatic improvement in cases of marked preoperative articular malalignment, loss of motion, and pain.[1,7,86]

DELAYED UNION AND NONUNION

Some fractures of the lateral condyle may go unrecognized or untreated for a prolonged period. Even in modern medical settings, elbow fractures may be treated as "sprains," and the diagnosis of a displaced lateral condylar fracture is not made, especially in young children. Thus, patients can present weeks later with a delayed union or months or even years later with a nonunited or malunited fracture fragment.

Delayed Union

Delayed union, in contrast to nonunion or malunion, occurs in a fracture in which the fracture fragments are in satisfactory position but union of the lateral condylar fragment to the metaphysis is delayed. Various biologic reasons have been suggested for delayed union of lateral condylar fractures, including poor circulation to the metaphyseal fragment[17] and bathing of the fracture site by articular fluid, which inhibits fibrin formation and subsequent callus formation.[26] Delayed union may indicate the need for increased stability at the fracture site, typically provided by pin or screw fixation. It is most likely that a combination of these factors, in addition to the constant tension forces exerted by the extensor musculature, is responsible for delayed union.

Delayed union is most common in patients treated nonoperatively. The symptoms and clinical examination determine the appropriate treatment. If on clinical examination the fragment is stable, the elbow is nontender, the range of elbow motion increases progressively, and the position of the fragment remains unchanged on radiographs, the fracture usually heals with continued nonoperative care (Fig. 17-23). Lateral spur formation or cubitus varus is relatively common with these late healing fractures. The need for further treatment depends on the presence of significant symptoms, limited motion, or risk of further displacement that may disrupt the joint surface and cause functional impairment. If there is any question as to the integrity of

Figure 17-22. A: Injury film of a 7-year-old child who sustained a fracture of the capitellum that spared the trochlea and was treated with cast immobilization alone. **B:** Radiograph taken 2 years later showed complete fusion of the condylar epiphysis to the metaphysis, with the development of a "bifid" condyle.

the joint surface, an MRI or arthrogram may help determine any joint incongruence and the need for surgical treatment.

Most minimally displaced fractures will ultimately unite with longer-term immobilization.[17] Percutaneous pinning or screw fixation can expedite the healing. For fractures treated with initial surgical management, delayed healing is more likely if there is residual displacement of more than 1 mm after fixation or if longer-than-usual intraoperative fluoroscopy time is required for reduction.[60]

Controversy exists as to whether elbow function can be improved by a late ORIF of the malaligned fracture fragment with delayed union. Delayed open reduction (>3 weeks after injury)

Figure 17-23. Delayed union and cubitus varus. **A:** Stage III lateral condylar fracture in a 7-year-old boy was treated in a cast. **B:** Seven months later, delayed union with malunion of the fracture and cubitus varus deformity was present.

Figure 17-24. Osteonecrosis of the lateral condyle after lateral condylar fracture in a 10-year-old boy. Early (**A**) and long-term (**B**) follow-up.

has a risk of osteonecrosis and further loss of elbow motion.[13,31,87] As previously discussed, osteonecrosis of the fragment is believed to result from the extensive soft tissue dissection necessary to reposition the fragment anatomically (Fig. 17-24). The key to preventing osteonecrosis is recognition of the course of the posterior blood supply to the lateral condyle. Only a small portion of the condyle is extra-articular, and the vessels that supply the lateral condylar epiphysis penetrate the condyle in a small posterior nonarticular area.[26] Careful late open reduction through a lateral approach generally is recommended to prevent displaced, painful nonunion and/or malunion.

Nonunion

If the fracture is displaced and is not united by 12 weeks, it is considered a nonunion.[17] True nonunion occurs most commonly in patients with progressive displacement of the fragment following initiation of nonoperative treatment or in patients with late presentation of a displaced fracture.

Nonunion can occur with or without angular deformity. Many patients with nonunions and minimal fragment displacement have no angulation and remain relatively asymptomatic with activities of daily living (Fig. 17-25). Weakness or pain can occur when the arm is used for high-performance activities. Because they are not significantly displaced, these fractures often can be stabilized with minimal extra-articular dissection using a combination of screw fixation and metaphyseal bone graft.

Nonunion with fragment displacement is more common after nonoperative treatment of unstable, type II or III fractures

Figure 17-25. Asymptomatic nonunion of a lateral condyle in a 19-year-old military recruit. Because the patient had a completely normal and asymptomatic range of motion in his nondominant extremity, operative stabilization was not thought to be necessary.

Figure 17-26. Minimally displaced lateral condylar fracture was treated nonoperatively and lost to follow-up. Patient returned 6 months later with a displaced nonunion.

(Fig. 17-26). If the fragment is mobile, it tends to migrate proximally, causing progression which in turn can be associated with the development of tardy ulnar nerve palsy (see Fig. 17-17). All of these nonunions have articular incongruity.

In the setting of nonunion, continued nonoperative treatment with immobilization will not achieve bony union. Stable internal fixation with percutaneously placed pins or cannulated screws has been recommended for impending, minimally displaced nonunions.[52] For late displaced nonunions with concomitant deformity, staged procedures have been described[52]: (1) ulnar nerve transposition with in situ fixation and bone grafting of the lateral condyle; followed by (2) distal humeral osteotomy, often with some shortening to take tension off the ulnar nerve, to correct angulation once the nonunion is healed and elbow ROM is regained. The use of a vascularized humeral periosteal free flap has been described in two patients to improve blood supply to the nonunion site; however, further study of this technique in a larger group of patients is necessary.[5] Surgical treatment of the nonunion deformity of the lateral condylar fragment is difficult and requires correction of two problems. First, articular cartilage of the displaced fragment may be opposing the distal humeral metaphysis, with resulting articular incongruity. Restoring articular alignment in this situation can be challenging and may not be possible without significant risk of osteonecrosis that comes with the extensive soft tissue dissection required to mobilize the fragment. The second problem is correcting the long-standing valgus angular deformity (Fig. 17-27).

To prevent progression of cubitus valgus deformity and subsequent ulnar nerve dysfunction, Shimada et al.[65] recommended osteosynthesis for nonunion of lateral humeral condylar fractures in children because union is easily achieved, the ROM is maintained, ulnar nerve function remains intact, and remodeling of the articular surfaces can be expected. They noted that bone grafting is essential to bridge the defect, to obtain congruity of the joint, and to promote union; damage to the blood supply should be avoided to prevent osteonecrosis. To avoid the development of osteonecrosis after delayed ORIF of acute fractures, Wattenbarger et al.[83] accepted malreduction rather than stripping the soft tissue off the lateral condylar fragment to achieve a more anatomic reduction. For fractures with more than 1 cm of displacement, the position of the fragment often was improved very little by surgery, but all fractures were united, alignment of the arm was good, and no child had developed osteonecrosis at an average 6-year follow-up.

Several authors including Tien et al.[78] described a technique that includes in situ compression fixation of the lateral condylar nonunion and a dome-shaped supracondylar osteotomy of the distal humerus through a single posterior incision.[1] They recommended this procedure for minimally displaced, established lateral condylar nonunions with a cubitus valgus deformity of 20 degrees or more, especially when the deformity is progressing, is complicated by a concurrent ulnar neuropathy, or is in a patient with elbow instability or elbow pain during sports activities. They listed as a contraindication to the procedure a lateral condylar nonunion associated with radiographic evidence of prominent displacement and rotation. In situ fixation of the nonunion was recommended because the extensive soft tissue stripping required for mobilization and reduction of the fracture fragments results in devascularization of the fragment, which can cause osteonecrosis, loss of motion, and persistent nonunion. Another study recommended fixation for in situ displaced nonunions,[54] touting good functional results, but cosmetic varus and valgus malalignment was common, necessitating corrective osteotomy in some.

Figure 17-27. With fracture through the capitellum sparing the trochlea, an angular deformity can be corrected with a closing wedge osteotomy.

We distinguish between fractures seen late (2–12 weeks after injury) and established nonunions (usually from 3 months to several years after injury).[69] In all late-presenting fractures, we strive to obtain fracture union without loss of elbow motion and avoid osteonecrosis of the lateral condyle through a careful ORIF.

Treating an established nonunion of a lateral humeral condylar fracture poses a more difficult dilemma. If no treatment is rendered, a progressive cubitus valgus deformity may occur with growth. Patients usually are asymptomatic initially, except for those with high-demand athletic or labor activities. A mild flexion contracture of the elbow is present, but the cubitus valgus deformity initially can be more esthetic than functional. The danger in delayed intervention is failure to recognize that late deformity and tardy ulnar nerve palsy can occur. If surgery is performed for an established nonunion, the potential risks of osteonecrosis and loss of elbow motion must be carefully considered. We believe the criteria outlined by Flynn et al.[17] are helpful in determining if surgical treatment is appropriate for an established nonunion:

• A large metaphyseal fragment
• Displacement of less than 1 cm from the joint surface
• An open, viable lateral condylar physis

It is also helpful to distinguish between three distinct clinical situations. First, for an established nonunion with a large metaphyseal fragment, minimal migration, and an open lateral condylar physis, we recommend modified open reduction, screw fixation, and a lateral extra-articular bone graft. This technique is markedly different from the surgical treatment of an acute lateral condylar fracture. The metaphyseal fragment of the lateral condyle and the distal humeral metaphysis are exposed, but no attempt is made to anatomically realign the articular surface. Intra-articular dissection and posterior dissection should be avoided to help prevent osteonecrosis and any further loss of elbow motion. The

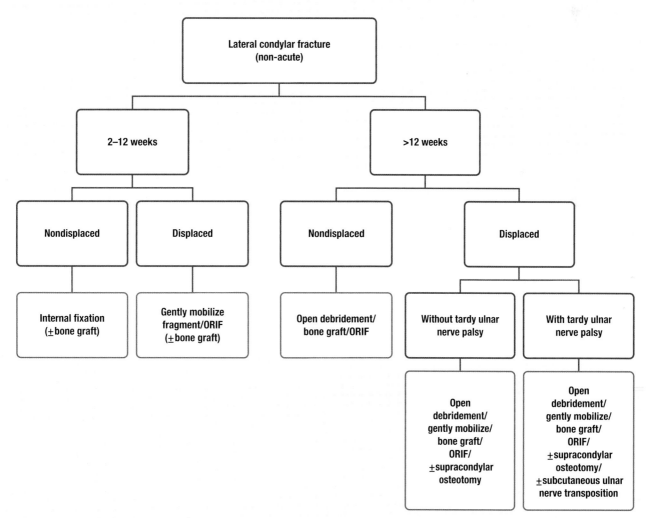

Algorithm 17-2. Authors' preferred treatment of nonunion.

Figure 17-28. A: Established nonunion with a large metaphyseal fragment. **B:** Complete healing after open reduction and internal fixation with bone grafting and cannulated screw fixation.

metaphyseal fragments are identified, and any interposed fibrous tissue is gently removed. The lateral condylar fragment usually can be moved distally a small distance for improved apposition and alignment. The metaphyseal fragments are firmly apposed, and a screw is used to fix the fragments with interfragmentary compression. Bone graft can be placed between the metaphyseal fragments before compression and then laterally after fixation. The elbow is immobilized in 80 to 90 degrees of flexion until motion is no longer a risk for displacement (Fig. 17-28).

Second, in patients with a nonunion who have esthetic concerns because of their malalignment but no functional complaints, treatment is similar to that for cubitus varus deformity after a supracondylar humeral fracture. If the patient and family desire, a supracondylar osteotomy can be performed.[43] Rigid internal fixation should be used if possible to allow early motion.

Third, patients with asymptomatic nonunion, cubitus valgus deformity, and symptomatic tardy ulnar nerve palsy can be treated with anterior transposition of the ulnar nerve; however, isolated ulnar nerve transposition rarely is done alone and usually is done in conjunction with corrective osteotomy with the goal of relieving tension on the ulnar nerve.

Capitellar Fractures

INTRODUCTION TO CAPITELLAR FRACTURES

Fractures of the capitellum involve only the true articular surface of the lateral condyle. This includes, in some instances, the articular surface of the lateral crista of the trochlea. In general, this fragment comes from the anterior portion of the distal articular surface. Capitellar fractures are rare in children and more likely seen in older adolescents.[21,32,41,51] However, anterior sleeve fractures of the lateral condyle have been reported in children as young as 8 years old (Fig. 17-29).[3,14] These anterior sleeve fractures involve a significant portion of the anterior articular surface, although technically they are not classified as pure capitellar fractures because they contain nonarticular epicondylar and metaphyseal portions in the fragment as well.

Capitellar fractures often are difficult to diagnose because there is little ossified tissue and should be considered in older adolescent patients who present with an elbow hemarthrosis.

CLASSIFICATION OF CAPITELLAR FRACTURES

Historically, two fracture patterns have been described. The first is the more common Hahn–Steinthal type, which usually contains a rather large portion of cancellous bone of the lateral condyle. The lateral crista of the trochlea also is often included (Fig. 17-30). The second, or Kocher–Lorenz type, is an articular

Figure 17-29. Fracture of the capitellum. **A:** Osteochondral fracture of the capitellum in an 8-year-old girl. Note the small fleck of bone (*arrows*), which indicates possible osteochondral fragment. **B:** Healed fracture with articular congruity, restoration of cartilage space, and no osteonecrosis. (Reprinted with permission from Drvaric DM, Rooks MD. Anterior sleeve fracture of the capitellum. *J Orthop Trauma.* 1990;4(2):188–192.)

fracture with little, if any, subchondral bone attached and may mimic a piece of articular cartilage from an underlying osteochondritis dissecans. This type of fracture is rare in children.[3,72]

Most recently, Murthy et al.[49] proposed a classification system to guide treatment: type I (anterior shear), nondisplaced (1A) or displaced (1B); type II (posterolateral shear), often associated with elbow dislocations; and type III, acute chondral shear injuries.

MECHANISMS OF INJURY FOR CAPITELLAR FRACTURES

The most commonly accepted mechanism of capitellar fractures is shearing of the anterior articular surface of the lateral condyle by the radial head.[21] The presence of elbow hyperextension or cubitus valgus seems to predispose the elbow to this fracture pattern. Because the mechanism is postulated to be a pushing off of the capitellum by the radial head, it stands to reason

Figure 17-30. Fracture of the capitellum in a 13-year-old girl. **A:** Injury film, lateral view, shows the large capitellar fragment lying anterior and proximal to the distal humerus. Both the radiocapitellar (*solid arrow*) and trochlear grooves (*open arrow*) are seen in the fragment. **B:** In the AP view, only a faint outline of the fragment is seen (*arrows*).

that there may be an associated radial head or neck fracture[32]; associated injuries of the proximal radius were reported in 31% of adults and children with capitellar fractures.[51] Elbow dislocations are also considered causative, especially with posterolateral shear fractures.[49]

ASSESSMENT OF CAPITELLAR FRACTURES

Often, swelling is minimal, and the presence of the fragment restricts flexion. If the fragment is large, it may be readily apparent on a lateral radiograph (Fig. 17-31). On an AP radiograph, however, the fragment may be hidden by the overlying distal metaphysis (see Fig. 17-30B). If the fragment is small, it often is difficult to see on plain radiographs. Oblique views may be necessary to show the fracture fragment. A high index of suspicion is needed to make the diagnosis. In younger children, arthrography or, more commonly, MRI may be required to diagnose this rare fracture. Often, advanced three-dimensional imaging modalities are used to confirm the diagnosis and plan operative reduction and fixation.

TREATMENT OPTIONS FOR CAPITELLAR FRACTURES

Nondisplaced fractures can be treated closed with immobilization, especially nondisplaced anterior shear fractures.[49] Closed reduction of displaced fractures is not likely to be successful as

A

B

C

Figure 17-31. **A, B:** Fracture of the capitellum in a 14-year-old boy. **A:** Lateral injury film shows large displaced capitellar fragment. **B, C:** After open reduction and fixation with two small cannulated screws through a lateral approach.

the fracture often is not reducible or is unstable after reduction. Fragment excision and open reduction and reattachment are the two most common forms of surgical treatment.

Excision of the Fragment

The fragment can be excised through an open arthrotomy. Excision can be successful in very young patients, late-presenting small fractures, and long-standing osteochondritis dissecans lesions that no longer reduce to the original donor site.[21] If excised, microfracture is added. In these circumstances, motion and rehabilitation can be initiated early. Even when large fragments are excised, joint instability does not appear to be a problem.[21] In patients in whom treatment is delayed, although the results are not as good as when treatment is provided immediately after injury, improvement in function can be expected, even with late excision. In patients with persistent symptoms and functional limitations after fragment excision, osteoarticular transplant (OATS) may be considered for reconstruction.

Reattachment of the Fragment

A large shear fracture fragment (types I and II) in an older child or adolescent is indicative of an intra-articular fracture, for which reduction is recommended. The fracture fixation is typically provided by wires or screws inserted through the posterior surface of the lateral condyle. Given their smaller dimension and paucity of subcentral bone, acute chondral fractures (type III) are most often repaired with bioabsorbable nails or buried interosseous screws. The major risk of ORIF is osteonecrosis of the reattached fragment. Satisfactory results have been reported with fixation with K-wires, Herbert screws, cannulated screws,[36] compression screws,[15,16] and even sutures.[72] An advantage of interosseous compression screw fixation is that it may not require later removal and allows earlier motion. Advantages cited for suture fixation include a low risk of growth arrest, sufficient stability to allow immediate postoperative motion, avoidance of implant removal, and facilitation of the acquisition of high-quality postoperative MR images to evaluate healing.

Authors' Preferred Treatment for Capitellar Fractures (Algorithm 17-3)

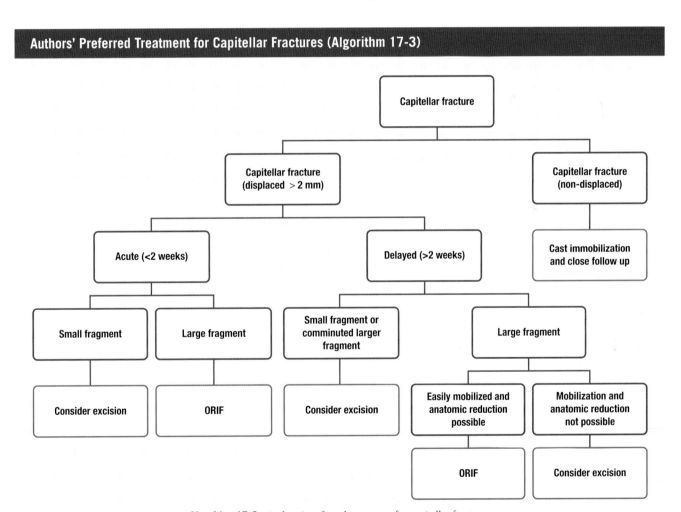

Algorithm 17-3. Authors' preferred treatment for capitellar fractures.

In acute fractures with large fragments, if an anatomic reduction can be achieved with a minimum of open manipulation or dissection, we prefer to reattach the fragment with two small headless compression screws inserted from posterior to anterior via a lateral approach. Headless compression screws are only feasible if enough bone is present in the capitellar fracture fragment to engage the screw threads. If the amount of bone in the capitellar fragment is limited, the screws can be placed from anterior to posterior, in which

case, countersunk, headed screws are utilized. If the fracture is chronic, comminuted, or with insufficient bone to accommodate screw threads, we excise the fragment, perform microfracture of the bony surface, and start early motion.

MANAGEMENT OF EXPECTED ADVERSE OUTCOMES AND UNEXPECTED COMPLICATIONS RELATED TO CAPITELLAR FRACTURES

The major complication is osteonecrosis of the fragment. This occurs only in fractures in which the capitellar fragment is retained. Posttraumatic degenerative arthritis can occur whether the

fragments are excised or retained. Many patients who are treated operatively or nonoperatively can expect to lose some ROM, but this loss is not always of functional or esthetic significance. It is important to emphasize to the parents before the onset of treatment that some motion may be lost regardless of the treatment method. Late reconstruction with OATS may be an option in patients with persistent pain or functional limitations after prior fixation or excision.

Annotated References

Reference	Annotation
Abed Y, Nour K, Kandil YR, El-Negery A. Triple management of cubitus valgus deformity complicating neglected nonunion of fractures of lateral humeral condyle in children: a case series. *Int Orthop.* 2018;42(2):375–384.	This study reported the outcomes of long-standing nonunion of the lateral humeral condyle treated with fixation of the nonunion site, dome osteotomy, and ulnar nerve transposition in 10 children. They noted that preservation of the blood supply of the nonunion fragment was necessary for success. None of their patients developed avascular necrosis.
Bauer AS, Bae DS, Brustowicz KA, Waters PM. Intra-articular corrective osteotomy of humeral lateral condyle malunions in children: early clinical and radiographic results. *J Pediatr Orthop.* 2013;33(1):20–25.	Lateral humeral condylar malunions are relatively uncommon. When present, the treatment is controversial. In this report of seven patients with elbow dysfunction due to lateral condylar malunions, the investigators describe their surgical technique, which includes intra-articular corrective osteotomy. They recommend careful preservations of soft tissue attachments to preserve the capitellar blood supply and suggest that Milch I fractures (those that extend lateral to the trochlea) might be more appropriate for this technique than Milch II fractures (those that extend into the trochlea).
Bernthal NM, Hoshino CM, Dichter D, et al. Recovery of elbow motion following pediatric lateral condylar fractures of the humerus. *J Bone Joint Surg Am.* 2011;93(9):871–877	In this prospective study of 141 lateral humeral condylar fractures, the total arc of elbow motion was limited in patients treated operatively for the first 18 weeks after injury as compared to those treated nonoperatively; however, beyond 18 weeks, ROM between the two groups was statistically similar. Older patients with more severe injuries and those with longer periods of immobilization recovered motion more slowly.
Das De S, Bae DS, Waters PM. Displaced humeral lateral condyle fractures in children: should we bury the pins? *J Pediatr Orthop.* 2012;32(6):573–578.	In a series of 235 children treated with smooth pins, 41 (17%) had exposed pins and 194 (83%) had buried pins. While there was no difference in healing rates, there was a higher rate of superficial wound infection with exposed pins (9.8% vs. 3.1%); however, buried pins had an overall higher complication rate including implant migration, skin breakdown, and pain. The mean cost savings for exposed pins was $3,442.
Gay JR, Love JG. Diagnosis and treatment of tardy paralysis of the ulnar nerve; based on a study of 100 cases. *J Bone Joint Surg Am.* 1947;29(4):1087–1097.	This "classic" article presents a series of 100 cases of tardy ulnar nerve palsy, 57 of which were attributed to sequelae of an "old fracture of the elbow." The authors discussed the diagnosis of the condition and the need for "prophylaxis" to identify and treat these injuries in childhood to prevent the progressive palsy. In this review, the authors also present 10 detailed case reports and discuss eight possible surgical treatments for this condition. The most common surgical technique used in this patient population was anterior transposition of the ulnar nerve.
Gilbert SR, MacLennan PA, Schlitz RS, Estes AR. Screw versus pin fixation with open reduction of pediatric lateral condyle fractures. *J Pediatr Orthop B.* 2016;25(2):148–152.	Forty-three patients with displaced lateral condyle fractures fixed with pins were compared to 43 with displaced fractures fixed with screws. Screw fixation led to a lower rate of nonunion (0) and faster return to motion. Screw fixation did require a second operative procedure to remove the screw.

Annotated References

Reference	Annotation
Koh SH, Seo SW, Kim KM, Shim JS. Clinical and radiographic results of lateral condylar fracture of distal humerus in children. *J Pediatr Orthop.* 2010;30(5):425–429.	A review of 175 patients with longer than 1 year of follow-up demonstrated that union can be reliably achieved with a variety of treatment options, and clinical outcomes are generally good. Cubitus varus and lateral overgrowth (spurring) were the most common residual deformities. Lateral spurring was more common with type III fractures and in those requiring ORIF.
Pennock AT, Salgueiro L, Upasani VV, et al. Closed reduction and percutaneous pinning versus open reduction and internal fixation for type II lateral condyle humerus fractures in children displaced >2 mm. *J Pediatr Orthop.* 2016;36:780–786.	A retrospective comparison of 74 patients treated with closed reduction and percutaneous pinning and open reduction internal fixation found that, while the time to union was the same in both groups, patients treated with closed reduction and pinning had shorter OR times and lower complication rates than those treated with ORIF.
Pribaz JR, Bernthal NM, Wong TC, Silva M. Lateral spurring (overgrowth) after pediatric lateral condyle fractures. *J Pediatr Orthop.* 2012;32(5):456–460.	Retrospective analysis of 212 consecutive lateral condylar fractures revealed that lateral spurring, defined as "an overgrowth of bone over the lateral aspect of the lateral condyle resulting in an irregularity of the metaphyseal flare," is extremely common after lateral humeral condylar fractures in children regardless of fracture type or treatment modality. Final outcome seems to be unaffected by the presence of the spurring aside from cosmetic concerns.
Shrestha S, Hutchison RL. Outcomes for late presenting lateral condyle fractures of the humerus in children: a case series. *J Clin Orthop Trauma.* 2020;11(2):251–258.	This retrospective study of 40 patients with lateral condylar fractures of the humerus that occurred more than 3 weeks prior revealed good results after ORIF. Children should be offered ORIF even if the fracture is older than 12 weeks.
Song KS, Kang CH, Min BW, et al. Closed reduction and internal fixation of displaced unstable lateral condylar fractures of the humerus in children. *J Bone Joint Surg Am.* 2008;90(12):2673–2681.	Pediatric lateral condyle fractures that were classified into five groups based on fracture pattern and displacement were used to develop a treatment algorithm. The use of the internal oblique radiograph provides the most accurate assessment of displacement. A prospective study of 63 unstable fractures was performed using this algorithm and found displaced fractures can be reduced closed and recommended ORIF if there was more than 2 mm residual displacement after attempted closed reduction.
Weiss JM, Graves S, Yang S, et al. A new classification system predictive of complications in surgically treated pediatric humeral lateral condyle fractures. *J Pediatr Orthop.* 2009;29(6):602–605.	The authors developed a classification system based on the amount of fracture displacement. They found that patients with more than 2-mm displacement with a disrupted cartilaginous hinge (type III fractures) had a threefold higher complication rate than those with more than 2-mm displacement and an intact cartilaginous hinge (type II fractures) as demonstrated on arthrogram.

REFERENCES

1. Abed Y, Nour K, Kandil YR, El-Negery A. Triple management of cubitus valgus deformity complicating neglected nonunion of fractures of lateral humeral condyle in children: a case series. *Int Orthop.* 2018;42(2):375–384.
2. Abzug JM, Dua K, Kozin SH, Herman MJ. Current concepts in the treatment of lateral condyle fractures in children. *J Am Acad Orthop Surg.* 2020;28(1):e9–e19.
3. Agins HJ, Marcus NW. Articular cartilage sleeve fracture of the lateral humeral condyle capitellum: a previously undescribed entity. *J Pediatr Orthop.* 1984;4(5):620–622.
4. Badelon O, Bensahel H, Mazda K, Vie P. Lateral humeral condylar fractures in children: a report of 47 cases. *J Pediatr Orthop.* 1988;8(1):31–34.
5. Barrera-Ochoa SS, Soldado F, Rodriguez-Baeza A, et al. Vascularized humeral periosteal flap to treat lateral humeral condyle nonunion: an anatomical study and report of two successfully-treated pediatric cases. *Microsurgery.* 2019;39(2):156–159.
6. Bast SC, Hoffer MM, Aval S. Nonoperative treatment for minimally and nondisplaced lateral humeral condyle fractures in children. *J Pediatr Orthop.* 1998;18(4):448–450.
7. Bauer AS, Bae DS, Brustowicz KA, Waters PM. Intra-articular corrective osteotomy of humeral lateral condyle malunions in children: early clinical and radiographic results. *J Pediatr Orthop.* 2013;33(1):20–25.
8. Bernthal NM, Hoshino CM, Dichter D, et al. Recovery of elbow motion following pediatric lateral condylar fractures of the humerus. *J Bone Joint Surg Am.* 2011;93(9):871–877.
9. Burnier M, Buisson G, Ricard A, et al. Diagnostic value of ultrasonography in elbow trauma in children: prospective study of 34 cases. *Orthop Traumatol Surg Res.* 2016;102(7):839–843.
10. Chessare JW, Rogers LF, White H, Tachdjian MO. Injuries of the medial epicondylar ossification center of the humerus. *AJR Am J Roentgenol.* 1977;129(1):49–55.
11. Das De S, Bae DS, Waters PM. Displaced humeral lateral condyle fractures in children: should we bury the pins? *J Pediatr Orthop.* 2012;32(6):573–578.
12. DeLee JC, Wilkins KE, Rogers LF, Rockwood CA. Fracture-separation of the distal humeral epiphysis. *J Bone Joint Surg Am.* 1980;62(1):46–51.
13. Dhillon KS, Sengupta S, Singh BJ. Delayed management of fracture of the lateral humeral condyle in children. *Acta Orthop Scand.* 1988;59(4):419–424.
14. Drvaric DM, Rooks MD. Anterior sleeve fracture of the capitellum. *J Orthop Trauma.* 1990;4(2):188–192.
15. Elkowitz SJ, Kubiak EN, Polatsch D, et al. Comparison of two headless screw designs for fixation of capitellum fractures. *Bull Hosp Jt Dis.* 2003;61(3–4):123–126.
16. Elkowitz SJ, Polatsch DB, Egol KA, et al. Capitellum fractures: a biomechanical evaluation of three fixation methods. *J Orthop Trauma.* 2002;16(7):503–506.
17. Flynn JC, Richards JF Jr, Saltzman RI. Prevention and treatment of nonunion of slightly displaced fractures of the lateral humeral condyle in children. An end-result study. *J Bone Joint Surg Am.* 1975;57(8):1087–1092.
18. Fontanetta P, Mackenzie DA, Rosman M. Missed, maluniting, and malunited fractures of the lateral humeral condyle in children. *J Trauma.* 1978;18(5):329–335.
19. Fornari ED, Suszter M, Roocroft J, et al. Childhood obesity as a risk factor for lateral condyle fractures over supracondylar humerus fractures. *Clin Orthop Relat Res.* 2013;471(4):1193–1198.
20. Foster DE, Sullivan JA, Gross RH. Lateral humeral condylar fractures in children. *J Pediatr Orthop.* 1985;5(1):16–22.
21. Fowles JV, Kassab MT. Fracture of the capitulum humeri. Treatment by excision. *J Bone Joint Surg Am.* 1974;56(4):794–798.
22. Gilbert SR, MacLennan PA, Schlitz RS, Estes AR. Screw versus pin fixation with open reduction of pediatric lateral condyle fractures. *J Pediatr Orthop B.* 2016;25(2):148–152.
23. Glotzbecker MP, Bae DS, Links AC, Waters PM. Fishtail deformity of the distal humerus: a report of 15 cases. *J Pediatr Orthop.* 2013;33(6):592–597.

24. Griffith JF, Roebuck DJ, Cheng JC, et al. Acute elbow trauma in children: spectrum of injury revealed by MR imaging not apparent on radiographs. *AJR Am J Roentgenol.* 2001;176(1):53–60.
25. Hamilton DA, Kalra K. Trochlear osteonecrosis after a nonoperative lateral humeral condyle fracture in a child. *J Am Acad Orthop Surg Glob Res Rev.* 2020;4(5):e1900101.
26. Haraldsson S. Osteochondrosis deformans juvenilis capituli humeri including investigation of intra-osseous vasculature in distal humerus. *Acta Orthop Scand Suppl.* 1959;38:1–232.
27. Haraldsson S. The intra-osseous vasculature of the distal end of the humerus with special reference to the capitulum; preliminary communication. *Acta Orthop Scand.* 1957;27(2):81–93.
28. Herring JA, Fitch RD. Lateral condylar fracture of the elbow. *J Pediatr Orthop.* 1986;6(6):724–727.
29. Horn BD, Herman MJ, Crisci K, et al. Fractures of the lateral humeral condyle: role of the cartilage hinge in fracture stability. *J Pediatr Orthop.* 2002;22(1):8–11.
30. Houshian S, Mehdi B, Larsen MS. The epidemiology of elbow fracture in children: analysis of 355 fractures, with special reference to supracondylar humerus fractures. *J Orthop Sci.* 2001;6(4):312–315.
31. Jakob R, Fowles JV, Rang M, Kassab MT. Observations concerning fractures of the lateral humeral condyle in children. *J Bone Joint Surg Br.* 1975;57(4):430–436.
32. Johansson J, Rosman M. Fracture of the capitulum humeri in children: a rare injury, often misdiagnosed. *Clin Orthop Relat Res.* 1980;146:157–160.
33. Kang S, Park SS. Predisposing effect of elbow alignment on the elbow fracture type in children. *J Orthop Trauma.* 2015;29(8):3253–3258.
34. Koh SH, Seo SW, Kim KM, Shim JS. Clinical and radiographic results of lateral condylar fracture of distal humerus in children. *J Pediatr Orthop.* 2010;30(5):425–429.
35. Landin LA, Danielsson LG. Elbow fractures in children. An epidemiological analysis of 589 cases. *Acta Orthop Scand.* 1986;57(4):309–312.
36. Letts M, Rumball K, Bauermeister S, et al. Fractures of the capitellum in adolescents. *J Pediatr Orthop.* 1997;17(3):315–320.
37. Levin H, Sangha G, Carey TP, Lim R. Fracture and nonaccidental injury: a case report of a lateral condylar fracture in a 13 months old. *Pediatr Emerg Care.* 2016;32(12):865–867.
38. Li WC, Xu RJ. Comparison of Kirschner wires and AO cannulated screw internal fixation for displaced lateral humeral condyle fracture in children. *Int Orthop.* 2012;36(6):1261–1266.
39. Liu CH, Kao HK, Lee WC, et al. Posterolateral approach for humeral lateral condyle fractures in children. *J Pediatr Orthop B.* 2016;25(2):153–158.
40. Liu TJ, Wang EB, Dai Q, et al. Open reduction and internal fixation for the treatment of fractures of the lateral humeral condyle with an early delayed presentation in children: a radiological and clinical prospective study. *Bone Joint J.* 2016;98-B(2):244–248.
41. Ma YZ, Zheng CB, Zhou TL, Yeh YC. Percutaneous probe reduction of frontal fractures of the humeral capitellum. *Clin Orthop Relat Res.* 1984;(183):17–21.
42. Major NM, Crawford ST. Elbow effusions in trauma in adults and children: is there an occult fracture? *AJR Am J Roentgenol.* 2002;178(2):413–418.
43. Masada K, Kawai H, Kawabata H, et al. Osteosynthesis for old, established nonunion of the lateral condyle of the humerus. *J Bone Joint Surg Am.* 1990;72(1):32–40.
44. Menkowitz M, Flynn JM. Floating elbow in an infant. *Orthopedics.* 2002;25(2):185–186.
45. Mintzer CM, Waters PM, Brown DJ, Kasser JR. Percutaneous pinning in the treatment of displaced lateral condyle fractures. *J Pediatr Orthop.* 1994;14(4):462–465.
46. Morin B, Fassier F, Poitras B, Labelle H. [Results of early surgical treatment of fractures of the lateral humeral condyle in children]. *Rev Chir Orthop Reparatrice Appar Mot.* 1988;74:129–131.
47. Morrissy RT, Wilkins KE. Deformity following distal humeral fracture in childhood. *J Bone Joint Surg Am.* 1984;66(4):557–562.
48. Moucha CS, Mason DE. Distal humeral epiphyseal separation. *Am J Orthop (Belle Mead NJ).* 2003;32(10):497–500.
49. Murthy PG, Vuillermin C, Naqvi MN, et al. Capitellar fractures in children and adolescents: classification and early results of treatment. *J Bone Joint Surg Am.* 2017;99(15):1282–1290.
50. Ormsby NM, Walton RDM, Robinson S, et al. Buried versus unburied Kirschner wires in the management of paediatric lateral condyle elbow fractures: a comparative study from a tertiary centre. *J Pediatr Orthop B.* 2016;25(1):69–73.
51. Palmer I. Open treatment of transcondylar T-fracture of the humerus. *Acta Chir Scand.* 1961;121:486–490.
52. Papandrea R, Waters PM. Posttraumatic reconstruction of the elbow in the pediatric patient. *Clin Orthop Relat Res.* 2000;(370):115–126.
53. Papavasiliou VA, Beslikas TA. Fractures of the lateral humeral condyle in children—an analysis of 39 cases. *Injury.* 1985;16(6):364–366.
54. Park H, Hwang JH, Kwon YU, Kim HW. Osteosynthesis in situ for lateral condyle nonunion in children. *J Pediatr Orthop.* 2015;35(4):334–340.
55. Pennock AT, Salgueiro L, Upasani VV, et al. Closed reduction and percutaneous pinning versus open reduction and internal fixation for type II lateral condyle humerus fractures in children displaced >2 mm. *J Pediatr Orthop.* 2016;36(8):780–786.
56. Petit P, Sapin C, Henry G, et al. Rate of abnormal osteoarticular radiographic findings in pediatric patients. *AJR Am J Roentgenol.* 2001;176(4):987–990.
57. Piskin A, Tomak Y, Sen C, Tomak L. The management of cubitus varus and valgus using the Ilizarov method. *J Bone Joint Surg Br.* 2007;89(12):1615–1619.
58. Pribaz JR, Bernthal NM, Wong TC, Silva M. Lateral spurring (overgrowth) after pediatric lateral condyle fractures. *J Pediatr Orthop.* 2012;32(5):456–460.
59. Rovinsky D, Ferguson C, Younis A, Otsuka NY. Pediatric elbow dislocation associated with a Milch type I lateral condyle fracture of the humerus. *J Orthop Trauma.* 1999;13(6):458–460.
60. Salgueiro L, Roocroft JH, Bastrom TP, et al. Rate and risk factors for delayed healing following surgical treatment of lateral condyle humerus fractures in children. *J Pediatr Orthop.* 2017;37(1):1–6.
61. Salter RB, Harris WR. Injuries involving the epiphyseal plate. *J Bone Joint Surg Am.* 1963;45:587–622.
62. Schlitz RS, Schwertz JM, Eberhardt AW, Gilbert SR. Biomechanical analysis of screws versus K-wires for lateral humeral condyle fractures. *J Pediatr Orthop.* 2015 35(8):e93–e97.
63. Shaerf DA, Vanhegan IS, Dattani R. Diagnosis, management and complications of distal humerus lateral condyle fractures in children. *Shoulder Elbow.* 2018;10(2):114–120.
64. Sharma JC, Arora A, Mathur NC, et al. Lateral condylar fractures of the humerus in children: fixation with partially threaded 4.0-mm AO cancellous screws. *J Trauma.* 1995;39(6):1129–1133.
65. Shimada K, Masada K, Tada K, Yamamoto T. Osteosynthesis for the treatment of nonunion of the lateral humeral condyle in children. *J Bone Joint Surg Am.* 1997; 79(2):234–240.
66. Shirley E, Anderson M, Neal K, Mazur J. Screw fixation of lateral condyle fractures: results of treatment. *J Pediatr Orthop.* 2015;35(8):821–824.
67. Shresta S, Hutchison RL. Outcomes for late presenting lateral condyle fractures of the humerus in children: a case series. *J Clin Orthop Trauma.* 2020;11(2):251–258.
68. Silva M, Cooper SD. Closed reduction and percutaneous pinning of displaced pediatric lateral condyle fractures of the humerus: a cohort study. *J Pediatr Orthop.* 2015;35(7):661–665.
69. Silva M, Paredes A, Sadlik G. Outcomes of ORIF >7 days after injury in displaced pediatric lateral condyle fracture. *J Pediatr Orthop.* 2017;37(1):7–13.
70. Skak SV, Olsen SD, Smaabrekke A. Deformity after fracture of the lateral humeral condyle in children. *J Pediatr Orthop B.* 2001;10(2):142–152.
71. So YC, Fang D, Leong JC, Bong SC. Varus deformity following lateral humeral condylar fracture in children. *J Pediatr Orthop.* 1985;5(5):569–572.
72. Sodl JF, Ricchetti ET, Huffman GR. Acute osteochondral shear fracture of the capitellum in a twelve-year-old patient. A case report. *J Bone Joint Surg Am.* 2008;90(3):629–633.
73. Song KS, Kang CH, Min BW, et al. Closed reduction and internal fixation of displaced unstable lateral condylar fractures of the humerus in children. *J Bone Joint Surg Am.* 2008;90(12):2673–2681.
74. Song KS, Shin YW, Oh CW, et al. Closed reduction and internal fixation of completely displaced and rotated lateral condyle fractures of the humerus in children. *J Orthop Trauma.* 2010;24(7):434–438.
75. Song KS, Waters PM. Lateral condylar humerus fractures: which ones should we fix? *J Pediatr Orthop.* 2012;32(Suppl 1):S5–S9.
76. Stans AA, Maritz NGJ, O'Driscoll SW, Morrey BF. Operative treatment of elbow contracture in patients 21 years of age or younger. *J Bone Joint Surg Am.* 2002;84(3):382–387.
77. Stein BE, Ramji AF, Hassanzadeh H, et al. Cannulated lag screw fixation of displaced lateral humeral condyle fractures is associated with lower rates of open reduction and infection than pin fixation. *J Pediatr Orthop.* 2017;37(1):7–13.
78. Tien YC, Chen JC, Fu YC, et al. Supracondylar dome osteotomy for cubitus valgus deformity associated with a lateral condylar nonunion in children. Surgical technique. *J Bone Joint Surg Am.* 2006;88(Suppl 1 Pt 2):191–201.
79. van Vugt AB, Severijnen RV, Festen C. Fractures of the lateral humeral condyle in children: late results. *Arch Orthop Trauma Surg (1978).* 1988;107(4):206–209.
80. Wadsworth TG. Premature epiphyseal fusion after injury of the capitulum. *J Bone Joint Surg Br.* 1964;46:46–49.
81. Wang YL, Chang WN, Hsu CJ, et al. The recovery of elbow range of motion after treatment of supracondylar and lateral condylar fractures of the distal humerus in children. *J Orthop Trauma.* 2009;23(2):120–125.
82. Waters PM, Bae DS. *Pediatric Hand and Upper Limb Surgery: A Practical Guide.* Lippincott Williams & Wilkins; 2012:316–337.
83. Wattenbarger JM, Gerardi J, Johnston CE. Late open reduction internal fixation of lateral condyle fractures. *J Pediatr Orthop.* 2002;22(3):394–398.
84. Weiss JM, Graves S, Yang S, et al. A new classification system predictive of complications in surgically treated pediatric humeral lateral condyle fractures. *J Pediatr Orthop.* 2009;29(6):602–605.
85. Wirmer J, Kruppa C, Fitze G. Operative treatment of lateral humeral condyle fractures in children. *Eur J Pediatr Surg.* 2012;22(4):289–294.
86. Yang WE, Shih CH, Lee ZL, et al. Anatomic reduction of old displaced lateral condylar fractures of the humerus in children via a posterior approach with olecranon osteotomy. *J Trauma.* 2008;64(5):1281–1289.
87. Zionts LE, Stolz MR. Late fracture of the lateral condyle of the humerus. *Orthopedics.* 1984;7:541–545.

18

Distal Humeral Physeal, Medial Condyle, Lateral Epicondylar, and Other Uncommon Elbow Fractures

Oduche Igboechi and Joshua M. Abzug

INTRODUCTION

The so-called TRASH lesions (*The Radiographic Appearance Seemed Harmless*) are rare injuries about the elbow that, although oftentimes underappreciated or acutely missed, can have serious long-term implications.[111] These typically occur in a very young patient prior to secondary ossification centers being visible, which would ordinarily aid with the diagnosis. Examples of TRASH lesion include distal humeral physeal fractures before the capitellum ossifies, medial condylar fractures before the trochlea ossifies, and osteochondral fractures in children less than 10 years old that lead to joint incongruity and instability.

Often, to accurately make the diagnosis and formulate a treatment plan, additional imaging modalities such as ultrasound, arthrography, and/or MRI scans are necessary. Usually these children have marked swelling, more than anticipated by the relatively benign radiographs This, in addition to appropriate knowledge of the pediatric elbow anatomy and timing of ossification centers, can help minimize negative outcomes. This chapter will cover many of the rare, potentially problematic injuries about the pediatric elbow.

Fractures Involving the Entire Distal Humerus

INTRODUCTION TO FRACTURES INVOLVING THE ENTIRE DISTAL HUMERUS

Originally thought to be a rare injury, fractures involving the entire distal humerus physis, also known as transphyseal humeral separations, have commonly been reported in the literature.[1,3,21,22,46,51,61,67,88,101,102,111] This injury pattern is often missed on initial assessment.[111] An ultrasound study showed that 56% may be missed on plain radiographs.[101] Delay in diagnosis even up to 1 week is not uncommon[2] and prolonged delay can have serious negative consequences to the child's long-term elbow function.

Most fractures involving the entire distal humeral physis occur before the age of 6 or 7 and are most common under the age of 3.[2,4,111] Younger the child is, the greater the relative volume of the distal humerus epiphysis. As the humerus matures, the physeal line progresses more distally, with a central V forming between the medial and lateral condylar physes (Fig. 18-1). Ashurst[5] believed that this V-shaped configuration of the physeal line helps protect the more mature distal humerus from physeal fractures.

ASSESSMENT OF FRACTURES INVOLVING THE ENTIRE DISTAL HUMERUS

A young child with any potential injury about their elbow needs to be assessed in a systematic manner. A thorough history is

Figure 18-1. A: Group A—AP view of a small infant who had a swollen left elbow after a difficult delivery. The displacement medially of the proximal radius and ulna (*arrows*) helps to make the diagnosis of a displaced total distal humeral physis. **B:** Normal elbow for comparison. **C:** Group B—AP view showing the posteromedial displacement of the distal fragment (*arrows*). The relationship between the ossification center of the lateral condyle and the proximal radius has been maintained. **D:** Group C—AP view with marked medial displacement of the distal fragment. **E:** Group C—lateral view of the same patient showing posterior displacement of the distal fragment. There is also a large metaphyseal fragment associated with the distal fragment (*arrow*).

important to obtain, including any past medical history of a potential skeletal dysplasia or bone metabolism abnormality. In addition, a thorough social history is needed to aid in determining if there is concern for nonaccidental trauma (NAT). Of note, transphyseal fractures less age 3 years are often misdiagnosed up to 78% of the time by the radiologist reading the acute radiograph and have a 13 times risk of NAT compared to a supracondylar fracture in the same age group.[18] When in doubt, appropriate evaluation for NAT is required, as presentation with a musculoskeletal fracture is second most common presentation after skin burns and bruising. The mechanism of injury, as well as timing of presentation compared to when injury occurred, is

important to make an accurate diagnosis. Less common infectious etiologies (elbow septic arthritis, distal humerus osteomyelitis) will also present with swelling, pain, and restricted arc of motion; so will inflammatory arthritides (Lyme disease, juvenile inflammatory arthritis). Nursemaid's elbow injuries also occur in the young and are reviewed in Chapter 17.

The physical examination should begin with observation of the appearance of the child's skin, looking for ecchymosis, open injuries, and the discoloration of the affected extremity, as well as the presence of any deformity. This skin assessment should not only be for the injured elbow but the entire body in the young child at risk for NAT. In addition, assessment of restricted range of active motion and hand neurologic function (intrinsic and extrinsic median and ulnar nerve and radial nerve extrinsic motor function) of the injured limb can often be evaluated by watching the child's movements. Palpation should begin on the lower extremities and contralateral uninjured upper extremity to ensure no other injuries are present. This also is reassuring to the child if there is not pain associated with this aspect of your examination before you move to the injured area. When beginning the palpation of the affected extremity, the examiner should start away from the elbow (i.e., at the hand or shoulder) and work toward the elbow, again ensuring there are no other injuries present. When palpating the injured elbow, it is important to assess it utilizing one or two fingers to isolate the exact location of the tenderness as opposed to grabbing the whole elbow with the examiner's hand. The radial pulse should be assessed when palpating the wrist region along with testing capillary refill of the digits to assess for vascular function.

MECHANISMS OF INJURY FOR FRACTURES INVOLVING THE ENTIRE DISTAL HUMERUS

The exact mechanism of this injury is usually a fall with outstretched limb but as mentioned can be secondary to NAT, especially in children less than 3 years of age, particularly those less than 2. A rare fracture mechanism is birth injuries associated with difficult deliveries.[2–6,24,32,50,108,111] During vaginal deliveries, this may occur as a result of labor forces and/or obstetrical maneuvers used to deliver the baby.[2] These fractures may also occur during cesarean sections when substantial traction and rotation are applied to the baby's arm.[2,50] In a study by Sherr-Lurie et al.,[91] only 2 of 92,882 patients sustained a traumatic transphyseal distal humerus separation during the birthing process. Siffert[93] and Kay[52] noted that the clinical appearance of these injured elbows at the time of delivery was not especially impressive. There was only moderate swelling and some crepitus.

DeLee et al.[22] noted a high incidence of confirmed or suspected NAT in their very young patients. Other reports have confirmed the frequency of NAT in infants and young children with these fractures, with up to 50% of these fractures in children under the age of 2 may be the result of NAT.[3,4,18,21,63,74,108,111] Crowe found a 13 times greater risk of NAT for children younger than 3 years of age who sustained a displaced transphyseal distal humeral fracture compared with displaced supracondylar humeral fractures. Therefore, clinicians should have a high index of suspicion for NAT, especially in the setting of a history of multiple injuries or an inconsistent history regarding the mechanism of injury.[2]

Bright[10] showed that a physis is more likely to fail with rotary shear forces than with pure bending or tension forces. Young infants have some residual flexion contractures of the elbow from intrauterine positioning, which prevents a hyperextension injury that results in supracondylar elbow fractures seen in older children. Rotary or shear forces on the elbow, which can be caused by NAT or birth trauma in young infants, are likely the mechanism for this injury in younger children. As these fractures are often confused with an elbow dislocation, it should be recognized that elbow dislocations are rare in this young age group because the cartilaginous physis is mechanically weaker than the bone ligament interface that would fail with an elbow dislocation.[2] In addition, elbow dislocations are often posterolaterally displaced and transphyseal fractures are usually posteromedially displaced.[18] In older children, a hyperextension force on an outstretched arm may cause the injury, which may occur from a fall from height or when an older child jumps on top of a younger child.[2,101] Abe et al.[1] reported 21 children, ranging in age from 1 to 11 years (average 5 years), with fracture separations of the distal humeral epiphysis, all of which were sustained in falls.

INJURIES ASSOCIATED WITH FRACTURES INVOLVING THE ENTIRE DISTAL HUMERUS

NAT should always be considered in children with a transphyseal distal humerus separation, especially a type A fracture pattern (see classification below), unless it occurs at birth. Type B and C injuries are often misdiagnosed as supraconylar or condylar fractures by emergent care radiologist and delivery team.[18] A young infant is unlikely to incur this type of injury spontaneously from the usual falls that occur during the first year of life.

Hariharan et al.[41] reported on 79 patients, all younger than 4 years of age. Forty-nine injuries resulted from accidental trauma, 21 from NAT, 6 from cesarean section, and 3 from vaginal delivery. With NAT occurring so frequently, it is imperative that other injuries commonly found in cases of NAT are considered, including bruising, bite marks, and scratches.[2,41]

If NAT is suspected, a bone scan and/or a skeletal survey is warranted, to look for metaphyseal corner fractures, rib fractures, or fractures at various stages of healing, and the possibility of head trauma should not be ignored. In a series of 16 patients with a transphyseal distal humerus separation evaluated with ultrasound, 10 (63%) had one or more additional humeral fractures (bucket handle fractures in 5 patients and condylar avulsion fractures in 6).[101] In addition, social services departments and child-abuse teams should be notified when NAT is suspected. Hariharan et al.[41] reported that child protective services were involved in 38% of surgically treated transphyseal humeral separations due to high suspicion of NAT.[41] Recognition of NAT and proper intervention can be life altering or even lifesaving for these children.

SIGNS AND SYMPTOMS OF FRACTURES INVOLVING THE ENTIRE DISTAL HUMERUS

In an infant less than 2 years of age, whose elbow is swollen secondary to trauma or suspected trauma, a fracture involving the entire distal humeral physis should be considered.[18] The newborn may be irritable or inconsolable.[2] Swelling, instability at the fracture site, limited range of motion, and/or lack of spontaneous movement (pseudoparalysis), all may suggest this injury.[2,81,101] In a young infant or newborn, swelling may be minimal with little crepitus, especially if the child presents in a somewhat delayed fashion when early abundant periosteal healing may already be present. Poland[83] described the crepitus as "muffled" crepitus in the acute phase because the fracture ends are covered with softer cartilage than the firm osseous tissue in other fractures about the elbow. Because of the large, wide fracture surfaces, there are fewer tendencies for tilting with distal fragment rotation, and the angular deformity can be less severe than that with supracondylar fractures. In older children, the elbow is often so swollen that a clinical assessment of the bony landmarks is impossible, and only radiographic evaluation can provide confirmation of the diagnosis.

IMAGING AND OTHER DIAGNOSTIC STUDIES FOR FRACTURES INVOLVING THE ENTIRE DISTAL HUMERUS

Confirming radiographic evidence of a distal humeral physeal separation can be difficult, especially if the ossification center of the lateral condyle is not visible in an infant. Radiographs of the entire extremity not centered on the elbow may lead to a missed diagnosis.[2] In a series of 16 patients evaluated with ultrasound, the diagnosis was missed in 9 (56%) patients, and 10 of 16 patients in this series did not have a true lateral radiograph.[101] The only relationship that can be determined is that of the primary ossification centers of the distal humerus to the proximal radius and ulna. One key component to the diagnosis on plain radiographs is recognizing that a line drawn along the shaft of the ulna is not aligned with the shaft of the humerus on the AP view.[2,81] The proximal radius and ulna maintain an anatomic relationship to each other but are usually displaced posteriorly and medially in relation to the distal humerus. Although theoretically, the distal fragment can be displaced in any direction, with rare exceptions, most fractures reported

have been displaced posteromedially. One series of 16 patients demonstrated medial displacement in 94% of cases and posterior displacement of the radius and ulna in 38%.[101] In a review of the literature including 33 cases, posteromedial displacement was identified in 64% of cases.[86] Comparison views of the opposite uninjured elbow may be helpful to determine the presence of posteromedial displacement (see Fig. 18-1A,B). A posterior fat pad sign is generally present while an anterior one is not.[2,33]

Distinguishing the injury from an elbow dislocation may be challenging. It should be remembered that elbow dislocations are rare in the peak age group for fractures involving the entire distal humeral physis. With elbow dislocations, the displacement of the proximal radius and ulna is almost always posterolateral, and the relationship between the proximal radius and lateral condylar epiphysis is disrupted.[2] Unfortunately, this can be especially difficult to assess in young children when the capitellum is not yet ossified (Fig. 18-2). In contrast, the anatomic relationship of the lateral condylar epiphysis with the radial head is maintained with a transphyseal distal humeral separation, even though the distal humeral epiphysis is displaced posterior and medial in relation to the metaphysis of the humerus. Once the lateral condylar epiphysis becomes ossified, displacement of the entire distal epiphysis is much more obvious.

Because they have a large metaphyseal fragment, type C fractures may be confused with either a low supracondylar fracture or a fracture of the lateral condylar physis. The key diagnostic point is the smooth outline of the distal metaphysis in fractures involving the entire distal physis. With supracondylar

Figure 18-2. Oblique (**A**) and AP (**B**) plain radiographs showing that the forearm is not aligned with the humerus, which is characteristic of a transphyseal distal humerus fracture. (Courtesy of Joshua Abzug, MD, Baltimore, MD.)

Figure 18-3. A 3-year-old girl fell off her bike and sustained a right lateral condyle fracture. Preoperative AP (**A**), internal oblique (**B**), and lateral (**C**) views. Postoperative AP (**D**) and lateral (**E**) views. (Copyright Joshua M. Abzug, MD, Baltimore, MD.)

fractures, the distal portion of the distal fragment has a more irregular border.

Differentiation from a fracture of the lateral condylar physis in an infant can be made on plain radiographs. With a displaced fracture of the lateral condylar physis, the relationship between the lateral condylar epiphysis and the proximal radius can be disrupted but may remain normal (Fig. 18-3). If the lateral crista of the trochlea is involved, the proximal radius and ulna may be displaced posterolaterally. Oblique radiographs or other advanced imaging may be necessary to distinguish these injuries. Misdiagnosis, even by pediatric radiologists, of transphyseal humeral physeal fractures is common in the acute setting.[18] Advanced imaging may be indicated.

If differentiation of this injury from an intra-articular fracture is uncertain, arthrography, ultrasound, and/or MRI may be helpful (Fig. 18-4).[2,74] In neonates and infants in whom ossification has not yet begun, ultrasonography can be used to identify the displaced epiphysis of the humerus without the need for sedation that is typically necessary for an MRI or arthrogram (Fig. 18-5).[23,52,73,101,108] In the review by Hariharan et al.,[41] all

(n = 79) patients had plain radiographs obtained, while 5% (n = 4) had an ultrasound and 5% (n = 4) had an MRI.

In a series of 16 patients in which 56% of the injuries were not identified on plain radiographs, ultrasound was performed in 12 of the patients and the diagnosis was made in all of them.[101] If the diagnosis is delayed, new periosteal bone forms around the distal humerus that will be seen on subsequent radiographs, and the whole epiphysis may remain displaced posteriorly and medially (Fig. 18-6).

CLASSIFICATION OF FRACTURES INVOLVING THE ENTIRE DISTAL HUMERUS

DeLee et al.[22] classified fractures of the entire distal humeral physis into three groups based on the degree of ossification of the lateral condylar epiphysis and the fracture pattern seen radiographically (see Fig. 18-1). Group A fractures occur in infants up to 12 months of age, before the secondary ossification center of the lateral condylar epiphysis appears (see Fig. 18-1A). They are usually Salter–Harris type I physeal

Figure 18-4. MRI demonstrating a transphyseal fracture of the distal humerus. Note the posterior displacement of the capitellar fragment such that the anterior humeral line does not intersect the capitellum. *Arrow* points to the capitellar fragment. (Copyright Joshua M. Abzug, MD, Baltimore, MD.)

injuries. This injury may be missed because of the lack of an ossification center in the lateral condylar epiphysis. Group B fractures occur most often in children 12 months to 3 years of age in whom there is definite ossification of the lateral condylar epiphysis (see Fig. 18-1C). Although there may be a small flake of metaphyseal bone (Salter–Harris II fracture), this essentially behaves as a type I Salter–Harris physeal injury. By definition, the fracture fragment is smaller than the lateral condylar ossification center. Group C fractures occur in older children, from 3 to 7 years of age, and result in a large metaphyseal fragment

Figure 18-5. Ultrasonography demonstrating the displaced distal humeral epiphysis. C, capitellum; H, humerus. (Copyright Joshua M. Abzug, MD, Baltimore, MD.)

Figure 18-6. The true nature of this injury as involving the entire distal humeral physis was not appreciated until periosteal new bone became visible 3 weeks after injury.

(Salter–Harris II fracture) that by definition is larger than the lateral condylar secondary ossification center and most commonly lateral but can be medial or posterior (see Fig. 18-1D,E).

Transphyseal distal humerus fractures are almost always extension-type injuries with the distal epiphyseal fragment displacing posterior to the metaphysis. A rare flexion type of injury can occur in which the epiphyseal fragment is displaced anteriorly. Stricker et al.[98] reported a coronal plane transcondylar (Salter–Harris type IV) fracture in a 3-year-old child that was initially diagnosed as a fracture of the lateral humeral condyle. No growth disturbance was evident 3 years after open reduction and pin fixation.

PATHOANATOMY AND APPLIED ANATOMY RELATING TO FRACTURES INVOLVING THE ENTIRE DISTAL HUMERUS

Distal humeral physeal injuries have similar anatomic considerations as supracondylar humerus fractures. However, because the patients who sustain this injury are often very young, diagnosis and treatment can be more challenging.

Because the fracture is distal, the fracture surfaces are broader than those proximally through the supracondylar region. This broader surface area of the fracture line may help prevent tilting of the distal fragment. Because the fracture lines do not involve the articular surface, development of joint incongruity with resultant long-term loss of elbow motion is unlikely if a malunion occurs.

The distal humeral epiphysis extends across to include the secondary ossification center of the medial epicondyle until about 6 to 7 years of age in girls and 8 to 9 years of age in boys. Thus, fractures involving the entire physeal line include the medial epicondyle up to these ages. In older children, only the lateral and medial condylar physeal lines are included.

A   **B**

Figure 18-7. **A:** At 1 year of age, the metaphysis has advanced only to the supracondylar ridges. **B:** By 4 years of age, the edge of the metaphysis has advanced well into the area of the epicondyles. (Copyright Joshua M. Abzug, MD, Baltimore, MD.)

Finally, it should be recognized that part of the blood supply to the medial crista of the trochlea courses directly through the physis. The blood supply to this area is vulnerable to injury, which may cause osteonecrosis in this part of the trochlea.

Because the physeal line is more proximal in young infants, it is nearer the center of the olecranon fossa (Fig. 18-7). A hyperextension injury in this age group is more likely to result in a physeal separation than a bony supracondylar fracture.[19]

TREATMENT OPTIONS FOR FRACTURES INVOLVING THE ENTIRE DISTAL HUMERUS

Treatment is first directed toward prompt injury recognition. Because the mechanism of injury may be associated with NAT, the child's home caregivers may delay seeking treatment. The goal of treatment is to obtain acceptable alignment before and up until the fracture heals over 2 to 3 weeks after injury. As stated previously, recognizing a child at risk for NAT and engaging appropriate professionals is an essential part of care for these children to prevent more serious injury in the future.

Simple splint or cast immobilization has been suggested by several authors.[4,22,61,78] However, many investigators have shown that cubitus varus develops after nonoperative treatment of these fractures.[1,21,22,46] De Jager and Hoffman[21] reported 12

fracture separations of the distal humeral epiphysis, 3 of which were initially diagnosed as fractures of the lateral condyle and 1 as an elbow dislocation. Because of the frequency of cubitus varus after this injury in young children, the authors recommended closed reduction and percutaneous pinning in children younger than 2 years of age. The carrying angle malalignment is corrected with reduction. Stability is assessed and often requires pin fixation to maintain alignment after reduction. Elbow arthrography is helpful for diagnostic purposes and to assess the reduction after fixation. (Fig. 18-8) An elbow arthrogram was performed in 87.3% (n = 69) of surgical cases in the review by Hariharan et al.[41] In a 2015 review of 33 cases identified in the literature, 12% underwent surgical treatment, 88% were treated nonoperatively, and 23 cases (69%) had an attempted reduction. In this review, 88% recovered the carrying angle and 80% range of motion with no differences in outcomes found between types of treatment.[86]

Several investigators have reported open reduction, usually performed owing to misdiagnosis as a displaced fracture of the lateral humeral condyle.[3,46,88] Mizuno et al.,[67] however, recommended primary open reduction because of their poor results with closed reduction. The authors approached the fracture posteriorly by removing the triceps insertion from the olecranon with a small piece of cartilage. An anterolateral approach may be more anatomic through the torn periosteum and less at risk for disruption of the posterior blood supply and intact soft tissues.

Figure 18-8. A 5-day-old boy who sustained a transphyseal separation during the birthing process. **A:** Intraoperative true AP fluoroscopic image of the elbow demonstrating the lack of alignment of the forearm and humeral shaft. **B, C:** Intraoperative arthrograms permit clear visualization of the distal humerus articular surface and aid in the pinning process. Intraoperative AP (**D**) and lateral (**E**) fluoroscopic images of the elbow demonstrating near anatomic alignment after reduction and pinning.

(continues)

F

G

Figure 18-8. (*Continued*) Postoperative AP (F) and lateral (G) radiographs of the elbow obtained at 3 weeks demonstrating abundant callus formation. (Courtesy of Joshua Abzug, MD, Baltimore, MD.)

If the fracture is more than 5 or 6 days old and the epiphysis is no longer mobile, manipulation should not be attempted given the risk of a growth arrest, and the elbow should be splinted for comfort. Many essentially untreated fractures remodel completely without any residual deformity if the distal fragment is only medially translocated and not tilted (Fig. 18-9). In the more displaced three-dimensional malunions, a later osteotomy may be indicated.

NONOPERATIVE TREATMENT OF FRACTURES INVOLVING THE ENTIRE DISTAL HUMERUS

Indications/Contraindications

Nonoperative Treatment of Fractures Involving the Entire Distal Humerus: INDICATIONS AND CONTRAINDICATIONS
Indications
• Minimal displacement • Neonate/small infants where anesthesia risks do not outweigh the benefits of surgical intervention
Relative Contraindication
• Markedly displaced fractures with prompt diagnosis

In neonates and very small infants in whom general anesthesia risks do not outweigh the benefits of surgical intervention, splint or cast immobilization can be used to treat these fractures but does carry a risk of extra-articular malunion. Late osteotomy may be required if fracture does not remodel.

Technique

The extremity is simply immobilized for 2 to 3 weeks in a long arm splint or cast with up to 90 degrees of elbow flexion with the forearm pronated.[2] The extremity is then externally stabilized with a swathe to limit movement and decrease pain.

Outcomes

Although outcome and function are usually good, some investigators have shown that cubitus varus can occur because of the posterior medial displacement of the fracture after nonoperative treatment of these injuries.[1,21,22,46] The rate of cubitus varus was noted to be 3 of 12,[22] 15 of 21,[1] and 5 of 7[46] in various series. In the series by Gilbert and Conklin, four patients were treated with immobilization alone, with three of them having residual deformity.[33] In a review of 33 cases identified in the literature, 88% were treated nonoperatively, and 23 cases (69%) had an attempted reduction. In this review, 88% recovered the carrying angle, 80% range of motion compared to the contralateral side, and no differences in outcomes were found between types of treatment.[86]

OPERATIVE TREATMENT OF FRACTURES INVOLVING THE ENTIRE DISTAL HUMERUS

Indications/Contraindications

In most infants and young children with a displaced fracture, external immobilization is usually not dependable in maintaining the reduction, and therefore, operative intervention is indicated. A contraindication to operative intervention is a neonate who is too medically unstable to undergo anesthesia in a timely manner following the fracture.

A, B   C

Figure 18-9. Remodeling of untreated fractures. **A:** AP view of a 2-year-old who had an unrecognized and untreated fracture of the distal humeral physis. The medial translocation is apparent. There was no varus or valgus tilting. **B:** Four years later, there had been almost complete remodeling of the distal humerus. A small supracondylar prominence (*arrow*) remains as a scar from the original injury. **C:** Clinical appearance 4 years after injury shows no difference in elbow alignment.

Closed Reduction and Percutaneous Pin Fixation

Preoperative Planning

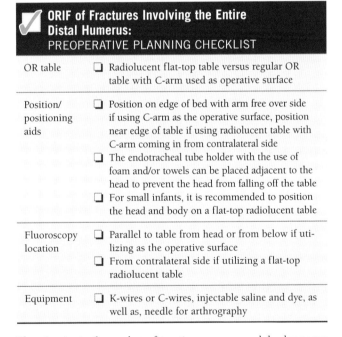

✓	**ORIF of Fractures Involving the Entire Distal Humerus:** PREOPERATIVE PLANNING CHECKLIST	
OR table	❏ Radiolucent flat-top table versus regular OR table with C-arm used as operative surface	
Position/ positioning aids	❏ Position on edge of bed with arm free over side if using C-arm as the operative surface, position near edge of table if using radiolucent table with C-arm coming in from contralateral side ❏ The endotracheal tube holder with the use of foam and/or towels can be placed adjacent to the head to prevent the head from falling off the table ❏ For small infants, it is recommended to position the head and body on a flat-top radiolucent table	
Fluoroscopy location	❏ Parallel to table from head or from below if utilizing as the operative surface ❏ From contralateral side if utilizing a flat-top radiolucent table	
Equipment	❏ K-wires or C-wires, injectable saline and dye, as well as, needle for arthrography	

Planning is similar to that of treating a supracondylar humerus fracture. In cases where the elbow is largely unossified, one must prepare for arthrography to aid with the diagnosis and to assess the reduction and fixation.

Positioning

The patient can be positioned two ways—on the edge of the table with the affected extremity free over the side of the table and with the base of the C-arm used as the operative surface; or on a radiolucent flat-top table on the edge of the table. The C-arm can be brought underneath the table from the contralateral side so that you can use the radiolucent table as the operative surface rather than the C-arm. Similarly, you can use a small radiolucent hand table or plexiglass support. If utilizing the C-arm as the operative surface, the endotracheal tube holder with the use of foam and/or towels can be placed adjacent to the head to prevent the head from falling off the table. Often the endotracheal tube is also positioned on the other side of the face to prevent interference.

Technique

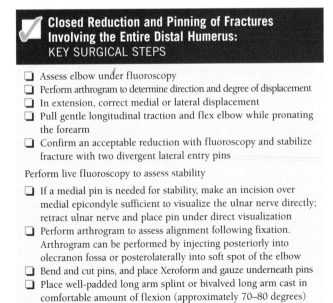

✓	**Closed Reduction and Pinning of Fractures Involving the Entire Distal Humerus:** KEY SURGICAL STEPS
	❏ Assess elbow under fluoroscopy ❏ Perform arthrogram to determine direction and degree of displacement ❏ In extension, correct medial or lateral displacement ❏ Pull gentle longitudinal traction and flex elbow while pronating the forearm ❏ Confirm an acceptable reduction with fluoroscopy and stabilize fracture with two divergent lateral entry pins

Perform live fluoroscopy to assess stability

❏ If a medial pin is needed for stability, make an incision over medial epicondyle sufficient to visualize the ulnar nerve directly; retract ulnar nerve and place pin under direct visualization
❏ Perform arthrogram to assess alignment following fixation. Arthrogram can be performed by injecting posteriorly into olecranon fossa or posterolaterally into soft spot of the elbow
❏ Bend and cut pins, and place Xeroform and gauze underneath pins
❏ Place well-padded long arm splint or bivalved long arm cast in comfortable amount of flexion (approximately 70–80 degrees)

Figure 18-10. Radiographs of a 3-year-old patient who sustained a transphyseal fracture of the distal humerus when they fell off of a bed. Preoperative AP (**A**) and attempted lateral (**B**) views, intraoperative fluoroscopic AP (**C**) and lateral (**D**) views following a closed reduction and percutaneous pinning with an arthrogram. (Copyright Joshua M. Abzug, MD, Baltimore, MD.)

Under general anesthesia, the elbow is initially manipulated while in extension to correct the medial displacement, and then the fragment is stabilized by flexing the elbow and pronating the forearm. When the forearm is supinated with the elbow flexed, the distal fragment tends to displace medially. This displacement is usually a pure medial horizontal translation without mediolateral coronal tilting. The fragment is secured with two bicortical, divergent lateral entry pins (Fig. 18-10).

Because of the swelling and immaturity of the distal humerus, the medial epicondyle is difficult to define as a distinct landmark, making it risky to attempt the percutaneous placement of a medial pin through the medial epicondyle. If a medial pin is necessary for stable fracture fixation, a medial incision should be made to allow direct observation of the medial epicondyle and the ulnar nerve. Usually, two or three smooth lateral pins (0.062 inches or smaller depending on size and age of patient) are used. In infants and young children with minimal ossification of the epiphyseal fragment, an intraoperative arthrogram should be obtained to help determine the quality of the reduction (see Fig. 18-8). The arthrogram is performed utilizing equal parts of injectable dye and injectable saline. A posterior portal can be utilized to limit potential iatrogenic injury to articular cartilage or extravasation that can make your arthrogram nondiagnostic.

In a recent study, Zhou et al.[117] described a procedure that uses ultrasonography to guide closed reduction of transphyseal fractures of the distal humerus. Under general anesthesia, ultrasonography is performed in two longitudinal sectional planes to show the lateral displacement of the distal end of the fracture and the posterior displacement of the distal end of the fracture. With this visualization, the reduction is performed with maneuvers similar to those required for a supracondylar humerus fracture. Subsequently, appropriately sized smooth K-wires are placed across the fracture site to stabilize the reduction. Outcomes were considered to be excellent in 77.78% of patients and good in 22.22% of patients, according to Flynn criteria. 7.4% of patients developed a cubitus varus deformity. There was no significant difference between the carrying angle of the uninjured side and the affected side at the final follow-up visit.[117]

Authors' Preferred Treatment for Fractures Involving the Entire Distal Humerus (Algorithm 18-1)

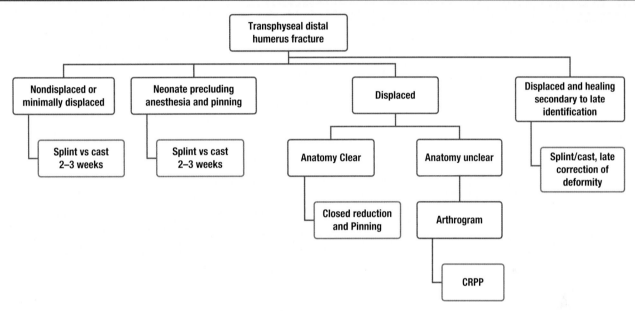

Algorithm 18-1. Authors' preferred treatment for fractures involving the entire distal humerus.

In neonates and infants in whom general anesthesia and percutaneous pin fixation is contraindicated, we typically simply immobilize the extremity in 90 degrees of flexion with the forearm pronated. The extremity is then externally stabilized with a splint.

In most infants and young children, external immobilization is usually not dependable in maintaining the reduction and therefore closed reduction with percutaneous pinning is performed, typically with the aid of an arthrogram (see Fig. 18-10). An intraoperative arthrogram will aid in determining the quality of the reduction in patients with limited ossification. If a medial pin is necessary for stable fracture fixation, a medial incision should be made, and the ulnar nerve identified and protected. Closed reduction, pinning, and arthrographic assessment are performed in neonates and very young children who can tolerate anesthesia safely.

If treatment is delayed more than 5 to 7 days and if the epiphysis is not freely movable, thus making it at risk of growth arrest if manipulated, the elbow is simply immobilized in a splint or cast. It is likely better to treat any resulting deformity later with a supracondylar osteotomy rather than to risk the complication of physeal injury or osteonecrosis of the epiphysis by performing a delayed manipulation or open reduction.

Postoperative Care

The extremity is immobilized for 3 weeks. After 3 weeks, the patient's cast/splint is removed, imaging is obtained, and the pins are removed in the office. There often is exuberant periosteal healing. The patient does not require further immobilization and active elbow motion is resumed. The patient is then followed until full motion is regained and until there is radiographic evidence of normal physeal and epiphyseal growth and if needed, fracture remodeling.

Fractures Involving the Entire Distal Humerus: POTENTIAL PITFALLS AND PREVENTIONS

Pitfalls	Preventions
Use medial pin, inaccurate placement, or iatrogenic ulnar nerve palsy	• Lateral entry pin placement • If medial pin is absolutely needed, make incision about the medial epicondyle and visualize directly and retract ulnar nerve posteriorly during pinning
Difficulty gauging reduction because of elbow being largely unossified	• Perform arthrogram to assess reduction
Loss of reduction	• Assess stability of fracture under live fluoroscopy following fixation • Ensure pins are bicortical and divergent in nature with at least 2 mm of separation at the fracture site

Because of the swelling and immaturity of the distal humerus, the ulnar nerve is at risk with placement of a medial pin. Making an incision and visualizing and retracting the ulnar nerve out of the way helps prevent iatrogenic injury. Quality of reduction is difficult to assess in small infants and young children and therefore an intraoperative arthrogram is utilized to ensure adequate reduction.

OUTCOMES

Abzug et al.[2] reported on 79 operatively managed transphyseal humeral separations over a 25-year period. Sixty-two percent were treated more than 24 hours after the initial injury. Closed reduction and percutaneous pinning was performed in most patients, with only two (2.5%) patients requiring open reduction and internal fixation. Eighty-seven percent of the patients underwent elbow arthrography. The most common pin size and pin configuration was 0.062 inch ($n = 44$, 59.5%) and lateral entry only ($n = 62$, 78%). In total, 11 complications (14%) were noted, including decreased range of motion ($n = 4$), cubitus varus/valgus ($n = 6$), and need for additional surgery ($n = 1$). One distal humeral osteotomy was performed in a case of cubitus varus.

Zhou et al. found no significant difference in functional outcomes for toddlers with transphyseal humerus fractures treated with open versus closed reduction and pinning.[118] Their cohort of 16 patients was all pain free with similar functional evaluation regardless of surgical procedure. The 10 patients who were old enough to assess had no significant difference in their Mayo elbow Performance Scores.

MANAGEMENT OF EXPECTED ADVERSE OUTCOMES AND UNEXPECTED COMPLICATIONS IN FRACTURES INVOLVING THE ENTIRE DISTAL HUMERUS

Fractures Involving the Entire Distal Humerus: COMMON ADVERSE OUTCOMES AND COMPLICATIONS

• Malunion/cubitus varus
• Neurovascular injuries (rare)
• Osteonecrosis of lateral condyle or trochlear epiphysis (rare)

MALUNION

Substantial cubitus varus deformity can occur after this injury (see Fig. 18-9B).[61,64] Because the fracture surfaces are wider with this injury than with supracondylar fractures, the distal fragment tends to tilt less, which seems to account for the lower incidence or severity of cubitus varus after this injury than after untreated supracondylar fractures. However, reduction and percutaneous pinning are recommended for acute fractures with displacement to prevent this complication. Oh et al. reported on 12 cases treated with operative and nonoperative treatment and 7 of 12 had residual cubitus varus.[76] Hariharan et al. reported 6 of 79 operatively managed went on to malunion. In the series of operatively managed by Zhou et al.,[118] the authors found that 50% of patients developed cubitus varus, but only one of eight was documented as severe. A delayed supracondylar humerus osteotomy may be indicated when there is insufficient remodeling. (See Chapter 14 for details of surgical techniques for osteotomies.)

NEUROVASCULAR INJURIES

Neurovascular injuries, either transient or permanent, are rare with transphyseal humerus fractures as opposed to the high incidence with supracondylar humerus fractures. This may be because the fracture fragments are covered with physeal cartilage and do not have sharp edges. In addition, the fracture fragments are usually not as markedly displaced as in supracondylar humerus fractures given the typically lower energy mechanism of injuries. Finally, the fracture displacement is usually posteromedial rather than posterolateral; posterolateral displacement puts tension on the median nerve and brachial artery.

NONUNION

Only one nonunion after a transphyseal humerus fracture has been reported, which occurred in a patient seen 3 months after the initial injury.[67] Because of the abundant vascularity and propensity for osteogenesis in this area, union is rapid even in patients who receive essentially no treatment.

OSTEONECROSIS

Osteonecrosis of the epiphysis of the lateral condyle or the trochlear epiphysis has rarely been reported after fractures of the entire distal humeral physis. Yoo et al.[115] reported eight patients with osteonecrosis of the trochlea after physeal fracture separations of the distal end of the humerus. Six of the eight fractures were diagnosed initially as medial condylar fractures, lateral condylar fractures, or traumatic elbow dislocations. All eight patients had rapid dissolution of the trochlea within 3 to 6 weeks after the injury, followed by the development of a medial or central condylar fishtail deformity. Oh et al. reported on 12 cases, and of the 7 cases that had cubitus varus, 6 had a partial defect of the medial condyle related to avascular necrosis.[76] Further discussion regarding the etiology of this complication is discussed in the section on osteonecrosis of the trochlea. Of note, the series of 79 fractures reported by Abzug et al. did not have any cases of avascular necrosis.[2]

SUMMARY, CONTROVERSIES, AND FUTURE DIRECTIONS FOR FRACTURES INVOLVING THE ENTIRE DISTAL HUMERUS

Transphyseal injuries of the distal humerus are rare. In young children, NAT should be suspected and the patient should be evaluated for associated injuries. This is imperative as it may be lifesaving. The injury should be distinguished from an elbow dislocation, which may be difficult to assess in the unossified elbow, but can be identified on close inspection of plain radiographs. In neonates or children in which anesthesia is contraindicated, simple immobilization can be used, but patients may heal in varus. In children who can undergo anesthesia, closed reduction and pin fixation, with the aid of an arthrogram, should be performed to improve alignment and minimize complications of cubitus varus. It is recommended to avoid late manipulation (after 5–7 days)[81] because of the danger of avascular necrosis, physeal injury, and/or growth disturbances. An arthrogram is often needed to adequately assess reduction and should be routinely performed.

Fractures Involving the Medial Condyle

INTRODUCTION TO FRACTURES INVOLVING THE MEDIAL CONDYLE

Fractures of the medial condyle can be thought of as the mirror image of lateral condyle fractures, which are more commonly encountered (see Chapter 17). Fractures involving the medial condyle have two components. The intra-articular component involves, in some manner, the trochlear articular surface. The extra-articular portion includes the medial metaphysis and medial epicondyle. Because the fracture line extends into the articular surface of the trochlea, these often are called *trochlear fractures*. For purposes of description in this chapter, fractures of the trochlea are those that include only the articular surface.

Fractures involving the medial condyle are rare in skeletally immature children, accounting for less than 1% of fractures involving the distal humerus.[47] Many of the large series of elbow fractures in the literature and early fracture texts do not mention these fractures as a separate entity. Blount[9] described only one such fracture in his classic text. In Faysse and Marion's[27] review of more than 2,000 fractures of the distal humerus in children, only 10 fractures involved the medial condyle. The more recent literature now has reports of medial condyle fractures in patients as young as 6 months of age, but most reports have these occurring in older children between 8 and 12 years, as the distal humeral growth plate closes.[28,121] These rare injuries are very problematic if they can occur before the trochlear secondary center of ossification appears. Diagnosis is difficult and may be missed. A high index of suspicion is necessary to avoid missing a displaced, intra-articular fracture in the young child (Fig. 18-11).

Figure 18-11. Intra-articular extension. **A:** Injury film of a 7-year-old girl who was initially suspected of having only a fracture of the medial epicondyle. In addition to moderate displacement, there was a significant metaphyseal fragment (*arrow*). **B:** An arthrogram revealed intra-articular components (*arrow*), which defined this injury instead as a fracture involving the medial condylar physis. (Courtesy of Carl McGarey, MD.)

A   **B**

Resultant malunion of the trochlear articular surface can be detrimental to long-term function.

Most series[79] show medial condylar fractures occurring somewhat later than lateral condylar fractures. A review of 40 patients in 11 series[14,26,31,38,77,79,84,100,109] in which the specific ages were given showed that 38 patients were in the age range of 8 to 14 years. Thus, this fracture seems to occur most often after the ossification centers of the medial condylar epiphysis begin to appear. As noted earlier, a medial condylar fracture can occur as early as 6 months of age; however, this is before any ossification of the distal humerus has appeared,[7,20] making the diagnosis extremely difficult and outcome poor if missed and not treated acutely with anatomic joint reduction and fracture stabilization.

ASSESSMENT OF FRACTURES INVOLVING THE MEDIAL CONDYLAR PHYSIS

MECHANISMS OF INJURY FOR FRACTURES INVOLVING THE MEDIAL CONDYLAR PHYSIS

Two separate mechanisms of injury can produce physeal fractures of the medial condyle. Ashurst's patients described falling directly on the point of their flexed elbow. This mechanism was also implicated in other reports.[7,14,39,84] In this mechanism, it is speculated that the semilunar notch's sharp edge of the olecranon splits the trochlea directly (Fig. 18-12A). This mechanism is also supported by recent case reports of a medial condyle fracture in the setting of a pre-existing fishtail deformity.[71,77]

In three more recent series,[13,29,31] many patients sustained a medial condyle fracture when they fell on their outstretched arms. The theory is that this is an avulsion injury caused by a valgus stress at the elbow (Fig. 18-12B). Fowles and Kassab[29] reported a patient with a concomitant valgus greenstick fracture of the olecranon associated with a fracture of the medial condyle. The authors believed this fracture provided further evidence that this was a valgus avulsion type of injury. Once the fragment becomes disassociated from the distal humerus, the forearm flexor muscles produce a sagittal anterior rotation of the fragment.

Yang et al. reported a case of delayed nonunion and displacement of a medial condyle fracture due to an initial missed diagnosis of a nondisplaced fracture, with subsequent excessive functional exercise, resulting in fragment displacement.[112]

INJURIES ASSOCIATED WITH FRACTURES INVOLVING THE MEDIAL CONDYLAR PHYSIS

As this fracture is rare, studies describing associated injuries are rare. Medial condylar physeal fractures have been reported in association with greenstick fractures of the olecranon and with true posterolateral elbow dislocations (Fig. 18-13).[7,20,29] Some investigators[7,20] found that NAT was more common in their younger patients with these fractures than with other elbow fractures. Regardless, the extremity should be evaluated for concomitant injuries about the forearm, wrist, and hand, and the radiographs should be inspected for additional fractures about the elbow.

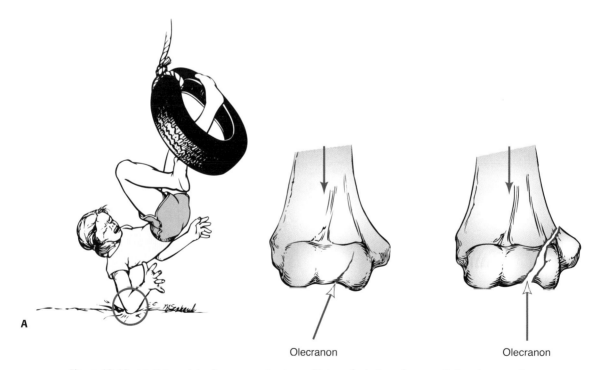

Figure 18-12. Medial condylar fracture mechanisms of injury. **A:** A direct force applied to the posterior aspect of the elbow causes the sharp articular margin of the olecranon to wedge the medial condyle from the distal humerus.

Olecranon   Olecranon

Figure 18-12. *(Continued)* **B:** Falling on the outstretched arm with the elbow extended and the wrist dorsiflexed causes the medial condyle to be avulsed by both ligamentous and muscular forces.

SIGNS AND SYMPTOMS OF FRACTURES INVOLVING THE MEDIAL CONDYLAR PHYSIS

Clinically, and on radiographs, a fracture of the medial condylar physis is most often confused with a fracture of the medial epicondyle.[56] In both fracture patterns, swelling is concentrated medially, and there may be valgus instability of the elbow joint. In a true intra-articular fracture, however, there is varus instability as well. Such is usually not the case with an isolated extra-articular fracture of the medial epicondyle. Ulnar nerve paresthesia may be present with both types of fractures. A high level of suspicion should be maintained for patients with a history of an elbow injury presenting with significant medial-sided edema, ecchymosis, and/or tenderness to palpation, even in the presence of benign radiographs.[111,121]

IMAGING AND OTHER DIAGNOSTIC STUDIES FOR FRACTURES INVOLVING THE MEDIAL CONDYLAR PHYSIS

In older children with a large metaphyseal fragment, involvement of the entire condyle is usually obvious on plain radiographs (Fig. 18-14A); an external oblique view of the elbow may make the fracture more easily identifiable and therefore should be obtained with a suspected medial condyle fracture. In younger children, in whom only the epicondyle is ossified, fracture of the medial condylar physis may be erroneously diagnosed as an isolated fracture of the medial epicondyle (Fig. 18-14B,C).[26,29]

In differentiating these two fractures, it is helpful to remember that medial epicondylar fractures are often associated with elbow dislocations, usually in a posterolateral direction, and that elbow dislocations are rare before ossification of the medial condylar epiphysis begins. With medial condylar physeal fractures, the elbow tends to subluxate posteromedially because of the loss of trochlear stability.

Any metaphyseal ossification with the epicondylar fragment suggests the presence of an intra-articular fracture of the medial condyle and is an indication for further evaluation. Often, the medial condyle and the medial epicondyle are markedly displaced as a unit. A positive posterior fat pad sign indicates that the injury has entered the elbow joint and a fracture of the medial condyle is likely.[42,96] Isolated fractures of the medial epicondyle are extra-articular and usually do not have a positive posterior fat pad sign unless it is associated with an elbow dislocation or spontaneous reduction of an elbow subluxation/dislocation.[81]

If the true location of the fracture line is questionable in a child younger than 8 to 10 years of age, with substantial medial elbow ecchymosis, ultrasound, arthrography, and/or MRI of the elbow should be performed.

CLASSIFICATION OF FRACTURES INVOLVING THE MEDIAL CONDYLAR PHYSIS

Classification, as with fractures of the lateral condylar physis, is based on the fracture line's location and the degree of the fracture's displacement.

Figure 18-13. An 8-year-old girl fell off a swing set and sustained a type III right medial condyle fracture with an associated elbow dislocation. Preoperative AP (**A**) and lateral (**B**) views. Postoperative AP (**C**), external oblique (**D**), and lateral (**E**) views. (Copyright Joshua M. Abzug, MD, Baltimore, MD.)

Figure 18-14. Missed medial condylar fracture. **A:** Initial film of a 6-year-old who was originally diagnosed as having a displaced fracture of the medial epicondyle (*arrows*). **B:** Normal side for comparison. **C:** Three months later, the patient continued to have a painful elbow, and there was ossification of the metaphysis (*arrow*) adjacent to the epicondyle.

Location of the Fracture Line

Milch[65] classified fractures of the medial condylar physis in adults into two types. In type I fractures, the fracture line traverses the apex of the trochlea. In type II fractures, it traverses more laterally through the capitulotrochlear groove. He believed that the origin of the fracture line depended on whether the radial head, as in type II, or the semilunar notch of the olecranon, as in type I, served as the impinging force for the abduction injury. Both fracture patterns occur in children (Fig. 18-15A), but type I fractures seem to be more common because the common physeal line, which serves as a point of weakness, ends in the apex of the trochlea.

Displacement of the Fracture

Kilfoyle[53] described three fracture displacement patterns that can be helpful in determining appropriate treatment (Fig. 18-15B). In type I, the fracture line in the medial condylar metaphysis extends down to the physis. He noted that some of these might represent incomplete supracondylar fractures. Unless there is a greenstick crushing of the medial supracondylar column, these fractures are usually nondisplaced, stable, and of no clinical significance. In type II, the fracture line extends into the medial condylar physis. The intra-articular portion, as it is in preosseous cartilage, is often not recognized. In this second type, the medial condylar fragment usually remains nondisplaced.

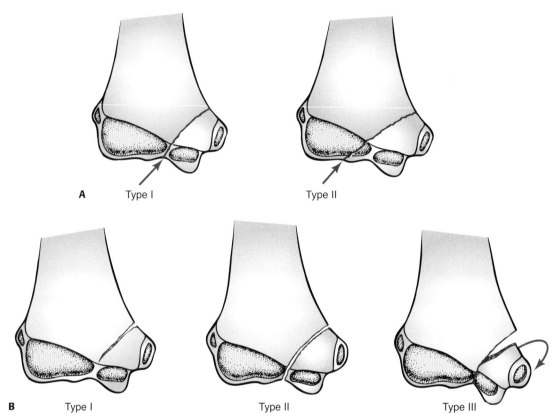

Figure 18-15. A: Medial condylar fracture patterns. In the Milch type I injury, the fracture line terminates in the trochlear notch (**left,** *arrow*). In the Milch type II injury, the fracture line terminates more laterally in the capitulotrochlear groove (**right,** *arrow*). **B:** Kilfoyle classification of displacement patterns. Degrees of displacement for fracture type I is an incomplete fracture that does not violate the joint but may hinge open; type II is a fracture that enters the joint but has less than 2-mm displacement; type III enters the joint and results in malangulation, malrotation, and articular displacement.

In type III fractures, the condylar fragment is both rotated and displaced. Some authors use a modification of Kilfoyle's classification based on the amount of displacement and describe it as nondisplaced (<2 mm), minimally displaced (2–4 mm), and displaced (>4 mm) similar to classifications of lateral condylar fractures.[45] Bensahel et al.[7] and Papavasiliou et al.[79] found that type III fractures, which accounted for only 25%, were more likely to occur in older adolescents, and type I fractures were more common in younger children. Fernandez et al.[28] found that type III fractures that occurred in older children always had the trochlea ossified. These studies also confirmed the correlation between the amount of displacement and the treatment method.

PATHOANATOMY AND APPLIED ANATOMY RELATING TO FRACTURES INVOLVING THE MEDIAL CONDYLAR PHYSIS

Fractures of the medial condylar physis involve both intra- and extraarticular components. They behave as Salter–Harris type IV physeal injuries, but not enough fractures have been described to show whether the fracture line courses through the secondary ossification center of the medial condylar epiphysis or whether it enters the common physeal line separating the lateral condylar ossification center from the medial condylar ossification center. This common physeal line terminates in the notch of the trochlea. The trochlea's lateral crista is ossified from the lateral condylar epiphysis. Only the medial crista is ossified by the secondary ossification center of the medial condylar epiphysis. This fracture is commonly described as a "mirror image" of the lateral condylar physeal injury and thus has characteristics of Salter–Harris type IV physeal injuries (Fig. 18-16). The complication that develops if the fracture is untreated is a nonunion, similar to that after lateral condylar physeal fracture, rather than a physeal fusion, as commonly occurs after alternative location Salter–Harris type IV injuries. The resultant deformity of a medial condylar nonunion is cubitus varus instead of the cubitus valgus deformity that occurs with nonunion of the lateral condyle. If the nonunion is displaced, the trochlea articular surface will heal incongruently.

Characteristically, the metaphyseal fragment includes the intact medial epicondyle along with the common flexor origin of the muscles of the forearm. These flexor muscles cause the loosened fragment to rotate so that the fracture surface is facing anteriorly and medially and the articular surface is facing posteriorly and laterally (Fig. 18-17).[14] Rotation of the fragment is especially accentuated

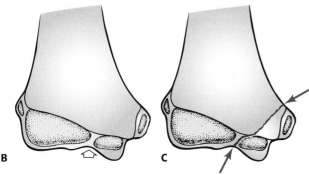

Figure 18-16. A: The AP radiograph of a 9-year-old boy demonstrates the location of the ossification centers. A common physeal line (*arrow*) separates the medial and lateral condylar physes. **B:** Relationship of the ossification centers to the articular surface. The common physis terminates in the trochlear notch (*arrow*). **C:** Location of the usual fracture line involving the medial condylar physis (*arrows*).

Figure 18-17. Displacement of the medial condyle. The pull of the forearm flexor muscles rotates the fragment so that the fracture surface is facing anteromedially and the articular surface is posterolateral.

when the elbow is extended. Chacha[14] also noted that often the lateral aspect of the common flexor origin and the anterior capsule of the joint were torn, permitting the fracture surface to commonly be reached through this anterior opening into the joint.

The blood supply to the medial epicondyle and medial metaphysis courses extra-articularly along with the medial flexor muscle groups. The blood supply to the lateral ossification center of the medial crista of the trochlea, however, must traverse the surface of the medial condylar physis. If the fracture line disrupts these small intra-articular vessels, disruption and subsequent circulation loss to the lateral portion of the medial crista can result, leading to osteonecrosis, collapse, and the development of a fishtail deformity.

TREATMENT OPTIONS FOR FRACTURES INVOLVING THE MEDIAL CONDYLAR PHYSIS

In Kilfoyle's displacement types I and II fracture patterns, enough residual internal stability is usually present to allow the fracture to be simply immobilized in a cast or long arm splint.[7,34,53,79] As with fractures of the lateral condylar physis, union may be slow. In fractures recognized and treated promptly, results have been satisfactory.[14,26,29] Because there is usually more displacement in older children, the results in this age group are not as satisfactory with closed treatment as those in younger children, who tend to have relatively nondisplaced or minimally displaced fractures.[7]

For displaced fractures, open reduction with internal fixation is the most often utilized treatment method.[7,13,29,31,53,79,82,84] The fracture fragment can be approached with a posteromedial incision that allows good exposure of both the fracture site and the ulnar nerve. Fixation is commonly achieved with smooth K-wires or with cannulated screws in older adolescents (Figs. 18-18 and 18-19). A minimum of two divergent K-wires are necessary due to the sagittal rotation forces exerted on the fracture fragment by the common flexor muscles. El Ghawabi[31] reported frequent delayed union and nonunion in fractures that were not rigidly stabilized.

NONOPERATIVE TREATMENT OF FRACTURES INVOLVING THE MEDIAL CONDYLAR PHYSIS

Indications/Contraindications

Nonoperative Treatment of Medial Condyle Fractures: INDICATIONS AND CONTRAINDICATIONS
Indications
• Nondisplaced fractures (Kilfoyle type I) • Minimally displaced fractures (some) (Kilfoyle type II)
Relative Contraindications
• Displaced fractures (Kilfoyle type III) • Fractures with increasing displacement upon close observation • Fractures in patients that will be noncompliant with close observation

Figure 18-18. A 5-year-old girl fell from a rocking horse and sustained a right medial condyle fracture. Preoperative AP (**A**) and lateral (**B**) views. **C:** Intraoperative photograph of the incision utilized for open reduction and internal fixation. Note the isolation of the ulnar nerve with a vessel loop and the utilization of a sterile tourniquet. Intraoperative fluoroscopic AP (**D**) and lateral (**E**) views following reduction and K-wire fixation. Note the utilization of the arthrogram with posterior portal placement of the needle. (Copyright Joshua M. Abzug, MD, Baltimore, MD.)

Figure 18-19. Medial condyle fracture fixed with cannulated screws to allow early range of motion.

Nondisplaced or minimally displaced fractures (Kilfoyle types I and II) can be treated nonoperatively with either splint or cast immobilization. However, close observation with weekly radiographs is necessary for a minimum of 2 weeks to ensure further displacement does not occur.

OPERATIVE TREATMENT OF FRACTURES INVOLVING THE MEDIAL CONDYLAR PHYSIS

Indications/Contraindications

For displaced fractures (Kilfoyle type III), operative fixation is recommended. In addition, minimally displaced fractures (Kilfoyle type II) that demonstrate instability and/or progressive displacement should be reduced anatomically and stabilized with fixation.

Open Reduction Internal Fixation of Medial Condyle Fracture

Preoperative Planning

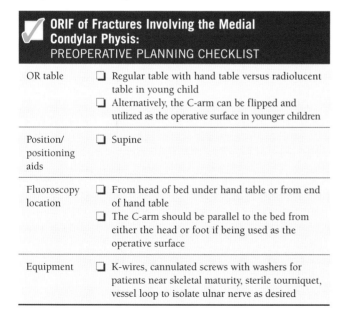

✓ **ORIF of Fractures Involving the Medial Condylar Physis:**
PREOPERATIVE PLANNING CHECKLIST

OR table	❏ Regular table with hand table versus radiolucent table in young child
	❏ Alternatively, the C-arm can be flipped and utilized as the operative surface in younger children
Position/ positioning aids	❏ Supine
Fluoroscopy location	❏ From head of bed under hand table or from end of hand table
	❏ The C-arm should be parallel to the bed from either the head or foot if being used as the operative surface
Equipment	❏ K-wires, cannulated screws with washers for patients near skeletal maturity, sterile tourniquet, vessel loop to isolate ulnar nerve as desired

Adequate radiographs, including an external oblique view, should be obtained to assess fracture morphology. At times, three-dimensional imaging is useful in operative planning, especially with late presentation or recognition.

Positioning

Although medial epicondyle fractures may be approached supine or prone,[35] typically the patient is positioned supine to approach a medial condyle fracture. A hand table is secured on the affected side. The extremity can be externally rotated through the shoulder to access the medial condyle, and the elbow is flexed to relax the flexor mass.

Surgical Approach

A posteromedial approach to the elbow that allows good exposure of both the fracture site and the ulnar nerve should be performed.

Technique

✓ **ORIF of Fractures Involving the Medial Condyle:**
KEY SURGICAL STEPS

- ❏ Application of sterile tourniquet
- Posteromedial incision over medial condyle
- ❏ Identify, isolate, and protect ulnar nerve
- Isolate and protect medial cutaneous nerves
- ❏ Debride fracture hematoma and identify fracture and articular surface
- ❏ Reduce fracture by decreasing tension of flexor mass by flexing elbow and wrist and pronating forearm
- ❏ Reduce fracture, ensuring an anatomic alignment at the articular surface
- ❏ Stabilize fracture with divergent K-wires (cannulated screws in older patients/adolescents)
- ❏ Apply long arm splint or bivalved long arm cast

After tourniquet control is obtained, an incision is centered over the medial condyle, in the region of the medial epicondyle. Often there is significant soft tissue swelling and displacement of the fracture fragment, which permits blunt dissection through the subcutaneous tissue to easily expose the fracture fragment. The medial brachial and antebrachial cutaneous nerves that transverse the field are protected. Care in the dissection avoids injury to the ulnar nerve, which sits posterior to the fragment but may be displaced by the fracture. The ulnar nerve is identified and protected to ensure that it is not entrapped in the reduced fracture and it is not iatrogenically injured by a pin or screw. The fracture site is irrigated and debrided of hematoma. The entire fracture line and articular surface should be identified to ensure accurate reduction of the articular surface. An army, navy, or other blunt retractor can be placed along the anterior surface of the capsule to aid in visualization. The fracture is reduced with the flexor-pronator soft tissue attachments left intact to lessen the risk of avascular necrosis. In the supine position, this requires flexion of the elbow and wrist with pronation of the forearm, which takes tension off of the condyle. The condyle is held in place, and K-wires are passed in a divergent manner to hold the fracture in place. Alternatively, cannulated screws with or without a washer can be used in older patients near skeletal maturity to allow more rigid fixation and early motion. Fluoroscopy should be utilized judiciously to ensure appropriate trajectories of the hardware. It is imperative to visualize the ulnar nerve while placing the hardware to ensure it is not injured or entrapped in the fracture site. Once the hardware is in place, the elbow must be brought through a range of motion to ensure the ulnar nerve will not be irritated by the hardware. In addition, direct visualization of the articular surface is imperative to ensure an anatomic alignment is present. The wound is now irrigated and the torniquet deflated.

Authors' Preferred Treatment for Fractures Involving the Medial Condylar Physis (Algorithm 18-2)

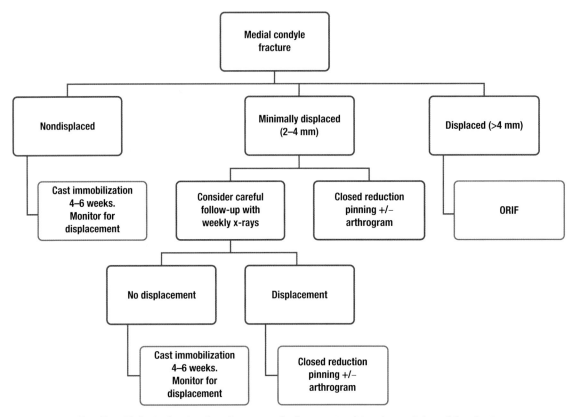

Algorithm 18-2. Authors' preferred treatment for fractures involving the medial condylar physis.

Kilfoyle type I nondisplaced fractures are treated with immobilization in a posterior splint with sidebars or a long arm cast. Follow-up radiographs, including an external oblique view, should be obtained at weekly intervals to ensure there is no late displacement. When there is good callus at the metaphyseal portion of the fracture line by 4 to 6 weeks, the splint/cast is removed and early active motion is initiated. The patient should be followed until there is symmetric range of motion and complete healing of the fracture line. Some type II fractures that maintain alignment can also be treated in the same manner; however, careful follow-up with weekly radiographs is imperative to ensure that the fragment has not moved.

Unstable Kilfoyle type II and type III displaced fractures should be reduced and stabilized with operative intervention.

This is usually difficult to do by closed methods because the swelling associated with this injury makes it hard to accurately identify the landmarks for pin placement and there is a substantial risk to the ulnar nerve with percutaneous pinning. As a result, it is recommended to proceed with an open reduction and internal fixation utilizing a posteromedial approach with identification and protection of the ulnar nerve. The posterior surface of the condylar fragment and the medial aspect of the medial crista of the trochlea should be avoided during the dissection as these are the blood supply sources to the ossific nuclei of the trochlea. Fixation with a minimum of two divergent pins should be in the metaphyseal segment if possible. Cannulated screw fixation can be utilized in adolescents near skeletal maturity to allow early protected range of motion.

Postoperative Care

Patients are immobilized largely dependent upon age, fracture pattern, and type of fixation. Nonoperatively treated fractures may be casted for 4 to 6 weeks, in a similar fashion to the treatment of lateral condyle fractures based on age, displacement, and the amount of healing. Those treated with K-wire fixation similarly will be casted for 4 to 6 weeks depending on healing, and the pins are often removed at 4 weeks if exposed, and can be removed any time after 6 weeks if they were buried. In patients treated with more rigid fixation, early (10–14 days) transition to a hinged elbow brace with protected range of motion is recommended.

Potential Pitfalls and Preventive Measures

Fractures Involving the Medial Condylar Physis: POTENTIAL PITFALLS AND PREVENTIONS

Pitfalls	Preventions
Progressive displacement of minimally displaced fracture leading to delayed union or malunion	• Monitor fractures treated nonoperatively with careful radiographic follow-up at weekly intervals
Disruption of blood supply leading to osteonecrosis	• Avoid dissection posteriorly on the medial aspect of the medial crista of the trochlea
Iatrogenic ulnar nerve injury	• Perform adequate exposure to identify and protect ulnar nerve during reduction and hardware fixation
Malunion	• Ensure adequate visualization of the articular surface

Nondisplaced or minimally displaced fractures should be monitored closely to ensure progressive displacement does not occur, which could lead to malunion, delayed union, or nonunion. When treating patients operatively, the posterior surface of the condylar fragment and the medial aspect of the medial crista of the trochlea should be avoided during the dissection because these are the blood supply sources to the ossific nuclei of the trochlea. The ulnar nerve should be identified and protected to avoid iatrogenic injury.

MANAGEMENT OF EXPECTED ADVERSE OUTCOMES AND UNEXPECTED COMPLICATIONS IN FRACTURES INVOLVING THE MEDIAL CONDYLAR PHYSIS

Fractures Involving the Medial Condylar Physis: COMMON ADVERSE OUTCOMES AND COMPLICATIONS

- Stiffness
- Ulnar neuropathy
- Delayed union
- Nonunion/malunion
- Cubitus varus

The major complication associated with medial condyles of the distal humerus is failure to make the proper diagnosis. This is especially true in younger children, in whom a medial condylar fracture can be confused with a displaced fracture of the medial epicondyle (see Fig. 18-14). When the diagnosis is uncertain, especially in a child with no ossification of the trochlea, examination with arthrography, ultrasound, and/or MRI is required (see Fig. 18-11). Leet et al.[57] reported complications in 7 of 21 medial condylar fractures, including osteonecrosis of the trochlea, nonunion, and loss of reduction leading to malunion. Untreated displaced fractures usually result in nonunion or malunion with cubitus varus deformity (Fig. 18-20).[29,109] Sugiura reported on a child, age 4, who was

Figure 18-20. Nonunion in addition to cubitus varus deformity. **A:** Original film of a 5-year-old girl who sustained an injury 1 year previously. The metaphyseal fragment (*arrow*) is attached to the medial epicondyle. **B:** Film taken 2 years later. Some ossification has developed in the medial condylar epiphysis (*arrow*). (Courtesy of Roy N. Davis, MD.)

A   B

treated nonoperatively and presented again at age 10 with severe varus deformity secondary to a medial condyle non-union.[100] Patients who sustain a nonunion are at high risk for loss of motion, function, pain, and eventual arthrosis. Ryu et al.[90] described a painful nonunion of the medial condyle in an adolescent that apparently resulted from a fracture when they were 3 years old. An osteotomy was performed to remove the nonunited section of bone, and an iliac crest bone graft was inserted and fixed with two screws. Union was obtained, and short-term follow-up demonstrated that the patient was able to participate in sports without pain. Delayed union has been reported in patients treated with inadequate fixation and those simply placed in a cast.[31,53]

Some disturbance of the vascular supply to the medial condylar fragment may occur during open reduction and internal fixation or at the time of initial injury. Several investigators have reported subsequent avascular changes in the medial crista of the trochlea.[29,31,53,79] Hanspal[38] reviewed Cothay's[17] original patient 18 years after delayed open reduction and found that despite some minimal loss of motion, the patient was asymptomatic. Radiographs, however, showed changes compatible with osteonecrosis of the medial condyle.

Both cubitus varus and valgus deformities have been reported in patients whose fractures united uneventfully. The valgus deformity appears to be caused by secondary stimulation or overgrowth of the medial condylar fragment. Some simple stimulation of the medial epicondyle's prominence may also produce the false appearance of a cubitus valgus deformity. Cubitus varus appears to result from decreased growth of the trochlea, possibly caused by a vascular insult.

The rate of nonunion after medial condyle fracture ranges between 8% and 33%.[28] Principles for treating nonunion of lateral condylar fractures are generally applicable to nonunions of the medial condyle (Fig. 18-21). Treatment options include open reduction and internal fixation, a lateral-based closing wedge osteotomy, or a supracondylar dome osteotomy. Open reduction and internal fixation achieves fragment stability but typically does not resolve residual elbow deformity and motion limitations. In contrast, an osteotomy typically results in fair-to-good resolution of symptoms with correction of the angular deformity.[28,99]

El Ghawabi[31] described one partial ulnar neuropathy occurring after this type of injury. The neuropathy almost completely recovered after anterior transposition of the ulnar nerve.

Sonohata et al.[97] reported a case of transient fishtail deformity in an 11-year-old boy who sustained a Kilfoyle type III fracture. He underwent open reduction and internal fixation with three K-wires 1 day after the injury. At 1 year postoperatively, he was found to have asymptomatic absorption of the trochlear groove and was diagnosed with a fishtail deformity. At 4 years postoperatively, there was significant remodeling of the trochlear groove with full painless range of motion. The authors believe that this transient fishtail deformity was due to improvement of ischemia of the trochlea after the medial condyle fracture, though they were uncertain if that was due to accurate reduction and fixation or due to the anatomy of the vascular supply of the medial condyle.

SUMMARY, CONTROVERSIES, AND FUTURE DIRECTIONS IN FRACTURES INVOLVING THE MEDIAL CONDYLAR PHYSIS

Medial condyle fractures about the distal humerus are rare. The key to their ultimate treatment is identifying them and making the correct diagnosis. The classification, radiographic assessment, and treatment goals are similar to lateral condyle fractures, which are encountered much more commonly. Although nondisplaced or minimally displaced fractures can be treated nonoperatively in a cast or splint, careful monitoring with weekly radiographs is required to identify further displacement and delayed union. When displaced, open treatment with identification of the ulnar nerve and direct visualization of the articular surface are needed. The fracture is reduced and stabilized while directly visualizing and protecting the ulnar nerve and ensuring the articular surface is reduced anatomically. The rate of complications is relatively high and may include osteonecrosis, elbow stiffness, malunion, and/or delayed union.

Fractures Involving the Lateral Epicondylar Apophysis

INTRODUCTION TO FRACTURES INVOLVING THE LATERAL EPICONDYLAR APOPHYSIS

Fracture of the lateral epicondylar apophysis is a rare injury, with only a few isolated injuries described, mostly in textbooks.[12,62,70,87,94,105,120]

ASSESSMENT OF FRACTURES INVOLVING THE LATERAL EPICONDYLAR APOPHYSIS

MECHANISMS OF INJURY FOR FRACTURES INVOLVING THE LATERAL EPICONDYLAR APOPHYSIS

In adults, the most common etiology is that of a direct blow to the lateral side of the elbow. In children, because the forearm extensor muscles originate from this area, it is believed that avulsion forces from these muscles can be responsible for some of these injuries.[70] Hasner and Husby[43] suggested that the location of the fracture line in relation to the origins of the various extensor muscles determines the degree of displacement that can occur (Fig. 18-22). If the proximal part of the fracture line lays between the origin of the common extensors and the extensor carpi radialis longus, there is usually little displacement. If the fracture lines enter the area of origin of the extensor carpi radialis longus, then considerable displacement can occur.

Figure 18-21. Nonunion of a medial condylar fracture in a 5-year-old girl. AP (**A**), external oblique (**B**), and lateral (**C**) views. (Copyright Joshua M. Abzug, MD, Baltimore, MD.)

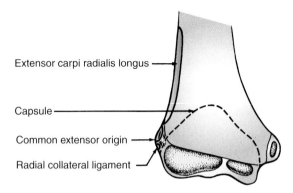

Extensor carpi radialis longus —

Capsule —

Common extensor origin —

Radial collateral ligament —

Figure 18-22. Soft tissue attachments. The origins of the forearm and wrist extensor muscles, radial collateral ligament, and outline of the capsule are shown in relation to the lateral epicondylar apophysis.

SIGNS AND SYMPTOMS OF FRACTURES INVOLVING THE LATERAL EPICONDYLAR APOPHYSIS

Patients will present similar to other elbow fractures, with pain and swelling in the elbow, with pain often localized to the lateral aspect of the distal humerus. As this fracture is so rare, associated injuries are not well described, though there are reported cases of concomitant elbow dislocation.[87]

IMAGING AND OTHER DIAGNOSTIC STUDIES FOR FRACTURES INVOLVING THE LATERAL EPICONDYLAR APOPHYSIS

Fractures can often be confused with normal anatomy of the lateral epicondyle.[94] The distal part of the epiphysis fuses with the capitellum before the proximal part unites with the adjacent

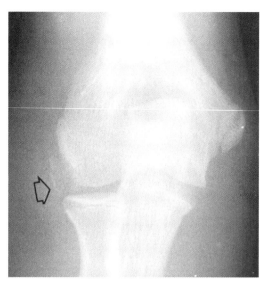

Figure 18-24. Avulsion injury. Avulsion of a portion of the lateral epicondyle in an adolescent (*arrow*). (Courtesy of R. Chandrasekharan, MD.)

humerus. This frequently results in the physis appearing like a fracture. Also, ossification of the epiphysis begins at the level of the capitellar physis and proceeds first to a typical sliver shape and then to a triangular shape. This natural separation can be confused with an avulsion fracture.[94] The key to determining true separation is looking beyond the osseous tissues for the presence of associated soft tissue swelling (Fig. 18-23). If the ossification center lies distal to the osteochondral border of the lateral condylar epiphysis, it should be considered displaced (Fig. 18-24). Comparison radiographs of the contralateral elbow can be used to aid in diagnosis.

A   **B**

Figure 18-23. Lateral swelling. **A:** Soft tissue swelling in the area of the lateral epicondylar apophysis (*arrows*) suggests an undisplaced fracture involving the apophysis. The fragmentation of the apophysis is caused by irregular ossification. **B:** A small avulsion of the lateral epicondyle (*open arrow*) in an adolescent who is almost skeletally mature. There was considerable soft tissue swelling in this area (*solid arrows*).

Figure 18-25. Lateral epicondylar apophysis. **A:** The cartilaginous apophysis occupies the wedge-shaped defect at the margin of the lateral condyle and metaphysis (*arrow*). The *dotted line* shows the margin of the cartilaginous apophysis. **B:** Ossification of the apophysis begins at the central portion of the wedge defect (*solid arrow*) and progresses both proximally and distally (*open arrows*) to form a triangular center.

PATHOANATOMY AND APPLIED ANATOMY RELATING TO FRACTURES INVOLVING THE LATERAL EPICONDYLAR APOPHYSIS

Because the presence of the lateral epicondylar apophysis is often misinterpreted as a small chip fracture, a thorough understanding of the anatomy and ossification process is essential for evaluating injuries in this area and distinguishing normal anatomy from pathoanatomy.

The lateral epicondylar apophysis is present for a considerable period but does not become ossified until the second decade. The best discussion of the anatomy of the ossification process is in a report by Silberstein et al.,[94] and much of the following discussion is paraphrased from their work. Just before ossification of the apophysis, the ossification margin of the lateral supracondylar ridge of the distal metaphysis curves abruptly medially toward the lateral condylar physis (Fig. 18-25). This process causes the osseous borders on the lateral aspect of the distal humerus to take the shape of the number 3. The central wedge of this defect contains the cartilaginous lateral epicondylar apophysis, which begins to ossify around 10 to 11 years of age. Ossification begins at the level of the lateral condylar physeal line and proceeds proximally and distally to form a triangle, with the apex directed toward the physeal line. The shape of the epicondylar apophyseal ossification center may also be in the form of a long sliver of bone with an irregular ossification pattern. Silberstein et al.[94] noted that the fracture line involving the lateral condylar physis often involves the proximal physeal line of the lateral epicondylar apophysis. Thus, this apophysis is almost always included with the lateral condylar fragment.

TREATMENT OPTIONS FOR FRACTURES INVOLVING THE LATERAL EPICONDYLAR APOPHYSIS

Unless the fragment is incarcerated within the joint,[62] treatment usually consists of simple immobilization for comfort. Although nonunion of the fragment can occur, this radiographic finding usually does not affect elbow function. Lateral column osteochondral nonunions can occur that represent chronic lateral ligament instability. Those patients are symptomatic, have functional limitations, and benefit from open repair. Yoon et al.[116] described their technique of arthroscopic repair of lateral epicondyle fractures, which they report has the added benefit of decreased postoperative scar formation and stiffness compared to open procedures.

MANAGEMENT OF EXPECTED ADVERSE OUTCOMES AND UNEXPECTED COMPLICATIONS IN FRACTURES INVOLVING THE LATERAL EPICONDYLAR APOPHYSIS

The rare major complication that has been described with fractures involving the lateral epicondylar apophysis is entrapment of the fragment within the elbow joint.[30,62] Lateral epicondylar malunion with residual elbow stiffness has also been described.[120]

SUMMARY, CONTROVERSIES, AND FUTURE DIRECTIONS RELATED TO FRACTURES INVOLVING THE LATERAL EPICONDYLAR APOPHYSIS

Fractures of the distal humerus lateral epicondyle are extremely rare. The radiographic appearance of the lateral epicondyle during growth can be confused with what appears to be a fracture. Unless there is entrapment of the fracture fragment in the joint or concern for elbow instability, treatment is nonoperative. Late nonunions with posterolateral instability will require open repair.

Fractures Involving the Trochlea/TRASH Lesions

Osteochondral fractures involving only the articular portion of the trochlea are extremely rare in skeletally immature children.[95,104,107,113,119] These lesions are also part of the constellation of fractures that make up TRASH lesions.[111]

Wang et al.[110] reported on 28 elbows in 28 pediatric patients with confirmed osteochondritis dissecans (OCD) of the humeral trochlea. They found that the most common symptoms at presentation were pain, crepitus, mechanical locking, and loss of motion. In most cases, advanced imaging with MRI was required to make the diagnosis, although retrospective analysis of the plain films showed signs of the OCD lesion in 18 of 28 of the radiographs. MRI analysis found associated capitellar OCD lesions in 16 of 28 patients.[110] Findings on radiographs can include a characteristic lucent lesion lateral to the apex of the trochlear grove or a pseudointercondylar notch sign.[85,114] Additional diagnostic ultrasonography can be performed using standard planes to detect TRASH lesions. However, diagnosis with ultrasound is dependent on the examiner's skill level and experience.[92]

Grant and Miller[36] reported on a 13-year-old boy who had a posterolateral dislocation of the elbow with marked valgus instability and fractures of the medial epicondyle and radial neck. When the elbow was explored to stabilize the epicondyle, a large osteochondral fragment from the medial crista of the trochlea was found lying between the two articular surfaces. The fragment was reduced and fixed, and a satisfactory result was obtained. Yano et al. describe a coronal shear fracture in a 7-year-old boy who had a trochlear shear fracture in the setting of a previously treated lateral epicondyle fracture at the age of 5.[113] Koëter et al.[55] described the surgical technique for treatment of a lateral condyle fracture and a dislocated trochlear shear injury in a 15-year-old male patient. The injury was repaired using an anterior neurovascular interval approach with a modified hedgehog-based technique for fixation. This patient achieved full range of motion at the 3-month follow-up appointment with no adverse outcomes.

Patel and Weiner[80] described OCD in two patients (three elbows) aged 12 and 14 years. In one patient, open biopsy was done because the osteochondral lesion was thought to be a neoplastic lesion. The other patient with bilateral lesions was treated conservatively with good results. Marshall et al.[59] reported osteochondral lesions of the trochlea in 18 young athletes ranging in age from 6 to 17 years; 10 of the 18 were throwing athletes and 2 were gymnasts. Based on MRI and MR arthrogram findings, injuries were classified as chondral/osteochondral injury/OCD lesions (13 patients) or trochlear osteonecrosis (5 patients). Ten of the 13 osteochondral lesions involved the lateral trochlea and were described as classic OCD; the three medial trochlear lesions were small (<6 mm) and were located on the posterior articular surface of the medial trochlea. Trochlear osteonecrosis in five patients was characterized by growth disturbance involving the ossification centers of the trochlea. The affected trochleas were misshapen and underdeveloped, and radiographs showed the secondary ossification centers to be fragmented, small, and sclerotic, or absent entirely. All five of the patients with osteonecrosis had histories of distal humeral fractures treated with K-wire fixation earlier in childhood (two lateral condylar fractures and a supracondylar, medial epicondylar, and medial condylar fracture). The authors suggested that

the athletic demands placed on the adolescent elbow revealed osteonecrosis from these earlier fractures.[59] The OCD lesions consistently occurred in the posteroinferior aspect of the lateral trochlea corresponding to a watershed zone of diminished vascularity, and the authors hypothesized that the lesions were caused by repeated forced elbow extension/hyperextension that led to impingement of the normal blood supply.[59] Small osteochondral lesions on the posteromedial trochlea were suggested to result from olecranon abutment occurring in an elbow with collateral ligament laxity or insufficiency.

In an older child who sustains an elbow dislocation and in whom there is some widening of the joint after reduction, an intra-articular osteochondral or chondral fracture of the trochlea, capitellum, or radial head should be suspected. Arthrography, MRI, or computed tomography–arthrography should be used for confirmation. Arthroscopy and debridement has been shown to be effective in treating capitellar OCD lesions, therefore, Ye et al.[114] described a similar surgical technique including arthroscopic ulnohumeral joint debridement and transolecranon microfracture to treat OCD of the humeral trochlea. This technique allows for minimal morbidity and reduces the need for olecranon osteotomy for exposure and repair. However, comparative outcomes following this procedure and other surgical procedures have not yet been performed.

Osteonecrosis of the Trochlea

INTRODUCTION TO OSTEONECROSIS OF THE TROCHLEA

Toniolo and Wilkins[106] reported a series of 30 cases collected over 20 years from various sources and suggested that osteonecrosis of the trochlea is probably one of the most unrecognized sequelae of injuries to the distal humerus. A systematic review of Hegemann disease and fishtail deformity identified 15 studies including 58 patients with fishtail deformity.[16] These patients had an average age of 7.8 years and were predominantly male (74%).[16] Because avascular necrosis of the trochlea is rare, or often unrecognized, the true incidence is unknown. Bronfen reported six cases in 288 displaced supracondylar humerus fractures.[11] McDonnell and Wilson reported four cases in a series of 53 supracondylar humerus fractures.[60] Narayanan described seven cases of which five children had type III supracondylar humerus fractures, one had a medial condyle fracture, and the other child a lateral condyle fracture.[72] Etier et al. described five additional cases after supracondylar humerus fractures.[25] Morito et al.[68] reported a case of Hegemann disease detected with a traumatic olecranon fracture in a 10-year-old boy practicing karate. His olecranon fracture was treated nonoperatively with subsequent resolution of osteonecrosis at final follow-up 2 years after the injury. Hamilton et al.[37] reported on a case of trochlear osteonecrosis in a 7-year-old who had sustained a minimally displaced lateral humeral condyle fracture treated nonoperatively at the age of 2 years. Glotzbecker et al. examined 15 cases of osteonecrosis of the trochlea, and during the same time period, more than 3,500 patients were treated operatively for a supracondylar or humeral condylar fracture at their institution.[34] This gives an incidence of less than 0.5% and does not include fractures treated nonoperatively, so some mild osteonecrosis cases may have been missed.

Three theories have been proposed to account for the posttraumatic changes that occur in the distal humerus after fractures in the vicinity of the trochlea: malunion, partial growth arrest, and vascular injury. The most common form follows some type of elbow trauma. In some cases, the trauma is occult or poorly defined.[8,9,49,60,69,115] It can occur after displaced or minimally displaced supracondylar humerus fractures, lateral condylar fractures, physeal separations, or medial condylar fractures, or may occur iatrogenically from excessive soft tissue stripping during operative exposure.[75,106] Posttraumatic trochlear osteonecrosis results in a spectrum of injury from simply a small defect of the trochlea (fishtail deformity) to complete destruction of the medial aspect of the distal humerus with a progressive varus deformity, decreased range of motion, and associated instability of the elbow. This spectrum of pathology is further described by Claessen et al.,[15] who propose using one nomenclature for this process: posttraumatic disturbance of the epiphysis of the humeral trochlea.

ASSESSMENT OF OSTEONECROSIS OF THE TROCHLEA

SIGNS AND SYMPTOMS OF OSTEONECROSIS OF THE TROCHLEA

Early there are often minimal, if any symptoms. It often may be 4 to 8 years after the initial injury when symptoms related to

the complication begin.[72] When symptoms are present, they can include pain and loss of motion secondary to joint incongruity, deformity, and locking, which is related to loose body formation and joint instability.[11,15,25,54,69,75]

The clinical signs and symptoms differ considerably between the two patterns of necrosis. Patients who have the type A (central defect) fishtail deformity usually do not develop any angular deformities. The severity of the fishtail deformity is related to the degree of necrosis and seems to dictate the severity of the symptoms. In children who have a pattern of total osteonecrosis of the trochlea, including part of the nonarticular surface, a progressive varus deformity usually develops. Because the entire medial trochlear surface is disrupted, significant loss of range of motion also develops. These deformities usually worsen esthetically and functionally as the child matures. The proximal ulna can sublux into the distal humerus defect causing impingement pain and osteochondral injury. Early degenerative joint disease with a loss of range of motion is the most common sequela in severe cases.

Some children with osteonecrosis of the trochlea develop late-onset ulnar neuropathy,[66,89,103] thought to be due to a multiplicity of factors, including joint malalignment, abnormal position of the ulnar nerve and triceps tendon, loss of protection by a deep ulnar groove, and the acute angle of entrance of the two heads of the flexor carpi ulnaris. Rarely, a patient may present with fracture (Fig. 18-26).[58]

CLASSIFICATION OF OSTEONECROSIS OF THE TROCHLEA

Osteonecrosis of the trochlea can appear as either a central defect (type A) or total hypoplasia manifest by complete absence of the trochlea (type B), depending on the extent of the vascular injury.

Type A—Fishtail Deformity

In the type A deformity, only the lateral portion of the medial crista or apex of the trochlea becomes involved in the necrotic process,

Figure 18-26. **A:** Twelve-year-old girl who had supracondylar humerus fracture treated with closed reduction and pinning at age of 5. She presented after a fall at age of 12 with a medial condyle fracture (**B**) that was treated with open reduction and internal fixation (**C**).
(continues)   **A**   **B**

C

Figure 18-26. *(Continued)*

which produces the typical fishtail deformity (Fig. 18-27). This more common pattern of necrosis seems to occur with very distal supracondylar fractures or with fractures involving the lateral condylar physis.

Type B—Malignant Varus Deformity

The type B deformity involves osteonecrosis of the entire trochlea and sometimes part of the metaphysis (Fig. 18-28). This type of necrosis has occurred as a sequela of fractures involving the entire distal humeral physis or fractures of the medial condylar physis[109] and can lead to a cubitus varus deformity in which the angulation progresses as the child matures.

IMAGING AND OTHER DIAGNOSTIC STUDIES FOR OSTEONECROSIS OF THE TROCHLEA

Radiographically, loss of motion is associated with subluxation of the radial head and ulna proximally into the defect.[34] With proximal migration of the ulna, the coronoid impinges anteriorly and the olecranon impinges posteriorly, leading to progressive loss of motion.[44] Proximal migration of the ulna, radial head escape, or the combination of both may all lead to loss of motion and osteochondral impingement. Plain radiographs can be used for diagnosis, but advanced imaging including the use

A   **B**

C   **D**

Figure 18-27. Fishtail deformity. **A, B:** Type A deformity. Osteonecrosis of only the lateral ossification center creates a defect in the apex of the trochlear groove. (**C**) AP and lateral (**D**) views of a right elbow fishtail deformity in a 14-year-old boy who previously sustained a supracondylar humerus fracture. (**C, D:** Copyright Joshua M. Abzug, MD, Baltimore, MD.)

Figure 18-28. Osteonecrosis of the entire trochlea. **A:** In this type B deformity, loss of blood supply from both the medial and lateral vessels results in osteonecrosis of the entire medial crista along with a portion of the metaphysis. **B:** Radiograph of a 4-year-old boy who sustained a type II physeal fracture involving the entire distal humeral physis. In this injury film, there is a large metaphyseal fragment on the medial side (*arrow*). **C:** As shown by the appearance 5 months later, a mild varus deformity is present because of an incomplete reduction. The ossification in the medial metaphyseal fragment has disappeared.

of MRI and/or CT can better characterize the deformity, assess osteochondral surfaces, and identify osteochondral loose bodies and arthrosis.[44,48,54] Because the trochlea generally ossifies between ages 7 and 10 years with fusion around age 12 to 17, early diagnosis is often not possible after the initial fracture, and explains why the diagnosis is often not made until several years after the initial injury.[72]

PATHOANATOMY AND APPLIED ANATOMY RELATING TO OSTEONECROSIS OF THE TROCHLEA

In Haraldsson's classic studies[39,40] of the blood supply of the distal humerus, it was demonstrated that the medial crista of the trochlea had two separate blood supply sources (Fig. 18-29). Neither has anastomoses with each other or with the other metaphyseal vessels. In the young infant, the vessels are small and lie on the surface of the perichondrium.

The lateral vessels supply the apex of the trochlea and the lateral aspect of the medial crista. These vessels cross the physis to enter the posterior aspect of the lateral trochlear ossification center. Their terminal branches lie just under the articular surface. Thus, they are particularly vulnerable to injury when the fracture line occurs through this area, as is typical in

fractures of the medial condylar physis, lateral condyle, or a T-condylar distal humeral fracture. By the same token, a fracture in the supracondylar area in which the fracture line is very distal or a total distal humeral physeal displacement can also disrupt the lateral trochlear epiphyseal vessels as they course along the surface of the metaphysis or at their entrance into the physeal plate. In a systematic review of 58 patients, 48% of patients had a preceding lateral condyle fracture, 31% had a supracondylar fracture, 3 patients had a capitellum fracture, 3 had a medial condyle fracture, and 4 patients had an unknown fracture.[16]

Another set of vessels enters medially through the nonarticulating surface of the trochlea. This set of vessels supplies the most medial aspect of the medial crista or the medial portion of the trochlear epiphysis. As shown in Haraldsson's studies,[39,40] there appear to be no anastomoses between the two sets of vessels supplying the trochlear epiphysis.

Ossification centers need blood supply for their appearance and development. Before these centers appear, the vessels are more superficial and less well defined. It is speculated that a lesion in these immature vessels in children leads only to a delay in the appearance of the centers. In older children, where there is already a well-defined ossification center, disruption produces a true bony osteonecrosis of one or both of the trochlea's ossification centers. This can result in a partial or total

Figure 18-29. Blood supply of the trochlea. **A:** Intraosseous vasculature in a 3-year-old boy. Only two small vessels supply the medial crista of the trochlea (*arrows*). The central portion of the crista appears avascular. **B:** In the lateral view through the medial crista of the trochlea, note that the vessels penetrate the physis posteriorly (*arrow*) to enter the epiphyseal cartilage. **C:** Close-up view showing the extent of the vascular supply of the trochlea. Note that no anastomoses are seen between these medial and lateral vessels. **D:** Lateral view through the medial crista of the trochlea. Note that the vessels penetrate the physis posteriorly (*arrow*) to enter the epiphyseal cartilage. **E:** Radiograph of a 12-year-old boy. The persistence of the two separate ossification centers (*arrows*) of the media crista is seen. The area supplied by the lateral vessel. (**A–D:** Reprinted from Haraldsson S. On osteochondrosis deformans juvenilis capituli humeri including investigation of intraosseous vasculature in distal humerus. *Acta Orthop Scand Suppl.* 1959;38:1–232, with permission.)

absence of further epiphyseal ossification, leading to either hypoplasia of the central or whole medial aspect of the trochlea, respectively.

TREATMENT OPTIONS FOR OSTEONECROSIS OF THE TROCHLEA

Descriptions of treatment options in the literature are extremely limited. In addition to observation and nonoperative care, proposed treatment options include arthroscopic debridement and removal of loose bodies, capsulotomy for contracture,[25,60,69] interposition arthroplasty for advanced arthrosis, surgical arrest of the remaining medial and/or lateral physis to prevent progressive fishtail deformity,[75] and/or osteotomy for persistent deformity.[75]

Because the osteonecrosis of the trochlea is a direct consequence of trauma to the vessels at the time of injury, there is no effective prevention or treatment of the primary necrosis. Treatment is aimed at only the sequelae of the osteonecrosis of the trochlea. If loss of range of motion is due to a significant disruption of the articular surface itself, the surgical options are limited. If the osteonecrosis of the trochlea has resulted in a varus deformity of the elbow, this deformity can be corrected with performance of a supracondylar osteotomy and an associated ulnar nerve transposition. The correction of the carrying angle may be esthetic without functional improvement. Surgical intervention carries the risk of increased stiffness due to the already limited elbow range of motion.

Small defects with minimal joint involvement can be observed.[34] In patients with extensive joint involvement, associated loss of motion, elbow stiffness, and/or loose bodies, arthroscopic debridement may help transiently improve symptoms, including pain and limited range of motion. However, as one would expect, symptoms often recur and long-term outcomes are unknown. Therefore, in patients who have limited deformity and mild symptoms, arthroscopic debridement can prove to be useful, particularly if there is limited medial and lateral growth of the distal humerus remaining. It may be the only salvage option for symptomatic patients with significant deformity and subluxation of the radial head.

If there is growth remaining in the medial or lateral physis, physeal closure may be of benefit in some patients. Nwakama et al.[75] have suggested that surgical closure of the lateral and/or medial portions of the physis to prevent progressive intracondylar notching can prevent proximal ulnar migration, impingement, and osteochondral injuries. Unfortunately, there are no studies that have outlined long-term follow-up from epiphysiodesis for this condition. However, this technique may be beneficial in patients with open physes, a mild deformity, and a congruent radiocapitellar joint.

ACKNOWLEDGMENT

The authors thank Dr. Michael Glotzbecker, who wrote this chapter in the previous edition, for a firm foundation to build from.

Annotated References

Reference	Annotation
Anari JB, Arkader A, Spiegel DA, Baldwin KD. Approaching unusual pediatric distal humerus fracture patterns. *J Am Acap Orthop Surg.* 2019;27(9):301–311.	Treatment philosophy for common and uncommon pediatric elbow fractures, including transphyseal humeral separation. Reviews clinical evaluation, imaging, and treatment principles.
Capo J, Khamsi B, Nourbakhsh A. Posterolateral instability of the elbow in an adolescent boy with a lateral epicondyle fracture: a case report. *Hand (NY).* 2011;6(1):71–75.	Multicenter prospective cohort of 19 patients with growth disturbance of the humeral trochlea assessing the similarities between Hegemann disease and fishtail deformities. The findings suggest that these represent a continuum of the same disease process.
Claessen FMAP, de Vos-Jakobs S, van den Bekerom MPJ, et al. Post-traumatic disturbance of the epiphysis of the humeral trochlea: a spectrum of pathology. *JSES Int.* 2020;4(4):1011–1017.	
Crowe M, Byerly L, Mehlman CT. Transphyseal distal humeral fractures: a 13-times-greater risk of non-accidental trauma compared with supracondylar humeral fractures in children less than 3 years of age. *J Bone Joint Surg.* 2022;104(13):1204–1211.	Retrospective double-cohort study comparing the incidence of NAT between transphyseal distal humeral fractures and supracondylar humeral fractures in children less than 3 years of age. The charts of 23 transphyseal distal humeral and 205 supracondylar humeral fracture cases were reviewed. NAT was the cause for 6 (26%) of the displaced transphyseal distal humeral fractures and 4 (2%) of the displaced supracondylar fractures. The associated risk of NAT was 13 times greater (95% confidence interval [CI], 4.05–43.7; $p < .001$) for children admitted for operative management of displaced transphyseal distal humeral fractures compared with those admitted for operative management of displaced supracondylar humeral fractures

84. Potter CM. Fracture-dislocation of the trochlea. *J Bone Joint Surg Br*. 1954;36-B(2): 250–253.

85. Pruthi S, Parnell SE, Thapa MM. Pseudointercondylar notch sign: Manifestation of osteochondritis dissecans of the trochlea. *Pediatr Radiol* 2009;39:180–183.

86. Ratti C, Guidani N, Riva G, et al. Transphyseal elbow fracture in newborn: review of literature. *Musculoskelet Surg*. 2015;99(Suppl 1):S99–S105.

87. Rincón D, Guzmén R, Camacho J, Abril C. Elbow dislocation and lateral epicondyle fracture in a five year-old girl. Case report. *Acta Ortop Mex*. 2014;28(6):369–373.

88. Rogers LF, Rockwood CA Jr. Separation of the entire distal humeral epiphysis. *Radiology*. 1973;106(2):393–400.

89. Royle SG, Burke D. Ulna neuropathy after elbow injury in children. *J Pediatr Orthop*. 1990;10(4):495–496.

90. Ryu K, Nagaoka M, Ryu J. Osteosynthesis for nonunion of the medial humeral condyle in an adolescent: a case report. *J Shoulder Elbow Surg*. 2007;16(3):e8–e12.

91. Sherr-Lurie N, Bialik GM, Ganel A, et al. Fractures of the humerus in the neonatal period. *Isr Med Assoc J*. 2011;13(6):363–365.

92. Shintani K, Hosomi R, Suzuki K, et al. Diagnostic imaging for elbow TRASH lesions in children and usefulness of ultrasonography using standard planes. *J Pediatr Orthop B*. 2023;32(6):557–564.

93. Siffert RS. Displacement of the distal humeral epiphysis in the newborn infant. *J Bone Joint Surg Am*. 1963;45:165–169.

94. Silberstein MJ, Brodeur AE, Graviss ER. Some vagaries of the lateral epicondyle. *J Bone Joint Surg Am*. 1982;64(3):444–448.

95. Singh AP, Dhammi IK, Jain AK, Jain S. Neglected isolated fracture of the trochlea humeri. *Chin J Traumatol*. 2010;13(4):247–249.

96. Skaggs DL, Mirzayan R. The posterior fat pad sign in association with occult fracture of the elbow in children. *J Bone Joint Surg Am*. 1999;81(10):1429–1433.

97. Sonohata M, Nakashima T, Suetsugi H, et al. Medial condyle fracture (Kilfoyle type III) of the distal humerus with transient fishtail deformity after surgery. *Case Rep Orthop*. 2017;2017:9053949.

98. Stricker SJ, Thomson JD, Kelly RA. Coronal-plane transcondylar fracture of the humerus in a child. *Clin Orthop Relat Res*. 1993;294:308–311.

99. Su HC, Chou SH, Ho HY, et al. Management of nonunion of humeral medial condyle fracture: a case series and review of the literature. *J Orthop Surg (Hong Kong)*. 2020;28(2):2309499020921755.

100. Sugiura H, Horii E, Koh S. Malunion of medial condyle fracture of the humerus: a case report. *J Pediatr Orthop B*. 2017;26:437–440.

101. Supakul N, Hicks RA, Caltoum CB, Karmazyn B. Distal humeral epiphyseal separation in young children: an often-missed fracture-radiographic signs and ultrasound confirmatory diagnosis. *AJR Am J Roentgenol*. 2015;204(2):W192–W198.

102. Sutherland DH. Displacement of the entire distal humeral epiphysis. *J Bone Joint Surg Am*. 1974;56:206.

103. Tanabu S, Yamauchi Y, Fukushima M. Hypoplasia of the trochlea of the humerus as a cause of ulnar-nerve palsy. Report of two cases. *J Bone Joint Surg Am*. 1985;67(1): 151–154.

104. Tomaru M, Osada D Tamai K, Taneichi H. Isolated coronal shear fracture of the nonossified humeral trochlea in a 7-year-old patient. *J Hand Surg Am*. 2018;43(2):191. e1–191.e5.

105. Toniolo RM, Wilkins KE. Apophyseal injuries of the distal humerus. In: Rockwood CA, Wilkinis KE, Beaty HB, eds. *Fractures in Children*. Lippincott Williams & Wilkins; 1996:819.

106. Toniolo RM, Wilkins KE. Avascular necrosis of the trochlea. In: Rockwood CA, Wilkinis KE, Beaty HB, eds. *Fractures in Children*. Lippincott Williams & Wilkins; 1996:822–830.

107. Tsukamoto N, Mae T, Hirabayashi K, et al. Isolated trochlea osteochondral fracture of the distal humerus in a 6-year-old patient surgically fixed using biodegradable pins: a case study with over 3 years of follow-up. *Trauma Case Rep*. 2022;40: 100666.

108. Varghese J, Teng M, Huang M, Balsam D. Birth injuries to growth plates: a sheep in wolves' clothing. *J Clin Ultrasound*. 2017;45:511–514.

109. Varma BP, Srivastava TP. Fractures of the medial condyle of the humerus in children: a report of four cases including the late sequelae. *Injury*. 1972;4:171–174.

110. Wang KK, Bixby SD, Bae DS. Osteochondritis dissecans of the humeral trochlea: characterization of a rare disorder based on 28 cases. *Am J Sports Med*. 2019; 47(9):2167–2173.

111. Waters PM, Beaty J, Kasser JR. Elbow "TRASH" (The Radiographic Appearance Seemed Harmless) lesions. *J Pediatr Orthop*. 2010;30(Suppl 2):S77–S81.

112. Yang L, Xia F, Guo JC, et al. Nonunion of humeral medial condyle fracture caused by excessive functional exercise: a case report and review of the literature. *BMC Musculoskel Disord*. 2022;23(1):964.

113. Yano K, Kaneshiro Y, Sakanaka H. Isolated osteochondral fracture of the trochlea in the coronal plane in a child before ossification of the trochlea: a case report and literature review. *J Hand Surg Am*. 2018;43:190.e1–190.e5.

114. Ye X, Ek ET, Wang KK. Arthroscopic ulnohumeral joint debridement and transolecranon microfracture for osteochondritis dissecans of the humeral trochlea. *Arthrosc Tech*. 2022;11(3):e285–e290.

115. Yoo CI, Suh JT, Suh KT, et al. Avascular necrosis after fracture-separation of the distal end of the humerus in children. *Orthopedics*. 1992;15(8):959–963.

116. Yoon S-H, Seo J-B, Kwak K-Y, Yoo J-S. Arthroscopic treatment of lateral epicondyle avulsion fracture of the elbow during adolescence: a technical note. *J Arthrosc Joint Surg*. 2020;7(3):157–160.

117. Zhou H, Zhang G, Li M, et al. Ultrasonography-guided closed reduction in the treatment of displaced transphyseal fracture of the distal humerus. *J Orthop Surg Res*. 2020;15(1):575.

118. Zhou W, Canavese F, Zhang L, Li L. Functional outcome of the elbow in toddlers with transphyseal fracture of the distal humerus treated surgically. *J Child Orthop*. 2019;13(1):47–56.

119. Zimmerman LJ, Jaurengui JJ, Aarons CE. isolated shear fracture of the humeral trochlea in an adolescent: a case report and literature review. *J Pediatr Orthop B*. 2015; 24:412–417.

120. Zionts LE, Mirzayan R. Elbow stiffness following malunion of a fracture of the lateral epicondyle of the humerus in a child: a case report. *J Bone Joint Surg Am*. 2002; 84(5):818–821.

121. Zukotynski BK, Alswang JM, Silva M. Medial condyle fractures of the humerus in the pediatric population: diagnostic challenges: a report of 3 cases. *JBJS Case Connect*. 2020;10(2):e0438.

19

Shoulder Dislocation and Fractures of the Proximal Humerus and Humeral Shaft

Donald S. Bae

Shoulder Dislocation

INTRODUCTION TO SHOULDER DISLOCATION

Historically, glenohumeral joint dislocations in skeletally immature patients were thought to be a rare occurrence.[141,147,373] Rowe's classic series of 500 glenohumeral joint dislocations from 1956 contained only 8 patients under 10 years of age, though 99 patients were reportedly between 10 and 20 years old.[307] Other published series similarly have documented shoulder instability in adolescents without specific reference to physeal status.[120,236,241,268,302] Prior studies in collegiate athletes have documented the incidence of shoulder instability to be approximately 1 per 10,000 athlete-exposures, and the incidence of dislocations has been reported to be 1.69 per 1,000 person-years in young adult military personnel.[275,276] A study of administrative databases in Ontario, Canada, documented an incidence of 1.64 per 1,000 person-years among patients between the ages of 10 and 16 years.[215] More recently, the incidence of 2/5 per 100,000 children between 0 and 14 years of age was reported in the United Kingdom.[391] Although these demographic data are limited, they do provide some insight into the expected range of glenohumeral joint instability rates in young, active people.

While the exact incidence of traumatic glenohumeral joint instability in skeletally immature patients remains unknown, there appears to be a rising frequency with which these injuries are occurring in older children and adolescents. Potential etiologies for this trend include increasing participation in higher-demand and higher-energy activities, younger age at first sports participation, and greater awareness among patients, families, and care providers. It is important to remember, however, that ligamentous laxity and shoulder subluxation may be a normal, nonpathologic finding in otherwise asymptomatic children and adolescents.[37] Indeed, there is published information to suggest that physical examination signs of glenohumeral joint instability may be seen in up to 50% of otherwise asymptomatic adolescents.[96]

ASSESSMENT OF SHOULDER DISLOCATION

MECHANISMS OF INJURY FOR SHOULDER DISLOCATION

In general, both traumatic and atraumatic glenohumeral joint instability may be seen. In traumatic instability, the predominant direction of humeral head dislocation is anterior. Typically, an anteriorly directed force applied to the humeral head with an abducted and externally rotated shoulder results in anterior dislocation. These injury mechanisms may be seen with sports participation, altercations, motor vehicle collisions, and even simple falls onto an outstretched upper extremity.[154] The spectrum of injury includes an anterior labral tear (Bankart lesion), glenohumeral joint capsular stretch, compression injury to the posterior humeral head (Hill–Sachs lesion), and/or anterior glenoid rim fracture.

Posterior dislocations are less common, representing 5% or less of all traumatic glenohumeral instability.[207] Typically patients dislocate with the affected shoulder forward flexed, internally rotated, and adducted. More commonly associated with higher-energy injury, posterior instability events may be seen after falls, sports collisions, motor vehicle collisions, seizures, or electroconvulsive therapy. As in adults, the diagnosis of posterior dislocation is often subtle, and a high index of suspicion is needed to avoid untimely or missed diagnosis.[139,364]

Atraumatic shoulder instability is common in children and adolescents. These situations are characterized by initially painless glenohumeral dislocation without antecedent or causative trauma and may be more commonly seen in patients with systemic ligamentous laxity and multidirectional instability.[45,250] Often, patients will report instability symptoms of other parts of the body, including the patellofemoral, ankle, and hip joints. Associations with connective tissue disorders may be seen, such as Ehlers–Danlos or Marfan syndrome, though these systemic diagnoses may yet to be made at the time of first dislocation. Atraumatic instability may be voluntary or involuntary, and both are thought to arise from selective activation of shoulder girdle muscles with inhibition of their antagonists (Fig. 19-1).[207] Spontaneous reduction is common, and if sedation or anesthesia is used, the glenohumeral joint typically reduces without need for manipulation.[302]

Finally, there are some pediatric patients who sustain glenohumeral joint dislocation due to neuromuscular pathology. In cases of arthrogryposis, brachial plexus birth injury, stroke, or cerebral palsy, muscle imbalance with or without glenohumeral joint dysplasia can lead to atraumatic dislocations, even in neonates or young children.[60,120,380] These situations must be distinguished from neonatal pseudodislocation, in which a traumatic displaced physeal fracture and radiographically unossified proximal humeral epiphysis may give the radiographic appearance of glenohumeral dislocation.

ASSOCIATED INJURIES WITH SHOULDER DISLOCATIONS

The axillary nerve is commonly injured in association with shoulder dislocations. Because of its circuitous course around the proximal humerus and inferior to the glenohumeral joint, as well as its relative tethering at the quadrilateral space, the axillary nerve may be stretched at the time of humeral head dislocation. As these are usually neuropraxic injuries, spontaneous recovery is typically seen, though recovery may take many months. In the event of complete axillary nerve injuries without spontaneous recovery after the expected period of time, the axillary nerve may be decompressed, repaired, grafted, or most often now treated with a partial radial to axillary motor nerve transfer to provide return of deltoid motor function.[9,62,94] Similarly, injuries to the axillary artery, though rare, have been reported in association with shoulder dislocation.[9] Prompt fracture reduction with or without arterial reconstitution should be performed in cases of vascular insufficiency and limb ischemia.

While less common than in adults, concomitant fractures of the proximal humerus (e.g., lesser tuberosity, greater tuberosity) or scapula (e.g., coracoid process, glenoid) may be seen with shoulder dislocation[59,87,301,368] (Fig. 19-2). Careful inspection

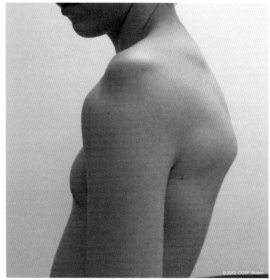

Figure 19-1. Clinical photographs of a preadolescent child with atraumatic multidirectional instability. **A:** Anterior view demonstrates obvious anteroinferior position of the humeral head. **B:** View of the lateral aspect depicts inferior humeral head position and the "sulcus" sign. (Courtesy of Children's Orthopaedic Surgery Foundation.)

Figure 19-2. Greater tuberosity fracture in setting of glenohumeral joint dislocation. **A:** AP view of the shoulder depicting an anteroinferior dislocation with fracture of the greater tuberosity (*arrow*). Axial (**B**) and coronal (**C**) CT images after closed reduction. The fracture line is still seen (*arrow*), but the greater tuberosity has reduced into anatomic position. (Courtesy of Children's Orthopaedic Surgery Foundation.)

Figure 19-3. A: Sensory distribution for the axillary nerve important in anterior dislocation. **B:** Deltoid muscle can be tested in acute anterior dislocation by grabbing the muscle belly with the right hand (*arrow*) while supporting the elbow with the left. The patient then can actively contract the deltoid by pushing the elbow against the examiner's hand (*arrow*) while the examiner feels the muscle contraction.

of plain radiographs is needed to assess for associated bony injuries. At times, three-dimensional imaging with computed tomography (CT) and/or magnetic resonance imaging (MRI) scan is required to make definitive diagnosis and decide on best treatment plan. While nondisplaced fractures may be effectively treated nonoperatively, displaced fractures may predispose to recurrent instability or functional limitations.[204]

SIGNS AND SYMPTOMS OF SHOULDER DISLOCATIONS

In cases of traumatic anterior glenohumeral joint dislocations, patients will present with pain, swelling, and limited shoulder motion. Typically the limb is held in slight abduction and external rotation, and often the patient will support the affected extremity with the contralateral hand. Careful inspection will reveal abnormal contour of the shoulder, with a prominent acromion, flattening, or concavity to the posterolateral shoulder girdle, and obvious prominence or fullness anteriorly in the area of the dislocated humeral head. Careful and comprehensive physical examination is critical to rule out concomitant neurologic injury. The axillary nerve is most commonly affected; sensation over the lateral aspect of the shoulder and deltoid muscle function is checked to assess axillary nerve function (Fig. 19-3). In cases in which there has been spontaneous reduction after an anterior instability event, the shoulder appears more normal in contour and glenohumeral motion is typically preserved, although often painful and with some anxiety. Patients will be guarded in active motion especially above shoulder height, resist extremes of abduction and external rotation, and demonstrate a positive apprehension test.[98,224,314,361]

Conversely, patients with traumatic posterior dislocations will present with a painful adducted and internally rotated shoulder. There is often flattening or concavity to the anterior aspect of the shoulder girdle, with palpable fullness posteriorly. Prominence of the superomedial scapular angle (the so-called

Putti sign) is often seen, and patients will resist attempts at passive shoulder motion, especially external rotation. Inability to passively externally rotate the shoulder or supinate the forearm should alert the examiner to the possibility of a posterior glenohumeral joint dislocation. Again, a comprehensive examination is performed to evaluate for associated neurovascular deficits.

Figure 19-4. Dramatic demonstration of inferior subluxation of the glenohumeral joint in a patient with multidirectional instability. The clinical correlate is the sulcus sign.

In neonates and infants, pseudodislocation may similarly present with pain, reluctance to move the affected upper limb, swelling, and asymmetric contour of the shoulder girdle. Occasionally, crepitus due to motion at the fracture site may be appreciated with gentle, small arc range of motion.

Children and adolescents with atraumatic and/or multidirectional instability present quite differently. In addition to the lack of causative or antecedent trauma, these patients may not have pain with joint subluxation or dislocation (see Fig. 19-1). Even with discomfort, patients will frequently report rapid resolution of pain after reduction. Examination will often elicit diffuse signs of ligamentous laxity, including hyperextension of the elbow, knee, and metacarpophalangeal joints.[266] Abnormally hyperelasticity and striae of the skin may be seen. Focused examination of the shoulder will demonstrate a positive sulcus sign and increased translation with anterior and posterior load-and-shift testing.[354] The sulcus sign refers to a concavity or indentation noted of the skin inferior to the acromion with manual longitudinal traction applied to the adducted arm (Fig. 19-4). Anterior and posterior load-and-shift tests are performed with the examiner standing behind or alongside the patient. While stabilizing the scapula with one hand, the humeral head is grasped and translated anteriorly and/or posteriorly with the examiner's other hand; translation of greater than 5 mm from center is thought to be an indicator of multidirectional instability. Though some patients are truly unstable in all directions, posteroinferior dislocations are most common. This pattern may be elicited with forward flexion and slight adduction, with joint reduction achieved with abduction. Patients with voluntary instability may demonstrate their condition by contracting the anterior deltoid and internal rotators while inhibiting the antagonistic muscles.

IMAGING AND OTHER DIAGNOSTIC STUDIES FOR SHOULDER DISLOCATION

Radiographic evaluation should include orthogonal views of the shoulder to assess for direction of dislocation, congruency of subsequent joint reduction, and presence of associated bony injuries. Anteroposterior (AP) and axillary views are preferred (Fig. 19-5). In the acutely injured or anxious, uncomfortable

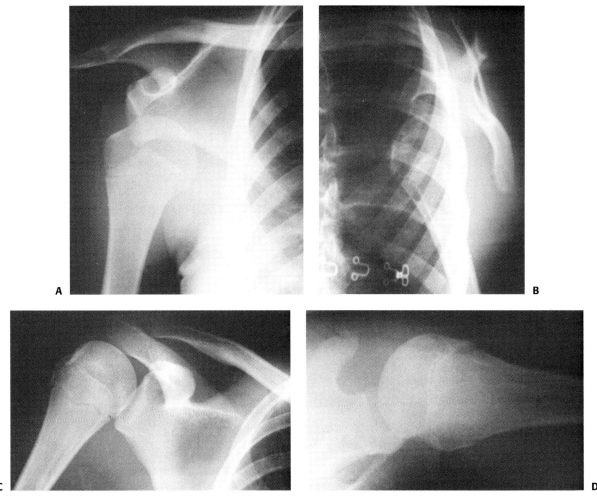

Figure 19-5. Anterior dislocation of the right shoulder in a 15-year-old girl. **A:** Note the typical subcoracoid position on the AP film. **B:** On a true scapular lateral film, note the anterior displacement of the humeral head. **C:** Postreduction film demonstrates a Hill–Sachs compression fracture in the posterolateral aspect of the humeral head. **D:** On the postreduction axillary film, note the posterolateral compression fracture of the humeral head.

Figure 19-6. MRI arthrogram of the left shoulder in a 14-year-old female with multidirectional instability. Axial (**A**) and coronal (**B**) images depict an intact labrum with a patulous capsule. (Courtesy of Children's Orthopaedic Surgery Foundation.)

child, alternative views including the transthoracic scapular Y, West Point lateral, or apical oblique projections may be performed.[115,125,338] AP views with the shoulder in internal rotation are not routinely required, but may allow for visualization of Hill–Sachs lesions of the humeral head.

In patients with recurrent instability or in whom the extent of injury needs to be assessed after the initial traumatic dislocation, advanced imaging may be performed. MRI will provide visualization of chondral, labral, capsular, and musculotendinous pathology. The addition of intra-articular contrast improves sensitivity for labral pathology and provides more detailed information regarding capsular patulousness; this is particularly helpful in patients with persistent, functionally limiting multidirectional instability in whom surgical treatment is being considered (Fig. 19-6). While CT and CT-arthrography are less helpful for soft tissue evaluation, they do provide the best modality to identify and quantify bony defects in the glenoid and humeral head[58,81,192] (Fig. 19-7). Enthusiasm for three-dimensional reconstructions of CT scans has increased, in efforts to characterize the extent of the Hill–Sachs lesions and determine if the humeral head is on or off the normal glenoid track. In 2007, Itoi introduced the concept of the glenoid track, which corresponds to the proportion of the glenoid upon which the humeral head articulates.[170] This track is approximately 83% the width of the best-fit circle drawn on the inferior glenoid. When the glenoid bone loss and Hill–Sachs lesion engage, the loss of bony contact results in dislocation.[389] Given the progressive ossification of the humeral head during skeletal maturation, care should be taken not to mistake normal ossification for Hill–Sachs lesions.[183] In children and adolescents in whom a large portion of the glenoid is incompletely ossified, careful inspection of the glenoid contour is needed to avoid missing bony lesions. Loss of the normal sclerotic margin of the glenoid has been proposed as a sign of bony defects of the anterior glenoid rim.[175]

Radiographic evaluation of patients with atraumatic multidirectional instability is similar, though a few points deserve mention. Though plain radiographs are typically normal, patients with congenital glenoid hypoplasia will have subtle rounding or convexity to the glenoid fossa, with or without scapular neck dysplasia.[60,69] As cited above, MRI-arthrography is a useful tool in assessing the capsular laxity and presence of pathologic lesions of the labrum in these patients.

CLASSIFICATION OF SHOULDER DISLOCATION

Classification of Shoulder Instability
Mechanism
Traumatic
Atraumatic
Direction
Anterior
Posterior
Inferior
Multidirectional
Chronicity
Acute
Recurrent
Chronic
Associated Conditions
None
Neuromuscular
Connective tissue

Figure 19-7. Bony glenoid deficiency in the setting of recurrent anterior instability in a 16-year-old male. **A:** AP radiograph depicts loss of the sclerotic margin of the anterior glenoid (*arrow*). **B:** Sagittal CT scan demonstrates loss of the antero-inferior glenoid. **C:** Three-dimensional reconstruction further highlights the loss of anteroinferior glenoid bone (*arrow*). (Courtesy of Children's Orthopaedic Surgery Foundation.)

In general, shoulder dislocations in children and adolescents are described according to the association with trauma, direction of instability, chronicity, and presence of underlying local or systemic disorders. Characterizing shoulder dislocations according to these categories is important and influences treatment decision making.

Shoulder dislocations may be traumatic or atraumatic in etiology. Direction of humeral instability may be anterior, posterior, inferior (luxatio erecta), or multidirectional. As in adults, perhaps 90% of traumatic dislocations in children and adolescents are anterior, with posterior dislocations occuring much less commonly and luxatio erecta described in case reports.[147,243,302] Furthermore, pathologic instability may include both subluxation or true dislocation. Dislocation refers to situations in which the humeral head moves completely out of the glenoid fossa, with no articular contact, and often with locking of the humeral head on the anterior or medial rim of the glenoid. Subluxation is defined as an incomplete dislocation characterized by pain, a feel of "looseness" or "slipping," and/or a "dead" feeling to the affected limb. Even traumatic subluxations have been associated with structural injury to the glenoid labrum and Hill–Sachs lesions of the humeral head.[277] These conditions must be distinguished from ligamentous laxity, which is typically asymptomatic.

Chronicity is generally classified as being acute, recurrent, or chronic. While a single episode of dislocation denotes acute instability, recurrent instability refers to multiple episodes. Chronic instability refers to unrecognized or untreated shoulder dislocations in which the humeral head is not reduced; it may be seen with congenital or neuromuscular conditions in children.

The presence or absence of associated systemic conditions—including collagen disorders such as Ehlers–Danlos syndrome, or congenital/neuromuscular syndromes such as cerebral palsy—is also a key consideration in diagnosis and management.

PATHOANATOMY AND APPLIED ANATOMY RELATING TO SHOULDER DISLOCATION

The anatomic development, structure, and growth of the proximal humerus are described in the section on proximal humerus fracture. The glenoid is a shallow, concave fossa with which the humeral head articulates. The radius of curvature of the humeral head is approximately three times that of the glenoid. As the glenohumeral articulation lacks substantial bony constraint, the shoulder is afforded near global range of motion, facilitating stable placement of the hand in space for upper limb function. A recent study by Yellin et al. suggests that adolescent patients with taller, narrower glenoids may be predisposed to glenohumeral instability.[392]

Given the relatively unconstrained bony architecture, the glenohumeral joint relies primarily on soft tissue capsuloligamentous structures for stability. The cartilaginous labrum runs along the rim of the glenoid, deepening the concavity and conferring stability. The glenohumeral ligaments are confluent with the labrum and are thickenings of the joint capsule. The inferior glenohumeral ligament has both anterior and posterior components. The anteroinferior glenohumeral ligament is taught and biomechanically contributes most stability in shoulder abduction and external rotation. Disruptions of the anteroinferior glenohumeral ligament or anteroinferior labrum (Bankart lesion) are most commonly seen with anterior traumatic instability (Fig. 19-8). Furthermore, traumatic instability may also cause elevation of the anterior labrum with the periosteum of the anterior glenoid neck, resulting in the so-called anterior labroligamentous periosteal sleeve avulsion (ALPSA).[263] The

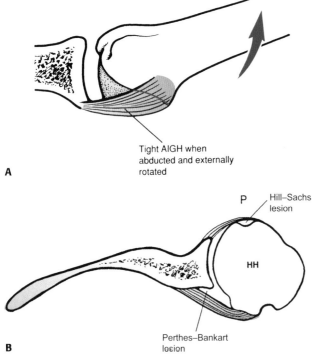

A

Tight AIGH when abducted and externally rotated

B

P — Hill–Sachs lesion

HH

Perthes–Bankart lesion

Figure 19-8. A: The tight anteroinferior glenohumeral ligament complex with the arm abducted and externally rotated (*arrow*). This ligament sling is the primary restraint against anterior instability of the shoulder. **B:** A cross-section in the transverse plane through the glenohumeral joint demonstrates the common lesions associated with anterior instability of the shoulder: Hill–Sachs lesion, Perthes–Bankart lesion, and redundant anteroinferior glenohumeral ligaments. HH, humeral head; P, posterior.

middle glenohumeral ligament (MGHL) is primarily responsible for stability in midabduction and external rotation, whereas the superior glenohumeral ligament resists inferior translation of the humeral head. This may explain the findings that symptomatic anterior instability in overhead throwing patients often involve pathology of the MGHL or superior labrum.[108]

On the humeral side, the joint capsule inserts along the anatomic neck of the humerus, except medially where the insertion lies more inferiorly along the proximal humeral metaphysis. Thus the proximal humeral physis is predominantly extracapsular, with exception of the very medial extent. Shoulder dislocation may result in detachment of the capsule from its humeral insertion, resulting in the so-called humeral avulsion of the glenohumeral ligament (HAGL) lesions.[386] Failure of recognition and repair of these HAGL lesions is a common cause of recurrent instability after surgical treatment.[289]

The glenohumeral joint is surrounded by the rotator cuff muscles, comprised of the supraspinatus, infraspinatus, teres minor, and subscapularis. While rotator cuff tears are uncommon in children, these musculotendinous units form a force couple with the larger surrounding shoulder girdle muscles (deltoid, pectoralis major, teres major, and latissimus dorsi) and serve as important dynamic secondary stabilizers of the shoulder. The dynamic stabilizing effects of the rotator cuff muscles are largely the focus of nonoperative rehabilitative programs for young patients with glenohumeral instability.[34]

TREATMENT OPTIONS FOR SHOULDER DISLOCATIONS

NONOPERATIVE TREATMENT OF SHOULDER DISLOCATIONS

Indications/Contraindications

Nonoperative Treatment for Shoulder Instability:
INDICATIONS AND CONTRAINDICATIONS

Indications

- Primary dislocation in patients willing to undergo physical therapy and accept risks of recurrent instability
- Multidirectional instability in setting of ligamentous laxity

Relative Contraindications

- Large bony glenoid fracture

Treatment options continue to evolve for shoulder instability in children and adolescents, though remain based on the classification system and considerations described above. Nonoperative treatment is typically recommended for acute traumatic dislocations as well as atraumatic multidirectional instability.

Closed reduction is performed for acute traumatic dislocations, and a host of reduction maneuvers have been described. Adequate analgesia and relaxation facilitates closed reduction, and both conscious sedation and intra-articular anesthetic

Figure 19-9. Techniques for closed shoulder reduction. A modification of the Hippocratic method uses a handheld sheet around the thorax (*arrow*) to provide countertraction (*arrow*).

Figure 19-10. The Stimson technique for closed shoulder reduction. With the patient in prone position, weight is hung from the wrist to distract the shoulder joint (*arrow*). Eventually, with sufficient fatigue in the shoulder musculature, the joint can be easily reduced.[349]

injection have been advocated. Multiple reports have suggested that intra-articular lidocaine injection is as safe and effective as intravenous sedation, with less cost and shorter length of stays.[57,240,253,257,372] Portable ultrasound makes accurate injection easier in the urgent care or emergency department setting. The method of traction–countertraction is advocated by many (Fig. 19-9). In this method, a bedsheet is looped around the axilla of the affected shoulder and passed superiorly and laterally to the contralateral shoulder. Longitudinal traction is applied to the affected upper extremity in line with the deformity, with countertraction provided by pull of the bedsheet. Steady, continuous traction will ultimately overcome the spasm of the shoulder girdle muscles, and the humeral head may be disimpacted and reduced. Others advocate modifications of the Milch maneuver.[76,249,250,267,337] In this technique, the patient is positioned supine and the affected limb supported. Gradual abduction and external rotation is used to achieve glenohumeral reduction. As this technique does not employ traction to overcome muscle spasm, it may be successfully performed without sedation.[312] Still others use the Stimson technique of reduction (Fig. 19-10).[349] With the patient in prone position and the affected limb hanging free over the edge of the stretcher, longitudinal traction is applied to the extremity by means of a weight attached to the wrist. As the spasm of the shoulder girdle muscles fatigues and is overcome, reduction is achieved spontaneously and relatively atraumatically. Additional scapular mobilization may assist with reduction using the Stimson technique.[196,242]

Posterior dislocations may be similarly reduced with traction–countertraction maneuvers. Furthermore, the addition of a laterally directed force on the proximal humeral diaphysis may assist in achieving reduction.[255] In the rare inferior dislocations (or luxation erecta), a two-step closed reduction maneuver has been advocated.[264] An anterior-directed force is applied

to the humeral shaft, converting the inferior dislocation to an anterior one. Subsequent external rotation will then achieve glenohumeral reduction. Closed reduction is the definitive management of luxatio erecta in most cases.[279]

Outcomes

Following closed reduction, patients are typically immobilized with a sling for comfort. There is no evidence that longer duration of sling immobilization with the shoulder in internal rotation reduces the risk of recurrent instability.[280] Recent work, however, has raised the question of whether immobilization with the shoulder in adduction and external rotation is preferred. Anatomically, 30 degrees or more of external rotation of the shoulder may tension the anterior soft tissues and "reduce" the torn anterior capsulolabral structures to a more anatomic position on the glenoid.[171,251] Dynamic MRI have demonstrated improved position of the displaced labrum with external rotation.[172,322,326,336] Subsequent clinical studies have demonstrated up to a 40% reduction in recurrent instability rates when external rotation bracing was used for 4 or more weeks.[169,170,353] These findings have not been universally reproducible; other investigators have failed to demonstrate reduction in recurrent instability with external rotation immobilization.[102,218,221,280,352] Regardless of the type or duration of immobilization after reduction of acute dislocation, physical therapy is typically recommended to improve the dynamic stability conferred by the rotator cuff and adjacent shoulder girdle muscles.[34]

Despite successful closed reduction and subsequent rehabilitation, there is a high risk of recurrent instability, particularly in young, active patients.[228] The available literature, however, is limited in quantifying the true recurrent dislocation rates in children and adolescents. Much of the previously published information consists of retrospective case series of both adult and pediatric patients with limited follow-up.

Rowe[306] previously reported recurrent anterior instability in 100% of children less than 10 years of age and 94% of patients between 11 and 20 years. Marans et al.[236] similarly reported universal recurrent instability in their series of 21 children following traumatic dislocations. Wagner and Lyne[371] reported an 80% recurrence in 10 patients with open physes. In a series of nine patients who sustained traumatic instability at a mean age of 12.3 years, Elbaum et al.[94] similarly reported recurrent instability in 71%. In their review of 154 traumatic dislocations, Vermeiren et al.[367] found a 68% recurrence rate in patients less than 20 years of age. More recently, Longo et al. reported the results of a systematic review of 693 patients aged 18 years or younger.[228] Recurrent instability was seen in 71% of shoulders with nonoperative care. In their literature review, Franklin and Weiss similarly found recurrence rates of greater than 70% in younger patients.[106] Higher rates of recurrent instability have been reported in higher-energy injuries as well as those associated with bony glenoid injuries.[248,295,300] Younger patients involved in overhead or contact sports have similarly been noted to have higher recurrent instability rates.[313] Indeed, in a mixed pediatric and adult population-based study of 654 patients, risk of recurrent instability increased 4% for every year of age under 40.[213]

Other reports, however, cite lower recurrence rates in younger patients. Rockwood[302] documented a 50% recurrence rate in patients between 13.8 and 15.8 years of age. Cordischi et al.[66] published their study of 14 patients between 10.9 and 13.1 years of age and reported that only 3 patients (21%) went on to surgical treatment for recurrent instability. In perhaps the largest study with the longest follow-up, Hovelius et al.[155] reported 25-year follow-up on 229 shoulders in 227 patients who sustained their first traumatic dislocation between 12 and 40 years of age. Of the 58 patients who sustained their primary dislocation between 12 and 19 years of age, 26% reported a single recurrence, and an additional 16% of shoulders stabilized over time (defined as no instability events in the last 10 years). Only 43% of patients underwent surgical stabilization procedures. Additional case reports and small case series exist of young patients without recurrent instability at midterm follow-up.[97,141]

OPERATIVE TREATMENT OF SHOULDER DISLOCATIONS

Arthroscopic Bankart Repair

Indications/Contraindications

Surgical treatment is considered in patients with functionally limiting recurrent instability as well as in high-demand, overhead, or contact athletes in whom the risk of recurrent instability after their primary event is unacceptably high. In general, patients considered for surgery should have failed attempts at physical therapy and rehabilitation. In patients with traumatic anterior shoulder dislocations, recurrent instability is due to injury to the anteroinferior labrum and adjacent glenohumeral joint capsule and ligaments. Surgical treatment is focused on repairing the torn labrum to its anatomic location on the glenoid rim.

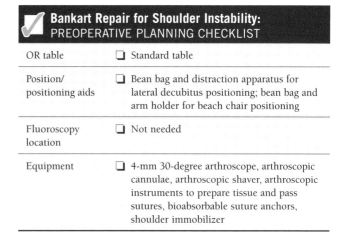

Bankart Repair for Shoulder Instability: PREOPERATIVE PLANNING CHECKLIST	
OR table	❏ Standard table
Position/ positioning aids	❏ Bean bag and distraction apparatus for lateral decubitus positioning; bean bag and arm holder for beach chair positioning
Fluoroscopy location	❏ Not needed
Equipment	❏ 4-mm 30-degree arthroscope, arthroscopic cannulae, arthroscopic shaver, arthroscopic instruments to prepare tissue and pass sutures, bioabsorbable suture anchors, shoulder immobilizer

Arthroscopic labral repair is the standard treatment for posttraumatic shoulder instability. Preoperative imaging should include plain radiographs of the affected shoulder to rule out associated bony lesions (e.g., glenoid fractures, Hill–Sachs lesions). MRI, with or without intra-articular contrast, is also helpful in determining the extent of labral injury and assessing for concomitant soft tissue injuries. Typical equipment required includes a standard 4-mm 30-degree arthroscope, arthroscopic cannulae, and surgical instruments used to mobilize and prepare the capsulolabral tissue (e.g., arthroscopic shavers, elevators, rasps, and suture passing devices). While a host of commercially available instruments are available, all provide the same fundamental arthroscopic capabilities. Suture anchors are also invaluable for arthroscopic labral repairs, and increasingly the standard is to use bioabsorbable suture anchors for intra-articular procedures.

Positioning

In general, arthroscopic stabilization may be performed in either the beach chair or lateral decubitus position (Fig. 19-11). Advantages of lateral decubitus position include ease of longitudinal and lateral distraction to assist in visualization and access to the axillary recess of the glenohumeral joint. Patients are placed with the unaffected shoulder down, allowing the thorax to fall posteriorly about 10 degrees, which will place the glenoid parallel to the ground. Care is taken to place an axillary roll for the unaffected down side to protect the contralateral brachial plexus and pad all bony prominences (e.g., contralateral fibular head to protect against peroneal nerve compression) to avoid excessive or prolonged compression of the peripheral nerves. The entire affected limb and shoulder girdle are prepped and draped into the surgical field. The limb is placed in balanced suspension with about 40 degrees of abduction and 10 to 20 degrees of forward flexion, typically with 7 to 10 lb of longitudinal and lateral distraction with the assistance of a limb holder. This allows for circumferential access to the shoulder girdle. Additional abduction–adduction and internal–external rotation may be employed during surgery for selective access and tensioning of soft tissues.

The modified beach chair position is also effective and commonly used. After placement of a roll or bump behind the patient between the scapulae, patients may be positioned with the affected limb and shoulder girdle off the edge of the table to allow circumferential access. The use of commercially available beach chairs, limb holders, and/or bean bags will assist with positioning.

Surgical Approach

The procedure begins with examination under anesthesia to assess pathologic instability anteriorly, posteriorly, and inferiorly. After intraoperative examination, the glenohumeral joint is insufflated with sterile saline solution and standard posterosuperior, anterosuperior, and anteroinferior arthroscopy portals are established. Viewing is traditionally performed from the posterosuperior portal, but moving the camera to the anterosuperior portal will allow for improved visualization of the anterior glenoid neck and anterior soft tissues, particularly in cases of long-standing instability where the labrum and capsule have scarred in a more medial position.

Technique

Bankart Repair for Shoulder Instability:
KEY SURGICAL STEPS

- ❏ Examination under anesthesia
- ❏ Establish arthroscopic portals
- ❏ Arthroscopic survey
- ❏ Mobilization of torn labrum and associated capsule
- ❏ Preparation of glenoid rim and glenoid neck
- ❏ Suture anchor placement in most inferior position of labral tear, just onto the chondral face of the glenoid
  - • Shuttle sutures through the adjacent capsulolabral tissue, effectuating an inferior-to-superior and medial-to-lateral shift
- ❏ Tie arthroscopic knot
- ❏ Repeat anchor placement, suture passage, and knot tying sequentially in more superior positions along the glenoid
- ❏ Minimum of three anchors are used
- ❏ Skin closure of portals with simple sutures
- ❏ Application of sling and swathe

Arthroscopic survey is performed to assess the extent of labral, capsular, and/or bony injury (Fig. 19-12). After confirmation of labral pathology, the capsulolabral complex is mobilized from its medialized position using arthroscopic elevators. The glenoid rim and medial glenoid neck in the region of the labral tear is similarly prepared with arthroscopic rasps or shavers in efforts to debride fibrinous tissue and prepare a bleeding bony bed for biologic healing. In a sequential fashion, arthroscopic suture anchors are placed from inferior to superior and sutures are shuttled through the capsulolabral complex.[293,327,363] Knots are tied in a sequential fashion, reapproximating the labrum to its anatomic location and retensioning the soft tissues. Suture anchors are also available which facilitate suture tensioning and tissue apposition without the need for manual knot tying. While a host of commercially available devices and techniques may be used, all conform to the standard principles of soft tissue mobilization, glenoid preparation, and repair of the soft tissue to the

glenoid rim, thus tensioning the anteroinferior capsule. More recently, there has been renewed enthusiasm for the addition of remplissage to fill the Hill–Sachs defect and minimize the risk of recurrent instability due to bony engagement.[161]

Latarjet Reconstruction

Indications/Contraindications

In patients with traumatic anterior shoulder dislocations, recurrent instability may also be due to bony fracture or insufficiency of the anteroinferior glenoid.[248,300] In these cases, soft tissue procedures alone may not address the underlying pathoanatomy and are prone to failure. This is particularly true in off-track lesions.[389] Surgical treatment in these situations typically involves restoring or augmenting the bony deficit of the glenoid. While several techniques have been advocated, transferring the coracoid process with its soft tissue attachments to the glenoid (the so-called Latarjet procedure) has increasingly become the standard of care.[281,285] Bony reconstructions such as the Latarjet procedure have also been advocated in patients with recurrent instability after prior failed soft tissue reconstruction.[185]

In addition to providing additional bony support for the articulating humeral head, the Latarjet procedure also stabilizes the glenohumeral joint by virtue of the fact that the conjoined tendon remains attached to the tip of the coracoid during transfer. These soft tissues act as a "sling" and provide additional anteroinferior stability. Stability is further conferred by preservation of the musculotendinous fibers of the subscapularis. This "triple effect" has been touted by Patte and Debeyre.[79,281,373]

Preoperative Planning

Latarjet Reconstruction for Shoulder Instability:
PREOPERATIVE PLANNING CHECKLIST

OR table	❏ Standard table
Position/ positioning aids	❏ Modified beach chair position
Fluoroscopy location	❏ Not needed
Equipment	❏ 90-degree oscillating saw, 3.5- or 4-mm cannulated screws

Though MRI is helpful in identifying and qualitatively assessing the extent of labral injury, Latarjet reconstructions are typically reserved for recurrent posttraumatic instability with associated glenoid loss or in those patients who have failed prior soft tissue stabilizations. In these situations, assessment of glenoid bone loss and possible engaging Hill–Sachs lesions is best done with CT three-dimensional reconstructions (see Fig. 19-7).

Most Latarjet reconstructions are performed via open deltopectoral approaches. Aside from the standard instruments and retractors used for open shoulder surgery, a few additional items are useful. A 90-degree oscillating saw blade will facilitate accurate and efficient coracoid osteotomy. Appropriate-sized cannulated screws—typically 4 mm in diameter and 30 to 34 mm in

Figure 19-11. Patient positioning for surgical procedures. **A, B:** Beach chair positioning allows for near circumferential access to the shoulder girdle. **C:** Lateral decubitus positioning with assistance of a bean bag. **D:** Use of longitudinal and/or lateral distraction will facilitate arthroscopic visualization. (Courtesy of Children's Orthopaedic Surgery Foundation.)

length—are used for fixation of the coracoid process to the anterior glenoid.

Positioning

The modified beach chair position is effective and commonly used. A roll or bump is placed behind the patient between the scapulae, to allow for scapular positioning and improved access to the glenoid neck. Patients are positioned with the affected limb and shoulder girdle off the edge of the table to allow circumferential access. The use of commercially available beach chairs, limb holders, and/or bean bags assist with positioning.

Surgical Approach

A standard deltopectoral approach is used. The incision is placed slightly more medial and superior than traditional deltopectoral approaches to the shoulder because of the need to expose the coracoid and medial glenoid neck. A vertical incision in Langer skin lines will maximize the aesthetics of the resultant scar. Superficial dissection will allow visualization of the deltopectoral interval, which is developed by taking the cephalic vein laterally with the deltoid. Deep dissection will allow visualization of the coracoid process, conjoined tendon, clavipectoral fascia, and subscapularis muscles.

Figure 19-12. Arthroscopic Bankart repair. **A:** Arthroscopic image of an anterior labral tear in the right shoulder of a 16-year-old male. The patient is positioned in the lateral decubitus position. **B:** Arthroscopic appearance after anterior labral repair, demonstrating reapproximation of the labral tissue to the glenoid rim. (Courtesy of Children's Orthopaedic Surgery Foundation.)

Technique

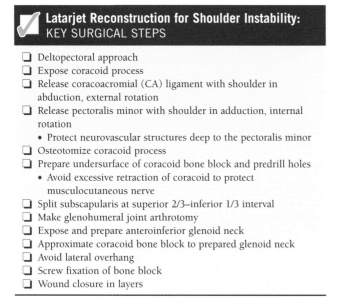

✓ **Latarjet Reconstruction for Shoulder Instability:**
KEY SURGICAL STEPS

❏ Deltopectoral approach
❏ Expose coracoid process
❏ Release coracoacromial (CA) ligament with shoulder in abduction, external rotation
❏ Release pectoralis minor with shoulder in adduction, internal rotation
  • Protect neurovascular structures deep to the pectoralis minor
❏ Osteotomize coracoid process
❏ Prepare undersurface of coracoid bone block and predrill holes
  • Avoid excessive retraction of coracoid to protect musculocutaneous nerve
❏ Split subscapularis at superior 2/3–inferior 1/3 interval
❏ Make glenohumeral joint arthrotomy
❏ Expose and prepare anteroinferior glenoid neck
❏ Approximate coracoid bone block to prepared glenoid neck
❏ Avoid lateral overhang
❏ Screw fixation of bone block
❏ Wound closure in layers

After initial dissection is performed, a spiked Hohmann retractor is placed superiorly over the coracoid process, with its tip just anterior to the origin of the coracoclavicular (CC) ligaments. The shoulder is abducted and externally rotated, placing the CA ligament under tension. The CA ligament is then divided approximately 1 to 2 cm from the coracoid, leaving a cuff of tissue that will be used later for capsular reconstruction. The shoulder is then adducted and internally rotated. The pectoralis minor insertion is then released off the coracoid process, being careful to protect the brachial plexus, which lies deep to the pectoralis minor. Following this, the coracoid is osteotomized at its flexure, or "knee," from medial to lateral. The use of

commercially available 90-degree microsagittal saws will facilitate coracoid osteotomy. The coracoid is then freed from the remaining surrounding soft tissue attachments, including the deep coracohumeral ligament, and mobilized while protecting the origin of the conjoined tendon. The undersurface of the coracoid is decorticated to expose bleeding cancellous bone. Two drill holes (typically 3.5–4 mm) are made in the coracoid to facilitate subsequent screw placement. Overzealous mobilization or retraction of the coracoid process is avoided, as the musculocutaneous nerve enters the coracobrachialis approximately 4 to 5 cm distal.

Direction is then turned to glenoid preparation. With the shoulder in adduction and external rotation, the subscapularis is split in line with its muscle fibers between the superior two-thirds and inferior one-third. This muscle-splitting technique preserves subscapularis integrity, contributing stability and minimizing iatrogenic injury to the axillary nerve. The plane between the subscapularis and underlying capsule is developed bluntly, and the glenohumeral joint line is identified. With the shoulder in neutral rotation, a vertical capsulotomy is made in the glenohumeral joint; this may be extended with a medial horizontal incision (in the shape of a sideways T) for improved exposure of the anteroinferior glenoid. With the shoulder internally rotated, a Fukuda or humeral head retractor is then placed into the glenohumeral joint. Exposure of the anteroinferior glenoid neck is then performed via subperiosteal elevation or debridement of the scar tissue and prior bony Bankart fragments. The recipient bed on the glenoid is then decorticated until punctate bleeding is seen.

The coracoid process is then passed through the subscapularis split and its previously decorticated deep surface is approximated to the anteroinferior glenoid neck. Care is made to position the coracoid bone block precisely; lateral overhang may result in joint incongruity and subsequent degenerative arthrosis or pain. After the coracoid is positioned, the previously placed drill holes are identified. Through these holes, the glenoid neck is drilled anterior to posteriorly in the path of anticipated screw passage. Measurements are taken, and screw fixation of the coracoid process to the glenoid is achieved with 3.5- or 4-mm screws (Fig. 19-13). Screws are typically 32 to 34 mm in older adolescents, though the size will vary according to patient to patient. The lateral portion of the glenohumeral capsule is then reapproximated to the cuff of prior CA ligament still attached to the coracoid, completing a capsular reconstruction. Wound closure is performed in layers including pectoralis major repair, though the subscapularis split need not be closed. Patients are placed in a sling and swathe postoperatively.

Arthroscopic Capsulorrhaphy

Indications/Contraindications

In patients with multidirectional instability which is painful and/or functionally limiting and has failed nonoperative treatment, arthroscopic capsulorrhaphy may be considered. As cited above, careful patient selection and preoperative counseling is critical, given the risk of recurrent instability and importance of postoperative therapy. Relative contraindications include patients with poorly controlled neuromuscular conditions, or those with cognitive or developmental delays limiting understanding and compliance with postoperative care.

Preoperative Planning

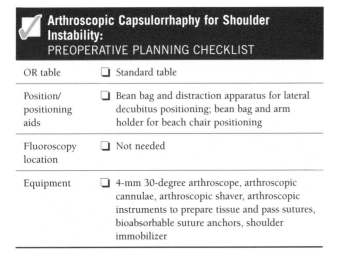

✓ Arthroscopic Capsulorrhaphy for Shoulder Instability: PREOPERATIVE PLANNING CHECKLIST	
OR table	❏ Standard table
Position/ positioning aids	❏ Bean bag and distraction apparatus for lateral decubitus positioning; bean bag and arm holder for beach chair positioning
Fluoroscopy location	❏ Not needed
Equipment	❏ 4-mm 30-degree arthroscope, arthroscopic cannulae, arthroscopic shaver, arthroscopic instruments to prepare tissue and pass sutures, bioabsorbable suture anchors, shoulder immobilizer

Preoperative planning and equipment is similar to arthroscopic Bankart repair, as described above. MRI-arthrography is particularly useful, as it may demonstrate areas of capsular redundancy and guide selective capsulorrhaphy.

Positioning

Arthroscopic capsulorrhaphy may be performed either in the lateral decubitus or modified beach chair positions. Given the need for circumferential access around the glenoid and glenohumeral joint, the addition of laterally directed distraction is

Figure 19-13. Intraoperative fluoroscopy images of the left shoulder following Latarjet reconstruction. **A:** Anteroposterior and (**B**) axillary projections depict screw fixation of the coracoid process, with care made not to lateralize the bone block. (Courtesy of Children's Orthopaedic Surgery Foundation.)

useful. This may be facilitated with the use of lateral traction, commercially available arm holders, or placement of a bump beneath the axilla.

Surgical Approach

Similar to arthroscopic Bankart repairs, the procedure begins with examination under anesthesia to assess pathologic instability anteriorly, posteriorly, and inferiorly. After glenohumeral joint is insufflated with sterile saline solution, standard posterosuperior, anterosuperior, and anteroinferior arthroscopy portals are established. Viewing is traditionally performed from the posterosuperior portal, but moving the camera to the anterosuperior portal and establishing a posterior working portal will allow for improved visualization and circumferential access to the glenohumeral joint capsule.

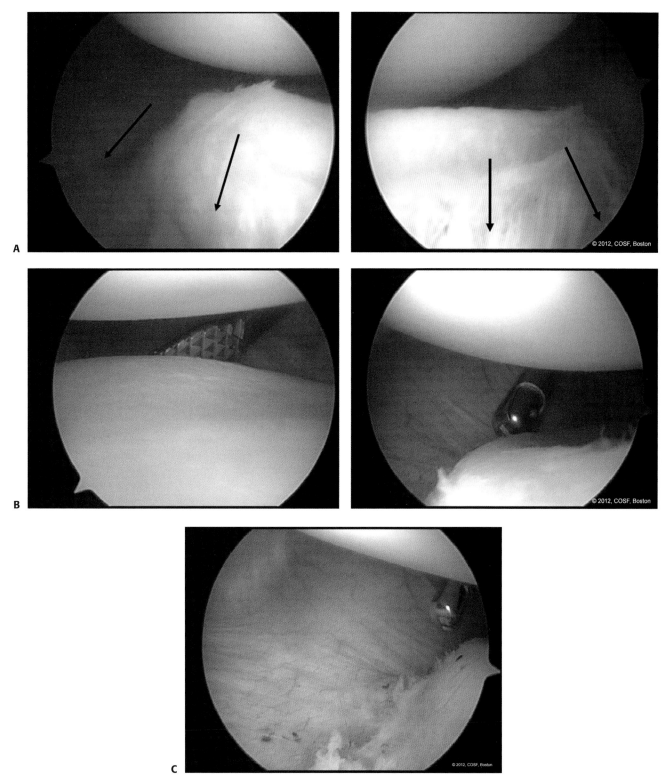

Figure 19-14. Arthroscopic capsulorrhaphy for multidirectional instability. **A:** Arthroscopic images depict redundant capsule (*arrows*), falling away from the glenoid rim and labrum. **B:** Tissue preparation may be performed with either rasps, shavers, or other devices to stimulate a bleeding response (**C**).

(*continues*)

Figure 19-14. *(Continued)* **D:** Suture passing devices are used in a "pinch-tuck" fashion to imbricate the redundant tissue. **E:** Arthroscopic view after posterior plication sutures has been passed. **F:** After sutures have been tied, note is made of plication of the capsule and loss of the capsular redundancy. (Courtesy of Children's Orthopaedic Surgery Foundation.)

Technique

Arthroscopic Capsulorrhaphy for Shoulder Instability:
KEY SURGICAL STEPS

- ☐ Examination under anesthesia
- ☐ Establish arthroscopic portals
- ☐ Arthroscopic survey
- ☐ Preparation and imbrication of posterior glenohumeral joint
  - Place arthroscope anterosuperiorly with working portal posteriorly
  - Stimulation of bleeding response in posterior capsule
  - Pass imbricating suture through capsule first, then through chondrolabral junction, beginning in most inferior position
  - May store sutures in anteroinferior portal to ease visualization and subsequent suture management
  - Pass additional plication sutures from inferior to superior
  - After all posterior sutures have been placed, tie in sequential fashion from inferior to superior
- ☐ Preparation and imbrication of anterior glenohumeral joint
  - Place arthroscope posteriorly and establish accessory portal anterosuperiorly
  - Stimulate redundant anterior capsule until bleeding response seen
  - Pass imbricating sutures through capsule and then chondrolabral junction, placating redundant tissue
  - Tie sutures as they are placed, inferiorly to superiorly
- ☐ Skin closure with simple sutures
- ☐ Application of sling and swathe

Arthroscopic survey is performed to assess the extent of capsular patulousness and rule out unrecognized labral and/or bony pathology (Fig. 19-14). As plication of the posterior capsule is typically more challenging, direction is first turned to the posterior aspect of the shoulder. The arthroscope is placed in the anterosuperior portal and a working portal established posteriorly. The redundant capsule adjacent to the glenoid rim is prepared using arthroscopic rasps or shavers until punctate bleeding is seen, in efforts to stimulate a healing response; care is made to avoid overzealous tissue preparation, as the tissue is thin and undesirable rents in the capsule may be created. Following this, imbricating sutures may be placed, beginning in the most inferior aspect of the joint. Typically, this is performed by passing a suture through capsular tissue approximately 1 cm from the labrum, and then passing the suture a second time from the capsule through the chondrolabral junction. Prior biomechanical studies have demonstrated that sutures passed through the chondrolabral junction of patients with an intact labrum are as strong as suture anchors.[290] This "pinch-tuck" suture will plicate the capsule when tied, reducing overall capsular volume. If knots are tied as the sutures are passed, the reduced capsular volume will often make subsequent suture placement more difficult; for this reason, consideration is made to pass all posterior sutures first before tying. After all posterior sutures are placed, they may be tied in sequential fashion from inferior to superior, completing the posterior capsulorrhaphy.

The arthroscope is then repositioned posteriorly and an accessory portal reestablished anterosuperiorly. The anteroinferior capsule is similarly prepared with rasps, shavers, or other instruments until punctate bleedings is seen. Plicating sutures are again passed in a "pinch-tuck" fashion, imbricating the redundant capsule to the intact glenoid labrum. These may be tied in series, completing the circumferential repair.

Open Capsulorrhaphy

Indications/Contraindications

Despite advances in arthroscopic surgical techniques, open soft tissue procedures may still be performed. Relative indications for open capsulorrhaphy include failed prior arthroscopic procedures, multidirectional instability in setting of capsular laxity without labral tear, and surgeon preference and/or experience. The principles of these procedures are similar to arthroscopic plication: Stability is conferred by tightening the redundant capsule, thus reducing joint volume and conferring stability.

Preoperative Planning

> ✓ **Open Capsulorrhaphy for Shoulder Instability:**
> PREOPERATIVE PLANNING CHECKLIST

OR table	❏ Standard table
Position/ positioning aids	❏ Modified beach chair position, limb holder if available
Fluoroscopy location	❏ Not needed
Equipment	❏ Shoulder retractors, nonabsorbable braided sutures

Preoperative planning similar to procedures described above.

Positioning

The modified beach chair position is used. Intraoperative positioning is aided by a limb holder.

Surgical Approach

A standard deltopectoral approach is used, with the skin incision beginning just lateral to the coracoid process and extending within Langer skin lines toward the axillary crease. The cephalic vein is typically retracted laterally with the deltoid. After the clavipectoral fascia is excised, the conjoined tendon

is carefully retracted medially to avoid excessive traction to the musculocutaneous nerve. This will allow direct visualization of the subscapularis and underlying glenohumeral joint capsule.

Technique

> ✓ **Open Capsulorrhaphy for Shoulder Instability:**
> KEY SURGICAL STEPS

❏ Deltopectoral approach
❏ Excise clavipectoral fascia
❏ Gentle retraction of conjoined tendon
❏ Subscapularis tenotomy, leaving cuff of tissue on lesser tuberosity for subsequent repair
  • Mobilize subscapularis after placement of traction sutures
❏ Perform T-shaped capsulotomy
❏ Imbricate capsule, advancing inferomedial capsular flap superolaterally, followed by repair of the superomedial flap inferomedially
  • Position limb in slight abduction and ~30 degrees external rotation to avoid overtightening
❏ Careful repair of subscapularis tenotomy using heavy braided nonabsorbable sutures
❏ Layered wound closure
❏ Sling-and-swathe immobilization

After the subscapularis is exposed, the limb is placed in adduction and external rotation. The lesser tuberosity is palpated and identified. A subscapularis tenotomy may then be performed 2 to 3 cm medial to its insertion on the lesser tuberosity, leaving a cuff of tissue laterally to allow for subsequent repair. Traction sutures are placed on the subscapularis tendon, which may then be mobilized and separated from the underlying glenohumeral joint capsule. In some situations, the upper two-thirds of the subscapularis may be divided, leaving a portion of the inferior musculotendinous unit intact. Another option is a subscapularis muscle-splitting approach, as described above.

Next, a T-shaped capsulotomy is created; a vertical incision is made laterally, with a subsequent transverse extension medially. The superomedial and inferomedial capsular flaps are then mobilized with suture tags. With the limb in the desired position of slight abduction and external rotation, the inferomedial limb is advanced and shifted superolaterally, repaired to the lateral capsule with multiple interrupted nonabsorbable sutures. This positioning preserves normal capsular laxity and lessens risk of degenerative arthrosis that can occur with surgical overtightening. The superomedial limb is then similarly advanced inferomedially and sewn to the lateral capsule, completing the capsulorrhaphy. Meticulous repair of the subscapularis tenotomy is performed with multiple braided nonabsorbable sutures. The subcutaneous tissues and skin are closed in layers, followed by application of a sling and swathe.

> ## Author's Preferred Treatment of Shoulder Dislocations (Algorithm 19-1)

Children and adolescents with traumatic, anterior shoulder dislocations are treated with prompt closed reduction and sling immobilization. Radiographs are obtained to confirm adequacy of glenohumeral reduction and

evaluate for possible bony glenoid fractures. In the majority of patients with purely soft tissue injuries—likely anteroinferior labral tears—physical therapy is initiated following brief immobilization. Return to sports is limited

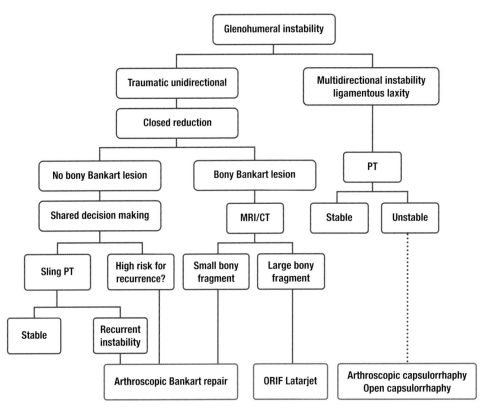

Algorithm 19-1. Author's preferred treatment for shoulder dislocation.

until patients have restoration of motion, strength, and proprioception.

Early in the postinjury period, patients and families are counseled regarding the risk of recurrent instability. In high-risk patients (e.g., contact or overhead athletes) or patients for whom the risk of recurrent instability is judged to be unacceptable, arthroscopic Bankart repair may be performed after primary dislocation.[134,272] In rare circumstances where patients wish to continue with high-risk activities despite known risk of recurrent instability (e.g., in-season contact athlete), functional bracing with orthoses limiting abduction and external rotation may be used.

Patients with bony Bankart lesions are further assessed with CT, and quantification is made of glenoid deficiency. Given the high risk of recurrent instability in the setting of glenoid bone loss, patients with small marginal lesions are offered arthroscopic repair. Patients with larger bony glenoid lesions are treated with open reduction and internal fixation (ORIF) versus Latarjet reconstruction, depending upon the integrity of the bony fragment.

Surgical stabilization of adolescents with recurrent unidirectional instability is typically performed via arthroscopic capsulolabral repair. Preoperative imaging with MRI-arthrography will better define the extent of labral injury and rule out unrecognized or attritional glenoid insufficiency. Latarjet reconstructions are performed in cases of glenoid bone loss or recurrent instability failing prior arthroscopic stabilizations.

Patients with atraumatic multidirectional instability in the setting of ligamentous laxity or other systemic conditions (e.g., hypermobility, Ehlers–Danlos, etc.) are treated with physical therapy, emphasizing strength, proprioception, biofeedback, and neuromuscular retraining of the entire shoulder girdle. In select patients where there is persistent, painful, or functionally limiting instability refractory to or precluding physical therapy, surgical treatment is considered. MRI-arthrography is obtained to characterize the extent and magnitude of capsular redundancy. Stabilization is performed via arthroscopic capsulorrhaphy, with appropriate postoperative immobilization and therapy.

Postoperative Care

Postoperatively, patients are sling immobilized for 4 weeks postoperatively. During the third and fourth postoperative weeks, patients initiate pendulum exercises only. Formal supervised physical therapy is begun after the fourth postoperative week, limiting forward flexion and lateral abduction in the plane of the scapula to 90 degrees and external rotation to 30 degrees. After the sixth postoperative week, motion and strengthening are advanced as tolerated. Sports participation is generally limited for 6 months postoperatively, provided full motion and strength has been restored.

Potential Pitfalls and Preventive Measures

Repair of Shoulder Instability:
POTENTIAL PITFALLS AND PREVENTIONS

Pitfall	Preventions
Failure to identify bony glenoid fractures	Careful evaluation of injury and postreduction radiographs including MRI and/or CT imaging
	Use of orthogonal radiographic images, including axillary view
Early recurrent instability after arthroscopic stabilization	Appropriate recognition of glenoid deficiency or large, engaging Hill–Sachs lesion requiring bony reconstruction
	Meticulous preparation, mobilization of capsulolabral tissue, particularly in the setting of an ALPSA lesion
	Appropriate suture passage and knot security
	Appropriate recognition of HAGL lesions
	Excessive, early at-risk activities and positioning
Early recurrent instability after stabilization for multidirectional instability	Comprehensive counseling regarding importance of therapy and nonoperative treatment modalities
	Appropriate patient selection
	Meticulous soft tissue preparation and plication

Potential pitfalls in the diagnosis and management of shoulder dislocations are described above. In general, early recurrent instability after nonoperative or surgical treatment is generally due to failure to recognize the pertinent pathoanatomy. Careful radiographic evaluation after primary or recurrent instability events is needed to recognize bony glenoid deficiency and guide appropriate management. Early recurrent instability after arthroscopic soft tissue procedures may be due to unrecognized glenoid deficiency, suboptimal mobilization and preparation of the capsulolabral tissue, untreated HAGL lesions, or technical errors in suture passage and knot security. Finally, recurrent instability after capsulorrhaphy for multidirectional instability may be due to unrecognized systemic connective tissue disorders, suboptimal tissue preparation and plication, or inappropriate patient selection.

Outcomes

As noted above, there is limited published information regarding the results of surgical stabilization for glenohumeral instability in children and adolescents. Much of the current understanding of the treatment outcomes is derived from applications of the adult experiences. A number of general observations may be gleaned from review of the existing retrospective case series. First, there has been an increase in the incidence of glenohumeral instability in younger patients, perhaps because of increasing activities and younger age of first sports participation, with expectation for high recurrence rates with nonoperative treatment alone.[80,121,155,355] Second, arthroscopic repairs have become increasingly common and preferred over open stabilization procedures.[235,295] Third, surgical stabilization of Bankart

lesions safely and effectively improves shoulder stability, with the risk of recurrence reduced to 5% to 25%.[2,46,211,328] Castagna et al.[46] reported the results of 65 patients between 13 and 18 years of age, treated with arthroscopic capsulolabral repair, all of whom were overhead or contact athletes. At mean 5-year follow-up, shoulder motion was restored and 81% had returned to their preinjury level of sports participation. Recurrent instability was reported in 21%, and recurrence was associated with choice of sports participation. In a report of 32 arthroscopic stabilizations in 30 patients under 18 years of age, Jones et al.[179] similarly reported high functional outcomes, though recurrent instability was noted in 12% to 19% of patients. Shymon et al. corroborated these results in a series of 99 patients treated with either open or arthroscopic Bankart repairs. Recurrent instability or need for secondary surgery was noted in 21% of patients, and no difference was seen based on surgical technique.[335] Egger et al. reported 31% recurrent instability in their ingle center review of 59 patients under 18 years of age.[92] Finally, bony procedures including the Latarjet coracoid transfer are safe and effective, with low risk of recurrent instability.[11,117,159] After a mean of 12 years of follow-up, Waltenspul found recurrent instability of only 6% in patients under 18 years of age following Latarjet reconstruction.[376]

MANAGEMENT OF ADVERSE OUTCOMES AND UNEXPECTED COMPLICATIONS RELATED TO SHOULDER DISLOCATIONS

Shoulder Dislocations:
COMMON ADVERSE OUTCOMES AND COMPLICATIONS

- Recurrent instability
- Neurovascular injury
- Chondrolysis
- Arthrosis

Adverse outcomes and complications occur infrequently with glenohumeral instability. As noted above, vascular injury is exceedingly rare, and the majority of neurologic injuries associated with traumatic dislocations represent neurapraxic traction injuries to the axillary nerve more commonly than brachial plexus, with expectation of spontaneous resolution over time. Nerve repairs or reconstructions are rarely needed and reserved for patients who fail to demonstrate progressive spontaneous recovery. Musculocutaneous nerve injuries can occur with excessive traction during open surgical exposure and reconstruction.

Chondrolysis has been increasingly reported in patients undergoing arthroscopic stabilizations for glenohumeral instability. Reports suggest that use of intra-articular analgesics (e.g., indwelling intra-articular pain catheters) is associated with chondrolysis, and for this reason are currently contraindicated.[321,324,341,383] Similarly, unexpected joint degeneration has been reported after thermal capsulorrhaphy and loose metallic suture anchors, likely related to thermal injury and third body wear of the articular cartilage, respectively.[65,85,122,181] Cartilage loss in a young, skeletally immature shoulder is a disastrous and yet unsolved complication. Avoidance of excessive heat and proper placement of bioabsorbable suture anchors may minimize these adverse events. Judicious placement of bone grafts and internal fixation, such as in the Latarjet procedure, is also critically important to minimize risk of early arthrosis.[158]

SUMMARY, CONTROVERSIES, AND FUTURE DIRECTIONS RELATED TO SHOULDER DISLOCATIONS

In summary, glenohumeral instability is common in children and adolescents. While closed reduction is easily performed after acute dislocations, there is a high risk of recurrent instability. In appropriately selected patients, arthroscopic or open soft tissue and/or bony stabilization procedures are safe and effective.

There is ongoing debate and controversy surrounding the indications for surgical stabilization after primary traumatic dislocation in the child or adolescent. Proponents of primary surgery point to the safety and efficacy of predominantly arthroscopic procedures in reducing recurrence risk and restoring stability and return of function. Furthermore, there is some evidence suggesting recurrent dislocations may lead to more extensive labral tears, development of glenoid insufficiency, and even arthrosis.[156,186] Many argue that surgical stabilization should be performed in higher-risk patients (e.g., young athletes involved in contact sports).[51,199] An expected-value decision analysis supports primary arthroscopic stabilization if recurrence risk above 32% and utility value of surgical intervention remains above 6.6.[21] Further investigation of the natural history of recurrent glenohumeral instability as well as prospective randomized trials of surgical versus nonoperative treatment is needed in the pediatric patient population.

Finally, as more information regarding the frequency and clinical significance of bony glenoid and humeral head defects becomes available, clarification of the indications for bony augmentation procedures (e.g., coracoid transfer, bone grafting) is needed. This is particularly relevant given the persistent risks of recurrent instability after arthroscopic Bankart repairs and the promising longer-term studies regarding the results of bony procedures.[58,157,159,175,192]

Proximal Humerus Fractures

INTRODUCTION TO PROXIMAL HUMERUS FRACTURES

Proximal humeral fractures are relatively uncommon injuries, with an estimated annual incidence of 1.2 to 4.4 per 1,000,

and representing less than 5% of all childhood fractures.[205,206,304] Given the metaphyseal location, thick periosteum, and proximity to the proximal humeral physis, there is tremendous healing and remodeling potential of proximal humerus fractures. Furthermore, given the robust, near-universal motion about the glenohumeral joint, little functional impairment may be seen even in cases of considerable bony malalignment. For these reasons, most proximal humeral fractures are amenable to nonoperative treatment.[135,278]

ASSESSMENT OF PROXIMAL HUMERUS FRACTURES

MECHANISMS OF INJURY FOR PROXIMAL HUMERUS FRACTURES

Proximal humerus fractures occur through a number of characteristic injury mechanisms. Birth-related fractures of the proximal humerus are not uncommon.[214] In general, hyperextension and/or rotational forces imparted on the upper limb during labor and delivery result in failure through the proximal humeral physis or metaphysis (Fig. 19-15).[75,137,214,233] Risk factors include difficult delivery, macrosomia, and breech presentation, but are not entirely predictive.[38,177] Indeed, proximal humerus fractures may occur during vaginal delivery of infants of all weights and sizes, implicating other maternal and perinatal factors.

In older children and adolescents, proximal humerus fractures are typically sustained from traumatic mechanisms, such as sports-related activities or motor vehicle collisions (Fig. 19-16). Direct trauma to the anterior or posterior aspect of the proximal humerus may result in fracture.[75,261,340] More commonly, indirect trauma via forces imparted on the upper limb during falls or nonphysiologic positioning may result in a proximal humeral fracture.[340] Indeed, Williams[385] postulated six distinct mechanisms by which proximal humerus fractures may be sustained: forced extension, forced flexion, forced extension with lateral or medial rotation, and forced flexion with lateral or medial rotation. Fractures may occur at the level of the proximal metaphysis or physis.

Figure 19-15. Hyperextension or rotation of the ipsilateral arm may result in a proximal humeral or physeal injury during birth.

A

B

Figure 19-16. **A:** Motor vehicle crashes may result in proximal humeral fracture due to blunt trauma to the shoulder region. **B:** Blunt trauma from contact sports may result in fracture of the proximal humerus in children.

Furthermore, the proximal humerus is a common location of pathologic fractures in children. Benign lesions—such as unicameral or aneurysmal bone cysts—and much less often malignant lesions (osteogenic sarcoma), commonly involve the proximal humerus and may first present in the setting of pathologic fracture.[3,273,299] Neuropathic conditions including Arnold–Chiari malformation, myelomeningocele, or syringomyelia have also been implicated in pathologic fractures of the proximal humerus.[10,225] Radiation therapy to the shoulder girdle may result in bony abnormalities predisposing to proximal humerus fracture.[90]

Finally, proximal humerus fractures may be seen in the setting of nonaccidental trauma and child abuse.[246,332] For this reason, careful assessment including comprehensive history and physical examinations is needed when assessing infants and young children with proximal humerus fractures.

INJURIES ASSOCIATED WITH PROXIMAL HUMERUS FRACTURES

Fractures of the proximal humerus may have concomitant dislocations of the glenohumeral joint, particularly with high-energy mechanisms of injury.[63,124,196,266,364,378] While radiographic pseudosubluxation may occur—due to fracture displacement and/or muscle imbalance—and resolve spontaneously, true joint dislocation may rarely be seen.[262,361] Glenohumeral joint dislocation may be anterior, posterior, or inferior, and concomitant intra-articular or apophyseal avulsion fractures may be seen.[258,305] All patients with proximal humerus fractures should be evaluated for concomitant glenohumeral joint reduction with appropriate radiographic imaging. A high index of suspicion is needed to avoid delayed or missed diagnosis. Ipsilateral fractures of the upper limb have also been reported, emphasizing the importance of a comprehensive physical examination and imaging of the entire humerus or upper limb as appropriate.[128,174,230]

Given the proximity to the brachial plexus and axillary vessels, proximal humerus fractures may be associated with neurovascular injury. Axillary nerve, radial nerve, and total brachial plexus palsies have been reported in the setting of displaced proximal humerus fractures.[6,89,165,364,369] These are typically seen in valgus injuries, in which the distal diaphyseal segment displaces medially and proximally into the region of the brachial plexus. While spontaneous neurologic recovery is seen in the majority of patients within 9 to 12 months, patients may develop a profound neurogenic pain syndrome.[165] Proximal humerus fractures associated with arterial injury and vascular insufficiency require emergent reduction and/or stabilization and vascular repair.[138,382] Associated injuries to the thorax, including rib fractures and pneumothorax, have also been reported.

SIGNS AND SYMPTOMS OF PROXIMAL HUMERUS FRACTURES

In neonates, the signs and symptoms of proximal humerus fractures may be subtle. Rarely will ecchymosis, swelling, or deformity be clinically apparent. Care providers will often report irritability or "fussiness" with handling or motion of the affected extremity. Often the absence of spontaneous movement of the upper limb—so-called pseudoparalysis—will alert the examiner to an underlying fracture. It is imperative to rule out undiagnosed septic arthritis or proximal humeral osteomyelitis in the neonate, as infections put the important proximal humerus physis at risk for growth arrest and glenohumeral joint of deformity.

In older children and adolescents, the clinical diagnosis is more obvious. Patients will present with pain, swelling, ecchymosis, and/or limited shoulder motion after traumatic injury. The limb is typically held against the body in adduction and internal rotation, and patients will guard against passive or active movement. Inspection will reveal asymmetry in the contour of the shoulder girdle compared with the contralateral, uninjured extremity. Subtle skin puckering may be seen, suggestive of soft tissue interposition in severely displaced fractures.[77] Careful evaluation of neurovascular status is critical to rule out concomitant nerve or vessel injury. Even in patients with considerable pain and guarding, axillary nerve function (sensation over the lateral deltoid, abduction of the shoulder) needs to be adequately assessed. Similarly, brachial plexus integrity may be assessed by distal motor sensory function without moving the injured limb.

Patients with associated posterior glenohumeral joint dislocation will posture with internal rotation and have limited or extremely painful passive external rotation. Associated fracture-dislocations involving the greater tuberosity and luxatio erecta will present with extreme abduction of the shoulder and elbow flexion.[195] Fractures of the lesser tuberosity and/or subscapularis disruption may be more subtle in presentation, though patients will have weak internal rotation, a positive lift-off sign, and often increased passive external rotation. These injuries can be missed acutely.[217,305,334,368]

IMAGING AND OTHER DIAGNOSTIC STUDIES FOR PROXIMAL HUMERUS FRACTURES

The proximal humeral epiphysis is not radiographically apparent until approximately 6 months of age, limiting the diagnostic utility of plain radiographs in the evaluation of neonates and infants.[200,271] In these very young patients, ultrasonography may provide meaningful diagnostic information.[29,104,160] MRI may also help distinguish between proximal humeral fracture and other potential causes of pseudoparalysis, such as osteomyelitis, septic arthritis, or glenohumeral joint instability in the setting of brachial plexus birth palsy, though MRI requires conscious sedation or general anesthesia.

Subtle radiographic signs of proximal humerus fracture in infants include asymmetric positioning of the proximal humeral metaphysis in relationship to the scapula and acromion, particularly when compared to images of the contralateral shoulder.[359] In patients with posteriorly displaced physeal fractures, the so-called "vanishing epiphysis" sign has been used to describe the apparent absence of the small epiphyseal ossification center, which lies behind the proximal metaphysis (Fig. 19-17).[191]

In older patients and adolescents, plain radiographs will confirm the diagnosis and characterize fracture pattern and displacement. Orthogonal views are necessary, and ideally AP and axillary views are obtained to assess for concomitant lesser tuberosity fracture or glenohumeral joint dislocation.[351] In appropriate axillary images, the humeral head normally resides between the acromion and coracoid process, concentrically reduced within the glenoid. Standardized assessment of plain radiographs will provide reliable measures of displacement and angulation, particularly when the epiphyseal margins of the humeral head fragment are identified and used.[33] Given the difficulty in obtaining axillary radiographs in the acutely injured child, a host of alternative radiographic views have been proposed, including the transthoracic scapular Y view, apical oblique view, and other variations.[115,338] In unusual situations in which adequate plain radiographs cannot be obtained, CT or MRI may be used. These advanced imaging modalities are particularly useful in cases of posterior glenohumeral fracture-dislocations, intra-articular fractures, or occult fractures.[14,124,311,358,360]

CLASSIFICATION OF PROXIMAL HUMERUS FRACTURES

Metaphyseal proximal humerus fractures occur most commonly in children between 5 and 12 years of age, and may be described according to their radiographic displacement and angulation (Fig. 19-18). It has been hypothesized that rapid

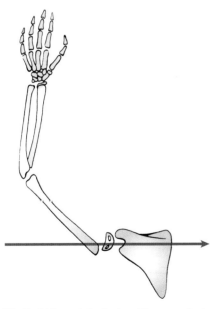

Figure 19-17. Vanishing epiphysis sign. The *arrow* depicts the direction of the x-ray beam.

Figure 19-18. Proximal humeral metaphyseal fracture in a 5-year-old male. (Courtesy of Children's Orthopaedic Surgery Foundation.)

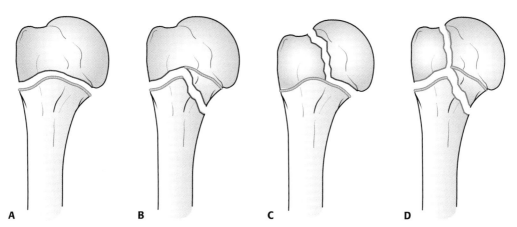

Figure 19-19. Physeal fractures of the proximal humerus. **A:** Salter–Harris type I. **B:** Salter–Harris type II. **C:** Salter–Harris type III. **D:** Salter–Harris type IV.

metaphyseal growth and thus relative porosity of the proximal humeral metaphysis contributes to the predilection to fracture in this age group.[75]

Physeal fractures are classified according to the Salter–Harris classification (Fig. 19-19).[315] Salter–Harris I injuries denote fractures through the physis and most commonly occur in patients under 5 years of age.[75,283] Salter–Harris II fractures exit through the metaphysis, often associated with an anterolateral bony fragment and are more commonly seen in older children and adolescents.[32,75,104,283] Salter–Harris III fractures are relatively rare and have been associated with concomitant glenohumeral dislocation. Salter–Harris IV fractures have not been reported in children.

Neer and Horwitz[261] proposed a classification system for pediatric proximal humerus fractures based on the amount of fracture displacement. In grade I fractures, there is up to 5 mm of displacement. Grade II fractures are displaced up to one-third of the cortical diameter of the humeral diaphysis. Grade III injuries have up to two-third displacement. Grade IV fractures have greater than two-thirds cortical diameter displacement. Angulation and malrotation are not specifically categorized in this classification system.

PATHOANATOMY AND APPLIED ANATOMY RELATING TO PROXIMAL HUMERUS FRACTURES

Care of proximal humerus fractures in children and adolescents is challenging for a number of reasons. First, given the robust remodeling potential in skeletally immature patients, there are variations in what is deemed "acceptable" deformity. Fracture reduction is often difficult, owing to the small size and deep location of the humeral head as well as the deforming muscle insertions on both the proximal and distal fracture fragments. Multiple reduction maneuvers and fixation options have been proposed, adding complexity to nonoperative or surgical decision making. Finally, the proximity of the zone of injury to adjacent neurovascular structures results in the potential for associated injuries and surgical risks. All of these considerations must be reconciled with evolving patient and family expectations regarding pain control, healing time, and functional return. For these reasons, understanding of the applied anatomy and pathoanatomy of proximal humerus fractures is critical.

The proximal humeral epiphysis does not become radiographically apparent until approximately 6 months of age.[200,271] Furthermore, the greater and lesser tuberosities have their own distinct secondary centers of ossification, which become visible at 1 to 3 years and 4 to 5 years of age, respectively.[271,317] The greater and lesser tuberosities coalesce between 5 and 7 years of age, and subsequently fuse to the rest of the humeral head between 7 and 13 years of age.

The proximal humeral physis ultimately contributes 80% of the longitudinal growth of the humerus.[25,287,288] There is some variation over time, however, as the proximal humeral physis contributes 75% of longitudinal growth of the humerus prior to 2 years of age but up to 90% of growth after the age of 11 years. In general, the proximal humeral physis closes at 14 to 17 years of age in females and between 16 and 18 years of age in males.[25,287,288,343]

The articular surface of the humeral head encompasses the medial aspect of the epiphysis as well as the proximal medial corner of the metaphysis (Fig. 19-20). The capsule of the glenohumeral joint correspondingly surrounds the articular surface. However, the proximal humeral physis is extracapsular and thus susceptible to injury. Indeed, most fractures of the proximal humerus involve the physis.[32,75,283] As with other growth plate injuries, proximal humeral physeal fractures typically occur through the zone of hypertrophy and provisional calcification, sparing the resting and proliferative zones. For these reasons, the typical Salter–Harris I and II injuries have tremendous remodeling potential and low risk for subsequent growth disturbance.[12,75,315]

The periosteum is thick and strong along the posteromedial aspect of the proximal humerus, but relatively weak anterolaterally, allowing for fracture fragment displacement. In cases of displaced fractures, interposed periosteum may block reduction attempts.[75,88,229]

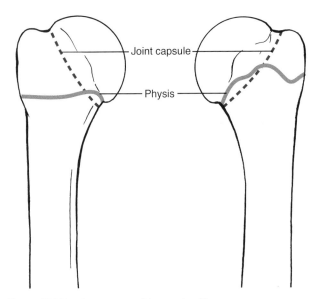

Figure 19-20. The anatomy of the proximal humerus.

A number of muscles insert on the proximal humerus, influencing fracture pattern, location, and characteristic displacement. Understanding of these dynamic influences is critical for successful fracture reduction. The subscapularis inserts anteriorly on the lesser tuberosity, whereas the supraspinatus, infraspinatus, and teres minor attach to the greater tuberosity and posterosuperior epiphysis. The deltoid tubercle lies more distally along the lateral aspect of the humeral diaphysis, and the pectoralis major and latissimus dorsi muscles insert along the anteromedial aspect of the metaphysis. In patients with physeal or metaphyseal fractures proximal to the pectoralis major insertion, the humeral head is abducted, flexed, and externally rotated by the action of the rotator cuff muscles, whereas the distal humeral diaphyseal segment is typically displaced proximally, medially, and into internal rotation. In metaphyseal fractures between the pectoralis major and deltoid insertions, the proximal fragment is adducted by the pull of the pectoralis major and the distal segment is pulled proximally and into abduction by the deltoid. For diaphyseal fractures distal to the deltoid insertion, the proximal fracture fragment is abducted by the deltoid and flexed by the pectoralis major, and the distal fragment is displaced proximally and medially by the biceps and triceps. Rarely, the subscapularis muscle may lead to displacement of an isolated fracture of the lesser tuberosity.

The vascularity of the proximal humerus arises from the axillary artery and its branches. In particular, the anterior and posterior humeral circumflex arteries supply the proximal humerus, whereas the humeral head derives most of its vascular supply from the arcuate artery, a branch of the ascending branch of the anterior humeral circumflex artery.[113,203] The posterior humeral circumflex artery supplies only a portion of the greater tuberosity and posteroinferior humeral head.[113]

Of the neurologic structures, the axillary nerve is the closest and most at risk of fractures and fracture-dislocations of the proximal humerus.[6,364] The axillary nerve arises from the posterior cord of the brachial plexus before it traverses the anterior aspect of the subscapularis muscle and passes just inferior to the glenohumeral joint. From there it passes through the quadrilateral space to innervate the deltoid and teres minor muscles and to supply sensation to the lateral aspect of the shoulder.

TREATMENT OPTIONS FOR PROXIMAL HUMERUS FRACTURES

NONOPERATIVE TREATMENT OF PROXIMAL HUMERUS FRACTURES

Indications/Contraindications

Nonoperative Treatment of Proximal Humerus Fractures: INDICATIONS AND CONTRAINDICATIONS
Indications
• Birth-related fractures
• Younger patients with stable or minimally displaced fractures
• Stress fractures
Relative Contraindications
• Open fractures
• Fractures with vascular or severe soft tissue injury
• Displaced intra-articular fractures
• Displaced tuberosity fractures
• Irreducible or unstable fractures in older adolescents with unacceptable alignment

Given their tremendous remodeling potential as well as the robust compensatory motion afforded by the shoulder joint, the vast majority of proximal humerus fractures may be treated by nonoperative means. Birth-related fractures of the proximal humerus may be successfully treated with simple pinning of the sleeve to the body or stockinette sling-and-swathe immobilization. Closed reduction is rarely needed in infants, and while ultrasonography may be used to confirm alignment, advanced imaging is almost always unnecessary. In these infants, healing is rapid and robust, typically within 2 to 3 weeks, and there is little concern for long-term aesthetic differences or functional limitations.[75,177]

Nondisplaced or minimally displaced fractures (Neer–Horwitz grades I and II) in older children and adolescents may also be treated with simple sling-and-swathe immobilization, with or without additional splinting (Fig. 19-21). As late fracture displacement is uncommon, prior reports suggest that serial radiographic evaluations are unnecessary and may impart additional cost and radiation exposure without clinical utility.[119] After confirmation of healing, patients may advance to motion and strengthening, with anticipation of excellent long-term results.[35,75] Similarly, stress fractures of the metaphysis or physis—such as seen from repetitive overuse sports activities,

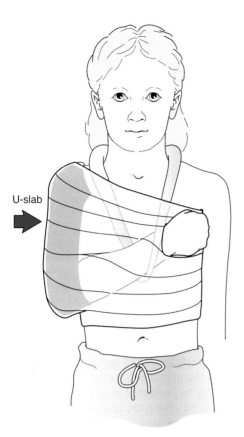

U-slab

Figure 19-21. Sling and swathe for immobilization of proximal humeral fracture. A plaster U-slab (*arrow*) may be added for additional splinting.

TABLE 19-1. Acceptable Alignment of Proximal Humerus Fractures		
Age	Angulation	Displacement
<5 years	70 degrees	100%
5–11 years	40–70 degrees	50–100%
>12 years	<40 degrees	<50%

neurologic conditions, metabolic bone disease, or local radiation therapy—may be successfully treated with rest, activity modification, and/or simple sling immobilization.[28,72,90]

With increasing age and skeletal maturity, remodeling capacity diminishes; therefore, the amount of "acceptable" deformity changes with age. Given the remodeling potential in patients less than 11 years of age, good-to-excellent results have been reported with nonoperative treatment regardless of fracture displacement.[75,208,261,340] Immobilization options include sling and swathe, Velpeau thoracobrachial bandages, hanging arm casts, and shoulder spica casts in the "saluting" and "Statue of Liberty" positions.[35,75,208]

There continues to be controversy, however, regarding what constitutes "acceptable" alignment in pediatric proximal humerus fractures, particularly in older children and adolescents. Much of the available information comes from historic retrospective case series, with little or no comparative outcome data available. Traditional recommendations have divided treatment recommendations according to patient age and fracture displacement (Table 19-1).[13,88,332] In patients less than 5 years of age, up to 70 degrees of angulation and 100% displacement is deemed acceptable. In patients between 5 and 11 years of age, 40 to 70 degrees of angulation and 50% to 100% displacement may be accepted. And in patients greater than 12 years of age with less growth and remodeling potential, less than

40 degrees and 50% translation should be accepted. Though these guidelines are generally accepted, appropriate clinical judgment weighing individual patient and provider factors should be made on a case-by-case basis.[13,75,88,208] For example, in overhead athletes requiring maximal shoulder abduction and forward flexion, less varus or apex anterior angulation may be tolerable, given concerns regarding acromial impingement and bony blocks to glenohumeral motion.

In patients older than 12 years, fracture reduction and immobilization is recommended for Neer–Horwitz grade III and IV injuries with unacceptable alignment.[13,52,75,208,261] Indeed a matched cohort analysis by Chaus et al. suggested incremental increased likelihood of suboptimal function with nonoperative management for each year over 12 years of age.[53] While a host of reduction maneuvers have been described, all adhere to the fundamental principles of reversing the deformity and counteracting the deforming forces. Most fractures may be reduced by applying longitudinal traction to the distal brachium, followed by abduction, flexion, and external rotation; this technique essentially brings the distal diaphyseal segment to the displaced humeral head. Often, initial adduction and internal rotation to relax the pectoralis major, followed by posteriorly directed pressure on the humeral diaphysis to correct the apex anterior angulation, will facilitate reduction.[173] Alternatively, reduction may be achieved by abduction, flexion to 90 degrees, and external rotation.[261] Still others advocate placing the limb in 135 degrees abduction and slight (30 degrees) flexion, followed by longitudinal traction and manual manipulation of the fracture fragments.[177] In cases of physeal fractures, gentle manipulation with the assistance of conscious sedation or general anesthesia should be considered to avoid excessively forceful manipulation and minimize the risk of iatrogenic physeal disturbance. After reduction, fracture stability needs to be assessed. Often the intact periosteum will stabilize the reduction and allow for immobilization at the patient's side. Typically, immobilization with sling and swathe or Velpeau thoracobrachial bandage is sufficient.[75]

Some fractures may not be reducible because of soft tissue interposition at the fracture site. Potential structural barriers to fracture realignment include the adjacent periosteum, glenohumeral joint capsule, and long head of biceps tendon.[13,88,173,229] In these situations, open reduction via a limited anterior deltopectoral approach may be needed to obtain appropriate reduction. Even in cases in which the bony alignment is improved to "acceptable" parameters but not anatomic, fracture healing and functional return may be expected; indeed, good functional

Figure 19-23. (*Continued*) Intraoperatively, the fracture is closed reduced with traction, abduction (**C**), and correction of the apex anterior angulation (**D**). **E:** Postoperative alignment after percutaneous pinning. **F:** Follow-up radiograph demonstrates improved alignment and bony healing. (Courtesy of Children's Orthopaedic Surgery Foundation.)

and then perform the appropriate reduction maneuver. Once the fracture is realigned, the pins may be simply advanced across the fracture site into the proximal fragment while holding the fracture reduced.

Once an adequate closed reduction has been achieved, the fracture is fixed with percutaneous smooth K-wires. Small stab incisions are made at or just proximal to the level of the deltoid tubercle, and careful blunt dissection is performed down to the lateral cortex of the humerus using a hemostat or narrow dissecting scissors. Injury to the axillary nerve may be avoided by placing the entry points for percutaneous pinning two times the height of the articular surface distal to the most proximal edge of the humerus.[308] Data from computer modeling studies of pediatric proximal humerus fractures suggest that pins entering laterally 4.4 and 8 cm distal to the superior

aspect of the humeral head at a coronal angle of 21 degrees allow for optimal pin placement.[245] More recently, Stavinoha et al. proposed the "one mountain, three valleys" concept.[346] If the height of the proximal humeral physis measured from the apex to the most lateral cortical point constitutes "one mountain" or "one valley" of distance, the axially nerve reliably ran one mountain above and three valleys below the lateral-most cortical point. Pins placed outside of this zone will safely avoid nerve injury.

After the first pin is placed, multiplanar fluoroscopic views are obtained to confirm appropriate alignment and implant placement. Following this, one or two additional pins are placed, again in a distal-lateral to proximal-medial direction. Parallel pin placement provides better biomechanics stability.[182] Care is made not to violate the subchondral surface of the humeral head and enter the glenohumeral joint. A drill hole at the entry site may make pin adjustment and placement easier and avoid inadvertent joint and/or adjacent soft tissue (brachial plexus) penetration. Once the desired alignment, depth, and stability are achieved, the pins are bent and cut either below the skin or outside the skin.[164] The limb is placed in a sling and swathe. Implants may be removed after radiographic evidence of healing is confirmed, typically 4 weeks after surgery.

Occasionally, additional fixation or assistance with closed reduction is needed. An antegrade pin entering the greater tuberosity and directed distally and medially may be considered, though is rarely necessary in pediatric patients. These pins should be placed with the limb in external rotation and directed to a point at least 2 cm inferior to the most medial aspect of the articular surface.[308] As cited earlier, if closed reduction is not successful, open reduction via a deltopectoral approach can be used, with pinning techniques performed in a similar fashion.

Intramedullary Fixation

Preoperative Planning

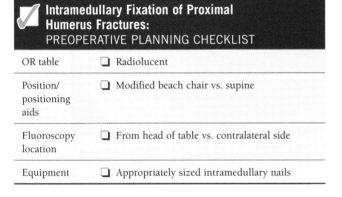

Intramedullary Fixation of Proximal Humerus Fractures: PREOPERATIVE PLANNING CHECKLIST	
OR table	❏ Radiolucent
Position/ positioning aids	❏ Modified beach chair vs. supine
Fluoroscopy location	❏ From head of table vs. contralateral side
Equipment	❏ Appropriately sized intramedullary nails

Intramedullary nailing is a common technique in the treatment of pediatric proximal humerus fractures.[39,54,55,184,286,292,323,387] Unlike adults, in whom solid reamed antegrade nails have been used, intramedullary fixation in children and adolescents typically involves retrograde passage of multiple flexible titanium elastic nails, Rush rods, or Enders nails. Adequate AP and lateral radiographs of the proximal humerus should be reviewed to assess fracture location, pattern, and displacement. Again, careful preoperative evaluation should be made to document neurovascular status, given the known risks of associate nerve injury. Appropriately sized flexible stainless steel or titanium intramedullary nails should be available. Similar to intramedullary fixation techniques of pediatric femur fractures, the selected nail diameter should be approximately 40% of the intramedullary canal dimension.

Positioning

Patient positioning should be predicated upon access to the shoulder girdle and upper limb and ease of fluoroscopic imaging. Use of the modified beach chair position will allow for easy manipulation, implant placement, and intraoperative imaging. In these cases, the fluoroscopy unit may be brought in from the head of the bed, allowing the surgeon to stand in the axilla or lateral to the affected shoulder and facilitating both AP and axillary views of the proximal humerus. Alternatively, patients may be positioned supine on a radiolucent table with a bump placed under the ipsilateral pelvis or between the scapulae. With supine positioning, the fluoroscopy unit may be brought in from the ipsilateral or contralateral side of the table.

Surgical Approach

Again, closed reduction of the proximal humerus fracture is performed using the maneuvers described above. If inadequate realignment is achieved, open reduction may be performed via a limited deltopectoral approach.

Technique

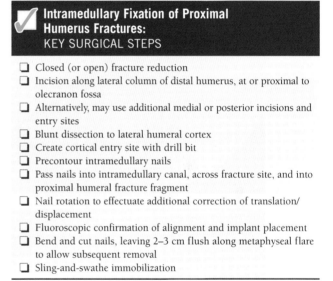

Intramedullary Fixation of Proximal Humerus Fractures: KEY SURGICAL STEPS

❏ Closed (or open) fracture reduction
❏ Incision along lateral column of distal humerus, at or proximal to olecranon fossa
❏ Alternatively, may use additional medial or posterior incisions and entry sites
❏ Blunt dissection to lateral humeral cortex
❏ Create cortical entry site with drill bit
❏ Precontour intramedullary nails
❏ Pass nails into intramedullary canal, across fracture site, and into proximal humeral fracture fragment
❏ Nail rotation to effectuate additional correction of translation/displacement
❏ Fluoroscopic confirmation of alignment and implant placement
❏ Bend and cut nails, leaving 2–3 cm flush along metaphyseal flare to allow subsequent removal
❏ Sling-and-swathe immobilization

Following fracture reduction, a longitudinal incision is made along the lateral column of the distal humerus at the level of the superior aspect of the olecranon fossa. Alternatively, medial column or posterior approaches may be used, splitting the triceps in the latter situation to gain access to the distal humerus and intramedullary canal above the olecranon fossa. Blunt dissection is performed through the subcutaneous tissues to the level of the distal humeral cortex (Fig. 19-24). Using a drill guide to protect the adjacent soft tissues, a 3.2- or 4.5-mm drill bit is used to create a cortical window in the lateral column; care is made to create this starting hole obliquely from distal-lateral to proximal-medial to facilitate subsequent nail passage. Appropriately sized intramedullary nails (typically 3–4 mm in diameter) are then prebent; if both nails are to be passed via a lateral entry point, one nail is bent in the shape of a gentle C and the other in the shape of a lazy S to of appropriate alignment and stability, the wound is closed in layers and the affected limb placed in a sling.

As noted above, avulsion fractures of the lesser tuberosity may occur in adolescents.[14] ORIF is recommended in patients with displaced injuries.[111,136,190,368] Similar patient positioning and surgical deltopectoral approach may be used. In general, the lesser tuberosity fracture fragment is easily identified, and

the attachment of the subscapularis tendon and muscle are preserved. Once fracture site on the proximal humerus is defined and debrided, bioabsorbable suture anchors may be placed in the donor site. Heavy, nonabsorbable sutures are then passed through the undersurface of the lesser tuberosity fracture fragment, exiting superficially. The fracture is then reduced, and the previously passed sutures are tied down, completing the repair.

Author's Preferred Treatment of Proximal Humerus Fractures (Algorithm 19-2)

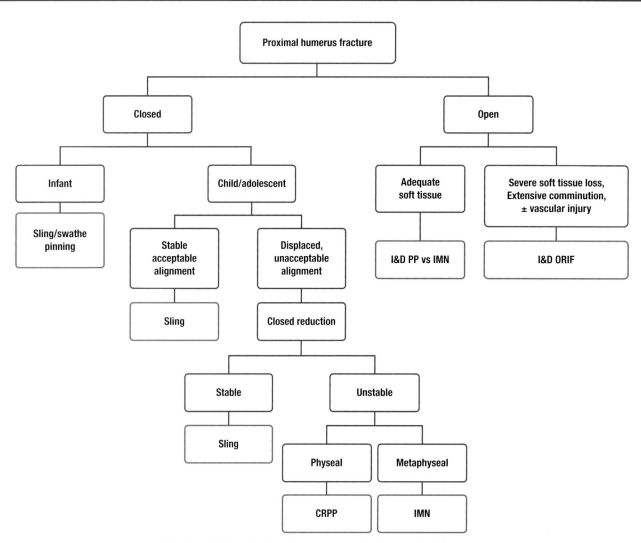

Algorithm 19-2. Author's preferred treatment for humeral shaft fracture.

Most proximal humerus fractures in children and adolescents can be successfully treated nonoperatively. In infants with birth-related fractures, immobilization with a stockinette or pinning of the sleeve to the trunk is simple and effective. Radiographic assessment of healing is performed at 4 to 6 weeks of age; immobilization is discontinued with evidence of clinical and radiographic healing.

In children and adolescents with closed proximal humerus fractures in acceptable deformity (see Table 19-1), simple sling immobilization is used. Serial radiographs are obtained to confirm adequate alignment. Bony union is typically obtained in 4 to 6 weeks, though clinically improvement and pain relief typically precedes radiographic healing. After confirmation of clinical and radiographic healing, range of motion and strengthening is advanced as tolerated.

In older children and adolescents with unacceptable radiographic alignment, initial closed reduction is performed with conscious sedation or general anesthesia. Careful radiographic evaluation of bony alignment and assessment of fracture stability is performed. Given the data suggesting that late displacement is a frequent occurrence following closed manipulation alone of severely displaced proximal humerus fractures in adolescents, a low threshold exists for fracture stabilization. For unstable injuries with deformity beyond what is anticipated to remodel with continued skeletal growth, fracture fixation is performed. Physeal fractures are treated with closed reduction and percutaneous smooth pin fixation; typically two retrograde pins will suffice. Pins may be bent and cut outside the skin, which facilitates subsequent removal and obviates the need for additional anesthesia. If pins are left outside the skin, patients are immobilized with sling and swathe or abduction pillow to prevent pin migration or pin-tract complications. In patients with metaphyseal fractures—in which there is still some metaphyseal bone on the proximal fracture fragment—intramedullary nailing is preferred (Fig. 19-25). Using the technique described above, appropriate flexible titanium intramedullary implants are prebent and inserted via a lateral entry point. Intramedullary nails are cut and left beneath the skin; attention to the trajectory and location of nail entry will allow the ends of the nails to lie flush against the metaphyseal flare of the distal humerus, avoiding unnecessary soft tissue irritation. Patients are placed in sling-and-swathe immobilization.

In cases of open fractures with adequate soft tissue coverage, open reduction and either pin or intramedullary nail fixation is performed after thorough irrigation and debridement of the open wound. In cases associated with excessive fracture comminution, vascular insufficiency, or severe soft tissue loss, internal fixation with plate-and-screw constructs is considered. Open reduction is similarly performed in closed injuries in which an acceptable reduction may not be achieved with manipulation, typically because of interposed soft tissue.[8,70,88]

Postoperative Care

Patients receiving nonoperative treatment of displaced proximal humeral fractures are followed weekly with radiographs to ensure confirm maintenance of alignment. Once there is evidence of clinical and radiographic healing, gentle shoulder pendulum and elbow range-of-motion exercises are begun. Immobilization is typically discontinued after 4 to 6 weeks. Sports participation is restricted until there is return of motion and strength, and patients/families are counseled regarding the risk of refracture.

Following surgical reduction and stabilization, sling immobilization is usually sufficient and continued until radiographic healing. With plate fixation, gentle pendulum and elbow range-of-motion exercises may be initiated once adequate comfort is achieved. In cases of intramedullary nail fixation, implants are typically removed at 6 months postoperatively.

A, B   **C**

Figure 19-25. Intramedullary fixation of a proximal humeral metaphyseal fracture. **A:** Preoperative radiograph depicting displacement and shortening. **B:** Postoperative radiographs depict bony healing. **C:** Radiograph after staged implant removal. (Courtesy of Children's Orthopaedic Surgery Foundation.)

Potential Pitfalls and Preventive Measures

Repair of Proximal Humerus Fractures:
POTENTIAL PITFALLS AND PREVENTIONS

Pitfall	Prevention
Failure to recognize fracture pattern	Appropriate orthogonal imaging
	Avoid varus and apex anterior angulation
	Individualized treatment
Difficulty with closed reduction	Understand, reverse deforming muscle actions
	Adequate analgesia/anesthesia
	Orthogonal fluoroscopic imaging
	Transition to open reduction if interposed soft tissue
Loss of alignment after reduction	Routine fracture fixation after closed reduction of severely displaced injuries in adolescents
	Preset pins into the distal fracture fragment first, then perform the reduction, then pass the pins across the fracture site with the shoulder abducted and/or externally rotated
Implant-related complications	Correct insertion of percutaneous pins
	Sling-and-swathe immobilization if percutaneous pins left out of skin

While the principles of treatment are seemingly straightforward, proximal humerus fractures present a number of challenges and potential pitfalls, particularly in the adolescent with severe displacement. First, assessment of what constitutes "acceptable deformity" can be challenging in the older pediatric patient population. Though guidelines exist on what constitutes adequate bony alignment, these recommendations are based on historical retrospective case series and expert opinion. The decision-making process is further challenged by changing patient functional demands and evolving parent/family expectations. Careful characterization of radiographic alignment in the context of patient demands is needed to ensure optimal outcomes. For example, less than 40 degrees of varus may be deemed permissible but might lead to limitations in abduction unacceptable to an overhead athlete. As in all pediatric orthopaedics, care should be individualized to account for these considerations.

Second, when indicated, closed reduction of severely displaced proximal humerus fractures is challenging. Awareness of the deforming muscular forces, adequate analgesia or anesthesia, and appropriate fluoroscopic imaging will facilitate successful closed manipulations. In cases where acceptable reduction cannot be achieved, open reduction should be pursued and any interposed periosteum or soft tissue extricated from the fracture site.

In addition, loss of reduction and further fracture displacement is common in older adolescents with severely displaced injuries. Careful assessment of fracture stability at the time of reduction and with serial radiographs is recommended. A low threshold should exist for percutaneous pin fixation or intramedullary nailing of severely displaced fractures to maintain bony alignment.

Furthermore, there are a number of potential pitfalls commonly encountered during surgical stabilization. Judicious percutaneous pin placement is imperative to avoid iatrogenic axillary nerve injury or inadvertent intra-articular penetration of the glenohumeral joint. Given the frequency with which pins cause soft tissue or infectious complications, adequate immobilization of the affected limb and timely pin removal are needed. Conversely, if intramedullary devices are used, appropriate entry point(s) and trajectory will prevent soft tissue irritation or migration of the implants.

Outcomes

Multiple published reports have suggested that surgical reduction and stabilization of displaced proximal humerus fractures is safe and effective in obtaining radiographic healing with improved bony alignment and minimal complications.[1,17,54,88,194] In patients with Neer–Horwitz grade III and IV injuries, improvement to grade I and II displacement may be expected.[88,164]

Kohler and Trillaud[194] have previously reported the clinical and radiographic outcomes of 52 patients at a mean of 5 years following proximal humerus fractures. Clinical results were "good" or "very good" in all cases, with little correlation to longer-term radiographic parameters. While the authors suggest that surgical intervention offers no advantages over nonoperative treatment, it should be noted that all surgical patients in their series underwent formal ORIF, with fixation including staples, pins, screws, and plate-and-screw constructs.

Beringer et al.[17] similarly advocated a nonoperative approach in their report of 48 patients with displaced proximal humerus fractures. All patients with longer-term follow-up reported no activity restrictions or limitations, and functional results did not correlate with radiographic findings. As three of the nine patients treated surgically had complications, the authors recommended nonsurgical treatment in the majority of cases.

Dobbs et al.[88] published their series of 29 patients treated for Neer–Horwitz grade III and IV fractures, of which 25 were treated with closed versus open reduction and pin or screw fixation. Most patients were greater than 15 years of age. Postoperatively, all patients improved to a grade I or II deformity, and there were no surgical complications. At a mean follow-up of 4 years, normal or near-normal motion and strength was seen in all patients. These findings support the efficacy and safety of surgical intervention for severely displaced injuries in older patients.

Chee et al.[54] presented their series of 14 patients, mean age 13 years, treated with single intramedullary flexible nail fixation for displaced proximal humerus fractures. All patients had full range of shoulder motion at final follow-up, supporting the author's assertion that intramedullary fixation is effective in select patients.

Kraus et al. reported on 40 adolescents treated with either percutaneous pinning or intramedullary fixation. At mean 5.8 years, functional outcomes as measured by DASH and Constant–Murley scores were excellent and radiographic alignment markedly improved.[198]

More recently, Lahdeoja et al. published longer-term outcomes of 209 adolescent patients treated for proximal humeral fractures. At mean 13-year follow-up, DASH and Simple Shoulder

Test (SST) scores for surgical patients did not differ from nonoperatively treated patients or population norms.[202] Similarly, Liebs et al. reported excellent longer-term function as assessed by the PedsQL and QuickDASH instruments in 190 children treated nonoperatively or with intramedullary flexible nails.[219]

MANAGEMENT OF EXPECTED ADVERSE OUTCOMES AND UNEXPECTED COMPLICATIONS RELATED TO PROXIMAL HUMERUS FRACTURES

Proximal Humerus Fractures:
COMMON ADVERSE OUTCOMES AND COMPLICATIONS

- Neurovascular injury
- Malunion/humerus varus
- Upper limb-length discrepancy
- Osteonecrosis
- Hypertrophic scar formation

While uncommon, complications of proximal humerus fractures may have considerable effect on shoulder girdle and upper limb function. Neurologic injury of the brachial plexus or peripheral nerves may be seen, particularly in severely displaced valgus injuries and the rare fracture-dislocation.[6,89,165,364,369] Most nerve palsies are diagnosed at the time of injury and represent neurapraxic injuries rather than true nerve transections. In general, these neurologic deficits will resolve spontaneously over 6 to 12 months but may be associated with neurogenic pain in the affected limb during recovery.[165] In patients with persistent nerve deficits without clinical signs of spontaneous recovery in the expected period of time, electrodiagnostic studies (electromyography and nerve conduction velocities) may be considered to characterize the location and severity of neurologic deficit. In rare situations, exploration with neurolysis, nerve repair, nerve grafting, or nerve transfers (i.e., radial motor branch of long head of triceps to axillary motor) may be necessary.[6,62] In chronic or late-presenting situations, salvage procedures such as tendon transfers or proximal humeral osteotomies may be considered to improve shoulder and upper limb function.[67,149,189,284]

Vascular insufficiency is a rare but potentially devastating complication of proximal humerus fractures. Treatment is predicated on prompt reduction, fracture stabilization, and reassessment of vascularity. In cases of persistent distal ischemia, appropriate exploration and vascular repair or reconstruction is needed.[165]

Humerus varus is another potential complication of proximal humerus fractures in children and adolescents. Humerus varus is characterized by a humeral neck-shaft angle of less than 140 degrees, a greater tuberosity cephalad to the superior aspect of the humeral head, and a reduced distance between the articular surface of the humeral head and the lateral cortex of the humerus.[193] The resultant varus angulation and prominent greater tuberosity leads to limitations in shoulder forward flexion and lateral abduction. Potential etiologies include varus malunion as well as partial physeal arrest following proximal humeral

physeal fracture. In cases of functionally limiting humerus varus, corrective osteotomy to restore more anatomic proximal humeral morphology may be performed (Fig. 19-26).[95,117,362]

Upper limb-length discrepancy may similarly be seen as a late sequela of physeal fractures.[12,75] Though more commonly reported in patients following operative reduction, physeal disturbance is likely due to the trauma associated with the initial injury rather than surgical intervention. Furthermore, prior reports have suggested that limb-length discrepancy is not correlated with the quality of initial fracture reduction.[12,261] Limb-length inequality has similarly been reported in patients with pathologic fractures of the proximal humerus through unicameral bone cysts.[148,256] In patients with functional limitations or predicted upper limb-length discrepancies of greater than 6 cm at skeletal maturity, limb-lengthening procedures may be considered.[153,212,282]

Osteonecrosis of the humeral head is much less common in children than adults.[238] In setting of confirmed osteonecrosis, revascularization and humeral head remodeling may be seen in skeletally immature patients, leading to satisfactory clinical outcomes.[378]

Finally, hypertrophic scar formation is commonly seen after surgical treatment of proximal humerus fractures, particularly following open reduction via a deltopectoral approach. Prior investigation has suggested this aesthetic difference may be psychologically troubling to adolescent patients.[116] For this reason, alternative, more aesthetic incisions in the axilla have been proposed.[126] Patients and families should be counseled about the possibility of hypertrophic scar formation from deltopectoral incisions or percutaneous pin sites prior to surgical intervention.

SUMMARY, CONTROVERSIES, AND FUTURE DIRECTIONS RELATED TO PROXIMAL HUMERUS FRACTURES

In summary, the majority of proximal humeral fractures may be effectively treated nonoperatively. In older adolescent patients with greater angulation and displacement, reduction and surgical stabilization is safe and effective in restoring radiographic alignment and shoulder motion. Future prospective, comparative investigation is needed to determine the criteria for reduction and fixation in older children and adolescents and characterize the patient-derived functional outcomes of these injuries in the long term.

Humerus Shaft Fractures

INTRODUCTION TO HUMERUS SHAFT FRACTURES

The humeral diaphysis is the location of 20% or less of all pediatric humerus fractures and 5% or less of all childhood skeletal injuries.[56,304] The incidence is estimated to be between 12 and 30 per 100,000 per year, and more recent

Figure 19-26. A: AP radiograph of a minimally displaced right proximal humeral physeal fracture in a 14-year-old male. **B:** Follow-up radiographs depicting humerus varus, characterized by a decreased neck-shaft angle and high-riding greater tuberosity resulting in limited shoulder abduction and bony impingement. **C:** Intraoperative image during corrective osteotomy, depicting percutaneous pin placement. **D:** Converging osteotomies (*arrows*) are made to create a lateral closing wedge osteotomy. **E:** Osteotomy fixed using percutaneous pins and a tension-band fixation construction. **F:** Follow-up radiographs demonstrating bony healing and restoration of more normal proximal humeral alignment. (Courtesy of Children's Orthopaedic Surgery Foundation.)

epidemiologic information from the United States suggests that this incidence has remained relatively constant despite population changes.[188,205] There is a bimodal distribution of ages of children who sustain humeral diaphyseal fractures, with the greatest frequency seen in infants and adolescents.[13]

ASSESSMENT OF HUMERUS SHAFT FRACTURES

MECHANISMS OF INJURY FOR HUMERUS SHAFT FRACTURES

Humeral shaft fractures may be due to a variety of injury mechanisms, each with its own set of clinical considerations.

Birth-related trauma is a frequent cause of humeral diaphyseal injury, with a reported incidence between 0.035% and 0.34%.[38,233] Macrosomia, breech presentation, and/or difficult delivery are thought to be potential risk factors. The humerus is at particular risk in situations where the upper limb is abducted above the newborn's head and must be delivered inferiorly after version and extraction.[233] Similarly, humerus fractures may occur in cases of shoulder dystocia with rotational maneuvers or posterior arm delivery.[216] Cesarean section delivery is not necessarily protective, and any forceful extraction may impart enough energy to cause a humerus fracture.[18,42,297]

Nonaccidental trauma may also manifest as humerus fracture in a child. Indeed, 12% of all fractures and up to 60% of new fractures stemming from nonaccidental trauma affect the humerus.[227,332]

While child abuse must be considered within the differential diagnosis of humeral diaphyseal fractures—particularly in children less than 3 years of age—only a minority of humeral shaft injuries in children are due to nonaccidental trauma.[332]

The most common mechanism of injury is direct or indirect force imparted upon the upper limb in the older child or adolescent. Direct blows to the brachium, falls onto an outstretched upper limb, motor vehicle collisions, and sports-related trauma may all result in diaphyseal fractures. Indeed, humeral shaft fractures have even been noted from throwing and other overuse activities, because of the rotational forces imparted upon the humerus during the throwing motion.[4,112,145,222,270]

INJURIES ASSOCIATED WITH HUMERUS SHAFT FRACTURES

Radial nerve palsies are commonly associated with humeral diaphyseal fractures and raise a number of treatment considerations and controversies.[13,74,93,142,231,234,303] Because of the anatomic proximity of the radial nerve to the mid- and distal humerus, the nerve may be contused, stretched, kinked, entrapped, or rarely transected with the initial injury and/or fracture displacement.[365] Furthermore, a delayed palsy may occur due to compression secondary to scar tissue, fracture callus, and even bone formation. It has been estimated that up to 20% of adult and 5% of pediatric humeral diaphyseal fractures will have associated radial nerve palsies.[24,231]

Clinically, radial nerve palsies may be categorized by the time of presentation. Primary radial nerve palsies occur at the time of injury and are clinically apparent at first evaluation. Secondary radial nerve palsies refer to deficits presumably sustained at the time of fracture reduction or manipulation, in patients in whom radial nerve function was initially intact.

Most published information suggests that the potential for spontaneous nerve recovery is high, with 78% to 100% of patients regaining radial nerve function with observation alone.[24,26,27,31,86,93,118,223,316] Indeed, in cases in which the primary radial nerve palsies were treated with immediate or early exploration, the vast majority of the time the nerve is found to be intact, though contused or tented over the displaced fracture fragments (Fig. 19-27).[123,231,330] In children, it has been hypothesized that the thicker periosteum may confer a protective effect on the radial nerve, reducing the risk of traumatic laceration or incarceration within the fracture site.

Radial nerve exploration should be performed in instances of open humeral diaphyseal fractures in which surgical debridement and stabilization is to be performed. If a true radial nerve laceration is encountered, options include tagging the nerve ends for subsequent identification and repair versus immediate primary neurorrhaphy.[105,350,357] Given the distance to reinnervation from a high radial nerve palsy, earlier repair when there are healthy appearing, noncontaminated nerve endings allows for the best anatomic and functional potential.[20]

In cases of primary radial nerve palsy, recommendations have been made for observation and exploration at 8 weeks to 6 months if there is failure of adequate recovery.[74,86,152] While these time-based guidelines are helpful, each patient must be considered individually, adhering to fundamental principles.[22] In general, if there is failure of adequate recovery after the anticipated time—based on the distance from the injury to distal points of reinnervation—surgical exploration should be considered. Physiologic studies have determined that following Wallerian degeneration, nerve growth will occur at a rate of an average of 1 mm per day.[350] For high radial nerve palsies, spontaneous resolution should entail an advancing Tinel sign, with sequential return of radial wrist extensors, central wrist extensors, digital extensors, and thumb extensors. In cases of late exploration where radial nerve lacerations are encountered, sural nerve grafting may be performed, with anticipation of functional return.[20,103,269,366]

There continues to be controversy regarding the optimal management of secondary radial nerve palsy. If nerve function is lost after fracture manipulation, observation alone is still supported by published data suggesting that spontaneous recovery will occur in the majority of patients.[24,27,86,201] Others advocate early exploration because of liability concerns and late extraction from fracture callus is much more difficult than early decompression. If radial nerve function is lost during the later period of fracture healing, careful consideration should be made regarding whether the nerve is entrapped within scar tissue, fracture callus, or bone.[91,390] Radiographs may depict an oval lucency corresponding to the bony foramen through which the nerve is running, the so-called Matev sign.[162,370] In these situations, surgical exploration and decompression should be performed.

SIGNS AND SYMPTOMS OF HUMERUS SHAFT FRACTURES

Clinical signs and symptoms will vary considerably depending upon the patient age and mechanism of injury.

In infants in whom a birth-related humerus fracture is suspected, a careful pre- and perinatal history should be obtained, specifically evaluating for macrosomia, prolonged or difficult labor and delivery, and history of shoulder dystocia. Additional historical information—such as whether the newborn will nurse from each breast—may guide the care provider to the correct diagnosis. Clinically, these infants will exhibit pseudoparalysis of the affected limb, holding or splinting the arm against the side. As distal neurologic function is intact, the infant will spontaneously grasp and move the digits and wrist. There will be reproducible tenderness, motion, and crepitus at the fracture site, though often little swelling or ecchymosis.

In older children who sustain traumatic or sports-related fractures, a careful history will provide insight into the mechanism of injury and any associated trauma. Details regarding the position of the upper limb, direction of forces imparted, and energy of injury will aid in clinical diagnosis. Patients will typically present with pain, swelling, ecchymosis, and guarding of the affected limb, with or without obvious deformity. The arm is typically held tightly against the body as the patient guards and protects the injured limb. Physical examination should include careful inspection of the overlying skin to assess for open wounds, ecchymosis, and skin tenting or dimpling. A thorough neurovascular examination is critical, particularly to assess potential injury of the radial nerve.[26,27,265,269]

Figure 19-27. A: AP radiograph of a 15-year-old female with an open humeral diaphyseal fracture and radial nerve palsy. **B:** Intraoperative radiograph depicting exposure via a lateral approach. The kinked and contused radial nerve (*long arrow*) displaced by the proximal fracture fragment (*short arrow*). **C:** After irrigation, debridement, and plate fixation of the fracture, the nerve can be seen decompressed overlying the implant. **D:** Postoperative radiograph depicting bony healing and implant placement. (Courtesy of Children's Orthopaedic Surgery Foundation.)

IMAGING AND OTHER DIAGNOSTIC STUDIES FOR HUMERUS SHAFT FRACTURES

Plain radiographs of the humerus will confirm the diagnosis and should be performed in all cases of suspected humeral diaphyseal fractures (Figs. 19-28 and 19-29). Orthogonal views should be obtained, as nondisplaced or incomplete greenstick fractures may occur in children. Appropriate lateral radiographs will demonstrate overlap or superimposition of the posterior supracondylar ridges of the medial and lateral epicondyles.[123]

In addition to confirming the diagnosis and characterizing its anatomic location and pattern, radiographs should be inspected

Figure 19-28. A, B: Radiographs depicting a humeral diaphyseal fracture in a 4-day-old infant with displacement and angulation. **C, D:** By 3 months of age, there is excellent bony healing and early remodeling. (Courtesy of Children's Orthopaedic Surgery Foundation.)

for associated lesions to evaluate for possible pathologic fractures.[273,347,356] The humerus is a common site for both benign and malignant lesions in skeletally immature patients, and care should be taken to identify an associated condition.

"Floating elbow" injuries may occur, particularly in the setting of higher-energy mechanisms.[345] In patients with ipsilateral wrist or forearm pain or swelling, radiographic evaluation of the elbow and forearm will allow for diagnosis of these associated injuries.

Finally, in cases of suspected nonaccidental trauma, a skeletal survey and bone scan may be performed to evaluate for the presence of other fractures at various stages of healing.

CLASSIFICATION OF HUMERUS SHAFT FRACTURES

Classification of humeral diaphyseal fractures remains largely descriptive. Anatomic location, fracture pattern, direction of displacement and/or angulation, and the presence of associated soft

tissue or ipsilateral skeletal injuries are used. While a classification system has been proposed by the Association for Study of Internal Fixation for humeral shaft fractures in adults, this has not been universally applied to the pediatric patient population, and questions persist over its interobserver reliability and clinical utility.[178,258]

PATHOANATOMY AND APPLIED ANATOMY RELATING TO HUMERUS SHAFT FRACTURES

While the humerus is a long, tubular bone, a number of anatomic features are worthy of note. First, the middiaphyseal region is triangular in cross-section and narrower than the adjacent proximal and distal metaphyseal regions. In children, the humerus is enveloped in thick periosteum and has a rich vascular supply; the primary nutrient artery enters at the

Figure 19-29. A: AP radiograph of a minimally displaced humeral diaphyseal fracture in a 13-year-old male. **B:** Radiograph in fracture brace, demonstrating maintenance of alignment. (Courtesy of Children's Orthopaedic Surgery Foundation.)

middiaphyseal level, though abundant accessory vessels supply the humeral shaft anteriorly and posteriorly.[44,123]

The deltoid tuberosity serves as the insertion of the deltoid and is located in the middiaphysis. The latissimus dorsi and teres major insert on the proximal aspect of the humerus, just medial to the bicipital groove. Conversely, the pectoralis major inserts along the anterior humerus lateral and distal to the bicipital groove. The coracobrachialis arises from the coracoid process and inserts along the middle third–distal third junction antero-medially. Distal and posterior to the deltoid tuberosity lies the so-called spiral groove, adjacent to which runs the radial nerve and from which the most proximal fibers of the brachialis originate. Similar to fractures of the proximal humerus, awareness of these muscle and soft tissue relationships helps explain typical fracture displacement patterns and guide reduction maneuvers.

The anatomic path of the radial nerve deserves special attention, given the frequency with which the nerve is injured with humeral diaphyseal fractures. While much of the published literature is derived from cadaveric data in adults, a few principles may be applied to the pediatric population. First, as the radial nerve arises from the posterior cord of the brachial plexus, it passes through the triangular interval, bounded by the teres major superiorly and the lateral and long heads of the triceps medially and laterally. The radial nerve is typically accompanied by the profunda brachii artery as it passes through the upper arm. The nerve travels along the spiral groove, but is typically not in direct contact with the posterior humeral cortex; instead, it is separated from the bone by muscular fibers.[43] In general, the radial nerve is located directly posterior to the humeral diaphysis at the level of the deltoid tuberosity, a useful anatomic relationship in cases of surgical fracture treatment.

The radial nerve continues distally and laterally, where it pierces the lateral intermuscular septum to enter the anterior compartment. Distally at the elbow, it may be found reliably in the brachialis–brachioradialis intermuscular interval.

The ulnar nerve runs in the medial aspect of the posterior compartment and does not give off any motor branches above the elbow. The median nerve travels just medial to the brachial artery in the distal half of the brachium.

TREATMENT OPTIONS FOR HUMERUS SHAFT FRACTURES

NONOPERATIVE TREATMENT OF HUMERUS SHAFT FRACTURES

Indications/Contraindications

Nonoperative Treatment of Humerus Shaft Fractures: INDICATIONS AND CONTRAINDICATIONS
Indications
• Birth-related fractures • Diaphyseal fractures with acceptable alignment • Stress fractures • Benign pathologic fractures
Relative Contraindications
• Open fractures • Associated vascular injury • Diaphyseal fractures with unacceptable alignment

Most humeral diaphyseal fractures in children are amenable to nonoperative care.[40,83] As the upper limb is not weight bearing, anatomic alignment of the humerus is not necessary for functional restoration. Furthermore, shoulder motion, elbow flexion-extension, and forearm rotation may effectively compensate for mild-to-moderate humeral deformity. Finally, there is considerable remodeling potential for humeral deformity in skeletally immature patients; indeed, even up to 30 degrees may remodel in the adolescent population.[74] For these reasons, up to 20 to 30 degrees of varus, 20 degrees of apex anterior angulation, 15 degrees of internal rotation, and bayonet apposition with 1 to 2 cm of shortening are deemed acceptable.[74,294] As with all guidelines, these parameters for "acceptable deformity" must be taken into their historical context, and individualized decisions should be made regarding the function demands and treatment goals of each patient. While limited information is available, recent comparisons of nonoperative and surgical treatment suggest that functional outcomes and return to activities are similar, though surgical stabilization may allow for less duration of immobilization.[40,41]

Birth-related fractures of the humeral diaphysis heal robustly and demonstrate profound remodeling potential. Indeed, 50% or greater remodeling may be seen within 1 to 2 years.[19] For this reason, simple immobilization to maximize comfort is sufficient, and no effort to achieve or maintain anatomic alignment is necessary.[150,163,333] A host of different treatment options have been proposed—ranging from sling and swathe, splinting, casting, traction, or simply pinning the sleeve of the affected arm to the body.[150,163,333] Concerns regarding immobilization and bony healing in excessive internal rotation may be addressed by immobilization of the upper extremity with elbow extension. This is particularly relevant in patients with concomitant brachial plexus birth palsies, in whom internal rotation contractures and external rotation weakness of the shoulder are common.[131,197,379]

Stress fractures of the humerus do occur and almost universally heal with appropriate rest, time, and activity modification.[4,112,222] Failure to allow for symptom-free healing may result in fracture completion and displacement.[4]

Sling-and-Swath Immobilization

Sling-and-swath immobilization is simple, safe, and effective for incomplete and minimally displaced fractures.[294] It may also be used for displaced fractures, though does not control apex anterior or varus angulation well, particularly in active and/or obese patients.[294,342] While the weight of the upper limb may be well supported, some patients find sling-and-swathe immobilization uncomfortable because of persistent motion at the fracture site.

Coaptation Splinting

Coaptation splinting (also referred to as U-plaster or sugar-tong splinting) has also been advocated in the treatment of humeral diaphyseal fractures.[393] The application of a coaptation splint is straightforward and is similar to that of sugar-tong splinting of the forearm (Fig. 19-30). A plaster splint, corresponding to the width of the brachium, is applied in a well-padded fashion from the

acromion superolaterally, around the olecranon distally, and back up to the level of the axilla medially. The splint may be gently molded to the upper arm and secured in place with an elastic bandage or wrap. Efforts should be made to advance the superolateral extension of the splint to the level of the neck, in efforts to prevent distal migration with gravity.[329] Others have recommended application of benzoin to the skin prior to splint placement and the use of a collar and cuff to prevent slippage.[150] Coaptation splinting has proven effective in children and is particularly useful in the acute setting as the plaster slab may be molded comfortably to the swollen limb.[74] However, as the initial swelling subsides, refitting or transitioning to other methods of immobilization may be needed. Furthermore, coaptation splinting is not as effective as other forms of immobilization at effectuating or maintaining reduction in cases of severe initial displacement.[150]

Traction

Both overhead and side-arm traction have been described for the treatment of humeral diaphyseal fractures.[150] Skin traction may be applied to the elbow, forearm, or hand. Alternatively, skeletal traction via an olecranon wingnut or transolecranon traction pin may be used.[7,16] Excessive or prolonged traction includes nonunion and elbow dislocation.[146] At present, because of patient and family demands, economic pressures, and wealth of alternative treatment options, the use of traction remains primarily of historic importance and is rarely used.

Hanging Casting

Hanging arm casts use both immobilization and gravity to impart stability and longitudinal traction to humerus fractures.[35] Long above-elbow casts are applied to the affected limb and supported by a sling or collar and cuff. Adjustments in sling/cuff placement may allow for correction of coronal and sagittal plane deformity, though rotational alignment is poorly controlled. While reported results demonstrate efficacy with this technique, compliance may be limited due to pain and difficulty maintaining an upright position, particularly in very young patients.[348] Furthermore, concerns regarding shoulder and elbow stiffness and internal rotation contractures persist.[61,298]

Functional Bracing

First described by Sarmiento et al.[319] in 1977, functional bracing of humeral diaphyseal fractures has been increasingly used in both children and adults.[50,130,331,374,378] In general, these functional braces confer a number of advantages over other nonoperative treatment options. In addition to providing external support via their clamshell design, when properly applied, functional braces may effectuate and maintain fracture reduction due to the hydraulic effect on the surrounding soft tissues (see Fig. 19-29). Furthermore, functional braces allow for elbow motion, minimizing the risk of late elbow contractures. While limited comparative information is available, there is data to suggest that functional bracing is superior to coaptation splinting and equally effective as locked intramedullary nailing in appropriately selected patients.[331,375]

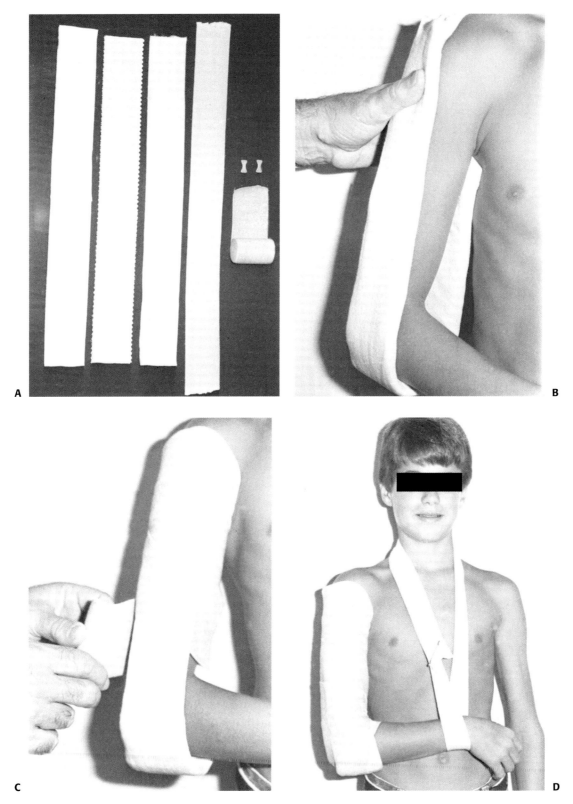

Figure 19-30. Coaptation splints with collar and cuff. **A:** The material used for a sugar-tong arm splint is two pieces of cast padding rolled out to the length of the plaster-of-Paris splint and applied to each side of the splint after it is wet. The splint is then brought into the tubular stockinette of the same width but 4 inches longer than the splint. **B:** The plaster splint is applied to the arm from the axilla up to the tip of the acromion. **C:** As the plaster is setting, the splint is molded to the arm. An elastic bandage holds the splint in place. **D:** Stockinette is applied and attached to the wrist to form a collar-and-cuff sling.

Prefabricated or custom-fit functional braces are used early in the course of treatment. Many patients will not tolerate functional bracing immediately and are temporarily supported in a sling and swathe or coaptation splint until the initial swelling subsides. Serial clinical visits and radiographic assessment are needed to ensure adequate brace fit and maintenance of radiographic alignment. Functional braces may even be used for comminuted extra-articular fractures of the distal third of the humerus, though occasionally brace extensions may need to assist in coronal plane control.[176,318] By design, functional braces for humerus fractures are not as effective in controlling apex anterior angulation, nor are they meant to support weight bearing of the affected upper limb.

OPERATIVE TREATMENT OF HUMERUS SHAFT FRACTURES

Indications/Contraindications

In general, indications for surgical treatment of humeral diaphyseal fractures include open fractures, fractures with vascular injury, floating elbow injuries (Fig. 19-31), and failure to achieve adequate alignment with nonoperative means. In addition, multitrauma and secondary radial nerve palsies (i.e., those occurring after closed fracture manipulation in patients in whom radial nerve function was initially intact) are deemed by many as relative indications for surgical exploration and fracture fixation. A host of options exist for surgical fracture

Figure 19-31. Floating elbow injury. **A:** AP radiograph depicting an open humeral diaphyseal fracture in a 10-year-old female. **B:** An ipsilateral radius fracture is also seen, consistent with a floating elbow injury. **C:** Postoperative radiograph after open irrigation and plate fixation of the humeral fracture. The radius fracture was also stabilized with internal fixation. (Courtesy of Children's Orthopaedic Surgery Foundation.)

fixation, including ORIF using plate-and-screw constructs, intramedullary nailing, and external fixation.[84,129,143,274]

Open Reduction and Internal Fixation

Preoperative Planning

☑ **ORIF of Humerus Shaft Fractures:** PREOPERATIVE PLANNING CHECKLIST	
OR table	❑ Radiolucent table or regular table with radiolucent hand table extension
Position/ positioning aids	❑ Supine
Fluoroscopy location	❑ From head of table as needed
Equipment	❑ 4.5 mm, 3.5 mm, or semitubular plates and screws
Tourniquet	❑ Sterile if needed

Preoperative planning for open reduction and plate-and-screw fixation includes appropriate AP and lateral radiographs of the humerus to assess fracture location, pattern, and displacement. The appropriate-sized implants should be determined in advance. While broad 4.5-mm dynamic compression plates are commonly used in adults, smaller 3.5-mm or semitubular plates are often used and sufficient for fixation of humeral diaphyseal fractures in children and adolescents, given the smaller size of the bone.[71,144,178,309] Furthermore, careful preoperative evaluation should be made to document neurovascular status, given the known risks of traumatic and iatrogenic radial nerve palsy associated with humeral diaphyseal fractures.

Positioning

Patient positioning is dependent in part on the planned surgical approach. In most instances, supine positioning is sufficient. In older children and adolescents, the affected limb may be placed on a radiolucent hand table to provide adequate access to both the surgeon and fluoroscopy unit. In the very young child, the patient and injured extremity may be positioned on a radiolucent fracture table. Even in cases in which a posterior surgical approach is to be used, supine positioning may be used with the limb adducted across the body. The fluoroscopy unit may be best positioned coming in from the head of the patient, allowing the surgeon to sit in the axilla and access the limb at all times.

Surgical Approach

A variety of different surgical approaches can be used. For distal humeral fractures, a posterior, triceps-splitting approach may be used.[151,259,384,394] Prone or lateral decubitus positioning may be helpful for this approach. After a posterior midline incision is made, dissection is performed down to the level of the triceps fascia, through the deep fascia. Skin flaps are elevated, exposing the triceps. The triceps tendon is split longitudinally in the midline, and this may be extended proximally in the interval between the long and lateral heads of the triceps. The deeper, medial head of the triceps may then be split and careful subperiosteal elevation is performed, exposing the humeral cortex. This approach is not extensile, and more proximal exposure is limited by the course of the radial nerve.

A traditional anterolateral approach is familiar to most surgeons and provides more extensile exposure.[15,151] In the supine position, a proximal deltopectoral incision is extended distally along the lateral aspect of the biceps. Proximally, the deltopectoral intermuscular interval is developed, retracting the cephalic vein laterally. More distally, the brachialis–brachioradialis interval is developed. Proximally, subperiosteal elevation will allow bony exposure. Distally, the brachialis muscle may be split longitudinally in the distal humeral shaft region, taking advantage of its dual innervation. The brachial artery and median and ulnar nerves are protected within the medial soft tissues. This exposure will not allow visualization or access to the radial nerve, which must be protected from overzealous retractor placement or drill/screw insertion posterior to the humerus.[388]

Alternatively, an extensile lateral or posterolateral approach will provide access to most of the humeral diaphysis as well as the radial nerve.[43,114,254] In the supine position, a lateral or posterolateral incision is created centered on the fracture site. Dissection is performed down to the level of the deep fascia and subcutaneous flaps elevated. The triceps fascia is incised just posterior to the lateral intermuscular septum, entering the posterior compartment of the brachium. The lateral head of the triceps is then elevated off the lateral intermuscular septum from distal to proximal. The radial nerve may then be identified, often surrounded by perineural fat, as it passes from the posterior to anterior compartments. Often the posterior antebrachial cutaneous nerve may be identified as it travels from proximal-posterior to distal-anterior more superficially; following this nerve proximally will allow for easy identification of the radial nerve proper. Other anatomic landmarks, including the apex of the triceps aponeurosis, have been used for radial nerve identification.[5] After the radial nerve is circumferentially dissected free, it may be isolated with a vessel loop and carefully retracted. Subperiosteal dissection will then allow for exposure of the humeral diaphysis.

Technique

☑ **ORIF of Humerus Shaft Fractures:** KEY SURGICAL STEPS
❑ Expose humeral diaphysis
❑ Identify and retract radial nerve, when applicable
❑ Anatomic reduction of humeral fracture
❑ Apply lateral plate, with care to protect the radial nerve
❑ Six cortices of fixation above and below the fracture site
❑ Layered wound closure
❑ Splint or cast immobilization

After the diaphysis is exposed and radial nerve identified and retracted, the fracture site is identified. Fracture hematoma is evacuated and the cortical fracture edges defined. Reduction may be performed under direct visualization, with interdigitation of the fracture edges restoring longitudinal alignment and proper rotation. The fracture is then fixed using appropriately sized plates for age and size of patient (3.5-mm compression plates, single or double-stacked semitubular plates), ideally obtaining six cortices of fixation above and below the fracture site using 3.5-mm cortical screws. Intraoperative fluoroscopy may be used to confirm anatomic reduction and appropriate implant placement. If the fracture site occurs adjacent to the radial nerve, care must be made to slide the plate beneath the nerve and avoid iatrogenic injury or kinking.

Intramedullary Fixation

Preoperative Planning

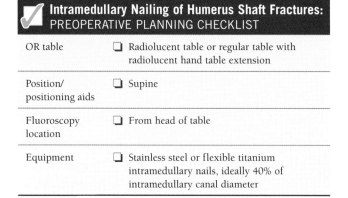

☑ **Intramedullary Nailing of Humerus Shaft Fractures:** PREOPERATIVE PLANNING CHECKLIST	
OR table	❏ Radiolucent table or regular table with radiolucent hand table extension
Position/ positioning aids	❏ Supine
Fluoroscopy location	❏ From head of table
Equipment	❏ Stainless steel or flexible titanium intramedullary nails, ideally 40% of intramedullary canal diameter

Preoperative planning for intramedullary nailing includes appropriate AP and lateral radiographs of the humerus to assess fracture location, pattern, and displacement. Again, careful preoperative evaluation should be made to document neurovascular status, given the known risks of traumatic and iatrogenic radial nerve palsy associated with humeral diaphyseal fractures. (In cases of radial nerve palsy, consideration should be given for formal open reduction and plate fixation, given the ability to simultaneously explore and decompress the radial nerve.) Appropriately sized flexible stainless steel or titanium intramedullary nails should be available. Similar to intramedullary fixation techniques of pediatric femur fractures, the selected nail diameter should be approximately 40% of the intramedullary canal dimension.

Positioning

In most cases, supine positioning is sufficient. In older children and adolescents, the affected limb may be placed on a radiolucent hand table to provide adequate access to both the surgeon and fluoroscopy unit. In the very young child, the patient and injured extremity may be supported by a radiolucent fracture table. The fluoroscopy unit may be best positioned coming in from the head of the patient, allowing the surgeon to sit in the axilla and access the limb at all times.

Surgical Approach

A theoretical advantage of intramedullary nailing of humeral diaphyseal fractures is the ability to achieve stable realignment via closed or indirect fracture reduction and minimally invasive

Figure 19-32. The Hackethal technique involves multiple smooth pins placed up the humeral shaft through a cortical window just above the olecranon fossa. The pins are placed until the canal is filled.

implant placement. Reduction and stabilization may be achieved efficiently, without need for extensive surgical dissection.[64,82,133] A host of surgical approaches may be used. Intramedullary implants (Enders nails, Rush rods, flexible titanium nails) may be inserted via a posterior approach. Through a small posterior incision and triceps-splitting approach to the posterior humeral cortex just proximal to the olecranon fossa, an oval corticotomy may be made, large enough to accommodate passage of two nails. Nails may then be inserted retrograde through this combined entry point. While two nails may be sufficient, some have advocated the Hackethal or "bouquet" technique, in which the canal is progressively filled with multiple pins to confer additional rigidity (Fig. 19-32).[124] This may be particularly useful in cases of segmental, comminuted, or pathologic fractures.

Alternatively, intramedullary nails may be placed via the lateral and/or medial columns of the distal humerus.[220,247] Small incisions may be made overlying the distal lateral and/or medial columns, at or above the level of olecranon fossa. Oval corticotomies are created at the site of nail entry to facilitate implant passage. Others have proposed insertion through the lateral and medial epicondyles via small drill holes. Care is made to retract and protect the posteromedial soft tissues—including the ulnar nerve—if a medial entry point is chosen. Nails may then be passed into the intramedullary canal and in a retrograde fashion to the fracture site.

Once fracture reduction is achieved, intramedullary nails may be atraumatically passed into the canal of the proximal fragment. Fluoroscopic guidance is helpful, and efforts should be made to avoid repeated false passage of the nails into the adjacent soft tissues. In general, two nails are sufficient, provided they are of appropriate diameter and symmetrically contoured to allow for appropriate angular correction and rotational control.[209,210,247]

While the experience in adults is well documented, at present there are limited indications for solid reamed intramedullary nailing of humeral diaphyseal fractures in skeletally immature patients. This is in part because of the risks of physeal disturbance, shoulder impingement, and the relative narrow dimensions of the intramedullary canal in younger patients.[68,132,168,239,296,303]

Technique

> **✓ Intramedullary Nailing of Humerus Shaft Fractures:**
> **KEY SURGICAL STEPS**
>
> ❑ Measure anticipated diameter and length of intramedullary nails
> ❑ Precontour intramedullary nails
> ❑ Create entry sites along lateral (and medial) column(s) of distal humerus
> ❑ Create cortical entry points for subsequent nail passage
> ❑ Introduce intramedullary nails and pass proximally to level of fracture site
> ❑ Closed reduction of humerus
>   • Fluoroscopic assistance
> ❑ Pass nails into intramedullary canal of proximal fragment, avoiding excessive false passage and trauma to the adjacent soft tissues
> ❑ Pass nails up to 1–2 cm distal to the proximal humeral epiphysis
> ❑ Bent and cut intramedullary nails beneath the skin
> ❑ Application of splint or sling after wound closure

Patients are positioned in the supine position. The appropriate-sized intramedullary implants (titanium elastic nails, Enders nails, Rush rods) are placed over the brachium, and fluoroscopy is used to determine the anticipated length of the intramedullary nail. The nails are then prebent into a gentle bow, with the apex centered at the level of the fracture site. If lateral column entry site only is to be used, the nails should be contoured into the shape of the letters C and S to maximize spread (and thus stability) at the level of the fracture site while still allowing for medial and lateral engagement of the proximal humeral metaphysis. If both medial and lateral column entry sites are planned, each nail will be prebent into a C shape.

A longitudinal incision is then created over the palpable lateral (and medial) column, just proximal to the olecranon fossa. Tourniquet control is not typically necessary. While epicondylar entry sites have been described, these have been associated with more frequent nail back-out.[133] Dissection is performed down to the level of the cortex. A small periosteal window may be elevated. Drill bits or awls may be used to create a cortical entry point, with care taken to orient the obliquity of the cortical tunnel along the anticipated trajectory of the nail. The intramedullary devices are then passed into the intramedullary canal of the distal fracture fragment to the level of the fracture. Fracture reduction is achieved through gentle closed manipulation, restoring length and correcting the angular deformity in the coronal and sagittal planes. Once fracture reduction is achieved, intramedullary nails may be atraumatically passed into the canal of the proximal fragment. A small bend at the leading tip of the intramedullary implant will facilitate engagement of the proximal fracture fragment. Fluoroscopic guidance is helpful, and efforts should be made to avoid repeated false passage of the nails into the adjacent soft tissues. In general, two nails are sufficient, provided they are of appropriate diameter and symmetrically contoured to allow for appropriate angular correction and rotational control.[209,210,247]

The implants are passed proximally into the proximal fragment until they lie 1 to 2 cm from the proximal humeral physis. At this time, the nails may be cut distally, leaving approximately 2 cm of length outside the cortex. If the nails were inserted with appropriate obliquity, the cut distal end of the nail would lie flush against the flare of the distal humeral metaphysis, avoiding symptomatic implant prominence yet still allowing for reliable implant retrieval. The entry wounds are closed in layers, and a long posterior splint, coaptation splint, or simple sling is applied.

External Fixation

Preoperative Planning

> **✓ External Fixation of Humerus Shaft Fractures:**
> **PREOPERATIVE PLANNING CHECKLIST**

OR table	❑ Radiolucent table
Position/ positioning aids	❑ Supine
Fluoroscopy location	❑ Ipsilateral side of table
Equipment	❑ Appropriate-sized external fixation pins, bars, rings

External fixation remains a treatment option for humeral shaft fractures, particularly in critically ill multitrauma patients or patients with severe open fractures associated with extensive soft tissue injury and/or bone loss.[47,78,187,291,310,339] Preoperative planning includes appropriate AP and lateral radiographs of the humerus to assess fracture location, pattern, displacement, and/or bone loss. Thorough documentation of preoperative neurovascular status is needed. For the multitrauma patient, communication with other care providers is important for care coordination and prioritization of injury treatment. In cases of severe soft tissue injury, appropriate consultation with plastic surgeons is recommended; this will allow for guidance regarding appropriate pin placement and planning of ultimate soft tissue coverage, if needed. Appropriately sized external fixator pins and bars should be available. While unilateral constructs are sufficient in most situations to provide stability, multiplanar or ring fixators may be employed, particularly if there are plans for subsequent lengthening, bone transport, or deformity correction.

Positioning

Patients may be positioned supine with the limb supported by a radiolucent table or hand table. Fluoroscopy units may be positioned on the ipsilateral side of the table, coming from the head or foot. Coordination should be made with other care providers in the multitrauma patient to allow adequate access to all anatomic regions necessitating care.

Surgical Approach

Surgical approaches are dictated by fracture characteristics, concomitant wounds and soft tissue injuries, and plans for future interventions. For a standard unilateral construct, pins may be inserted using percutaneous approaches via small incisions and careful spreading through the underlying soft tissues. Understanding of the cross-sectional anatomy of the brachium is important to avoid potential neurovascular injury.

Technique

> ### ✔ External Fixation of Humerus Shaft Fractures:
> ### KEY SURGICAL STEPS
>
> ❑ Identify fracture location and pattern
> ❑ Preassemble external fixator frame with planned pin-to-bar/ring clamps
> ❑ Small stab incisions made in skin at desired pin sites
> ❑ Blunt dissection through the subcutaneous tissues to level of humeral cortex
> ❑ Insert threaded pins (should be coplanar if unilateral fixator used)
> ❑ Provisionally connect the pins to the bar/ring
> ❑ Reduce or realign fracture
> ❑ Tighten pin-to-bar/ring connections
> ❑ Evaluate final alignment and construct with fluoroscopy or full-length radiographs of the humerus

Once the patient is positioned and the fracture location and pattern identified, the configuration of the ultimate external fixator construct is determined. Biomechanically, maximal spread of pins in both the proximal and distal fracture fragments will allow for the most rigid construct. If a unilateral frame is to be applied, preassembly of the bar with pin-to-bar clamps may facilitate coplanar placement of pins; indeed, the pin-to-bar clamps may be used as a "drill guide" during pin placement.

In a sequential fashion, the skin is incised at the site of pin placement and gentle, blunt dissection is performed through the subcutaneous tissues to the level of the humeral cortex. Appropriately sized threaded pins may then be drilled into the humerus, and use of cannulae or drill guides will protect the adjacent soft tissues and minimize the risk of iatrogenic neurovascular injury. This is particularly true for the radial nerve when lateral pins are placed in the mid- to distal diaphysis.

After pins are placed and connected to the external fixator bar, the fracture may be aligned in the desired position and stabilized. The addition of a second bar, while not always necessary, will improve bending rigidity of the construct.

Author's Preferred Treatment of Humerus Shaft Fractures (Algorithm 19-3)

Most humeral shaft fractures in children and adolescents can be successfully treated nonoperatively. In infants with birth-related fractures, immobilization with a stockinette or pinning of the sleeve to the trunk is simple and effective. Radiographic assessment of healing is performed at 4 to 6 weeks of age; immobilization is discontinued after confirmation of clinical and radiographic healing.

In children and adolescents with closed humeral diaphyseal fractures, stable injuries (e.g., torus or minimally displaced greenstick fractures) may be treated with simple sling immobilization. Patients with displaced fractures typically present with considerable pain, swelling, and ecchymosis. In these situations, gentle fracture realignment of the fracture may be performed with conscious sedation or general anesthesia, followed by application of a well-molded coaptation splint. Patients may be transitioned to a fracture brace at 1 to 2 weeks postinjury, after the initial swelling and discomfort has subsided. Serial radiographs are obtained to monitor fracture alignment and bony healing. Bony union is typically obtained by 6 weeks, after which immobilization is discontinued and activities advanced.

Similar nonoperative treatment is advocated for patients with closed injuries and acceptable alignment who present with radial nerve palsies. Even after bony union is achieved, serial clinical checks are performed monthly to monitor nerve recovery. An advancing Tinel sign and sequential motor recovery, beginning with wrist extension and progressing to digital and thumb extension, portend a favorable prognosis and spontaneous recovery. In general,

nerve regeneration progresses 1 mm per day, and calculation of the distance from the fracture site to the sites of distal muscle innervation will allow for prediction of time to motor recovery. Surgical exploration with radial nerve decompression, repair, or reconstruction is considered after 3 to 6 months without evidence of any neurologic recovery.

Surgical intervention is indicated in cases of open fractures, fractures with vascular or severe soft tissue injury, and fractures in unacceptable alignment. Surgery is also considered for patients with failure of appropriate radial nerve recovery or new radial nerve palsies after fracture manipulation.

For most humeral diaphyseal fractures proximal to the distal metadiaphysis and without intercondylar extension that are treated surgically, formal open reduction and plate fixation is preferred. An extensile lateral or posterolateral approach is used, as it allows safe access to up to 90% of the humeral diaphysis.[114] As surgery is often performed in the setting of radial nerve palsy, the lateral approach confers the additional advantage of allowing identification, mobilization, and/or repair of the radial nerve.[43,114,254]

Intramedullary nailing may be considered in patients without preoperative radial nerve palsy and transverse or short oblique (i.e., "length stable") fracture patterns. While the principles of intramedullary fixation are well established and the results well documented, closed nailing does not allow for visualization or decompression of the radial nerve.

Algorithm 19-3. Author's preferred treatment for humeral shaft fractures.

Postoperative Care

Patients receiving nonoperative treatment of humeral diaphyseal fractures are followed weekly with radiographs in splint or fracture brace to ensure adequate fit, monitor neurovascular function, and confirm radiographic alignment. In patients with associated radial nerve palsies, evaluation for an advancing Tinel sign and sequential motor recovery is performed. Once there is evidence of clinical and radiographic healing, gentle shoulder pendulum and elbow range-of-motion exercises are begun. Immobilization is typically discontinued after 6 weeks. Sports participation is restricted until there is return of motion and strength, and patients/families are counseled regarding the risk of refracture.

Following surgical reduction and stabilization, sling immobilization is usually sufficient and continued until radiographic healing. With plate fixation, gentle elbow range-of-motion exercises may be initiated once adequate comfort is achieved. In cases of intramedullary nail fixation, implants are typically removed at 6 months postoperatively.

Potential Pitfalls and Preventative Measures

Repair of Humerus Shaft Fractures: POTENTIAL PITFALLS AND PREVENTIONS	
Pitfall	**Prevention**
Malalignment of distal fractures (nonoperative)	Extensions of fracture brace
	Use of long-arm casts/splints
Malalignment of distal fractures (surgical)	Avoid percutaneous pinning
	Use of plates or IM nails
	Bicolumnar fixation
	Supplement with cast/splint immobilization
Radial nerve injury during ORIF	Careful dissection and mobilization
	Position plate beneath nerve
	Direct visualization of nerve with insertion of plate/screws
	Avoid excessive nerve retraction
Complications of IM nailing	Lateral entry above olecranon fossa
	Appropriate vector for nail insertion

While the techniques described above are well established, a number of potential pitfalls may be encountered during the treatment of diaphyseal fractures. First, nonoperative treatment of distal diaphyseal fractures may be challenging, given the anatomic location and relative limited amount of distal humerus that may be incorporated into a fracture brace or splint.[100] In these situations, use of medial and lateral extensions of conventional fracture brace may be needed to provide better control of coronal plane and rotational alignment. Alternatively, long-arm casts or long posterior splints may be used to provide stability and maintain alignment until clinical and radiographic healing occurs. Careful clinical and radiographic monitoring is needed, due to the tendency for varus malalignment and the limited capacity for remodeling of very distal humeral deformity.[30]

Similarly, surgical treatment of distal diaphyseal fractures may provide several challenges (Fig. 19-33).[100] Closed reduction and percutaneous pinning techniques commonly used for supracondylar humerus fractures may not provide adequate stability, as the more proximal fracture location results in medial and lateral entry pins that cross at the fracture site (Fig. 19-34). This may result in longer operative times, loss of fixation with late deformity, and loss of motion. Alternative treatments include open plating or intramedullary nailing via medial and lateral epicondyle entry sites (Fig. 19-35). With a medial epicondylar entry, the ulnar nerve needs to be identified and protected. When open plate or intramedullary nail fixation is chosen, consideration should be made for stabilization of both the medial and lateral columns to provide maximal control and minimize risk for late instability. In cases where bicolumnar fixation is not possible, supplementation with long-arm casts or other external immobilization is suggested.

A © 2012, COSF, Boston   © 2012, COSF, Boston   **B**

Figure 19-33. A: Intraoperative image depicting a comminuted, open distal humerus fracture in a 3-year-old boy after a motorcycle injury. **B:** Intraoperative image after lateral column plate fixation, sparing the distal humeral physes.

(continues)

Figure 19-33. (*Continued*) **C:** Given single-column fixation, some loss of fixation is seen. Internal fixation was supplemented with spica cast immobilization. **D:** Final radiographs demonstrate appropriate bony healing and alignment. (Courtesy of Children's Orthopaedic Surgery Foundation.)

During ORIF via a lateral or posterolateral approach, care of the radial nerve is paramount. Identification of the posterior brachial cutaneous nerve and/or the characteristic fat stripe along the lateral aspect of the triceps will enable radial nerve identification during surgical exposures. Often the radial nerve must be mobilized to allow for implant placement between the humeral cortex below and the radial nerve above. Adequate direct visualization of plate placement and screw insertion is imperative to minimize the risk of iatrogenic nerve injury (Fig. 19-36).

Figure 19-34. A, B: Distal humeral diaphyseal fracture in a 19-month-old treated with closed reduction and percutaneous pinning.

C, D   E

Figure 19-34. (*Continued*) **C:** The pins cross at the fracture site with decreased stability and some loss of position. **D, E:** The ultimate outcome was good.

Figure 19-35. Ideally, pin fixation for distal humeral diaphyseal–metaphyseal junction fractures involves pins placed in intramedullary fashion up the medial and lateral columns.

Figure 19-36. Intraoperative radiograph depicting radial nerve placement beneath a previously applied lateral plate. (Courtesy of Children's Orthopaedic Surgery Foundation.)

Finally, a few maneuvers may aid in the intramedullary nailing of humeral diaphyseal fractures. Lateral column entry provides easy surgical access and minimizes risk to the ulnar nerve. If this is chosen, nails should be precontoured into the shape of a C and S to allow for maximal spread at the fracture site and engagement of the proximal humeral fracture fragment. Creating the cortical entry point above the olecranon fossa with the appropriate distal-lateral to proximal-medial vector will allow the nail to sit against the metaphyseal flare of the lateral column when cut; this will facilitate subsequent retrieval and minimize the soft tissue irritation commonly caused by epicondylar entry points.

Outcomes

Overall, reported clinical results are good after surgical treatment of humeral diaphyseal fractures using both intramedullary nailing and open plate fixation techniques.[15,68,133,143,168,303,348]

MANAGEMENT OF EXPECTED ADVERSE OUTCOMES AND UNEXPECTED COMPLICATIONS RELATED TO HUMERUS SHAFT FRACTURES

Humerus Shaft Fractures:
COMMON ADVERSE OUTCOMES AND COMPLICATIONS

- Radial nerve palsy
- Malunion
- Nonunion
- Limb-length discrepancy
- Stiffness

Radial nerve palsies are commonly seen with humeral diaphyseal fractures. As discussed above, these nerve injuries may be primary or secondary. Secondary radial nerve injuries may result from a host of mechanisms, including excessive fracture manipulation resulting in neurapraxia, nerve incarceration within the fracture site or subsequent fracture callus, or rarely direct nerve injury or transection during fracture manipulation or implant placement. These inadvertent neurologic complications may be seen with both nonoperative and surgical treatment. There continues to be controversy regarding the initial management of immediate secondary nerve palsies, though it is clear that failure of spontaneous recovery after an appropriate period of observation should prompt surgical exploration, decompression, and/or nerve reconstruction.[107,377] In addition to radial nerve injuries, ulnar and median nerve injuries have been reported.[232,311]

Compartment syndrome of the brachium is relatively rare, in part because of anatomic differences in fascial strength, ability to avoid extreme positioning during fracture immobilization, and fracture characteristics.[23,36,109,127] Patients with associated ipsilateral upper extremity fractures or vascular injuries are at higher risk.

Vascular injuries, including brachial artery transection, are uncommon but mandate prompt evaluation and intervention to restore vascularity to the upper limb.[244] In cases in which vascular repair or reconstruction is needed, fracture stability with external or internal fixation is needed to protect and facilitate vascular repair.

Functionally limiting malunion is uncommon in pediatric humeral diaphyseal fractures. As cited previously, 20 to 30 degrees of varus and 20 degrees of apex anterior angulation may be accepted, with often little aesthetic differences and functional consequence.[74,95,294,345] Up to 15 degrees of internal rotation is also well tolerated.[74] Patients younger than 6 years of age will remodel most angular deformity, and obese patients—though more prone to malunion given the challenges of immobilization—may hide their resultant deformity better.[152,309] Because of the remodeling potential, compensatory motion at the shoulder, elbow, and forearm, and lack of functional deficits, corrective osteotomies for humeral diaphyseal malunions are rarely necessary.

While more commonly reported in adults, nonunion of humeral diaphyseal fractures may rarely occur in children and adolescents (Fig. 19-37).[105] Risk factors may include excessive soft tissue injury, vascular insufficiency, segmental bone defects, or underlying bone abnormalities, such as osteogenesis imperfecta. Treatment principles for humeral nonunion in children have been extrapolated from adult orthopaedics.[99,140,258] In cases of hypertrophic nonunions, treatment is predicated on provision of bony stability, typically with ORIF. In cases of atrophic nonunions, ORIF with debridement of the pseudarthrosis back to bleeding bone and use of autogenous bone grafting is

Figure 19-37. Radiograph depicting an atrophic humeral diaphyseal nonunion in a skeletally mature adolescent previously treated with screw and cerclage wire fixation of an open humeral diaphyseal fracture. (Courtesy of Children's Orthopaedic Surgery Foundation.)

advised.[146] Alternative treatments include external fixation and the Ilizarov technique.[48,166,167] In cases of pathologic fractures or systemic bone abnormalities—such as osteogenesis imperfecta—intramedullary implants are preferred.[110] In rare situations, a vascularized fibula graft is appropriate to provide bony alignment, stability, and healing.[180]

Limb-length discrepancy may result from prior humeral diaphyseal fracture, though clinically up to 6 to 8 cm of shortening may be well tolerated without functional loss. As with other long bone fractures, overgrowth may occur following humerus fracture, though the magnitude is often minimal (<1 cm).[320] In cases of considerable limb-length discrepancy and functional compromise, humeral lengthening via distraction osteogenesis using unilateral or multiplanar ring fixators may be performed.[48,49,73,282]

Finally, while loss of shoulder and/or elbow motion is common with both nonoperative and surgical treatment of humeral diaphyseal fractures in adults, persistent stiffness is uncommon in pediatric patients.[146] Judicious initiation of early range of motion will aid to minimize the risk of this complication.

SUMMARY, CONTROVERSIES, AND FUTURE DIRECTIONS RELATED TO HUMERUS SHAFT FRACTURES

In summary, most humeral diaphyseal fractures may be effectively treated nonoperatively. In older patients with greater deformity, surgical reduction and stabilization will result in reliable bony healing and improved radiographic alignment. Controversy continues regarding the optimal management of secondary radial nerve palsies as well as the relative indications for intramedullary nailing versus open reduction and plate fixation of displaced humeral shaft fractures. Future prospective, comparative investigation is needed to determine the optimal surgical management of these injuries.

Annotated References

Reference	Annotation
Beaty JH. Fractures of the proximal humerus and shaft in children. *Instr Course Lect*. 1992;41:369–372.	Instructional course lecture with guidelines regarding parameters of acceptable radiographic alignment for pediatric proximal humerus fractures.
Canavese F, Marengo L, Cravino M, et al. Outcome of conservative versus surgical treatment of humeral shaft fracture in children and adolescents: comparison between nonoperative treatment (Desault's bandage), external fixation and elastic stable intramedullary nailing. *J Pediatr Orthop*. 2017; 37(3):e156–e163.	Comparative retrospective analysis of 36 patients treated with simple immobilization, external fixation, or flexible intramedullary nailing of humeral diaphyseal fractures. While surgical patients required less duration of immobilization and improved radiographic alignment, DASH scores and return to sports rates were similar among treatment groups.
Dobbs MB, Luhmann SL, Gordon JE, et al. Severely displaced proximal humeral epiphyseal fractures. *J Pediatr Orthop*. 2003;23(2):208–215.	Retrospective case series of children and adolescents with severely displaced (Neer–Horwitz 3 or 4) proximal humeral fractures. The authors identify risk of late displacement after initial closed reduction in adolescents, as well as soft tissue impediments to closed reduction.
Handoll HH, Almaiyah MA, Rangan A. Surgical versus non-surgical treatment for acute anterior shoulder dislocation. *Cochrane Database Syst Rev*. 2004;2004(1):CD004325.	Cochrane database review regarding the treatment of acute traumatic shoulder dislocation, suggesting surgical stabilization after primary dislocation may be beneficial in young male contact athletes.
Hovelius L, Olofsson A, Sandström B, et al. Nonoperative treatment of primary anterior shoulder dislocation in patients forty years of age and younger: a prospective twenty-five-year follow-up. *J Bone Joint Surg Am*. 2008;90(5):945–952.	Long-term follow-up of young patients treated nonoperatively for traumatic shoulder dislocations, characterizing risk of recurrent instability and rates of subsequent surgical stabilization.
Khan A, Samba A, Pereira B, Canavese F. Anterior dislocation of the shoulder in skeletally immature patients: comparison between non-operative treatment versus open Latarjet's procedure. *Bone Joint J*. 2014;96-B(3): 354–359.	In this retrospective case series of skeletally immature patients, surgical stabilization with the Latarjet procedure was effective in reducing risk of recurrent instability and allowing patients to return to preinjury activities.
Kraus T, Hoermann S, Ploder G, et al. Elastic stable intramedullary nailing versus Kirschner wire pinning: outcome of severely displaced proximal humeral fractures in juvenile patients. *J Shoulder Elbow Surg*. 2014;23(10):1462–1467.	Excellent functional outcomes and radiographic alignment were achieved with either percutaneous pinning or elastic intramedullary nails for juvenile proximal humeral fractures.
Longo UG, van der Linde JA, Loppini M, et al. Surgical versus nonoperative treatment in patients up to 18 years old with traumatic shoulder instability: a systematic review and quantitative synthesis of the literature. *Arthroscopy*. 2016;32(5):944–952.	Systematic review from 15 published articles of 705 shoulders in patients 18 years of age or younger. Overall recurrent dislocation rate with nonoperative and surgical treatment was 71.3% vs. 17.5%, respectively.
Neer CS 2nd, Horwitz BS. Fractures of the proximal humeral epiphysial plate. *Clin Orthop Relat Res*. 1965;41:24–31.	Classic paper with description of classification of proximal humeral fractures in pediatric and adolescent patients.

REFERENCES

1. Abbot S, Proudman S, Ravichandran B, Williams N. Predictors of outcomes of proximal humerus fractures in children and adolescents: a systematic review. *J Child Orthop.* 2022;16:347–354.
2. Ahmed I, Ashton F, Robinson CM. Arthroscopic Bankart repair and capsular shift for recurrent anterior shoulder instability: functional outcomes and identification of risk factors for recurrence. *J Bone Joint Surg Am.* 2012;94:1308–1315.
3. Ahn JI, Park JS. Pathological fractures secondary to unicameral bone cysts. *Int Orthop.* 1994;18:20–22.
4. Allen ME. Stress fracture of the humerus. A case study. *Am J Sports Med.* 1984;12:244–245.
5. Arora S, Goel N, Cheema GS, et al. A method to localize the radial nerve using the "apex of triceps aponeurosis" as a landmark. *Clin Orthop Relat Res.* 2011;469:2638–2644.
6. Artico M, Salvati M, D'Andrea V, et al. Isolated lesion of the axillary nerve: surgical treatment and outcome in 12 cases. *Neurosurgery.* 1991;29:697–700.
7. Badhe NP, Howard PW. Olecranon screw traction for displaced supracondylar fractures of the humerus in children. *Injury.* 1998;29:457–460.
8. Bahrs C, Zipplies S, Ochs BG, et al. Proximal humeral fractures in children and adolescents. *J Pediatr Orthop.* 2009;29:238–242.
9. Baratta JB, Lim V, Mastromonaco E, Edillon EL. Axillary artery disruption secondary to anterior dislocation of the shoulder. *J Trauma.* 1983;23:1009–1011.
10. Barber DB, Janus RB, Wade WH. Neuroarthropathy: an overuse injury of the shoulder in quadriplegia. *J Spinal Cord Med.* 1996;19:9–11.
11. Barry TP, Lombardo SJ, Kerlan RK, et al. The coracoid transfer for recurrent anterior instability of the shoulder in adolescents. *J Bone Joint Surg Am.* 1985;67:383–387.
12. Baxter MP, Wiley JJ. Fractures of the proximal humeral epiphysis. Their influence on humeral growth. *J Bone Joint Surg Br.* 1986;68:570–573.
13. Beaty JH. Fractures of the proximal humerus and shaft in children. *Instr Course Lect.* 1992;41:369–372.
14. Bedoya MA, Barrera CA, Bencardino JT, Ho-Fung V. Humeral lesser tuberosity avulsion fractures - magnetic resonance imaging characteristics in the pediatric population. *Pediatric Radial.* 2021;51:1421–1430.
15. Bell MJ, Beauchamp CG, Kellam JK, McMurtry RY. The results of plating humeral shaft fractures in patients with multiple injuries. The Sunnybrook experience. *J Bone Joint Surg Br.* 1985;67:293–296.
16. Berghausen T, Leslie BM, Ruby LK, Zimbler S. The severely displaced pediatric supracondylar fracture of humerus treated by skeletal traction with olecranon pin. *Orthop Rev.* 1986;15:510–515.
17. Beringer DC, Weiner DS, Noble JS, Bell RH. Severely displaced proximal humeral epiphyseal fractures: a follow-up study. *J Pediatr Orthop.* 1998;18:31–37.
18. Bhat BV, Kumar A, Oumachigui A. Bone injuries during delivery. *Indian J Pediatr.* 1994;61:401–405.
19. Bianco AJ, Schlein AP, Kruse RL, Johnson EW Jr. Birth fractures. *Minn Med.* 1972;55:471–474.
20. Birch R. Lesions of peripheral nerves: the present position. *J Bone Joint Surg Br.* 1986;68:2–8.
21. Bishop JA, Crall TS, Kocher MS. Operative versus nonoperative treatment after primary traumatic anterior glenohumeral dislocation: expected-value decision analysis. *J Shoulder Elbow Surg.* 2011;20:1087–1094.
22. Bishop J, Ring D. Management of radial nerve palsy associated with humeral shaft fracture: a decision analysis model. *J Hand Surg Am.* 2009;34:991–996.
23. Blakemore LC, Cooperman DR, Thompson GH, et al. Compartment syndrome in ipsilateral humerus and forearm fractures in children. *Clin Orthop Relat Res.* 2000;(376):32–38.
24. Bleeker WA, Nijsten MW, ten Duis HJ. Treatment of humeral shaft fractures related to associated injuries. A retrospective study of 237 patients. *Acta Orthop Scand.* 1991;62:148–153.
25. Bortel DT, Pritchett JW. Straight-line graphs for the prediction of growth of the upper extremities. *J Bone Joint Surg Am.* 1993;75:885–892.
26. Böstman O, Bakalim G, Vainionpää S, et al. Immediate radial nerve palsy complicating fracture of the shaft of the humerus: when is early exploration justified? *Injury.* 1985;16:499–502.
27. Böstman O, Bakalim G, Vainionpää S, et al. Radial palsy in shaft fracture of the humerus. *Acta Orthop Scand.* 1986;57:316–319.
28. Boyd KT, Batt ME. Stress fracture of the proximal humeral epiphysis in an elite junior badminton player. *Br J Sports Med.* 1997;31:252–253.
29. Broker FH, Burbach T. Ultrasonic diagnosis of separation of the proximal humeral epiphysis in the newborn. *J Bone Joint Surg Am.* 1990;72:187–191.
30. Brug E, Winckler S, Klein W. Distal diaphyseal fracture of the humerus. *Unfallchirurg.* 1994;97:74–77.
31. Bumbasirevic M, Lesic A, Bumbasirevic V, et al. The management of humeral shaft fractures with associated radial nerve palsy: a review of 117 cases. *Arch Orthop Trauma Surg.* 2010;130:519–522.
32. Burgos-Flores J, Gonzalez-Herranz P, Lopez-Mondejar JA, et al. Fractures of the proximal humeral epiphysis. *Int Orthop.* 1993;17:16–19.
33. Burke MC, Minnock C, Robbins CB, et al. Intraobserver and interobserver reliability of radiographic analysis of proxima humerus fractures in adolescents. *J Pediatr Orthop.* 2019;39(2):e125–e129.
34. Burkhead WZ Jr, Rockwood CA Jr. Treatment of instability of the shoulder with an exercise program. *J Bone Joint Surg Am.* 1992;74:890–896.
35. Caldwell JA. Treatment of fractures in the Cincinnati General Hospital. *Ann Surg.* 1933;97:161–176.
36. Cameron SE. Acute compartment syndrome of the triceps. A case report. *Acta Orthop Scand.* 1993;64:107–108.
37. Cameron KL, Duffey ML, DeBerardino TM, et al. Association of generalized joint hypermobility with a history of glenohumeral joint instability. *J Athl Train.* 2010;45:253–258.
38. Camus M, Lefebvre G, Veron P, Darbois Y. Obstetrical injuries of the newborn infant. Retrospective study apropos of 20,409 births. *J Gynecol Obstet Biol Reprod (Paris).* 1985;14:1033–1043.
39. Canavese F, Athlani L, Marengo L, et al. Evaluation of upper-extremity function following surgical treatment of displaced proximal humerus fractures in children. *J Pediatr Orthop B.* 2014;23:144–149.
40. Canavese F, Marengo L, Cravino M, et al. Outcome of conservative versus surgical treatment of humeral shaft fracture in children and adolescents: comparison between nonoperative treatment (Desault's bandage), external fixation and elastic stable intramedullary nailing. *J Pediatr Orthop.* 2017;37:e156–e163.
41. Canavese F, Marengo L, Samba A, et al. Evaluation of upper extremity function of displaced diaphyseal humeral fractures in children treated by elastic stable intramedullary nailing: preliminary results. *J Pediatr Orthop B.* 2016;25:399–405.
42. Canpolat FE, Köse A, Yurdakök M. Bilateral humerus fracture in a neonate after cesarean delivery. *Arch Gynecol Obstet.* 2010;281:967–969.
43. Carlan D, Pratt J, Patterson JMM, et al. The radial nerve in the brachium: an anatomic study in human cadavers. *J Hand Surg Am.* 2007;32:1177–1182.
44. Carroll SE. A study of the nutrient foramina of the humeral diaphysis. *J Bone Joint Surg Br.* 1963;45-B:176–181.
45. Carter C, Sweetnam R. Recurrent dislocation of the patella and of the shoulder. Their association with familial joint laxity. *J Bone Joint Surg Br.* 1960;42-R:721–727.
46. Castagna A, Delle Rose G, Borroni M, et al. Arthroscopic stabilization of the shoulder in adolescent athletes participating in overhead or contact sports. *Arthroscopy.* 2012;28:309–315.
47. Catagni MA, Lovisetti L, Guerreschi F, et al. The external fixation in the treatment of humeral diaphyseal fractures: outcomes of 84 cases. *Injury.* 2010;41:1107–1111.
48. Cattaneo R, Catagni MA, Guerreschi F. Applications of the Ilizarov method in the humerus. Lengthenings and nonunions. *Hand Clin.* 1993;9:729–739.
49. Cattaneo R, Villa A, Catagni MA, Bell D. Lengthening of the humerus using the Ilizarov technique. Description of the method and report of 43 cases. *Clin Orthop Relat Res.* 1990;(250):117–124.
50. Caviglia H, Garrido CP, Palazzi FF, Meana NV. Pediatric fractures of the humerus. *Clin Orthop Relat Res.* 2005;(432):49–56.
51. Chahal J, Marks PH, Macdonald PB, et al. Anatomic Bankart repair compared with nonoperative treatment and/or arthroscopic lavage for first-time traumatic shoulder dislocation. *Arthroscopy.* 2012;28:565–575.
52. Chan D, Petricciuolo F, Maffulli N. Fracture of the humeral diaphysis with extreme rotation. *Acta Orthop Belg.* 1991;57:427–429.
53. Chaus GW, Carry PM, Pishkenari AK, Hadley-Miller N. Operative versus nonoperative treatment of displaced proximal humeral physeal fractures: a matched cohort. *J Pediatr Orthop.* 2015;35:234–239.
54. Chee Y, Agorastides I, Garg N, et al. Treatment of severely displaced proximal humeral fractures in children with elastic stable intramedullary nailing. *J Pediatr Orthop B.* 2006;15:45–50.
55. Chen CY, Chao EK, Tu YK, et al. Closed management and percutaneous fixation of unstable proximal humerus fractures. *J Trauma.* 1998;45:1039–1045.
56. Cheng JC, Shen WY. Limb fracture pattern in different pediatric age groups: a study of 3,350 children. *J Orthop Trauma.* 1993;7:15–22.
57. Cheok CY, Mohamad JA, Ahmad TS. Pain relief for reduction of acute anterior shoulder dislocations: a prospective randomized study comparing intravenous sedation with intra-articular lidocaine. *J Orthop Trauma.* 2011;25:5–10.
58. Cho SH, Cho NS, Rhee YG. Preoperative analysis of the Hill–Sachs lesion in anterior shoulder instability: how to predict engagement of the lesion. *Am J Sports Med.* 2011;39:2389–2395.
59. Choi YS, Potter HG, Scher DM. A shearing osteochondral fracture of the humeral head following an anterior shoulder dislocation in a child. *HSS J.* 2005;1:100–102.
60. Chung SM, Nissenbaum MM. Congenital and developmental defects of the shoulder. *Orthop Clin North Am.* 1975;6:381–392.
61. Ciernik IF, Meier L, Hollinger A. Humeral mobility after treatment with hanging cast. *J Trauma.* 1991;31:230–233.
62. Coene LN, Narakas AO. Operative management of lesions of the axillary nerve, isolated or combined with other nerve lesions. *Clin Neurol Neurosurg.* 1992;94(Suppl):S64–S66.
63. Cohn BT, Froimson AI. Salter 3 fracture dislocation of glenohumeral joint in a 10-year-old. *Orthop Rev.* 1986;15:403–404.
64. Confalonieri N, Simonatti R, Ramondetta V, Centanni L. Intramedullary nailing with a Rush pin in the treatment of diaphyseal humeral fractures. *Arch Putti Chir Organi Mov.* 1990;38:395–403.
65. Coobs BR, LaPrade RF. Severe chondrolysis of the glenohumeral joint after shoulder thermal capsulorrhaphy. *Am J Orthop (Belle Mead NJ).* 2009;38:E34–E37.
66. Cordischi K, Li X, Busconi B. Intermediate outcomes after primary traumatic anterior shoulder dislocation in skeletally immature patients aged 10 to 13 years. *Orthopedics.* 2009;32(9).
67. Covey DC, Riordan DC, Milstead ME, Albright JA. Modification of the L'Episcopo procedure for brachial plexus birth palsies. *J Bone Joint Surg Br.* 1992;74:897–901.
68. Crolla RM, de Vries LS, Clevers GJ. Locked intramedullary nailing of humeral fractures. *Injury.* 1993;24:403–406.
69. Currarino G, Sheffield E, Twickler D. Congenital glenoid dysplasia. *Pediatr Radiol.* 1998;28:30–37.
70. Curtis RJ Jr. Operative management of children's fractures of the shoulder region. *Orthop Clin North Am.* 1990;21:315–324.
71. Dabezies EJ, Banta CJ II, Murphy CP, d'Ambrosia RD. Plate fixation of the humeral shaft for acute fractures, with and without radial nerve injuries. *J Orthop Trauma.* 1992;6:10–13.

72. Dal Monte A, Andrisano A, Manfrini M, Zucchi M. Humeral lengthening in hypoplasia of the upper limb. *J Pediatr Orthop.* 1985;5:202–207.

73. Dalldorf PG, Bryan WJ. Displaced Salter-Harris type I injury in a gymnast. A slipped capital humeral epiphysis? *Orthop Rev.* 1994;23:538–541.

74. Dameron TB Jr, Grubb SA. Humeral shaft fractures in adults. *South Med J.* 1981; 74:1461–1467.

75. Dameron TB Jr, Reibel DB. Fractures involving the proximal humeral epiphyseal plate. *J Bone Joint Surg Am.* 1969;51:289–297.

76. Danzl DF, Vicario SJ, Gleis GL, et al. Closed reduction of anterior subcoracoid shoulder dislocation. Evaluation of an external rotation method. *Orthop Rev.* 1986; 15:311–315.

77. Davarinos N, Ellanti P, Khan Bhambro KS, Keogh P. Skin puckering an uncommon sign of underlying humeral neck fracture: a case report. *Ir J Med Sci.* 2011;180: 731–733.

78. De Bastiani G, Aldegheri R, Renzi Brivio L. The treatment of fractures with a dynamic axial fixator. *J Bone Joint Surg Br.* 1984;66:538–545.

79. de Beer J, Burkhart SS, Roberts CP, et al. The congruent-arc Latarjet. *Tech Shoulder Surg.* 2009;10:62–67.

80. Deitch J, Mehlman CT, Foad SL, et al. Traumatic anterior shoulder dislocation in adolescents. *Am J Sports Med.* 2003;31:758–763.

81. d'Elia G, Di Giacomo A, D'Alessandro P, Cirillo LC. Traumatic anterior glenohumeral instability: quantification of glenoid bone loss by spiral CT. *Radiol Med.* 2008;113:496–503.

82. DeLong WG Jr, Born CT, Marcelli E, et al. Ender nail fixation in long bone fractures: experience in a level I trauma center. *J Trauma.* 1989;29:571–576.

83. Denard A Jr, Richards JE, Obremskey WT, et al. Outcome of nonoperative vs operative treatment of humeral shaft fractures: a retrospective study of 213 patients. *Orthopedics.* 2010;33(8).

84. Denies E, Nijs S, Sermon A, Broos P. Operative treatment of humeral shaft fractures. Comparison of plating and intramedullary nailing. *Acta Orthop Belg.* 2010;76: 735–742.

85. Dhawan A, Ghodadra N, Karas V, et al. Complications of bioabsorbable suture anchors in the shoulder. *Am J Sports Med.* 2012;40:1424–1430.

86. Di Filippo P, Mancini GB, Gillio A. Humeral fractures with paralysis of the radial nerve. *Arch Putti Chir Organi Mov.* 1990;38:405–409.

87. Dimakopoulos P, Panagopoulos A, Kasimatis G, et al. Anterior traumatic shoulder dislocation associated with displaced greater tuberosity fracture: the necessity of operative treatment. *J Orthop Trauma.* 2007;21:104–112.

88. Dobbs MB, Luhmann SL, Gordon JE, et al. Severely displaced proximal humeral epiphyseal fractures. *J Pediatr Orthop.* 2003;23:208–215.

89. Drew SJ, Giddins GE, Birch R. A slowly evolving brachial plexus injury following a proximal humeral fracture in a child. *J Hand Surg Br.* 1995;20:24–25.

90. Edeiken BS, Libshitz HI, Cohen MA. Slipped proximal humeral epiphysis: a complication of radiotherapy to the shoulder in children. *Skeletal Radiol.* 1982;9: 123–125.

91. Edwards P, Kurth L. Postoperative radial nerve paralysis caused by fracture callus. *J Orthop Trauma.* 1992;6:234–236.

92. Egger AC, Willimon SC, Busch MT, et al. Arthroscopic Bankart repair for adolescent anterior shoulder instability: clinical and imaging predictors of revision surgery and recurrent subjective instability. *Am J Sports Med.* 2023;51:877–884.

93. Ekholm R, Ponzer S, Törnkvist H, et al. Primary radial nerve palsy in patients with acute humeral shaft fractures. *J Orthop Trauma.* 2008;22:408–414.

94. Elbaum R, Parent H, Zeller R, Seringe R. Traumatic scapulo-humeral dislocation in children and adolescents. Apropos of 9 patients. *Acta Orthop Belg.* 1994;60: 204–209.

95. Ellefsen BK, Frierson MA, Raney EM, Ogden JA. Humerus varus: a complication of neonatal, infantile, and childhood injury and infection. *J Pediatr Orthop.* 1994;14:479–486.

96. Emery RJ, Mullaji AB. Glenohumeral joint instability in normal adolescents. Incidence and significance. *J Bone Joint Surg Br.* 1991;73:406–408.

97. Endo S, Kasai T, Fujii N, et al. Traumatic anterior dislocation of the shoulder in a child. *Arch Orthop Trauma Surg.* 1993;112:201–202.

98. Farber AJ, Castillo R, Clough M, et al. Clinical assessment of three common tests for traumatic anterior shoulder instability. *J Bone Joint Surg Am.* 2006;88:1467–1474.

99. Fattah HA, Halawa EE, Shafy TH. Non-union of the humeral shaft: a report on 25 cases. *Injury.* 1982;14:255–262.

100. Fayssoux RS, Stankovits L, Domzalski ME, Guille JT. Fractures of the distal humeral metaphyseal-diaphyseal junction in children. *J Pediatr Orthop.* 2008;28:142–146.

101. Fernandez FF, Eberhardt O, Langendörfer M, Wirth T. Treatment of severely displaced proximal humeral fractures in children with retrograde elastic stable intramedullary nailing. *Injury.* 2008;39:1453–1459.

102. Finestone A, Milgrom C, Radeva-Petrova DR, et al. Bracing in external rotation for traumatic anterior dislocation of the shoulder. *J Bone Joint Surg Br.* 2009;91:918–921.

103. Fisher TR, McGeoch CM. Severe injuries of the radial nerve treated by sural nerve grafting. *Injury.* 1985;16:411–412.

104. Fisher NA, Newman B, Lloyd J, Mimouni F. Ultrasonographic evaluation of birth injury to the shoulder. *J Perinatol.* 1995;15:398–400.

105. Foster RJ, Swiontkowski MF, Bach AW, Sack JT. Radial nerve palsy caused by open humeral shaft fractures. *J Hand Surg Am.* 1993;18:121–124.

106. Franklin CC, Weiss JM. The natural history of pediatric and adolescent shoulder dislocation. *J Pediatr Orthop.* 2019;39(Suppl 1):S50–S52.

107. Friedman RJ, Smith RJ. Radial-nerve laceration twenty-six years after screw fixation of a humeral fracture. A case report. *J Bone Joint Surg Am.* 1984;66:959–960.

108. Funakoshi T, Takahashi T, Shimokobe H, et al. Arthroscopic findings of the glenohumeral joint in symptomatic anterior instabilities: comparison between overhead throwing disorders and traumatic shoulder dislocation. *J Shoulder Elbow Surg.* 2023;32:776–785.

109. Gaffney D, Slabaugh M. Deltoid compartment syndrome after antegrade humeral nailing. *J Orthop Trauma.* 2009;23:229–231.

110. Gamble JG, Rinsky LA, Strudwick J, Bleck EE. Non-union of fractures in children who have osteogenesis imperfecta. *J Bone Joint Surg Am.* 1988;70:439–443.

111. Garrigues GE, Warnick DE, Busch MT. Subscapularis avulsion of the lesser tuberosity in adolescents. *J Pediatr Orthop.* 2013;33:8–13.

112. Garth WP Jr, Leberte MA, Cool TA. Recurrent fractures of the humerus in a baseball pitcher. A case report. *J Bone Joint Surg Am.* 1988;70:305–306.

113. Gerber C, Schneeberger AG, Vinh TS. The arterial vascularization of the humeral head. An anatomical study. *J Bone Joint Surg Am.* 1990;72:1486–1494.

114. Gerwin M, Hotchkiss RN, Weiland AJ. Alternative operative exposures of the posterior aspect of the humeral diaphysis with reference to the radial nerve. *J Bone Joint Surg Am.* 1996;78:1690–1695.

115. Geusens E, Pans S, Verhulst D, Brys P. The modified axillary view of the shoulder, a painless alternative. *Emerg Radiol.* 2006;12:227–230.

116. Giebel G, Suren EG. Injuries of the proximal humeral epiphysis. Indications for surgical therapy and results. *Chirurg.* 1983;54:406–410.

117. Gill TJ, Waters P. Valgus osteotomy of the humeral neck: a technique for the treatment of humerus varus. *J Shoulder Elbow Surg.* 1997;6:306–310.

118. Gjengedal E, Slungaard U. Treatment of humeral fractures with and without injury to the radial nerve. A follow-up study. *Tidsskr Nor Laegeforen.* 1981;101(31):1746–1749.

119. Gladstein AZ, Schade AT, Howard AW, Camp MW. Reducing resource utilization during non-operative treatment of pediatric proximal humerus fractures. *Orthop Traumatol Surg Res.* 2017;103:115–118.

120. Goldberg BJ, Nirschl RP, McConnell JP, Pettrone FA. Arthroscopic transglenoid suture capsulolabral repairs: preliminary results. *Am J Sports Med.* 1993;21: 656–664.

121. Good CR, MacGillivray JD. Traumatic shoulder dislocation in the adolescent athlete: advances in surgical treatment. *Curr Opin Pediatr.* 2005;17:25–29.

122. Good CR, Shindle MK, Kelly BT, et al. Glenohumeral chondrolysis after shoulder arthroscopy with thermal capsulorrhaphy. *Arthroscopy.* 2007;23:797.e1–e5.

123. Gray DJ, Gardner E. The prenatal development of the human humerus. *Am J Anat.* 1969;124:431–445.

124. Gregg-Smith SJ, White SH. Salter-Harris III fracture-dislocation of the proximal humeral epiphysis. *Injury.* 1992;23:199–200.

125. Gudinchet F, Naggar L, Ginalski JM, et al. Magnetic resonance imaging of nontraumatic shoulder instability in children. *Skeletal Radiol.* 1992;21:19–21.

126. Guibert L, Allouis M, Bourdelat D, et al. Fractures and slipped epiphyses of the proximal humerus in children. Place and methods of surgical treatment. *Chir Pediatr.* 1983;24:197–200.

127. Gupta A, Sharma S. Volar compartment syndrome of the arm complicating a fracture of the humeral shaft. A case report. *Acta Orthop Scand.* 1991;62:77–78.

128. Guven M, Akman B, Kormaz T, et al. "Floating arm" injury in a child with fractures of the proximal and distal parts of the humerus: a case report. *J Med Case Rep.* 2009;3:9287.

129. Hackethal KH. Die Bundel-Nagelung. *Experimentelle und Klinische Studie über eine Neuartige Methode der Markraum-Schienung Langer Röhrenknochen.* Springer-Verlag; 1961.

130. Hackstock H. Functional bracing of fractures. *Orthopade.* 1988;17:41–51.

131. Hale HB, Bae DS, Waters PM. Current concepts in the management of brachial plexus birth palsy. *J Hand Surg Am.* 2010;35:322–331.

132. Hall RF Jr. Closed intramedullary fixation of humeral shaft fractures. *Instr Course Lect.* 1987;36:349–358.

133. Hall RF Jr, Pankovich AM. Ender nailing of acute fractures of the humerus. A study of closed fixation by intramedullary nails without reaming. *J Bone Joint Surg Am.* 1987;69:558–567.

134. Handoll HH, Almaiyah MA, Rangan A. Surgical versus non-surgical treatment for acute anterior shoulder dislocation. *Cochrane Database Syst Rev.* 2004; 2004(1):CD004325.

135. Hannonen J, Hyvönen H, Korhonen L, et al. The incidence and treatment trends of pediatric proximal humerus fractures. *BMC Musculoskelet Disord.* 2019;20:571.

136. Harper DK, Craig JG, van Holsbeeck MT. Apophyseal injuries of the lesser tuberosity in adolescents: a series of five cases. *Emerg Radiol.* 2013;20:33–37.

137. Harris BA Jr. Shoulder dystocia. *Clin Obstet Gynecol.* 1984;27:106–111.

138. Hasan SA, Cordell CL, Rauls RB, Eidt JF. Brachial artery injury with a proximal humerus fracture in a 10-year-old girl. *Am J Orthop (Belle Mead NJ).* 2009;38:462–466.

139. Hawkins RJ, Koppert G, Johnston G. Recurrent posterior instability (subluxation) of the shoulder. *J Bone Joint Surg Am.* 1984;66:169–174.

140. Healy WL, White GM, Mick CA, et al. Nonunion of the humeral shaft. *Clin Orthop Relat Res.* 1987;(219):206–213.

141. Heck CC. Anterior dislocation of the glenohumeral joint in a child. *J Trauma.* 1981;21:174–175.

142. Heckler MW, Bamberger HB. Humeral shaft fractures and radial nerve palsy: to explore or not to explore...That is the question. *Am J Orthop (Belle Mead NJ).* 2008;37:415–419.

143. Heim D, Herkert F, Hess P, Regazzoni P. Surgical treatment of humeral shaft fractures—the Basel experience. *J Trauma.* 1993;35:226–232.

144. Henley MB, Monroe M, Tencer AF. Biomechanical comparison of methods of fixation of a midshaft osteotomy of the humerus. *J Orthop Trauma.* 1991;5:14–20.

145. Hennigan SP, Bush-Joseph CA, Kuo KN, Bach BR Jr. Throwing-induced humeral shaft fracture in skeletally immature adolescents. *Orthopedics.* 1999;22:621–622.

146. Hermichen HG, Pfister U, Weller S. Influence of the treatment of fractures on the development of pseudoarthroses of the humerus shaft. *Aktuelle Traumatol.* 1980;10:137–142.

147. Hernandez A, Drez D. Operative treatment of posterior shoulder dislocations by posterior glenoidplasty, capsulorrhaphy, and infraspinatus advancement. *Am J Sports Med.* 1986;14:187–191.

148. Herring JA, Peterson HA. Simple bone cyst with growth arrest. *J Pediatr Orthop.* 1987;7:231–235.
149. Hoffer MM, Phipps GJ. Closed reduction and tendon transfer for treatment of dislocation of the glenohumeral joint secondary to brachial plexus birth palsy. *J Bone Joint Surg Am.* 1998;80:997–1001.
150. Holm CL. Management of humeral shaft fractures. Fundamental nonoperative technics. *Clin Orthop Relat Res.* 1970;71:132–139.
151. Hoppenfeld S, deBoer P, Buckley R. The humerus. In: *Surgical Exposures in Orthopaedics: The Anatomic Approach.* 4th ed. Lippincott Williams & Wilkins; 2009:74–110.
152. Hosner W. Fractures of the shaft of the humerus. An analysis of 100 consecutive cases. *Reconstr Surg Traumatol.* 1974;14(0):38–64.
153. Hosny GA. Unilateral humeral lengthening in children and adolescents. *J Pediatr Orthop B.* 2005;14:439–443.
154. Hovelius L. Anterior dislocation of the shoulder in teen-agers and young adults. Five-year prognosis. *J Bone Joint Surg Am.* 1987;69:393–399.
155. Hovelius L, Olofsson A, Sandström B, et al. Nonoperative treatment of primary anterior shoulder dislocation in patients forty years of age and younger: a prospective twenty-five-year follow-up. *J Bone Joint Surg Am.* 2008;90:945–952.
156. Hovelius L, Saeboe M. Neer Award 2008: Arthropathy after primary anterior shoulder dislocation–223 shoulders prospectively followed up for twenty-five years. *J Shoulder Elbow Surg.* 2009;18:339–347.
157. Hovelius L, Sandström B, Olofsson A, et al. The effect of capsular repair, bone block healing, and position on the results of the Bristow-Latarjet procedure (study III): long-term follow-up in 319 shoulders. *J Shoulder Elbow Surg.* 2012;21:647–660.
158. Hovelius L, Sandström B, Saebö M. One hundred eighteen Bristow-Latarjet repairs for recurrent anterior dislocation of the shoulder prospectively followed for fifteen years: study II-the evolution of dislocation arthropathy. *J Shoulder Elbow Surg.* 2006;15:279–289.
159. Hovelius L, Vikerfors O, Olofsson A, et al. Bristow-Latarjet and Bankart: a comparative study of shoulder stabilization in 185 shoulders during a seventeen-year follow-up. *J Shoulder Elbow Surg.* 2011;20:1095–1101.
160. Howard CB, Shinwell E, Nyska M, Meller I. Ultrasound diagnosis of neonatal fracture separation of the upper humeral epiphysis. *J Bone Joint Surg Br.* 1992;74: 471–472.
161. Hughes JL, Bastrom T, Pennock AT, Edmonds EW. Arthroscopic Bankart repairs with and without remplissage in recurrent adolescent anterior shoulder instability with Hill–Sachs deformity. *Orthop J Sports Med.* 2018;6:2325967118813981.
162. Hugon S, Daubresse F, Depierreux L. Radial nerve entrapment in a humeral fracture callus. *Acta Orthop Belg.* 2008;74:118–121.
163. Husain SN, King EC, Young JL, Sarwark JF. Remodeling of birth fractures of the humeral diaphysis. *J Pediatr Orthop.* 2008;28:10–13.
164. Hutchinson PH, Bae DS, Waters PM. Intramedullary nailing versus percutaneous pin fixation of pediatric proximal humerus fractures: a comparison of complications and early radiographic results. *J Pediatr Orthop.* 2011;31:617–622.
165. Hwang RW, Bae DS, Waters PM. Brachial plexus palsy following proximal humerus fracture in patients who are skeletally immature. *J Orthop Trauma.* 2008;22: 286–290.
166. Ilizarov GA. *Transosseous Osteosynthesis.* Springer-Verlag; 1992.
167. Ilizarov GA, Shevtsov VI. Bloodless compression-distraction osteosynthesis in the treatment of pseudarthroses of the humerus. *Voen Med Zh.* 1974;(6):27–31.
168. Ingman AM, Waters DA. Locked intramedullary nailing of humeral shaft fractures: implant design, surgical technique, and clinical results. *J Bone Joint Surg Br.* 1994;76:23–29.
169. Itoi E, Hatakeyama Y, Kido T, et al. A new method of immobilization after traumatic anterior dislocation of the shoulder: a preliminary study. *J Shoulder Elbow Surg.* 2003;12:413–415.
170. Itoi E, Hatakeyama Y, Sato T, et al. Immobilization in external rotation after shoulder dislocation reduces the risk of recurrence. A randomized controlled trial. *J Bone Joint Surg Am.* 2007;89:2124–2131.
171. Itoi E, Hatakeyama Y, Urayama M, et al. Position of immobilization after dislocation of the shoulder. A cadaveric study. *J Bone Joint Surg Am.* 1999;81:385–390.
172. Itoi E, Sashi R, Minagawa H, et al. Position of immobilization after dislocation of the glenohumeral joint. A study with use of magnetic resonance imaging. *J Bone Joint Surg Am.* 2001;83:661–667.
173. Jaberg H, Warner JJ, Jakob RP. Percutaneous stabilization of unstable fractures of the humerus. *J Bone Joint Surg Am.* 1992;74:508–515.
174. James D, Heinrich SD. Ipsilateral proximal metaphyseal and flexion supracondylar humerus fractures with an associated olecranon avulsion fracture. *Orthopedics.* 1991;14:713–716.
175. Jankauskas L, Rüdiger HA, Pfirrmann CWA, et al. Loss of the sclerotic line of the glenoid on anteroposterior radiographs of the shoulder: a diagnostic sign for an osseous defect of the anterior glenoid rim. *J Shoulder Elbow Surg.* 2010;19:151–156.
176. Jawa A, McCarty P, Doornberg J, et al. Extra-articular distal-third diaphyseal fractures of the humerus. A comparison of functional bracing and plate fixation. *J Bone Joint Surg Am.* 2006;88:2343–2347.
177. Jeffery CC. Fracture separation of the upper humeral epiphysis. *Surg Gynecol Obstet.* 1953;96:205–209.
178. Johnstone DJ, Radford WJ, Parnell EJ. Interobserver variation using the AO/ASIF classification of long bone fractures. *Injury.* 1993;24:163–165.
179. Jones KJ, Wiesel B, Ganley TJ, Wells L. Functional outcomes of early arthroscopic Bankart repair in adolescents aged 11 to 18 years. *J Pediatr Orthop.* 2007;27: 209–213.
180. Jupiter JB. Complex non-union of the humeral diaphysis. Treatment with a medial approach, an anterior plate, and a vascularized fibular graft. *J Bone Joint Surg Am.* 1990;72:701–707.
181. Kaar TK, Schenck RC Jr, Wirth MA, Rockwood CA Jr. Complications of metallic suture anchors in shoulder surgery: a report of 8 cases. *Arthroscopy.* 2001;17:31–37.
182. Kaya M, Karahan N. The effect of different pin configurations on cyclic stability in pediatric proximal humerus fracture fixation: a Sawbones model study. *Injury.* 2022;53:1824–1828.
183. Kelly A, Heath MR, Amoroso EE, et al. Normal humeral head ossification in pediatric and adolescent shoulders can mimic Hill–Sachs lesions: a magnetic resonance imaging-based study. *J Pediatric Orthop.* 2022;42:e143–e148.
184. Khan A, Athlani L, Rousset M, et al. Functional results of displaced proximal humerus fractures in children treated by elastic stable intramedullary nail. *Eur J Orthop Surg Traumatol.* 2014;24:165–172.
185. Khan A, Samba A, Pereira B, Canavese F. Anterior dislocation of the shoulder in skeletally immature patients: comparison between non-operative treatment versus open Latarjet's procedure. *Bone Joint J.* 2014;96-B:354–359.
186. Kim DS, Yoon YS, Yi CH. Prevalence comparison of accompanying lesions between primary and recurrent anterior dislocation in the shoulder. *Am J Sports Med.* 2010;38:2071–2076.
187. Kim NH, Hahn SB, Park HW, Yang IH. The Orthofix external fixator for fractures of long bones. *Int Orthop.* 1994;18:42–46.
188. Kim SH, Szabo RM, Marder RA. Epidemiology of humerus fractures in the United States: nationwide emergency department sample, 2008. *Arthritis Care Res (Hoboken).* 2012;64:407–414.
189. Kirkos JM, Papadopoulos IA. Late treatment of brachial plexus palsy secondary to birth injuries: rotational osteotomy of the proximal part of the humerus. *J Bone Joint Surg Am.* 1998;80:1477–1483.
190. Klasson SC, Vander Schilden JL, Park JP. Late effect of isolated avulsion fractures of the lesser tubercle of the humerus in children. Report of two cases. *J Bone Joint Surg Am.* 1993;75:1691–1694.
191. Kleinman PK, Akins CM. The "vanishing" epiphysis: sign of Salter type I fracture of the proximal humerus in infancy. *Br J Radiol.* 1982;55(659):865–867.
192. Kodali P, Jones MH, Polster J, et al. Accuracy of measurement of Hill–Sachs lesions with computed tomography. *J Shoulder Elbow Surg.* 2011;20:1328–1334.
193. Kohler L. *Roentgenology.* 2nd ed. Balliere, Tindall, and Cox; 1935.
194. Kohler R, Trillaud JM. Fracture and fracture separation of the proximal humerus in children: report of 136 cases. *J Pediatr Orthop.* 1983;3:326–332.
195. Kothari K, Bernstein RM, Griffiths HJ, et al. Luxatio erecta. *Skeletal Radiol.* 1984;11:47–49.
196. Kothari RU, Dronen SC. Prospective evaluation of the scapular manipulation technique in reducing anterior shoulder dislocations. *Ann Emerg Med.* 1992;21: 1349–1352.
197. Kozin SH. Correlation between external rotation of the glenohumeral joint and deformity after brachial plexus birth palsy. *J Pediatr Orthop.* 2004;24:189–193.
198. Kraus T, Hoermann S, Ploder G, et al. Elastic stable intramedullary nailing versus Kirschner wire pinning: outcome of severely displaced proximal humeral fractures in juvenile patients. *J Shoulder Elbow Surg.* 2014;23:1462–1467.
199. Kuhn JE. Treating the initial anterior shoulder dislocation—an evidence-based medicine approach. *Sports Med Arthrosc Rev.* 2006;14:192–198.
200. Kuhns LR, Sherman MP, Poznanski AK, Holt JF. Humeral-head and coracoid ossification in the newborn. *Radiology.* 1973;107:145–149.
201. Kwasny O, Maier R, Kutscha-Lissberg F, Scharf W. Treatment procedure in humeral shaft fractures with primary or secondary radial nerve damage. *Unfallchirurgie.* 1992;18:168–173.
202. Lähdeoja T, Pakkasjärv N, Aronen P, et al. Outcomes at a mean of 13 years after proximal humeral fracture during adolescence. *J Bone Joint Surg.* 2023. doi: 10.2106/JBJS.22.01131
203. Laing PG. The arterial supply of the adult humerus. *J Bone Joint Surg Am.* 1956; 38-A:1105–1116.
204. Lal H, Bansal P, Sabharwal VK, et al. Recurrent shoulder dislocations secondary to coracoid process fracture: a case report. *J Orthop Surg (Hong Kong).* 2012;20: 121–125.
205. Landin LA. Epidemiology of children's fractures. *J Pediatr Orthop B.* 1997;6:79–83.
206. Landin LA. Fracture patterns in children. Analysis of 8,682 fractures with special reference to incidence, etiology and secular changes in a Swedish urban population 1950–1979. *Acta Orthop Scand Suppl.* 1983;202(Suppl):1–109.
207. Langlais T, Hardy MB, Lavoue V, et al. Recurrent posterior shoulder instability starting in childhood and adolescence. *Bone Joint J.* 2020;102-B:1760–1766.
208. Larsen CF, Kiaer T, Lindequist S. Fractures of the proximal humerus in children. Nine-year follow-up of 64 unoperated on cases. *Acta Orthop Scand.* 1990;61: 255–257.
209. Lascombes P, Haumont T, Journeau P. Use and abuse of flexible intramedullary nailing in children and adolescents. *J Pediatr Orthop.* 2006;26:827–834.
210. Lascombes P, Nespola A, Poircuitte JM, et al. Early complications with flexible intramedullary nailing in childhood fracture: 100 cases managed with precurved tip and shaft nails. *Orthop Traumatol Surg Res.* 2012;98:369–375.
211. Lawton RL, Choudhury S, Mansat P, et al. Pediatric shoulder instability: presentation, findings, treatment, and outcomes. *J Pediatr Orthop.* 2002;22:52–61.
212. Lee FY, Schoeb JS, Yu J, et al. Operative lengthening of the humerus: indications, benefits, and complications. *J Pediatr Orthop.* 2005;25:613–616.
213. Leland DP, Bernard CD, Keys LK, et al. An age-based approach to anterior shoulder instability in patients under 40 years old: analysis of a US population. *Am J Sports Med* 2020;48(1):56–62.
214. Lemperg R, Liliequist B. Dislocation of the proximal epiphysis of the humerus in newborns. *Acta Paediatr Scand.* 1970;59:377–380.
215. Leroux T, Ogilvie-Harris D, Veillette C, et al. The epidemiology of primary anterior shoulder dislocations in patients aged 10 to 16 years. *Am J Sports Med.* 2015;43:2111–2117.
216. Leung TY, Stuart O, Suen SSH, et al. Comparison of perinatal outcomes of shoulder dystocia alleviated by different type and sequence of manoeuvers: a retrospective review. *BJOG.* 2011;118:985–990.

217. Levine B, Pereira D, Rosen J. Avulsion fractures of the lesser tuberosity of the humerus in adolescents: review of the literature and case report. *J Orthop Trauma.* 2005;19:349–352.
218. Liavaag S, Brox JI, Pripp AH, et al. Immobilization in external rotation after primary shoulder dislocation did not reduce the risk of recurrence: a randomized controlled trial. *J Bone Joint Surg Am.* 2011;93:897–904.
219. Liebs TR, Rompen I, Berger SM, Ziebarth K. Health-related quality of life after conservatively and surgically-treated paediatric proximal humeral fractures. *J Child Orthop.* 2021;15(3):204–214.
220. Ligier JN, Metaizeau JP, Prévot J. Closed flexible medullary nailing in pediatric traumatology. *Chir Pediatr.* 1983;24:383–385.
221. Limpisvasti O, Yang BY, Hosseinzadeh P, et al. The effect of glenohumeral position on the shoulder after traumatic anterior dislocation. *Am J Sports Med.* 2008;36:775–780.
222. Linn RM, Kriegshauser LA. Ball thrower's fracture of the humerus. A case report. *Am J Sports Med.* 1991;19:194–197.
223. Liu G-Y, Zhang C-Y, Wu H-W. Comparison of initial nonoperative and operative management of radial nerve palsy associated with acute humeral shaft fractures. *Orthopedics.* 2012;35:702–708.
224. Lo IK, Nonweiler B, Woolfrey M, et al. An evaluation of the apprehension, relocation, and surprise tests for anterior shoulder instability. *Am J Sports Med.* 2004;32:301–307.
225. Lock TR, Aronson DD. Fractures in patients who have myelomeningocele. *J Bone Joint Surg Am.* 1989;71:1153–1157.
226. Loder RT. Pediatric polytrauma: orthopaedic care and hospital course. *J Orthop Trauma.* 1987;1:48–54.
227. Loder RT, Bookout C. Fracture patterns in battered children. *J Orthop Trauma.* 1991;5:428–433.
228. Longo UG, van der Linde JA, Loppini M, et al. Surgical versus nonoperative treatment in patients up to 18 years old with traumatic shoulder instability: a systematic review and quantitative synthesis of the literature. *Arthroscopy.* 2016;32:944–952.
229. Lucas JC, Mehlman CT, Laor T. The location of the biceps tendon in completely displaced proximal humerus fractures in children: a report of four cases with magnetic resonance imaging and cadaveric correlation. *J Pediatr Orthop.* 2004;24:249–253.
230. Macfarlane I, Mushayt K. Double closed fractures of the humerus in a child. A case report. *J Bone Joint Surg Am.* 1990;72:443.
231. Machan FG, Vinz H. Humeral shaft fracture in childhood. *Unfallchirurgie.* 1993;19:166–174.
232. Macnicol MF. Roentgenographic evidence of median-nerve entrapment in a greenstick humeral fracture. *J Bone Joint Surg Am.* 1978;60:998–1000.
233. Madsen ET. Fractures of the extremities in the newborn. *Acta Obstet Gynecol Scand.* 1955;34:41–74.
234. Mahabier KC, Vogels LMM, Punt BJ, et al. Humeral shaft fractures: retrospective results of non-operative and operative treatment of 186 patients. *Injury.* 2013;44:427–430.
235. Malhotra A, Freudmann MS, Hay SM. Management of traumatic anterior shoulder dislocation in the 17- to 25-year age group: a dramatic evolution of practice. *J Shoulder Elbow Surg.* 2012;21:545–553.
236. Marans HJ, Angel KR, Schemitsch EH, Wedge JH. The fate of traumatic anterior dislocation of the shoulder in children. *J Bone Joint Surg Am.* 1992;74:1242–1244.
237. Markel DC, Donley BG, Blasier RB. Percutaneous intramedullary pinning of proximal humeral fractures. *Orthop Rev.* 1994;23:667–671.
238. Martin RP, Parsons DL. Avascular necrosis of the proximal humeral epiphysis after physeal fracture. A case report. *J Bone Joint Surg Am.* 1997;79:760–762.
239. Marty B, Käch K, Candinas D, et al. Results of intramedullary nailing in humerus shaft fractures. *Helv Chir Acta.* 1993;59:681–685.
240. Matthews DE, Roberts T. Intraarticular lidocaine versus intravenous analgesic for reduction of acute anterior shoulder dislocations. A prospective randomized study. *Am J Sports Med.* 1995;23:54–58.
241. Matton D, Van Looy F, Geens S. Recurrent anterior dislocations of the shoulder joint treated by the Bristow-Latarjet procedure. Historical review, operative technique and results. *Acta Orthop Belg.* 1992;58:16–22.
242. McNamara RM. Reduction of anterior shoulder dislocations by scapular manipulation. *Ann Emerg Med.* 1993;22:1140–1144.
243. McNeil EL. Luxatio erecta. *Ann Emerg Med.* 1984;13:490–491.
244. McQuillan WM, Nolan B. Ischemia complicating injury. A report of thirty-seven cases. *J Bone Joint Surg Br.* 1968;50:482–492.
245. Mehin R, Mehin A, Wickham D, Letts M. Pinning technique for shoulder fractures in adolescents: computer modelling of percutaneous pinning of proximal humeral fractures. *Can J Surg.* 2009;52:E222–E228.
246. Merten DF, Kirks DR, Ruderman RJ. Occult humeral epiphyseal fracture in battered infants. *Pediatr Radiol.* 1981;10:151–154.
247. Metaizeau JP, Ligier JN. Surgical treatment of fractures of the long bones in children. Interference between osteosynthesis and the physiological processes of consolidation. Therapeutic indications. *J Chir (Paris).* 1984;121(8–9):527–537.
248. Milano G, Grasso A, Russo A, et al. Analysis of risk factors for glenoid bone defect in anterior shoulder instability. *Am J Sports Med.* 2011;39:1870–1876.
249. Milch H. Treatment of dislocation of the shoulder. *Surgery.* 1934;3:732–740.
250. Milch H. The treatment of recent dislocations and fracture-dislocations of the shoulder. *J Bone Joint Surg Am.* 1949;31A:173–180.
251. Miller BS, Sonnabend DH, Hatrick C, et al. Should acute anterior dislocations of the shoulder be immobilized in external rotation? A cadaveric study. *J Shoulder Elbow Surg.* 2004;13:589–592.
252. Miller MC, Redman CN, Mistovich RJ, et al. Single-screw fixation of adolescent salter-ii proximal humeral fractures: biomechanical analysis of the "one pass door lock" technique. *J Pediatr Orthop.* 2017;37:e342–e346.
253. Miller SL, Cleeman E, Auerbach J, Flatow EL. Comparison of intra-articular lidocaine and intravenous sedation for reduction of shoulder dislocations: a randomized, prospective study. *J Bone Joint Surg Am.* 2002;84-A:2135–2139.
254. Mills WJ, Hanel DP, Smith DG. Lateral approach to the humeral shaft: an alternative approach for fracture treatment. *J Orthop Trauma.* 1996;10:81–86.
255. Mimura T, Mori K, Matsusue Y, et al. Closed reduction for traumatic posterior dislocation of the shoulder using the "lever principle": two case reports and a review of the literature. *J Orthop Surg (Hong Kong).* 2006;14:336–339.
256. Moed BR, LaMont RL. Unicameral bone cyst complicated by growth retardation. *J Bone Joint Surg Am.* 1982;64:1379–1381.
257. Moharari RS, Khademhosseini P, Espandar R, et al. Intra-articular lidocaine versus intravenous meperidine/diazepam in anterior shoulder dislocation: a randomised clinical trial. *Emerg Med J.* 2008;25:262–264.
258. Muller M, Allgower M, Schneider R, et al. *Manual of Internal Fixation.* 3rd ed. Springer-Verlag; 1991.
259. Nauth A, McKee MD, Ristevski B, et al. Distal humeral fractures in adults. *J Bone Joint Surg Am.* 2011;93:686–700.
260. Neer CS II. Involuntary inferior and multidirectional instability of the shoulder: etiology, recognition, and treatment. *Instr Course Lect.* 1985;34:232–238.
261. Neer CS II, Horwitz BS. Fractures of the proximal humeral epiphysial plate. *Clin Orthop Relat Res.* 1965;41:24–31.
262. Nelson G, Brown C, Liu RW. No incidence of glenohumeral joint dislocation in a review of 220 paediatric proximal humerus fractures. *J Child Orthop.* 2018;12(5):493–496.
263. Neviaser TJ. The anterior labroligamentous periosteal sleeve avulsion lesion: a cause of anterior instability of the shoulder. *Arthroscopy.* 1993;9:17–21.
264. Nho SJ, Dodson CC, Bardzik KF, et al. The two-step maneuver for closed reduction of inferior glenohumeral dislocation (luxatio erecta to anterior dislocation to reduction). *J Orthop Trauma.* 2006;20:354–357.
265. Noaman H, Khalifa AR, El-Deen MA, Shiha A. Early surgical exploration of radial nerve injury associated with fracture shaft humerus. *Microsurgery.* 2008;28:635–642.
266. Obremskey W, Routt ML Jr. Fracture-dislocation of the shoulder in a child: case report. *J Trauma.* 1994;36:137–140.
267. O'Connor DR, Schwarze D, Fragomen AT, Perdomo M. Painless reduction of acute anterior shoulder dislocations without anesthesia. *Orthopedics.* 2006;29:528–532.
268. O'Driscoll SW, Evans DC. Contralateral shoulder instability following anterior repair. An epidemiological investigation. *J Bone Joint Surg Br.* 1991;73:941–946.
269. Ogawa BK, Kay RM, Choi PD, Stevanovic MV. Complete division of the radial nerve associated with a closed fracture of the humeral shaft in a child. *J Bone Joint Surg Br.* 2007;89:821–824.
270. Ogawa K, Yoshida A. Throwing fracture of the humeral shaft. An analysis of 90 patients. *Am J Sports Med.* 1998;26:242–246.
271. Ogden JA, Conlogue GJ, Jensen P. Radiology of postnatal skeletal development: the proximal humerus. *Skeletal Radiol.* 1978;2:153–160.
272. Olds M, Donaldson K, Ellis R, Kersten P. In children 18 years and under, what promotes recurrent shoulder instability after traumatic anterior shoulder dislocation? A systematic review and meta-analysis of risk factors. *Br J Sports Med.* 2016;50:1135–1141.
273. Ortiz EJ, Isler MH, Navia JE, Canosa R. Pathologic fractures in children. *Clin Orthop Relat Res.* 2005;(432):116–126.
274. Ouyang H, Xiong J, Xiang P, et al. Plate versus intramedullary nail fixation in the treatment of humeral shaft fractures: an updated meta-analysis. *J Shoulder Elbow Surg.* 2013;22:387–395.
275. Owens BD, Agel J, Mountcastle SB, et al. Incidence of glenohumeral instability in collegiate athletics. *Am J Sports Med.* 2009;37:1750–1754.
276. Owens BD, Dawson L, Burks R, Cameron KL. Incidence of shoulder dislocation in the United States military: demographic considerations from a high-risk population. *J Bone Joint Surg Am.* 2009;91:791–796.
277. Owens BD, Nelson BJ, Duffey ML, et al. Pathoanatomy of first-time, traumatic, anterior glenohumeral subluxation events. *J Bone Joint Surg Am.* 2010;92:1605–1611.
278. Pahlavan S, Baldwin KD, Pandya NK, et al. Proximal humerus fractures in the pediatric population: a systematic review. *J Child Orthop.* 2011;5:187–194.
279. Patel DN, Zuckerman JD, Egol KA. Luxatio erecta: case series with review of diagnostic and management principles. *Am J Orthop (Belle Mead NJ).* 2011;40:566–570.
280. Paterson WH, Throckmorton TW, Koester M, et al. Position and duration of immobilization after primary anterior shoulder dislocation: a systematic review and meta-analysis of the literature. *J Bone Joint Surg Am.* 2010;92:2924–2933.
281. Patte D, Debeyre J. Luxations recidivantes de l'epaule. *Encycl Med Chir Paris-Technique chirurgicale Orthopedie.* 1980;44265(4).
282. Peterson HA. Surgical lengthening of the humerus: case report and review. *J Pediatr Orthop.* 1989;9:596–601.
283. Peterson HA, Madhok R, Benson JT, et al. Physeal fractures: part 1. Epidemiology in Olmsted County, Minnesota, 1979–1988. *J Pediatr Orthop.* 1994;14:423–430.
284. Phipps GJ, Hoffer MM. Latissimus dorsi and teres major transfer to rotator cuff for Erb's palsy. *J Shoulder Elbow Surg.* 1995;4:124–129.
285. Piasecki DP, Verma NN, Romeo AA, et al. Glenoid bone deficiency in recurrent anterior shoulder instability: diagnosis and management. *J Am Acad Orthop Surg.* 2009;17:482–493.
286. Pogorelić Z, Kadić S, Milunović KP, et al. Flexible intramedullary nailing for treatment of proximal humerus and humeral shaft fractures in children: a retrospective series of 118 cases. *Orthop Traumatol Surg Res.* 2017;103:765–770.
287. Pritchett JW. Growth and predictions of growth in the upper extremity. *J Bone Joint Surg Am.* 1988;70:520–525.
288. Pritchett JW. Growth plate activity in the upper extremity. *Clin Orthop Relat Res.* 1991;(268):235–242.
289. Provencher MT, Ghodadra N, Romeo AA. Arthroscopic management of anterior instability: pearls, pitfalls, and lessons learned. *Orthop Clin North Am.* 2010;41:325–337.
290. Provencher MT, Verma N, Obopilwe E, et al. A biomechanical analysis of capsular plication versus anchor repair of the shoulder: can the labrum be used as a suture anchor?. *Arthroscopy.* 2008;24:210–216.

20

Clavicle and Scapula Fractures and Acromioclavicular and Sternoclavicular Injuries

Benton E. Heyworth

Midshaft Clavicle Fractures

INTRODUCTION

The clavicle is one of the most commonly fractured bones in children, representing 5% to 15% of all pediatric fractures.[90] The most common location for a clavicle fracture is the midshaft of the bone, accounting for up to 80% of fractures.[29,90,93,97] Despite this high incidence, relatively little literature exists regarding management and outcomes of pediatric clavicle fractures. Much of the literature cited throughout this chapter is therefore extrapolated from scientific studies of adult clavicle fractures. However, there is an increasing trend for operative fixation in adults and older children.[117,135] Therefore, more scientific investigations regarding the management of clavicle fractures in children are being performed, the results of which are of utmost importance to elucidation of future treatment algorithms for this younger population. An adolescent clavicle fracture study group was formed specifically to address the paucity of age-specific investigations regarding the optimal treatments for different adolescent subpopulations.[29] Until a more methodologically rigorous and comprehensive body of evidence emerges regarding the optimal treatment approach in children and, in particular, adolescents, clavicle fractures are one of the most controversial areas in pediatric orthopaedics and sports medicine.

ASSESSMENT OF MIDSHAFT CLAVICLE FRACTURES

MECHANISMS OF INJURY FOR MIDSHAFT CLAVICLE FRACTURES

Clavicle fractures are common in children from birth to skeletal maturity, with different mechanisms of injury accounting for fractures in different age groups.

involved in high-energy mechanisms of injury. The vessel can spasm, have a thrombosis from blunt trauma, or rarely have a penetrating injury. Assessment of the radial pulse should be symmetric and if there is any concern for injury of the vessel, further diagnostic evaluation with advanced imaging should be performed.

IMAGING AND OTHER DIAGNOSTIC STUDIES FOR MIDSHAFT CLAVICLE FRACTURES

Initial imaging of a suspected clavicle fracture includes plain radiographs of the clavicle in two projections. Typically, a standard anteroposterior (AP) radiograph and a cephalic tilt view, ranging from 15-degree cephalad to 45-degree cephalad, are obtained (Fig. 20-3). These images provide visualization of the shoulder girdle region as well as the upper lung fields, both of which should be assessed for additional injuries. However, if clinical suspicion is present for additional injuries, dedicated series of the suspected part(s) should be obtained.

Clavicle fractures are often detected on chest x-rays obtained for trauma patients, and rarely require additional imaging, if the general fracture pattern and approximate shortening can be assessed for completely displaced fractures. Advanced imaging is rarely needed to evaluate clavicle fractures, as the fracture pattern, displacement, and presence of comminution can almost always be assessed on plain films. As described in greater detail below, fractures or suspected dislocations about the sternoclavicular joint are frequently assessed with computed tomography (CT) scans, but midshaft fractures, which are much more common, benefit from such imaging only in the case of a suspected or possible fracture nonunion or possible refracture through a healing fracture. Distal fractures are assessed by CT scans at times to decide on degree and direction of displacement that might indicate need for operative intervention.

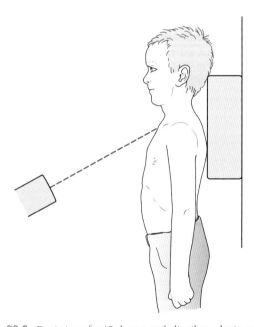

Figure 20-3. Depiction of a 45-degree cephalic tilt to obtain an additional view of the clavicle.

CLASSIFICATION OF MIDSHAFT CLAVICLE FRACTURES

Clavicle fractures are usually described based on the location of the fracture, the fracture pattern, and the presence or absence of displacement. Thus, clavicle fractures are either medial, midshaft, or lateral; nondisplaced or displaced; open or closed; comminuted or simple. Displaced fractures can be qualified as partially displaced, when the two fracture fragments of a two-part fracture are still in contact, with or without angulation, whereas completely displaced fractures have fracture fragments that are not in contact with each other, or are three- or four-part fractures with comminution. The description of partially displaced fractures with angulation benefit from a measurement of the degree of angulation, as increasing angulation has been associated with a greater risk of refracture in some studies.[35,75] For completely displaced fractures, a measurement of the degree of "shortening," as measured in millimeters (mm), has been used more commonly in adult clavicle fracture studies. For example, some authors have contended that shortening of more than 14 or 20 mm may be associated with poorer outcomes with nonoperative treatment, when compared with lesser amounts of shortening. As a result, many have considered 20 mm as a potential threshold or an indication for surgery. However, important studies by Schulz et al.[108] and Bae et al.[8] have suggested that even fractures with more than 15 to 20 mm of shortening are not associated with functional limitations in adolescents treated nonoperatively. Moreover, new research suggests that traditional measurement techniques may grossly overestimate the "true" shortening of the clavicle, by not accounting for the oblique nature of clavicle fractures.[71] Thus, we believe that additional research is warranted before adult-based metrics are applied to the young who have greater healing and remodeling capacity. Classifications that go beyond this descriptive scheme, such as the AO classification,[34] have been proposed to evaluate clavicle fractures, but none are widely utilized, as they are either purely descriptive of fracture location[3] or cumbersome with multiple types and subtypes.[34]

OUTCOME MEASURES FOR MIDSHAFT CLAVICLE FRACTURES

No specific outcome scores have been widely used to assess results following pediatric clavicle fractures, though the American Shoulder and Elbow Society (ASES) score, the Disability of the Arm, Shoulder, and Hand (DASH) Score, the QuickDASH, and the Constant Shoulder Score have been utilized. The creation of a novel Pediatric and Adolescent Shoulder and Elbow Survey (Pedi-ASES) has stemmed from research demonstrating that adult shoulder outcome scores are associated with poor validity and comprehensibility. The Pedi-ASES may represent a future standard for use in pediatric and adolescent shoulder research.[45]

PATHOANATOMY AND APPLIED ANATOMY RELATED TO MIDSHAFT CLAVICLE FRACTURES

The clavicle, also referred to as the collar bone, is an S-shaped bone that lies along the subcutaneous border of the anterior aspect of the shoulder girdle. An anterior convexity is present medially to permit the passage of the brachial plexus and axillary vessels from the neck region into the upper arm, whereas laterally there is an anterior concavity.

Development of the clavicle begins at 5 and a half weeks' gestation via intramembranous ossification, and by 8 weeks, the bone has developed into its S-shaped configuration. Postnatally, the clavicle continues to grow at a steady rate until age 12, increasing approximately 8.4 mm per year.[78] After 12 years of age, the clavicle grows approximately 2.6 mm per year in females and 5.4 mm per year in males. Thus, 80% of the final clavicle length is reached by age 9 in females and age 12 in males.[78] While some authors have cited these findings to suggest limited remodeling capacity for fractures in adolescents,[73] other studies have demonstrated the ongoing ossification of the clavicle until age 25, as it is known to be the last bone in the body to complete its ossification process.[36] As a result, the final 20% of clavicular growth may be clinically enough to allow substantial remodeling, including in older adolescents. Along these lines, Pennock et al. demonstrated considerable remodeling capacity in adolescents of various ages between 10 and 18 years old.[95] In their study of 98 adolescents with mean radiographic follow-up of 3.4 years, the authors demonstrated that 85% of adolescents aged under 14 years and 54% of patients aged 14 years or older at the time of injury demonstrated "complete" or "near-complete" remodeling, with improvement in each of three different radiographic parameters, including clavicular length/fracture shortening, superior displacement, and angulation of the original completely displaced fracture.

Medially, the clavicle articulates with the sternum, forming the sternoclavicular joint, whereas laterally the bone ends in an articulation with the acromion, forming the AC joint. The medial inferior aspect of the clavicle is the site of attachment of the costoclavicular ligament, whereas laterally on the inferior aspect there is the conoid tubercle and trapezoid line, the sites of attachment for the conoid and trapezoid ligaments, respectively.

All these ligaments slant posteriorly as they approach the clavicle, and therefore when the clavicle elevates and the ligaments are put on stretch, the clavicle rotates posteriorly. In addition, these ligaments provide significant stability at both ends of the clavicle, thus making fractures in the middle third of the clavicle more likely.

The pectoralis major originates from the medial aspect of the clavicle as well as the sternum and inserts onto the humerus at the intertubercular groove, whereas the deltoid originates from the lateral aspect of the clavicle as well as the acromion and scapular spine to insert onto the humerus at the deltoid tuberosity. In addition, the sternocleidomastoid and sternohyoid muscles originate from the clavicle whereas the trapezius and subclavius insert onto the clavicle.

TREATMENT OPTIONS FOR MIDSHAFT CLAVICLE FRACTURES

The mainstay of treatment of pediatric and adolescent clavicle fractures is nonoperative, allowing the fracture to form callous and heal in situ, even if significant displacement is present (Fig. 20-4).[8] It is well agreed upon that nondisplaced or partially displaced fractures, even those that are moderately angulated in an apex-superior pattern, should be treated nonoperatively. Fractures that should proceed directly to operative intervention include open fractures, fractures with severe skin tenting associated with blanching, hypovascular skin, or skin "at risk" for necrosis (i.e., skin with pallor or clear dysvascularity), and fractures with associated neurovascular injuries clearly affecting motor function or blood supply to the upper extremity. Decreased sensation in the skin of the chest wall distal to the fracture may be reported and likely stems from contusions or stretch injuries to the superficial supraclavicular sensory nerves. While case reports of supraclavicular nerve branches entrapped

Figure 20-4. **A:** Radiograph of a moderately displaced diaphyseal right clavicular fracture. **B:** Radiograph of the healed fracture with abundant callus formation, demonstrating the potential of remodeling with growth. (Reprinted with permission from Waters PM, Bae DS, eds. *Pediatric Hand and Upper Limb Surgery: A Practical Guide.* Wolters Kluwer; 2012.)

in fracture callus have been published,[55] and may benefit from surgical exploration and neurolysis, at least in the setting of persistently severe symptoms, these represent the minority of cases, and chest wall numbness does not represent an independent indication for surgery. Monitoring over the course of 2 or 3 months after injury may represent a reasonable period to assess the resolution of sensory symptoms associated with a completely displaced or comminuted fracture. Of course, these same nerves are at risk for injury during primary surgical fixation.

NONOPERATIVE TREATMENT

Nonoperative treatment of clavicle fractures is performed by immobilizing the child's shoulder girdle, typically with a sling. Younger children may benefit from a sling and swath, at least in the first several days postinjury, primarily to improve comfort levels. While more traditional figure-of-eight dressings or shoulder immobilizers can be utilized, these are more cumbersome and have not been shown to provide improved results. Neonates who sustain a clavicular fracture during the birthing process can be immobilized with a swath technique, such as placing cast padding or a soft elastic bandage around the torso and arm, but, due to the speed of callus formation, can usually be discontinued within 1 week.

Follow-up radiographs are obtained at the 2-week, 6-week, and 3-month postinjury intervals until fracture union occurs. A 2-week postinjury radiograph allows for confirmation of maintenance of the fracture alignment or degree of shortening seen at the time of injury, as some nondisplaced fractures can displace in the early postinjury phase. Such a visit will also allow for a progression to use of the sling only when ambulating or at school, while the sling can often be discontinued as comfort allows when at home, from the 2-week to the 6-week period. A 6-week visit frequently shows significant callus formation stabilizing the fracture, which can allow for discontinuation of the sling, with an understanding that refractures can occur with falls or premature return to sports.[19] However, noncontact fitness and sports activities can usually be allowed at 6 weeks, provided there is intermediate healing. Strength training, including upper body weightlifting, can be progressed as symptoms allow, with most patients having no symptoms at the 6-week postinjury visit. Return to contact sports may be pursued if 3-month radiograph has confirmed advanced callous formation or bony bridging. Calder et al. have suggested that follow-up radiographs are unnecessary in pediatric patients, given the near-universal expected fracture healing rate in a child.[19] This may be a reasonable approach to those under 13 years old, depending on the activity level of the patient. However, in adolescent athletes, radiographs are routinely obtained by many until union is established to assess the appropriate timing of return to sports with decreased refracture risk.[19]

Outcomes and Return to Sport

Despite the high incidence of pediatric clavicle fractures and the fact that most of these fractures are treated nonoperatively, little data exist regarding the outcomes of these injuries. Union rates from 95% to 100% have been reported with nonoperative

treatment.[41,60,126] Most nondisplaced fractures have demonstrated union by 4 to 8 weeks of time, whereas displaced fractures take longer, approximately 10 to 12 weeks.[126]

Overall, most patients have excellent outcomes and are able to return to their activities without limitations. A small percentage of patients treated nonoperatively with significant fracture displacement may have subjective complaints of pain with prolonged activity, easy fatiguability, axillary pain, or drooping shoulders with bony prominence.[126] Bae et al. evaluated a group of 16 patients with displaced (>2 cm) middiaphyseal clavicle fractures treated nonoperatively. All fractures united with no meaningful loss of shoulder motion or abduction–adduction strength by isokinetic testing. The vast majority of patients had low DASH and pain Visual Analog Scores (VAS) that were very low, means of 4.9 and 1.6, respectively. Notably, 1 patient of 16 required a corrective osteotomy, but this must be understood as a rare event in the context of retrospective study performed at a tertiary care regional referral center.[8] The authors concluded that routine surgical fixation for displaced, nonsegmental clavicle fractures may not be justified based on concerns regarding shoulder motion and strength alone. In recent years, a series of studies have emerged that have further substantiated nonoperative treatment as the gold standard of care for adolescents, even those with completely displaced fractures. Ng et al.[88] retrospectively assessed 606 midshaft fractures in adolescents, 263 of which were completely displaced. They identified only one case of nonunion (0.4%), a 3.2% rate of refracture (all of which subsequently healed with nonoperative treatment), and high patient-reported outcome (PRO) and satisfaction scores, concluding that relative surgical indications utilized in adult fractures are not applicable to adolescents. Similarly, Risser et al.[102] retrospectively compared outcomes of 61 and 48 adolescents with displaced midshaft fractures treated nonoperatively and operatively and found no difference in PROs, only one case of nonunion with nonoperative treatment (1.6%), and no clear indication for performing surgery in the adolescent age group. Swarup et al.[118] also performed a retrospective assessment of 43 operatively treated and 36 nonoperatively treated adolescent clavicle fractures, with no instances of nonunion and similar PROs and refracture rates. In one of the few prospective, comparative cohort studies in the literature, and the largest adolescent level 2 study to date, Heyworth et al. prospectively assessed the complications and outcomes of 416 completely displaced midshaft clavicle fractures in patients 10 to 18 years old.[46] All patients were followed through the bony healing period, with over two-thirds (68%) providing 2-year follow-up PROs. While there was no statistically significant difference in functional outcomes between the operative and nonoperative cohorts, surgical patients had significantly more complications and more unexpected subsequent surgeries following initial treatment. Compared with adult studies and systematic reviews citing rates of nonunion and symptomatic malunion in the range of 15% and 10%, respectively, the large cohort followed by Heyworth et al. showed exceedingly low rates of complications such as nonunion (0.4%), delayed union (1.9%), symptomatic malunion (0.4%), and refracture (2.6%), with no differences in these between treatment cohorts.[46] While some authors cite the advantage of a faster recovery with operative treatment, this young cohort had uneventful return to activities that was not shown to be different between cohorts. Notably, another study of 47 high school athletes in South Carolina demonstrated that nonoperatively treated clavicle fracture patients returned to sport 40% faster than those treated with surgery.[2] Another retrospective study assessing cohorts of operatively and nonoperatively treated midshaft clavicle fractures of 55 pediatric or adolescent fractures each demonstrated no difference in full return to activities or QuickDASH scores.[4] Interestingly, 22% of the nonoperative group sustained refractures, which is a higher rate than that reported in comparable subpopulations, while 27% of the operative group underwent secondary surgery for removal of implants.

Indications/Contraindications

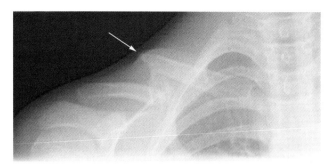

Figure 20-5. Radiograph of a segmental right diaphyseal fracture causing skin tenting (*arrow*) and subsequent compromise. Note the vertical nature of the segmental fragment. (Reprinted with permission from Waters PM, Bae DS, eds. *Pediatric Hand and Upper Limb Surgery: A Practical Guide*. Wolters Kluwer; 2012.)

Nonoperative Treatment of Midshaft Clavicle Fractures:
INDICATIONS AND CONTRAINDICATIONS

Indications

- Nondisplaced fractures
- Partially displaced fractures (without severe angulation)
- Completely displaced fractures without severe shortening (<3 cm)

Contraindications

- Open fractures
- Fractures associated with neurovascular injury

Relative Contraindications

- "Floating shoulder" injury pattern (concomitant completely displaced fractures of clavicle and humeral shaft or glenoid neck)
- Fractures associated with severe skin tenting (blanching, hypovascular, skin at risk for necrosis)
- Fractures associated with polytrauma injury (multiple extremity fractures for which earlier upper extremity weight bearing would be highly beneficial to global health and mobility goals)

OPERATIVE TREATMENT OF MIDSHAFT CLAVICLE FRACTURES

Absolute indications for operative treatment of clavicle fractures in the pediatric and adolescent population include open fractures and fractures associated with neurovascular injury. Additional relative indications may include fractures with severe skin tenting/compromise (Fig. 20-5), floating shoulder injuries, and fractures associated with polytrauma, in which multiple extremities are compromised and stabilization of the clavicle may greatly enhance or speed rehabilitation goals. Floating shoulder injuries involving displaced midshaft clavicle fractures and fractures of the glenoid neck or humeral shaft treated by open reduction internal fixation (ORIF) of the clavicle alone can be sufficient as ligamentotaxis can reduce the other fracture via the coracoclavicular (CC) ligament.[9]

A subset of displaced adult fractures treated nonoperatively have been shown to heal with malunion that can cause changes to shoulder mechanics. These alterations may lead to pain with overhead activities, decreased strength, and decreased endurance.[79] Therefore, multiple studies have investigated the benefit of operative fixation versus nonoperative management of displaced midshaft clavicle fractures. The most impactful of such studies was a randomized controlled trial of an adult Canadian population with a mean age of 33.5 years, in which the operative cohort was shown to have improved functional outcome measures and lower rates of nonunion and symptomatic malunion than the nonoperative cohort.[20] A subsequent meta-analysis evaluating the results of randomized clinical trials that compared nonoperative and operative treatment in adults confirmed a significantly higher nonunion and symptomatic malunion rate in the nonoperative group. In addition, patients treated with operative intervention had earlier functional return.[80] The recent studies in adolescents[46,88,102,118] have elucidated that these adult findings are not clearly transferable to adolescents, and randomized controlled trials in other adult populations[106,127] have suggested that the indications for surgery are more limited in adult populations than suggested by the Canadian study. Clearly, younger children, especially less than age 13 years, have the potential to remodel even a foreshortened, displaced fracture. The approach to older adolescents remains a shared decision-making process with families of young athletes, with considerations toward the severity of the fracture pattern, the sports played, and the tolerance level for a malunion that is likely to demonstrate a full return to function. Importantly, to date, no studies in adolescent populations have demonstrated clear superiority of operative treatment over nonoperative treatment, given the significantly lower rates of nonunion and symptomatic malunion in adolescents, relative to adults, and there now exists data to share with parents that are applicable to their adolescent sons and daughters. With some concern that surgery, on average, actually increases the risk of complications and unexpected subsequent surgeries, the pediatric orthopaedic community may have a responsibility to emphasize the importance of protecting our children from such risks, though more nuanced and substratified research is needed to confirm the comparative findings in various adolescent subpopulations.

Open Reduction and Internal Fixation or Intramedullary Fixation

Preoperative Planning

☑	**Operative Treatment of Midshaft Clavicle Fractures:** PREOPERATIVE PLANNING CHECKLIST
OR table	❑ Standard table capable of going into beach chair position
Position/ positioning aids	❑ Supine beach chair position with head and neck tilted away ❑ Bump placed behind the scapula
Fluoroscopy location	❑ Surgeon's preference (may be ipsilateral or contralateral to fracture)
Equipment	❑ Surgeon's choice of implant (precontoured 3.5-mm clavicle plates or dual/orthogonal 2.4-mm minifragment plates, which have been shown to have lower rates of implant removal)
Draping	❑ Shoulder girdle, entire clavicle, and ipsilateral limb are prepped and draped into the field to allow for visualization traction and manipulation ❑ Medially, the ipsilateral sternoclavicular joint should be included in the operative field

As with any internal fixation procedure, it is imperative to have the desired implants available before proceeding to the OR. Options for treatment of pediatric and adolescent clavicle fractures include anatomically designed manufacturer-precontoured clavicle plates, standard nonlocking and locking plates, and intramedullary devices including pins, wires, screws, and elastic nails.

Intramedullary fixation has the potential benefits of requiring less soft tissue stripping at the fracture site, better aesthetics with smaller skin incisions, easier implant removal, less potential for implant irritation, and less bony weakness following implant removal compared with plate fixation. However, the ability to resist torsional forces is less with intramedullary fixation compared with plating, which can result in fracture of the intramedullary implant (Fig. 20-6). Furthermore, the potential for nonblocking intramedullary devices to migrate is a major concern for many surgeons, thus limiting its usage. More modern intramedullary devices with locking potential have decreased concerns regarding migration of traditional Kirschner-wire (K-wire) constructs but are more likely to require secondary implant removal surgeries to avoid soft tissue irritation at the posterolateral clavicle entry sites.

Thus, the locking intramedullary implants are preferred by some, but not only do they have a higher risk of undergoing removal in a young population, there is also risk of disabling the locking mechanism in the setting of a refracture, with a potentially catastrophic phenomenon of inability to remove a portion of the implant without more invasive bony interventions. Eisenstein et al.[28] reported difficulty advancing a 2-mm nail beyond the lateral 2 to 3 cm of the distal segment in seven adolescent clavicle fractures, as well as a removal of implant rate of 57%.

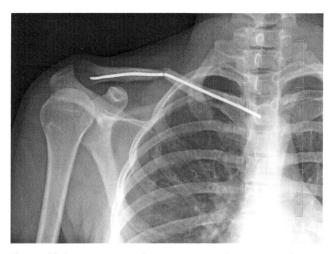

Figure 20-6. Radiograph of a right midshaft clavicular fracture treated with an intramedullary elastic nail, which subsequently went on to fracture. (Reprinted with permission from Waters PM, Bae DS, eds. *Pediatric Hand and Upper Limb Surgery: A Practical Guide.* Wolters Kluwer; 2012.)

If plate fixation is being planned, one must determine what the preferred location of the plate will be, anteroinferior or superior. Anteroinferior plates have the advantage of performing drilling in a posterosuperior direction, and thus the drill is not directed toward the surrounding neurovascular structures. In addition, the plate may be less prominent in this location. However, the anterior position of the plate may compromise the soft tissue reattachment of the important pectoralis major muscle complex. Superior placement of the plate is both technically easier and allows for better resistance of the biomechanical forces acting to displace the fracture.

Positioning

Options for positioning during ORIF of clavicle fractures include using the beach chair position (i.e., ~60 degrees), having the patient supine, or different degrees of torso elevation in between the two, that is, "sloppy beach chair" positioning (e.g., ~45 degrees). With either position, a bump may be placed behind the scapula to bring the fracture fragments forward for ease of dissection.

Surgical Approach

ORIF is performed via a direct surgical approach to the clavicle using a skin incision that follows Langer lines. To avoid problems by having the incision directly over the plate, as well as to improve aesthetics, incise the skin on the inferior aspect of the clavicle,[24] or even up to 1 to 2 cm distal to the clavicle, with proximal dissection to the fracture site. Once the skin is incised, the platysma is dissected, revealing the underlying cutaneous supraclavicular nerves as they cross the clavicle, which should be identified and protected to avoid chest wall numbness, dysesthesias, or neuromas. Meticulous subperiosteal dissection is then carried out to expose the fracture site while ensuring maintenance of the soft tissue attachments to any malrotated or segmental fracture fragments. Preservation of the integrity of the periosteum, which may be torn at the site of the fracture, is critical to the postfixation closure of this layer, which will aid in optimization of bone healing and minimization of hardware irritation. The posteroinferior periosteal sleeve also protects the underlying neurovascular structures.

Intramedullary fixation is performed by making a similar approach using a small incision over the fracture site to expose only the ends of fracture fragments. An additional percutaneous incision is placed over the superolateral part of the clavicle to place the intramedullary device in an antegrade manner.

Technique

Open Reduction and Internal Fixation

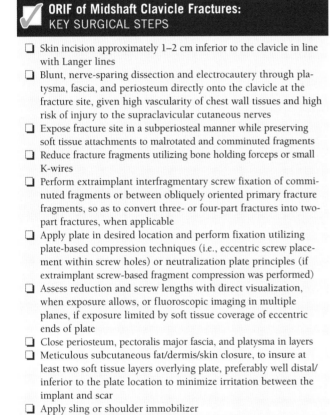

✓ ORIF of Midshaft Clavicle Fractures:
KEY SURGICAL STEPS

- ❏ Skin incision approximately 1–2 cm inferior to the clavicle in line with Langer lines
- ❏ Blunt, nerve-sparing dissection and electrocautery through platysma, fascia, and periosteum directly onto the clavicle at the fracture site, given high vascularity of chest wall tissues and high risk of injury to the supraclavicular cutaneous nerves
- ❏ Expose fracture site in a subperiosteal manner while preserving soft tissue attachments to malrotated and comminuted fragments
- ❏ Reduce fracture fragments utilizing bone holding forceps or small K-wires
- ❏ Perform extraimplant interfragmentary screw fixation of comminuted fragments or between obliquely oriented primary fracture fragments, so as to convert three- or four-part fractures into two-part fractures, when applicable
- ❏ Apply plate in desired location and perform fixation utilizing plate-based compression techniques (i.e., eccentric screw placement within screw holes) or neutralization plate principles (if extraimplant screw-based fragment compression was performed)
- ❏ Assess reduction and screw lengths with direct visualization, when exposure allows, or fluoroscopic imaging in multiple planes, if exposure limited by soft tissue coverage of eccentric ends of plate
- ❏ Close periosteum, pectoralis major fascia, and platysma in layers
- ❏ Meticulous subcutaneous fat/dermis/skin closure, to insure at least two soft tissue layers overlying plate, preferably well distal/inferior to the plate location to minimize irritation between the implant and scar
- ❏ Apply sling or shoulder immobilizer

For these patients, we use the beach chair position and make our skin incision approximately 1 cm inferior to the clavicle, to prevent scar formation in the area of eventual plate location. Following a nerve-sparing approach to dissection to the level of the periosteum, sharp dissection through the periosteum allows for exposure of the fracture fragments. Reduction is performed utilizing bone holding forceps, and either plate-based compression techniques are used or extraimplant interfragmentary screw fixation is performed for comminuted fragments or between obliquely oriented primary fracture fragments. It is imperative to restore the length and contour of the clavicle during the reduction process. Because comminuted fractures are among the more common fractures that, overall, undergo

operative fixation, interfragmentary fixation of a free fragment with a 2.0- or 2.7-mm lag screw is helpful in turning a three-part or four-part fracture into a two-part fracture amenable to plate placement. Once the reduction is anatomic, the plate is applied on the superior aspect of the clavicle. During drilling and screw placement, we protect the surrounding neurovascular structures by placement of blunt Homan retractors or a malleable retractor inferior to the clavicle. Following provisional plate placement, fluoroscopic biplanar imaging and/or direct visualization is utilized to assess the fracture reduction, screw lengths, and central screw placement, given that eccentric screw placement, particularly at the far-medial or far-lateral plate position, risks refracture with any return to contact sports. Compression techniques with eccentric drilling within the oblique holes of the plate are considered critical to an anatomic final reduction and optimization of healing rates. The wound is then thoroughly irrigated and the periosteum closed. We favor closure of the overlying fascial layer and platysma layer, to optimize soft tissue coverage over the subcutaneous plate. Final assessment of the supraclavicular nerves is performed to be certain they are intact and without entrapment. A meticulous dermal layer and subcuticular closure is then performed to obtain the best cosmetic result possible and decrease the chance of wound complications. Sterile dressings are applied followed by placement of the patient into a simple shoulder sling.

Intramedullary Fixation

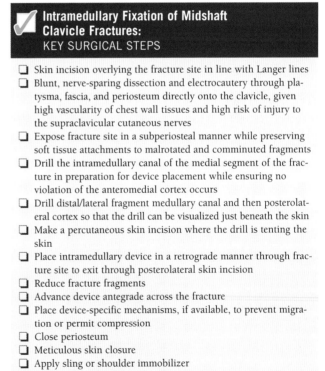

✓ Intramedullary Fixation of Midshaft
Clavicle Fractures:
KEY SURGICAL STEPS

- ❏ Skin incision overlying the fracture site in line with Langer lines
- ❏ Blunt, nerve-sparing dissection and electrocautery through platysma, fascia, and periosteum directly onto the clavicle, given high vascularity of chest wall tissues and high risk of injury to the supraclavicular cutaneous nerves
- ❏ Expose fracture site in a subperiosteal manner while preserving soft tissue attachments to malrotated and comminuted fragments
- ❏ Drill the intramedullary canal of the medial segment of the fracture in preparation for device placement while ensuring no violation of the anteromedial cortex occurs
- ❏ Drill distal/lateral fragment medullary canal and then posterolateral cortex so that the drill can be visualized just beneath the skin
- ❏ Make a percutaneous skin incision where the drill is tenting the skin
- ❏ Place intramedullary device in a retrograde manner through fracture site to exit through posterolateral skin incision
- ❏ Reduce fracture fragments
- ❏ Advance device antegrade across the fracture
- ❏ Place device-specific mechanisms, if available, to prevent migration or permit compression
- ❏ Close periosteum
- ❏ Meticulous skin closure
- ❏ Apply sling or shoulder immobilizer

A skin incision is made overlying the fracture site in line with Langer lines. The platysma is dissected, and supraclavicular cutaneous nerves are identified and protected. The fracture site is exposed in a subperiosteal manner. The soft tissue attachments to malrotated and comminuted fragments are preserved.

The intramedullary canal of the medial fracture fragment is drilled in preparation for device placement, with care taken to ensure no violation of the anteromedial cortex occurs. The distal fragment medullary canal and then the posterolateral cortex are drilled so that the drill can be visualized just beneath the skin. A percutaneous skin incision is made where the drill is tenting the skin. The intramedullary device is placed in a retrograde manner through fracture site to exit through posterolateral skin incision. Fracture fragments are reduced, and the device is advanced in an antegrade manner across the fracture. If available, device-specific mechanisms are placed to prevent migration or permit compression. The periosteum, overlying fascial layers, platysma layer, and skin are closed. A sling or shoulder immobilizer is applied.

Author's Preferred Treatment for Midshaft Clavicle Fractures (Algorithm 20-1)

[1]Shared decision-making approach, based on latest evidence, including slightly increased refracture risk;[95] may be relevant to contact athletes
[2]Assessment of true shortening should be achieved with 'cortex to corresponding cortex' technique, rather than 'end to end' technique[97a]
[3]Shared decision-making approach, based on latest evidence, including a low risk of symptomatic malunion; may be relevant

Algorithm 20-1. Authors' preferred treatment for midshaft clavicle fractures.

Most pediatric and adolescent clavicle fractures are treated nonoperatively with initial immobilization. In general, full-time use of the sling, other than for bathing, is advised during the first 2 weeks after injury. From 2 weeks postinjury, at which time an office-based visit can allow for confirmation of early fracture healing, initial callus formation, and reported improvement in overall patient comfort, to 6 weeks postinjury, adolescents may be allowed to remove the sling when at home. However, it is generally advisable to continue sling use when out of the house and at school, given that symptoms are usually quite minimal, but risk of early refracture or disruption of callus formation can occur. At 6 weeks postinjury, the sling is discontinued altogether, and patients are allowed to return to noncontact sports and sports training, including weight-based strength training and push-ups. Contact athletes may feel that they can return to their sport as well, but are generally held out of sports, such as football, hockey, rugby, lacrosse, and wrestling until 3 months postinjury, when repeat radiographs will confirm advanced bony healing. Overall, formal physical therapy is rarely utilized or needed, but can be initiated at any time, particularly if patients feel any symptoms of asymmetry or scapular dyskinesis at their 3-month postinjury evaluation. Operative treatment is performed for open fractures, those associated with neurologic or vascular injury, multiple refractures, and significantly displaced fractures in athletes

that are symptomatic and show absent callus formation 6 weeks to 3 months postinjury (Fig. 20-7). For completely displaced fractures with severe shortening clearly greater than 30 mm, or severely comminuted fractures, a shared decision-making process is pursued with the patient and family. Based on research demonstrating exceedingly low nonunion rates and symptomatic malunion rates in adolescents, even in the face of significant shortening, nonoperative treatment is recommended. For such fractures in the dominant arm of high-level baseball pitchers and other overhead or throwing athletes, consideration of the low risk of a potential symptomatic malunion, which may alter the short-term biomechanics of the throwing motion, may be discussed. When families favor operative treatment, plate fixation is recommended over intramedullary fixation, provided there is awareness of a relatively high (~18%) rate of potential plate irritation and the need for secondary removal surgery.

Figure 20-7. A: Radiograph of a displaced, segmental right diaphyseal clavicle fracture. **B:** Incision in line with Langer lines, ensuring protection of the supraclavicular cutaneous nerves as the exposure is performed. **C:** Plate placement on the superior aspect of the clavicle while preserving the supraclavicular cutaneous nerves. **D:** Postoperative radiograph of the anatomically reduced fracture. Note the interfragmentary screw that was utilized to convert this fracture from three fragments to two. (Reprinted with permission from Waters PM, Bae DS, eds. *Pediatric Hand and Upper Limb Surgery: A Practical Guide.* Wolters Kluwer; 2012.)

Postoperative Care

Whether ORIF or intramedullary fixation is performed, the post-operative rehabilitation protocol generally matches that of non-operatively treated fracture, with 2 weeks of full-time sling use and 4 subsequent weeks of partial sling use (when out of the house and at school). At the 6-week postoperative visit, clinical examination is used to assess shoulder range of motion and possible tenderness at the fracture site and radiographs in two planes are obtained to assess bone healing. If the examination and radiographs are consistent with healing, the patient is permitted to begin noncontact sports and sports training, including weight training and push-ups. Full return to contact sports is generally reserved for the 3-month time point, as early refracture through the fracture site, within the plate, can occur if the fracture is incompletely healed. After 3 months postoperatively, refracture can still occur, but is more likely to be localized just adjacent to the plate, or through the most eccentric screw site, particularly if this was not drilled in the central position of the shaft, highlighting the importance of biplanar fluoroscopic guidance or confirmation of screw position, particularly in the axillary (AP) plane.

Potential Pitfalls and Preventive Measures

Midshaft Clavicle Fractures: SURGICAL PITFALLS AND PREVENTIONS	
Pitfall	**Prevention**
Neurovascular injury/ pneumothorax	• Utilize subperiosteal dissection at fracture site • Place retractors inferiorly when drilling from superior to inferior direction, take extra measures to prevent inferior "plunging" of drill bit
Delayed union/ nonunion	• Maintain soft tissue attachments to comminuted or malrotated fragments
Malunion	• Achieve adequate exposure to assess fracture reduction and plate placement • Anatomically reduce and stabilize segmental fractures
Implant-related symptoms	• Inferior/distal incision placement, superiorly directed soft tissue dissection with superior plate placement (or, for fractures benefiting from anterior plate placement, utilize superior/proximal incision placement)

The most dreaded intraoperative complication would be damage to a neurovascular structure or creation of a pneumothorax. Both of these exceedingly rare complications can be prevented by utilizing meticulous technique during the exposure of the fracture fragments and drilling/screw placement during the plate application. When exposing the primary fracture fragments at the fracture site, it is important to stay subperiosteal to create a layer between the bone and surrounding neurovascular structures. However, for three- and four-part fractures with comminuted fragments, maintenance of subperiosteal attachments should be pursued. Maintenance of soft tissue attachments to comminuted or malrotated small fragments will also aid the surgeon in the reduction process. Furthermore, if these fragments are completely devoid of soft tissue attachments, devitalization may cause bony union to be delayed or not occur.

Whether the drilling and screw placement is more central in the fracture site (usually subperiosteal dissection), or more eccentric, where the periosteum can usually be maintained, retractors can be under the clavicle or gently, after meticulous blunt dissection, under the inferior periosteum, to avoid damaging the neurovascular structures.

Wound complications can be prevented by utilizing the inferior skin incision rather than a direct approach to the clavicle. In addition, a meticulous layered closure at the end of the procedure will permit the best cosmetic outcome while minimizing the chance of wound issues.

Outcomes

Despite the high incidence of pediatric clavicle fractures and the fact that the vast majority of these fractures are treated nonoperatively, limited data exist regarding the outcomes of these injuries. In general, union rates from 95% to 100% have been reported with nonoperative treatment.[41,62,126] A recent study of 185 adolescent clavicle fractures with a median age of 14.4 years, 38% of which were completely displaced, demonstrated only 1 case of nonunion and 1 delayed union, with the majority demonstrating good-to-excellent functional outcomes measure scores.[99]

In addition, several small series have recently emerged regarding operative treatment. Mehlman et al. performed a retrospective review of 24 children in China with a mean age of 12 years who underwent operative treatment of completely displaced clavicle shaft fractures. In their series, there were no nonunions and no infections. Twenty-one of the 24 patients were able to return to unrestricted sports activity. Three complications were reported including two patients who had scar sensitivity and one patient who had a transient ulnar nerve neurapraxia. However, all patients underwent implant removal on an elective basis, so the implications or sequelae of retained implants could not be ascertained.[81] A more recent retrospective study from authors from the same institution included a comparison of 55 patients treated operatively to 55 patients treated nonoperatively. Ames et al.[4] reported a 27% rate of implant removal in the surgical cohort, while the nonoperative group demonstrated a 22% refracture rate, which is higher than rates described in prospective efforts.

Namdari et al. also performed a retrospective review of 14 skeletally immature patients who underwent ORIF of displaced midshaft clavicle fractures. No nonunions occurred in the cohort, but eight patients had numbness about the surgical site, and four patients underwent hardware removal.[84]

Vander Have et al. performed a retrospective comparative study evaluating nonoperative versus operative treatment of mid shaft clavicle fractures in adolescents, though the two cohorts were not matched. The authors reviewed the course of 43 fracture patients, 25 of which were treated nonoperatively and 17 were treated operatively. No nonunions occurred in either group, but five symptomatic malunions occurred in the nonoperative group, four of which were treated with a corrective osteotomy. All complications in the operative group were related to the prominence of the implant. In fact, a longer-term study from the same institution performed by Li et al.[72] followed the course of 37 fractures in 36 adolescent operative patients who demonstrated a 46% rate of major complications and 86% overall complications, which included 59% implant prominence/irritation, 16% chest wall numbness, 5% wound dehiscence or infection, 3% peri-implant refracture, 3% refracture through screw holes after implant removal, and 42% secondary implant removal surgery. These data are more consistent with those of the prospective study by Heyworth et al.,[46] which showed a significantly higher risk of clinically significant complications and unexpected surgery with operative treatment, when compared with nonoperative treatment of completely displaced clavicle fractures.

A comparative study of over 650 clavicle fractures in patients 10 to 18 years old retrospectively reviewed at a large regional pediatric trauma center demonstrated a nonunion rate of 0.2% in fractures treated nonoperatively, and a symptomatic malunion rate of 2%.[45] The authors demonstrated a significantly higher complication rate (16.2%) in fractures treated operatively, compared with those treated nonoperatively (5.2%). The results of Li et al. corroborated these findings in a smaller, single-site study, in which there was a 43% major complication rate in 37 adolescents treated with plate fixation, the most common of which was secondary surgery for symptomatic plate removal.[72]

Most nondisplaced fractures have union by 4 to 8 weeks of time, whereas displaced fractures may take longer, approximately 10 weeks.[126] A retrospective multicenter investigation of all nonunion cases reported at nine pediatric hospitals over an 11-year period was performed by an adolescent clavicle fracture study group. The investigation yielded only 25 total cases, all of which were successfully treated with surgery, which speaks about the ability to effectively treat this exceedingly rare complication, should it arise following nonoperative treatment. Thus, most pediatric patients treated with a simple sling have excellent outcomes and are able to return to their activities without limitations. A small percentage of patients treated nonoperatively with significant fracture displacement may have subjective complaints of pain with prolonged activity, easy fatigability, axillary pain, or drooping shoulders with bony prominence.[126] However, Bae et al. evaluated a group of 16 patients with displaced (>2 cm) middiaphyseal clavicle fractures treated nonoperatively. All fractures united with no meaningful loss of shoulder motion or abduction–adduction strength by isokinetic testing. Most patients had low DASH and pain VAS that were very low, means of 4.9 and 1.6, respectively. Only 1 patient out of 16 required a corrective osteotomy.[8] The authors concluded that routine surgical fixation for displaced, nonsegmental clavicle fractures may not be justified based on concerns regarding shoulder motion and strength alone in the face of shortening. A similar study by Schulz et al. demonstrated no functional outcome deficits, when compared with the uninjured limb, in 16 adolescent patients with a minimum of 1 cm shortening and a mean of 14 mm of shortening of a displaced clavicle fracture, when assessed more than 2 years following nonoperative treatment.

The largest series of operative fractures in adolescents is that prospectively assessed in the previously mentioned level 2 multicenter series.[46] The Function After Adolescent Clavicle

Trauma and Surgery (FACTS) Study Group reported good to excellent 2-year results in most patients, in the form of PROs, reliable healing, and return to sport rates in 125 patients 10 to 18 years old who underwent ORIF of completely displaced midshaft fractures. However, the overall complication rate, when including sensory changes in the clavicle, chest wall, or shoulder region, was 43%. When those level 1 complications, which did not have a clinically significant impact on the patient's course or plan of care, were excluded, the complication rate was 21%, with a 10% rate of unexpected subsequent surgery, both of which were significantly higher than that reported for the cohort of adolescents treated nonoperatively.

Clearly, further investigation with substratified cohort analyses of subsets of adolescents, particularly overhead athletes, is required to better determine the optimal treatment for all adolescents or risk factors for possible pain or functional compromise in the minority of pediatric patients who develop nonunion, symptomatic malunion, or other complications following clavicle shaft fractures, based on the two different treatment options.

MANAGEMENT OF EXPECTED ADVERSE OUTCOMES AND UNEXPECTED COMPLICATIONS RELATED TO MIDSHAFT CLAVICLE FRACTURES

Midshaft Clavicle Fractures:
COMMON ADVERSE OUTCOMES AND COMPLICATIONS

- Hardware prominence
- Malunion
- Nonunion
- Wound complications

Patients who have implant prominence can be successfully treated by removal of their hardware.[81,84,126] If a patient initially treated by nonoperative measures develops a symptomatic malunion, corrective osteotomy has been shown to be successful in eliminating symptoms (Fig. 20-8).[126] In the Vander Have series, all patients who underwent corrective osteotomy of their malunion went on to union and resolution of their symptoms.[126] The rate of nonunion is exceedingly low in this younger population. Pennock et al.[95] investigated all cases of midshaft clavicle nonunion over an 11-year period at nine different pediatric centers, finding only 25 total cases, suggesting a rate of less than 0.25% per institution per year. Interestingly, the only risk factor for nonunion identified by the multicenter study group was refracture. All but one case had uneventful healing when treated operatively. Hughes et al.[49] performed a systematic review of all cases published prior to that multicenter study, identifying only 21 cases in the world literature, with similar conclusions about the extreme rarity and the effectiveness of surgical intervention when it arises in association with symptoms. Treatment can be successfully performed by subsequent ORIF with a stable construct. On rare occasions, a vascularized bone or corticoperiosteal flap may be necessary (Fig. 20-9).

Figure 20-8. **A:** Intraoperative photograph depicting the middiaphyseal malunion. **B:** Intraoperative photograph showing the osteotomy has been performed in the plane of maximal deformity. **C:** Intraoperative photograph following reduction and plating of the malunion. (Reprinted with permission from Waters PM, Bae DS, eds. *Pediatric Hand and Upper Limb Surgery: A Practical Guide.* Wolters Kluwer; 2012.)

SUMMARY, CONTROVERSIES, AND FUTURE DIRECTIONS RELATED TO MIDSHAFT CLAVICLE FRACTURES

Most pediatric and adolescent midshaft clavicle fractures can be treated successfully with nonoperative measures. ORIF should be performed for the rare open fracture, fractures with skin at risk of necrosis, and fractures with nerve or vascular injury. Future prospective studies are underway to better determine the

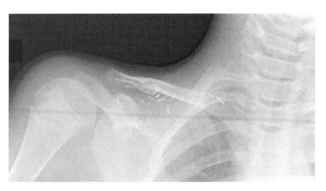

Figure 20-9. Radiograph of a healed clavicle fracture following treatment of a symptomatic nonunion with a vascularized fibula graft. (Reprinted with permission from Waters PM, Bae DS, eds. *Pediatric Hand and Upper Limb Surgery: A Practical Guide.* Wolters Kluwer; 2012.)

potential benefits and complications of operative fixation versus nonoperative treatment in adolescents.

Distal Clavicle Fractures

INTRODUCTION TO DISTAL CLAVICLE FRACTURES

Distal clavicle fractures account for 10% to 30% of all clavicle fractures, thus making it the second most common site for a clavicle fracture, after midshaft clavicle fractures.[104] Minimal studies exist regarding the treatment and outcomes of these fractures for pediatric and adolescent patients. Therefore, the information presented here will mainly be extrapolated from the adult literature and our experience.

ASSESSMENT OF DISTAL CLAVICLE FRACTURES

MECHANISMS OF INJURY FOR DISTAL CLAVICLE FRACTURES

Akin to midshaft clavicle fractures, distal clavicle fractures are typically the result of a direct blow to the shoulder girdle or a fall onto the distal aspect of the clavicle.[104] Direct blows typically occur in adolescents involved in collision-type sports such as football or lacrosse. When a fall is the mechanism of injury, direct contact from the ground is made against the acromion with the arm typically held in an adducted position. The force is transmitted from the acromion across the AC joint to the distal end of the clavicle.

INJURIES ASSOCIATED WITH DISTAL CLAVICLE FRACTURES

Common injuries associated with distal clavicle fractures include additional fractures about the shoulder girdle including proximal humerus and scapular fractures, thus constituting a floating shoulder–type injury. In addition, rib fractures, lung injuries including contusions, and brachial plexus injuries may occur concomitantly. Finally, cervical spine injuries must be ruled out in collision or high-energy mechanisms of injury.

SIGNS AND SYMPTOMS OF DISTAL CLAVICLE FRACTURES

Patients who sustain distal clavicle fractures present with pain about the involved shoulder, especially with any attempt at movement of the arm. Paresthesias may be present if a concomitant brachial plexus injury has occurred.

Physical examination should begin by observing for obvious swelling, ecchymosis, and/or bony prominence or skin tenting, which may be present if there is a completely displaced fracture with superior displacement of the medial fragment and drooping of the unsupported shoulder girdle due to disruption of the strut function of the clavicle. The area posterior to the AC joint should be palpated, as a posteriorly displaced proximal fragment may be entrapped in the trapezius muscle, and is critical to treatment decision making. In addition, palpation of the entire upper extremity, hemithorax, and cervical spine should be performed to identify the location of maximal tenderness as well as additional areas that may have sustained a concomitant injury. A complete neurovascular examination should be performed to evaluate for rare brachial plexus injury. Patients involved in high-energy mechanisms should have a complete head-to-toe survey performed by the orthopaedic physician as well as either a member of the trauma team or the emergency room physician.

IMAGING AND OTHER DIAGNOSTIC STUDIES FOR DISTAL CLAVICLE FRACTURES

Initial imaging should be performed by obtaining plain radiographs of the shoulder, including a true AP view and a cephalic tilt view, which may be performed most commonly with a 15-degree cephalic or 45-degree cephalic tilt.[136] Due to the significance of assessing posterior displacement of the medial fragment relative to the acromion or distal fragment, the axillary lateral view is of critical importance, and should be pursued, even if it requires assistance from a member of the clinical team, with gentle, gradual abduction of the arm to facilitate a clear view of the shoulder. A CT scan may be diagnostic for intra-articular fractures, which

may require operative intervention for best results, and can be helpful to assess the precise degree and direction of the displaced medial fragment, the position of which will determine the need for surgery when physical examination and the axillary view do not allow for a clear assessment.

CLASSIFICATION OF DISTAL CLAVICLE FRACTURES

The most commonly used classification scheme for distal clavicle fractures is that proposed by Neer[86] and modified by Craig.[25] This classification scheme includes five types based on the relationship of the fracture line to the CC ligaments, the AC ligaments, and the physis. Most lateral clavicle fractures in the skeletally immature patients are periosteal disruptions in which the bone displaces away from the periosteal sleeve whereas the CC ligaments remain attached to the intact inferior portion of the periosteum.

Type I fractures occur distal to the CC ligaments but do not involve the AC joint. Minimal displacement occurs due to the proximal fragment being stabilized by the intact CC ligaments and the distal fragment being stabilized by the AC joint capsule, the AC ligaments, and the deltotrapezial fascia.

Type II fractures are subdivided into type IIA and type IIB fractures, with type IIA fractures occurring medial to the CC ligaments and type IIB fractures occurring between the CC ligaments with concomitant injury to the conoid ligament. In type IIA injuries, the proximal fragment loses the stability provided by the CC ligaments and displaces superiorly out of the periosteal sleeve. In contrast, the distal fragment remains stable because of the attachments of the AC joint capsule, AC ligaments, and the CC ligament(s). This remains true for type IIB fractures as well, because even though the conoid ligament is disrupted, the trapezoid ligament remains attached.

Type III fractures occur distal to the CC ligaments and extend into the AC joint. As these fractures do not disrupt the ligamentous structures, minimal displacement is the norm.

Type IV fractures occur in skeletally immature patients and involve a fracture medial to the physis. The epiphysis and physis remain uninjured and attached to the AC joint. However, significant displacement can occur between the physis and metaphyseal fragment, as the CC ligaments are attached to the shaft. This is especially true if the periosteal sleeve is disrupted. In essence, this is analogous to a type IIA fracture.

Type V fractures have a fracture line that leaves a free-floating inferior cortical fragment attached to the CC ligaments with an additional fracture line dividing the distal clavicle from the remainder of the clavicle. Therefore, neither the proximal nor distal fragment is attached to the CC ligaments. The end result is instability with the potential for significant displacement of the distal end of the proximal fragment.

OUTCOME MEASURES FOR DISTAL CLAVICLE FRACTURES

No outcome measures have been specifically applied to pediatric distal clavicle fractures. Commonly utilized measures for adult distal clavicle fractures include the ASES score, the DASH Score, the QuickDASH, and the Constant Shoulder Score. The recent publication of a novel Pedi-ASES demonstrated that adult shoulder outcome scores such as the DASH and ASES surveys are associated with poor validity and comprehensibility in pediatric populations, and this new metric, when more comprehensively validated, may emerge as a future standard for use in pediatric and adolescent shoulder research.[45]

PATHOANATOMY AND APPLIED ANATOMY RELATED TO DISTAL CLAVICLE FRACTURES

The distal aspect of the clavicle forms the articulation with the scapula via the AC joint. Ligamentous connections between this portion of the clavicle and the scapula include the AC ligaments and CC ligaments. The CC ligaments include the trapezoid ligament, located more laterally with an attachment to the distal clavicle approximately 2 cm from the AC joint, and the conoid ligament, located more medially with an attachment to the distal clavicle approximately 4 cm from the AC joint.[101] The presence of these ligamentous attachments and the AC joint capsule permits fluid scapulothoracic motion.[10]

Stability of the clavicle in the horizontal/AP plane is provided by the AC ligaments, whereas stability in the vertical/superoinferior plane is provided by the CC ligaments. This stability permits the definition of the CC space, the space between the coracoid process and the undersurface of the clavicle, which should be 1.1 to 1.3 cm.

TREATMENT OPTIONS FOR DISTAL CLAVICLE FRACTURES

NONOPERATIVE TREATMENT OF DISTAL CLAVICLE FRACTURES

Indications/Contraindications

Nonoperative Treatment of Distal Clavicle Fractures: INDICATIONS AND CONTRAINDICATIONS

Indications

- Nondisplaced and minimally displaced fractures (type I and type III fractures)

Relative Contraindications

- Open fractures
- Fractures with associated skin compromise
- Fractures with concomitant neurovascular injury requiring surgical intervention

Most distal clavicle fractures in the pediatric and adolescent population can be managed nonoperatively with immobilization alone as long as significant displacement is not present. Typically, this is universally true for type I and type III fractures. However, types II, IV, and V fractures may have significant displacement with subsequent skin tenting, bony prominence, or instability present about the shoulder girdle. Contraindications to nonsurgical management include open fractures, fractures associated with skin necrosis, and fractures with concomitant neurovascular injury requiring surgical intervention. Due to the relative thickness of the soft tissues overlying the AC joint region, skin tenting causing skin at risk of necrosis associated with distal clavicle fractures is rare, compared to that of the more subcutaneous position of the bone in the diaphyseal region. Displaced fractures in the pediatric and adolescent population (types II, IV, and V) should be treated on an individual basis depending on the patient's age, the amount of displacement, and the patient's activities.

Technique

The standard approach to nonoperative treatment includes use of a sling for approximately 6 weeks or sling and swath for the first 1 to 2 weeks, with progression to a simple sling when comfort levels allow. After 4 to 6 weeks, active range of motion may begin. Radiographs are taken at the 6-week follow-up visit to assess healing and progress to functional activities, though full contact in sports such as ice hockey, football, and lacrosse should generally be delayed until 2 to 3 months, after advanced bony bridging is observed radiographically.

Outcomes

Nonoperative treatment of nondisplaced or minimally displaced distal clavicle fractures typically has excellent outcomes with successful union occurring and patients able to return to full activities. While types I and III fractures have been shown to go on to delayed-onset symptomatic AC joint arthrosis in the adult literature, this has not been replicated in pediatric studies.

Treatment of significantly displaced distal clavicle fractures is somewhat controversial, due to a relatively high nonunion rate reported in the adult literature. In a retrospective review performed by Neer,[85] all patients with type II distal clavicle fractures treated nonoperatively had either a delayed union (67%) or a nonunion (33%). Edwards et al.[26] treated 20 patients with type II distal clavicle fractures nonoperatively and had a 45% delayed union rate and a 30% nonunion rate. Additional studies have shown similar nonunion rates ranging from 25% to 44% for type II fractures treated nonoperatively.[91,104,105] In contrast, all type II fractures treated surgically with ORIF have gone on to union.[26,85] While nonunion of significantly displaced pediatric distal clavicle fractures may be considered to be a more common occurrence than nonunion of pediatric midshaft clavicle fractures, it still represents a rare event, and operative considerations revolve more around concerns of symptomatic malunion and altered shoulder biomechanics with overhead sports or activities.

OPERATIVE TREATMENT OF DISTAL CLAVICLE FRACTURES

Indications/Contraindications

Absolute indications for operative treatment of distal clavicle fractures include open fractures, fractures with significant skin compromise, displaced intra-articular extension, and fractures with associated neurovascular injuries that require operative intervention. Additional relative indications may include significantly displaced fractures in competitive athletes and adolescents, entrapment in the trapezius muscle, floating shoulder–type injuries, and patients with polytrauma. The most common indication for surgical treatment of distal clavicle fractures in the pediatric population is significant posterior displacement that suggests complete discontinuity of the proximal fragment and/or trapezial entrapment, in which case diffuse soft tissue swelling may be seen over the AC joint region with severe pain with any attempted shoulder motion. Children and younger adolescents are unlikely to experience disruption of the CC ligaments, given that the thick periosteum generally remains attached to the underlying ligamentous complex. Nevertheless, the proximal fragment may alternatively tear through the superior periosteum with enough force to generate severe superior displacement and bony prominence.

Open Reduction and Internal Fixation

Preoperative Planning

✓ ORIF of Distal Clavicle Fractures:
PREOPERATIVE PLANNING CHECKLIST

OR table	❏ Standard table capable of going into beach chair position
Position/ positioning aids	❏ Beach chair position with head and neck tilted away or supine ❏ Bump placed behind the scapula ❏ Leave plenty of sterile standing space above the shoulder adjacent to the head
Fluoroscopy location	❏ Contralateral side of fracture
Equipment	❏ Nonabsorbable suture, anatomic distal clavicle plates, hook plates, minifragment, or modular hand-locking plates
Draping	❏ Entire shoulder girdle region and ipsilateral limb are prepped and draped into the field to allow for traction and manipulation ❏ Medially, the ipsilateral sternoclavicular joint should be included in the operative field

It is necessary to determine preoperatively what the plan for fixation is going to be as numerous techniques can be performed to stabilize the distal clavicle. Ideally, multiple options are available at the time of surgical intervention including various nonabsorbable suture options, specialty distal clavicle locking plates, and hook plates. The position the patient will be in during the procedure needs to be discussed with the anesthesiologist and OR staff, especially if the beach chair position is being used.

Positioning

The patient can be positioned in either the beach chair position (i.e., ~60 degrees of head elevation) with the head and neck

tilted away, a "sloppy beach chair" position (i.e., 45 degrees of head elevation), or supine on a radiolucent table. With either position, a bump should be placed behind the scapula. The entire shoulder girdle, beginning at the medial edge of the clavicle, and the entire limb should be prepped and draped in the operative field to allow for movement of the limb which facilitates fracture reduction and fixation. A sterile area above the shoulder adjacent to the head is maintained to allow for the surgeon to work both inferior and superior to the clavicle and shoulder.

Surgical Approach

An incision in Langer skin lines over the distal third of the clavicle and AC joint should be made. Once the skin is divided, the subcutaneous tissue, fascia, and periosteum are incised to maintain a thick flap. Subperiosteal dissection is then carried out from nonfractured clavicle out to the fracture site to expose the fracture fragments.

Technique

✓ ORIF of Distal Clavicle Fractures:
KEY SURGICAL STEPS

- ❏ Skin incision over distal one-third of clavicle and acromion in line with Langer lines
- ❏ Electrocautery through subcutaneous tissue, fascia, and periosteum directly onto the clavicle
- ❏ Expose fracture site in a subperiosteal manner while preserving the AC and CC ligaments
- ❏ Reduce fracture fragments with reduction clamps and temporary K-wire fixation if necessary
- ❏ Apply distal clavicle plate on superior aspect of distal clavicle
- ❏ Assess reduction and screw lengths with direct visualization and/ or fluoroscopic imaging in multiple planes
- ❏ Repair periosteum to tighten CC and AC ligaments. Rarely, apply supplemental fixation to CC ligaments utilizing suture around coracoid and clavicle if fixation is marginal
- ❏ Irrigate wound and close periosteum
- ❏ Meticulous skin closure with absorbable suture
- ❏ Apply sling or shoulder immobilizer

The implant choice will depend on the age and size of the patient, as well as the size and location of the fracture fragments. Fixation with low-profile anatomic distal locking plates can be used for older adolescents with fractures that have a distal fracture fragment large enough to accommodate multiple screws, which may be locking screws or a combination of cortical and locking screws. If there is not adequate bone on the distal fragment or in the rare case of a complete AC joint dislocation with no distal bony fragment, a hook plate may be used (Fig. 20-10) but has the disadvantage of requiring secondary surgery for hardware removal once healing is confirmed. Younger adolescents or preadolescents with robust periosteum may require only suture-based fixation, with three potential fixation constructs: (1) suture repair of the periosteum only, in cases in which a thick enough cuff of superior periosteum can provide adequate stabilization of the proximal fragment; (2) suture repair in which high-strength nonabsorbable figure-of-eight

Figure 20-10. **A:** Radiograph of a displaced intra-articular lateral clavicle fracture where the lateral aspect of the medial fragment was entrapped in the trapezius muscle. **B:** Postoperative radiograph demonstrating fixation utilizing a hook plate. Removal of the implant is planned. (Reprinted with permission from Waters PM, Bae DS, eds. *Pediatric Hand and Upper Limb Surgery: A Practical Guide.* Wolters Kluwer; 2012.)

sutures are placed through the thick inferior periosteum/CC ligament complex and wrapped around the clavicle or through small superior-to-inferior drill holes through the distal aspect of the proximal fragment, with overlying superior periosteal repair; or (3) suture repair through small drill holes in the distal and proximal bone fracture fragments, with overlying superior periosteal repair. For younger patients with smaller clavicle sizes who undergo plate fixation, utilization of modular hand instrumentation or minifragment locking plates (Synthes, Inc., West Chester, PA) may be warranted. Distal radius plate fixation has also been suggested by placement of the 2.4-mm locking screws in the distal clavicle fragment.[56]

K-wire fixation is rarely utilized but should be supplemented with a dorsal tension band, utilizing either suture or wire. Threaded wires are also rarely used, but have been described to lessen the risk of K-wire migration.[6,57,70,74]

Additional fixation of the CC ligaments has been suggested to decrease the chance of nonunion in adults and may be applicable to the older adolescent. This has been performed utilizing suture or soft tissue tendon grafts.[129] In addition, arthroscopic techniques, utilizing suture, the Tightrope system (Arthrex, Naples, FL), or a double-button device, to stabilize the CC ligaments have also been reported in adults.[13,22,92,98] Some authors have proposed placement of a screw between the coracoid and

clavicle; however, this requires screw removal following fracture union.[26,31,53,73,134] Neither of these techniques is used very often in children or adolescents.

Operative treatment of distal clavicle fractures has excellent results with regard to union rates, especially in children and adolescents. The most common postoperative complication is implant irritation requiring secondary removal surgery. Because utilization of smooth wires about this region can lead to migration of the wires into areas including the lung, abdomen, spine, trachea, and vascular structures, smooth K-wires should be avoided if possible; or, can be left outside of the skin and removed at 4 weeks.[100,124] Tension band wiring is particularly prone to symptoms requiring a second procedure for removal. Using nonabsorbable suture as a tension band can lessen the risk of implant irritation but suture granulomas can also be irritating and require subsequent removal at times.[68]

Union rates with plate fixation have been reported to be as high as 100%.[19] Two studies have found that hook plate usage in adults yielded higher rates of return to work and sports participation and a lower complication rate than other techniques,[33,68] but a more recent study showed superior outcomes and lower complications with distal locking plates, compared with hook plates.[30] We advocate removal of the hook plate in an adolescent when the fracture is healed to avoid secondary complications.

Authors' Preferred Treatment for Distal Clavicle Fractures

Our preferred technique is to treat nearly all distal clavicle fractures in the pediatric and adolescent populations with nonoperative measures. Patients are placed into a sling for 6 weeks and then advanced to active range of motion, presuming union has occurred. Operative intervention is reserved

for open fractures, fractures with skin compromise, fractures with associated neurovascular injury requiring operative intervention, displaced intra-articular fractures, and significantly displaced fractures, especially those displaced posteriorly with entrapment in trapezius muscle.

A direct approach to the fracture site is performed using a Langer skin line. Following sharp incision of the skin, electrocautery is utilized to divide the subcutaneous tissue, fascia, and periosteum. A periosteal elevator or scalpel is then used to elevate the periosteum off of the clavicle while preserving the AC and CC ligament attachments. The fracture fragments are then exposed and irrigated free of hematoma and debris in preparation for reduction.

For younger adolescents and preadolescents, if the superior periosteum is found to be robust enough, reduction of the proximal fragment and suture repair of the periosteum is preferred. If the stability of this construct appears questionable, high-strength nonabsorbable figure-of-eight sutures are placed through the thick inferior periosteum/CC ligament complex and wrapped around the clavicle or placed through small superior-to-inferior drill holes through the distal aspect of the proximal fragment, with additional overlying superior periosteal repair. For older adolescents, fixation of a distal clavicle fracture is may be performed using an anatomically contoured distal clavicular locking plate and screw construct, assuming there is enough bone laterally for stable fixation. If the fragment is too small for these implants, we attempt to perform fixation utilizing minifragment or modular hand-locking plates (Synthes, Inc., West Chester, PA). In this sub-population, we use anatomically contoured distal clavicular locking plates when feasible. If the fragment is too small for these implants, we attempt to perform fixation utilizing minifragment or modular hand-locking plates (Synthes, Inc.,

West Chester, PA). We do not routinely supplement our plate fixation with suture around the coracoid and clavicle unless the fixation was marginal. The periosteal repair is generally sufficient for ligamentous and soft tissue stability.

For patients aged 13 years and under, or if plate fixation is not an option, interosseous suture fixation of the fracture fragments represents a viable and effective option, using high-strength no. 2 braided sutures (Fig. 20-11). We have not found it necessary to place suture around the coracoid and clavicle to obtain union in the pediatric and adolescent populations. Intraosseous suture fixation can be supplemented with sutures placed into the inferior periosteal complex overlying the CC ligaments, either with a figure-of-eight or Mason–Allen-type configuration. The two limbs of sutures from this soft tissue fixation construct can be fed through drill holes in the clavicle overlying this location in the periosteal complex, or around the clavicle. Moreover, anterior and/or posterior sutures placed through the clavicle to the adjacent thick periosteum may further reinforce this non–implant-mediated stabilization, preventing the risk of implant-related symptoms and subsequent removal surgery. Hook plates are utilized as a last resort in the setting of an older adolescent without adequate distal fragment bone to accommodate screws, as they require a second procedure for removal in all cases. However, they are made available during all procedures, in case adequate fixation is unable to be obtained without them. In general, the hook plate would be used in an appropriately sized adolescent.

Postoperative Care

Postoperatively, patients are placed in a sling for 6 weeks. When suture-only fixation is pursued in the younger adolescent or preadolescent, a sling and swath is generally favored. When solid rigid plate fixation is achieved, immobilization is removed several times a day for pendulum exercises. Following union of the fracture, active shoulder range of motion and strengthening is initiated. Contact sports participation is usually avoided for 3 months.

Potential Pitfalls and Preventive Measures

Distal Clavicle Fractures:
SURGICAL PITFALLS AND PREVENTIONS

Pitfall	Preventions
Nonunion/ hardware failure	Ensure adequate fixation in distal fragment
	Supplement fixation with suture and prolonged immobilization until healed
Screw penetration into AC joint	Directly visualize joint and utilize fluoroscopy in multiple planes following plate fixation

Nonunion or hardware failure can occur if there is inadequate fixation of the distal clavicular fragment or excessive activity

early. In addition, it is imperative to avoid screw penetration into the AC joint, which can be assessed with direct visualization and/or utilizing fluoroscopy in multiple planes.

MANAGEMENT OF EXPECTED ADVERSE OUTCOMES AND UNEXPECTED COMPLICATIONS RELATED TO DISTAL CLAVICLE FRACTURES

Distal Clavicle Fractures:
COMMON ADVERSE OUTCOMES AND COMPLICATIONS

- Implant prominence
- Hardware migration
- Nonunion
- Symptomatic malunion

The most common complication of treatment of operative distal clavicle fractures is related to symptomatic implants, which is easily remedied by removal of hardware. Nonunion and symptomatic malunions are best managed by performing ORIF of the fracture. In rare cases of minimal distal fragment bone or bony erosion, the distal fragment can be excised and the AC joint reconstructed using a modified Weaver–Dunn procedure, where

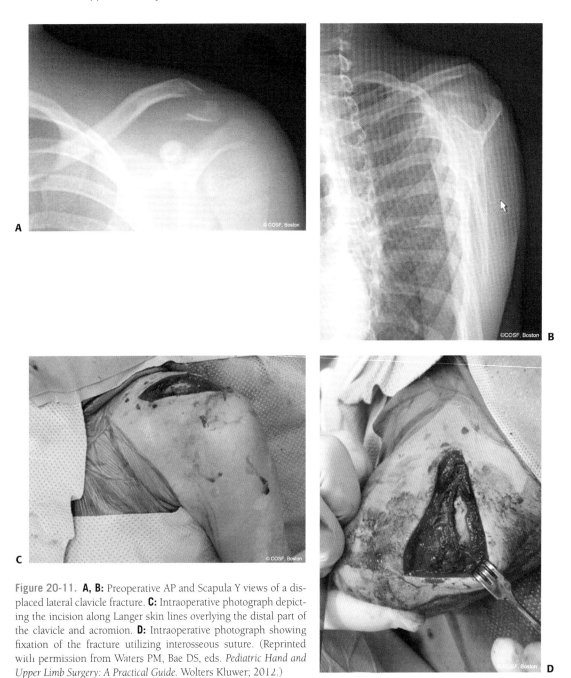

Figure 20-11. **A, B:** Preoperative AP and Scapula Y views of a displaced lateral clavicle fracture. **C:** Intraoperative photograph depicting the incision along Langer skin lines overlying the distal part of the clavicle and acromion. **D:** Intraoperative photograph showing fixation of the fracture utilizing interosseous suture. (Reprinted with permission from Waters PM, Bae DS, eds. *Pediatric Hand and Upper Limb Surgery: A Practical Guide.* Wolters Kluwer; 2012.)

the coracoacromial ligament is transferred to the distal end of the remaining clavicle.[5] However, this represents a more historical option for adults rarely applied in this younger population.

SUMMARY, CONTROVERSIES, AND FUTURE DIRECTIONS RELATED TO DISTAL CLAVICLE FRACTURES

Most of the literature available on distal clavicle fractures is for the adult population. Typically, if a child or adolescent sustains a fracture in this region, immobilization alone is sufficient to obtain a successful outcome. In older adolescents, highly competitive athletes, or instances of severe posterior or superior displacement, operative intervention may be warranted. Suture-based periosteal repair or fixation in younger adolescents or preadolescents avoids hardware-related complications, but adequate stability must be ensured through meticulous technique. Utilization of a plate and screw construct also typically yields excellent results with a rapid return to function, a very high union rate, and a low complication rate. Further studies evaluating the treatment and outcomes of these fractures in the pediatric and adolescent are needed.

Scapula Fractures

INTRODUCTION TO SCAPULA FRACTURES

Scapula fractures are uncommon accounting for 1% of all fractures in adults with an even lower incidence in children.[40,120] Fractures involving the scapular body are most common, accounting for approximately 45% of scapula fractures. The remainder of fractures involve the glenoid neck (25%), glenoid cavity (10%), acromion process (8%), coracoid process (7%), and scapular spine (5%).[77,120] Very rarely, scapulothoracic dissociation can occur.[87] Because of the low incidence of scapular fractures, mostly case report and retrospective small case series literature exist on their treatment and outcomes in the pediatric and adolescent populations.

ASSESSMENT OF SCAPULA FRACTURES

MECHANISMS OF INJURY FOR SCAPULA FRACTURES

When scapula body fractures occur in children, they are likely the result of either high-energy mechanisms, such as a fall from a height, ATV accidents or motor vehicle accidents, or the result of nonaccidental injury.[18,111] Bullock et al.[18] showed that scapula fractures had the highest risk of abuse for any fracture other than rib/sternum fractures, and when they were present, they were more than twice as likely to be associated with child abuse than not.

Glenoid fractures most commonly occur due to a direct force on the lateral shoulder, such as that occur during a fall or a collision sport. The force is transmitted to the humeral head, which then is driven into the glenoid surface. An alternative mechanism of injury is a fall onto a flexed elbow. The position of the arm at the time of injury will determine whether an anterior or posterior rim fracture occurs.

Acromion fractures occur due to a direct blow to the lateral aspect of the shoulder, which typically occurs during a fall or a collision in sport.[77] It is imperative to recognize that complete failure of the epiphyses to fuse is a normal anatomic variant known as os acromiale and should not be mistaken for a fracture. If necessary, comparison radiographs of the contralateral side can be obtained to confirm this.

Coracoid fractures occur due to the pull of either the AC ligaments or the conjoint tendon. When the AC ligaments avulse the coracoid from the remainder of the scapula, the fracture occurs at the physis through the base of the coracoid and upper quarter of the glenoid. In contrast, when the conjoint tendon avulses the coracoid from the scapula, the fracture occurs through the tip of the coracoid.

INJURIES ASSOCIATED WITH SCAPULA FRACTURES

Whether scapula fractures occur due to high-energy mechanisms or nonaccidental trauma, associated injuries are common, including life-threatening injuries. Such injuries include closed head injuries, pneumo- or hemothorax, rib fractures, ruptured viscera, and concomitant long-bone fractures.[40,120] An analysis of high-energy pediatric scapula fractures due to motorized vehicle accidents found a higher Injury Severity Score (ISS) in the scapula fracture patients compared with a cohort of patients with similar high-energy motor vehicle accidents that did not have scapula fractures.[110] Almost half of all children admitted to the hospital for nonaccidental trauma have at least one fracture and approximately one-third had a diagnosis of contusion.[18] Concomitant neurovascular injury may also occur involving the brachial plexus, subclavian artery/vein, or axillary vessels. Finally, additional fractures or dislocations can occur about the shoulder girdle, particularly clavicle fractures, leading to a floating shoulder.[110]

SIGNS AND SYMPTOMS OF SCAPULA FRACTURES

Because of the large amount of force required to sustain a scapula fracture, a complete head-to-toe survey should be performed by either the trauma team or emergency room physician. Associated rib fractures or lung injury may cause difficulty breathing, whereas ruptured viscera will lead to an acute abdomen. In cases of suspected nonaccidental trauma, a complete evaluation needs to be performed including a head CT scan, an ophthalmologic examination, a skeletal survey, and a social work consultation.

Patients with scapula fractures will often complain of significant pain about their chest, back, and shoulder region. Numbness may be present because of concomitant brachial plexus injury or significant swelling. Observation for significant swelling and ecchymosis should begin the examination. Subsequently, a complete neurovascular examination of the involved upper extremity is necessary. Palpation should then be performed to determine the location of maximal tenderness as well as additional areas of tenderness, as concomitant shoulder girdle fractures can be present. A secondary survey should be performed by the orthopaedic surgeon to ensure there are no additional musculoskeletal injuries.

IMAGING AND OTHER DIAGNOSTIC STUDIES FOR SCAPULA FRACTURES

Scapula fractures may initially be discovered on the chest x-ray obtained during the trauma workup; however, additional imaging is necessary to fully evaluate the fracture. Plain radiographs including true AP and lateral scapula views as well as a glenohumeral axillary view should be obtained when a scapula fracture is suspected. In addition, because of the significant amount of overlying bony and soft tissue structures, a CT scan will enable the surgeon to fully understand the fracture pattern. The addition of reconstructions, including three-dimensional reconstructions, will aid in preoperative planning if operative intervention is being considered.

CLASSIFICATION OF SCAPULA FRACTURES

Scapula fractures are classified according to the fracture location within the scapula: body, glenoid cavity, glenoid neck, acromion, and coracoid. In addition, scapulothoracic dissociation is a term utilized to describe complete separation of the scapula from the posterior chest wall.

Glenoid Neck Fractures:
CLASSIFICATION

Type	Description
I	Displaced <1 cm and angulated <40 degrees
II	Displaced >1 cm and angulated >40 degrees

Glenoid neck fractures are further classified based on their displacement and angulation. A type I fracture is displaced less than 1 cm and angulated less than 40 degrees, whereas a type II fracture has more than 1 cm of displacement and is angulated greater than 40 degrees.[39] Type I fractures account for 90% of glenoid neck fractures.[137]

Glenoid Cavity Fractures:
CLASSIFICATION

Type	Description
Ia	Fracture involving the anterior glenoid rim
Ib	Fracture involving the posterior glenoid rim
II	Transverse fracture line that divides the superior and inferior aspects of the glenoid and then exits inferiorly through the lateral scapular border
III	Fracture line dividing the superior and inferior aspects of the glenoid, but exits superiorly near or through the scapular notch
IV	Fracture line dividing the superior and inferior aspects of the glenoid, but exits medially through the medial border of the scapula
Va	More than one fracture line involving a combination of types II and IV fractures
Vb	More than one fracture line involving a combination of types III and IV fractures
Vc	More than one fracture line involving a combination of types II, III, and IV fractures
VI	Severely comminuted fractures

Glenoid cavity fractures are classified into six types based on the location of the fracture within the glenoid cavity and their severity (Fig. 20-12).[38,50] Type I fractures involve either the anterior (type Ia) or posterior (type Ib) aspect of the glenoid rim. Type II fractures have a transverse fracture line that divides the superior and inferior aspects of the glenoid and then exits inferiorly through the lateral scapular border. Types III and IV fractures also begin with a fracture line dividing the superior and inferior aspects of the glenoid, but type III fractures exit superiorly near or through the scapular notch and type IV fractures exit medially through the medial border of the scapula. Type V fractures have more than one fracture line involving a combination of types II to IV and are further sub-classified into a, b, and c. Type Va fractures are a combination of type II and IV fractures; type Vb fractures are a combination of types III and IV fractures; and type Vc fractures are a

combination of types II, III, and IV fractures. Finally, type VI fractures are severely comminuted fractures.

OUTCOME MEASURES FOR SCAPULA FRACTURES

No specific outcome measures exist for the evaluation of scapula fractures. Results in the adult literature utilize subjective complaints of pain, fracture displacement, residual deformity, nonunion, and development of posttraumatic arthritis as determinants for success.[27,60,65,89] Specific pediatric outcomes have not been developed but the goals of outcome are the same: restoration of motion, function, and strength without long-term limitations and/or pain.

PATHOANATOMY AND APPLIED ANATOMY RELATED TO SCAPULA FRACTURES

The scapula is a flat bone on the posterior aspect of the chest wall, covered almost entirely by muscle due to it having 17 muscular attachments on it. Only the dorsal aspect of the scapular spine and acromion are subcutaneous, and thus the remainder of the bone is deep and well protected from low-energy mechanisms of injury. Three articulations occur with the scapula; the acromion articulates with the clavicle at the AC joint; the proximal humerus articulates with the glenoid at the glenohumeral joint; and the posterior chest wall articulates with the anterior scapula to make up the scapulothoracic articulation.

TREATMENT OPTIONS FOR SCAPULA FRACTURES

NONOPERATIVE TREATMENT OF SCAPULA FRACTURES

Indications/Contraindications

Nonoperative Treatment of Scapula Fractures:
INDICATIONS AND CONTRAINDICATIONS

Indications

- Nondisplaced or minimally displaced scapula body fractures
- Acromion fractures
- Coracoid fractures with <2 cm of displacement
- Glenoid fractures with <1 cm of displacement and 40 degrees of angulation
- Glenoid cavity fractures with <5 mm of intra-articular displacement
- Severely comminuted glenoid fractures unable to support stable fixation

Relative Contraindications

- Open fractures
- Fractures with associated neurovascular injuries requiring surgical intervention
- Glenoid cavity fractures with >5 mm of intra-articular displacement
- Large glenoid rim fractures with associated proximal humerus subluxation/dislocation
- Type II glenoid neck fractures

Most scapula fractures can be treated nonoperatively with immobilization alone, no matter what part of the scapula the fracture

Figure 20-12. Schematic depicting the six types of glenoid cavity fractures.

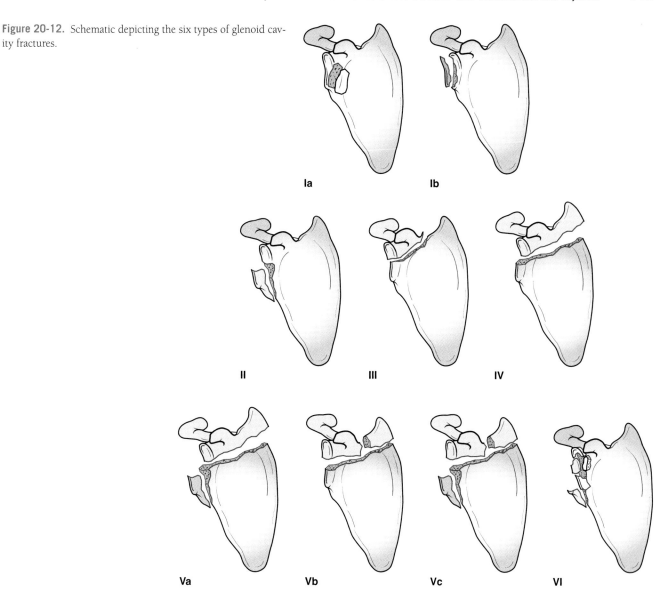

involves. Exceptions include open fractures, fractures with associated neurovascular injuries requiring operative intervention, scapulothoracic dissociation, large glenoid rim fractures with associated proximal humerus subluxation/dislocation, type II glenoid neck fractures, and glenoid cavity fractures with displacement of more than 5 mm.[60,87] All of these are very rare in children but need not be missed.

Techniques

A sling or shoulder immobilizer is used for 3 to 6 weeks depending on patient, injury severity, and healing. When there is sufficient healing and reduction in pain, rehabilitation progresses from pendulum exercises to full range of motion and strengthening. Return to sports is usually 8 to 12 weeks after injury.

Outcomes

No large studies exist regarding the outcomes of children treated for scapula fractures. In the adult literature, most patients obtain fracture union and have minimal to no pain with good functional outcomes expected.[40,89] Similarly, most reports indicate children do well with this rare injury.

OPERATIVE TREATMENT OF SCAPULA FRACTURES

Indications/Contraindications

Operative indications for scapula fractures are limited in the pediatric and adolescent populations but include open fractures, fractures with associated neurovascular injuries requiring operative intervention, scapulothoracic dissociation, large glenoid rim fractures with associated proximal humerus subluxation/dislocation, type II glenoid neck fractures, coracoid process fractures with greater than 2 cm of displacement, and glenoid cavity fractures with displacement greater than 5 mm.[60,87] Floating shoulder injuries involving the midshaft of the clavicle and the glenoid neck can be treated by ORIF of the clavicle as the glenoid neck will reduce via ligamentotaxis provided by the intact CC ligament.[9] Similarly, floating shoulder injuries involving fractures of the glenoid neck, midshaft of the clavicle, and scapula spine will heal by ORIF of the clavicle and scapula spine due to ligamentotaxis provided by the intact CC and/or coracoacromial ligaments.[9] Nonoperative management with immobilization should be used for the remainder of injuries.

Open Reduction and Internal Fixation

Preoperative Planning

✓ ORIF of Scapula Fractures: PREOPERATIVE PLANNING CHECKLIST	
OR table	❏ Flattop Jackson table or standard OR table with the ability to go into beach chair position depending on the approach being utilized
Position/ positioning aids	❏ Lateral decubitus in bean bag or beach chair
Fluoroscopy location	❏ Contralateral side of fracture
Equipment	❏ 2.7-mm or 3.5-mm plate/screw constructs; heavy nonabsorbable suture
Draping	❏ U-drapes

The position of the patient and necessary implants will depend on which part of the scapula is fractured. Typically, it is necessary to utilize plates that can be bent and twisted to match the shape of the scapula. Advanced imaging with three-dimensional reconstruction is helpful in planning for ORIF of scapula fractures.

Positioning

Patient positioning will depend on the location of the fracture within the scapula and subsequently the approach being used. If anterior exposure is necessary, the patient is placed in the beach chair position and a standard deltopectoral approach is performed. Posterior exposure is performed by having the patient in the lateral decubitus position in a bean bag, allowing the shoulder and trunk to droop slightly forward.

Surgical Approach

Anterior access to the glenoid and coracoid is performed through a standard deltopectoral approach. An incision is made along the deltopectoral groove from the coracoid proximally and carried 10 to 15 cm distally. Sharp dissection is carried out through the skin and the cephalic vein is identified in the deltopectoral groove. Subsequently, the deltoid is retracted laterally and the pectoralis major medially. The cephalic vein can be taken in either direction. Deep, the short head of the biceps and the coracobrachialis are identified and retracted in a medial direction. Access to the anterior aspect of the shoulder joint is now easily obtained. Typically, to have adequate exposure of the glenoid, the subscapularis must be taken down and a retractor placed in the glenohumeral joint to retract the humeral head.

If a posterior approach to the glenoid is being performed, a vertical incision is made overlying the posterior glenoid and full-thickness skin flaps are raised. Exposure of the glenoid is performed by splitting the deltoid longitudinally in line with its fibers. The infraspinatus and teres minor are now visible. These muscles can be partially or completely detached, or the interval between them can be utilized, depending on the amount of exposure necessary. Alternatively, a transverse incision can be performed along the length of the scapula spine, extending to the posterior corner of the acromion. The deltoid is then detached from its origin on the scapular spine and the plane between the deltoid and infraspinatus is identified and developed. Identification of the teres minor is now performed and the plane between the teres minor and infraspinatus is developed. By retracting the infraspinatus superiorly and the teres minor inferiorly, the posterior aspect of the glenoid and scapula neck is now exposed. The glenohumeral joint capsule can be incised longitudinally along the edge of the scapula to gain access to the joint.

Technique

✓ ORIF of Scapula Fractures: KEY SURGICAL STEPS
Posterior Glenoid Cavity Fractures and Glenoid Neck Fractures
❏ Lateral decubitus position using bean bag
❏ Prep and drape entire upper extremity and hemithorax
❏ Posterior approach with arm abducted
❏ Retract posterior part of deltoid superolaterally without detaching its origin or insertion—the muscle can be detached if needed for improved visualization
❏ Identify and explore interval between the teres minor and infraspinatus by retracting the teres minor inferiorly and infraspinatus superiorly
❏ Detach infraspinatous insertion if necessary and incise capsule if fixing a glenoid cavity fracture
❏ Reduce fragment utilizing K-wires as joysticks and provisional fixation
❏ Fix fragment with either interfragmentary screws or plate/screw construct
Anterior Glenoid Cavity Fractures
❏ Beach chair position with Mayfield headrest
❏ Prep and drape entire upper extremity and hemithorax
❏ Standard deltopectoral approach
❏ Place stay sutures in subscapularis and detach muscle from humerus
❏ Longitudinal incision to enter glenohumeral joint
❏ Place Fuduka retractor on humeral head to expose glenoid
❏ Reduce fragment utilizing intact labrum or K-wires as joysticks and provisional fixation
❏ Fix fragment with either interfragmentary screws or plate/screw construct
Displaced Coracoid Process Fractures
❏ Beach chair position with Mayfield headrest
❏ Prep and drape entire upper extremity and hemithorax
❏ Standard deltopectoral approach
❏ Identify and protect musculocutaneous nerve
❏ Fix large coracoid process fractures with interfragmentary screw fixation
❏ Fix small coracoid process fractures using heavy nonabsorbable suture through the conjoint tendon and pass through a drill hole in the intact coracoid process

Displaced glenoid neck fractures are approached through the posterior approach with placement of a plate along the posterior aspect of the glenoid and extending down along the lateral angle of the scapula. Operative treatment of type Ib, type II, and type IV glenoid cavity fractures is also performed via a posterior approach. The infraspinatus can remain attached during fixation of type Ib fractures, whereas detachment is necessary for types II and IV fractures. Fixation of type Ib fragments is typically performed using two interfragmentary screws, whereas types II and IV fractures typically require plate and screw fixation.

An anterior deltopectoral approach is used to perform ORIF of type Ia and III glenoid cavity fractures as well as coracoid fractures displaced greater than 2 cm. Fixation is achieved with interfragmentary screws for type Ia and large coracoid process fractures if the fragment is large enough, whereas plate and screw fixation is typically necessary for type III fractures. Alternatively, suture anchors can be used to stabilize type Ia fragments and small coracoid process fractures can be reattached with the conjoint tendon utilizing heavy nonabsorbable suture placed in a Bunnell fashion through the tendon and passed through a drill hole in the intact coracoid process. Arthroscopic fixation of type Ia fractures can also be performed by using suture anchor fixation to the intact labral attachment of the fragment.[116]

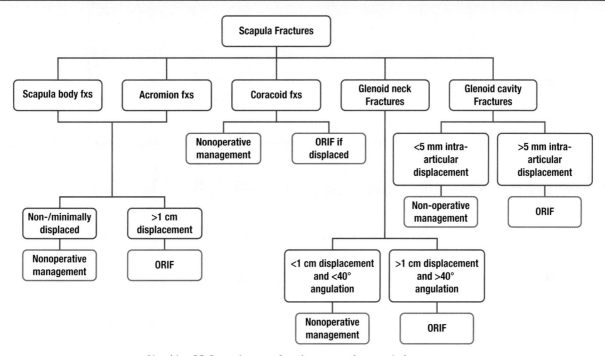

Authors' Preferred Treatment for Scapula Fractures (Algorithm 20-2)

Algorithm 20-2. Authors' preferred treatment for scapula fractures.

Most pediatric and adolescent scapula fractures are treated nonoperatively with immobilization for 3 to 4 weeks followed by pendulum exercises and progressed to active range of motion as tolerated. This includes scapula body fractures, acromion fractures, coracoid process fractures, and glenoid neck and cavity fractures without significant displacement. Operative treatment is reserved for open fractures and glenoid cavity fractures with significant size and/or displacement leading to glenohumeral subluxation/dislocation. Coracoid process fractures displaced greater than 2 cm are also treated with ORIF.

Our preference is to perform arthroscopic reduction of type Ia glenoid cavity fractures and ORIF for the remainder of glenoid cavity fractures and glenoid neck fractures requiring operative fixation. We routinely obtain three-dimensional CT scans to aid in preoperative planning and determination of the best surgical approach to utilize based on the fracture pattern.

Postoperative Care

Postoperatively, patients are placed in a sling or shoulder immobilizer for 3 to 6 weeks. Subsequently, pendulum exercises are performed followed by advancement to active range of motion based on radiographic union and pain. Strengthening and contact sports are not permitted for a minimum of 3 months postoperatively.

Scapula Fractures: SURGICAL PITFALLS AND PREVENTIONS	
Pitfall	**Prevention**
Neurovascular injury	Avoid overly vigorous retraction
Persistent glenohumeral subluxation/dislocation	Obtain near-anatomic (<2-mm incongruity) of glenoid cavity fragments

Care must be taken during ORIF when retracting structures about the shoulder region, as vigorous retraction can damage neurovascular structures. For example, the musculocutaneous nerve is at risk during excessive medial retraction about the glenohumeral joint/coracoid.

It is necessary to obtain a near-anatomic reduction of the articular surface during ORIF of glenoid cavity fractures as residual displacement of more than 2 mm leads to poorer outcomes.[60] Furthermore, failure to reduce large glenoid cavity fragments may lead to persistent glenohumeral subluxation/dislocation.

Outcomes

No data exist regarding the outcomes of pediatric and adolescent patients treated with ORIF for scapula fractures. The adult literature has demonstrated that the results of operative fixation of glenoid cavity fractures depend on near-anatomic restoration of joint alignment. If residual incongruity is less than 2 mm, good-to-excellent results can be expected for 80% to 90% of patients. Furthermore, posttraumatic arthritis will be minimal.[60]

MANAGEMENT OF EXPECTED ADVERSE OUTCOMES AND UNEXPECTED COMPLICATIONS RELATED TO SCAPULA FRACTURES

Scapula Fractures: COMMON ADVERSE OUTCOMES AND COMPLICATIONS
• Nonunion
• Symptomatic malunion
• Glenohumeral subluxation/dislocation

Nonunion and symptomatic malunion can occur following treatment of scapular body fractures nonoperatively.[52,82] Nonunions can be addressed by performing ORIF with good-to-excellent results expected. In addition, significant displacement associated with glenoid neck fractures has been shown to be a poor prognostic indicator. Therefore, fixation of fractures with more than 1 cm of displacement or angulation greater than 40 degrees will yield improved outcomes.[27,65,89] Finally, large glenoid rim fractures should be addressed operatively to prevent subluxation/dislocation of the glenohumeral joint.

SUMMARY, CONTROVERSIES, AND FUTURE DIRECTIONS RELATED TO SCAPULA FRACTURES

Scapula fractures are rare injuries that occur due to high-energy mechanisms or nonaccidental trauma. Conservative treatment with immobilization yields excellent outcomes in the vast majority of cases. However, it is important to recognize fractures that can potentially lead to adverse outcomes and complications. Advanced imaging with CT scans, including three-dimensional reconstruction, can aid the surgeon by providing better understanding of the fracture pattern. Operative fixation should be performed for fractures about the glenoid with significant displacement or those leading to glenohumeral subluxation/dislocation. Because of the rarity of these fractures, it is likely that future multicenter studies will be necessary to provide information regarding the best treatments and their outcomes for pediatric and adolescent scapula fractures.

Acromioclavicular Dislocations

INTRODUCTION TO ACROMIOCLAVICULAR DISLOCATIONS

While AC dislocations are common in adults, they are rare in children. Injuries that appear to disrupt the AC joint in a child may actually be an epiphyseal separation of the distal clavicle termed a "pseudodislocation," rather than a true AC joint disruption.[107] However, older adolescents can sustain true AC dislocations, especially those involved in competitive sports participation.[59] Treatment of these injuries, especially complete dislocations, remains somewhat controversial and is based on individual patient demands.

ASSESSMENT OF ACROMIOCLAVICULAR DISLOCATIONS

MECHANISMS OF INJURY FOR ACROMIOCLAVICULAR DISLOCATIONS

AC joint injuries typically occur due to a direct blow to the acromion with the shoulder adducted, as can occur during collision sports, or due to a fall onto the superolateral aspect of the shoulder. The result of this blow is inferior and medial movement of the acromion while the clavicle remains stable because of the sternoclavicular joint ligaments.[103] Propagation of the force to the CC ligaments and deltotrapezial fascia can occur following complete disruption of the AC ligaments.[107] Indirect force can also result in injury to the AC joint, as occurs during a fall onto an outstretched hand or elbow.[112]

INJURIES ASSOCIATED WITH ACROMIOCLAVICULAR DISLOCATIONS

As with any injury to the shoulder region, the entire shoulder girdle must be examined for a concomitant injury. Anterior sternoclavicular dislocations or additional scapula, humerus, or clavicle fractures can occur simultaneously if enough force was present at the time of impact. In addition, brachial plexus or cervical spine injuries may be present, especially if the injury occurred during a collision sport, such as football.

SIGNS AND SYMPTOMS OF ACROMIOCLAVICULAR DISLOCATIONS

Patients with AC dislocations usually complain of pain in the shoulder region localized to the AC joint area. Numbness and tingling may be present because of swelling or concomitant cervical spine/brachial plexus injury. Sometimes, they only complain of a "bump" in the region.

The physical examination should begin by observation of the shoulder region with the patient in an upright position, which permits the weight of the arm to make any deformity more apparent. Swelling, ecchymosis, abrasions, and skin tenting should be noted. Palpation overlying the AC joint will cause significant discomfort and should be reserved until the end of the examination. Additional areas that should be palpated first include the proximal humerus, the midshaft and medial clavicle, the sternoclavicular joint, and the cervical spine. A thorough neurologic examination should be performed to assess for concomitant brachial plexus or cervical spine injury. Most displaced distal clavicle fractures are malpositioned superiorly and have both visual and palpable deformities. However, some displace posteriorly, get entrapped in the trapezius muscle, and have a palpable prominence and tenderness medial and posterior to the acromion. These type IV injuries may be hard to diagnose unless examined specifically.

Once an AC injury is suspected, the joint should be assessed for stability if possible. Typically, this needs to be done after the acute pain has subsided, approximately 5 to 7 days following the injury. Horizontal and vertical stabilities can be assessed and potentially the joint can be reduced by closed means. This is performed by stabilizing the clavicle with one hand and using the other hand to place an upward force under the ipsilateral elbow. Once the joint is reduced in the coronal plane, the midshaft of the clavicle can be grasped and translated in an anterior and posterior direction to assess horizontal stability.[112]

IMAGING AND OTHER DIAGNOSTIC STUDIES FOR ACROMIOCLAVICULAR DISLOCATIONS

Plain radiographs are the initial imaging modality of choice and should include a true AP view of the shoulder, an axillary lateral view of the shoulder, and a Zanca view to better visualize the AC joint. The Zanca view is performed with the patient in an upright position, allowing the injured arm to hang by the weight of gravity, and aiming the x-ray beam 10 to 15 degrees cephalad.[136] In addition, stress views can be performed, to differentiate between types II and III injuries, by having the patient hold a weight in each hand, with a single radiograph of the bilateral clavicles obtained. The posterior fracture dislocation (type IV) is often difficult to recognize by plain radiographs and may require a CT scan for accurate diagnosis.

CLASSIFICATION OF ACROMIOCLAVICULAR DISLOCATIONS

The classic description of AC injuries for adults is that of Tossy et al.[123] and Allman[3] which was subsequently modified by Rockwood and colleagues (Fig. 20-13).[130] Type I injuries have normal radiographs with the only finding being tenderness to palpation over the AC joint due to a sprain of the AC ligaments. Type II injuries have disruption of the AC ligaments and a sprain of the CC ligaments. The radiographs show a widened AC joint with slight vertical displacement demonstrated by a mild increase in the CC space. Type III injuries have disruption of the AC and CC ligaments with the radiographs showing the clavicle displaced superiorly relative to the acromion by 25% to 100% the width of the clavicle. Type IV injuries have disruption of the AC and CC ligaments as well as the deltopectoral fascia which allows for the clavicle to be posteriorly displaced into or through the trapezius muscle. Type V injuries have disruption of the AC and CC ligaments as well as the deltopectoral fascia with concomitant injury to the deltoid and trapezius muscle attachments to the clavicle. These injuries present with the clavicle displaced greater than 100% and lying in the

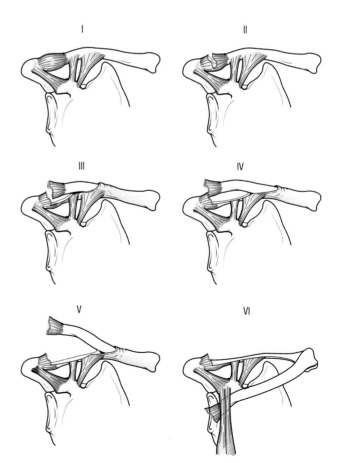

Figure 20-13. Schematic depicting the Rockwood classification of acromioclavicular joint injuries.

subcutaneous tissue. Type VI injuries have disruption of the AC ligaments and deltopectoral fascia, but the CC ligaments remain intact. This occurs due to a high-energy mechanism of injury that causes the shoulder to be hyperabducted and externally rotated. The end result is that the clavicle lies subacromial or subcoracoid, with a resultant decrease in the CC distance seen on radiographs.

The classification mentioned above has been modified for the pediatric and adolescent populations, as true AC injuries are rare during skeletal immaturity compared with fractures of the distal clavicle. Typically, the clavicle itself displaces out of the periosteal sleeve, leaving the periosteum attached to the CC and AC ligaments. The resultant clavicle injuries are then analogous to the six types described for the adult classification.

OUTCOME MEASURES FOR ACROMIOCLAVICULAR DISLOCATIONS

Typically, results of AC injuries have been reported based on subjective outcomes, the development of AC osteoarthritis, and range of motion. No outcome measures have been specifically applied to pediatric AC injuries. Commonly utilized measures for adult AC joint injuries include the ASES score, the DASH Score, the QuickDASH, and the Constant Shoulder Score. The recent publication of a novel Pedi-ASES demonstrated that adult shoulder outcome scores such as the DASH and ASES surveys are associated with poor validity and comprehensibility in pediatric populations, and this new metric, when more comprehensively validated, may emerge as a future standard for use in pediatric and adolescent shoulder research.[44]

PATHOANATOMY AND APPLIED ANATOMY RELATED TO ACROMIOCLAVICULAR DISLOCATIONS

The AC joint is formed by the distal end of the clavicle and medial aspect of the acromion with a fibrocartilaginous disk between them. It is an important contribution to the superior shoulder suspensory complex, a bone–soft tissue ring composed of the glenoid, coracoid, CC ligaments, distal clavicle, AC joint, and acromion (Fig. 20-14). This complex maintains a normal relationship between the scapula, upper extremity, and axial skeleton to permit fluid scapulothoracic motion. While the clavicle does rotate some relative to the acromion through the AC joint, most motion occurs synchronously.

The ligamentous structures about the AC joint provide most stability, with a smaller component provided by the muscular attachments of the anterior deltoid onto the clavicle and trapezius onto the acromion. Horizontal stability is provided by the AC ligaments that reinforce the joint capsule, mainly the posterior and superior ligaments.[63] Vertical stability is provided by the CC ligaments, including the conoid ligament medially and trapezoid ligament laterally. The normal distance between the coracoid and the clavicle, the CC space, should be 1.1 to 1.3 cm.

TREATMENT OPTIONS FOR ACROMIOCLAVICULAR DISLOCATIONS

NONOPERATIVE TREATMENT OF ACROMIOCLAVICULAR DISLOCATIONS

Nonoperative treatment of types I and II AC injuries is uniformly accepted. However, treatment of type III injuries remains somewhat controversial. The vast majority of types IV, V, and VI injuries should be treated surgically to reduce the AC joint and restore stability to the superior shoulder suspensory complex. Absolute contraindications to nonoperative treatment include open injuries and injuries with associated neurovascular injury requiring operative intervention.

Techniques

Nonoperative treatment is performed using immobilization in a sling or shoulder immobilizer for 2 to 4 weeks. Following the

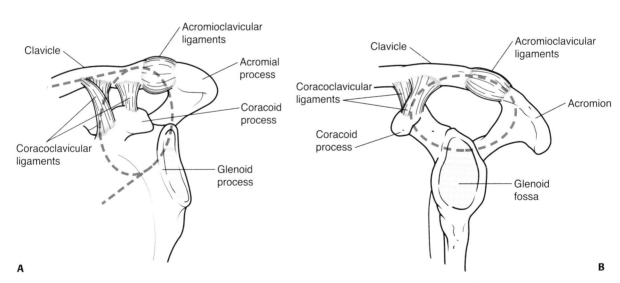

Figure 20-14. Schematic of the superior shoulder suspensory complex. **A:** Frontal view. **B:** Lateral view.

period of immobilization and resolution of the pain, patients are gradually progressed from pendulum exercises to active range of motion. Strengthening is begun once range of motion is equal to the uninjured side. Contact sports are avoided for 6 to 12 weeks following injury to allow for complete ligamentous healing and for prevention of converting an incomplete injury (type II) to a complete injury (type III).[112]

Little published data exist regarding the nonoperative treatment of types I and II injuries in the pediatric and adolescent populations. The adult literature has demonstrated a 9% to 30% rate of pain and limitation of activities with closed treatment of type I injuries and a 23% to 42% rate for closed treatment of type II injuries, some of which required surgical intervention.[15,83] Children and adolescents seem to do better in terms of pain and restoration of function but it has not been studied extensively.

Treatment of type III injuries remains controversial because of the outcomes demonstrated in the adult literature. Bannister et al.[11] found that injuries with 2 cm or more of displacement treated nonsurgically had 20% good or excellent results compared with 70% in the surgically treated group. However, a study involving athletes and laborers with type III injuries treated nonoperatively showed that they were able to recover adequate strength and endurance to return to their preinjury activities.[132] A meta-analysis by Phillips et al.[96] supported nonoperative treatment of type III injuries as patients treated surgically had a higher complication rate, with patients treated nonoperatively able to return to work and preinjury activities faster.

Indications/Contraindications

Nonoperative Treatment of Acromioclavicular Dislocations:
INDICATIONS AND CONTRAINDICATIONS

Indications

- Type I injuries
- Type II injuries

Relative Contraindications

- Open injuries
- Injuries with associated neurovascular injuries requiring operative treatment

---

OPERATIVE TREATMENT OF ACROMIOCLAVICULAR DISLOCATIONS

Indications/Contraindications

Indications for operative treatment of AC injuries include complete disruptions of the joint, leading to true dislocations in adolescents or fracture dislocations in the pediatric population, mainly types IV, V, and VI injuries. The most common operative indication in the young is a type IV injury with displacement and entrapment in the trapezius muscle posteriorly. In addition, an injury that is open or has a concomitant neurovascular injury requiring operative intervention should be treated operatively. As noted above, the treatment of type III injuries is somewhat controversial.

Preoperative Planning

✓ ORIF of Acromioclavicular Dislocations:
PREOPERATIVE PLANNING CHECKLIST

OR table	❏ Standard table capable of going into beach chair position
Position/ positioning aids	❏ Beach chair position with adequate sterile space above the shoulder adjacent to the head
Fluoroscopy location	❏ Contralateral side
Equipment	❏ Implants may include hook plate, cannulated screws, K-wires, heavy nonabsorbable suture, hamstring autograft, allograft

---

Treatment of AC injuries surgically requires planning to ensure that the appropriate equipment is available. If implants are being utilized, these may include a hook plate, cannulated screws, K-wires, or heavy nonabsorbable suture. Reconstruction of the ligaments, however, requires either planning to obtain hamstring tendon autograft or having tendon allograft available.

Positioning

Whether open reduction or ligament reconstruction is being performed, the beach chair position is utilized. A bump is placed behind the scapula to bring the acromion into a more anterior position.

Surgical Approach

A direct approach to the AC joint is used by making an incision along the lateral clavicle and anterior aspect of the joint in Langer skin lines. Sharp dissection is carried out through the skin only. Subsequently, electrocautery is utilized the remainder of the way down to bone so that hemostasis and dissection can occur simultaneously. It is easiest to incise the periosteum of the distal clavicle and acromion before entering the joint. It is imperative to avoid disruption of the CC ligaments in type VI injuries as they are intact. The AC and CC ligaments as well as the deltopectoral fascia are disrupted in types II, IV, and V injuries in the skeletally mature patients; they are attached to the periosteum in younger patients.

Technique

✓ ORIF of Acromioclavicular Dislocations:
KEY SURGICAL STEPS

- ❏ Skin incision in Langer line directly anterior to acromioclavicular joint
- ❏ Electrocautery down to distal clavicle and acromion
- ❏ Reduce acromioclavicular joint
- ❏ Repair periosteum and ligamentous structures and assess stability
- ❏ Use hook plate if joint remains unstable for segmental fractures or intra-articular fractures
- ❏ Place lateral end of hook plate under acromion and facilitate AC joint reduction by placing medial part of plate on clavicle
- ❏ Place bicortical screws in medial part of hook plate
- ❏ Irrigate wound and close
- ❏ Plate removal 2–3 months postoperatively

Once the dissection has exposed the AC joint, an open reduction of the joint is performed. Type IV injuries necessitate carefully extracting the distal clavicle from the trapezius muscle, type V injuries require reducing the distal clavicle from the subcutaneous tissue, and type VI injuries require removing the distal clavicle from beneath the coracoid process. Once the distal clavicle is reduced to the level of the acromion, temporary pin fixation across the AC joint may be necessary to hold the reduction. As the periosteum is torn but still attached to the acromion, once the clavicle is reduced, simple repair of the periosteum and ligamentous structures may be all that is required in the pediatric population.

If the patient is older and a hook plate is being used, the lateral end of the plate is placed deep to the acromion and the medial side is placed on the clavicle, which will facilitate joint reduction and maintenance of the reduction. Bicortical screws are now placed into the clavicle to hold the plate in place.

Ligament reconstruction and/or augmentation have been performed, via various methods, as the primary method of treatment for the injury in adults. Fortunately, these operations are rare in the acute setting for adolescents. More often these reconstructions are in chronic, painful AC separations in adults. Both semitendinosus autograft and allograft can be used as a loop around the coracoid and clavicle[54] or placed through bone tunnels in the coracoid and clavicle and secured with interference screws.[76] The interference screws are placed at the locations of the CC ligaments in an attempt to restore normal anatomy.

CC screw placement or loops of heavy nonabsorbable suture/Dacron tape around the coracoid and clavicle has also been used to treat AC injuries, either by itself or in conjunction with ligament reconstruction. Screw placement requires removal whereas the loop technique can lead to suture cutout or aseptic foreign body reactions.[16,115] The modified Weaver–Dunn procedure has been performed in arthritic situations by resecting the distal end of the clavicle, detaching the coracoacromial ligament from the deep surface of the acromion, and transferring it to the distal end of the clavicle. Again, this is very rarely performed in children and adolescents.

Author's Preferred Treatment for Acromioclavicular Dislocations

We treat all types I and II AC injuries as well as most type III injuries nonoperatively, with immobilization in a sling or shoulder immobilizer for 2 to 4 weeks followed by early restoration of range of motion. Contact sports are avoided for at least 6 to 12 weeks. The vast majority of types IV, V, and VI injuries are treated operatively. Once the distal clavicle is exposed, we determine whether repair of the periosteum and ligamentous structures surrounding the clavicle is sufficient or if a plate is required. The vast majority can be treated with periosteal repair over the reduced clavicle. Most often operative repair is for type IV fracture–dislocations with entrapment in the trapezius. Hook plates are most commonly utilized in older patients with fractures that are either segmental or intra-articular. Following plate placement, the periosteum and ligamentous structures are repaired.

Postoperative Care

Postoperatively, patients are placed in either a sling or shoulder immobilizer for 4 to 6 weeks. Pendulum exercises are then begun followed by gentle active range of motion below shoulder level for 6 to 8 weeks. At 8 weeks, full active range of motion is permitted. If a hook plate or CC screw was placed, it is removed with sufficient healing, usually at approximately 12 weeks. Contact sports are avoided for a minimum of 3 months following operative intervention.

Potential Pitfalls and Preventive Measures

Acromioclavicular Dislocations:
SURGICAL PITFALLS AND PREVENTIONS

Pitfall	Preventions
Missing a type IV injury	Careful assessment of the radiographs
	Adequate lateral radiograph
	Utilize physical examination to aid in the diagnosis
	CT scan

One of the biggest pitfalls when treating AC injuries is failure to recognize a type IV injury. Although types V and VI injuries are fairly obvious on AP plain radiographs, type IV injuries, because of their posterior displacement, may not be readily apparent. Furthermore, lateral views may be inadequate or difficult to obtain, thus making it easy to miss a type IV injury. A high index of clinical suspicion, careful examination, and often a CT scan are necessary for accurate diagnosis and appropriate surgical treatment.

Outcomes

No studies have specifically evaluated the treatment of AC injuries in the pediatric and adolescent populations. In our experience, operative treatment of types IV, V, and VI injuries has yielded excellent outcomes in the majority of patients. Restoration of joint congruity and stability permits rapid return to function. However, we do not have long-term data to determine how many patients develop degenerative arthritis.

MANAGEMENT OF EXPECTED ADVERSE OUTCOMES AND UNEXPECTED COMPLICATIONS RELATED TO ACROMIOCLAVICULAR DISLOCATIONS

Acromioclavicular Dislocations:
COMMON ADVERSE OUTCOMES AND COMPLICATIONS

- Posttraumatic arthritis
- Persistent instability
- Symptomatic hardware
- Pin migration
- Persistent pain
- Suture cutout
- Aseptic foreign body reaction

Development of degenerative arthritis can be treated by distal clavicle resection. However, the results of this are not favorable if the CC ligaments are disrupted as instability will ensue.[23] Persistent instability following closed treatment of an AC joint injury can be treated with ligament reconstruction or augmentation.

Complications related to open reduction include migration of pins, symptomatic implants, and persistent pain. As noted earlier, usage of synthetic material can lead to suture cutout or aseptic foreign material reaction. Any technique that passes material around the coracoid may lead to coracoid fracture or injury to the musculocutaneous nerve.

SUMMARY, CONTROVERSIES, AND FUTURE DIRECTIONS RELATED TO ACROMIOCLAVICULAR DISLOCATIONS

AC injuries are relatively rare in the pediatric and adolescent populations. The injury patterns are classified similar to the adult population. However, in the young, the periosteum tears permitting the clavicle to displace while the periosteal attachment to the acromion and coracoid remains intact. Treatment can be immobilization alone for injuries that are not widely displaced, but operative intervention should be performed for significantly displaced injuries. Restoration of normal anatomy by reduction of the AC joint, suture repair of the periosteum, and ligamentous repair as needed can yield excellent outcomes in the pediatric population while avoiding utilization of metal implants. Future studies are necessary to assess outcomes of these injuries in the pediatric and adolescent populations.

Sternoclavicular Fracture-Dislocations

INTRODUCTION TO STERNOCLAVICULAR FRACTURE-DISLOCATIONS

Injuries to the sternoclavicular joint are rare, representing less than 5% of shoulder girdle injuries.[51] These injuries occur secondary to high-energy mechanisms and therefore can be associated with life-threatening complications. Historically, treatment by observation has occurred in the pediatric and adolescent populations. More recent trends are to operatively reduce and stabilize acute posterior fracture-dislocations to restore anatomy and improve functional outcomes.

ASSESSMENT OF STERNOCLAVICULAR FRACTURE-DISLOCATIONS

MECHANISMS OF INJURY FOR STERNOCLAVICULAR FRACTURE-DISLOCATIONS

A significant amount of force is required to disrupt the sternoclavicular joint because of the numerous surrounding ligaments

as well as the stability provided by the rib cage. Therefore, high-energy mechanisms, such as motor vehicle accidents and sports participation, result in over 80% of injuries.[17] Sports injuries are the most common mechanism of injury (71%), with football, rugby, and wrestling being the most commonly involved sports.[119] Motor vehicle collisions may result in either an anterior or posterior force across the joint with a resultant anterior or posterior dislocation or fracture/dislocation. A direct lateral blow to the shoulder with the shoulder extended will result in the more common anterior dislocation. Posterior dislocations can result from indirect force transferred to the shoulder girdle when the shoulder is adducted and flexed. Alternatively, a direct anterior-to-posterior blow to the medial clavicle is another mechanism for posterior sternoclavicular dislocation during sports participation.[42] Of note, most cases of anterior sternoclavicular instability are atraumatic and associated with ligamentous laxity.

INJURIES ASSOCIATED WITH STERNOCLAVICULAR FRACTURE-DISLOCATIONS

Because of the high-energy mechanisms that cause posterior sternoclavicular injuries, associated chest wall injuries do occur such as rib fractures. In addition, the trachea, esophagus, lungs, or great vessels may be compressed. Dysphagia or dyspnea is present in up to 30% of patients.[119] Patients may also experience a brachial plexopathy. Life-threatening injuries, including vessel laceration, stroke, pneumomediastinum, or even death can occur but are rare. Very rarely, the entire clavicle may dislocate from both the sternoclavicular joint and AC joint, thus constituting a floating shoulder. It is imperative to carefully evaluate the entire shoulder girdle for concomitant fractures or dislocations.

SIGNS AND SYMPTOMS OF STERNOCLAVICULAR FRACTURE-DISLOCATIONS

Patients who sustain sternoclavicular joint injuries present with complaints of pain localized to the sternoclavicular joint. Additional subjective complaints may include shortness of breath, dyspnea, dysphagia, odynophagia, or hoarseness.[128] If an associated brachial plexopathy is present, patients may report the presence of paresthesias and/or weakness in the ipsilateral arm.

Objective evaluation will demonstrate a significant amount of swelling and ecchymosis present, so much so, that it may be difficult to determine the direction of the dislocation.[42] Anterior dislocations may exhibit prominence of the medial clavicle, which is more easily appreciated with the patient supine (Fig. 20-15).[42] In contrast, the corner of the sternum may be palpable in cases of posterior dislocation, as the medial clavicle is displaced posteriorly. However, at times, the posterior fracture dislocation can be more subtle than expected as the swelling can mimic normal sternoclavicular alignment on cursory examination.

Passive range of motion of the ipsilateral shoulder will cause pain and may elicit the sensation of instability. It is imperative that a formal trauma team or emergency room physician evaluation occurs to rule out associated life-threatening injuries. Signs of venous congestion and arterial insufficiency to the involved extremity or neck region may be present due to compression of vessels.

Figure 20-15. Clinical photograph demonstrating an anterior sterno-clavicular dislocation. This was more easily identified once the patient was lying supine. (Reprinted with permission from Waters PM, Bae DS, eds. *Pediatric Hand and Upper Limb Surgery: A Practical Guide.* Wolters Kluwer; 2012.)

IMAGING AND OTHER DIAGNOSTIC STUDIES FOR STERNOCLAVICULAR FRACTURE-DISLOCATIONS

As with any injury, plain radiographs are the initial imaging modality performed. The routine AP chest radiograph may demonstrate asymmetry of the sternoclavicular articulations or clavicle lengths. However, these studies can be quite difficult to interpret because of the overlap of the medial clavicle, lungs, ribs, sternum, and spine (Fig. 20-16).

Specific radiographic views to evaluate the sternoclavicular joint have been described to overcome these obstacles. Heinig described a tangential view of the sternoclavicular joint which

is obtained by laying the patient supine and placing the cassette behind the opposite shoulder. The beam is then angled coronally, parallel to the longitudinal axis of the opposite clavicle (Fig. 20-17A). Hobbs[47] proposed taking a 90-degree cephalo-caudal lateral view, by having the patient seated and flexed over a table while the beam is directed through the cervical spine (Fig. 20-17B). Finally, the serendipity view described by Rockwood is performed by placing the cassette behind the chest and angling the x-ray beam 40 degrees cephalad while it is centered on the sternum, thus providing a view of both sternoclavicular joints (Fig. 20-17C).[131] In cases of anterior dislocation, the affected side will appear superiorly displaced, whereas in cases of posterior dislocation, the affected side will appear inferiorly displaced (Fig. 20-18).

Despite these described plain radiographic views, the easiest way to evaluate the sternoclavicular joint is with CT scan that provides a three-dimensional view of the joint (Fig. 20-19). In addition to assessment of the sternoclavicular joint, one can evaluate the adjacent soft tissue structures including the esophagus, trachea, lungs, and brachiocephalic vessels. Distinction between a physeal fracture and a true dislocation may also be possible if the secondary center has ossified.

Magnetic resonance imaging (MRI) can also be used to evaluate the sternoclavicular joint as well as the surrounding soft tissues. The integrity of the costoclavicular ligaments and intra-articular disk may be possible.[42] A recent study by Tytherleigh-Strong et al.[125] described the utility of MRI in 13 adolescent patients, with the specific advantage of differentiating between true dislocations, which are isolated ligamentous injuries, and the more common physeal fracture-dislocation at the proximal clavicle.[125] More pointedly, they cited the advantage of MRI allowing for assessment of physeal injuries with some residual bone contact between the fragments, which they were able

A

B

C

Figure 20-16. A: Apparent normal anteroposterior (AP) view of the clavicle. **B:** Serendipity view demonstrating asymmetry of the sternoclavicular joint with a posterior dislocation on the right. **C:** CT scan clearly showing the right posterior sternoclavicular dislocation. (Reprinted with permission from Waters PM, Bae DS, eds. *Pediatric Hand and Upper Limb Surgery: A Practical Guide.* Wolters Kluwer; 2012.)

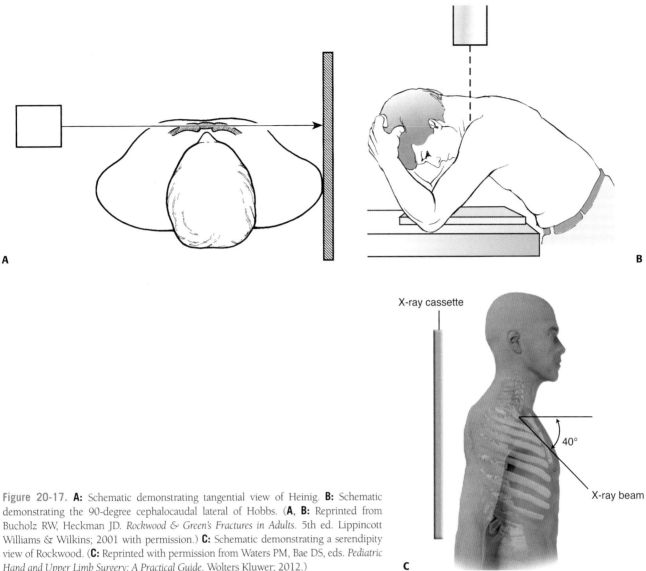

Figure 20-17. **A:** Schematic demonstrating tangential view of Heinig. **B:** Schematic demonstrating the 90-degree cephalocaudal lateral of Hobbs. (**A, B:** Reprinted from Bucholz RW, Heckman JD. *Rockwood & Green's Fractures in Adults.* 5th ed. Lippincott Williams & Wilkins; 2001 with permission.) **C:** Schematic demonstrating a serendipity view of Rockwood. (**C:** Reprinted with permission from Waters PM, Bae DS, eds. *Pediatric Hand and Upper Limb Surgery: A Practical Guide.* Wolters Kluwer; 2012.)

X-ray cassette

40°

X-ray beam

Figure 20-18. **A:** Serendipity radiograph showing a left posteriorly dislocated sternoclavicular joint. Note that the affected side appears inferiorly displaced. **B:** CT scan of the same patient clearly showing the left posterior dislocation.

A   B

Figure 20-19. A: CT scan showing a posterior dislocation of the right sternoclavicular joint. **B:** Three-dimensional reconstruction makes the injury more apparent.

to therefore treat nonoperatively with success. While a small series, this work creates some opportunity for this nonradiation modality, at least at centers where there may be better access to MRI, being a reasonable surrogate to CT images. Despite the potential to gain additional information, at most centers CT scan is recommended over MRI scan to evaluate acute injuries because of its speed and availability, particularly the setting of any symptoms suggestive of mediastinal compromise.

CLASSIFICATION OF STERNOCLAVICULAR FRACTURE-DISLOCATIONS

Sternoclavicular dislocations are classified based on the direction of displacement, anterior or posterior, as well as the chronicity of the injury, acute or chronic. The injury needs to be defined as a dislocation (displacement between the epiphysis and the sternum) or a fracture (displacement through the physis with the epiphysis still articulating with sternum). In addition, a sprain, rather than a true dislocation, may occur leading to subluxation.

OUTCOME MEASURES FOR STERNOCLAVICULAR FRACTURE-DISLOCATIONS

No specific outcome scores exist that specifically evaluate sternoclavicular joint injuries. Results reported have assessed subjective complaints of pain, recurrence of instability, return to function,

and utilization of adult shoulder outcome measures, such as the ASES score, the simple shoulder test, and Rockwood scores.

PATHOANATOMY AND APPLIED ANATOMY RELATED TO STERNOCLAVICULAR FRACTURE-DISLOCATIONS

The sternoclavicular joint is a true diarthrodial joint comprising the medial clavicle and clavicular notch of the sternum. Thus, this joint is the only connection between the axial skeleton and the upper extremity. However, less than 50% of the clavicular head articulates with the clavicular notch of the sternum, resulting in little bony congruity. Stability is therefore provided by the multiple ligamentous and muscular attachments, including the sternocleidomastoid, pectoralis major, and sternohyoid muscles. The ligamentous structures include anterior and posterior sternoclavicular ligaments which reinforce the joint capsule as well as the interclavicular (connects both medial ends of the clavicle) and costoclavicular ligaments (between the inferior aspect of the clavicle and the superior costal cartilage of the adjacent rib). In addition, there is an intra-articular disk that is attached to the superoposterior part of the clavicular articular surface and inferiorly to the costocartilaginous junction of the first rib (Fig. 20-20). The greatest

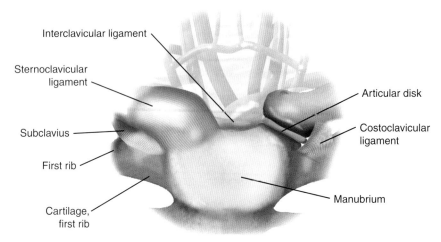

Interclavicular ligament

Sternoclavicular ligament

Subclavius

First rib

Cartilage, first rib

Articular disk

Costoclavicular ligament

Manubrium

Figure 20-20. Schematic drawing of the sternoclavicular joint. Note the numerous ligamentous structures that provide stability. (Reprinted with permission from Waters PM, Bae DS, eds. *Pediatric Hand and Upper Limb Surgery: A Practical Guide.* Wolters Kluwer; 2012.)

amount of stability with regard to anterior translation is provided by the posterior capsule and sternoclavicular ligaments. The greatest stability with regard to posterior translation is provided by the posterior capsule.[113,114]

The medial epiphysis of the clavicle does not ossify until approximately 18 to 20 years of age and closes between 22 and 25 years of age. Therefore, sternoclavicular injuries occurring in pediatric and adolescent patients are difficult to discern radiographically between fractures and dislocations. Operative treatment of posterior sternoclavicular injuries has taught us that dislocations and physeal fractures have near-equivalent incidence rather than the previous teaching that most posterior sternoclavicular injuries were physeal fractures. Although the medial physis contributes approximately 80% of longitudinal growth of the clavicle, the degree of remodeling possible from a physeal fracture is uncertain. Clearly, remodeling cannot occur with a dislocation.

TREATMENT OPTIONS FOR STERNOCLAVICULAR FRACTURE-DISLOCATIONS

NONOPERATIVE TREATMENT OF STERNOCLAVICULAR DISLOCATIONS

Indications/Contraindications

Nonoperative Treatment of Sternoclavicular Fracture-Dislocations:
INDICATIONS AND CONTRAINDICATIONS

Indications

• Atraumatic anterior dislocations

Relative Contraindications

• Acute posterior dislocations with associated neurovascular injury, dyspnea, dysphagia, odynophagia, or hoarseness

An atraumatic anterior dislocation should be treated nonoperatively. Some have advocated closed reduction maneuvers be performed for acute posterior fracture-dislocations due to potential stability of reduction and/or remodeling of the medial clavicle.[131] Acute posterior dislocations with associated neurovascular injury, dyspnea, dysphagia, odynophagia, or hoarseness should clearly be treated with open reduction. We advocate that all posterior fracture-dislocations should be treated operatively.

Techniques

Closed treatment of a nondisplaced injury consists of sling immobilization for approximately 3 weeks followed by gradual return to activities. Attempted closed reduction of anterior dislocations can be performed by placing a posteriorly directed force over the medial clavicle as the scapula is retracted by utilization of a bump placed between the shoulders. Subsequently, the patient is placed in a figure-of-eight strap or Velpeau-type sling for 6 weeks.[42] Successful reduction can often be obtained; however, recurrent instability is common.

Closed reduction of a posterior dislocation is performed by placing the patient supine on an OR table with a thick bump placed between the scapulae to extend the shoulders and the involved arm off the edge of the table. The ipsilateral arm is then abducted in line with the clavicle, with traction applied, while an assistant applies countertraction and stabilizes the patient. Traction is continued and increased and the arm is brought into extension as the joint reduces.[42] Alternatively, the arm can be placed in adduction while posterior pressure is applied to the shoulder which levers the clavicle over the first rib to permit reduction of the joint. If these maneuvers fail, a sterile towel clip can be used to percutaneously grasp the medial clavicle and draw it anteriorly while traction is applied to the ipsilateral limb. An audible snap is typically noted as the joint reduces.[42]

Closed reductions of posterior sternoclavicular injuries are at risk for mediastinal hemorrhage and hemodynamic compromise. Therefore, closed reductions are performed in the controlled setting of the operating suite with vascular surgery standby. In addition, the orthopaedic concern with closed reduction is recurrent instability.[37,43,128]

Outcomes

Most patients treated with immobilization alone for anterior dislocations yield good outcomes, despite the high rates of recurrent instability. Those patients who develop symptoms following closed treatment of anterior dislocations may achieve relief of symptoms with physical therapy to promote scapular retraction and avoid provocative positions. If therapy is unsuccessful, ligament reconstruction can be performed with reasonable outcomes anticipated.[7,113]

Posterior fracture-dislocations that are reduced by closed means have been reported by some to be stable following reduction,[43] whereas others have shown recurrent instability does occur.[37,43,67,128] If the reduction is maintained over time, return to full activities can be expected in the majority of patients.[119] A recent meta-analysis of sternoclavicular dislocations assessing results in 92 patients, many of whom were older adolescents (16–19 years of age), concluded that acute dislocations warranted attempted closed treatment, with open treatment being reserved for cases of failed reduction with closed means.[109] However, the authors pooled anterior and posterior dislocations, which most experts approach in very different ways, and did not account for the large portion of physeal fracture-dislocations that are more common in the pediatric population.

OPERATIVE TREATMENT OF STERNOCLAVICULAR FRACTURE-DISLOCATIONS

Indications/Contraindications

Although many surgeons have attempted closed treatment of posterior fracture-dislocations with either immobilization alone or closed reduction followed by immobilization, recurrent instability can occur leading to symptomatic patients who require operative intervention.[12] Therefore, the majority of patients with acute traumatic posterior sternoclavicular fracture-dislocations are currently treated operatively. Operative intervention provides symptomatic relief, restores anatomy, and decreases the chance of late complications including recurrent instability and degenerative arthritis.[128]

Additional indications for operative treatment include patients with symptomatic acute or chronic anterior dislocations who have failed conservative measures and symptomatic patients with chronic posterior dislocations. Contraindications to operative intervention include those patients with asymptomatic anterior dislocations or patients with atraumatic recurrent anterior instability.

Open Reduction and Internal Fixation

Preoperative Planning

> ✓ **ORIF of Sternoclavicular Fracture-Dislocations:**
> PREOPERATIVE PLANNING CHECKLIST

OR table	❏ Standard table capable of going into beach chair position
Position/ positioning aids	❏ Beach chair position with Mayfield head positioner and a bump behind the scapula
Fluoroscopy location	❏ Contralateral side, if used
Equipment	❏ Heavy nonabsorbable suture, drill ❏ General surgery or thoracic surgery backup

It is imperative to be familiar with the anatomy surrounding the sternoclavicular joint as well as the bony articulation of the medial clavicle and clavicular notch of the sternum. Having a general surgeon or thoracic surgeon available to assist the orthopaedic surgeon in case of hemodynamic compromise is essential during the reduction maneuver or open reduction.

Positioning

Patients undergoing any procedure involving the sternoclavicular joint are placed in the modified beach chair position with a large bump or rolled towel placed between the scapulae to provide scapular retraction. The entire limb and hemithorax including the contralateral sternoclavicular joint, medial clavicle, and chest is prepped and draped into the operative field. The sternum to upper abdomen is prepped and draped in case an emergency median sternotomy is required (Fig. 20-21).

Surgical Approach

A transverse incision is made through the skin from the medial aspect of the clavicle over the ipsilateral sternoclavicular joint in Langer lines. The subcutaneous tissue and platysma are divided, utilizing electrocautery. The supraclavicular nerves are protected if in the operative field. The periosteum of the midportion of the clavicle is elevated and a bone clamp is applied to the clavicle for control. The anterior periosteum is delicately divided over the posteriorly displaced clavicle until either the epiphysis or sternum is reached depending on whether it is a dislocation or a physeal fracture (Fig. 20-22). Typically, the

Figure 20-21. Intraoperative photograph showing the area that should be prepped and draped into the sterile field. (Reprinted with permission from Waters PM, Bae DS, eds. *Pediatric Hand and Upper Limb Surgery: A Practical Guide.* Wolters Kluwer; 2012.)

posterior periosteum of the clavicle and the posterior joint capsule are intact, providing a protective layer between the bony injury and mediastinal structures.

Technique

> ✓ **ORIF of Sternoclavicular Fracture-Dislocations:**
> KEY SURGICAL STEPS

❏ Prep and drape the entire limb and hemithorax, including contralateral sternoclavicular joint, chest, and upper abdomen
❏ Transverse skin incision in Langer lines from the diaphysis of the clavicle to the sternoclavicular joint
❏ Divide subcutaneous tissue and platysma in line with skin incision. Protect the supraclavicular nerves.
❏ Expose clavicle and sternum and incise periosteum working from lateral to medial on clavicle and from midline to lateral on sternum
❏ Evaluate the sternoclavicular joint to determine whether a true dislocation or physeal fracture occurred
❏ Reduce dislocation/fracture with aid of a fracture reduction clamp
❏ Converse with anesthesia to ensure hemodynamic stability of patient
❏ Place drill holes in anterior epiphysis and metaphysis for physeal fractures or anterior epiphysis and sternum for dislocations
❏ Pass heavy nonabsorbable suture in a figure-of-eight fashion and tie
❏ Reapproximate periosteum with heavy suture
❏ Irrigate and close wound in sequential layers
❏ Immobilize patient in sling and swathe or shoulder immobilizer

Following exposure of the physeal fracture or sternoclavicular dislocation, a gentle reduction is performed utilizing the aid of a fracture reduction clamp. Once the clavicle is brought anteriorly, it is important to converse with the anesthesiologist to ensure that the patient remained hemodynamically stable. An anatomic reduction is now performed ensuring that the clavicular head is anatomically seated in the clavicular notch of the sternum.

Figure 20-22. A: Marking of the anatomy prior to incision. The *dashed lines* represent the posterior dislocation of the right sternoclavicular joint. **B:** Identification and preservation of the supraclavicular nerves. **C:** Exposure of the medial clavicle and sternoclavicular joint following periosteal elevation. (Reprinted with permission from Waters PM, Bae DS, eds. *Pediatric Hand and Upper Limb Surgery: A Practical Guide.* Wolters Kluwer; 2012.)

Following anatomic reduction of either the fracture or dislocation, drill holes are made in the anterior metaphysis and epiphysis of the clavicle in cases of a fracture or the anterior epiphysis and sternum in cases of a dislocation. Placement of malleable retractors between the bone and posterior periosteum is helpful in preventing the drill from entering the mediastinum. Heavy nonabsorbable suture is then passed in a figure-of-eight fashion to provide the necessary stability (Fig. 20-23). The periosteum is then reapproximated with heavy suture to provide added stability, especially with a true dislocation as it provides indirect repair of the costoclavicular and sternoclavicular ligaments. Stability is now assessed by ranging the ipsilateral shoulder and limb. Once stability is satisfactory, the wound is irrigated and closed in sequential layers.

Authors' Preferred Treatment for Sternoclavicular Fracture-Dislocations

We treat acute atraumatic anterior dislocations with immobilization alone for 1 to 4 weeks followed by gradual return to function. If patients experience recurrent instability, therapy is initiated. Operative intervention is reserved for patients with persistent symptoms and typically involves reconstruction of the ligaments.

Acute posterior dislocations are treated operatively with ORIF, usually with suture-based "fixation" constructs being sufficient to maintain the stability of the reduced joint in the early postoperative weeks, during which the ligaments heal and scar. Chronic posterior dislocations that are symptomatic are treated with ligament reconstruction utilizing allograft. Rarely, medial clavicle resection is required in painful chronic dislocations that have deformity of the bone and early arthritis of the joint.

Postoperative Care

Postoperatively, patients are placed in either a sling and swathe or shoulder immobilizer for 4 to 6 weeks. Subsequently, range-of-motion exercises are begun. Strengthening is permitted at 3 months postoperatively. Return to sports is dependent on full motion and strength, usually 3 to 6 months postoperatively.

Figure 20-23. A: Drill holes created in the anteromedial clavicle and sternum in cases of true dislocations or anteromedial clavicular metaphysis and clavicular epiphysis in cases of physeal fracture. **B:** Heavy nonabsorbable suture placed through the drill holes in a figure-of-eight fashion. **C:** Anatomic joint reduction following tying of the sutures. (Reprinted with permission from Waters PM, Bae DS, eds. *Pediatric Hand and Upper Limb Surgery: A Practical Guide.* Wolters Kluwer; 2012.)

Potential Pitfalls and Preventive Measures

Sternoclavicular Fracture-Dislocations:
SURGICAL PITFALLS AND PREVENTIONS

Pitfall	Prevention
Overreduction of clavicle into clavicular notch of sternum	Be knowledgeable about the bony anatomy of the sternoclavicular joint
Osteolysis from Dacron	Utilize heavy (braided no. 2) nonabsorbable or partially nonabsorbable suture
K-wire migration	Avoid K-wires

It is imperative to be familiar with the sternoclavicular bony alignment as overreduction of the clavicle into the clavicular notch of the sternum can occur. In addition, utilization of Dacron tape may cause osteolysis. Pins may migrate and therefore should be avoided.

Outcomes

The outcomes following ORIF of posterior sternoclavicular dislocations or medial clavicle physeal fractures in pediatric and adolescent patients have been quite favorable in most reported cases.[12,37,64,122,128] In a retrospective review by Waters et al.,[128] all patients treated with open reduction and suture fixation of their posterior sternoclavicular joint fracture dislocation had restoration of joint stability and shoulder motion with full return to activities. Similar findings were reported by Goldfarb et al.[37] with all patients returning to their preinjury function including sports participation. Lee et al. recently published a series that included 40 patients treated operatively, of which 1 patient had a recurrent dislocation on postoperative day 1 that was addressed immediately. None of the other patients had a subsequent dislocation. It is important to note that none of the patients required reconstruction of the sternoclavicular or costoclavicular ligaments to maintain stability.[67]

The best evidence regarding these injuries is from a recent meta-analysis that showed that 96% of patients treated with ORIF had full pain-free range of motion without recurrence.[119]

MANAGEMENT OF EXPECTED ADVERSE OUTCOMES AND UNEXPECTED COMPLICATIONS IN STERNOCLAVICULAR FRACTURE-DISLOCATIONS

Sternoclavicular Fracture-Dislocations:
COMMON ADVERSE OUTCOMES AND COMPLICATIONS

- Failure of closed treatment
- Persistent pain
- Recurrent instability

Attempts at closed reduction may be unsuccessful, leading to the necessity to perform an ORIF. Studies have shown that the success of closed reduction greatly reduces beyond 24 to 48 hours from the time of injury.[67,119] Therefore, one may consider proceeding directly to ORIF if the patient presents greater than 48 hours from the initial injury.

Recurrent instability following acute repair is relatively rare but can occur, especially if the sternoclavicular joint is overreduced. Patients will present with persistent pain and a sense of instability. Treatment with ligament reconstruction can be performed utilizing semitendinosus autograft or allograft passed in a figure-of-eight fashion similar to the suture utilized during the acute repair. Ideally, the parallel strands of the tendon graft are passed on the "instability side" to minimize the risk of recurrent instability occurring again.

Alternatively, as a salvage procedure, medial clavicle resection arthroplasty can be performed with supplemental ligament reconstruction or soft tissue interposition. Approximately 1 cm of medial clavicle is excised in an oblique fashion to preserve the inferior ligamentous attachments. The intra-articular disk can be passed into the medullary canal of the clavicle by detaching its superior end while preserving the inferior attachments. Sutures are passed through drill holes in the superior clavicle and tied over a bony bridge (Fig. 20-24). Additional stability can be provided by sutures passed between the costoclavicular ligament and the clavicle. In a case series by Ting et al. on surgical care for patients, this rare complication revealed pain reduction and improved function.[121]

The results of treatment for recurrent anterior instability have been reported by Bae et al. in a retrospective review.[7] Sixty percent of patients had stable, pain-free joints following the procedure. No patients developed instability following their treatment. Many still had some minor limitations of function or persistent pain.

Figure 20-24. A: Schematic demonstrating the technique of medial clavicular resection arthroplasty. **B:** Intraoperative photograph of a patient with recurrent anterior sternoclavicular instability with resultant pain due to a deformed and irreducible clavicular head. **C:** Intraoperative photograph following medial clavicular head resection and intramedullary passage of the intra-articular disk ligament. (Reprinted with permission from Waters PM, Bae DS, eds. *Pediatric Hand and Upper Limb Surgery: A Practical Guide.* Wolters Kluwer; 2012.)

SUMMARY, CONTROVERSIES, AND FUTURE DIRECTIONS RELATED TO STERNOCLAVICULAR FRACTURE-DISLOCATIONS

Although sternoclavicular joint injuries are relatively rare, they do occur, even in the pediatric and adolescent populations. As high-energy mechanisms cause sternoclavicular injuries, associated damage to critical mediastinal structures can occur, and therefore, a thorough evaluation is necessary to avoid missing an associated life-threatening injury. Most anterior dislocations can be treated with immobilization alone, whereas acute posterior injuries are typically treated with operative intervention yielding excellent results.

Annotated References

Reference	Annotation
Lee JT, Nasreddine AY, Black EM, et al. Posterior stenoclavicular joint injuries in skeletally immature patients. *J Pediatr Orthop.* 2014;34(4); 369–375.	Retrospective case series of 48 patients treated for a posterior sternoclavicular joint injury.
Shannon SF, Hernandez NM, Sems SA, et al. High-energy pediatric scapula fractures and their associated injuries. *J Pediatr Orthop.* 2019;39(7): 377–381.	This is the largest series of pediatric scapula fractures that investigates the associated injuries, the morbidity, and the mortality.
Tepolt F, Carry PM, Heyn PC, Miller NH. Posterior sternoclavicular joint injuries in the adolescent population: a meta-analysis. *Am J Sports Med.* 2014;42(10):2517–2524.	Meta-analysis reviewing associated injuries and outcomes of posterior sternoclavicular joint injuries in the adolescent population.

REFERENCES

1. Abbot AE, Hannafin JA. Stress fracture of the clavicle in a female lightweight rower. A case report and review of literature. *Am J Sports Med.* 2001;29:370–372.
2. Ahearn BM, Shanley E, Thigpen CA, et al. Factors influencing time to return to sport following clavicular fractures in adolescent athletes. *J Shoulder Elbow Surg.* 2021;30(7S):S140–S144.
3. Allman FL Jr. Fractures and ligamentous injuries of the clavicle and its articulation. *J Bone Joint Surg Am.* 1967;49:774–784.
4. Ames TD, Mehlman CT, Toy R, Parikh SN. Comparative effectiveness of nonoperative versus operative treatment of completely displaced clavicle shaft fractures among children. *Orthopedics.* 2022;45(6):373-377.
5. Anderson K. Evaluation and treatment of distal clavicle fractures. *Clin Sports Med.* 2003;22:319–326.
6. Badhe SP, Lawrence TM, Clark DI. Tension band suturing for the treatment of displaced type 2 lateral end clavicle fractures. *Arch Orthop Trauma Surg.* 2007;127: 25–28.
7. Bae DS, Kocher MS, Waters PM, et al. Chronic recurrent anterior sternoclavicular joint instability: results of surgical management. *J Pediatr Orthop.* 2006;26:71–74.
8. Bae DS, Shah AS, Kalish LA, et al. Shoulder motion, strength, and functional outcomes in children with established malunion of the clavicle. *J Pediatr Orthop.* 2013;33(5):544–550.
9. Bahk MS, Kuhn JE, Galatz LM, et al. Acromioclavicular and sternoclavicular injuries and clavicular, glenoid, and scapular fractures. *J Bone Joint Surg Am.* 2009;91: 2492–2510.
10. Banerjee R, Waterman B, Padalecki J, Robertson W. Management of distal clavicle fractures. *J Am Acad Orthop Surg.* 2011;19:392–401.
11. Bannister GC, Wallace WA, Stableforth PG, Hutson MA. The management of acute acromioclavicular dislocation: a randomized prospective controlled trial. *J Bone Joint Surg Br.* 1989;71:848–850.
12. Baumann M, Vogel T, Weise K, et al. Bilateral posterior sternoclavicular dislocation. *Orthopedics.* 2010;33:510.
13. Baumgarten KM. Arthroscopic fixation of a type II-variant, unstable distal clavicle fracture. *Orthopedics.* 2008;31.
14. Beall MH, Ross MG. Clavicle fracture in labor: risk factors and associated morbidities. *J Perinatol.* 2001;21:513–515.
15. Bergfield JA, Andrish JT, Clancy WG. Evaluation of the acromioclavicular joint following first- and second-degree sprains. *Am J Sports Med.* 1978;6:153–159.
16. Boldin C, Frankhauser F, Ratschek M, Haller-Schober EM. Foreign-body reaction after reconstruction of complete acromioclavicular dislocation using PDS augmentation. *J Shoulder Elbow Surg.* 2004;13:99–100.
17. Buckley BJ, Hayden SR. Posterior sternoclavicular dislocation. *J Emerg Med.* 2008;34:331–332.
18. Bullock DP, Koval KJ, Moen KY, et al. Hospitalized cases of child abuse in America: who, what, when, and where. *J Pediatr Orthop.* 2009;29:231–237.
19. Calder JD, Solan M, Gidwani S, et al. Management of paediatric clavicle fractures—is follow-up necessary? An audit of 346 cases. *Ann R Coll Surg Engl.* 2002;84: 331–333.
20. Candian Orthopaedic Trauma Society. Nonoperative treatment compared with plate fixation of displaced midshaft clavicular fractures. A multicenter, randomized clinical trial. *J Bone Joint Surg Am.* 2007;89(1):1–10.
21. Chang DC, Knight V, Ziegfeld S, et al. The tip of the iceberg for child abuse: the critical roles of the pediatric trauma service and its registry. *J Trauma.* 2004;57:1189–1198.
22. Checcia SL, Doneux PS, Miyazaki AN, et al. Treatment of distal clavicle fractures using an arthroscopic technique. *J Shoulder Elbow Surg.* 2008;17:395–398.
23. Corteen DP, Teitge RA. Stabilization of the clavicle after distal resection: a biomechanical study. *Am J Sports Med.* 2005;33:61–67.
24. Coupe BD, Wimhurst JA, Indar R, et al. A new approach for plate fixation of midshaft clavicular fractures. *Injury.* 2005;36:1166–1171.
25. Craig EV. Fractures of the clavicle. In: Rockwood CA Jr, Green DP, Bucholz RW, Heckman JD, eds. *Rockwood and Green's Fractures in Adults.* 4th ed. Lippincott-Raven; 1996:1009–1193.
26. Edwards DJ, Kavanagh TG, Flannery MC. Fractures of the distal clavicle: a case for fixation. *Injury.* 1992;23:44–46.
27. Edwards SG, Whittle AP, Wood GW II. Nonoperative treatment of ipsilateral fractures of the scapula and clavicle. *J Bone Joint Surg Am.* 2000;82:774–780.
28. Eisenstein ED, Misenhimer JJ, Kotb A, et al. Management of displaced midshaft clavicle fractures in adolescent patients using intramedullary flexible nails: a case series. *J Clin Orthop Trauma.* 2018;9(Suppl 1):S97–S102.
29. Ellis HB, Li Y, Bae DS, et al. Descriptive epidemiology of adolescent clavicle fractures: results from the FACTS (Function after Adolescent Clavicle Trauma and Surgery) prospective, multicenter cohort study. *Orthop J Sports Med.* 2020; 8(5):2325967120921344.
30. Erdle B, Izadpanah K, Jaeger M, et al. Comparative analysis of locking plate versus hook plate osteosynthesis of Neer type IIB lateral clavicle fractures. *Arch Orthop Trauma Surg.* 2017;137(5):651–662.
31. Fazal MA, Saksena J, Haddad FS. Temporary coracoclavicular screw fixation for displaced distal clavicle fractures. *J Orthop Surg (Hong Kong).* 2007;15:9–11.
32. Ferraz IC, Papadimitriou NG, Sotereanos DG. Scapular body nonunion: a case report. *J Shoulder Elbow Surg.* 2002;11:98–100.
33. Flinkkilä T, Ristiniemi J, Hyvönen P, Hämäläinen M. Surgical treatment of unstable fractures of the distal clavicle: a comparative study of Kirschner wire and clavicular hook plate fixation. *Acta Orthop Scand.* 2002;73:50–53.
34. Fracture and dislocation compendium. Orthopedic Trauma Association Committee for Coding and Classification. *J Orthop Trauma* 1996;10(Suppl 1):1–154.
35. Furey MJ, Zdero R, McKee MD. Clavicular refracture at the site of angular malunion in young athletes. *J Orthop Trauma.* 2017;31(4):e130–e132.
36. Gausden EB, Fabricant PD. Management of clavicle fractures in adolescents: a critical analysis review. *JBJS Rev.* 2018;6(9):e4.
37. Goldfarb CA, Bassett GS, Sullivan S, Gordon JE. Retrosternal displacement after physeal fracture of the medial clavicle in children treatment by open reduction and internal fixation. *J Bone Joint Surg Br.* 2001;83:1168–1172.
38. Goss TP. Fractures of the glenoid cavity. *J Bone Joint Surg Am.* 1992;74:299–305.
39. Goss TP. Fractures of the glenoid neck. *J Shoulder Elbow Surg.* 1994;3:42–52.
40. Goss TP. Scapular fractures and dislocations: diagnosis and treatment. *J Am Acad Orthop Surg.* 1995;3:22–33.

41. Grassi FA, Tajana MS, D'Angelo F. Management of midclavicular fractures: comparison between nonoperative treatment and open intramedullary fixation in 80 patients. *J Trauma.* 2001;50:1096–1100.

42. Groh GI, Wirth MA. Management of traumatic sternoclavicular injuries. *J Am Acad Orthop Surg.* 2011;19:1–7.

43. Groh GI, Wirth MA, Rockwood CA Jr. Treatment of traumatic posterior sternoclavicular dislocations. *J Shoulder Elbow Surg.* 2011;20:107–113.

44. Heyworth BE, Cohen L, von Heideken J, et al. Validity and comprehensibility of outcome measures in children with shoulder and elbow disorders: creation of a new Pediatric and Adolescent Shoulder and Elbow Survey (Pedi-ASES). *J Shoulder Elbow Surg.* 2018;27:1162–1171.

45. Heyworth BE, May C, Carsen S, et al. Outcomes of operative and non-operative treatment of adolescent mid-diaphyseal clavicle fractures. *Orthop J Sports Med.* 2014;2(2 Suppl):2325967114S00064.

46. Heyworth BE, Pennock AT, Li Y, et al. Two-year functional outcomes of operative vs nonoperative treatment of completely displaced midshaft clavicle fractures in adolescents: results from the prospective multicenter FACTS study group. *Am J Sports Med.* 2022;50(11):3045–3055.

47. Hobbs DW. Sternoclavicular joint: a new axial radiographic view. *Radiology.* 1968;90:801.

48. Hsu T-Y, Hung F-C, Lu Y-J, et al. Neonatal clavicular fracture: clinical analysis of incidence, predisposing factors, diagnosis, and outcome. *Am J Perinatol.* 2002;19:17–21.

49. Hughes K, Kimpton J, Wei R, et al. Clavicle fracture nonunion in the paediatric population: a systematic review of the literature. *J Child Orthop.* 2018;12(1):2–8.

50. Ideberg R, Grevsten S, Larsson S. Epidemiology of scapular fractures: incidence and classification of 338 fractures. *Acta Orthop Scand.* 1995;66:395–397.

51. Jaggard MKJ, Gupte CM, Gulati V, Reilly P. A comprehensive review of trauma and disruption to the sternoclavicular joint with the proposal of a new classification system. *J Trauma.* 2009;66:576–584.

52. Jeray KJ. Acute midshaft clavicular fracture. *J Am Acad Orthop Surg.* 2007;15:239–248.

53. Jin CZ, Kim HK, Min BH. Surgical treatment for distal clavicle fracture associated with coracoclavicular ligament rupture using a cannulated screw fixation technique. *J Trauma.* 2006;60:1358–1361.

54. Jones HP, Lemos MJ, Schepsis AA. Salvage of failed acromioclavicular joint reconstruction using autogenous semitendinosus tendon from the knee. Surgical technique and case report. *Am J Sports Med.* 2001;29:234–237.

55. Jupiter JB, Leibman MI. Supraclavicular nerve entrapment due to clavicular fracture callus. *J Shoulder Elbow Surg.* 2007;16(5):e13–e14.

56. Kalamaras M, Cutbush K, Robinson M. A method for internal fixation of unstable distal clavicle fractures: early observations using a new technique. *J Shoulder Elbow Surg.* 2008;17:60–62.

57. Kao FC, Chao EK, Chen CH, et al. Treatment of distal clavicle fracture using Kirschner wires and tension-band wires. *J Trauma.* 2001;51:522–525.

58. Kaplan B, Rabinerson D, Avrech OM, et al. Fracture of the clavicle in the newborn following normal labor and delivery. *Int J Gynaecol Obstet.* 1998;63:15–20.

59. Kaplan LD, Flanigan DC, Norwig J, et al. Prevalence and variance of shoulder injuries in elite collegiate football players. *Am J Sports Med.* 2005;33:1142–1146.

60. Kavanagh BF, Bradway JK, Cofield RH. Open reduction and internal fixation of displaced intra-articular fractures of the glenoid fossa. *J Bone Joint Surg Am.* 1993;75:479–484.

61. Kellum E, Creek A, Dawkins R, et al. Age-related patterns of injury in children involved in all-terrain vehicle accidents. *J Pediatr Orthop.* 2008;28(8):854–858.

62. Khan LAK, Bradnock TJ, Scott C, Robinson CM. Fractures of the clavicle. *J Bone Joint Surg Am.* 2009;91:447–460.

63. Klimkiewicz JJ, Williams GR, Sher JS, et al. The acromioclavicular capsule as a restraint to posterior translation of the clavicle: a biomechanical analysis. *J Shoulder Elbow Surg.* 1999;8:119–124.

64. Koch MJ, Wells L. Proximal clavicle physeal fracture with posterior displacement: diagnosis, treatment, and prevention. *Orthopedics.* 2012;35:e108–e111.

65. Labler L, Platz A, Weishaupt D, Trentz O. Clinical and functional results after floating shoulder injuries. *J Trauma.* 2004;57:595–602.

66. Lam MH, Wong GY, Lao TT. Reappraisal of neonatal clavicular fracture: relationship between infant size and risk factors. *J Reprod Med.* 2002;47:903–908.

67. Lee JT, Nasreddine AY, Black EM, et al. Posterior sternoclavicular joint injuries in skeletally immature patients. *J Pediatr Orthop.* 2014;34(4):369–375.

68. Lee YS, Lau MJ, Tseng YC, et al. Comparison of the efficacy of hook plate versus tension band wire in the treatment of unstable fractures of the distal clavicle. *Int Orthop.* 2009;33:1401–1405.

69. Levine MG, Holroyde J, Wood JR Jr, et al. Birth trauma: incidence and predisposing factors. *Obstet Gynecol.* 1984;63:792–295.

70. Levy O. Simple, minimally invasive surgical technique for treatment of type 2 fractures of the distal clavicle. *J Shoulder Elbow Surg.* 2003;12:24–28.

71. Li Y, Donohue KS, Robbins CB, et al; Function After Adolescent Clavicle Trauma and Surgery (FACTS) Multicenter Study Group. Reliability of radiographic assessments of adolescent midshaft clavicle fractures by the FACTS multicenter study group. *J Orthop Trauma.* 2017;31(9):479–484.

72. Li Y, Helvie P, Farley FA, et al. Complications after plate fixation of displaced pediatric midshaft clavicle fractures. *J Pediatr Orthop.* 2018;38(7):350–353.

73. Macheras G, Kateros KT, Savvidou OD, et al. Coracoclavicular screw fixation for unstable distal clavicle fractures. *Orthopedics.* 2005;28:693–696.

74. Mall JW, Jacobi CA, Philipp AW, Peter FJ. Surgical treatment of fractures of the distal clavicle with polydioxanone suture tension band wiring: an alternative osteosynthesis. *J Orthop Sci.* 2002;7:535–537.

75. Masnovi ME, Mehlman CT, Eismann EA, Matey DA. Pediatric refracture rates after angulated and completely displaced clavicle shaft fractures. *J Orthop Trauma.* 2014;28(11):648–652.

76. Mazzocca AD, Santangelo SA, Johnson ST, et al. A biomechanical evaluation of an anatomical coracoclavicular ligament reconstruction. *Am J Sports Med.* 2006;34:236–246.

77. McGahan JP, Rab GT, Dublin A. Fractures of the scapula. *J Trauma.* 1980;20:880–883.

78. McGraw MA, Mehlman CT, Lindsell CJ, Kirby CL. Postnatal growth of the clavicle: birth to 18 years of age. *J Pediatr Orthop.* 2009;29:937–943.

79. McKee MD, Wild LW, Schemitsch EH. Midshaft malunions of the clavicle. *J Bone Joint Surg Am.* 2003;85-A:790–797.

80. McKee RC, Whelan DB, Schemitsch EH, McKee MD. Operative versus nonoperative care of displaced midshaft clavicular fractures: a meta-analysis of randomized clinical trials. *J Bone Joint Surg Am.* 2012;94A:675–684.

81. Mehlman CT, Yihua G, Bochang C, Zhigang W. Operative treatment of completely displaced clavicle shaft fractures in children. *J Pediatr Orthop.* 2009;29:851–855.

82. Michael D, Fazal MA, Cohen B. Nonunion of a fracture of the body of the scapula: case report and literature review. *J Shoulder Elbow Surg.* 2001;10:385–386.

83. Mouhsine E, Garofalo R, Crevoisier X, Farron A. Grade I and II acromioclavicular dislocations: results of conservative treatment. *J Shoulder Elbow Surg.* 2003;12:599–602.

84. Namdari S, Ganley TJ, Baldwin K, et al. Fixation of displaced midshaft clavicle fractures in skeletally immature patients. *J Pediatr Orthop.* 2011;31:507–511.

85. Neer CS II. Fracture of the distal clavicle with detachment of the coracoclavicular ligaments in adults. *J Trauma.* 1963;3:99–110.

86. Neer C II. Fractures and dislocations of the shoulder. In: Rockwood CA Jr, Green DP, eds. *Fractures in Adults.* JB Lippincott; 1984:711–712.

87. Nettrour LF, Krufky EL, Mueller RE, Raycroft JF. Locked scapula: intrathoracic dislocation of the inferior angle. A case report. *J Bone Joint Surg Am.* 1972;54:413–416.

88. Ng N, Nicholson JA, Chen P, et al. Adolescent mid-shaft clavicular fracture displacement does not predict nonunion or inferior functional outcome at long-term follow-up. *Bone Joint J.* 2021;103-B(5):951–957.

89. Nordqvist A, Petersson C. Fracture of the body, neck, or spine of the scapula: a long-term follow-up study. *Clin Orthop Relat Res.* 1992;283:139–144.

90. Nordqvist A, Petersson C. The incidence of fractures of the clavicle. *Clin Orthop Relat Res.* 1994;300:127–132.

91. Norqvist A, Petersson C, Redlund-Johnell I. The natural course of lateral clavicle fracture: 15 (11–21) year follow-up of 110 cases. *Acta Orthop Scand.* 1993;64:87–91.

92. Nourissat G, Kakuda C, Dumontier C, et al. Arthroscopic stabilization of Neer type 2 fracture of the distal part of the clavicle. *Arthroscopy.* 2007;23:e1.e1–e4.

93. Nowak J, Mallmin H, Larsson S. The aetiology and epidemiology of clavicular fractures. A prospective study during a two-year period in Uppsala, Sweden. *Injury.* 2000;31:353–358.

94. Pandya NK, Baldwin K, Wolfgruber H, et al. Child abuse and orthopaedic injury patterns: analysis at a level I pediatric trauma center. *J Pediatr Orthop.* 2009;29:618–625.

95. Pennock AT, Bastrom TP, Boutelle KE, et al; FACTS Study Group. Bony remodeling of adolescent displaced clavicle fractures: a FACTS study [published correction appears in *Am J Sports Med.* 2023:3635465231168388]. *Am J Sports Med.* 2023;51(4):871–876.

96. Phillips AM, Smart C, Groom AF. Acromioclavicular dislocation. Conservative or surgical therapy. *Clin Orthop Relat Res.* 1998;353:10–17.

97. Postacchini F, Gumina S, De Santis P, Albo F. Epidemiology of clavicle fractures. *J Shoulder Elbow Surg.* 2002;11:452–456.

98. Pujol N, Philippeau JM, Richou J, et al. Arthroscopic treatment of distal clavicle fractures: a technical note. *Knee Surg Sports Traumatol Arthrosc.* 2008;16:884–886.

99. Randsborg PH, Fuglesang HFS, Røtterud JH, et al. Long-term patient-reported outcome after fractures of the clavicle in patients aged 10 to 18 years. *J Pediatr Orthop.* 2014;34(4):393–399.

100. Regel JP, Pospiech J, Aalders TA, Ruchholtz S. Intraspinal migration of a Kirschner wire 3 months after clavicular fracture fixation. *Neurosurg Rev.* 2002;25:110–112.

101. Renfree KJ, Riley MK, Wheeler D, et al. Ligamentous anatomy of the distal clavicle. *J Shoulder Elbow Surg.* 2003;12:355–359.

102. Riiser MO, Molund M. Long-term functional outcomes and complications in operative versus nonoperative treatment for displaced midshaft clavicle fractures in adolescents: a retrospective comparative study. *J Pediatr Orthop.* 2021;41(5):279–283.

103. Rios CG, Arciero RA, Mazzocca AD. Anatomy of the clavicle and coracoid process for reconstruction of the coracoclavicular ligaments. *Am J Sports Med.* 2007;35:811–817.

104. Robinson CM, Cairns DA. Primary nonoperative treatment of displaced lateral fractures of the clavicle. *J Bone Joint Surg Am.* 2004;86:778–782.

105. Robinson CM, Court-Brown CM, McQueen MM, Wakefield AE. Estimating the risk of nonunion following nonoperative treatment of a clavicular fracture. *J Bone Joint Surg Am.* 2004;86:1359–1365.

106. Robinson CM, Goudie EB, Murray IR, et al. Open reduction and plate fixation versus nonoperative treatment for displaced midshaft clavicular fractures: a multicenter, randomized, controlled trial. *J Bone Joint Surg Am.* 2013;95A:1576–1584.

107. Rockwood CA Jr, Williams GR Jr. Disorders of the acromioclavicular joint. In: Rockwood CA, Matsen FA, eds. *The Shoulder.* 3rd ed. WB Saunders; 1998:483–553.

108. Schulz J, Moor M, Roocroft J, et al. Functional and radiographic outcomes of nonoperative treatment of displaced adolescent clavicle fractures. *J Bone Joint Surg Am.* 2013;95:1159–1165.

109. Sernandez H, Riehl J. Sternoclavicular joint dislocation: a systematic review and meta-analysis. *J Orthop Trauma.* 2019;33(7):e251–e255.

110. Shannon SF, Hernandez NM, Sems SA, et al. High-energy pediatric scapula fractures and their associated injuries. *J Pediatr Orthop.* 2019;39(7):377–381.

111. Shannon SF, Hernandez NM, Sems SA, et al. Pediatric orthopaedic trauma and associated injuries of snowmobile, ATV, and dirtbike accidents: a 19-year experience at a level 1 pediatric trauma center. *J Pediatr Orthop.* 2018;38(8):403–409.

112. Simovitch R, Sanders B, Ozbaydar M, et al. Acromioclavicular joint injuries: diagnosis and management. *J Am Acad Orthop Surg.* 2009;17:207–219.

113. Spencer EE, Kuhn JE, Huston LJ, et al. Ligamentous restraints to anterior and posterior translation of the sternoclavicular joint. *J Shoulder Elbow Surg.* 2002;11:43–47.
114. Spencer EE Jr, Kuhn JE. Biomechanical analysis of reconstructions for sternoclavicular joint instability. *J Bone Joint Surg Am.* 2004;86:98–105.
115. Stewart AM, Ahmad CS. Failure of acromioclavicular reconstruction using Gore-Tex graft due to aseptic foreign-body reaction and clavicle osteolysis: a case report. *J Shoulder Elbow Surg.* 2004;13:558–561.
116. Sugaya H, Kon Y, Tsuchiya A. Arthroscopic repair of glenoid fractures using suture anchors. *Arthroscopy.* 2005;21:635.
117. Suppan CA, Bae DS, Donohue KS, et al. Trends in the volume of operative treatment of midshaft clavicle fractures in children and adolescents: a retrospective, 12-year, single-institution analysis. *J Pediatr Orthop B.* 2016;25(4):305–309.
118. Swarup I, Maheshwer B, Orr S, et al. Intermediate-term outcomes following operative and nonoperative management of midshaft clavicle fractures in children and adolescents: internal fixation may improve outcomes. *JBJS Open Access.* 2021;6(1):e20.00036.
119. Tepolt F, Carry PM, Heyn PC, Miller NH. Posterior sternoclavicular joint injuries in the adolescent population: a meta-analysis. *Am J Sports Med.* 2014;42:2517–2524.
120. Thompson DA, Flynn C, Miller PW, Fischer RP. The significance of scapular fractures. *J Trauma.* 1985;25:974–977.
121. Ting BL, Bae DS, Waters PM. Chronic posterior sternoclavicular joint fracture dislocations in children and young adults: results of surgical management. *J Pediatr Orthop.* 2014;34:542–547.
122. Tompkins M, Bliss J, Villarreal R, Solga P. Posterior sternoclavicular disruption with ipsilateral clavicle fracture in a nine-year-old hockey player. *J Orthop Trauma.* 2010;24:e36–e39.
123. Tossy JD, Mead MC, Sigmond HM. Acromioclavicular separations: useful and practical classification for treatment. *Clin Orthop Relat Res.* 1963;28:111–119.
124. Tsai CH, Hsu HC, Huan CY, et al. Late migration of threaded wire (Schanz screw) from right distal clavicle to the cervical spine. *J Chin Med Assoc.* 2009;72:48–51.
125. Tytherleigh-Strong G, Cuthbert R, Poutoglidou F, Tang Q. Magnetic resonance imaging in the management of significantly displaced adolescent posterior sternoclavicular joint injuries. *J Pediatr Orthop.* 2023;43(5):e374–e382.
126. Vander Have KL, Perdue AM, Caird MS, Farley FA. Operative versus nonoperative treatment of midshaft clavicle fractures in adolescents. *J Pediatr Orthop.* 2010;30:307–312.
127. Virtanen KJ, Remes V, Pajarinen J, et al. Sling compared with plate osteosynthesis for treatment of displaced midshaft clavicular fractures: a randomized clinical trial. *J Bone Joint Surg Am.* 2012;94A:1546–1553.
128. Waters PM, Bae DS, Kadiyala RK. Short-term outcomes after surgical treatment of traumatic posterior sternoclavicular fracture-dislocations in children and adolescents. *J Pediatr Orthop.* 2003;23:464–469.
129. Webber MC, Haines JF. The treatment of lateral clavicle fractures. *Injury.* 2000;31:175–179.
130. Williams GR Jr, Nguyen VD, Rockwood CA Jr. Classification and radiographic analysis of acromioclavicular dislocations. *Appl Radiol.* 1989;18:29–34.
131. Wirth MA, Rockwood CA Jr. Acute and chronic traumatic injuries of the sternoclavicular joint. *J Am Acad Orthop Surg.* 1996;4:268–278.
132. Wojtys EM, Nelson G. Conservative treatment of Grade III acromioclavicular dislocations. *Clin Orthop Relat Res.* 1991;268:112–119.
133. Wu CD, Chen YL. Stress fracture of the clavicle in a professional baseball player. *J Shoulder Elbow Surg.* 1998;7:164–167.
134. Yamaguchi H, Arakawa H, Kobayashi M. Results of the Bosworth method for unstable fractures of the distal clavicle. *Int Orthop.* 1998;22:366–368.
135. Yang S, Werner BC, Gwathmey FW Jr. Treatment trends in adolescent clavicle fractures. *J Pediatr Orthop.* 2015;35(3):229–233.
136. Zanca P. Shoulder pain: involvement of the acromioclavicular joint. (Analysis of 1,000 cases). *Am J Roentgenol Radium Ther Nucl Med.* 1971;112:493–506.
137. Zdravkovic D, Damholt VV. Comminuted and severely displaced fractures of the scapula. *Acta Orthop Scand.* 1974;45:60–65.

Cervical Spine Injuries in Children

Rajiv Iyer and Douglas Brockmeyer

Cervical Spine Injury

INTRODUCTION TO CERVICAL SPINE INJURY

Cervical spine fractures in children are relatively rare, accounting for only 1% of all pediatric fractures and 2% of all spinal injuries.[29,62,68,69,78,157,171] The incidence is estimated to be 7.4 in 100,000 per year[16,87,111,139]; however, that may be misleading because some injuries are not detected or are detected only at autopsy.

Cervical spine fractures and injuries in children younger than 8 years of age tend to occur in the upper cervical spine, whereas older children and adolescents tend to have injuries involving either the mid or lower cervical spine.[81,86,128,131,132] The upper cervical spine in young children is more prone to injury because of its anatomic and biomechanical properties.[168,169] The immature cervical spine is hypermobile because of relative ligamentous laxity, horizontally positioned facet joints, and a relatively large head to body size ratio. These anatomical characteristics change the fulcrum of motion to the upper cervical spine. With age, anatomical spine maturation leads to a lower fulcrum and an increased prevalence of lower cervical spine injuries, similar to adult patterns.

Cervical spine injuries associated with neurologic deficits are infrequent in children. When the neurologic deficits are incomplete, there tends to be a better prognosis for recovery in children than in adults.[13,43,51,52,122,164,166] Complete neurologic deficits, regardless of patient age, tend to have a poor prognosis for recovery, and are indicative of the severity and magnitude of injury.[55,110,134] Death from cervical spine injuries tends to be related to the level of injury and the associated injuries. Higher cervical spine injuries (e.g., atlanto-occipital dislocation) in younger children are associated with the highest mortality rate.[17,125,126] Children with significant cervical spine injuries may have associated severe head injuries, also leading to an increase in mortality. In a study of 61 pediatric deaths related to spinal cord injuries, 89% of fatalities occurred at the scene, and most were related to high cervical cord injuries in patients who had sustained multiple injuries.[71]

MECHANISM OF INJURY FOR CERVICAL SPINE INJURY

The mechanism of injury in the cervical spine varies with age. To begin with, infants are at risk during birth and early development because of their lack of head control. Injuries associated with breech delivery usually are in the lower cervical spine or upper thoracic spine and are thought to result from traction forces, whereas injuries associated with cephalic delivery usually occur in the upper cervical spine and are thought to result from rotation. Skeletal spine injury from obstetric trauma is probably underreported because the infantile spine is largely cartilaginous and difficult to evaluate with radiographs, especially if the injury is through the cartilage or cartilage–bone interface. A cervical spine injury should be considered in an infant who is floppy at birth, especially after a difficult delivery. Flaccid paralysis, with areflexia, usually is followed by a typical pattern of hyperreflexia once spinal cord shock is over.

Most cervical spine injuries in infants not related to birth trauma are caused by child abuse or inflicted injury.[88] In toddlers and young children, most cervical spine injuries result from falls, motor vehicle accidents, or being struck by a vehicle.[23,66,115] Distraction-type injuries to the upper cervical spine occur in toddlers in forward-facing car seats. During sudden deceleration maneuvers, the head continues forward while the remainder of the body is strapped in the car seat, resulting in injury.[64,94] As children become adolescents, the prevalence of sports injuries increases, as does the risk of spinal cord injury.[47,56,98,104] Once driving age is reached, the prevalence of motor vehicle accidents increases substantially and parallels that of adults.

INJURIES ASSOCIATED WITH CERVICAL SPINE INJURY

Patients with suspected cervical spine injuries should be thoroughly evaluated according to established Advanced Trauma Life Support and trauma protocols. During the primary and secondary surveys, as well during follow-up evaluation, other associated injuries may also be discovered. Facial injuries, thoracolumbar spine injuries, and traumatic brain injuries are commonly seen with cervical spine injuries because of their anatomical proximity and vulnerability to injury mechanisms.[39,124,145] In cases where intubation is required, an important role of the spine specialist is to facilitate this being done safely, often fiberoptically, to avoid any additional neurologic injury when securing the airway.

SIGNS AND SYMPTOMS OF CERVICAL SPINE INJURY

The most common presenting symptom in patients with a cervical spine injury is neck pain. Other complaints, such as headache, inability to move the neck, subjective feelings of instability, and neurologic symptoms, all warrant complete evaluation. Infants may present with unexplained respiratory distress, motor weakness, or hypotonia, which warrant further evaluation. In patients with head and neck trauma, distraction injuries, or altered levels of consciousness, there is a high likelihood of a cervical spine injury, and these children need to be thoroughly evaluated before cervical spine clearance.[113] The presence of an occult cervical spine injury in an uncooperative or obtunded patient needs to be considered.[130,144]

RADIOGRAPHIC CLEARANCE OF THE CERVICAL SPINE IN THE TRAUMA SETTING

In pediatric trauma hospitals, as well as adult centers taking care of pediatric trauma, an algorithmic approach or protocol is a critical part of injury assessment and cervical spine clearance. According to the American College of Surgeons, each pediatric trauma center is responsible for developing its own protocol.[4,44] Ideally, an algorithm for cervical spine clearance identifies all important injuries, facilitates removal of provisional cervical spinal motion restriction in an expeditious manner, and limits the patient's exposure to ionizing radiation, all while using health care resources responsibly. In a recent multidisciplinary, multicenter, consensus-based effort, the Pediatric Cervical Spine Clearance Working Group used a modified Delphi approach to create a comprehensive algorithm for pediatric cervical spine clearance.[77] Central to the protocol is the use of the National Emergency X-Radiography Utilization Study (NEXUS) criteria to clear the cervical spine in patients without using plain x-rays.[83] Furthermore, the adoption of computed tomography (CT) as a key part of the initial evaluation of the cervical spine in severely injured children is recommended. The panel concluded that the risk of missed injury outweighed the risk of increased radiation exposure from CT in the evaluation of cervical injury in a severely injured patient. Further advanced imaging, such as magnetic resonance imaging (MRI), may be used in a supporting role, depending upon the initial x-ray and CT findings.

IMAGING OF CERVICAL SPINE INJURY

Plain Radiographs

Plain x-rays are useful in the evaluation of mild to moderate pediatric cervical spine injuries. The NEXUS criteria are useful to help determine whether a cervical spine x-ray is needed at all.[83] The criteria include (1) the presence of midline spinal tenderness, (2) a focal neurologic deficit, (3) an altered level of consciousness, (4) intoxication, or a (5) distracting injury. If none of those five criteria are present, the cervical spine may be cleared with 99% sensitivity, according to one validation study.[82]

Dynamic flexion/extension x-rays may also aid in the evaluation of the cervical spine injuries and can be considered, along with MRI, as one of the gold standards for cervical spine clearance. They are commonly performed in the emergency room after an initial neutral x-ray is taken and interpreted as normal. They can be helpful in evaluating for cervical subluxation due to ligamentous injury; however, in the setting of acute trauma, many patients are unable to normally move their neck because of pain, and therefore flexion/extension x-rays cannot be performed. In that case, the patient is typically placed in a hard cervical collar and seen back in 1 to 2 weeks for evaluation, with

TABLE 21-1. Classification of Odontoid Fractures

Type	Illustration	Description
I		At level of the synchondrosis
IA	Type IA	Displacement less than 10%
IVB	Type IB	Displacement 10–100%
IC	Type IC	Displacement more than 100%
II	Type II	Fractures above the level of the synchondrosis

Adapted from Hosalkar HS, et al. Fractures of the odontoid in children with an open basilar synchondrosis. *J Bone Joint Surg Br.* 2009;91(6):789–796, permission conveyed through Copyright Clearance Center, Inc.

Figure 21-1. Pseudosubluxation of C2 on C3. In flexion, the posterior element of C2 should normally align itself with the posterior elements C1 and C3. The relationship of the body of C2 with the body of C3 gives the appearance of subluxation; however, the alignment of the posterior elements of C1 to C3 confirms pseudosubluxation.

flexion/extension x-rays done at that time. One study, however, tracked the compliance of cervical collar use and physician follow-up after trauma and found it to be quite low.[80]

Knowledge of the anatomic ossification centers and radiographic variations that occur in children is important. The absence of normal cervical lordosis, an increase in the prevertebral soft tissue space, and subluxation of C2 on C3 are all anatomic variations that may be normal in children.[36] Ossification centers also may be confused with fractures, most commonly in evaluation of the dens. Conversely, a fracture can also be mistaken for a normal synchondrosis. The presence of a synchondrosis at the base of the odontoid can be distinguished from a fracture based on the age of the patient and the location of synchondrosis well below the facet joints. For a list, please refer to Table 21-1 and Figure 21-1.

Computed Tomography

Cervical spine CT is an extremely helpful tool in the evaluation of pediatric cervical spine injuries. It is especially useful in the evaluation of the severely injured child. As mentioned previously, CT is the cornerstone of the Pediatric Cervical Spine Clearance Working Group's evaluation of the cervical spine in the setting of severe injuries.[77] It immediately provides information regarding spinal column injury and alignment, as well as the possibility of spinal cord injury. It is highly sensitive to predicting spinal instability and can be used while establishing a cervical Subaxial Injury Classification (SLIC) score for an injured child.[134] For further information, please refer to the section regarding cervical spine classification schemes.

Magnetic Resonance Imaging

Cervical spine MRI is also very helpful in the diagnosis of spinal cord injury and is supportive to CT in establishing the diagnosis of spinal instability. Its ability to detect spinal ligamentous damage is useful in making the diagnosis of injuries such as

atlanto-occipital dislocation (AOD) and pure subaxial ligamentous injury.[30] However, the sensitivity of MRI may also predispose it to a high rate of false-positive findings. Care must be taken not to overinterpret all MRI findings to mean instability, and physicians must use appropriate diagnostic judgment. Furthermore, MRI can also be used as part of establishing the SLIC score for pediatric cervical spine injuries.[134]

RADIOGRAPHIC EVALUATION OF THE SPINE BY LEVEL

Atlanto-Occipital Joint

The primary tool to evaluate the atlanto-occipital (AO) joint is CT. It is very difficult to evaluate a patient with AOD with plain x-ray because of the inability to see the joint in sufficient detail. Furthermore, the fact is that most children evaluated for AOD have experienced severe injuries and require an initial trauma CT scan for evaluation. The sagittal and coronal CT reconstructions are the primary images used to evaluate the AO joint. According to Pang's work in 2007, the condyle-C1 interval, or CCI, should measure less than 3.0 mm (Fig. 21-2).[129] A CCI greater than 3.5 mm is suspicious for AOD and should be investigated further with MRI. The cervical MRI supports or rules out the diagnosis of AOD if the CCI is found to be abnormal. Extensive work has been published investigating normal CCIs by age. In general, the CCI decreases over time, but at early ages (0–3 years), the cartilaginous endplates of the AO joint may artificially increase the CCI because cartilage cannot be seen on CT.[141] In general, a CCI greater than 4.0 mm, either unilaterally or bilaterally, is consistent with AOD. MRI can frequently show evidence of abnormal signal within the AO joint or complete disruption of the capsule in AOD. Other findings, such as tectorial membrane or

Figure 21-2. CCI in the sagittal (**A**) and coronal (**B**) planes. Four points (*arrowheads*) equidistant from each other are picked for measurement of the joint interval to compensate for the slight unevenness of the joint space. A CCI of greater than 3.5 mm is suggestive of atlanto-occipital dislocation (AOD) and should be investigated with MRI. A CCI greater than 4.0 mm is strong evidence for AOD. (Reprinted with permission from Pang D, et al. Atlanto-occipital dislocation. Part 2: the clinical use of (occipital) condyle–C1 interval, comparison with other diagnostic methods, and the manifestation, management, and outcome of atlanto-occipital dislocation in children. *Neurosurgery*. 2007;61(5):995–1015.)

posterior ligamentous injury, are supportive of, but not pathognomonic of, AOD. The use of other imaging parameters, such as Power ratio or the basion-dens interval, are either outdated or misleading in the pediatric population because of their high rate of false-negative and false-positive findings.[129]

Atlantoaxial Joint

The atlantoaxial (AA) joint is seen well with plain x-ray and CT. MRI has a supportive role in investigating the AA joint in the setting of trauma. The atlantodental interval (ADI) and the space available for the spinal cord are two useful measurements for its evaluation (Fig. 21-3). While the cutoff for normal ADI in adults is considered 3 mm, a generally accepted cutoff in young children is 5 mm. The ADI is easily measured on flexion and extension x-rays and is helpful in determining instability of the AA joint. In very young children, extension views may sometimes give the appearance of subluxation of the anterior portion of the atlas over the unossified dens, but this represents a pseudosubluxation and not instability.[45] Fracture and/or

subluxations of C1 to C2 should be further investigated with CT angiography to rule out the possibility of vertebral artery injury.

Upper Cervical Spine

Anterior displacement of C2 to C3 or C3 to C4 up to 3 mm is a common radiographic finding in children on static or dynamic cervical spine x-rays. This finding may be present up to approximately 11 years of age. The posterior line of Swischuk and Rowe[142] has been used to differentiate pathologic subluxation from normal anatomic variation; this line is drawn from the anterior cortex of the spinous process of C1 to the spinous process of C3. The anterior cortex of the spinous process of C2 should lie within 3 mm of this line; if the distance is more than this, a true subluxation should be suspected. Widening of the spinous processes between C1 and C2 of more than 10 mm also is indicative of a ligamentous injury and should be evaluated by further imaging studies such as MRI.[16] Fracture and/or subluxations of the upper cervical spine or transverse foramina should also be investigated with CT angiography to rule out the possibility of a vertebral artery injury.

Lower Cervical Spine

Plain x-rays and CT are the most useful studies in evaluating children for lower cervical spine injuries. Plain x-rays are usually taken in the setting of mild to moderate trauma, whereas CT is used in the setting of severe trauma. Again, MRI is used mainly in a supportive role to help establish a precise diagnosis. Fracture and/or subluxations of the lower cervical spine or transverse foramina should also be investigated with CT angiography to rule out the possibility of a vertebral artery injury.

TREATMENT OPTIONS FOR CERVICAL SPINE INJURY

INITIAL MANAGEMENT AND TRANSPORT OF PATIENTS WITH SUSPECTED CERVICAL SPINE INJURY

The initial management of a child with a suspected cervical spine injury is critical to avoiding further injury to the cervical spine and spinal cord.[50] The initial management of any child thought to have a cervical spine injury starts with immobilization in the field. Extraction from an automobile or transport to the hospital may cause damage to the spinal cord in a child with an unstable cervical spine injury if care is not taken to properly immobilize the neck before moving the patient.

The use of backboards in pediatric trauma patients deserves special attention because of the anatomic differences between children and adults. Compared with adults, children have a disproportionately larger head with respect to the body. This anatomic relationship causes a child's cervical spine to be placed in flexion if immobilization is done on a standard backboard. Herzenberg et al.[79] reported 10 children under the age of 7 years whose cervical spines had anterior angulation or translation on radiograph when they were placed on a standard backboard (Fig. 21-4A,B). Unnecessary flexion can be avoided by using a

Figure 21-3. The ADI and the space available for cord are used in determining atlantoaxial instability. The Wackenheim clivus-canal line is used to determine atlanto-occipital injury, while the McRae and McGregor lines are used in the measurement of basilar impression. (Modified from Copley LA, Dormans JP. Cervical spine disorders in infants and children. *J Am Acad Orthop Surg.* 1998;6(4):204–214. With permission.)

backboard with a recess into which the head can be lowered or by supporting the body with two mattresses and the head with only one mattress, allowing the cervical spine to assume a neutral position (Fig. 21-4C,D). Children younger than 8 years of age should be immobilized on a backboard using one of these techniques.[41,123]

Cervical collars supplement backboards for immobilization in the trauma setting. Further displacement of an unstable cervical injury may occur during resuscitation. Any manipulation of the cervical spine, even during intubation, must be done with caution and with the assumption that the patient has an unstable cervical spine injury until proven otherwise.

Figure 21-4. A: Adult immobilized on a standard backboard. **B:** Young child on a standard backboard. The relatively large head forces the neck into a kyphotic position. Such flexion can be avoided by using a modified backboard that has a cutout to the recess of the occiput, obtaining better supine cervical alignment (**C**) or by using a modified backboard that has a double-mattress pad (**D**) to raise the chest, obtaining better supine cervical alignment. (Reprinted with permission from Herzenberg JE, et al. Emergency transport and positioning of young children who have an injury of the cervical spine: the standard blackboard may be hazardous. *J Bone Joint Surg Am.* 1989;71(1):15–22.)

After initial evaluation and stabilization by the trauma team, the physical evaluation of any patient with a suspected cervical spine injury should begin with inspection. Head trauma is associated with a high incidence of cervical spine injuries, so external signs of head trauma should be noted.[5,127] Soft tissue abrasions or shoulder-harness marks on the neck from a seatbelt may be clues to an underlying cervical spine injury.[63]

The next step in the evaluation is palpation of the cervical spine for tenderness, muscle spasm, and overall alignment. The most prominent levels should be the spinous processes at C2, C3, and C7. Anterior palpation should focus on the presence of tenderness or swelling in the cervical area.

A neurologic examination should be done next, which can sometimes be difficult in pediatric patients because of either lack of cooperation or the fact the patient might be intubated, sedated, and chemically paralyzed. Strength, sensation, reflexes, and proprioception should be documented if possible. In patients who are uncooperative because of age or altered mental status, repeat examinations can be important; however, the initial neurologic examination should be documented even if it entails only gross movements of the extremities. The evaluation of rectal sphincter tone, bulbocavernosus reflex, and perianal sensation are important, especially in obtunded patients and patients with partial or complete neurologic injuries, regardless of age. Patients who are cooperative and awake can be asked to perform supervised cervical flexion, extension, rotation, and lateral bending. Uncooperative or obtunded patients should not have any manipulation of the neck until their cervical spine has undergone radiographic clearance.

NONOPERATIVE TREATMENT OF CERVICAL SPINE INJURY

Cervical Collars

Many cervical spine injuries may be managed with a hard cervical collar. For example, patients with mild cervical spine injuries, such as strains and sprains, who cannot be radiographically cleared in the emergency room, may require a period of immobilization until their pain and muscle spasm subside. Typically, they are encouraged to visit a physician's office to formally clear their spine after a period of time, but as mentioned before, there is a relatively low compliance with this strategy.[80]

For more severe injuries or in special circumstances, a custom molded cervical orthosis may be used. An advantage to custom devices is the ability to use lightweight thermoplastic materials that are molded to each patient's anatomy. These devices can be extended to the thorax if necessary to provide further support for lower cervical spine injuries.

Halo Orthoses

A halo orthosis can also be used for the treatment of selected cervical spine injuries, especially in the craniocervical region (Fig. 21-5). A halo device typically can be used in children down to 1 year of age, but caution must be used because of the immature nature of the skull.[22,146,161] Thin skull osteology requires placing more pins, sometimes up to eight, as well as reducing the applied torque to the pins. The halo ring can be used alone to apply traction for cervical reduction or with a vest for definitive

Figure 21-5. A: Halo ring and vest. **B:** Closeup of halo pin placement, with eight pins total—four in the front and four in the back—avoiding the thinnest part of the temporal bone.

immobilization of an unstable cervical spine injury. Prefabricated vests are available in various sizes. Infants, toddlers, and children can all be accommodated, with size measurements based on the circumference of the chest at the xiphoid process.

Halo orthoses can be used safely, but their complication rate is relatively high. In one pediatric series, the complication rate related to the use of a halo was 68%; however, all patients were able to wear the halo until fracture healing occurred or arthrodesis was achieved.[40] The most common complications in this series were superficial pin track infection and pin loosening. Other complications that occur less frequently include dural penetration, supraorbital nerve injury, unsightly pin scars, and deep infection.[14,48]

Methylprednisolone

In the setting of acute spinal cord injury, older studies have found that neurologic outcomes in adults are improved with the administration of high-dose methylprednisolone within the first 8 hours after injury.[25–28] However, recent studies have shown little or no benefit of high-dose methylprednisolone for acute spinal cord injury, as well as increased complications such as pneumonia.[2,24,58] Only a few studies examined the use of methylprednisolone for spinal cord injury in pediatric patients.[10,37,38] In one study by Caruso et al.,[38] 354 pediatric patients with acute spinal cord injuries were evaluated. The authors determined that methylprednisolone was not only unreliably administered according to protocol, but those who received steroids were significantly more likely to have complications than those who did not. Currently, high-dose methylprednisolone is only recommended as a treatment option for acute spinal cord injury. This recommendation is supported by a recent multidisciplinary consensus report.[77]

OPERATIVE TREATMENT OF CERVICAL SPINE INJURY

The injured cervical spine should be immobilized with a hard cervical collar during transport to the operating room and the operating table. During intubation, manual in-line stabilization is the most widely accepted technique for immobilization. This technique consists of grasping the mastoid processes with the fingertips with no traction being applied and then cupping the occiput in the palm of the hands.[61,106] Studies have confirmed the clinical safety of orotracheal intubation by direct laryngoscopy with manual in-line stabilization in patients with cervical spine injury.[147,151] After intubation, spinal cord monitoring is frequently used during surgery. Typically, a total intravenous anesthetic is used to avoid interfering with the monitoring potentials. Motor-evoked potentials and somatosensory-evoked potentials are the most commonly used neuromonitoring techniques, although others, such as brainstem-evoked potentials or D-wave monitoring, may also be used in select circumstances.

Positioning and Approach

The two primary intraoperative positions for cervical spine stabilization are prone and supine. Prone procedures may be aided by the use of a Jackson table, but this is not mandatory. The cervical collar is typically kept on during positioning. Often, a three-pin Mayfield head holder or halo ring is applied when the patient is still supine and then fixed to the table once the patient is prone. The patient is turned using a log-roll technique maintaining axial alignment. Intraoperative fluoroscopy is used to verify proper alignment of the cervical spine after the patient is prone. For supine procedures, Halter traction is frequently used to maintain axial alignment and help restore sagittal deformities.

The two most common surgical approaches for treatment of pediatric cervical spine instability are the midline posterior approach and Smith–Robinson-style anterior approach. The posterior approach is most commonly used for craniocervial stabilization but is highly adaptable and can be extended down to the thoracic spine if necessary. This approach has been previously well described in the literature, including its pitfalls and preventions in pediatric patients.

Posterior Approach to Cervical Spine Injury: PITFALLS AND PREVENTIONS

Pitfall	Prevention
Autofusion of all exposed vertebrae	• Avoid exposure of vertebrae not planned in fusion
Vertebral artery injury with lateral dissection at C1	• Avoid more than 8 mm lateral dissection at C1 in <2-year-olds, 10 mm in 2–8-year-olds, and 12 mm in older children
Inadequate lordosis correction in posterior-only approach	• Consider anterior fusion first for correction of lordosis

Anterior cervical exposures are performed with the patient supine through a small mid-cervical horizontal incision. Localization of the incision is aided by the use of intraoperative fluoroscopy. The approach has been well described in the literature but in essence is carried out by dissecting between the omohyoid and sternocleidomastoid muscles down the longus colli and prevertebral fascia. In the process, the carotid artery is retracted laterally and the trachea and esophagus are retracted medially. Once the target vertebrae are identified, distracting pins are placed in the appropriate vertebral bodies, with decompression, reduction, instrumentation, and fusion carried out as necessary.

Anterior Approach to Cervical Spine Injury: KEY SURGICAL STEPS

- Patient placed supine in halter traction (5–20 lb, as appropriate)
- Incision localized using fluoroscopy
- Anterior horizontal incision made
- Dissection carried out between omohyoid and sternocleidomastoid muscles down to longus colli
- Self-retaining retractors placed into wound
- Vertebral levels confirmed with fluoroscopy, distraction posts placed appropriately, and reduction maneuvers performed if necessary
- Discectomy and/or corpectomy performed at appropriate levels
- Appropriate arthrodesis placed (allograft, autograft, or cage)
- Plating performed with screw fixation as appropriate
- Closure in standard fashion

Occipitocervical Injuries

INTRODUCTION TO OCCIPITAL CONDYLAR FRACTURES

Occipital condylar fractures in children are rare, and their diagnosis requires a high index of suspicion.[116,120] The initial trauma CT scan in severely injured patients typically detects condylar injuries, but in less severely injured patients who do not undergo CT, it may be harder to diagnose. The true incidence of occipital condylar fractures in pediatric patients is not known, as most reported cases are in adult patients.[92] Several reports of occipital condylar fractures in children indicate an incidence of up to 1%[72,107,120]; however, prevalences reported in other CT-based studies are much higher, ranging from 4% to 19%.[19,20,103]

An occipital condyle fracture may be caused by axial loading with a component of ipsilateral flexion or by extreme rotation and lateral bending with avulsion fracture involving the alar ligament.

Many patients with occipital condylar fractures have associated head injuries.[3,116,163] Associated cranial nerve deficits may occur but are relatively rare. Damage to the hypoglossal nerve (cranial nerve XII) can occur as the nerve passes through the hypoglossal canal that is located above the middle third of the occipital condyle.[93]

ASSESSMENT OF OCCIPITAL CONDYLAR FRACTURES

The clinical presentation of occipital condylar fractures is variable. Pain and tenderness in the posterior occipitocervical region or torticollis may be the only complaints, whereas other patients may have significant neurologic deficits.[170]

As mentioned previously, plain radiographs often do not clearly show occipital condylar fractures, and CT is necessary to establish the diagnosis. Tuli et al.[162] recommended that a CT scan be obtained in the following circumstances: presence of isolated lower cranial nerve deficits, associated head injury or basal skull fracture, or persistent neck pain despite normal radiographs.

The two most common classifications schemes for occipital condylar fractures were published by Anderson and Montesano in 1988[7] and Tuli et al. in 1997.[162] In essence, the classification schemes can be used simultaneously, with MRI and CT used to detect potentially unstable injuries.

☑ Occipital Condylar Fractures:
ANDERSON AND MONTESANO CLASSIFICATION

Type	Description	Biomechanics
I	Impaction	Results from axial loading; ipsilateral alar ligament may be compromised, but stability is maintained by contralateral alar ligament and tectorial membrane
II	Skull base extension	Extends from occipital bone via condyle to enter foramen magnum; stability is maintained by intact alar ligaments and tectorial membrane
III	Avulsion	Mediated via alar ligament tension; associated disruption of tectorial membrane and contralateral alar ligament may cause instability

☑ Occipital Condylar Fractures:
CLASSIFICATION BY DISPLACEMENT AND STABILITY[162]

Type	Description	Biomechanics
1	Nondisplaced	Stable
2A	Displaced (≥2 mm of osseous separation)	Stable; no radiographic, CT, or MRI evidence of occipitoatlantoaxial instability of ligamentous disruption
2B	Displaced (≥2 mm of osseous separation)	Unstable; positive radiographic, CT, or MRI evidence of occipitoatlantoaxial instability or ligamentous disruption

TREATMENT OF OCCIPITAL CONDYLAR FRACTURES

Stable occipital condylar fractures (Anderson and Montesano types I and II, Tuli types 1 and 2A) are typically treated with a rigid cervical collar. Unstable injuries (Anderson and Montesano type III fracture, Tuli type 2B fracture) should most often be treated with a halo orthosis. Rarely, occipitocervial fusion is necessary, and would only occur in the setting of concomitant AOD.

Atlanto-Occipital Instability

ATLANTO-OCCIPITAL DISLOCATION

AOD was once thought to be a rare fatal injury found only at the time of autopsy (Fig. 21-6).[11,21,25,34,153] This injury is now being recognized more often, and children frequently survive with good to excellent outcomes.[48,54,156] This increase in the survival

A, B   **C**

Figure 21-6. X-ray (**A**), CT (**B**), and MRI (**C**) of a patient with atlanto-occipital dislocation.

rate may be due to increased awareness, improved emergency care, and better resuscitation/spinal immobilization methods used by emergency personnel.

AOD occurs in sudden acceleration and deceleration accidents, such as motor vehicle or pedestrian–vehicle accidents. The head is thrown forward, and this can cause sudden craniovertebral separation.[1] It may also occur if the patient is thrown from the vehicle.

The atlanto-occipital joint is a condylar joint that has little inherent bony stability. Stability is mainly provided by the occipitoatlantal capsular ligaments.[136] Secondary stabilizers of the OA joint are the alar ligaments and tectorial membrane.

ASSOCIATED INJURIES AND SIGNS AND SYMPTOMS OF ATLANTO-OCCIPITAL INSTABILITY

Although patients with this injury have a history of trauma, some may have no neurologic deficits. Others, however, may have symptoms such as cranial nerve injury, vomiting, headache, torticollis, or motor or sensory deficits.[34,35,42,74,85,133] Closed head injury and facial trauma are frequently associated with atlanto-occipital instability. The high association of closed head injures may mask other physical findings. A small amount of blood in the subarachnoid space surrounding the brainstem on the trauma CT scan in a patient with evidence of an upper spinal cord injury is strongly indicative of AOD. Similarly, unexplained weakness or difficulty in weaning off a ventilator after a closed head injury may be indicative of AOD.

IMAGING FOR ATLANTO-OCCIPITAL INSTABILITY

As mentioned previously, the use of CT and the measurement of the CCI described by Pang et al.[128] have greatly improved the ability to detect AOD in pediatric trauma patients. A CCI greater than 3.5 mm should be investigated further with MRI and a CCI greater than 4.0 mm should be considered strong evidence for true AOD. MRI is useful in the support of the diagnosis, as abnormal signal intensity is frequently seen within the OA joint. Other MRI findings may include tectorial membrane injury, posterior interspinous ligament injury, and alar ligament injury.

CLASSIFICATION OF ATLANTO-OCCIPITAL INSTABILITY

Prior classification schemes divided AOD into three types: longitudinal distraction with axial occipital separation, rotational injury, and anterior or posterior occipital displacement with respect to the atlas. With the use of the CCI on CT to diagnose AOD, these references are for historical interest only.

TREATMENT OPTIONS FOR ATLANTO-OCCIPITAL INSTABILITY

Because AOD is primarily a ligamentous injury, nonoperative treatment is typically unsuccessful. Although there are examples of halo stabilization in AOD, others have found persistent atlanto-occipital instability after halo immobilization. Therefore,

surgical stabilization is the recommended treatment for most cases of AOD.[89,158] Modern techniques in pediatric spine surgery have evolved significantly in the past few decades, and posterior rigid occipitocervical instrumentation from occiput to C2 is the preferred approach.[31,73,143] Attempting to perform an isolated occipitoatlantal fusion is fraught with technical difficulty and places abnormal stress on the adjoining AA joint after O-C1 fusion. Similarly, it has been shown that instrumenting C1 within an occiput-to-C2 construct is unnecessary, as it does not lead to higher fusion rate. Bone and wire techniques, often supplemented with a halo orthosis, are still sometimes used in selected circumstances, but it has been shown they have higher rates of fusion failure.[73,143]

The choice of C2 instrumentation is dictated by the patient's size and anatomy. The first choice is typically top-loading C2 pars screws, but close evaluation of the size and position of the vertebral artery notch is necessary.[31] If the C2 pars anatomy is inadequate or undesirable, C2 translaminar may be considered as a backup particularly in very young children.[110] Another option is using a C2 pedicle screw, although this is often not a viable option in pediatrics due to the size or trajectory of the C2 pedicle. Several options exist for occipital fixation portion of the procedure. A variety of top-loading occipital plates exist, as well as plate-rods that extend down directly to C2 (Fig. 21-7).

Either autologous rib or iliac crest bone graft may be harvested depending upon the surgeon's preference. Local harvest of split-thickness occipital bone has also been described, although this is not a preferred option in young children because of the thinness of their bone. It is recommended that the bone graft is compressed against the occiput and posterior portion of C2 using either screws or cables (or both) to aid in the fusion process. The use of recombinant human bone morphogenetic protein has also been described but may not be necessary in healthy patients with normal bone.

Postoperatively, the patient is placed in a hard cervical collar until CT evidence of successful fusion takes place, which is typically 3 to 4 months after surgery. Alternatively, in smaller children, or when there are concerns about the robustness of the fixation, a halo orthosis can be used for reinforcement.

Plate and Rod Fixation of Occiput to C2

This technique uses an occipital plate that attaches to a rod for fixation.

Plate and Rod Fixation of Occiput to C2: KEY SURGICAL STEPS

- Expose the occiput and spinous processes of the upper cervical vertebrae
- Position plate in midline of occiput, remove bone with burr as necessary to lay flat
- Drill holes in occiput and tap
- Insert screws and provisionally tighten
- Place C2 pars screws
- Bend rod to allow attachment to occipital plate
- Place rods into implants and tighten
- Perform final tightening of occipital plate set screws
- Perform arthrodesis with structural autograft (preferred) or allograft.

Initial postoperative   **12 years later**   C

A, B

Figure 21-7. A: Illustration of posterior occipitocervical fusion with instrumentation from occiput to C2 along with rib autografts. Maxillofacial screws are used to secure the rib graft in place at the subocciput. The star marks the area of C2 pars screw placement. **B:** Immediate postoperative x-ray after occipitocervical fusion for AOD in an 18-month-old patient. **C:** Twelve-year follow-up x-ray from the same patient depicting normal occipitocervical alignment. (**A:** Courtesy of the Department of Neurosurgery, University of Utah.)

C1–C2 Injuries

ASSESSMENT OF FRACTURES OF THE ATLAS

A fracture of the ring of C1 (Jefferson fracture) is a rare injury and accounts for fewer than 5% of all cervical spine fractures in children.[9,18] This fracture is caused by an axial load applied to the head.[91,108,160] The force is transmitted through the occipital condyles to the lateral masses of C1, causing a disruption in the ring of C1, usually in two places, with fractures occurring in both the anterior and posterior rings.[46] In children, an isolated single fracture of the ring can occur with the remaining fracture hinging on a synchondrosis.[15,97] This is an important distinction in children because fractures often occur through a normal synchondrosis. In addition, there can be plastic deformation of the ring with no evidence of a fracture.[12,91,140,159] This distinction can be seen on plain radiographs and CT scan, with fractures appearing through what appears to be normal physes. CT scan usually is the best imaging modality for making the diagnosis. As the lateral masses separate, the transverse ligament may be ruptured or avulsed, resulting in C1 and C2 instability.[114] The classic signs of an atlas fracture in a child are neck pain, cervical muscle spasm, decreased range of motion, and head tilt.[91] Children often hold their heads with their hands to relieve pain.

IMAGING AND OTHER DIAGNOSTIC STUDIES OF FRACTURES OF THE ATLAS

CT is the preferred imaging modality to diagnose atlas fracture. Occasionally, a C1 fracture may be found via anteroposterior x-ray using the rule of Spence, which states that radiographic evidence of lateral mass displacement (i.e., the distance that the C1 lateral masses extend beyond the C2 superior articular processes) greater than 6.9 mm may indicate both a torn transverse ligament and need for surgical management. The validity of this "rule," however, has often been called into question and probably needs to be retired.[100] Injury to the transverse ligament may be from intrinsic rupture or an avulsion of the ligamentous attachment to C1. MRI is useful in determining the integrity of the transverse ligament and detecting fractures through the normal synchondroses of the atlas. With a fracture through a synchondrosis, associated edema and hemorrhage are seen on MRI.[101]

Other cervical spine fractures may be present with an atlas fracture, and MRI should be carefully scrutinized to identify other fractures.[70,109]

CLASSIFICATION OF FRACTURES OF THE ATLAS

Treatment algorithms for Jefferson fractures are based on the integrity of the transverse ligament. These fractures are considered potentially unstable if the transverse ligament is disrupted.

Dickman Classification of Unstable Atlas Fractures Based on Transverse Ligament		
Type	Description	Treatment
I	Intrinsic tear of the transverse ligament	C1–C2 fusion
II	Bony avulsion at tubercle on C1 lateral mass	Halo vest successful in 75%

TREATMENT OPTIONS FOR FRACTURES OF THE ATLAS

NONOPERATIVE TREATMENT OF FRACTURES OF THE ATLAS

Nonoperative Treatment of Fractures of the Atlas: INDICATIONS AND CONTRAINDICATIONS

Indication

- Stable atlas fracture

Relative Contraindication

- Intrasubstance tear of transverse ligament (TAL)

Most atlas fractures are stable fractures and treatment consists of immobilization in an external orthosis. Occasionally, a Minerva or halo brace may be required for severe injuries. The length of immobilization necessary is debatable, but typically 8 weeks is prescribed. The final decision to remove the brace is based on documented healing by CT imaging and no instability on flexion and extension x-rays.

OPERATIVE TREATMENT OF FRACTURES OF THE ATLAS

Surgery is rarely necessary to stabilize these fractures but may be indicated if there is clear documentation of a transverse ligament tear along with significant C1 to C2 subluxation. In that case, atlantoaxial instrumentation and fusion is necessary to stabilize this injury.

Odontoid Fracture

INTRODUCTION TO ODONTOID FRACTURE

Odontoid fractures are relatively common fractures of the cervical spine in children, occurring at an average age of 4 years.[50,67,150] In adults, they are generally classified as type 1 fractures occurring through the tip of the odontoid process, type 2 fractures occurring through the neck of the odontoid process, and type 3 fractures, which involve the body of the C2 vertebra. Odontoid fractures account for approximately 10% of all cervical spine fractures and dislocations in children. In children, the dentocentral synchondrosis ossifies around 7 to 9 years of life, and thus, odontoid fractures in young individuals may occur through the synchondrosis itself. The dentocentral synchondrosis is a cartilage line at the base of the odontoid process, and injury may be analogous to a physeal or Salter–Harris type I injury. Careful neurologic assessment and multimodal imaging are important in the evaluation of an odontoid fracture, as these features help determine the decision to pursue conservative or surgical management of these injuries.

ASSESSMENT OF ODONTOID FRACTURE

MECHANISM OF INJURY OF ODONTOID FRACTURE

Fracture of the odontoid process is often associated with head trauma; in children, this frequently occurs due to motor vehicle accidents, falls from a height, and other mechanisms of sufficient impact and velocity such as sports-related injuries.[149] Odent et al.[124,125] reported that 8 of 15 fractures in children were the result of motor vehicle accidents, with the child fastened in a forward-facing seat. Odontoid fractures are typically caused by hyperflexion or hyperextension of the upper cervical spine, and children have a higher propensity for such injuries given their relatively large head size in proportion to their torso.

IMAGING AND OTHER DIAGNOSTIC STUDIES FOR ODONTOID FRACTURE

Although odontoid fractures are detectable on plain radiographs, CT imaging allows for careful delineation of the type of odontoid fracture present. It also provides detailed information regarding fracture line morphology and the degree of displacement and angulation of the fractured odontoid process in the supine position and demonstrates the relevant bony architecture for surgical planning purposes. Three-dimensional reconstructions of the spine are afforded by CT imaging, which allows for careful assessment of the type of fracture present, and the relative cortication of bony surfaces to determine fracture acuity as compared with congenital variants.

MRI is important in understanding the extent of ligamentous injury, the presence or absence of a transverse ligament injury or avulsion, posterior ligamentous complex (PLC) integrity, atlanto-occipital joint morphology or the presence of a joint effusion, and the status of the high cervical spinal cord itself. The transverse ligament is the primary stabilizer of the odontoid against forward displacement and may be involved in the setting of an odontoid fracture. Secondary stabilizers consist of the apical and alar ligaments, which arise from the tip of the odontoid and insert on the base of the skull. These also stabilize the atlanto-occipital joint indirectly. The normal distance from the anterior cortex of the dens to the posterior cortex of the anterior ring of C1 is 3 mm in adults and 4.5 mm in children. In children, if the distance is more than 4.5 mm, disruption of the transverse ligament is presumed. Acute rupture of the transverse ligament is rare and reportedly occurs in fewer than 10% of pediatric cervical spine injuries.[112] However, avulsion of the attachment of the transverse ligament to C1 may occur instead of rupture of the transverse ligament, and careful inspection of both C1 and MRI studies should be undertaken when evaluating such injuries.

CLASSIFICATION OF ODONTOID FRACTURE

Odontoid fractures have been classified in adults by location.[6] Type I (<5%) occurs at the tip of dens at the insertion of alar ligament that connects the dens to the occiput. Type II (>60%) is a fracture at the base of the dens at its attachment to the body of C2. Type III (30%) involves a fracture through the body of C2. Although this classification is mostly useful in older children and adolescents once the dentocentral synchondrosis has fused, many odontoid fractures in children occur through the synchondrosis of C2. Hosalkar et al.[84] proposed a classification system based on the extent of displacement of the odontoid process from the vertebral body (Table 21-1).

TREATMENT OPTIONS FOR ODONTOID FRACTURE

NONOPERATIVE TREATMENT OF ODONTOID FRACTURE

Nonoperative treatment may be appropriate in some odontoid fractures when the likelihood of bony or ligamentous healing is expected without the need for surgical reduction or stabilization. Surgery may be avoided in children with such injuries in accordance with the concept that bony healing rates with conservative treatment in children are superior to those in adults.[65] Type 1 odontoid fractures often can be managed with observation and use of a rigid orthosis; however, it is imperative to ensure that no coexisting craniocervical injury such as an AOD is present. Similarly, for some type 3 odontoid fractures, nonoperative treatment can be pursued after careful patient and imaging evaluation if the fracture is deemed stable. More controversy exists with type 2 odontoid fractures, as the fracture lies in a region of C2 thought to have less robust blood supply and, thus, nonunion rates are higher when treated nonoperatively.[148] However, this occurrence is thought to be an issue occurring with more advanced adult age. In children, healing rates of type 2 odontoid fractures is likely higher than in adults, although there is a lack of strong literature on this topic.[95] For significantly displaced odontoid fractures, closed reduction (usually extension

or slight hyperextension of the neck) may be necessary prior to external immobilization, but this is not commonly needed. Immobilization in the form of a halo vest, custom rigid cervical orthosis, Minerva brace, SOMI (sternal occipital mandibular immobilizer) brace, or others may be used. Follow-up evaluation approximately 8 weeks after injury should be planned, and evidence of bony healing can be assessed directly on CT imaging and on flexion/extension lateral radiographs.

OPERATIVE TREATMENT OF ODONTOID FRACTURE

For odontoid fractures that are thought to be unstable, surgical treatment is often pursued. Anterior odontoid screw placement can be attempted if the fracture morphology is appropriate, the transverse ligament is intact, and patient anatomy is suitable to achieve the angle required for screw placement (e.g., no barrel chest). Traditionally, placement of an anterior compression screw for odontoid fractures involves use of biplanar fluoroscopy, but as intraoperative adaptive technologies continue to evolve, CT-based navigation, and other technologies may play an increasing role in the operative approach to such injuries.[137] Intraoperative reduction can often be achieved under anesthesia, and high cervical alignment should be carefully evaluated to confirm reduction of the fracture.

Posterior C1 to C2 spinal instrumentation and fusion is used more commonly than an anterior approach in children (Fig. 21-8). Even in young children, AA arthrodesis in the modern era of rigid spinal fixation typically consists of C1 lateral mass fixation and C2 instrumentation with pars, pedicle, or translaminar screws. Another approach is placement of bilateral C1 to C2 transarticular screws with posterior interspace bone grafting. Table 21-2 lists a multitude of fusion techniques for C1 to C2, including those involving wiring and/or cabling.

Figure 21-8. A: A 15-year-old boy was in a motor vehicle collision and suffered a type 2 odontoid fracture as evaluated on CT. **B:** MRI demonstrated an intact transverse ligament and no spinal cord injury. **C:** He was trialed in a rigid cervical orthosis and, because of persistent instability, underwent a C1 to C2 fusion with bilateral transarticular screws and iliac crest allograft with cabling.

TABLE 21-3. Posterior Fusion Techniques

Atlantoaxial Fusion

Gallie[60]

- Advantage: One wire passed beneath lamina of C1
- Disadvantage: Wire may cause unstable C1 vertebra to displace posteriorly and fuse in dislocated position

Brooks and Jenkins[33]

- Advantage: Greater resistance to rotational movement, lateral bending, and extension
- Disadvantage: Requires sublaminar wires at C1 and C2

Harms and Melcher

- Advantage: Individual placement of polyaxial screws simplifies technique and involves less risk to C1–C2 facet joint and vertebral artery
- Disadvantage: Possible irritation of the C2 ganglion from instrumentation

Magerl and Seeman[105]

- Advantage: Significant improvement in fusion rates over traditional posterior wire stabilization and bone grafting techniques
- Disadvantage: Technically demanding and must be combined with Gallie or Brooks fusion for maximum stability

Occipitocervical Fusion

- Required when other bony anomalies occur at occipitocervical junction

Wertheim and Bohlman[167]

- Wires passed through outer table of skull at occipital protuberance instead of through inner and outer tables near foramen magnum
- Lessens risk of danger to superior sagittal and transverse sinuses (which are cephalad to occipital protuberance)

Koop et al.[99]

- No internal fixation used
- Autogenous corticocancellous iliac bone graft

Dormans et al.[49]

- Stable fixation is achieved by exact fit of autogenous iliac crest bone graft and fixation of the spinous process with button wire and fixation of the occiput with wires through burr holes
- Can be used in high-risk patients (Down syndrome) with increased stabilization and shorter immobilization time

Contoured Rod, Screw, or Contoured Plate Fixation

- Has the advantage of achieving immediate stability of the occipitocervical junction

Preoperative Planning

Preoperative imaging often consists of plain radiographs, CT scan, and sometimes MRI or CTA of the cervical spine. If significant subluxation of C1 to C2 is present, this can add complexity and difficulty to transarticular screw placement. It is imperative to understand the bilateral vertebral artery course prior to attempting transarticular fusion at the C1 to C2 joint. It has been reported that a high-riding vertebral artery may preclude placement of transarticular screws in approximately 11% of cases.[32]

Figure 21-11. Wires are passed under the lamina of the atlas and through the spine of the axis and tied over the graft. This method is used most frequently. (Reprinted with permission from Fielding JW, et al. Spine fusion for atlanto-axial instability. *J Bone Joint Surg Am.* 1976;58(3):400–407.)

Technique

 Atlantoaxial Arthrodesis With Posterior C1–C2 Transarticular Screw Fixation:
KEY SURGICAL STEPS

- ❏ Expose the spine from the dorsal surface of C1 as well as the C2 lamina bilaterally, without violating the C2–C3 facet joint
- ❏ Using the C2 inferior facet as landmark, the drill entry point is 2 mm lateral to the medial edge and 2 mm above the inferior border of the C2 facet
- ❏ Tap hole and place threaded screw of the appropriate length and diameter across C1–C2 joint on both sides
- ❏ Harvest bone graft from posterior iliac crest or use structural allograft fashioned to the appropriate size
- ❏ Perform C1–C2 fusion using either Brooks or Gallie technique

The patient is placed prone with the head held in a Mayfield skull clamp or with a halo ring attached to the Mayfield attachment. Under fluoroscopic guidance, proper alignment of the AA joint is confirmed. The upper thoracic spine should be included in the surgical field during preparation to allow for percutaneous placement of the transarticular screw, if needed. Percutaneous screw placement may be necessary because of the cephalad orientation of the C1 to C2 transarticular screw.

The spine is exposed in a subperiosteal fashion, including the dorsal surface of C1, the bilateral C2 laminae, and the bilateral C2 pars. Care should be used not to violate the C2 to C3 joint capsules. The C2 inferior facet is used as the landmark for screw entry: the entry point is 2 mm lateral to the medial edge and 2 mm above the inferior border of the C2 facet. The drill trajectory is angled toward the midpoint of the ipsilateral C2 pars. On the lateral fluoroscopic radiograph, the drill trajectory is adjusted toward the posterior cortex of the anterior arch of C1. Percutaneous placement of C1 to C2 transarticular screws may be necessary if the intraoperative AA alignment precludes drilling or placement of screws through the operative incision. After cannulation, tapping and screw placement are performed, with attention paid on fluoroscopy that these maneuvers do not result in C1 becoming more distanced from C2, which may imply that the instrument has not entered the previously cannulated tract within C1 at the level of the C1 to C2 joint. After placement of bilateral C1 to C2 transarticular screws, a bone graft is harvested from the posterior iliac crest or fashioned from structural allograft. A traditional posterior C1 to C2 fusion is performed after the contact points at C1 and C2 are decorticated, and this is completed through either the modified Gallie or the Brooks technique.

To perform the modified Gallie fusion, a cable or wire is passed ipsilaterally in the C1 sublaminar space, through the interspinous space under C2, sublaminar under the contralateral C1 lamina, and back through the interspinous space of C2 to C3. The graft is held in place and tensioned appropriately (see Fig. 21-11).

Postoperative Care

The patient is typically immobilized in a rigid cervical collar only, although halo or Minerva use can be considered if there are any concerns about the strength of the construct.

Potential Pitfalls and Preventive Measures

The disadvantages of this technique are potential injury to the vertebral artery, its technical difficulty, and the requirement for sublaminar wire and fusion (Brooks or Gallie technique).

HANGMAN'S FRACTURE

INTRODUCTION TO HANGMAN'S FRACTURE

Bilateral fracture of the pars interarticularis of C2, also known as traumatic spondylolisthesis, or hangman's fractures, can occur in both adults and children.[138] This injury probably occurs more frequently in the younger age group because of the disproportionately large head and underdeveloped musculature of young children. The possibility of child abuse also must be ruled out.[96,140,165]

ASSESSMENT OF HANGMAN'S FRACTURE

MECHANISM OF INJURY FOR HANGMAN'S FRACTURE

The mechanism of injury is forced hyperextension and axial loading.

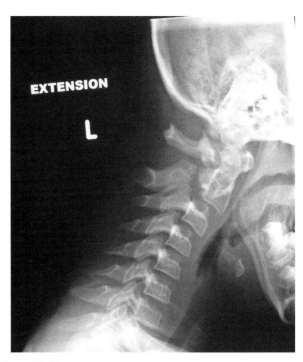

Figure 21-12. Lateral radiograph of patient with traumatic C2 spondylolisthesis (hangman's fracture).

ASSOCIATED INJURIES AND SIGNS AND SYMPTOMS OF HANGMAN'S FRACTURE

Facial and head injuries may be associated. Patients present with neck pain and resist any movement of the head and neck. There should be a history of trauma (Fig. 21-12).

IMAGING AND OTHER DIAGNOSTIC STUDIES FOR HANGMAN'S FRACTURE

Radiographs reveal lucency anterior to the pedicles of the axis, usually with some forward subluxation of C2 on C3. One must be sure this is a fracture and not a persistent synchondrosis of the axis.[97,121,155] Differentiating a persistent synchondrosis from a fracture may be difficult. Several radiographic findings can help distinguish congenital spondylolysis from a hangman's fracture. With congenital spondylolysis, there should be a symmetrical osseous gap with smooth, clearly defined cortical margins; no prevertebral soft tissue swelling should be observed; and there should be no signs of instability. Often, small foci of ossification are seen in the defect. CT scans show the defect to be at the level of the neurocentral synchondrosis. MRI does not show any edema or soft tissue swelling that typically is present with a fracture.[165,117]

CLASSIFICATION OF HANGMAN'S FRACTURE

The classification by Effendi et al.,[53] which was modified by Levine and Edwards[102] and later by Müller et al.,[118] is based on the severity of associated soft tissue injuries.

Classification of Hangman's Fracture (Levine and Edwards[102])

Type	Fracture Characteristics	Mechanism of Injury	Stability
I	Bilateral pars fracture, <3-mm anterior C2–C3 subluxation, intact C2–C3 discoligamentous complex	Pure hyperextension–axial loading	Stable
II	Discoligamentous injury at C2–C3 with displacement of the pars fracture and anterior translation of the C2 body	Combination hyperextension–axial loading with secondary anterior flexion–compression	Unstable
IIa	Minimal displacement, severe angulation (hinging from anterior longitudinal ligament)	Flexion–distraction	Unstable
III	Fracture of the pars interarticularis with C2–C3 facet dislocations	Flexion–compression	Very unstable

Müller et al.[118] subclassified type II fractures as flexion, extension, and listhesis. Type III is a fracture of the pars interarticularis with C2 to C3 facet dislocations. This classification is for adult patients and may not be completely applicable to pediatric patients.[123]

TREATMENT OPTIONS FOR HANGMAN'S FRACTURE

NONOPERATIVE TREATMENT OF HANGMAN'S FRACTURE

Nonoperative Treatment of Hangman's Fracture:
INDICATIONS AND CONTRAINDICATIONS

Indication

• Stable fracture

Relative Contraindications

• Nonunion
• Documented instability

Treatment of stable hangman's fractures should be with immobilization in a Minerva cast, halo, or cervical orthosis for 8 to 12 weeks. Pizzutillo et al.[138] reported that four of five patients healed with immobilization.

OPERATIVE TREATMENT OF HANGMAN'S FRACTURE

If union does not occur or there is documented instability, a posterior or anterior arthrodesis can be done to stabilize this fracture. Anterior approaches would typically entail an anterior cervical discectomy and fusion at C2 to C3. Posterior stabilization would

often involve C1 to C3 posterior spinal instrumentation and fusion with or without instrumentation at C2 itself.

Subaxial (C3–C7) Injuries

INTRODUCTION TO SUBAXIAL (C3–C7) INJURIES

Although cervical spine injuries are the most common spinal injuries in the pediatric population, adult patterns of osseous injury in the subaxial spine (C3–C7) are rare in children and infants[59,90,111,152] and most often resemble adult injuries in the adolescent age group. Although operative injuries to the subaxial cervical spine are rare in children, a high degree of suspicion for such injuries should be maintained in children evaluated for high-impact mechanisms of injury, because the consequences of missed cervical spinal injuries can lead to high patient morbidity. In addition to careful assessment of bony fractures in children, a careful direct or indirect assessment of potential ligamentous compromise should be undertaken, as these elements may play a more important role than bone architecture alone in providing stability of the cervical spine through its range of motion.

Depending on the size and anatomy of the patient, standard anterior and posterior instrumentation techniques with modern rigid fixation can often be used in subaxial spine fractures or dislocations in children.

CLASSIFICATION OF POSTERIOR LIGAMENTOUS DISRUPTION

Classifying injuries of the cervical spine can be helpful in guiding the approach for treatment. The SLIC and severity score identifies three major injury characteristics to describe subaxial cervical injuries: fracture morphology, discoligamentous complex (DLC) integrity, and patient neurologic status (Table 21-4).[134] Although no scoring system supersedes the clinical discretion of the treating surgeon, these features help guide the treatment team toward nonoperative or operative intervention. This scoring system was validated in the adult population, and while more work is required with regard to the reliability and validity of the SLIC score in the management of cervical spine injuries in children, it does provide some useful guidance across ages.

Posterior Ligamentous Disruptions

ASSESSMENT OF DLC/PLC DISRUPTIONS

MECHANISM OF INJURY FOR DLC DISRUPTION

DLC/PLC disruption can occur with a flexion or distraction injury to the cervical spine

TABLE 21-4. Subaxial Injury Classification (SLIC) System	
Characteristic	Points
Morphology	
No abnormality	0
Compression	1
Burst	2
Distraction (e.g., facet perch, hyperextension)	3
Rotation/translation (e.g., facet dislocation, unstable teardrop, or advanced-stage flexion compression injury)	4
DLC	
Intact	0
Indeterminate (e.g., isolated interspinous widening, MRI signal change only)	1
Disrupted (e.g., widening of anterior disc space, facet perch or dislocation, kyphotic deformity)	2
Neurologic Status	
Intact	0
Root injury	1
Complete cord injury	2
Incomplete cord injury	3
Ongoing cord compression (in setting of a neurologic deficit)	+1

Reproduced with permission from Patel JC, et al. Subaxial cervical spine trauma classification: The Subaxial Injury Classification system and case examples. *Neurosurg Focus.* 2008;25:E8.

ASSOCIATED INJURIES AND SIGNS AND SYMPTOMS OF DLC/PLC DISRUPTION

Intervertebral disc disruption, facet fracture, and other ligamentous disruptions may be associated with this injury. The patient usually has point tenderness at the injury site and complaints of neck pain.

IMAGING AND OTHER DIAGNOSTIC STUDIES FOR PLC DISRUPTION

Initial radiographs may be unremarkable except for loss of normal cervical lordosis. This may be a normal finding in young children, but adolescents should be evaluated for possible ligamentous injury. Widening or splaying of the posterior interspinous distance is suggestive of PLC disruption. Guidelines for instability in children have not been fully developed. CT imaging is useful in further characterizing the bony injury present. MRI is also extremely useful in characterizing the degree of PLC disruption. Importantly, the PLC is comprised generally of the supraspinous and interspinous ligaments, as well as the ligamentum flavum. In the cervical spine, the complex between the intervertebral disc as well as the PLC is known as

the discoligamentous complex, or DLC. High-resolution imaging of cervical spine injuries can help detect gross disruption of these ligaments, the presence of absence of a compressive hematoma, and ligamentous strain.

TREATMENT OPTIONS FOR DLC DISRUPTION

Treatment considerations for DLC disruption should account for the presence or absence of cervical spine fractures and patient neurologic status. At this time, there is no universally accepted definition of a "stable" versus "unstable" ligamentous injury.

Isolated PLC disruption is rare but possible. Isolated "single-column" ligamentous injuries are often considered "stable," and treatment includes pain control, the use of an external orthosis, physical therapy, and close observation with or without serial imaging. Often, patients are evaluated at a time interval after the injury to determine whether any clinical or radiographic evidence of instability is present (i.e., continued severe neck pain, excess motion, or subluxation on a flexion–extension radiograph). The SLIC scoring system can be useful in putting DLC/PLC disruption into context with the overall injury pattern and the patient's neurologic status to help guide treatment decisions in terms of operative or nonoperative intervention. However, each clinical decision should be tailored to an individual patient's presentation, radiographic characteristics, and clinical evaluation.

Compression Fracture

ASSESSMENT OF COMPRESSION FRACTURE

Compression fractures are isolated anterior column injuries that are generally considered "stable."

MECHANISM OF INJURY FOR COMPRESSION FRACTURE

Compression fractures, the most common fractures of the subaxial spine in children, are caused by flexion and axial loading that result in a loss of vertebral body height, which may be more pronounced in the anterior vertebral body, producing a wedge-like injury.

IMAGING AND OTHER DIAGNOSTIC STUDIES FOR COMPRESSION FRACTURE

Compression fractures are often detected on a lateral plain radiograph, and this finding alone does not generally necessitate advanced imaging with CT or MRI. Given the naturally convex midvertebral endplates in children, it can be difficult to distinguish between physiologic wedging and wedge compression fractures, which makes obtaining a history and physical examination important in understanding the likelihood of a truly

Figure 21-14. Anteroposterior and lateral radiographs and CT scan of patient with a minimally displaced burst fracture of C5.

TREATMENT OPTIONS FOR BURST FRACTURE

NONOPERATIVE TREATMENT OF BURST FRACTURE

Nonoperative management of a cervical burst fracture may be considered in a child with no neurologic symptoms, reasonable cervical alignment, and minimal discoligamentous disruption. Close follow-up is recommended if the conservative management route is undertaken. Nonoperative treatment typically consists of rigid external orthosis with a cervical collar that may be custom fit for children, as well as a halo vest.

OPERATIVE TREATMENT OF BURST FRACTURE

Operative treatment of a cervical burst fracture often consists of an anterior approach for vertebral corpectomy of the affected level, with interbody grafting and anterior plating (Fig. 21-15). In some occasions, a burst fracture may be associated with disruption of the posterior elements, which may prompt anterior and posterior stabilization.

Spondylolysis and Spondylolisthesis

ASSESSMENT OF TRAUMATIC SPONDYLOLYSIS AND SPONDYLOLISTHESIS

Traumatic spondylolysis refers to fracture of the pars interarticularis. This type of injury at the level of C2 is known as a hangman's fracture and has been described earlier in this chapter (see page 755). Such injury is uncommon in the subaxial spine but is theoretically possible. In the setting of a discoligamentous injury with associated bilateral pars interarticularis fractures, traumatic spondylolisthesis can occur, also referred to as vertebral subluxation. These injuries are uncommon in younger children that have not achieved a mature spinal ossification pattern. However, ring apophyseal disruption and significant ligamentous injuries (Chance fracture) or facet dislocation can cause similar vertebral body subluxation or dislocation.

TREATMENT OPTIONS FOR SPONDYLOLYSIS AND SPONDYLOLISTHESIS

NONOPERATIVE TREATMENT OF SPONDYLOLYSIS AND SPONDYLOLISTHESIS

Treatment consists of immobilization in a cervical orthosis or halo brace. Evidence of spinal instability and subluxation (spondylolisthesis) may warrant surgical intervention, but evaluation should occur on a patient-by-patient basis after careful clinical and radiographic review. Importantly, physiologic pseudosubluxation, especially at the C2 to C3 disc space, can be seen in young children and adolescents, with a prevalence of up to 20%.[57]

OPERATIVE TREATMENT OF SPONDYLOLYSIS AND SPONDYLOLISTHESIS

Surgical stabilization is recommended for unstable fractures, with persistent and debilitating deformity, in patients with neurologic deficits, or for cases featuring nonunion after nonoperative measures.

Posterior Arthrodesis for Subaxial Injuries

Positioning

The patient is placed prone on chest rolls or a Jackson frame using a Mayfield skull clamp or Gardner–Wells tongs, with associated head rest (horseshoe) or a halo ring with appropriate stabilizing pads with or without traction.

A, B   **C**

Figure 21-15. A: A 9-year-old boy suffered from a trampoline injury which resulted in a C4 burst fracture seen on sagittal and axial CT imaging. MRI revealed spinal canal narrowing and evidence of spinal cord edema (**B**), which, together with painful dysesthesia and upper extremity weakness on clinical evaluation, prompted urgent surgery for anterior cervical corpectomy with cage and plate placement as seen on plain radiography (**C**).

Technique

> **✓ Posterior Arthrodesis for Subaxial Injuries:**
> KEY SURGICAL STEPS

- ❑ Expose the chosen spinous processes and posterior elements with a midline incision
- ❑ Carefully place spinal implants (mostly lateral mass fixation in the subaxial cervical spine) based on preoperative evaluation of the imaging, with caution to avoid injury to the vertebral artery and exiting nerve root; may use real-time imaging with fluoroscopy to aid in implant placement
- ❑ Roughen the cortical and joint surfaces when possible to create fusion surface
- ❑ Place corticocancellous bone graft or local autograft if performing a decompression
- ❑ Close wound in layers

Posterior Arthrodesis With Lateral Mass Screw Fixation

Modern rigid fixation techniques with lateral mass screw placement (or rarely, cervical pedicle screw placement) are most commonly used for subaxial cervical spine stabilization from a posterior approach. This involves a posterior midline incision and subperiosteal exposure of the lamina and lateral masses/facet joints of the intended levels of instrumentation and arthrodesis. Several techniques of lateral mass screw fixation for the lower cervical spine have been described. They differ primarily in entry point location for the screws and in trajectory of screw placement; both are acceptable forms of lateral mass fixation.

Positioning

The patient is placed prone using a Mayfield skull clamp, Gardner–Wells tongs (often with underlying horseshoe), or a halo ring with appropriate stabilizing pads or halo with traction bale and longitudinal traction weight.

Technique

Roy–Camille Technique

> **✓ Posterior Arthrodesis With Lateral Mass Screw Fixation (Roy–Camille):**
> KEY SURGICAL STEPS

- ❑ Place entry point for screw at center of rectangular posterior face of lateral mass
- ❑ Drill perpendicular to posterior wall to a safe depth
- ❑ Exit point should be at junction of lateral mass and transverse process for additional pullout strength

The entry point for the screw is at the center of the rectangular posterior face of the lateral mass or can be measured 5 mm medial to the lateral edge and midway between the facets included in the fusion joints (Fig. 21-16A). The drill is directed perpendicular to the posterior wall of the vertebral body with a 10-degree lateral angle (Fig. 21-16B). This trajectory establishes an exit point slightly lateral to the vertebral artery and below the exiting nerve root. The lateral mass depth from C3 to C6 ranges from 6 to 14 mm. An adjustable drill guide set to the appropriate depth is used and can be gradually increased if local anatomy permits. Pullout strength of the screw may be increased with bicortical fixation.

Figure 21-19. CT shows placement of screws.

Figure 21-20. Lateral (**left**) and anteroposterior (**right**) views of completed C1 to C2 fixation with C1 lateral mass screws connected to C2 laminar screws (lateral view). (With permission from Leonard JR, Wright NM. Pediatric atlantoaxial fixation with bilateral, crossing C2 translaminar screws: Technical note. *J Neurosurg Pediatr.* 2006;104:59–63.)

Potential Pitfalls and Preventive Measures

See page 753 for potential pitfalls with posterior approaches.

Anterior Arthrodesis

In pediatric patients and adolescents, the technique of anterior instrumentation and fusion is similar to that used in adults, with some modifications in unique cases. The anatomy of the vertebral body should be evaluated preoperatively to determine whether anterior plates and screws may be used. Traditional plating systems use bilaterally placed vertebral body screws. In children with small bony architecture, a single-screw plating system could be used.

ACKNOWLEDGMENTS

The authors thank William C. Warner and Daniel J. Hedequist, who wrote the chapter on cervical spine injuries in the previous edition, on which this revision is based.

Annotated References

Reference	Annotation
Alexiades NG, Shao B, Braga BP, et al. Development of best practices in the utilization and implementation of pediatric cervical spine traction: a modified Delphi study. *J Neurosurg Pediatr.* 2021;27(6):649–660.	A recent paper describing a Delphi-driven approach to the use of cervical spine traction in children
AuYong N, Piatt J Jr. Jefferson fractures of the immature spine. Report of 3 cases. *J Neurosurg Pediatr.* 2009;3(1):15–19.	Article describing Jefferson fracture correlate morphology in the young spine
Beckmann NM, Chinapuvvula NR, Zhang X, West OC. Epidemiology and imaging classification of pediatric cervical spine injuries: 12-year experience at a level 1 trauma center. *AJR Am J Roentgenol.* 2020;214(6):1359–1368.	Useful study describing the epidemiology of cervical spine injuries in children with blunt trauma, including injury classifications by age cohort
Brockmeyer DL, Sivakumar W, Mazur MD, et al. Identifying factors predictive of atlantoaxial fusion failure in pediatric patients: lessons learned from a retrospective Pediatric Craniocervical Society study. *Spine (Phila Pa 1976).* 2018;43(11):754–760.	Article evaluating factors associated with fusion failure for atlantoaxial abnormalities in children
Brockmeyer DL, York JE, Apfelbaum RI. Anatomical suitability of C1-2 transarticular screw placement in pediatric patients. *J Neurosurg.* 2000;92(1 Suppl):7–11.	Article describing considerations for placement of transarticular screws for C1–C2 instrumentation and arthrodesis in children
Dastagirzada YM, Alexiades NG, Kurland DB, et al. Developing consensus for the management of pediatric cervical spine disorders and stabilization: a modified Delphi study. *J Neurosurg Pediatr.* 2023;31(1):32–42.	A recent article identifying consensus statements by orthopaedic and neurologic surgeons for the management of children with cervical spine disorders
Eleraky MA, Theodore N, Adams M, et al. Pediatric cervical spine injuries: report of 102 cases and review of the literature. *J Neurosurg.* 2000;92(1 Suppl):12–17.	Single-institution study describing cervical spine injuries in children and their neurosurgical management, as well as a thorough review of the literature to date

Annotated References

Reference	Annotation
Herman MJ, Brown KO, Sponseller PD, et al. Pediatric cervical spine clearance: a consensus statement and algorithm from the Pediatric Cervical Spine Clearance Working Group. *J Bone Joint Surg Am.* 2019;101(1):e1.	A consensus Delphi-driven statement from a multidisciplinary group of pediatric cervical spine trauma experts that outlines an evidence-based approach to cervical spine clearance
Hewes HA, Ravindra VM, Ryan S, et al. The fate of the cervical collar: an observational pilot study investigating follow-up care after emergency department discharge in children with mild traumatic neck injuries. *Pediatr Emerg Care.* 2023;39(4):274–278.	A single-center study describing low compliance of cervical spine collar use in children after mild traumatic neck injuries
Pang D, Nemzek WR, Zovickian J. Atlanto-occipital dislocation: part 1–normal occipital condyle-C1 interval in 89 children. *Neurosurgery.* 2007;61(3):514–521.	The original description of using the condyle–C1 interval (CCI) in the evaluation and management of atlanto-occipital dislocation
Patel AA, Dailey A, Brodke DS, et al. Subaxial cervical spine trauma classification: the Subaxial Injury Classification system and case examples. *Neurosurg Focus.* 2008;25(5):E8.	Article describing a useful classification system for subaxial injuries that has been subsequently validated in the pediatric population

REFERENCES

1. Ahmed R, Traynelis VC, Menezes AH. Fusions at the craniovertebral junction. *Childs Nerv Syst.* 2008;24(10):1209–1224.
2. Ahuja CS, Schroeder GD, Vaccaro AR, Fehlings MG. Spinal cord injury: what are the controversies? *J Orthop Trauma.* 2017;31(Suppl 4):S7–S13.
3. Alcelik I, Manik KS, Sian PS, Khoshneviszadeh SE. Occipital condylar fractures: review of the literature and case report. *J Bone Joint Surg Br.* 2006;88(5):665–669.
4. Alexiades NG, Shao B, Braga BP, et al. Development of best practices in the utilization and implementation of pediatric cervical spine traction: a modified Delphi study. *J Neurosurg Pediatr.* 2021;27(6):649–660.
5. American Academy of Orthopaedic Surgeons, Committee on Pediatric Orthopaedics. *Trauma of the Cervical Spine. Position Statement.* American Academy of Orthopaedic Surgeons, Committee on Pediatric Orthopaedics; 1990.
6. Anderson LD, D'Alonzo RT. Fractures of the odontoid process of the axis. *J Bone Joint Surg Am.* 1974;56(8):1663–1674.
7. Anderson PA, Montesano PX. Morphology and treatment of occipital condyle fractures. *Spine (Phila Pa 1976).* 1988;13(7):731–736.
8. Anissipour AK, Agel J, Bellabarba C, Bransford RJ. Cervical facet dislocations in the adolescent population: a report of 21 cases at a level 1 trauma center from 2004 to 2014. *Eur Spine J.* 2017;26(4):1266–1271.
9. Apple JS, Kirks DR, Merten DF, Martinez S. Cervical spine fractures and dislocations in children. *Pediatr Radiol.* 1987;17(1):45–49.
10. Arora B, Suresh S. Spinal cord injuries in older children: is there a role for high-dose methylprednisolone? *Pediatr Emerg Care.* 2011;27(12):1192–1194.
11. Aufdermaur M. Spinal injuries in juveniles: necropsy findings in twelve cases. *J Bone Joint Surg Br.* 1974;56B(3):513–519.
12. AuYong N, Piatt J Jr. Jefferson fractures of the immature spine. Report of 3 cases. *J Neurosurg Pediatr.* 2009;3(1):15–19.
13. Baron EM, Loftus CM, Vaccaro AR, Dominique DA. Anterior approach to the subaxial cervical spine in children: a brief review. *Neurosurg Focus.* 2006;20(2):E4.
14. Baum JA, Hanley EN Jr, Pullekines J. Comparison of halo complications in adults and children. *Spine (Phila Pa 1976).* 1989;14(3):251–252.
15. Bayar MA, Erdem Y, Ozturk K, Buharali Z. Isolated anterior arch fracture of the atlas: child case report. *Spine (Phila Pa 1976).* 2002;27(2):E47–E49.
16. Beckmann NM, Chinapuvvula NR, Zhang X, West OC. Epidemiology and imaging classification of pediatric cervical spine injuries: 12-year experience at a level 1 trauma center. *AJR Am J Roentgenol.* 2020;214(6):1359–1368.
17. Benzel EC, Zhang DH, Iannotti C, et al. Occipitocervical fusion in an infant with atlantooccipital dislocation. *World Neurosurg.* 2012;78(6):715.e17–e24.
18. Birney TJ, Hanley EN Jr. Traumatic cervical spine injuries in childhood and adolescence. *Spine (Phila Pa 1976).* 1989;14(12):1277–1282.
19. Bloom AI, Neeman Z, Floman Y, et al. Occipital condyle fracture and ligament injury: imaging by CT. *Pediatr Radiol.* 1996;26(11):786–790.
20. Bloom AI, Neeman Z, Slasky BS, et al. Fracture of the occipital condyles and associated craniocervical ligament injury: incidence, CT imaging and implications. *Clin Radiol.* 1997;52(3):198–202.
21. Bohlman HH. Acute fractures and dislocations of the cervical spine. An analysis of three hundred hospitalized patients and review of the literature. *J Bone Joint Surg Am.* 1979;61(8):1119–1142.
22. Bono CM. The halo fixator. *J Am Acad Orthop Surg.* 2007;15(12):728–737.
23. Booth TN. Cervical spine evaluation in pediatric trauma. *AJR Am J Roentgenol.* 2012;198(5):W417–W425.
24. Bowers CA, Kundu B, Hawryluk GW. Methylprednisolone for acute spinal cord injury: an increasingly philosophical debate. *Neural Regen Res.* 2016;11(6):882–885.
25. Bracken MB. Pharmacological treatment of acute spinal cord injury: current status and future projects. *J Emerg Med.* 1993;11(Suppl 1):43–48.
26. Bracken MB. Treatment of acute spinal cord injury with methylprednisolone: results of a multicenter, randomized clinical trial. *J Neurotrauma.* 1991;8(Suppl 1):S47–S50.
27. Bracken MB, Shepard MJ, Collins WF, et al. A randomized, controlled trial of methylprednisolone or naloxone in the treatment of acute spinal-cord injury: results of the Second National Acute Spinal Cord Injury Study. *N Engl J Med.* 1990;322(20):1405–1411.
28. Bracken MB, Shepard MJ, Collins WF Jr, et al. Methylprednisolone or naloxone treatment after acute spinal cord injury: 1-year follow-up data: results of the second National Acute Spinal Cord Injury Study. *J Neurosurg.* 1992;76(1):23–31.
29. Bransford RJ, Alton TB, Patel AR, Bellabarba C. Upper cervical spine trauma. *J Am Acad Orthop Surg.* 2014;22(11):718–729.
30. Brockmeyer DL, Ragel BT, Kestle JRW. The pediatric cervical spine instability study: a pilot study assessing the prognostic value of four imaging modalities in clearing the cervical spine for children with severe traumatic injuries. *Childs Nerv Syst.* 2012;28(5):699–705.
31. Brockmeyer DL, Sivakumar W, Mazur MD, et al. Identifying factors predictive of atlantoaxial fusion failure in pediatric patients: lessons learned from a Retrospective Pediatric Craniocervical Society Study. *Spine (Phila Pa 1976).* 2018;43(11):754–760.
32. Brockmeyer DL, York JE, Apfelbaum RI. Anatomical suitability of C1-2 transarticular screw placement in pediatric patients. *J Neurosurg.* 2000;92(1 Suppl):7–11.
33. Brooks AL, Jenkins EB. Atlanto-axial arthrodesis by the wedge compression method. *J Bone Joint Surg Am.* 1978;60(3):279–284.
34. Bucholz RW, Burkhead WZ. The pathological anatomy of fatal atlanto-occipital dislocations. *J Bone Joint Surg Am.* 1979;61(2):248–250.
35. Burkus JK, Deponte RJ. Chronic atlantoaxial rotatory fixation correction by cervical traction, manipulation, and bracing. *J Pediatr Orthop.* 1986;6(5):631–635.
36. Caffey J. The whiplash shaken infant syndrome: manual shaking by the extremities with whiplash-induced intracranial and intraocular bleedings, linked with residual permanent brain damage and mental retardation. *Pediatrics.* 1974;54(4):396–403.
37. Cage JM, Knox JB, Wimberly RL, et al. Complications associated with high-dose corticosteroid administration in children with spinal cord injury. *J Pediatr Orthop.* 2015;35(7):687–692.
38. Caruso MC, Daugherty MC, Moody SM, et al. Lessons learned from administration of high-dose methylprednisolone sodium succinate for acute pediatric spinal cord injuries. *J Neurosurg Pediatr.* 2017;20(6):567–574.
39. Chu MW, Soleimani T, Evans TA, et al. C-spine injury and mandibular fractures: lifesaver broken in two spots. *J Surg Res.* 2016;206(2):386–390.
40. Chugh S, Kamian K, Depreitere B, Schwartz ML. Occipital condyle fracture with associated hypoglossal nerve injury. *Can J Neurol Sci.* 2006;33(3):322–324.
41. Chung S, Mikrogianakis A, Wales PW, et al. Trauma association of Canada Pediatric Subcommittee National Pediatric Cervical Spine Evaluation Pathway: consensus guidelines. *J Trauma.* 2011;70(4):873–884.
42. Collalto PM, DeMuth WW, Schwentker EP, Boal DK. Traumatic atlanto-occipital dislocation. Case report. *J Bone Joint Surg Am.* 1986;68(7):1106–1109.
43. Copley LA, Dormans JP. Cervical spine disorders in infants and children. *J Am Acad Orthop Surg.* 1998;6(4):204–214.
44. Dastagirzada YM, Alexiades NG, Kurland DB, et al. Developing consensus for the management of pediatric cervical spine disorders and stabilization: a modified Delphi study. *J Neurosurg Pediatr.* 2022;31(1):32–42.
45. de Beer JD, Hoffman EB, Kieck CF. Traumatic atlantoaxial subluxation in children. *J Pediatr Orthop.* 1990;10(3):397–400.
46. Dettling SD, Morscher MA, Masin JS, Adamczyk MJ. Cranial nerve IX and X impairment after a sports-related Jefferson (C1) fracture in a 16-year-old male: a case report. *J Pediatr Orthop.* 2013;33(3):e23–e27.
47. Deutsch RJ, Badawy MK. Pediatric cervical spine fracture caused by an adult 3-point seatbelt. *Pediatr Emerg Care.* 2008;24(2):105–108.

48. Dormans JP, Criscitiello AA, Drummond DS, Davidson RS. Complications in children managed with immobilization in a halo vest. *J Bone Joint Surg Am.* 1995;77(9):1370–1373.
49. Dormans JP, Drummond DS, Sutton LN, et al. Occipitocervical arthrodesis in children: a new technique and analysis of results. *J Bone Joint Surg Am.* 1995;77(8):1234–1240.
50. Duhem R, Tonnelle V, Vinchon M, et al. Unstable upper pediatric cervical spine injuries: report of 28 cases and review of the literature. *Childs Nerv Syst.* 2008;24(3):343–348.
51. Easter JS, Barkin R, Rosen CL, Ban K. Cervical spine injuries in children, part I: mechanism of injury, clinical presentation, and imaging. *J Emerg Med.* 2011;41(2):142–150.
52. Easter JS, Barkin R, Rosen CL, Ban K. Cervical spine injuries in children, part II: management and special considerations. *J Emerg Med.* 2011;41(3):252–256.
53. Effendi B, Roy D, Cornish B, et al. Fractures of the ring of the axis: a classification based on the analysis of 131 cases. *J Bone Joint Surg Br.* 1981;63-B(3):319–327.
54. Ehlinger M, Charles Y-P, Adam P, et al. Survivor of a traumatic atlanto-occipital dislocation. *Orthop Traumatol Surg Res.* 2011;97(3):335–340.
55. Eleraky MA, Theodore N, Adams M, et al. Pediatric cervical spine injuries: report of 102 cases and review of the literature. *J Neurosurg.* 2000;92(1 Suppl):12–17.
56. Elgamal EA, Elwatidy S, Zakaria AM, Abdel-Raouf AA. Spinal cord injury without radiological abnormality (SCIWORA). A diagnosis that is missed in unconscious children. *Neurosciences (Riyadh).* 2008;13(4):437–440.
57. Fedorchuk C, Comer RD, Stockwell TL, et al. Prevalence of cervical spondylolisthesis in the sagittal plane using radiographic imaging in a pediatric population: a cross sectional analysis of vertebral subluxation. *J Radiol Case Rep.* 2021;15(6):1–18.
58. Fehlings MG, Wilson JR, Cho N. Methylprednisolone for the treatment of acute spinal cord injury: counterpoint. *Neurosurgery.* 2014;61 Suppl 1:36–42.
59. Finch GD, Barnes MJ. Major cervical spine injuries in children and adolescents. *J Pediatr Orthop.* 1998;18(6):811–814.
60. Gallie WE. Fractures and dislocations of the cervical spine. *Am J Surg.* 1939;46:495–499.
61. Gerling MC, Davis DP, Hamilton RS, et al. Effects of cervical spine immobilization technique and laryngoscope blade selection on an unstable cervical spine in a cadaver model of intubation. *Ann Emerg Med.* 2000;36(4):293–300.
62. Ghanem I, El Hage S, Rachkidi R, et al. Pediatric cervical spine instability. *J Child Orthop.* 2008;2(2):71–84.
63. Ghatan S, Ellenbogen RG. Pediatric spine and spinal cord injury after inflicted trauma. *Neurosurg Clin N Am.* 2002;13(2):227–233.
64. Givens TG, Polley KA, Smith GF, Hardin WD Jr. Pediatric cervical spine injury: a three-year experience. *J Trauma.* 1996;41(2):310–314.
65. Godard J, Hadji M, Raul JS. Odontoid fractures in the child with neurological injury. Direct anterior osteosynthesis with a cortico-spongious screw and literature review. *Childs Nerv Syst.* 1997;13(2):105–107.
66. Goldstein RY, Sunde CD, Assaad P, et al. Location of the vertebral artery at C1 in children: how far out laterally can one safely dissect? *J Bone Joint Surg Am.* 2014;96(18):1552–1556.
67. Griffiths SC. Fracture of odontoid process in children. *J Pediatr Surg.* 1972;7(6):680–683.
68. Hadley MN. Occipital condyle fractures. *Neurosurgery.* 2002;50(3 Suppl):S114–S119.
69. Hadley MN, Zabramski JM, Browner CM, et al. Pediatric spinal trauma: review of 122 cases of spinal cord and vertebral column injuries. *J Neurosurg.* 1988;68(1):18–24.
70. Hall JE, Simmons ED, Danylchuk K, Barnes PD. Instability of the cervical spine and neurological involvement in Klippel-Feil syndrome: a case report. *J Bone Joint Surg Am.* 1990;72(3):460–462.
71. Halsey JN, Hoppe IC, Marano AA, et al. Characteristics of cervical spine injury in pediatric patients with facial fractures. *J Craniofac Surg.* 2016;27(1):109–111.
72. Hamoud K, Abbas J. A new technique for stabilization of injuries at C2-C3 in young children. *Injury.* 2014;45(11):1791–1795.
73. Hankinson TC, Avellino AM, Harter D, et al. Equivalence of fusion rates after rigid internal fixation of the occiput to C-2 with or without C-1 instrumentation. *J Neurosurg Pediatr.* 2010;5(4):380–384.
74. Haque A, Price AV, Sklar FH, et al. Screw fixation of the upper cervical spine in the pediatric population. Clinical article. *J Neurosurg Pediatr.* 2009;3(6):529–533.
75. Harms J, Melcher RP. Posterior C1-C2 fusion with polyaxial screw and rod fixation. *Spine (Phila Pa 1976).* 2001;26(22):2467–2471.
76. Henriques T, Cunningham BW, Olerud C, et al. Biomechanical comparison of five different atlantoaxial posterior fixation techniques. *Spine (Phila Pa 1976).* 2000;25(22):2877–2883.
77. Herman MJ, Brown KO, Sponseller PD, et al. Pediatric cervical spine clearance: a consensus statement and algorithm from the Pediatric Cervical Spine Clearance Working Group. *J Bone Joint Surg Am.* 2019;101(1):e1.
78. Herzenberg JE, Hensinger RN. Pediatric cervical spine injuries. *Trauma Q.* 1989;5:73–81.
79. Herzenberg JE, Hensinger RN, Dedrick DK, Phillips WA. Emergency transport and positioning of young children who have an injury of the cervical spine: the standard backboard may be hazardous. *J Bone Joint Surg Am.* 1989;71(1):15–22.
80. Hewes HA, Ravindra VM, Ryan S, et al. The fate of the cervical collar: an observational pilot study investigating follow-up care after emergency department discharge in children with mild traumatic neck injuries. *Pediatr Emerg Care.* 2023;39(4):274–278.
81. Hofbauer M, Jaindl M, Hochtl LL, et al. Spine injuries in polytraumatized pediatric patients: characteristics and experience from a Level I trauma center over two decades. *J Trauma Acute Care Surg.* 2012;73(1):156–161.
82. Hoffman JR, Mower WR, Wolfson AB, et al. Validity of a set of clinical criteria to rule out injury to the cervical spine in patients with blunt trauma. National Emergency X-Radiography Utilization Study Group. *N Engl J Med.* 2000;343(2):94–99.
83. Hoffman JR, Wolfson AB, Todd K, Mower WR. Selective cervical spine radiography in blunt trauma: methodology of the National Emergency X-Radiography Utilization Study (NEXUS). *Ann Emerg Med.* 1998;32(4):461–469.
84. Hosalkar HS, Greenbaum JN, Flynn JM, et al. Fractures of the odontoid in children with an open basilar synchondrosis. *J Bone Joint Surg Br.* 2009;91(6):789–796.
85. Hosono N, Yonenobu K, Kawagoe K, et al. Traumatic anterior atlanto-occipital dislocation: a case report with survival. *Spine (Phila Pa 1976).* 1993;18(6):786–790.
86. Jain A, Brooks JT, Rao SS, et al. Cervical fractures with associated spinal cord injury in children and adolescents: epidemiology, costs, and in-hospital mortality rates in 4418 patients. *J Child Orthop.* 2015;9(3):171–175.
87. Jarvers JS, Herren C, Jung MK, et al. Pediatric cervical spine injuries-results of the German multicenter CHILDSPINE study. *Eur Spine J.* 2023;32(4):1291–1299.
88. Jauregui JJ, Perfetti DC, Cautela FS, et al. Spine injuries in child abuse. *J Pediatr Orthop.* 2019;39(2):85–89.
89. Joaquim AF, Ghizoni E, Tedeschi H, et al. Upper cervical injuries – a rational approach to guide surgical management. *J Spinal Cord Med.* 2014;37(2):139–151.
90. Jones E, Hensinger R. Cervical spine injuries in children. *Contemp Orthop.* 1982;5:17–23.
91. Judd DB, Liem LK, Petermann G. Pediatric atlas fracture: a case of fracture through a synchondrosis and review of the literature. *Neurosurgery.* 2000;46(4):991–994.
92. Junewick JJ. Pediatric craniocervical junction injuries. *AJR Am J Roentgenol.* 2011;196(5):1003–1010.
93. Kaiser R, Mehdian H. Permanent twelfth nerve palsy secondary to C0 and C1 fracture in patient with craniocervical pneumatisation. *Eur Spine J.* 2021;30(2):381–384.
94. Kapapa T, Tschan CA, König K, et al. Fracture of the occipital condyle caused by minor trauma in a child. *J Pediatr Surg.* 2006;41(10):1774–1776.
95. Kim W, O'Malley M, Kieser DC. Noninvasive management of an odontoid process fracture in a toddler: case report. *Global Spine J.* 2015;5(1):59–62.
96. Kleinman PK, Shelton YA. Hangman's fracture in an abused infant: imaging features. *Pediatr Radiol.* 1997;27(9):776–777.
97. Kobets AJ, Nakhla J, Biswas A, et al. Isolated synchondrosis fracture of the atlas presenting as rotatory fixation of the neck: case report and review of literature. *Surg Neurol Int.* 2016;7(Suppl 42):S1092–S1095.
98. Kokoska ER, Keller MS, Rallo MC, Weber TR. Characteristics of pediatric cervical spine injuries. *J Pediatr Surg.* 2001;36(1):100–105.
99. Koop SE, Winter RB, Lonstein JE. The surgical treatment of instability of the upper part of the cervical spine in children and adolescents. *J Bone Joint Surg Am.* 1984;66(3):403–411.
100. Kopparapu S, Mao G, Judy BF, Theodore N. Fifty years later: the "rule of Spence" is finally ready for retirement. *J Neurosurg Spine.* 2022:1–8.
101. Korinth MC, Kapser A, Weinzierl MR. Jefferson fracture in a child: illustrative case report. *Pediatr Neurosurg.* 2007;43(6):526–530.
102. Levine AM, Edwards CC. The management of traumatic spondylolisthesis of the axis. *J Bone Joint Surg Am.* 1985;67(2):217–226.
103. Lewis SJ, Canavese F, Keetbaas S. Intralaminar screw insertion of thoracic spine in children with severe spinal deformities: two case reports. *Spine (Phila Pa 1976).* 2009;34(7):E251–E254.
104. Liu JK, Decker D, Tenner MS, et al. Traumatic arteriovenous fistula of the posterior inferior cerebellar artery treated with endovascular coil embolization: case report. *Surg Neurol.* 2004;61(3):255–260.
105. Magerl F, Seeman P. Stable posterior fusion of the atlas and axis by transarticular screw fixation. In: Kehr P, Weidner A, eds. *Cervical Spine.* Springer-Verlag; 1985:322–327.
106. Maheshwaran S, Sgouros S, Jeyapalan K, et al. Imaging of childhood torticollis due to atlanto-axial rotatory fixation. *Childs Nerv Syst.* 1995;11(12):667–671.
107. Majernick TG, Bieniek R, Houston JB, Hughes HG. Cervical spine movement during orotracheal intubation. *Ann Emerg Med.* 1986;15(4):417–420.
108. Manson N, An H. Halo placement in the pediatric and adult patient. In: Vaccaro A, Barton E, eds. *Operative Techniques in Spine Surgery.* Saunders; 2008:13.
109. Mayfield JK, Erkkila JC, Winter RB. Spine deformities subsequent to acquired childhood spinal cord injury. *Orthop Trans.* 1981;63:1401–1411.
110. Mazur MD, Sivakumar W, Riva-Cambrin J, et al. Avoiding early complications and reoperation during occipitocervical fusion in pediatric patients. *J Neurosurg Pediatr.* 2014;14(5):465–475.
111. McClain R, Clark C, El-Khoury GY. C6–C7 dislocation in a neurologically intact neonate: a case report. *Spine (Phila Pa 1976).* 1989;14:125–127.
112. McGrory BJ, Klassen RA, Chao EY, et al. Acute fractures and dislocations of the cervical spine in children and adolescents. *J Bone Joint Surg Am.* 1993;75(7):988–995.
113. McKay SD, Al-Omari A, Tomlinson LA, Dormans JP. Review of cervical spine anomalies in genetic syndromes. *Spine (Phila Pa 1976).* 2012;37(5):E269–E277.
114. Mesfin A, Nesterenko SO, Al-Hourani KG, et al. Management of hangman's fractures and a subaxial compression fracture in two children with osteogenesis imperfecta. *J Surg Orthop Adv.* 2013;22(4):326–329.
115. Millington PJ, Ellingsen JM, Hauswirth BE, Fabian PJ. Thermoplastic Minerva body jacket: a practical alternative to current methods of cervical spine stabilization: a clinical report. *Phys Ther.* 1987;67(2):223–225.
116. Miz GS, Engler GL. Atlanto-axial subluxation in Larsen's syndrome: a case report. *Spine (Phila Pa 1976).* 1987;12(4):411–412.
117. Mondschein J, Karasick D. Spondylolysis of the axis vertebra: a rare anomaly simulating hangman's fracture. *AJR Am J Roentgenol.* 1999;172(2):556–557.
118. Muller EJ, Wick M, Muhr G. Traumatic spondylolisthesis of the axis: treatment rationale based on the stability of the different fracture types. *Eur Spine J.* 2000;9(2):123–128.

119. Nigrovic LE, Rogers AJ, Adelgais KM, et al. Utility of plain radiographs in detecting traumatic injuries of the cervical spine in children. *Pediatr Emerg Care.* 2012;28(5): 426–432.

120. Nitecki S, Moir CR. Predictive factors of the outcome of traumatic cervical spine fracture in children. *J Pediatr Surg.* 1994;29(11):1409–1411.

121. Nordstrom RE, Lahdenranta TV, Kaitila II, Laasonen EM. Familial spondylolisthesis of the axis vertebra. *J Bone Joint Surg Br.* 1986;68(5):704–706.

122. Norman MC, Wedderburn LC. Fetal spinal cord injury with cephalic delivery. *Obstet Gynecol.* 1973;42(3):355–358.

123. Nuckley DJ, Van Nausdle JA, Eck MP, Ching RP. Neural space and biomechanical integrity of the developing cervical spine in compression. *Spine (Phila Pa 1976).* 2007;32(6):E181–E187.

124. Odent T, Langlais J, Glorion C, et al. Fractures of the odontoid process: a report of 15 cases in children younger than 6 years. *J Pediatr Orthop.* 1999;19(1):51–54.

125. Oluigbo CO, Gan YC, Sgouros S, et al. Pattern, management and outcome of cervical spine injuries associated with head injuries in paediatric patients. *Childs Nerv Syst.* 2008;24(1):87–92.

126. Orenstein JB, Klein BL, Gotschall CS, et al. Age and outcome in pediatric cervical spine injury: 11-year experience. *Pediatr Emerg Care.* 1994;10(3):132–137.

127. Orenstein JB, Klein BL, Ochsenschlager DW. Delayed diagnosis of pediatric cervical spine injury. *Pediatrics.* 1992;89(6 Pt 2):1185–1188.

128. Pang D, Nemzek WR, Zovickian J. Atlanto-occipital dislocation. Part 2: The clinical use of (occipital) condyle-C1 interval, comparison with other diagnostic methods, and the manifestation, management, and outcome of atlanto-occipital dislocation in children. *Neurosurgery.* 2007;61(5):995–1015.

129. Pang D, Nemzek WR, Zovickian J. Atlanto-occipital dislocation. Part 1: normal occipital condyle-C1 interval in 89 children. *Neurosurgery.* 2007;61(3):514–521.

130. Pang D, Pollack IF. Spinal cord injury without radiographic abnormality in children: the SCIWORA syndrome. *J Trauma.* 1989;29(5):654–664.

131. Pang D, Wilberger JE Jr. Spinal cord injuries without radiographic abnormalities in children. *J Neurosurg.* 1982;57(1):114–129.

132. Panjabi MM, White AA III, Johnson RM. Cervical spine mechanics as a function of transection of components. *J Biomech.* 1975;8(5):327–336.

133. Panjabi MM, White AA III, Keller D, et al. Stability of the cervical spine under tension. *J Biomech.* 1978;11(4):189–197.

134. Patel AA, Dailey A, Brodke DS, et al. Subaxial cervical spine trauma classification: the Subaxial Injury Classification system and case examples. *Neurosurg Focus.* 2008;25(5):E8.

135. Pehler S, Jones R, Staggers JR, et al. Clinical outcomes of cervical facet fractures treated nonoperatively with hard collar or halo immobilization. *Global Spine J.* 2019;9(1):48–54.

136. Phuntsok R, Ellis BJ, Herron MR, et al. The occipitoatlantal capsular ligaments are the primary stabilizers of the occipitoatlantal joint in the craniocervical junction: a finite element analysis. *J Neurosurg Spine.* 2019;30(5):593–601.

137. Pisapia JM, Nayak NR, Salinas RD, et al. Navigated odontoid screw placement using the O-arm: technical note and case series. *J Neurosurg Spine.* 2017;26(1):10–18.

138. Pizzutillo PD, Rocha E, D'Astous J, et al. Bilateral fractures of the pedicle of the second cervical vertebra in the young child. *J Bone Joint Surg Am.* 1986;68:892–896.

139. Platzer P, Jaindl M, Thalhammer G, et al. Cervical spine injuries in pediatric patients. *J Trauma.* 2007;62(2):389–396.

140. Ranjith RK, Mullett JH, Burke TE. Hangman's fracture caused by suspected child abuse: a case report. *J Pediatr Orthop B.* 2002;11(4):329–332.

141. Ravindra VM, Riva-Cambrin J, Horn K, et al. A 2D threshold of the condylar-C1 interval to maximize identification of patients at high risk for atlantooccipital dislocation using computed tomography. *J Neurosurg Pediatr.* 2017;19(4):458–463.

142. Reilly CW, Leung F, Synchondrosis fracture in a pediatric patient. *Can J Surg.* 2005;48(2):158–159.

143. Robinson LC, Anderson RCE, Brockmeyer DL, et al. Comparison of fusion rates based on graft material following occipitocervical and atlantoaxial arthrodesis in adults and children. *Oper Neurosurg (Hagerstown).* 2018;15(5):530–537.

144. Ruff SJ, Taylor TK. Hangman's fracture in an infant. *J Bone Joint Surg Br.* 1986; 68(5):702–703.

145. Ruge JR, Sinson GP, McLone DG, Cerullo LJ. Pediatric spinal injury: the very young. *J Neurosurg.* 1988;68:25–30.

146. Samartzis D, Shen FH, Herman J, Mardjetko SM. Atlantoaxial rotatory fixation in the setting of associated congenital malformations: a modified classification system. *Spine (Phila Pa 1976).* 2010;35(4):E119–E127.

147. Savage JG, Fulkerson DH, Sen AN, et al. Fixation with C-2 laminar screws in occipitocervical or C1-2 constructs in children 5 years of age or younger: a series of 18 patients. *J Neurosurg Pediatr.* 2014;14(1):87–93.

148. Schatzker J, Rorabeck CH, Waddell JP. Fractures of the dens (odontoid process): an analysis of thirty-seven cases. *J Bone Joint Surg Br.* 1971;53(3):392–405.

149. Schwartz GR, Wright SW, Fein JA, et al. Pediatric cervical spine injury sustained in falls from low heights. *Ann Emerg Med.* 1997;30(3):249–252.

150. Seimon LP. Fracture of the odontoid process in young children. *J Bone Joint Surg Am.* 1977;59(7):943–948.

151. Sharma BS, Mahajan RK, Bhatia S, Khosla VK. Collet-Sicard syndrome after closed head injury. *Clin Neurol Neurosurg.* 1994;96(2):197–198.

152. Sherk HH, Schut L, Lane JM. Fractures and dislocations of the cervical spine in children. *Orthop Clin North Am.* 1976;7(3):593–604.

153. Shirasaki N, Okada K, Oka S, et al. Os odontoideum with posterior atlantoaxial instability. *Spine (Phila Pa 1976).* 1991;16(7):706–715.

154. Singh B, Cree A. Laminar screw fixation of the axis in the pediatric population: a series of eight patients. *Spine J.* 2015;15(2):e17–e25.

155. Smith JT, Skinner SR, Shonnard NH. Persistent synchondrosis of the second cervical vertebra simulating a hangman's fracture in a child. Report of a case. *J Bone Joint Surg Am.* 1993;75(8):1228–1230.

156. Spitzer R, Rabinowitch JY, Wybar KC. A Study of the abnormalities of the skull, teeth and lenses in Mongolism. *Can Med Assoc J.* 1961;84(11):567–572.

157. Sponseller P, Herzenberg J. Cervical spine injuries in children. In: Clark C, CDvorak J, Ducker T, eds. *The Cervical Spine.* Lippincott-Raven; 1998:357–371.

158. Swischuk LE. Spine and spinal cord trauma in the battered child syndrome. *Radiology.* 1969;92(4):733–738.

159. Taylor AR. The mechanism of injury to the spinal cord in the neck without damage to vertebral column. *J Bone Joint Surg Br.* 1951;33-B(4):543–547.

160. Tolhurst SR, Vanderhave KL, Caird MS, et al. Cervical arterial injury after blunt trauma in children: characterization and advanced imaging. *J Pediatr Orthop.* 2013;33(1): 37–42.

161. Tolo VT, Weiland AJ. Unsuspected atlas fracture and instability associated with oropharyngeal injury: case report. *J Trauma.* 1979;19(4):278–280.

162. Tuli S, Tator CH, Fehlings MG, Mackay M. Occipital condyle fractures. *Neurosurgery.* 1997;41(2):368–376.

163. Uchiyama T, Kawaji Y, Moriya K, et al. Two cases of odontoid fracture in preschool children. *J Spinal Disord Tech.* 2006;19(3):204–207.

164. Utheim NC, Josefsen R, Nakstad PH, et al. Occipital condyle fracture and lower cranial nerve palsy after blunt head trauma: a literature review and case report. *J Trauma Manag Outcomes.* 2015;9:2.

165. van Rijn RR, Kool DR, de Witt Hamer PC, Majoie CB. An abused five-month-old girl: hangman's fracture or congenital arch defect? *J Emerg Med.* 2005;29(1): 61–65.

166. Wang X, Fan CY, Liu ZH. The single transoral approach for os odontoideum with irreducible atlantoaxial dislocation. *Eur Spine J.* 2010;19(Suppl 2):S91–S95.

167. Wertheim SB, Bohlman HH. Occipitocervical fusion. Indications, technique, and long-term results in thirteen patients. *J Bone Joint Surg Am.* 1987;69(6):833–836.

168. Wetzel FT, La Rocca H. Grisel's syndrome. *Clin Orthop Relat Res.* 1989;(240):141–152.

169. White AA III, Johnson RM, Panjabi MM, Southwick WO. Biomechanical analysis of clinical stability in the cervical spine. *Clin Orthop Relat Res.* 1975;(109):85–96.

170. White P, Al-Mahfoudh R. The role of conservative management in incidental os odontoideum. *World Neurosurg.* 2016;88:695.e615–695.e617.

171. Yadav A, Singh A, Verma R, et al. Pediatric cervical spine injuries. *Asian J Neurosurg.* 2022;17(4):557–562.

172. Yeom JS, Buchowski JM, Kim HJ, et al. Postoperative occipital neuralgia with and without C2 nerve root transection during atlantoaxial screw fixation: a post-hoc comparative outcome study of prospectively collected data. *Spine J.* 2013;13(7):786–795.

22

Thoracolumbar Spine Fractures

Kenneth D. Illingworth and David L. Skaggs

INTRODUCTION TO THORACOLUMBAR SPINE FRACTURES

Fractures of the thoracic and lumbar spine in pediatric patients are relatively uncommon,[74] as the inherent elasticity and mobility of the pediatric spine protects children. The mechanisms of injury vary with age.[75] These fractures can be broadly grouped as compression, burst, flexion-distraction, and fracture-dislocations. The treatment principles are based on the mechanism of injury and the stability of the fracture. Clarifying the stability of any given fracture can be challenging, and controversy remains in determining which fractures require surgical stabilization. Understanding the mechanism of injury, the neurologic status,[5,28] and associated injuries[6,33,37,49,53,71] is important to guide treatment of pediatric thoracolumbar fractures. In trauma patients, thoracolumbar fractures are more common in older children and adolescents, and there is a low mortality rate and infrequent need for operative stabilization.[77] The goals of treatment are to provide skeletal stability to protect against spinal cord injury (SCI) and to maximize the potential for recovery of spinal cord function if an SCI is present. These two goals may be analyzed separately when both instability and SCI exist.

ASSESSMENT OF THORACOLUMBAR SPINE FRACTURES

MECHANISMS OF INJURY OF THORACOLUMBAR SPINE FRACTURES

One of the most important aspects of treating pediatric thoracolumbar spinal fractures is understanding the mechanism of injury.

A, B   C

Figure 22-1. **A:** Sagittal thoracic MRI of a 3-year-old girl who sustained a three-column unstable chance fracture with complete thoracic cord injury after nonaccidental trauma. Sitting PA (**B**) and lateral (**C**) radiographs demonstrating stabilization with posterior spinal fusion and instrumentation. Fixed pedicle screws were used to decrease implant prominence. (Used with permission of Kenneth D. Illingworth, MD.)

Spine trauma, just like appendicular trauma, should raise concern for child abuse or nonaccidental injury in infants and young children, especially those who are not yet ambulatory (Fig. 22-1).[22,45]

Motor vehicle accidents may be the most common cause of spinal column injury in all age groups.[6] The type of seat belt restraint has clear implications in the mechanism of force transferred to the spine, with the lap belt a common cause of both intra-abdominal and spinal injuries.[33,49,71,76,86] Addition of a shoulder strap or child seat with a five-point frontal harness limits flexion of the torso with frontal impact accidents and protects the spine (and other vital organs) from injury.

Falls from a height generally result in axial loading of the spine, which may result in a compression fracture (anterior column injury) or burst fracture (anterior and middle column injury), depending on the degree of flexion of the trunk at the time of impact. These fracture patterns are possible with any mechanism associated with axial compression and can also occur with motor vehicle accidents and sporting injuries. Compression of the vertebra when the trunk is flexed creates the greatest forces in the anterior aspect of the vertebra, leading more commonly to anterior column wedging (compression fracture). This is in contrast to axial compression when the trunk is in an extended position, which loads the vertebral body more symmetrically. Fractures in this case often collapse with radial expansion and fracture both the anterior and middle columns of the vertebral body (burst fracture). Displacement of the vertebral body fragments into the spinal canal may cause injury or compression of the neurologic elements.[34]

If the magnitude of injury sustained seems out of proportion to the force applied, the possibility of an insufficiency fracture due to weak bone should be considered. Osteoporotic insufficiency fractures, common in the elderly, are rare in children; however, several disease states may predispose children to these injury patterns. Chronic corticosteroid use associated with the management of many pediatric rheumatologic and oncologic diseases often leads to osteoporosis and increased risk of compression fractures. In addition, primary lesions of the bone, such as Langerhans histiocytosis or bone cysts, can weaken thoracic vertebrae.[29] Other tumors and infections warrant consideration when nontraumatic compression fractures are identified.[56,73]

INJURIES ASSOCIATED WITH THORACOLUMBAR SPINE FRACTURES

Both mechanism of injury and fracture pattern should raise suspicion for associated injuries, for the spine and other organ systems. First, any vertebral fracture should be considered a significant risk factor for a vertebral fracture at another level, with a 32% rate of concomitant injuries in one series.[52] The traumatic force required to create one fracture is often enough to result in one or more additional fractures at other locations.

The lap belt mechanism of injury is well known to create flexion-distraction injuries of the spine but also is associated with intra-abdominal injury (Fig. 22-2).[71] Compressed between the seat belt and the spinal column, the aorta, intestinal viscera, and abdominal wall musculature are at risk for laceration. Abdominal injuries are present in almost 50% of pediatric patients with Chance fractures (three-column injuries of the spine) (Fig. 22-3).[60] Ecchymosis on the anterior abdomen is suggestive of intra-abdominal injury that warrants further evaluation with advanced imaging (Fig. 22-4).[6,86] A high index of suspicion is required, as missed injuries may be life threatening.[49]

Figure 22-2. A lap belt used for a child can create a point of rotation about which the spine is flexed with an abrupt stop. This is a common mechanism for creating both intra-abdominal and flexion-distraction spinal injuries.

Associated injury to the spinal cord has obvious significance and may be present with many fracture patterns. Disruption of the stability of the spinal column or bony intrusion into the spinal canal may result in compromise of neurologic function (Fig. 22-5). All patients with a known spinal column fracture or dislocation warrant a careful neurologic examination.

Overall, most pediatric patients with thoracolumbar fractures are neurologically intact (85%), and less commonly present with SCIs (incomplete in 5% and complete in 10%).[24] Similarly, patients with a traumatic neurologic deficit require a careful evaluation of the spinal column integrity. There are, however, a subset of patients who present with SCI without radiographic abnormality (SCIWORA).[62,63] The concept of SCIWORA was popularized by Pang and Wilberger[63] who described their experience at the University of Pittsburgh. They noted a series of patients presenting with traumatic SCIs that were not evident on plain radiographs or tomograms. Several mechanisms to explain these findings have been proposed, including spinal cord stretch and vascular disruption/infarction. Magnetic resonance imaging (MRI) studies have confirmed patterns of both cord edema and hemorrhage in such cases.[31,89,100] Important additional facts about SCIWORA include the finding that some patients had a delayed onset of

Figure 22-3. A 12-year-old boy involved in a high-speed MVC had a positive lap belt sign. **A:** Sagittal MRI demonstrating unstable three-column injury with complete disruption of the posterior ligamentous complex. **B, C:** Trauma CT scans demonstrated pneumoperitoneum and hemoperitoneum requiring emergent exploratory laparotomy with ruptured small bowel. (Used with permission of David L. Skaggs, MD.)

Figure 22-4. A seatbelt sign may be subtle, as in this example of horizontal ecchymosis in the setting of a soft tissue L2–L3 chance fracture. **A:** In this case, the injury was missed on the initial radiology reading, and the clinical picture helped establish the diagnosis. **B:** Circle demonstrates horizontal ecchymosis across the abdomen consistent with a seatbelt sign. (Used with permission of Kenneth D. Illingworth, MD.)

Figure 22-5. A: Lumbar CT scans showing three-column bony injury with fragment retropulsion, severe canal stenosis, and (**B**) neurologic compromise. (Used with permission of Lindsay M. Andras, MD.)

their neurologic deficits. Transient neurologic symptoms were persistent in many who later developed a lasting deficit. In addition, the younger patients (<8 years old) had more severe neurologic involvement.[8] Although these injuries may not be visible on plain radiographs, nearly all will have some evidence of soft tissue injury of the spine on more sensitive MRI studies.[31] The term SCIWORA is less relevant in the era of routine MRI, which should be obtained in all patients with neurologic compromise or SCI.[42]

SIGNS AND SYMPTOMS OF THORACOLUMBAR SPINE FRACTURES

Careful evaluation of a patient with a potential traumatic spinal injury is critical. The ABCs of resuscitation (airway, breathing, circulation) are performed while maintaining cervical and thoracolumbar spine precautions. After stabilizing the cardiorespiratory systems, symptoms of pain, numbness, and tingling should be sought if the patient is old enough and alert enough to cooperate. Pain in the back is often not appreciated when other distracting injuries exist, and the patient is immobilized on a backboard. Maintaining initial axial stabilization of the spine is vital to preventing possible further neurologic injury. One must take into account the relative size of a child's head during transport and backboard immobilization, often with the occiput needing to be recessed into the backboard. Examination of the back must not be forgotten and is performed by logrolling the patient. Visual inspection, along with palpation, should seek areas of swelling, deformity, ecchymosis, and/or tenderness that may provide a clue to the presence of an injury. Clinically, the ability to diagnose a thoracolumbar spine fracture in pediatric trauma patients has been demonstrated to have an 87% sensitivity and 75% specificity.[39,77] Hence, routine screening radiographs of any patients suspected of having a thoracolumbar spine injury should be performed, to minimize the likelihood of missing an injury.

Neurologic examination provides information on the integrity of the spinal cord. The age of the patient may limit the thoroughness of this assessment, but some indication of sensory and motor function should be sought. In cases of spinal cord deficit, a detailed examination of the strength of appropriate muscle groups, sensory levels, and rectal tone will need to be serially compared over time and the quality of the documentation cannot be overemphasized. The prognosis for recovery is significantly better if the SCI is incomplete (SCI with some preserved motor or sensory function below the injury level).[15,94] The status of the neurologic function over time may lead to important treatment decisions regarding the necessity and timing of surgical intervention. A progressive neurologic deficit in the setting of an unstable spine or neurologic compression usually warrants urgent surgical attention, with the understanding there may be many factors to consider; whereas an improving status may suggest a less urgent approach. In cases of spinal shock, one must weigh the pros and cons to early surgical intervention and observation for return of bulbocavernosus reflex, to determine the true extent of the neurologic injury.

IMAGING AND OTHER DIAGNOSTIC STUDIES FOR THORACOLUMBAR SPINE FRACTURES

Following a careful clinical examination of all patients with a suspected spinal injury, plain radiographs are obtained first. An alert, cooperative patient without pain or tenderness in the back can be cleared without radiographs. However, any patient with a significant mechanism of injury (e.g., motor vehicle accident, fall from >10 feet, cervical or head injury) requires thoracolumbar spine radiographs if they have spinal tenderness, are obtunded, or have a distracting injury. Initial films should include supine anteroposterior (AP) and lateral views of the thoracic and lumbar spine. In addition, because of the strong association between cervical spine fractures and thoracolumbar spine fractures after blunt or vehicular trauma, routine imaging of the entire spine is indicated when a cervical fracture is identified.[97]

Plain radiographs often show relatively subtle findings. On AP radiographs, soft tissue shadows may be widened by paravertebral hematoma. The bony anatomy is viewed to evaluate for loss of height of the vertebral body as compared with adjacent levels. Similar comparisons can be made regarding interpedicular distance and interspinous spacing (Fig. 22-6).[10] Lateral radiographs give important information about the sagittal plane: anterior vertebral wedging, vertebral collapse, posterior element distraction, or fracture. Scrutiny of the plain radiographs is always prudent; however, the computed tomography (CT) scan will nearly always be used to clarify any suspected fractures. Antevil et al.[3] reported the sensitivity of plain radiographs to be 70% (14 of 20 patients) for spine trauma, whereas the sensitivity was 100% for CT scanning (34 of 34 patients).

CT is now a standard component of the evaluation of many trauma patients. Multidetector scanners allow rapid assessment with axial, coronal, and sagittal images for patients with plain radiographic abnormalities. The axial images are best for evaluating the integrity of the spinal canal in cases of a burst fracture, whereas the sagittal views will demonstrate vertebral body compression as well as posterior element distraction or fracture. In addition, major dislocations easily seen on plain radiographs will be better understood with regard to the space left in the spinal canal for the neurologic elements. The amount of spinal canal compromise has been correlated with the probability of neurologic deficit.[57] In addition, three-dimensional reconstructions are invaluable for assessing fracture patterns and determining surgical planning.

MRI is the modality of choice for evaluating the discs, spinal cord, and posterior ligamentous structures.[42,48,88] Although more challenging to obtain in a multiply injured patient, this study is mandatory in patients with a neurologic deficit to assess the potential cause of cord/neurologic dysfunction. The MRI can distinguish areas of spinal cord hemorrhage and edema. Assessment of the posterior ligamentous complex (PLC) is critical in differentiating stable and unstable burst fractures, as well as flexion-distraction injuries. Although subject to overinterpretation, MRI has been shown to modify the diagnosis made by plain radiographs and CT and correlates very well with intraoperative findings of the structural integrity of the posterior soft tissues (Fig. 22-7).[48,68]

Figure 22-6. A: AP chest radiograph of 5-year-old involved in a motor vehicle collision and admitted for pneumothorax. A three-column unstable thoracic spine injury was identified based on the asymmetrical pedicle distances on the AP chest radiograph. CT (**B**) and MRI (**C**) confirmed diagnosis which required surgical stabilization. (Used with permission of Kenneth D. Illingworth, MD.)

Figure 22-7. A, B: A 4-year-old who was involved in an MVC and sustained a three-column chance fracture with evidence of posterior ligamentous disruption on the MRI. One can also appreciate the extensive subcutaneous hematoma superficial to the fascia. **C:** Intraoperative photos confirm complete ligamentous disruption down to the level of bone. (Used with permission of Kenneth D. Illingworth, MD.)

CLASSIFICATION OF THORACOLUMBAR SPINE FRACTURES

Several classification systems have been developed for thoracolumbar spine fractures. The most commonly used in practice today include: Denis three-column,[21] Thoracolumbar Injury Classification and Severity Score (TLICS),[91] and the AO Spine Thoracolumbar Spine Injury Classification System.[91]

Denis (Three-Column System): CLASSIFICATION

- Compression fracture
- Burst fracture
- Flexion-distraction injuries
- Fracture-dislocation

Designed primarily with the adult spine fracture patterns in mind, the Denis classification translates well for the categorization of most pediatric thoracolumbar injuries.[47] Based on theories of stability related to the three-column biomechanical concept of the spine (anterior, middle, posterior columns), the Denis classification in its simplest form includes compression, burst, flexion-distraction, and fracture-dislocations (Fig. 22-8).

Compression fractures are the most common thoracolumbar spine fracture pattern.[13,36] The vertebral body loses height anteriorly compared with the posterior wall. The anterior aspect of the vertebral body is involved, but the middle column (posterior wall) of the vertebral body is by definition intact. Axial load with flexion is the common mechanism. Depending on the degree and direction of flexion, the wedging may vary between the coronal and sagittal planes (Fig. 22-9). The percentage of lost height defines the severity of compression fractures, which rarely have an associated neurologic deficit. However, the fractures are often associated with similar or occasionally more severe fractures at adjacent or distant levels. Contiguous compression fractures, each of a modest degree, together may result in a substantial

A   Compression

B   Burst

C   Flexion-distraction

D   Fracture-dislocation

Figure 22-8. Denis classification of thoracolumbar fractures. **A:** Compression fracture: This injury results in mild wedging of the vertebra primarily involving the anterior aspects of the vertebral body. The posterior vertebral height and posterior cortex remain intact. **B:** Burst fracture: A burst fracture involves both the anterior and middle columns with loss of height throughout the vertebral body. There may be substantial retropulsion of the posterior aspect of the vertebra into the spinal canal. In addition, posterior vertebral fractures and/or ligamentous injury may occur. **C:** Flexion-distraction injuries: This fracture, which occurs commonly with a seat belt injury mechanism, results in posterior distraction with disruption of the ligaments and bony elements of the posterior column, commonly extending into the anterior columns with or without compression of the most anterior aspects of the vertebra. **D:** Fracture-dislocation: These complex injuries involve marked translation of one vertebra on another with frequently associated SCI as a result of translations through the spinal canal.

Figure 22-9. Compression fractures. **A:** PA view demonstrates wedging in the coronal plane. **B:** The more commonly recognized compression fractures involve wedging primarily in the sagittal plane with loss of anterior vertebral height. *Arrow* indicates vertebral body wedging in the coronal and sagittal plane respectively.

kyphotic deformity. Because the cause of these injuries, such as a fall, are fairly common, it is at times necessary to determine if a wedged vertebra seen radiographically represents an acute compression fracture, sequelae of Scheuermann kyphosis, anatomic variant with delayed ossification, or a remote injury. Clinical examination can localize pain to the site of the fracture in acute injuries; however, MRI or bone scan can be used to confirm acute fracture based on signal changes and increased isotope uptake.

Burst fractures likely represent a more severe form of compression fracture that extends posteriorly in the vertebral body to include the posterior wall (middle column). Axial compression is the primary mechanism, although posterior element fractures may also occur. Laminar fractures have been known to entrap the dural contents. The fractures are most common in the lower thoracic and upper lumbar levels. Associated neurologic injury is related to the severity of injury (greater injury index scores correlate with greater frequency of SCI[51] and the degree of spinal canal encroachment by retropulsed bony fragments).[34] SCI at the thoracolumbar junction may result in conus medullaris syndrome or cauda equina syndrome. Careful examination of the perineal area is required to identify these spinal lesions.

Flexion-distraction injuries are especially relevant to the pediatric population because this classic lap belt injury is more frequent in backseat passengers, particularly when a shoulder strap or five-point harness is lacking. Motor vehicle accidents are the primary cause of this injury. The lap belt, which restrains the pelvis in adults, may ride up onto the abdomen in children. Chance, and later Smith, described how with a frontal impact, the weight of the torso is driven forward, flexing over the restraining belt (see Fig. 22-2). With the axis of rotation in front of the spine, distractive forces are placed on the posterior elements, with variable degrees of

anterior vertebral compression. This three-column injury is generally unstable. The disruption of the posterior elements may occur entirely through the bone (Chance; Fig. 22-10) or ligamentous (Smith; see Fig. 22-7) elements, although many times the fracture propagates through both soft and bony tissues.

The injury is most obvious on lateral radiographs; however, if no fracture exists, widening of the interspinous distance may be the only finding on a lateral radiograph (Fig. 22-11). Studies have demonstrated the difficulty in appropriately diagnosing this injury in children, many presenting with a delayed diagnosis or misdiagnosis after an average of 3 months in one series.[1] Standard axial CT imaging may also miss this injury because the plane of injury lies within the plane of imaging. One classic finding in ligamentous flexion-distraction injuries is the "empty facet" sign (Fig. 22-12). When the inferior articular process of the superior vertebra is no longer in contact with the superior articular process of the inferior vertebra, the facet appears empty in the axial CT image. Sagittal reconstructions are most revealing, and MRI will provide information about the integrity of the PLC. A large subcutaneous hematoma is almost always present in a fresh chance fracture, which can be noted by physical exam as well as MRI. Identification of a purely intravertebral flexion-distraction fracture is important, as this may alter the treatment compared with those with severe ligamentous injury.

Fracture-dislocations of the spinal column result from complex severe loading mechanisms. These are by definition unstable injuries with a component of shearing and/or rotational displacement. A special note in the pediatric population is the documentation of this injury pattern in young patients exposed to nonaccidental trauma.[22,45,50]

Figure 22-10. A: Bony chance fractures have distraction of the posterior elements through bone, not the interspinous ligament. This is much less common than a soft tissue chance fracture. **B:** MRI confirms intact posterior ligamentous complex. (Used with permission of David L. Skaggs, MD.)

Thoracolumbar Injury:
CLASSIFICATION AND SEVERITY SCORE

Category	Points
1. Injury morphology	
a. Compression/burst	1/+1
b. Translational/rotation	3
c. Distraction	4
2. Neurologic status	
a. Intact	0
b. Nerve root injury	2
c. Cord/conus medullaris	
Incomplete	3
Complete	2
Cauda equina	3
3. Posterior ligamentous complex	
a. Intact	0
b. Injury suspected	2
c. Injured	3

The TLICS system, introduced by the Spine Trauma Study Group in 2005, was developed to streamline injury assessment and guide surgical decision making.[91] The system assigns numerical values to each injury based on the categories of morphology of injury, integrity of the PLC, and neurologic involvement. The numerical scores are then summated to produce an injury severity score, which is, in turn, used to guide treatment. A score of greater than or equal to 5 suggests operative treatment of the patient due to significant instability, whereas a score of less than or equal to 3 suggests nonoperative treatment. A patient with a score of 4 may be treated either operatively or nonoperatively. In the setting of multiple fractures, the injury with the greatest TLICS score is used to guide treatment. This system has demonstrated good-to-excellent inter- and intraobserver reliability and has been shown to be easily taught, learned, and incorporated into clinical practice.[38,67,82] Multiple studies have recently shown the TLICS classification to be valid and useful for determining treatment decisions in the pediatric population.[19,20,80–82]

AO Spine Thoracolumbar Spine Injury Classification System

Type	Description
A	Compression injury
A0	Minor injuries (transverse process/spinous process)
A1	Wedge compression
A2	Split or pincer type
A3	Incomplete burst
A4	Complete burst
B	Posterior or anterior tension band injury
B1	Monosegmental bony posterior tension band
B2	Posterior tension band disruption
B3	Hyperextension injury
C	Failure of all elements (dislocation)—translation or displacement

Figure 22-11. A, B: Lateral radiographs demonstrating increased interspinous distance on a missed three-column chance fracture. **C, D:** Intraoperative photos confirm increased interspinous distance and facet diastasis. (Used with permission of Kenneth D. Illingworth, MD.)

A   B

Figure 22-12. A: "Empty facet sign" characteristic of a soft tissue chance fracture. Normally, there would be both superior and inferior facets present in a transverse CT cut, but with separation of the posterior elements, only the superior facet is visualized. **B:** In contrast, this is an image of normal facet joints at an uninjured level in the same patient. (Used with permission of David L. Skaggs, MD.)

The AO Spine Thoracolumbar Spine Injury Classification System was published in 2013.[90] Recent studies have shown high statistical correlation between the AO Spine thoracolumbar (TL) spine injury classification and TLICS, and to intraoperative evaluation of the PLC, suggesting that the AO Spine TL spine injury classification is applicable to the pediatric population.[59] Despite both classifications being valid in the pediatric population, there are varying reports on which is superior in this population.[19,81]

OUTCOME MEASURES FOR THORACOLUMBAR SPINE FRACTURES

SCIs in children have remarkable potential for recovery.[65,94] In a study from a major metropolitan trauma center, complete SCIs were associated with fatal injuries in one-third and no neurologic recovery in another third, whereas most of the remaining one-third of patients made improvements that ultimately allowed functional ambulation. Less surprisingly, nearly all patients with incomplete SCI made some improvement over time.[94] This ability to recover, even from complete injuries, has led some to suggest more aggressive attempts at spinal cord decompression in the early course of treatment,[27,64] whereas others have suggested a period of "spinal cord rest" with observation.[51] In adults, early fracture fixation has been shown to be beneficial, minimizing respiratory morbidity and decreasing days in the intensive care setting and length of hospital stay.[7] There are certainly no controlled series of pediatric patients treated by both approaches to support either hypothesis. The data do, however, suggest a more optimistic view regarding the potential recovery of traumatic SCIs in children compared with adults.

Spinal column structural integrity should be assessed in all cases of injury because the functional capacity of the vertebral elements to protect the spinal cord will continue to be required. This evaluation may be performed with functional radiographs, such as flexion-extension views (Fig. 22-13) or with an MRI evaluation of associated soft tissue injuries that may coexist with more obvious bony fractures. Several methods of estimating spinal column stability have been proposed including the three-column concept of Denis.[21] Based on division into anterior, middle, and posterior columns, injuries to all three of these sagittal columns have been considered an unstable injury pattern. Plain radiography with a CT scan is appropriate for evaluating the bony elements. An MRI is often required to elucidate the nature of the disc and ligamentous injuries.[32,42] MRI is extremely sensitive and, given the brightness of edema fluid on T2 images, may be overinterpreted. A study correlating MRI and intraoperative surgical findings, however, demonstrated high levels of both sensitivity and specificity in the MRI evaluation of posterior soft tissue injuries (see Fig. 22-7).[48]

The ultimate treatment goal is a stable spinal column. This often requires surgical treatment in unstable fracture patterns. In contrast, most stable injuries can be managed nonoperatively. There are particular exceptions to these generalizations, of course. At times, the associated SCI or a substantial associated deformity may alter the treatment approach to an otherwise mechanically stable injury. The presence of a complete

A   B

Figure 22-13. A: A 15-year-old boy with unrecognized unstable chance fracture after an MVC. He had continued pain 6 months after injury. **B:** Flexion lumbar radiograph confirmed unstable spine injury with widening of the interspinous space and widening of the posterior disc space indicating complete ligamentous injury without healing. (Used with permission of David L. Skaggs, MD.)

SCI in a child younger than 10 years is also a determinant that may affect treatment strategies. The incidence of paralytic spinal deformity (scoliosis) is nearly 100% in such cases, and a long-instrumented fusion will likely be required at some point (Fig. 22-14).[2,66] Depending on the fracture pattern and age of the patient, it may be prudent to include much of the thoracic and lumbar spine in the initial instrumented fusion.[54] This strategy, if employed, should be reserved for older children as to not restrict thoracic/pulmonary growth. However, in the patient without neurologic deficit, there is evidence that the use of posterior stabilization of thoracolumbar fractures using nonfusion methods followed by removal of metal implants within an appropriate period appears to be a safe, viable option.[18,44]

PATHOANATOMY AND APPLIED ANATOMY RELATED TO THORACOLUMBAR SPINE FRACTURES

The thoracic and lumbar spine links the upper and lower extremities through the torso. The 12 thoracic and 5 lumbar vertebrae are joined by intravertebral discs and strong ligaments, both anteriorly and posteriorly. The bony architecture of the vertebrae varies, with the smaller thoracic vertebrae having

a more shingled overlapping configuration compared with the lumbar segments. The thoracic facets are oriented in the coronal plane, whereas those in the lumbar spine lie in the sagittal plane (Fig. 22-15).

Mobility is less in the thoracic spine owing to the adjacent and linked rib cage as well as the smaller intervertebral discs. The ribs make an important connection between the vertebra with each rib head articulating across a given disc space. This contrasts with the relatively mobile lumbar segments, which have thick intravertebral discs that permit substantial flexion-extension, lateral bending, and axial rotation motion. The junction between the stiffer thoracic spine and more flexible lumbar spine is a region of frequent injury because of this transition between two regions which have differing inherent flexibility.

Ligamentous components include the anterior and posterior longitudinal ligaments, facet capsules, ligamentum flavum, as well as the interspinous and supraspinous ligaments. Together, these structures limit the motion between vertebrae to protect the neurologic elements. The anterior longitudinal ligament is rarely disrupted in flexion injuries but may be rendered incompetent by extension loading or a severe fracture-dislocation. On the contrary, flexion is the primary mechanism of injury to the PLC—supraspinous and interspinous, facet capsule, and ligamentum flavum. The healing capacity of the completely torn

Figure 22-14. A 5-year-old boy who sustained a complete spinal cord injury at the cervicothoracic junction requiring posterior spinal fusion and instrumentation. Within 2 years of injury, he developed progressive paralytic scoliosis with pelvic obliquity and sitting imbalance. (Used with permission of Kenneth D. Illingworth, MD.)

PLC is limited, though substantially better in the pediatric population compared with adults, whereas bony fractures are more likely to heal with resultant stability.

The neural anatomy varies over the length of the thoracolumbar spine as well. The space within the canal is largest in the lumbar spine. The spinal cord traverses the entirety of the thoracic spine and typically terminates as the conus medullaris

at the L1 or L2 level. The cauda equina occupies the dural tube below this level, and injuries below L1 are generally less likely to lead to permanent neurologic deficit. This is not to say that compression at this level cannot be serious, and careful examination of the perineum for sensation as well as rectal tone is important in the evaluation of potential conus medullaris and cauda equina syndromes.

Treatment Options for Thoracolumbar Spine Fractures

COMPRESSION FRACTURES

NONOPERATIVE TREATMENT OF COMPRESSION FRACTURES

Indications/Contraindications

These are nearly always stable injuries, although examination of the posterior soft tissues is required to rule out any more severe flexion-distraction injury. If there is concern for a higher energy injury, a CT scan is required to rule out a burst fracture or posterior element involvement. Indications for nonoperative treatment are intact posterior soft tissues and kyphosis less than 30 degrees. The presence of disrupted posterior soft tissues implies the injury is more significant, such as a chance fracture, which is more likely to require operative intervention given the three-column injury.

Techniques

An isolated compression fracture without neurologic involvement is the most common thoracolumbar fracture pattern and can nearly always be treated with immobilization with rest and activity modification. Molding a thoracolumbosacral orthosis (TLSO) into slight hyperextension at the fracture site will limit flexion, provides pain relief, and reduces further loading of the

Figure 22-15. Difference in lumbar facet orientation (**A**) and thoracic facet orientation (**B**) with ideal starting point for pedicle screw insertion. (Used with permission of Kenneth D. Illingworth, MD.)

Figure 22-16. A 7-year-old boy treated with a Jewett hyperextension brace for a compression fracture. (Used with permission of Kenneth D. Illingworth, MD.)

fracture. Alternatively, a less-constricting hyperextension brace is often well tolerated (Fig. 22-16).

Outcomes

Most fractures heal in 4 to 6 weeks without significant additional collapse, and radiographs should be obtained to follow the sagittal alignment. Long-term studies have suggested modest remodeling capacity of compression fractures occurring in childhood.[40,69,85] Asymmetric growth at the end plates seems to allow some correction in the wedged alignment over time in the skeletally immature patient. Long-term results of compression fractures have been generally favorable, although fractures of the end plates can be associated with later disc degeneration.[43]

Osteoporosis of a variety of etiologies may affect children and adolescents to a degree that predisposes them to insufficiency fractures that are most often compression fractures (Fig. 22-17). Multilevel fractures are more frequent in this setting, and problematic kyphosis may develop. Differentiating new from old fractures can be difficult if serial radiographs are not available. An MRI can be used to define fracture acuity based on the amount of edema present within each vertebral body. A TLSO or hyperextension brace for a period of time longer than typically used for simple compression fracture healing may be necessary to prevent progressive kyphosis, though treating the primary cause of the osteopenia is critical to maintaining normal alignment in such cases. Evaluation by a Pediatric Endocrinologist and possibly assessment of bone density by dual-energy x-ray absorptiometry (DEXA) are advised.

Figure 22-17. Lumbar spine radiograph demonstrating multiple compression fractures in a child on chronic corticosteroids.

OPERATIVE TREATMENT OF COMPRESSION FRACTURES

Indications/Contraindications

If the kyphosis associated with compression fractures markedly alters local sagittal alignment, surgical treatment may be considered. For example, 30 to 40 degrees of additional relative kyphosis than would be anticipated for that region of the spine. This is most frequent in multiple adjacent compression fractures that together create unacceptable focal region of relative kyphosis. Single-level compression fractures rarely require surgical stabilization.

Surgical Procedures

The preferred surgical treatment of such fractures is generally a posterior compression instrumentation construct that spans one or two levels above and below the affected vertebrae. Anterior surgical treatment is rarely required. The intact posterior vertebral wall provides a fulcrum to achieve kyphosis correction. The preferred method of posterior fixation is pedicle screw constructs, with hooks used as needed to supplement fixation. A posterior fusion over the instrumented segments ensures a lasting stable correction. Although some have advocated for balloon vertebroplasty with calcium phosphate cement in adult patients as a potentially viable option to treat compression fractures this remains an area of controversy.[46,92,93] There are some case reports of vertebroplasty in pediatric patients with nontraumatic compression fractures.

However, there is a lack of comparative studies demonstrating benefit and given the potential risks of cement extravasation the authors currently do not advise this.[12,35,58]

BURST FRACTURES

NONOPERATIVE TREATMENT OF BURST FRACTURES

The treatment and classification of this fracture pattern are controversial areas of spinal trauma management. There are burst fractures that can be easily managed nonoperatively in a brace and others that collapse further, resulting in increased deformity unless surgically stabilized. Defining the characteristics of stable and unstable burst fractures has been attempted by several authors.[21,55,91] An additional compounding variable in the treatment algorithm is SCI and neurologic compromise, which is more frequent with burst fractures than with compression fractures.

Indications/Contraindications

In cases which are neurologically intact, defining stable and unstable burst fractures has been attempted based on the degree of comminution, loss of vertebral height, kyphotic wedging, and integrity of the PLC. A load-sharing classification system assigns points based on comminution, fragment apposition, and kyphosis.[55] Although the Denis classification suggests that all burst fractures are unstable because of the involvement of at least two columns, it is clear that in many cases the addition of a third-column injury is required to result in a truly unstable condition. Vertebral body translation of greater than 3.5 mm has been demonstrated to predict PLC injury.[70] Some advocate differentiating stable and unstable burst fractures solely on the integrity of the PLC.[84,99] Yet, some may argue addition of PLC, by definition, makes a three-column injury and not an isolated burst fracture.

Techniques

When a burst fracture is deemed stable, it must be done so on a presumptive basis. In these patients, a Jewett hyperextension brace (see Fig. 22-16) or TLSO can be used with the goal of allowing an upright position and ambulation.[84] Frequent radiographic and neurologic follow-up is necessary to identify early failures. Depending on the age of the patient and severity of the fracture, immobilization is suggested for a duration of 2 to 4 months.

Outcomes

Studies of immature patients treated for burst fractures are uncommon,[47] yet much of the adult literature provides valuable information about the outcomes to expect following nonoperative treatment. Most of these fractures in adults heal with little change in kyphosis and function and minimal, if any, residual pain.[30] It is reasonable to expect adolescent patients to heal at least as well and probably even faster. Wood et al.[99] compared operative and nonoperative treatment in a prospective randomized study of patients with burst fractures who were neurologically intact with a normal PLC. The radiologic and functional outcomes were not substantially different, and these authors concluded that nonoperative treatment should be considered when the PLC and neurologic function are intact.[99] Functional outcome does not appear to correlate with the degree of spinal kyphosis, although long-term studies of scoliosis treatment do suggest that an alteration of sagittal alignment may be detrimental (flat back syndrome) in the long term.

OPERATIVE TREATMENT OF BURST FRACTURES

Indications/Contraindications

Fractures with three-column involvement, neurologic deficit, concomitant musculoskeletal injury, and thoracic/abdominal injury precluding the use of a brace are all considered indications for surgical management of burst fractures. Contraindications mainly center on medical conditions (coexisting or new) which make surgical intervention too risky.

Surgical Procedure

When surgical treatment is selected, either an anterior or posterior approach can be used, although this also remains controversial. Anterior stabilization generally involves discectomy/corpectomy and strut grafting that spans the fractured vertebra. Stabilization with a plate or dual-rod system is appropriate. Posterior options include pedicle screw fixation one or two levels above and below the fractured vertebra. Advances in the application of posterior instrumentation for thoracolumbar fractures have demonstrated encouraging, early outcomes with fracture stabilization without fusion and in minimally invasive surgical techniques.[83,95,96] The presence of a dural tear due to the retropulsed posterior wall fragment may also play a role when deciding how to approach the fracture.

The decision to proceed anteriorly or posteriorly for the surgical treatment of a burst fracture is largely dictated by surgeon preference and, to some degree, the features of the fracture, and degree of neurologic involvement. There has been an increased trend to posterior approaches to these injuries. Posterior approaches are familiar to all surgeons and can easily be extended over many levels. In addition, a transforaminal lumbar interbody fusion (TLIF) can be performed if anterior interbody support is deemed beneficial to construct stability. Decompression of the spinal cord can be achieved by indirect or direct methods. Restoration of the sagittal alignment frequently leads to spontaneous repositioning of the posteriorly displaced vertebral body fracture fragments. If additional reduction of posterior wall fragments is required, direct fracture reduction can be accomplished with a posterolateral or transpedicular decompression.[27] This also allows additional anterior column bone grafting that may add structural integrity and speed fracture healing.

The anterior approach allows direct canal decompression through a corpectomy of the fractured vertebra. Structural strut

Figure 22-18. Burst fracture. **A:** This teenage patient presented with loss of vertebral body height associated with a motorcycle accident after jumping more than 20 feet. His neurologic examination was intact. **B:** CT scan confirmed a burst fracture component with very little retropulsion into the spinal canal. This appeared to be a stable injury and was initially managed with an orthosis. **C, D:** There was poor compliance with the orthosis and further collapse. **E, F:** Given the lack of compliance and progressive kyphosis, the patient underwent anterior reconstruction with an iliac crest strut graft and plating.

grafting restores the integrity of the anterior column. With this graft, a load-sharing anterior plate or rod system completes the reconstruction. This approach deals most directly with the pathology, which in burst fractures lies within the anterior and middle vertebral columns (Fig. 22-18). Proponents of the anterior approach cite better biomechanical stabilization of the unstable spine, better correction of segmental kyphosis, and less loss of correction postoperatively.[78,79,98] In adults, a combined anterior and posterior approach may provide the best stability and sagittal alignment, especially in very unstable injuries. However, the increased morbidity with this approach is likely why it is not routinely used in the pediatric/adolescent patient population.[72]

FLEXION-DISTRACTION INJURIES (CHANCE FRACTURES)

NONOPERATIVE TREATMENT OF FLEXION-DISTRACTION INJURIES (CHANCE FRACTURES)

Indications/Contraindications

The treatment of flexion-distraction injuries is dictated by the injury pattern and the associated abdominal injuries. In general, these fractures are reduced by an extension moment that can be maintained with either a brace or internal fixation. A hyperextension brace is ideal for younger patients (<~10 years) with a primary bony injury pattern and no significant intra-abdominal injuries. However, unacceptable kyphosis may be an indication for surgical treatment. As described above, the posterior disruption may pass through ligaments or joint capsules in a purely soft tissue plane of injury or traverse an entirely bony path. The distinction is important, because bony fractures have the potential for primary bony union, whereas the severe ligamentous injuries are less likely to heal with lasting stability without surgical intervention.

Technique

Hyperextension cast for very young or noncompliant patients. TLSO or Jewett hyperextension brace as detailed for compression and burst fractures.

Outcomes

Nonoperative treatment has been demonstrated to be effective in selected patients. The most frequent problem with the nonoperative approach has been progression of the kyphotic deformity.[1,4]

OPERATIVE TREATMENT OF FLEXION-DISTRACTION INJURIES (CHANCE FRACTURES)

Indications/Contraindications

The greater the degree of ligamentous/facet disruption, the more likely the need for stabilization with an arthrodesis of the injured motion segment. In addition, the greater the degree of kyphosis, the more likely posttraumatic progressive kyphosis will become a problem.[4] Healing of posterior ligamentous disruption is not reliable, though in very young children it may be possible (Fig. 22-19).

Surgical Procedure

Options for internal fixation include posterior wiring in very young children (supplemented with a brace) and segmental fixation in a primarily compressive mode (see Fig. 22-1). Most young children can be successfully managed with modern posterior pedicle screw instrumentation. In some cases, one may utilize smaller fixed pedicle screws or cervical instrumentation depending on patient size (Fig. 22-20). This approach can decrease the injury kyphosis and maintain sagittal alignment during the healing process. Operative treatment has been demonstrated to have a good clinical outcome in 84% of pediatric patients, compared with 45% in the nonoperative group.[4]

FRACTURE-DISLOCATIONS

OPERATIVE TREATMENT OF FRACTURE-DISLOCATIONS

Indications/Contraindications

These highly unstable injuries always require surgical stabilization. When the spinal cord function remains intact, instrumented fusion gives the greatest chance for maintaining cord function. On the other hand, if a complete SCI has occurred, internal fixation will aid in the rehabilitation process, allowing early transfers and upright sitting.

Surgical Procedure

The typical procedure is a posterior instrumented fusion that extends at least two levels above and below the level of injury to

A, B   **C**

Figure 22-19. Sagittal CT scan (**A**) and MRI (**B**) of an unstable chance fracture with posterior ligamentous disruption at L1–L2. **C:** To try and preserve as much lumbar motion as possible, a single-level posterior spinal fusion and instrumentation was chosen. (Used with permission of David L. Skaggs, MD.)

Figure 22-20. **A, B:** An 8-month-old child presented with an incomplete SCI and a thoracolumbar fracture-dislocation due to non-accidental trauma. The malalignment of the vertebral segments is noted on both the AP and lateral projections. **C:** The MRI demonstrated a three-column injury with a fracture through the vertebral endplate. **D, E:** The patient had an open reduction and instrumentation with pedicle screw fixation using a 3.5-mm cervical system.

ensure restoration of alignment and stability. In cases of SCI below the age of 10 years, a longer fusion may be considered to reduce the incidence and severity of subsequent paralytic scoliosis. However, one must consider remaining thoracic growth and pulmonary development when considering longer thoracic fusions in young children. Early thoracic fusions inhibit pulmonary development and increase morbidity.[41] Those injured after the adolescent growth spurt are at low risk for late deformity if the fracture is well aligned at the time of initial fixation (Fig. 22-21).

SPECIAL FRACTURES

END PLATE FRACTURES

End plate fractures are growth plate fractures similar to a Salter I or Salter II fractures of long bones. It is thus a unique pediatric injury that does not occur in adults. There is almost always a history of a specific inciting event, such as kicking a soccer ball or landing in a gymnastics competition with sudden pain and sometimes hearing a "pop." The mechanism is thought to be related to flexion with a portion of the posterior corner of the vertebral body (ring apophysis) fracturing and displacing posteriorly into the spinal canal. Symptoms may mimic disc herniation, although the offending structure is bone and cartilage rather than disc material.[23,25]

This injury is rarely noted on x-rays, and often misread on MRI as a bulging disc. The diagnosis is confirmed with CT, usually best visualized on a sagittal cut (Fig. 22-22).

On physical examination, the patients are in very significant pain, to the point where physicians at times wonder if they are exaggerating the pain. The pain is consistent with nerve roots being tented across the bony edge of a fresh fracture. While historically some have suggested observation will eventually lead to resolution, this is rarely if ever clinically tolerated. Injections are unlikely to help, and physical therapy is contraindicated as it is

Figure 22-21. A: Skeletally mature 15-year-old girl was involved in an MVC and sustained complete spinal cord injury at the thoracolumbar junction with multilevel burst fractures and U-type sacral fracture. **B:** Patient underwent T10-pelvic posterior spinal fusion and instrumentation without signs of proximal deformity progression 2 years after surgery. (Used with permission of Kenneth D. Illingworth, MD.)

likely to exacerbate pain with little hope of benefit. Treatment is removal of the fracture fragment through a laminectomy. A TLSO for 4 to 6 weeks postoperatively allows for rapid healing of this growth plate injury.

FACET FRACTURES

Lumbar and sacral facet fractures have been described as a likely underrecognized source of low back pain, particularly in young athletes.[61,87] The mechanism of injury is repetitive hyperextension with or without twisting that places stress on the facets. Given the mechanism of injury, the fractures are often seen in conjunction with spondylolysis (Fig. 22-23). At times, the patient may remember a specific event in which the back pain started, but more frequently it is a chronic pain. An acute history tends to be more localized and those with chronic pain may have a wider distribution of pain. On physical examination, the pain is reproduced with hyperextension while standing, often indistinguishable from spondylolysis-type pain. This should produce localized back pain at the area of the facet fracture. If there is no back pain reproduced with hyperextension,

one should be very hesitant to attribute the back pain to a facet fracture, or other posterior element etiology. The fractures are almost never seen on plane radiographs, and they are quite often missed by MRI. CT is the gold standard, and three-dimensional reconstructions are helpful both for identification of the fracture and surgical approach (Fig. 22-24). Injections may be beneficial for confirming the pain generator, however false negatives are possible. Injections and/or conservative care is unlikely to relieve the patient symptoms long term. In theory, an intra-articular fracture could cause joint damage, which would suggest removing this fragment sooner rather than later would help prevent arthritis and long-term pain.

Treatment of an isolated lumbar or sacral facet fracture is surgical removal.[61] This can usually be accomplished through about a 16-mm incision using either a minimally invasive retractor set or standard retractors. Having the three-dimensional CT scan in the operating room is very helpful. At times, a bit of normal facet must be removed to see the fragment. At the time of surgery, the fragment is clearly mobile and usually surrounded by some inflammatory tissue. Removal tends to cause immediate pain relief and the patient may return to normal activities as tolerated.

Figure 22-22. A: A 14-year-old girl felt a pop while kicking a soccer ball and had severe back pain. Months of steroid injections did nothing to relieve her pain. She was unable to walk or go to school. *Red arrow* demonstrates L4 inferior end plate fracture on MRI. **B:** CT scan confirmed diagnosis of an end plate fracture. Surgical removal of the intracanal fragment adjacent to nerve roots relieved pain and the patient was able to return to soccer within a few weeks. *White arrow* more clearly demonstrates same injury on CT. (Used with permission of David L. Skaggs, MD.)

Figure 22-23. Sagittal CT scans of the lumbosacral junction demonstrating bilateral L5 spondylolysis with bilateral facet fractures of the inferior articular process of L4. (Used with permission of David L. Skaggs, MD.)

Figure 22-24. Sagittal CT scan (**A**) and 3D CT scan (**B**) of a left L4/L5 facet fracture of the inferior articular process of L4. **C:** The facet fracture is not seen on lumbar MRI. (Used with permission of David L. Skaggs, MD.)

Authors' Preferred Treatment for Thoracolumbar Spine Fractures (Algorithm 22-1)

Algorithm 22-1. Author's preferred treatment for thoracolumbar spine fractures.

Compression Fractures

Nearly all compression fractures are managed nonoperatively in an off-the-shelf TLSO brace. Occasionally, a fracture is too proximal for such an orthosis and an extension to the chin/occiput is required. For fractures proximal to T6, a cervicothoracic orthosis (CTO) brace is used. These fractures typically heal within 4 to 6 weeks, when the immobilization can be discontinued. Activities should be limited for an additional 4 to 6 weeks. Compression fractures with more than 50% loss of anterior vertebral height are considered for surgical correction with posterior instrumentation, especially in the setting of significant acute kyphosis. Compression fractures associated with neurologic injury, although rare, are managed surgically to allow for early rehabilitation and optimize neurologic recovery.

Burst Fractures

Our preferred approach to neurologically intact patients with burst fractures is nonoperative treatment. If the neurologic status is normal and the posterior soft tissues are intact, a TLSO is used for 8 to 12 weeks. As with compression fractures, anterior column height loss with significant acute kyphosis is an indication for consideration of surgical intervention. An anterior decompression/corpectomy could be performed for canal compromise, especially with greater than 50% of posterior canal retropulsion with neurologic deficits. In the lumbar spine, posterior instrumentation with the restoration of normal sagittal profile and some distraction can reduce the fracture and open up the canal assuming the posterior ligament is intact, which it should be for a pure burst fracture. In addition, in the lumbar spine, from a posterior approach one can access the canal through a laminotomy or laminectomy for direct tamping of the retropulsed fragment.

Flexion-Distraction Injuries

Our treatment of chance fractures is based on two findings: associated abdominal injuries and the presence of a ligamentous component to the fracture. If either exists, surgical treatment is the preferred approach. A well-molded brace in extension is appropriate for fractures that transverse an entirely bony plane without intra-abdominal pathology or injury to the PLC. A thigh extension may be incorporated into the cast for greater control of lumbar lordosis. Surgical treatment is by a posterior approach with segmental pedicle screw instrumentation. Number of levels depends on the injury and location. For lumbar level Chance fractures we will try to preserve as many motion segments as possible.

Fracture-Dislocations

Surgical stabilization is the treatment of choice for all fracture-dislocations with or without neurologic injury. The timing of such intervention depends on the associated injuries and the ability of the patient to tolerate surgical intervention; however, stabilization as early as possible is preferred, with consideration to associated injuries and operating room team optimization. SCI nearly always complicates the management of these injuries, and a deteriorating neurologic examination makes surgical treatment of the spine an emergency that should be treated as quickly as possible.

POTENTIAL PITFALLS AND PREVENTIVE MEASURES FOR THORACOLUMBAR SPINE FRACTURE

Thoracolumbar Spine Fracture: PITFALLS AND PREVENTIONS

Pitfall	Prevention
Delay in diagnosis or missed associated injuries	• Through physical examination. • Serial physical examination with clear documentation. • Early advanced imaging (CT and/or MRI). • Image the entire spine to identify additional levels of spinal injury.
Deteriorating neurologic status	• Understand the mechanics of the injury to develop a treatment plan. • Serial neurologic exams to monitor spinal cord function. • Early surgical intervention to minimize neurologic deterioration and prolonged neurologic injury.
Deformity progression	• Follow nonoperative patients closely to ensure compliance and maintained alignment. • Do not assume interspinous ligaments will heal and prevent kyphosis. • Anticipate development of spinal deformity in SCI in patients <10 years and treat accordingly.

SUMMARY, CONTROVERSIES, AND FUTURE DIRECTIONS RELATED TO THORACOLUMBAR SPINE FRACTURES

Several areas of controversy remain with regard to the management of pediatric thoracolumbar fractures and associated SCI. These include both nonoperative and operative methods of treatment. Investigations into the benefits of steroids, cooling

Steroid Treatment

Methylprednisolone sodium succinate (MPSS) has been studied as a pharmacologic adjunct that may be given to patients with acute SCI to improve neurologic recovery. It became the standard of care in adults, despite a lack of evidence supporting clinical benefit.[9] Recent studies in adolescent and pediatric patients have demonstrated increased complication rates associated with steroids, which is consistent with older studies.[11,14,26] A systematic review and consensus-based expert panel recommended that there was no evidence to support the use of neuroprotective approaches for the treatment of acute SCI in children.[65] A recent Delphi study amongst pediatric spine experts recommended for the use of steroids only for injury after intradural surgery and not for acute traumatic spinal cord injuries, or spinal cord injuries from extradural procedures.[17]

therapy, or other neuroprotective techniques in mitigating the effects of the secondary phase of SCI that follows the acute trauma have been mixed. The timing and necessity of spinal decompression for an SCI also remains debated. Traditional teaching suggests no benefit to decompression when a complete SCI exists. This may be true, but if early decompression of an incomplete SCI is beneficial, and there are experimental data to suggest it is,[64] then it may be impossible to determine early on if the patient has an incomplete injury but remains in spinal shock. Spinal shock may last for 24 hours, leaving an incomplete SCI patient completely unresponsive with regard to spinal cord function. Early surgery has been documented to shorten the intensive care unit stays and length of hospitalizations, shorten time on mechanical ventilation support, and lower overall complication rates in patients with SCI and thoracolumbar spine injuries.[16]

In pediatric patients with SCI, it is difficult to argue against spinal cord decompression if the MRI documents persistent compression in the setting of an SCI. Pediatric patients have a substantial potential for recovery,[65] and reducing pressure on the neural elements may be important in maximizing functional recovery. There is little controversy if spinal cord function is deteriorating in a patient with a known compressive lesion. This is an emergency that warrants decompression by either an anterior and/or posterior approach. Realignment of the spinal column and removal of fragments from the canal are required. The exact surgical approach depends on the location of offending structures and the nature of the spinal instability.

ACKNOWLEDGMENTS

The authors thank Peter O. Newton and Vidyadhar V. Upasani, who wrote the chapter in the 9th edition on which this revision is based.

Annotated References

Reference	Annotation
Bellabarba C, Fisher C, Chapman JR, et al. Does early fracture fixation of thoracolumbar spine fractures decrease morbidity and mortality? *Spine (Phila Pa 1976).* 2010;35(9):S138–S145.	Systematic review of articles published from 1990 to 2008 that concluded that patients with unstable thoracic fractures should undergo early (<72 hours) stabilization of their injury to reduce morbidity, and possibly mortality.
Caruso MC, Daugherty MC, Moody SM, et al. Lesson learned from administration of high-dose methylprednisolone sodium succinate for acute pediatric spinal cord injuries. *J Neurosurg Pediatr.* 2017;20(6):567–574.	Single-center review of 354 patients concluding that pediatric patients who received high-dose methylprednisolone sodium succinate for acute spinal cord injury were significantly more likely to experience complications.
Denis F. The three column spine and its significance in the classification of acute thoracolumbar spinal injuries. *Spine (Phila Pa 1976).* 1983;8(8):817–831.	Classic article that reviewed 412 thoracolumbar injuries to classify them into four different categories: compression fractures, burst fracture, seat-belt–type injuries, and fracture dislocations.
Lee HM, Kim HS, Kim DJ, et al. Reliability of magnetic resonance imaging in detecting posterior ligament complex injury in thoracolumbar spinal fractures. *Spine (Phila Pa 1976).* 2000;25(16):2079–2084.	Prospective study of 34 patients with thoracolumbar spinal fractures that demonstrated that fat-suppressed T2-weighted sagittal sequence is a highly sensitive, specific, and accurate method of evaluating posterior ligamentous complex injury.
Mahan ST, Mooney DP, Karlin LI, Hresko MT. Multiple level injuries in pediatric spinal trauma. *J Trauma.* 2009;67(3):537–542.	Single-center retrospective review of 195 patients that found that pediatric spine injuries are more common in patients over age 8 and that these patients are more likely to have multiple levels of injury (similar to the adult population).
Pang D, Wilberger JE Jr. Spinal cord injury without radiographic abnormalities in children. *J Neurosurg.* 1982;57(1):114–129.	Retrospective review of 24 children treated between 1960 and 1980 with spinal cord injury without radiographic abnormality. This article reports on the proposed mechanism of injury and the grim long-term prognosis for neurologic recovery in their cohort.
Radcliff K, Su BW, Kepler CK, et al. Correlation of posterior ligamentous complex injury and neurological injury to loss of vertebral body height, kyphosis, and canal compromise. *Spine (Phila Pa 1976).* 2012;37(13):1142–1150.	Retrospective case-control study which demonstrated that loss of vertebral body height and local kyphosis were not predictive of posterior ligamentous complex (PLC) injury. Translation greater than 3.5 mm was associated with PLC injury.
Vaccaro AR, Lehman RA Jr, Hulbert RJ, et al. A new classification of thoracolumbar injuries: the importance of injury morphology, the integrity of the posterior ligamentous complex, and neurologic status. *Spine (Phila Pa 1976).* 2005;30(20):2325–2333.	Proposed the Thoracolumbar Injury Classification and Severity Score (TLICS) to facilitate clinical decision making and improve communication between providers regarding these complex injuries.
Weinstein JN, Collalto P, Lehmann TR. Thoracolumbar "burst" fractures treated conservatively: a long-term follow-up. *Spine (Phila Pa 1976).* 1988;13(1):33–38.	Retrospective review of 42 patients followed for an average of 20 years concluding that nonoperative treatment of thoracolumbar burst fractures is a viable alternative in patients without neurologic deficit and can lead to acceptable long-term results.

REFERENCES

1. Andras LM, Skaggs KF, Badkoobehi H, et al. Chance fractures in the pediatric population are often misdiagnosed. *J Pediatr Orthop.* 2019;39(5):222–225.
2. Angelliaume A, Bouty A, Sales De Gauzy J, et al. Post-trauma scoliosis after conservative treatment of thoracolumbar spinal fracture in children and adolescents: results in 48 patients. *Eur Spine J.* 2016;25(4):1144–1152.
3. Antevil JL, Sise MJ, Sack DI, et al. Spiral computed tomography for the initial evaluation of spine trauma: a new standard of care? *J Trauma.* 2006;61(2):382–387.
4. Arkader A, Warner WC, Tolo VT, et al. Pediatric chance fractures: a multicenter perspective. *J Pediatr Orthop.* 2011;31(7):741–744.
5. Augutis M, Levi R. Pediatric spinal cord injury in Sweden: incidence, etiology and outcome. *Spinal Cord.* 2003;41(6):328–336.
6. Beaunoyer M, St-Vil D, Lallier M, Blanchard H. Abdominal injuries associated with thoracolumbar fractures after motor vehicle collision. *J Pediatr Surg.* 2001;36(5):760–762.
7. Bellabarba C, Fisher C, Chapman JR, et al. Does early fracture fixation of thoracolumbar spine fractures decrease morbidity and mortality? *Spine (Phila Pa 1976).* 2010;35(9):S138–S145.
8. Bosch PP, Vogt MT, Ward WT. Pediatric spinal cord injury without radiographic abnormality (SCIWORA): the absence of occult instability and lack of indication for bracing. *Spine (Phila Pa 1976).* 2002;27(24):2788–2800.
9. Bracken MB. Methylprednisolone in the management of acute spinal cord injuries. *Med J Aust.* 1990;153(6):368.
10. Caffaro MFS, Avanzi O. Can the interpedicular distance reliably assess the severity of thoracolumbar burst fractures? *Spine (Phila Pa 1976).* 2012;37(4):E231–E236.
11. Cage JM, Knox JB, Wimberly RL, et al. Complications associated with high-dose corticosteroid administration in children with spinal cord injury. *J Pediatr Orthop.* 2015;35(7):687–692.
12. Cardarelli-Leite L, Rassekh SR, D'Ortenzio R, Heran MKS. Vertebroplasty as a palliative treatment option for intractable pain in pediatric patients with spinal tumors. *Pediatr Blood Cancer.* 2021;68(12):e29307.
13. Carreon LY, Glassman SD, Campbell MJ. Pediatric spine fractures: a review of 137 hospital admissions. *J Spinal Disord Tech.* 2004;17(6):477–482.
14. Caruso MC, Daugherty MC, Moody SM, et al. Lessons learned from administration of high-dose methylprednisolone sodium succinate for acute pediatric spinal cord injuries. *J Neurosurg Pediatr.* 2017;20(6):567–574.
15. Catz A, Thaleisnik M, Fishel B, et al. Recovery of neurologic function after spinal cord injury in Israel. *Spine (Phila Pa 1976).* 2002;27(16):1733–1735.
16. Chipman JG, Deuser WE, Beilman GJ. Early surgery for thoracolumbar spine injuries decreases complications. *J Trauma.* 2004;56(1):52–57.
17. CreveCoeur TS, Alexiades NG, Bonfield CM, et al. Building consensus for the medical management of children with moderate and severe acute spinal cord injury: a modified Delphi study. *J Neurosurg Spine.* 2023:1–4.

18. Cui S, Busel GA, Puryear AS. Temporary percutaneous pedicle screw stabilization without fusion of adolescent thoracolumbar spine fractures. *J Pediatr Orthop.* 2016;36(7):701–708.

19. Dauleac C, Mottolese C, Beuriat PA, et al. Superiority of thoracolumbar injury classification and severity score (TLICS) over AOSpine thoracolumbar spine injury classification for the surgical management decision of traumatic spine injury in the pediatric population. *Eur Spine J.* 2021;30(10):3036–3042.

20. Dawkins RL, Miller JH, Menacho ST, et al. Thoracolumbar injury classification and severity score in children: a validity study. *Neurosurgery.* 2019;84(6):E362–E367.

21. Denis F. The three column spine and its significance in the classification of acute thoracolumbar spinal injuries. *Spine (Phila Pa 1976).* 1983;8(8):817–831.

22. Diamond P, Hansen CM, Christofersen MR. Child abuse presenting as a thoracolumbar spinal fracture dislocation: a case report. *Pediatr Emerg Care.* 1994;10(2):83–86.

23. Dietemann JL, Runge M, Badoz A, et al. Radiology of posterior lumbar apophyseal ring fractures: report of 13 cases. *Neuroradiology.* 1988;30(4):337–344.

24. Dogan S, Safavi-Abbasi S, Theodore N, et al. Thoracolumbar and sacral spinal injuries in children and adolescents: a review of 89 cases. *J Neurosurg.* 2007;106(6):426–433.

25. Epstein NE, Epstein JA. Limbus lumbar vertebral fractures in 27 adolescents and adults. *Spine (Phila Pa 1976).* 1991;16(8):962–966.

26. Galandiuk S, Raque G, Appel S, Polk HC Jr. The two-edged sword of large-dose steroids for spinal cord trauma. *Ann Surg.* 1993;218(4):419–425.

27. Gambardella G, Coman TC, Zaccone C, et al. Posterolateral approach in the treatment of unstable vertebral body fractures of the thoracic-lumbar junction with incomplete spinal cord injury in the paediatric age group. *Childs Nerv Syst.* 2003;19(1):35–41.

28. Garcia RA, Gaebler-Spira D, Sisung C, Heinemann AW. Functional improvement after pediatric spinal cord injury. *Am J Phys Med Rehabil.* 2002;81(6):458–463.

29. Garg S, Mehta S, Dormans JP. Langerhans cell histiocytosis of the spine in children. Long-term follow-up. *J Bone Joint Surg Am.* 2004;86(8):1740–1750.

30. Gnanenthiran SR, Adie S, Harris IA. Nonoperative versus operative treatment for thoracolumbar burst fractures without neurologic deficit: a meta-analysis. *Clin Orthop Relat Res.* 2012;470(2):567–577.

31. Grabb PA, Pang D. Magnetic resonance imaging in the evaluation of spinal cord injury without radiographic abnormality in children. *Neurosurgery.* 1994;35(3):406–414.

32. Green RAR, Saifuddin A. Whole spine MRI in the assessment of acute vertebral body trauma. *Skeletal Radiol.* 2004;33(3):129–135.

33. Griffet J, Bastiani-Griffet F, El-Hayek T, et al. Management of seat-belt syndrome in children: gravity of 2-point seat-belt. *Eur J Pediatr Surg.* 2002;12(1):63–66.

34. Hashimoto T, Kaneda K, Abumi K. Relationship between traumatic spinal canal stenosis and neurologic deficits in thoracolumbar burst fractures. *Spine (Phila Pa 1976).* 1988;13(11):1268–1272.

35. Hoashi JS, Thomas SM, Goodwin RC, et al. Balloon kyphoplasty for managing intractable pain in pediatric pathologic vertebral fractures. *J Pediatr Orthop.* 2017;37(4):e286–e291.

36. Holmes JF, Miller PQ, Panacek EA, et al. Epidemiology of thoracolumbar spine injury in blunt trauma. *Acad Emerg Med.* 2001;8(9):866–872.

37. Inaba K, Kirkpatrick AW, Finkelstein J, et al. Blunt abdominal aortic trauma in association with thoracolumbar spine fractures. *Injury.* 2001;32(3):201–207.

38. Joaquim AF, de Almeida Bastos DC, Jorge Torres HH, Patel AA. Thoracolumbar injury classification and injury severity score system: a literature review of its safety. *Global Spine J.* 2016;6(1):80–85.

39. Junkins EP Jr, Stotts A, Santiago R, Guenther E. The clinical presentation of pediatric thoracolumbar fractures: a prospective study. *J Trauma.* 2008;65(5):1066–1071.

40. Karlsson MK, Moller A, Hasserius R, et al. A modeling capacity of vertebral fractures exists during growth: an up-to-47-year follow-up. *Spine (Phila Pa 1976).* 2003;28(18):2087–2092.

41. Karol LA, Johnston C, Mladenov K, et al. Pulmonary function following early thoracic fusion in non-neuromuscular scoliosis. *J Bone Joint Surg Am.* 2008;90(6):1272–1281.

42. Kerslake RW, Jaspan T, Worthington BS. Magnetic resonance imaging of spinal trauma. *Br J Radiol.* 1991;64(761):386–402.

43. Kerttula LI, Serlo WS, Tervonen OA, et al. Posttraumatic findings of the spine after earlier vertebral fracture in young patients: clinical and MRI study. *Spine (Phila Pa 1976).* 2000;25(9):1104–1108.

44. Kim YM, Kim DS, Choi ES, et al. Nonfusion method in thoracolumbar and lumbar spinal fractures. *Spine (Phila Pa 1976).* 2011;36(2):170–176.

45. Kleinman PK, Marks SC. Vertebral body fractures in child abuse: radiologic-histopathologic correlates. *Invest Radiol.* 1992;27(9):715–722.

46. Korovessis P, Repantis T, Petsinis G, et al. Direct reduction of thoracolumbar burst fractures by means of balloon kyphoplasty with calcium phosphate and stabilization with pedicle-screw instrumentation and fusion. *Spine (Phila Pa 1976).* 2008;33(4):E100–E108.

47. Lalonde F, Letts M, Yang JP, Thomas K. An analysis of burst fractures of the spine in adolescents. *Am J Orthop (Belle Mead NJ).* 2001;30(2):115–120.

48. Lee HM, Kim HS, Kim DJ, et al. Reliability of magnetic resonance imaging in detecting posterior ligament complex injury in thoracolumbar spinal fractures. *Spine (Phila Pa 1976).* 2000;25(16):2079–2084.

49. Letts M, Davidson D, Fleuriau-Chateau P, Chou S. Seat belt fracture with late development of an enterocolic fistula in a child: a case report. *Spine (Phila Pa 1976).* 1999;24(11):1151–1155.

50. Levin TL, Berdon WE, Cassell I, Blitman NM. Thoracolumbar fracture with listhesis: an uncommon manifestation of child abuse. *Pediatr Radiol.* 2003;33(5):305–310.

51. Limb D, Shaw DL, Dickson RA. Neurological injury in thoracolumbar burst fractures. *J Bone Joint Surg Br.* 1995;77(5):774–777.

52. Mahan ST, Mooney DP, Karlin LI, Hresko MT. Multiple level injuries in pediatric spinal trauma. *J Trauma.* 2009;67(3):537–542.

53. Mann DC, Dodds JA. Spinal injuries in 57 patients 17 years or younger. *Orthopedics.* 1993;16(2):159–164.

54. Mayfield JK, Erkkila JC, Winter RB. Spine deformity subsequent to acquired childhood spinal cord injury. *J Bone Joint Surg Am.* 1981;63(9):1401–1411.

55. McCormack T, Karaikovic E, Gaines RW. The load sharing classification of spine fractures. *Spine (Phila Pa 1976).* 1994;19(15):1741–1744.

56. Meehan PL, Viroslav S, Schmitt EW Jr. Vertebral collapse in childhood leukemia. *J Pediatr Orthop.* 1995;15(5):592–595.

57. Meves R, Avanzi O. Correlation between neurologic deficit and spinal canal compromise in 198 patients with thoracolumbar and lumbar fractures. *Spine (Phila Pa 1976).* 2005;30(7):787–791.

58. Missiuna PC, Sarraj M, Bosakhar B, et al. Vertebroplasty for treatment of steroid-induced osteoporotic vertebral compression fractures in an adolescent with Duchenne muscular dystrophy. *HSS J.* 2021;17(2):223–226.

59. Mo AZ, Miller PE, Troy MJ, et al. The AOSpine thoracolumbar spine injury classification system: a comparative study with the thoracolumbar injury classification system and severity score in children. *OTA Int.* 2019;2(4):e036.

60. Mulpuri K, Reilly CW, Perdios A, et al. The spectrum of abdominal injuries associated with chance fractures in pediatric patients. *Eur J Pediatr Surg.* 2007;17(5):322–327.

61. Nazareth A, Andras LM, Illingworth KD, et al. Outcomes of operatively managed lumbar and sacral facet fractures in pediatric athletes: a case series. *J Pediatr Orthop.* 2022;42(1):e45–e49.

62. Pang D, Pollack IF. Spinal cord injury without radiographic abnormality in children: the SCIWORA syndrome. *J Trauma.* 1989;29(5):654–664.

63. Pang D, Wilberger JE Jr. Spinal cord injury without radiographic abnormalities in children. *J Neurosurg.* 1982;57(1):114–129.

64. Papadopoulos SM, Selden NR, Quint DJ, et al. Immediate spinal cord decompression for cervical spinal cord injury: feasibility and outcome. *J Trauma.* 2002;52(2):323–332.

65. Parent S, Mac-Thiong JM, Roy-Beaudry M, et al. Spinal cord injury in the pediatric population: a systematic review of the literature. *J Neurotrauma.* 2011;28(8):1515–1524.

66. Parisini P, Di Silvestre M, Greggi T. Treatment of spinal fractures in children and adolescents: long-term results in 44 patients. *Spine (Phila Pa 1976).* 2002;27(18):1989–1994.

67. Patel AA, Vaccaro AR. Thoracolumbar spine trauma classification. *J Am Acad Orthop Surg.* 2010;18(2):63–71.

68. Pizones J, Izquierdo E, Alvarez P, et al. Impact of magnetic resonance imaging on decision making for thoracolumbar spine fracture diagnosis and treatment. *Eur Spine J.* 2011;20(3):390–396.

69. Pouliquen JC, Kassis B, Glorion C, Langlais J. Vertebral growth after thoracic or lumbar fracture of the spine in children. *J Pediatr Orthop.* 1997;17(1):115–120.

70. Radcliff K, Su BW, Kepler CK, et al. Correlation of posterior ligamentous complex injury and neurological injury to loss of vertebral body height, kyphosis, and canal compromise. *Spine (Phila Pa 1976).* 2012;37(13):1142–1150.

71. Reid AB, Letts RM, Black GB. Pediatric chance fractures: association with intra-abdominal injuries and seatbelt use. *J Trauma.* 1990;30(4):384–391.

72. Reinhold M, Knop C, Beisse R, et al. Operative treatment of 733 patients with acute thoracolumbar spinal injuries: comprehensive results from the second, prospective, internet-based multicenter study of the Spine Study Group of the German Association of Trauma Surgery. *Eur Spine J.* 2010;19(10):1657–1676.

73. Ribeiro RC, Pui CH, Schell MJ. Vertebral compression fracture as a presenting feature of acute lymphoblastic leukemia in children. *Cancer.* 1988;61(3):589–592.

74. Roche C, Carty H. Spinal trauma in children. *Pediatr Radiol.* 2001;31(10):677–700.

75. Ruge JR, Sinson GP, McLone DG, Cerullo LJ. Pediatric spinal injury: the very young. *J Neurosurg.* 1988;68(1):25–30.

76. Rumball K, Jarvis J. Seat-belt injuries of the spine in young children. *J Bone Joint Surg Br.* 1992;74(4):571–574.

77. Santiago R, Guenther E, Carroll K, Junkins EP Jr. The clinical presentation of pediatric thoracolumbar fractures. *J Trauma.* 2006;60(1):187–192.

78. Sasso RC, Best NM, Reilly TM, McGuire RA Jr. Anterior-only stabilization of three-column thoracolumbar injuries. *J Spinal Disord Tech.* 2005;18:S7–S14.

79. Sasso RC, Renkens K, Hanson D, et al. Unstable thoracolumbar burst fractures: anterior only versus short-segment posterior fixation. *J Spinal Disord Tech.* 2006;19(4):242–248.

80. Savage JW, Moore TA, Arnold PM, et al. The reliability and validity of the thoracolumbar injury classification system in pediatric spine trauma. *Spine (Phila Pa 1976).* 2015;40(18):E1014–E1018.

81. Schömig F, Taheri N, Kalaf H, et al. Validation of the TLICS and AOSpine injury score for surgical management of paediatric traumatic spinal injuries. *Arch Orthop Trauma Surg.* 2023;143(4):2011–2017.

82. Sellin JN, Steele WJ III, Simpson L, et al. Multicenter retrospective evaluation of the validity of the thoracolumbar injury classification and severity score system in children. *J Neurosurg Pediatr.* 2016;18(2):164–170.

83. Shen WJ, Liu TJ, Shen YS. Nonoperative treatment versus posterior fixation for thoracolumbar junction burst fractures without neurologic deficit. *Spine (Phila Pa 1976).* 2001;26(9):1038–1045.

84. Shen WJ, Shen YS. Nonsurgical treatment of three-column thoracolumbar junction burst fractures without neurologic deficit. *Spine (Phila Pa 1976).* 1999;24(4):412–415.

85. Singer G, Parzer S, Castellani C, et al. The influence of brace immobilization on the remodeling potential of thoracolumbar impaction fractures in children and adolescents. *Eur Spine J.* 2016;25(2):607–613.

86. Sivit CJ, Taylor GA, Newman KD, et al. Safety-belt injuries in children with lap-belt ecchymosis: CT findings in 61 patients. *AJR Am J Roentgenol.* 1991;157(1):111–114.

87. Skaggs DL, Avramis I, Myung K, Weiss J. Sacral facet fractures in elite athletes. *Spine (Phila Pa 1976)*. 2012;37(8):E514–E517.

88. Sledge JB, Allred D, Hyman J. Use of magnetic resonance imaging in evaluating injuries to the pediatric thoracolumbar spine. *J Pediatr Orthop*. 2001;21(3): 288–293.

89. Trigylidas T, Yuh SJ, Vassilyadi M, et al. Spinal cord injuries without radiographic abnormality at two pediatric trauma centers in Ontario. *Pediatr Neurosurg*. 2010; 46(4):283–289.

90. Vaccaro AR, Oner C, Kepler CK, et al. AOSpine thoracolumbar spine injury classification system: fracture description, neurological status, and key modifiers. *Spine (Phila Pa 1976)*. 2013;38(23):2028–2037.

91. Vaccaro AR, Lehman RA Jr, Hulbert RJ, et al. A new classification of thoracolumbar injuries: the importance of injury morphology, the integrity of the posterior ligamentous complex, and neurologic status. *Spine (Phila Pa 1976)*. 2005;30(20):2325–2333.

92. Verlaan JJ, van de Kraats EB, Oner FC, et al. Bone displacement and the role of longitudinal ligaments during balloon vertebroplasty in traumatic thoracolumbar fractures. *Spine (Phila Pa 1976)*. 2005;30(16):1832–1839.

93. Verlaan JJ, van de Kraats EB, Oner FC, et al. The reduction of endplate fractures during balloon vertebroplasty: a detailed radiological analysis of the treatment of burst fractures using pedicle screws, balloon vertebroplasty, and calcium phosphate cement. *Spine (Phila Pa 1976)*. 2005;30(16):1840–1845.

94. Wang MY, Hoh DJ, Leary SP, et al. High rates of neurological improvement following severe traumatic pediatric spinal cord injury. *Spine (Phila Pa 1976)*. 2004;29(13):1493–1497.

95. Wang ST, Ma HL, Liu CL, et al. Is fusion necessary for surgically treated burst fractures of the thoracolumbar and lumbar spine? A prospective, randomized study. *Spine (Phila Pa 1976)*. 2006;31(23):2646–2652.

96. Wild MH, Glees M, Plieschnegger C, Wenda K. Five-year follow-up examination after purely minimally invasive posterior stabilization of thoracolumbar fractures: a comparison of minimally invasive percutaneously and conventionally open treated patients. *Arch Orthop Trauma Surg*. 2007;127(5):335–343.

97. Winslow JE III, Hensberry R, Bozeman WP, et al. Risk of thoracolumbar fractures doubled in victims of motor vehicle collisions with cervical spine fractures. *J Trauma*. 2006;61(3):686–687.

98. Wood KB, Bohn D, Mehbod A. Anterior versus posterior treatment of stable thoracolumbar burst fractures without neurologic deficit: a prospective, randomized study. *J Spinal Disord Tech*. 2005;18:S15–S23.

99. Wood K, Buttermann G, Mehbod A, et al. Operative compared with nonoperative treatment of a thoracolumbar burst fracture without neurological deficit. A prospective, randomized study. *J Bone Joint Surg Am*. 2003;85(5):773–781.

100. Yucesoy K, Yuksel KZ. SCIWORA in MRI era. *Clin Neurol Neurosurg*. 2008;110(5):429–433.

Pelvic and Acetabular Fractures

Julia S. Sanders and Wudbhav N. Sankar

as they exit the pelvis.[70,90] A thorough neurologic examination of the lower extremities, including motor and sensory testing, and assessment of sphincter tone and perianal sensation should be routine in all patients with displaced fractures. Magnetic resonance imaging (MRI) is sometimes helpful to assess the integrity of the lumbosacral plexus. The superior gluteal nerve, the obturator nerve, sacral roots, and incomplete lumbosacral trunk injuries in particular are sometimes difficult to diagnose and may not be recognized until days to weeks after injury. Neurophysiologic studies are indicated in the recovery phase if deficits persist.

Thromboembolic events, including venous thromboembolism (VTE) and pulmonary embolism, are uncommon in children, even in those with significant trauma. The current use of anticoagulation regimens varies greatly between institutions.[22,27] A clinical tool to predict the risk of developing VTE in pediatric trauma patients has been tested in a multisite trial and represents an initial step toward the development of the specific VTE protocols for pediatric trauma patients.[48]

SIGNS AND SYMPTOMS OF PELVIC AND ACETABULAR FRACTURES

A full systematic examination of the child with a pelvic or acetabular injury is indicated. The patient will often be first seen in the trauma bay by a multidisciplinary trauma team. Other life threatening issues may prevent a complete examination immediately, and the patient's mental status may be impaired. Secondary examinations after the patient is stabilized are critical to identify lesser injuries that may not have been as obvious initially.

Evaluation of a child with a suspected pelvic injury should begin with the assessment of the airway, breathing, and circulatory status, as with any polytraumatized patient. The Glasgow Coma Score (GCS) is one method for assessing the patient's mental status; the reliability of the clinical examination is diminished for patients with a GCS less than 13 and aids in identifying patients with a closed head injury. Aside from the primary pelvic evaluation, careful examination of the head, neck, and spine should be performed to assess for obvious spinal or head injury. A careful neurovascular examination, including evaluation of peripheral pulses in the lower extremities, should be part of the initial survey in all patients when possible. Documentation of the function of the muscles innervated by the lumbosacral plexus and the skin supplied by its sensory branches is sometimes difficult to fully assess in the acute setting but is especially important to perform for patients with possible severe pelvic trauma. A secondary survey, after stabilization of cardiovascular status and provisional treatment of obvious injuries, should include a careful repeat evaluation of the axial skeleton and extremities as well as a follow-up neurovascular evaluation.

After the primary survey, the evaluation specific to pelvic injuries begins with a complete inspection of the pelvis and perineum to evaluate for lacerations and ecchymosis. The child should be gently logrolled to facilitate a complete inspection. The Morel–Lavallee lesion (a degloving injury in which

Figure 23-2. Clinical photograph of a Morel–Lavellee lesion, the result of an underlying unstable pelvic fracture. This is an internal degloving injury in which the skin and subcutaneous fat are sheared off the underlying muscle. (Courtesy of Samir Mehta, MD.)

the skin and subcutaneous fat is sheared from the underlying muscle, creating a large space where a hematoma can form) may be identified (Fig. 23-2). A careful genitourinary evaluation must be performed because of the intimate relationship between the pelvis, bladder, and urethra. Rectal examination has historically been recommended for children with significantly displaced pelvic fractures or if there is any blood in the perineal area. A more recent study, however, revealed that a digital rectal examination has high specificity but low sensitivity for bowel injury and should not be used alone as a screening tool.[83,84]

Pelvic landmarks, including the anterosuperior iliac spine, crest of the ilium, SI joints, and symphysis pubis should be palpated.[41] Manual manipulation should be performed carefully when needed. The maneuvers are often painful and if performed too vigorously may further displace the fracture or stimulate further intrapelvic bleeding. Pushing posteriorly on the anterosuperior iliac crest produces pain at the fracture site as the pelvic ring is opened. Compressing the pelvic ring by squeezing the right and left iliac wings together also causes pain, and crepitation may be felt if a pelvic fracture is present. Pressure downward on the symphysis pubis and posteriorly on the SI joints causes pain and possibly motion if there is a disruption.

Pain with range of motion of the extremities, especially the hip joint, may indicate acetabular involvement or pelvic ring instability as well as other fractures or tendon and ligament injuries. Passive gentle flexion, abduction, and external rotation of the hip, known as the FABER test, will elicit pain in the posterior buttock and hip in cases of SI joint injury.

While classified as pelvic fractures, avulsion injuries present differently than the more serious pelvic ring disruptions and are seen in the outpatient setting more frequently than in the trauma bay. Avulsion fractures of the pelvis typically result in localized swelling and tenderness at the site of the avulsion fracture, often after a specific acute injury. Hip motion may be limited because of guarding, and pain may be mild or marked. In the case of repetitive stress injury, pain and limitation of motion are gradually progressive. In patients with ischial avulsions, pain at the ischial tuberosity can be elicited by flexing the hip and extending the knee (straight-leg raising). Patients may also have pain while sitting or moving on the involved tuberosity. Avulsion fractures of the anterior inferior iliac spine (ASIS), and iliac apophysis, in the acute setting, present with localized pain at these sites and tenderness to palpation over the affected apophysis.

IMAGING AND OTHER DIAGNOSTIC STUDIES FOR PELVIC AND ACETABULAR FRACTURES

Following initial stabilization of the child, all polytraumatized patients and those with suspected pelvic or acetabular trauma should undergo an AP radiograph of the pelvis as part of the initial trauma series. Once the primary survey is completed and the patient is stable, region-specific radiographs should be obtained of any area with signs of trauma on secondary assessment.

Additional views, including the inlet/outlet and Judet views, are useful for further evaluation of pelvic ring injuries (Fig. 23-3). The inlet view is obtained by directing the x-ray beam caudally at an angle of 60 degrees to the x-ray plate. The inlet view is best for the determination of posterior displacement of a hemipelvis or rami fractures, as well as plastic deformity due to lateral compression. The outlet view is obtained by directing the x-ray beam in a cephalad direction at an angle of 45 degrees to the x-ray plate. The outlet view best demonstrates superior displacement of the hemipelvis or vertical shifting of the anterior pelvis. Internal and external rotation views (also called Judet or oblique views) are primarily obtained when an acetabular fracture is identified (Fig. 23-4).

Figure 23-3. Schematic representing the direction of the incident x-ray beam for (**A**) inlet projection and (**B**) outlet projection of the pelvic ring. **C:** Inlet projection of the pelvic ring. **D:** Outlet projection of the pelvic ring.

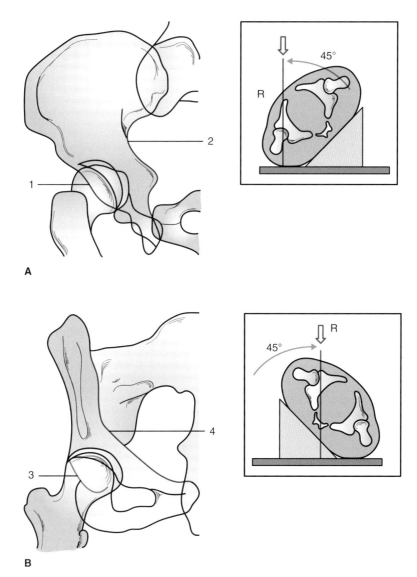

Figure 23-4. A: Iliac oblique (external) view. 1 indicates the anterior wall, 2 the posterior column. **B:** Obturator oblique (internal) view. 3 indicates the posterior wall, 4 the anterior column.

A number of studies have tried to identify clinical criteria that would effectively rule out the need for pelvic radiographs in childhood trauma patients.[32,43,45] Children being evaluated after blunt trauma, who have a GCS score of 13 or higher but are without abdominal pain, an abnormal abdominal or pelvic examination, femur deformity, hematuria, or hemodynamic instability, constitute a low-risk population for pelvic fracture, with less than 0.5% risk rate.[28] This population may not require routine pelvic imaging. The value of these criteria for avoiding radiation to the pelvis is a noble effort but its efficacy has not yet been established and most polytraumatized children do not meet these criteria.

Computed tomography (CT) is the best modality to evaluate the bony pelvis, especially the details of potential injury of the SI joints, sacrum, and acetabulum. Most authors agree that CT is indicated if there is doubt about the diagnosis on the plain radiographs or if operative intervention is planned.

Plain radiographs alone, however, allow classification of most pelvic fracture patterns routinely seen in children equally as well as CT.[5] For those with potential operative fractures, however, CT better defines the type of fracture and the degree and direction of displacement. CT imaging also can detect retained intra-articular bony fragments which may prevent concentric reduction of the hip joint for patients with concomitant hip dislocations or fracture patterns with intra-articular extension (Fig. 23-5).[10,25,58,87] This information is crucial for determining the best treatment option and selection of the operative approach.[54] Three-dimensional CT reconstructions can give an excellent view of the overall bony fracture pattern but often underestimate the magnitude of cartilaginous fragments, especially of posterior wall fractures in children. Many trauma centers routinely obtain CT scans of the abdomen and pelvis to assess patients for possible visceral injuries.

Figure 23-5. A: Postreduction anteroposterior pelvis radiograph of a 12-year-old with the left hip appearing nonconcentric. **B:** CT scan showing a bony fragment from the posterior wall impeding reduction.

MRI currently has a minimal role in evaluation of the acute trauma patient, although this practice may evolve with quicker sequencing and better access. MRI is better than CT in delineating soft tissue injuries and does not emit ionizing radiation. Cartilaginous structures, such as posterior wall fractures associated with traumatic hip dislocations, or nonacute fractures, such as occult stress fractures or avulsion fractures, may be diagnosed more readily with MRI.[31,72] An MRI is recommended as an adjunctive imaging study for all pediatric acetabular fractures because MRI discloses the true size of largely cartilaginous posterior wall fragments in children (Fig. 23-6).[72] Particularly following a traumatic hip dislocation, any bony "fleck"

Figure 23-6. A: Postreduction radiograph of a left hip dislocation in a 12-year-old boy. **B:** CT scan demonstrates small ossified posterior wall fragments. **C:** Sagittal MRI demonstrates 90% posterior wall involvement with intra-articular step-off (*arrow*). (Reprinted by permission from Springer Nature: Rubel IF, et al. MRI assessment of the posterior acetabular wall fracture in traumatic dislocation of the hip in children. *Pediatr Radiol.* 2002;32(6):435–439. Copyright © 2002 Springer-Verlag.)

visualized on postreduction CT scans or radiographs warrants an MRI, as it may represent a larger posterior labral osteochondral avulsion.[6]

Radioisotope bone scan is rarely indicated but may be useful for the identification of occult pelvic fractures or other acute injuries in children and adults with head injuries or multiple-system injuries.[88]

In children with avulsions of the pelvis, radiographs will usually show displacement of the affected apophysis. Avulsion injuries affect secondary centers of ossification before the center is fused with the pelvis, primarily in children of ages 11 to 17 years.[85] Comparison views of the contralateral apophysis, or the routine use of an AP pelvis x-ray instead of a view of the affected side only, help to ensure that what appears to be an avulsion fracture is not, in reality, a normal adolescent variant. Radiographs of children with delayed presentations of these injuries may demonstrate callus formation and these findings can occasionally mimic a malignant process. In this scenario, MRI is helpful in distinguishing these pathologies from each other.

CLASSIFICATION OF PELVIC AND ACETABULAR FRACTURES

Pelvic Fracture Classification

Pediatric Classification

Pelvic Fractures in Children:
MODIFIED TORODE AND ZIEG CLASSIFICATION

I. Avulsion fractures
II. Iliac wing fractures
   a. Separation of the iliac apophysis
   b. Fracture of the bony iliac wing
III. Stable ring disruptions
   a. Simple anterior ring fractures involving pubic rami or pubic symphysis
   b. Stable anterior and posterior ring fractures
IV. Unstable ring disruptions
   a. "Straddle" fractures, characterized by bilateral inferior and superior pubic rami fractures
   b. Fractures involving the anterior pubic rami or pubic symphysis and the posterior elements (e.g., SI joint, sacral ala)
   c. Fractures that create an unstable segment between the anterior ring of the pelvis and the acetabulum

The original Torode and Zieg[101] classification based on plain radiographs, and its most recent modification based on radiographs and CT scans,[54] is the most commonly used classification of pediatric pelvic fractures. To create this classification, the authors reviewed the radiographs of 141 children with pelvic fractures and classified the injuries on the basis of the fracture pattern as well as their associated prognosis. The classification defines type I (avulsion fractures), type II (iliac wing fractures), type III (simple ring fractures), and type IV (ring disruptions) fracture patterns. The modified scheme, published 27 years after the original classification from the same institution, is identical to the earlier scheme

but additionally divides type III "stable" simple ring injuries into IIIA (anterior-only ring fractures) and IIIB (anterior and posterior ring fractures) (Fig. 23-7). The morbidity, mortality, and complications are all greatest in the type IV group with "unstable" ring disruptions, but it should be emphasized that one "stable" pattern, type IIIB, also is associated with higher transfusion rates and morbidity compared with the other "stable" patterns. This classification does not include acetabular fractures.

Silber and Flynn[86] reviewed radiographs of 133 children and adolescents with pelvic fractures and classified them into two groups: immature (Risser 0 and all physes open) and mature (closed triradiate cartilage). These authors suggested that, in the immature group, management should focus on the associated injuries because the pelvic fractures rarely required surgical intervention compared with the group with mature pelvises. Fractures in the mature group were best classified utilizing adult pelvic fracture schemes and treated according to management principles utilized for adult patients.[8,64,88] This classification emphasizes the concept that pelvic ring injury patterns reflect the patient's skeletal maturity and not their chronologic age, an important factor to consider when evaluating and managing these injuries.

Adult Classifications

Pelvic Fractures in Adults:
TILE AND PENNAL CLASSIFICATION

A. Stable fractures
   A1. Avulsion fractures
   A2. Undisplaced pelvic ring or iliac wing fractures
   A3. Transverse fractures of the sacrum and coccyx
B. Partially unstable fractures
   B1. Open-book fractures
   B2. Lateral compression injuries (includes triradiate injury)
   B3. Bilateral type B injuries
C. Unstable fractures of the pelvic ring
   C1. Unilateral fractures
      C1-1. Fractures of the ilium
      C1-2. Dislocation or fracture-dislocation of the SI joint
      C1-3. Fractures of the sacrum
   C2. Bilateral fractures, one type B and one type C
   C3. Bilateral type C fractures

Pennal et al.[65] classified adult pelvic fractures according to the direction of force producing the injury: (a) AP compression, (b) lateral compression with or without rotation, and (c) vertical shear. This classification was modified and expanded by Tile et al.[98] Burgess et al.[10] further modified the Pennal system and incorporated subsets to the lateral compression and AP compression groups to quantify the amount of force applied to the pelvic ring. These authors also created a fourth category, combined mechanical injury, to include injuries resulting from combined forces that may not be strictly categorized according to the classification scheme of Pennal.

Figure 23-7. The modified Torode and Zieg classification. **Torode I** (avulsion fractures): avulsion of the bony elements of the pelvis, invariably a separation through or adjacent to the cartilaginous growth plate. **Torode II** (iliac wing fractures): resulting from a direct lateral force against the pelvis, causing a disruption of the iliac apophysis or an infolding fracture of the wing of the ilium. **Torode III-A** (simple anterior ring fractures): This group involved only children with stable anterior fractures involving the pubic rami or pubic symphysis. **Torode III-B** (stable anterior and posterior ring fractures): This new group involved children with both anterior and posterior ring fractures that were stable. **Torode IV** (unstable ring disruption fractures): This group of children had unstable pelvic fractures, including ring disruptions, hip dislocations, and combined pelvic and acetabular fractures. (Reprinted with permission from Shore BJ, et al. Pediatric pelvic fracture: A modification of a preexisting classification. *J Pediatr Orthop.* 2012;32(2):162–168.)

Pelvic Fractures in Adults:
OTA/AO CLASSIFICATION

A. Stable fractures
B. Rotationally unstable fractures, vertically stable
C. Rotationally and vertically unstable fractures
   C1. Unilateral posterior arch disruption
      C1-1. Iliac fracture
      C1-2. Sacroiliac fracture-dislocation
      C1-3. Sacral fracture
   C2. Bilateral posterior arch disruption, one side vertically unstable
   C3. Bilateral injury, both unstable

The Tile classification has been incorporated into the Orthopaedic Trauma Association (OTA)/AO classification, which is divided into bone segments, types, and groups.[68] The OTA/AO system classifies pelvic fractures on the basis of stability versus instability, and surgical indications are based on the fracture types. Surgery is rarely indicated for type A fractures, whereas anterior and/or posterior surgical stabilization may be indicated for type B and C fractures. Numerous subtypes are included and are beyond the scope of this chapter.

In general, the basic classifications—(a) mature or immature pelvis and (b) stable or unstable fracture—can be useful for making treatment decisions. However, published data suggests significant discrepancy in treatment choice for similar fracture patterns, indicating the need for improved algorithms for decision making.[59] Hemodynamic parameters are a primary concern for management of pelvic injuries regardless of the specific pattern. From the standpoint of orthopaedic management, however, if there is an extremely misshapen pelvic ring, a displaced posterior ring injury, or a displaced triradiate fracture, the injury should be considered unstable and will likely require

Figure 23-8. Triradiate cartilage in the pediatric acetabulum. **A:** Normal triradiate cartilage. **B:** Salter–Harris type I fracture.

surgical intervention regardless of the patient's age or the specific classification of the injury.

Acetabular Fracture Classification

Pediatric Classifications

Bucholz et al.[9] classified pediatric acetabular fractures based on the Salter–Harris classification (Fig. 23-8). Their classification system is used to help determine the prognosis of a triradiate cartilage injury that may result in a deformity of the acetabulum with growth. The anatomy of the triradiate is such that the superior weight-bearing portion of the acetabulum is separated from the inferior third by the superior arms of the triradiate cartilage. These superior arms are usually the ones involved in a fracture. In the Bucholz classification, a type I or II injury occurs from a traumatic force to the ischial ramus, pubic ramus, or proximal femur, resulting in a shearing force through the superior arms of the triradiate cartilage. If there is a metaphyseal bone fragment, this is a type II fracture. A type V injury is a crush injury to the physis.[9,45] Watts described four types of acetabular fractures in children: (i) small fragments that most often occur with dislocation of the hip, (ii) linear fractures that occur in association with pelvic fractures without displacement and usually are stable, (iii) linear fractures with hip joint instability, and (iv) fractures secondary to central fracture-dislocation of the hip.[108]

Adult Acetabular Classification

Acetabular fractures in children can also be described similarly to those in adults, which are usually classified by the system of Judet et al.[40] and Letournel and Judet.[50] A more comprehensive system is the AO fracture classification, which groups all fractures into A, B, and C types with increasing severity. Type A acetabular fractures involve a single wall or column; type B fractures involve both columns (transverse or T-types) and a portion of the dome remains attached to the intact ilium; and type C fractures involve both columns and separate the dome fragment from the axial skeleton by a fracture through the ilium.

OUTCOME MEASURES FOR PELVIC AND ACETABULAR FRACTURES

Outcome data have been assessed by several functional assessments; these outcome measures are not specific to pelvic fractures but are broadly applied outcome measures for traumatized patients. Measures used to evaluate the quality of life in trauma patients include the Child Health Questionnaire (CHQ), the Functional Independence Measure, the Impact of Family Scale,[72] and the Health-Related Quality of Life (HRQOL) scale.[71] Longer-term patient-reported outcomes in adults after pelvic fractures demonstrate significant decrease in both quality of life and physical functioning.[4] While increasing asymmetry has been associated with symptoms such as lumbar pain, Trendelenburg sign, and leg length discrepancy in pediatric patients high-quality long-term patient-reported outcomes are yet to be published.[90]

PATHOANATOMY AND APPLIED ANATOMY RELATED TO PELVIC AND ACETABULAR FRACTURES

PELVIC AND ACETABULAR DEVELOPMENT

The pelvis of a child arises from three primary ossification centers: the ilium, ischium, and pubis. The three centers meet at the triradiate cartilage and fuse at approximately 12 to 14 years of age (Fig. 23-9).[69] The pubis and ischium fuse inferiorly at the pubic ramus at 6 or 7 years of age. Occasionally, at approximately the time of fusion of the ischium to the pubis, an asymptomatic lucent area is noted on radiographs in the midportion of the inferior pubic ramus, termed the ischiopubic synchondrosis. It is often bilateral, fuses completely in most children, and may be confused with an acute or stress fracture of the pelvis, or tumor or infection (Fig. 23-10).

Secondary centers of ossification arise in the iliac crest, ischium, anterosuperior iliac spine, anteroinferior iliac spine, pubic tubercle, angle of the pubis, ischial spine, and the lateral wing of the sacrum; the first four centers listed are most important for understanding of pelvic avulsion fractures. Secondary ossification of the iliac crest is first seen at age 13 to 15 years and fuses to the ilium by age 15 to 17 years. This ossification pattern progresses from anterior to posterior (or lateral to medial when viewed on AP radiographs) and its time course of progression to fusion is the basis of Risser staging of skeletal maturity. The secondary ossification center of the ischium is first seen at 15 to 17 years and fuses at 19 years of age, although in some young adults it may fuse as late as 25 years of age. The ASIS develops as an apophysis of the anterior iliac crest at 13 years of age and fuses sometime around age 15. A center of ossification appears at the anteroinferior iliac spine at approximately 14 years, fusing at 16 years of age.[64,69,108] Knowledge about the location, age of appearance, and fusion of the secondary centers are important in differentiating these centers from fractures and avulsion injuries. Chondro-osseous growth also occurs through "physes" in the pubis at the area adjacent to the symphysis pubis, in the

Figure 23-9. A: Triradiate-acetabular cartilage complex viewed from the lateral side, showing the sites occupied by the iliac, ischial, and pubic bones. **B:** Normal acetabular cartilage complex of a 1-day-old infant. The ilium, ischium, and pubis have been removed with a curette. The lateral view shows the cup-shaped acetabulum. (Reprinted with permission from Ponseti IV. Growth and development of the acetabulum in the normal child: Anatomical, histological, and roentgeno-graphic studies. *J Bone Joint Surg Am.* 1978;60(5):575–585.)

Figure 23-10. AP pelvis of 14-year-old girl demonstrating an asymptomatic ischiopubic synchondrosis (*white arrows*) and a healing ASIS avulsion (*black arrow*). (Used with permission of the Children's Orthopaedic Center, Los Angeles.)

ilium adjacent to the SI joint, and to a lesser extent in the lateral sacrum; symphyseal separations and SI joint injuries in children may represent fractures through these growth areas as opposed to ligamentous disruptions.[64]

The acetabulum contains the shared physes of the ilium, ischium, and pubis that merge to become the triradiate cartilage. Interstitial growth in the triradiate part of the cartilage complex causes the acetabulum to expand during growth and causes the pubis, ischium, and ilium to enlarge as well. The concavity of the acetabulum develops in response to the presence of a spherical head. The depth of the acetabulum increases during development as the result of interstitial growth in the acetabular cartilage, appositional growth of the periphery of this cartilage, and periosteal new bone formation at the acetabular margin.[69] The triradiate cartilage of the acetabulum closes at approximately 12 years of age in girls and 14 years of age in boys.[102] At puberty, three secondary centers of ossification appear in the hyaline cartilage surrounding the acetabular cavity. The os acetabuli, which is the epiphysis of the pubis, forms the anterior wall of the acetabulum. The epiphysis of the ilium, the acetabular epiphysis,[69,107] forms a large part of the superior wall of the acetabulum. The small secondary center of the ischium is rarely seen. The os acetabuli, the largest part, starts to develop at approximately 8 years of age and expands to form the major portion of the anterior wall of the acetabulum; it unites with the pubis at approximately 18 years of age. The acetabular epiphysis develops in the iliac acetabular cartilage at approximately 8 years and fuses with the ilium at 18 years of age, forming a substantial part of the superior acetabular joint surface (Fig. 23-11). The secondary center of the ischium, the

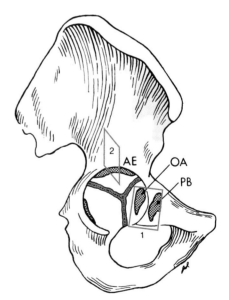

Figure 23-11. Right innominate bone of an adolescent. The os acetabuli (OA) is shown within the acetabular cartilage adjoining the pubic bone (PB); the acetabular epiphysis (AE), within the acetabular cartilage adjoining the iliac bone; and another small epiphysis (not labeled), within the acetabular cartilage adjoining the ischium (left). (Reprinted with permission from Ponseti IV. Growth and development of the acetabulum in the normal child. Anatomical, histological, and roentgeno-graphic studies. *J Bone Joint Surg Am.* 1978;60(5):575–585.)

smallest of the three, develops in the ninth year, unites with the acetabulum at 17 years, and contributes very little to acetabular development. These secondary centers are sometimes confused with avulsion fractures or loose bodies in the hip joint.

CHILD VERSUS ADULT PELVIS

As mentioned previously, there are important anatomic differences between the pelvis of a child and that of an adult:

* Greater bone plasticity and ligament elasticity that permit more bone deformation and greater mobility of the SI joints and symphysis pubis with trauma
* Thick periosteum, structural cartilage components, including the triradiate cartilage, that also permit more mobility of the ring but are susceptible to growth disturbance
* The presence of bone-cartilage apophyses toward the end of skeletal growth that are susceptible to avulsion fractures from violent contraction of attached muscles

Because of some of these differences, the pediatric pelvis is better able to absorb energy without significant displacement. Minimally displaced fractures and single breaks of the ring are frequently seen in pediatric pelvic fractures, a finding opposed to the traditional concept of a mandatory "double break" in the ring seen in adult fractures.[64] Plastic deformity can result in severe deformation of the pelvic ring and can make restoration of the normal anatomy challenging, even with surgical intervention. Most importantly, a child may sustain a higher-energy injury than suspected from the bony injury, making it crucial that the surgeon be aware that even minor pelvic fractures may be associated with other potentially serious injuries.

Pelvic Fractures

AVULSION FRACTURES (TORODE AND ZIEG TYPE I)

TREATMENT OPTIONS FOR AVULSION FRACTURES

Nonoperative Treatment of Avulsion Fractures

Of pelvic avulsion fractures reported in two large published series,[76] approximately 37% were avulsions of the anteroinferior iliac spine, 31% were ischial tuberosity avulsions, 25% were avulsions of the anterosuperior iliac spine, and 6% were iliac crest avulsions. Some athletes experience more than one avulsion fracture over the course of their development. Most pelvic avulsion fractures in children heal satisfactorily with nonoperative management, including rest, careful extremity positioning to minimize muscle stretch, partial weight bearing on crutches for 2 or more weeks, and physical therapy after symptoms improve. Typically, children resume normal activities by 6 to 8 weeks (Fig. 23-12). Two small series of adolescents with pelvic avulsion fractures treated conservatively concluded that nonsurgical treatment was successful in all patients, and all patients returned to preinjury activity levels.

Operative Treatment of Ischial Avulsion Fractures

Surgical treatment of ASIS and AIIS fractures has been described but is rarely indicated. While most pelvic avulsion fractures heal without surgical treatment, however, some fracture types, specifically, avulsion of the ischial tuberosity, and less so of the AIIS, require surgery. In one series of 198 competitive adolescent athletes with pelvic avulsion fractures, 3 were treated operatively,[71] corroborating the findings of another recent series of 228 fractures in which 3% required surgery.[76] In this later series, the authors reported that 14% of patients with avulsion fractures report pain greater than 3 months in duration and that AIIS avulsion fractures are 4.47 times more likely to have chronic pain greater than 3 months compared with all other types; additionally, 5 nonunions required surgery: 4 ischial tuberosity avulsions and 1 AIIS avulsion. Sinikumpu et al. reported on a series of 32 pelvic avulsion fractures treated operatively with a mean displacement of 3.4 cm. This included predominantly AIIS avulsions (11/34) and ischial avulsions (11/34). Eighty-one percent of patients reported good or excellent outcomes and were able to return to their preinjury activity level by an average of 3 months after surgery.[89] In this series, there were no differences in functional outcome with early (<3 months) versus late treatment. Ischial avulsion fractures have been associated with a higher incidence of functional disability and inability to return to competitive athletic activity compared with other types.[95] In one long-term follow-up study of 12 patients with ischial avulsions, 8 reported significant reduction in athletic ability and 5 had persistent local symptoms.[75] Because many have satisfactory outcomes without surgery, indications for surgical management are not clear nor is the best operative technique established. Some authors have recommended consideration for open reduction and internal fixation (ORIF) of those rare acute avulsion fractures displaced more than 1 to 2 cm (Fig. 23-13)[53,76] because of concern for late complications, but the authors have rarely found this necessary. Excision of the apophyseal fragment and takedown of nonunion and fixation are options in the chronic pain and disability. Other indications for late surgery include painful prominence after healing, concern for labral involvement,[38] and painful anterior hip impingement from heterotopic bone after healing.[56]

Open Reduction and Internal Fixation of Avulsion Fractures

Preoperative Planning

Open Reduction and Internal Fixation of Ischial Avulsion Fractures: PREOPERATIVE PLANNING CHECKLIST

OR table	❏ Fluoroscopic table such as a Jackson table
Position/ positioning aids	❏ Prone
Fluoroscopy location	❏ *Opposite the side of injury*
Equipment	❏ Screw set including 4.5- to 6.5-mm screws with washers ❏ Cables, wires, and/or suture anchors available as a backup

Figure 23-12. A: A 13-year-old who suffered an ASIS avulsion fracture (*arrow*) while kicking a football. He experienced sudden pain and initially was unable to walk. On standard AP view of the pelvis, the fracture is difficult to visualize. **B:** The avulsion of the ASIS (*arrow*) is much easier to appreciate on the iliac oblique view. **C:** One month after injury, there is significant healing present (*arrow*). (Courtesy of David L. Skaggs, MD.)

Technique

 Open Reduction and Internal Fixation of Ischial Avulsion Fractures:
KEY SURGICAL STEPS

❏ Prone position with the hip and knee slightly flexed.
❏ 7- to 10-cm incision is made along the gluteal crease.
❏ The gluteus maximus/hamstrings plane is developed and the hamstring muscles are then traced to the fracture site.
❏ Identify the bony fragment with the hamstrings attached, ensuring protection of the sciatic nerve.
❏ The fragment is reduced more easily with the hip extended and the knee slightly flexed.
❏ The fragment is stabilized with cancellous screws, with or without washers.
❏ If necessary, additional fixation with suture anchors, cables, or wires can be used.

Postoperative Care

After surgery, the patient is permitted to sit up with the hips and knees slightly flexed to decrease stress on the hamstrings. Initially made non–weight bearing, patients may progress to full weight bearing in 3 to 6 weeks. At 12 weeks postoperatively, the patient may resume full activities.

ISOLATED ILIAC WING FRACTURES (TORODE AND ZIEG TYPE II)

Direct trauma may fracture the wing of the ilium, but isolated iliac wing fractures are relatively rare, with a reported incidence of 5% to 14% in children with fractures of the pelvis.[86] However, iliac wing fractures often occur in conjunction with other fractures of the pelvis, and thus the overall incidence of iliac wing fractures is significantly higher than the incidence of isolated iliac wing fractures (Fig. 23-14).

The patient with an iliac wing fracture typically presents with pain that is located over the wing of the ilium, which worsens with trunk rotation or hip abduction. On examination, motion at the fracture site may be noted. A painful Trendelenburg gait may be present because of spasm of the hip abductor muscles. Plain radiographic diagnosis is sometimes difficult. A fracture of the wing of the ilium may be overlooked on an underexposed radiograph of the pelvis in which the ilium is poorly visualized, appearing only as a large area of radiolucency. CT is useful to delineate the fracture pattern and displacement in situations where surgery is being considered. Displacement of the fracture usually occurs laterally, but it may also occur medially or proximally. Severe displacement is rare

Figure 23-13. **A:** A painful ischial apophyseal nonunion in an athlete. **B:** Fixation of the apophysis. **C:** Healed apophysis after implant removal. (Courtesy of Dr. David C Scher, MD, Hospital for Special Surgery, NY.)

Figure 23-14. Stable fracture of the left iliac wing with associated anterior ring fractures.

because the iliac wing is tethered by the abdominal muscles, the hip abductors, and thick periosteum.

Treatment of an iliac wing fracture is mostly dictated by the associated injuries such as abdominal trauma. Symptomatic treatment is all that is necessary for most iliac wing fractures and typically includes pain management and partial weight bearing on crutches for comfort until the symptoms are completely resolved. Regardless of comminution or displacement, these fractures usually unite without complications. Open reduction and fixation with screws alone or plate–screw constructs are rarely indicated, except for large fragments with severe displacement. These fractures may also require fixation if the fracture extends into the acetabulum or the SI joint and is displaced.

OTHER STABLE FRACTURES

FRACTURES OF THE SACRUM

Sacral fractures constitute a very small fraction of pelvic fractures reported in children. Rieger and Brug reported two sacral

Figure 23-15. A: An example of an AP pelvic radiograph where the sacral fracture is not well visualized. **B:** CT scan of the patient showing the sacral fracture.

fractures and seven SI fracture-dislocations in 54 patients. Nine of 166 patients (5.4%) with pelvic fractures in the series by Silber et al.[88] had associated sacral fractures, none with nerve root involvement. Sacral fractures are probably more common than reported but may be missed because these injuries are sometimes obscured by the anterior ring of the bony pelvis and the soft tissue shadows of the abdominal viscera on plain radiographs, and are rarely displaced.

There are two general types of sacral injuries. Spinal-type injuries may present as a crush or compression-type injury, with vertical foreshortening of the sacrum or horizontal fractures across the sacrum. These fractures may be significant because sacral nerve root injury may result in the loss of bowel and bladder function. Alar-type injuries are vertical fractures through the alae or sacral foraminae. It is important to note that these fractures may represent the posterior break of the double ring fracture, an indicator of potential pelvic ring instability. In cases where the pelvic ring is disrupted, small compression fractures or avulsion fragments of the sacral periphery at the SI joint may be seen but the body and ala are intact.

The presence of sacral fractures may be suggested clinically. Pain, swelling, and tenderness over the sacrum posteriorly are present in some injuries. Digital rectal examination performed in patients with sacral fractures may reveal step-offs, fracture fragments, rectal tears, and urethral disruptions. Because digital rectal examination in pediatric trauma patients has a high false-negative rate, however, its usefulness is questionable and is not routinely performed in all centers.[84]

As suggested above, sacral fractures are sometimes difficult to diagnose on plain radiographs. AP and outlet views of the pelvis and a lateral view of the sacrum are best for identifying these injuries. Occasionally, the fracture line is oblique, but most are transverse with minimal displacement and occur through a sacral foramen, which is the weakest part of the body of the sacrum. Minimal disruption of the cortical rim of the foramen and offset of the lateral edge of the body of the sacrum are subtle indicators of a sacral fracture. Lateral views are helpful if there is anterior displacement, which is rare. CT and MRI scans are best for identification of sacral fractures missed on plain radiographic images.[25,82,87] In one study comparing radiographs with CT scans in a consecutive series of 103 pediatric

trauma patients with pelvic radiographs and pelvic CT scans, only three sacral fractures were identified with plain radiographs whereas nine sacral fractures were identified with CT (Fig. 23-15).[25] Sacral fractures are generally managed nonsurgically with pain management and protected weight bearing for comfort; weight bearing as tolerated is generally permitted because most are stable patterns. In rare cases, sacral nerve roots encroached upon by fracture displacement or fracture fragments may require surgical decompression. Sacral avulsion fractures and chondro-osseous injuries of the sacrum associated with SI joint fracture-dislocations generally are managed as part of the treatment for the SI joint injury with open or closed reduction of the SI joint and percutaneous SI or transiliac–transsacral screw fixation. Open reduction and fixation of isolated sacral fractures, however, is rarely necessary in children.

FRACTURES OF THE COCCYX

Many children fall on the tailbone and have subsequent pain. The possibility of fracture must be entertained. Because the coccyx is made up of multiple small segments composed of cartilage and bone, is obscured by soft tissue, and naturally has a "crook" or apex posterior angulation of the distal segments, it is difficult to determine on radiographs whether a coccygeal fracture has occurred. These fractures rarely have associated injuries other than localized pain at the injury site. Clinically, patients describe immediate, severe pain in the area of the coccyx. Pain on defecation may be present as well as pain on rectal examination. Because radiographic identification is difficult, clinical confirmation of the diagnosis may be made by digital rectal examination though palpation outside of the rectum is usually sufficient. Exquisite pain may be elicited and an abnormal mobility of the coccygeal fragments may be noted. Acute, severe symptoms typically abate in 1 to 2 weeks, but chronic, mild-to-moderate discomfort can persist in some patients for weeks or even months. Lateral radiographs of the coccyx with the hips flexed maximally may reveal an obvious fracture in some cases (Fig. 23-16), but apex posterior angulation of the coccyx is a normal variant and should not be falsely interpreted as a fracture or dislocation. CT and MRI may be helpful in differentiating between physes and fracture lines and also help to

Figure 23-16. Lateral radiograph with the hips maximally flexed reveals a displaced coccygeal fracture in a 14-year-old boy.

rule out other possible etiologies of the pain such as neoplasm or intrapelvic pathology. Treatment is symptomatic initially and consists of activity restriction and a pressure-relieving cushion for sitting, with an expectation of resolution in 4 to 6 weeks for acute fractures. Some rare pediatric patients have chronic pain that persists for several months, probably better described by the diagnosis of "coccydynia." Symptomatic treatments, injections, and coccygectomy are some management options with good results in adolescents.[24]

STRESS FRACTURES OF THE PELVIS

Stress fractures of the pelvis are rare in children but do occur in adolescents and young adults from chronic, repetitive stress, most commonly from sports activities such as running. These may occur through the sacrum and pubic rami and pelvic apophyses. Stress fractures of the sacrum have been described rarely in adolescent runners, volleyball players, and pregnant women who present primarily with low back pain.[61,82] Chronic low-grade groin and pubic pain that worsens with activities, especially distance running, are presenting signs of stress fractures of the pubic rami, most commonly at a site in the inferior ramus adjacent to the pubis. Patients with hip dysplasia who undergo periacetabular osteotomies are also at greater risk for stress rami fractures after surgery.[29] Stress fractures of the iliac crest apophysis of adolescent athletes have also been reported.[32] Radiographs often reveal no evidence of fracture initially but a small amount of periosteal reaction may become obvious after 4 to 6 weeks of symptoms. MRI is the best test to identify stress fractures of the pelvis. Alternatively, technetium bone scan may reveal increased uptake early in the course of symptoms.[36]

Figure 23-17. Radiograph of the pelvis of a 9-year-old child. Although the differentiation could not be made between a fracture and fusion of the right ischiopubic ossification at the time of radiograph, the patient had no symptoms and the mass was considered a variant of normal development.

Treatment should consist of avoiding the stressful activity and limited weight bearing for 4 to 6 weeks.

Stress fracture of the ischiopubic synchondrosis may also occur. This diagnosis is rare, however, and must be differentiated from ischiopubic osteochondritis, infections, and neoplasms. The ischiopubic synchondrosis usually closes between 4 and 7 years of age.[43] Caffey and Ross[42] noted that bilateral fusion of the ischiopubic synchondrosis is complete in only 6% of children at 4 years of age but is seen in 83% of children by 12 years of age. Children at an average of 7 years who present with vague groin or buttock pain, mild tenderness or fullness at the ischiopubic junction, and radiographs that reveal hyperostosis at the junction likely have ischiopubic osteochondritis or van Neck disease, a self-limited process that resolves with fusion of the synchondrosis.[64,107] Remember that in older children, those with a history suggestive of infection or neoplasm, or those who participate in repetitive stress activities such as distance running, with findings of hyperostosis of the ischiopubic synchondrosis on radiographs, should be ruled out for other diagnoses such as osteomyelitis, tumors, and stress fractures. Further diagnostic evaluation includes MRI of the pelvis, technetium bone scan, and blood work based on the clinical setting (Fig. 23-17).

SIMPLE RING FRACTURES (TORODE AND ZIEG TYPE IIIA AND IIIB)

Using the original Torode and Zieg classification scheme, simple ring injuries constitute up to 56% of all pelvic fractures in children,[68,74] with the majority resulting from motor vehicles striking pedestrians.[86] Many of these reported injuries were breaks in the anterior pelvic ring and were single ramus fractures, most commonly fractures of the superior ramus (Fig. 23-18).[47] With the increased use of CT scans to define these injuries, however, it became apparent that not all stable pelvic ring injuries are the same with regard to fracture pattern, mechanism, associated

Figure 23-18. A: Stable superior pubic ramus fracture. The patient was allowed full weight bearing as tolerated. **B:** Radiographs show complete fracture union and remodeling.

injuries, or prognosis. To reflect important differences among the types of simple ring injuries, Shore et al.[80] modified the Torode and Zieg scheme. In the modified classification, type III stable or simple ring fractures are subdivided into types IIIA and IIIB. Type IIIA fractures are defined as simple anterior ring fractures and type IIIB fractures are stable anterior and posterior ring fractures. This distinction is critical because type IIIB injuries are associated with an increased need for blood transfusions, an increased length of hospital stay, more frequent admissions to the ICU, and more associated injuries compared with type IIIA fractures.

NONOPERATIVE TREATMENT OF SIMPLE RING FRACTURES

Patients with these injuries typically present with pain and tenderness along the pubic rami. Weight bearing is difficult or impossible secondary to pain, and hip range of motion is often limited because of muscle guarding around the hip. The pelvic ring is grossly stable to rocking and compression but, for patients with type IIIB injuries, tenderness along the sacrum and SI joints may be elicited with palpation. Pelvic inlet and outlet radiographic views, or more commonly a CT scan, are used to distinguish type IIIA from type IIIB fractures.

Most stable ring fractures require no surgical intervention for management of the pelvic ring injury because, by definition, the pelvic ring is stable. For patients with type IIIB fractures, monitoring of cardiovascular status and blood loss and management of associated injuries are priorities compared to pelvic fracture management. Most patients with type III fractures, however, require only symptomatic treatment. Pain control and mobilization out of bed with non–weight bearing or protected weight bearing as dictated but the status of associated injuries when present is important for the initial 1 to 2 weeks after injury. For fractures with significant displacement or asymmetry, surgical intervention should be considered. After pelvic ring healing has progressed and the pain has diminished, progressive weight bearing is permitted. Most children with type III pelvic fractures return to full activities within 6 to 8 weeks of the initial injury, unless associated comorbidities influence recovery.

Special Situations

Fractures of the Two Ipsilateral Rami

Fractures of the ipsilateral superior and inferior pubic rami made up 18% of pediatric pelvic fractures in one series of 120 pediatric pelvic fractures.[11] Although these fractures are generally stable, they may be associated with injuries of the abdominal viscera, especially the genitourinary system (e.g., bladder rupture).[11] A careful examination of the perineum, rectal examination, and a cystourethrogram may be indicated to fully assess these injuries. Because these fractures typically unite without surgical treatment, most are treated nonsurgically, except when severe displacement has occurred.

Fractures of the Body of the Ischium

Fracture of the body of the ischium near the acetabulum is extremely rare in children. The fracture occurs from external force to the ischium, most commonly in a fall from a considerable height. The fracture usually is minimally displaced and management consists of symptomatic treatment and progressive weight bearing (Fig. 23-19).

Widening of the Symphysis Pubis

Isolated injuries to the symphysis pubis are rare because these typically occur in association with disruption of the posterior ring, at or near the SI joint most commonly. Although significant force is necessary to disrupt or fracture the symphysis pubis in children, isolated disruption of the symphysis pubis can occur.[108] Clinically, exquisite pain is present anteriorly at the symphysis. The lower extremities may lie externally rotated when the patient is supine. Motion of the hips in flexion, abduction, external rotation, and extension is restricted and painful (FABER sign). Pain associated with a pubic diastasis is often improved by side lying compared with supine positioning.[108]

Radiographs and CT imaging may reveal subluxation or widening of the symphysis or in the bone of the anterior ring just adjacent to it and vertical or AP offset of the two sides of the symphysis.[93] Although some elasticity of the pubic symphysis

Figure 23-19. **A:** Nondisplaced fracture (*curved arrow*) through left ischium and contralateral pubic ramus fracture. **B:** Follow-up radiograph shows mild displacement and incongruity of the acetabulum and complete healing of the superior pubic ramus fracture. Either displacement of the fracture fragments or premature closure of the triradiate cartilage could have contributed to the incongruity of the femoral head in the acetabulum.

Figure 23-21. Radiograph of the pelvis after plating of the pubic symphysis that also includes acetabular fixation.

is normal in children and adolescents, diastasis greater than or equal to 2.5 cm or rotational deformity greater than 15 degrees suggests significant instability and is an indication for reduction.[17] There is a normal variation of the width of the symphysis in children as measured on radiographs, because the pubic bones at the symphysis are composed of ischiopubic cartilage with a thickness that varies with age, making the extent of traumatic separation difficult to evaluate. Watts[108] suggested obtaining radiographs with and without lateral compression of the pelvis to detect abnormalities, with greater than 1 cm of difference in the width of the symphysis pubis between the two views indicating a symphyseal separation. Examination under anesthesia

under fluoroscopy with internal rotation, external rotation, and axial stress on both lower extremities has been demonstrated to assist with assessment of occult pelvic ring instability and surgical decision making in adult patients.[73,109] Imaging must also be carefully scrutinized to detect SI joint disruptions and triradiate cartilage fractures, both of which may occur in association with symphysis pubis separation (Fig. 23-20).[61]

Treatment of an isolated injury of the symphysis pubis with less than 2 cm of diastasis is generally symptomatic, similar to that described above for other stable pelvic ring injuries. Wider diastasis is best treated with closed reduction and external fixation or ORIF (with either suture or plate and screw constructs) of the symphysis through an anterior Pfannenstiel incision (Fig. 23-21). Because this injury in children is often through the cartilage of the pubis at the symphysis, and not disruption of symphyseal ligaments, healing is more reliable and rapid compared with adults.

Figure 23-20. **A:** Fracture adjacent to the symphysis pubis with symphysis pubis separation. **B:** CT scan showing no posterior instability.

Figure 23-22. A 4 year old with a pelvic fracture primarily with posterior involvement. **A:** Pelvic outlet radiograph showing a posterior injury at the sacroiliac joint. **B:** CT scan showing the minimal posterior SI widening. **C:** CT scan showing no anterior ring injury.

Fractures Near or Through the Sacroiliac Joint

The type IIIB fracture pattern is the most common injury pattern that is associated with stable, nondisplaced or minimally displaced fractures near or through the SI joints. The anatomy of the child's SI joint complex is different from that of an adult in several important ways. In children, disruptions tend to be incomplete because, while the anterior ligaments may tear, the thick posterior ligamentous complex prevents complete disruption in most cases. In addition, the SI joint may separate not through the joint but instead through the chondro-osseous "physis" of the medial ilium or, less commonly, the lateral sacrum of the growing child.[64] These fractures are clinically impossible to separate from ligamentous SI joint disruption and often are not identified on radiographs, making this a CT diagnosis.[11] Axial imaging by CT reveals subtle asymmetry of the rotation of the iliac wings, SI joint space widening, and a metaphyseal fracture line or tiny avulsion fragments of the ilium where the physeal fracture line exits out of metaphyseal bone just adjacent to the SI joint.[64] The "crescent" fracture is an iliac wing fracture that also occurs adjacent to the SI joint and is characterized by a metaphyseal fracture that exits posteriorly out of the ilium from the SI joint, creating a posterior iliac fragment that remains attached to the intact posterior ligaments; the surgeon must distinguish this pattern because it may reflect rotational instability of the injury.[91] Inlet/outlet pelvic views and coronal CT images reveal subtle distal SI joint step-off (Fig. 23-22) and anterior SI joint widening. Minimally displaced SI joint injuries are rarely associated with vascular or nerve root injuries. These injuries are treated conservatively with a short period of bed-to-chair

non–weight bearing for comfort, typically 4 to 6 weeks or, in rare cases, with a spica cast.

RING DISRUPTION: UNSTABLE FRACTURE PATTERNS (TORODE AND ZIEG TYPE IV)

Unstable pelvic fractures in children and adolescents constitute a small percentage of all pelvic fractures in pediatric patients. These are classified as Torode and Zieg type IV injuries and may have multiple fracture patterns. In one series of pelvic ring fractures, type IV injuries represented 10% of all pelvic fractures seen.[85] Most of these injuries result from high-velocity trauma, such as motor vehicle collisions and pedestrians being struck by motor vehicles. Children older than 12 years of age and those with closed triradiate cartilages[86] are more likely to sustain these types of fractures compared with younger patients with open triradiate cartilages. Blood transfusions, intensive care unit lengths of stay, and surgical interventions, among other parameters, are generally increased in patients with type IV fractures compared with other types of pelvic fractures, as is the incidence of death.[85]

Type IV fractures are typically divided into three subcategories:

1. Double anterior ring disruptions. This injury subtype includes bilateral inferior and superior pubic rami fractures (the straddle or floating injury) and disruptions of the pubis with an associated second break in the anterior ring.

2. Anterior and posterior pelvic ring (double ring) disruptions with instability and displacement, including vertical displacement (Malgaigne type). The anterior disruptions may be rami fractures or symphysis pubis disruption. Posterior ring injuries include fractures of the sacrum or ilium and disruptions through or adjacent to the SI joints.

3. Multiple crushing injuries that produce at least two severely comminuted fractures located at any site in the pelvic ring. These fractures may also be associated with acetabular fractures.

BILATERAL FRACTURES OF THE INFERIOR AND SUPERIOR PUBIC RAMI

Bilateral fractures of the inferior and superior pubic rami may occur in a fall while straddling a hard object, bilateral compression of the pelvis, or by sudden impact while riding a motorized cycle. The floating fragment usually is displaced superiorly, pulled in this direction by the rectus abdominis muscles.[108] As with ipsilateral superior and inferior pubic rami fractures, which may occur by similar mechanisms, bladder or urethral disruptions[13,90] are commonly associated injuries that must be ruled out in patients with this type of pelvic fracture.

Radiographically, an inlet/outlet views or CT scan most accurately determine the degree and direction of displacement. Bilateral fractures of the inferior and superior pubic rami (straddle fractures) or disruption of the symphysis pubis with unilateral fractures of the rami are two fracture patterns that result in a floating anterior segment of the pelvic ring. Although this floating anterior arch is inherently unstable (Fig. 23-23), the posterior ring is usually not disrupted except, in some cases, by stable fractures of the sacrum or ilium.

Treatment

Because in most cases the posterior ring is intact and the anterior fractures are not displaced, treatment is similar to that described for type IIIB injuries. After associated injuries have been diagnosed and managed appropriately, treatment initially includes bed rest and pain control. Skeletal traction is unnecessary, and a pelvic binder is contraindicated because of the possibility that compression will cause medial displacement of the ilium.[64,108] Protected weight bearing with progression to full weight bearing and unrestricted activities is then permitted as pain improves. In children, pelvic ring healing occurs reliably in 6 to 8 weeks for most injuries. Bone remodeling can be expected over the ensuing months. Surgical treatment of the superior ramus fractures with reduction and fixation with cannulated screws or plating techniques is rarely necessary to treat children but may be indicated in adolescents with significant displacement, or in patients with associated genitourinary injuries.

ANTERIOR AND POSTERIOR RING DISRUPTIONS

Double breaks in the pelvic ring, in which fractures occur both anterior and posterior to the acetabulum (Fig. 23-24), result in instability of the pelvis in many cases, especially when the posterior ring injury is displaced. These injuries result from a variety of mechanisms. Lateral compression patterns are the most common in skeletally immature patients, but other possible causes of injury are anterior to posterior forces, indirect forces transmitted proximally along the femoral shaft with the hip fixed in extension and abduction, and combined mechanisms of injury in which the pelvis is subject to multiple forces from different directions.[62,64] The injury patterns are best classified according to the AO-OTA scheme which may be applied to children's injuries.[68,78]

Double breaks in the pelvic ring, especially those with displacement, represent the most dangerous type of pelvic fracture in children.[23,85,88,101] These unstable fractures are often accompanied by retroperitoneal and intraperitoneal bleeding and are most likely to be associated with severe, life-threatening hemorrhage. Concomitant abdominal injury is also significantly more likely to occur in patients with unstable pelvic fractures compared to those with stable pelvic fractures.[23,85,88,101]

Aside from the physical signs usually associated with pelvic fractures, leg length discrepancy and asymmetry of the pelvis

Figure 23-23. Example of a straddle fracture.

Figure 23-24. An unstable pelvis fracture with fractures in both the anterior and posterior ring of the pelvis. The left hemipelvis is displaced and rotated.

Figure 23-25. A potentially unstable pelvic fracture with anterior and posterior injury. **A:** The radiograph shows left superior and inferior rami fractures. **B:** The CT scan shows a minimally displaced fracture adjacent to the sacroiliac joint. This is also an example where both CT and plain radiographs can be used to evaluate the injury and help decide on displacement and treatment. This patient was treated nonoperatively with follow-up, making sure there was no displacement.

may be present. Apparent leg length discrepancy is seen in patients with vertical or cephalad displacement of the fractured hemipelvis. Internal or external rotation of the unstable hemipelvis may appear as asymmetry of the iliac crests.

Inlet and outlet radiographs and CT scan reveal the degree and direction of pelvic displacement and determine the exact fracture pattern and associated plastic deformity. Anterior ring disruption may be the result of rami fractures or symphyseal separation. The posterior ring disruption may occur through the SI joint, with the majority causing tearing of the anterior ligaments but sparing the stronger and thicker posterior complex, although complete ligamentous disruptions do occur. More commonly, however, especially in younger children, the posterior ring disruption occurs through the chondro-osseus junction of the ilium or sacrum adjacent to the SI joint, as mentioned above.

Treatment

Initial treatment is focused on cardiovascular resuscitation with fluids and blood products and stabilization of the child's overall condition before treatment of the pelvic fractures.[37,91] Pelvic binders or sheets, placed circumferentially across the greater trochanters to limit pelvic ring expansion with severe hemorrhage, may be used safely in larger children and adolescents with similar indications and precautions as in adults. Some injuries caused predominantly by lateral compression forces, however, may not be amenable to this because compression may increase the pelvic deformity. Embolization of arterial vessels is also an option for uncontrolled bleeding but is rarely necessary since most bleeding is venous in origin.[20] The search for other sites of hemorrhage must be undertaken before attributing hemodynamic instability to the pelvic trauma in these younger children.

Minimally Displaced Fractures

Treatment of the AP pelvic ring injury varies based on the fracture pattern, degree of displacement, and the age and condition of the child. Most fractures with minimal displacement, some of which are type IV injuries, or more commonly type IIIB injuries,

are treated symptomatically by pain control, weight-bearing restrictions, and close radiographic follow-up for displacement (Fig. 23-25). Spica casting can be used in the younger children to improve the comfort of the patient and to prevent weight bearing, after cardiovascular parameters and associated injures have been stabilized. In some cases, older children and adolescents with minimally displaced fractures benefit from fixation to lessen pain associated with the fracture and facilitate mobilization.

Displaced Fractures

Nonoperative Treatment

Historically, operative treatment of pelvic fractures in children has not been routinely used for the following reasons[23,39,88]:

- Severe hemorrhage from the pelvic fracture is unusual in children, making operative pelvic stabilization to control bleeding rarely necessary.
- The thick periosteum and ligaments about the pelvis in children limit displacement and stabilize the fracture to some degree, limiting fracture fragment mobility and facilitating healing so that nonsurgical treatment is well tolerated by patients, and prolonged immobilization is not necessary for fracture healing.
- Remodeling may occur in skeletally immature patients, reducing the need to achieve anatomic alignment of some fractures.

Techniques

Nonoperative treatment for unstable pelvic fractures historically included bed rest and spica cast immobilization, neither of which significantly improves fracture alignment. Skeletal traction can be used to improve alignment of fractures with vertical displacement. Longitudinal traction is applied through a pin placed in the distal femur with weights similar to those utilized for femoral shaft reduction. Traction is applied for a minimum of 2 to 4 weeks to achieve some stability of the injury, after which the child may be placed in a spica cast or kept on bed rest until further healing allows safe mobilization. Skeletal traction cannot improve alignment of symphyseal "open book" injuries, severe SI disruptions with widening or posterior displacement, or fractures with rotational deformities of the hemipelvis. This treatment modality is no longer regularly utilized due to prolonged hospitalization and immobility.

Outcomes

Despite the fact that the classic assumptions and observations regarding unstable pelvic fractures are generally correct, the published outcomes of nonsurgical treatments have not been uniformly satisfactory. Nierenberg et al.[61] reported excellent or good results after conservative treatment of 20 unstable pelvic fractures in children, despite radiographic evidence of deformity. These authors concluded that treatment guidelines for unstable pelvic fractures are not the same for children as for adults, and recommended that external or internal fixation should be used only when conservative methods fail.[61] Another study, however, found that a third of 15 skeletally immature patients with unstable fractures treated nonoperatively had chronic pain at follow-up.[57] Similar findings were shown in another large series of unstable pediatric pelvic fractures treated nonsurgically with a mean of 7.4 years follow-up. In this study, about one-fourth of patients had musculoskeletal complaints at follow-up, including leg length discrepancy, back pain, and SI ankylosis.[94] In addition, these authors identified important nonorthopaedic complications, including 23 patients with genitourinary abnormalities, such as incontinence and erectile dysfunction, and 31 patients with psychiatric diagnoses such as posttraumatic stress disorder and major depression. These authors stressed the importance of minimizing prolonged hospital stays, addressing urologic needs fully, and anticipating the need for mental health support.

In addition to the advantages of improved mobilization, anatomic or near-anatomic realignment of pelvic fractures likely improves outcomes. Residual pelvic ring asymmetry, specifically vertical displacement of the hemipelvis and SI joint malalignment, and acetabular malrotation leading to altered hip coverage and mechanics do not reliably remodel after fracture healing and have been associated with poor long-term outcomes such as leg length discrepancy, hip pain, back pain, scoliosis, and SI arthrosis in children.[45,77,90] Pelvic obliquity and asymmetry has also been associated with pelvic floor dysfunction and pain. In one long-term follow-up study of 17 children with unstable pelvic fractures treated nonoperatively, 8 patients had pelvic asymmetry at follow-up.[77] Of these eight patients, five had functional deformities, including scoliosis and leg length discrepancies that resulted in chronic back pain. In another study, Smith et al.[90] followed 20 patients with open triradiate cartilages who were treated for unstable pelvic fractures for a mean of 6.5 years. Pelvic asymmetry was quantified on an AP pelvis radiograph by measuring the difference in length (in centimeters) between two diagonal lines drawn from the border of the SI joint to the contralateral triradiate cartilage. Eighteen patients were treated operatively with external fixation, internal fixation, or a combination of both; pelvic asymmetry was less than 1 cm in 10 of 18 patients. At follow-up, the authors noted that pelvic asymmetry did not remodel to any significant degree,

even in younger patients. Based on the Short Musculoskeletal Function Assessment (SMFA) questionnaire, patients with 1 cm or less of pelvic asymmetry had significantly less back and SI pain, and better SMFA outcome scores than those patients with pelvic asymmetry greater than 1 cm. In addition, all patients with greater than 1.1 cm of pelvic asymmetry had three or more of the following: nonstructural scoliosis, lumbar pain, a Trendelenburg sign, or SI joint tenderness and pain. The authors concluded that fractures associated with at least 1.1 cm of pelvic asymmetry following closed reduction should be treated with open reduction and internal or external fixation to improve alignment and the long-term functional outcome.[90]

Operative Treatment

Because of concerns for poor outcomes based on prior experience with nonsurgical treatment of unstable pediatric pelvic fractures, modern evidence supports the safety and efficacy of surgical treatment for displaced and unstable pelvic fractures in children and adolescents. Karunaker et al.[42] surgically managed 18 unstable pelvic and acetabular fractures in children younger than 16 years of age using the principles of anatomic realignment and stable fixation routinely applied to adults. All patients healed by 10 weeks after surgery and had recovered full function with minimal residual pain at follow-up. No significant complications occurred, notably no cases of premature triradiate cartilage closure or SI joint abnormalities. They recommended operative intervention in skeletally immature patients with significant deformity of the pelvis at the time of injury to prevent late morbidities.[42] Others have drawn similar conclusions based on their experience with surgical management of unstable pediatric pelvic disruptions.[1,68,78,100]

Indications/Contraindications

The exact indications for surgical treatment are not clearly delineated in the literature but have become less controversial over time. Holden et al.[37] determined, after a review of the literature prior to 2006, that fractures with more than 2 cm of displacement must be reduced and stabilized in children. Others have suggested that pelvic asymmetry greater than or equal to 1.1 cm is an indication for reduction. Silber et al.,[88] in one review of 166 children with pelvic fractures, recommended that all patients with closed triradiate cartilages, regardless of age, be treated as adults with anatomic realignment and stable fixation. Anatomic realignment and fixation is recommended by others for all displaced pelvic ring fractures regardless of age, utilizing similar parameters applied to adults with displaced and unstable pelvic ring injuries.[1,68,78,100]

Preoperative Planning

Because surgery for pelvic ring reduction and fixation in children is rare, one may consider including an experienced orthopaedic traumatologist, in conjunction with a pediatric orthopaedic surgeon, using techniques more commonly needed in adults but modified for children. These modifications include implants sized appropriately for children and techniques that preserve, as much as possible, the potential for growth. Perioperative care is best accomplished with a multidisciplinary team that is familiar with pediatric anesthesia and critical care and includes pediatric trauma nursing, child support services, and pediatric rehabilitation.

The timing of surgery is based on the needs of the individual patient. Although uncommon, emergency placement of external or internal fixation may be necessary to achieve cardiovascular stability, such as with an open book pelvis fracture not stabilized by a pelvic binder. Complex surgery was historically thought to represent a "second hit" to the traumatized patient that further incited inflammatory processes and challenges the body's ability to respond to the stress of surgery. In adults, the concept of "damage control orthopaedics"[19] favors delaying surgery until concomitant injuries have been managed and after a period of cardiovascular stability. A recent study demonstrated that systemic inflammatory response syndrome (SIRS) occurs in children as well as adults, but for unknown reasons, acute respiratory distress and lung injury are less common.[2] Therefore the timing of surgery should be determined by the condition of the patient and the team's judgment.

Many different surgical strategies and techniques may be utilized to achieve reduction and stability. The surgical team must carefully plan which technique or combination of techniques is best for the individual patient. Stabilization of the anterior ring may be accomplished with external fixation, symphyseal and/or rami plate or suture fixation, or screw fixation of the rami and anterior column (Fig. 23-26). Options for posterior stabilization include SI screw fixation and plate fixation (Fig. 23-27).

Figure 23-26. This radiographic series highlights treatment of an unstable pelvic fracture with hemodynamic instability. **A:** Anteroposterior pelvic radiograph of a 12-year-old boy who was a pedestrian hit by a car. There is a wide symphysis and a displaced fracture adjacent to the left sacroiliac joint. The towel clips seen on radiograph are to hold a sheet (sling) around the pelvis to help temporarily control hemorrhage. **B:** CT scan showing the displaced posterior injury. **C:** Pelvic radiograph after an anterior external fixation was placed urgently to stabilize the pelvis. This along with resuscitation stabilized the hemodynamic status. **D:** Once the patient had stabilized, the external fixation was converted to anterior internal fixation with a plate on the symphysis pubis and the posterior instability was treated with a sacroiliac screw.

Figure 23-27. A 6-year-old boy who was struck by a school bus. He had a pneumothorax and a pelvic fracture. AP pelvis (**A**) and initial CT scan (**B**) show an unstable type IV fracture with vertical displacement of the hemipelvis. He was placed in traction during resuscitation (**C**) with realignment of the fracture. After stabilization 6 days after injury, he underwent closed reduction, SI screw fixation, and application of an external fixator. Postoperative radiograph (**D**) of the pelvis and CT scan (**E**) show near-anatomic reduction.

Because these techniques are discussed in detail in the companion to this text, *Rockwood and Wilkins' Fractures in Adults*, this section will discuss only the two most commonly used techniques for children, external fixation and SI screw fixation.

External Fixation

External fixation is used to stabilize an unstable fracture with anterior ring separation or anterior fractures and for control of pelvic ring volume emergently in some AP ring disruptions. This technique maintains reduction, decreases pain, facilitates mobilization out of bed, and may be better tolerated by older children than spica casting.[21,44] External fixation, however, may not effectively control the posterior ring for all fracture patterns. Anterior external fixation may be achieved by placing one or two pins in the supra-acetabular bone on each side of the pelvis (Fig. 23-28)[74] or by placing one to two pins into each iliac crest and spanning these pin clusters with an external frame, ideally

Figure 23-28. Fixation of an unstable pelvic fracture with external fixation. One or two pins are placed in the iliac wing. The starting point is 1 to 2 cm posterior to the anterosuperior iliac spine. An anterior-to-posterior supra-acetabular pin may also be used.

one that allows access to the abdomen and enough mobility to allow sitting.

Preoperative Planning

 Placement of Pelvic External Fixation in Children:
PREOPERATIVE PLANNING CHECKLIST

OR table	❏ Fluoroscopic table such as flat top Jackson table
Position/ positioning aids	❏ Supine with a small bolster under the sacrum
Fluoroscopy	❏ Position for either side of the table. Confirm ability to obtain AP, inlet, outlet, and oblique views of the pelvis
Equipment	❏ 4-, 4.5-, 5-mm half pins ❏ Radiolucent external fixation frame

Technique

 Placement of Pelvic External Fixation in Children:
KEY SURGICAL STEPS

- ❏ Complete prep and drape of the abdomen above the umbilicus, pelvis, and lower extremities
- ❏ For placement of iliac crest pins:
  - Small transverse incision over iliac crest for each pin. The first incision is made 2 cm posterior to AIIS
  - Split the iliac apophysis and locate the metaphyseal bone between the iliac tables
  - Drill path between the tables perpendicular to the iliac crest; confirm position with fluoroscopy
  - Place pin (self-drilling screws may be placed directly through apophysis)
  - Place second pin 2 cm posterior to the first along the iliac crest; place a total of 2–3 pins per side
  - The inner or outer table of the pelvis may be palpated to ensure pin is wholly in bone
  - Construct frame that allows access to the abdomen
- ❏ For placement of supra-acetabular pins
  - Small longitudinal incision 2 cm proximal to the joint just medial to an imaginary line drawn between AIIS and ASIS
  - Bluntly dissect to the supra-acetabular bone
  - Drill path perpendicular to the bone; confirm position with fluoroscopy using oblique views
  - Place pin
  - A single pin may be placed per side or second pin may be placed just superior and in line with the first
  - Construct frame that allows access to the abdomen and hip flexion
- ❏ Loosen frame to allow for closed reduction under fluoroscopic guidance: provisional reduction held manually before pin placement may facilitate the process
- ❏ Confirm reduction and final tightening of the frame

Postoperative Care

After frame placement, patients may be out of bed to a chair if pelvic ring stability is acceptable and the associated injuries permit mobilization. Half-pin care is typically initiated within 4 to 7 days of surgery and continues until the frame is removed. Care regimens vary but daily cleaning is typically recommended. By 4 to 6 weeks after placement, limited weight bearing is started.

Weight bearing in the frame may be possible for some patients but typically for children, it is not fully instituted until removal of the frame, which is typically done in the operating room 6 to 10 weeks after application.

Symphyseal Plating

Symphyseal plating is a good alternative to anterior ring fixation in some children and adolescents.[21] This fixation choice is less bulky than external fixation and can often be performed at the time of other procedures for associated urogenital or abdominal injuries. The approach and technique are identical to that utilized for adult symphyseal plating, except that the plate size must be selected appropriately based on the size of the child. The best choice is a rigid plate–screw construct, such as a 3.5-mm reconstruction plate, but small and less bulky choices may be indicated for smaller patients.

Sacroiliac Reduction and Screw Fixation

Posterior ring injuries in children are typically SI joint disruptions, either from a true joint disruption or from fractures of the ilium, fractures of the iliac, or sacral chondro-osseous zones that extend into or are adjacent to the SI joint, or sacral fractures. Indications for surgical treatment of these injuries are unstable ring injuries with combined anterior and posterior instability and posterior ring fractures with displacement greater than about 1 cm, although, as noted above, the amount of acceptable displacement is controversial. Closed reduction, or limited open reduction, with percutaneous stabilization is an important strategy for pelvic fracture management in children and is the first option when addressing displaced fractures.[1,78] Open reduction and plate fixation of posterior ring injuries is indicated when closed reduction and screw fixation techniques cannot achieve adequate realignment or stable fixation. Adequate visualization can often be achieved through an anterior approach utilizing the "lateral window."

Preoperative Planning

 Placement of SI Screw Fixation:
PREOPERATIVE PLANNING CHECKLIST

OR table	❏ Fluoroscopic table such as flat top Jackson table
Position/ positioning aids	❏ Supine with a small bolster under the sacrum ❏ Place leads for neuromonitoring of the lower extremity on the affected side
Fluoroscopy	❏ Position for either side of the table. Confirm ability to obtain AP, inlet, outlet, lateral, and oblique views of the pelvis
Equipment	❏ 4.5–6.5-mm fully threaded cannulated screws ❏ Pelvic plate system (as backup) ❏ Setup for femoral traction pin placement ❏ Setup to perform open reduction and fixation of the SI joint if necessary

Before considering this technique, the CT scan of the pelvis must be carefully scrutinized to determine if the fracture pattern is amenable to closed reduction. Specifically, it is important to determine if comminution or severe displacement may prevent reduction or risk of soft tissue or neurovascular entrapment or injury. The CT scan is helpful to assess the sacral anatomy of the individual patient, which may vary widely, to determine the ideal entry position and safe trajectory. In the pediatric patient, the narrow corridor for safe screw placement makes the procedure difficult but safe placement of percutaneous SI screws can be achieved[78,94] and has been reported in children as young as 6 years of age.[1] If transiliac–transsacral fixation is necessary, the S2 corridor is often more amenable than the S1 corridor. When a concomitant anterior pelvic injury is present, it may be necessary to stabilize it prior to fixation of the posterior injury, although the strategy varies based on the fracture pattern and displacement.

Technique

 Placement of SI Screws:
KEY SURGICAL STEPS

❑ Careful analysis of preoperative CT scan to review sacral anatomy and safe zones for screw placement
❑ Complete prep and drape of the abdomen above the umbilicus, pelvis, and lower extremities. Achieve provisional reduction of the SI joint
❑ Identify starting point:
  • Utilize the outlet view to obtain AP of the sacrum to provisionally mark skin incision start point
  • Obtain a perfect lateral view of the S1 body; the greater sciatic notches should overlap completely on the ideal lateral view of the sacrum. Mark the skin in the lateral plane along your first provisional line (the entry point is typically at the intersection of the long axis of the femur and a vertical line drawn posteriorly for the ASIS)
❑ Place the guidewire on to the lateral ilium and confirm position with fluoroscopy
❑ Advance guidewire, confirming position as you proceed to prevent entering the sacral foramen, the neural canal, and penetrating the anterior cortex of the S1 body: neuromonitoring is checked to assure safe passage
❑ After confirming the final position of the guidewire to the midline of the sacrum or just past the midline, the length is measured and the guidewire is overdrilled
❑ The screw is advanced over a washer to the level of the lateral ilium
❑ Multiplane fluoroscopy is utilized to confirm reduction and stability. A second SI screw, on rare occasions, is indicated; the need for anterior ring fixation is then determined
❑ After completion of the procedure, neuromonitoring confirms that no injury has occurred to the lumbosacral plexus or L5 nerve
❑ Reduction techniques:
  • To reduce vertical displacement, longitudinal traction is applied through the leg manually, or by a traction bow attached to a distal femoral traction pin
  • Posterior and rotational displacement may be reduced manually or by applying force through a T-handled chuck on a half-pin placed in the iliac crest away from potential incision sites
  • Open reduction may be required, most commonly anteriorly

Postoperative Care

If the pelvic ring is stable after fixation, cast immobilization is not necessary. The patient may be out of bed to a chair after surgery. Weight bearing is restricted for a minimum of 6 weeks

before gradual progression. SI screws are not typically removed in adults. Although the growth consequences of SI joint fixation in younger children are not fully understood, it is our preference to remove screws after healing in this younger age group.

Open Reduction and Plate Fixation

Like adults, open reduction and plating of SI joint disruptions and fractures of the posterior ring are also sometimes indicated, most commonly when adequate reduction cannot be achieved with closed manipulative techniques, such as with large vertical displacement of the hemipelvis. This technique can be done either through an anterior retroperitoneal approach or via a posterior approach. The choice of implants is based on the size of the patient and the fracture type. Safe and effective plate fixation of unstable pelvic injuries has been reported in toddlers using 3.5-mm plating systems and adult techniques.[93]

SEVERE CRUSH INJURIES AND OPEN FRACTURES

Crush injuries of the pelvis and open fractures are relatively rare. In patients with crushing injuries, distortion of the pelvic ring is severe, resulting in multiple breaks in both the anterior and posterior pelvis as well as the acetabulum and triradiate cartilage. These uncommon injuries are nearly always associated with serious concomitant injuries, particularly thoracoabdominal and genitourinary abnormalities (Fig. 23-29). Neurologic injuries of the lumbosacral plexus and vascular injuries are also common associated findings. Risk of massive hemorrhage is

A

B

Figure 23-29. A: Open pelvic fracture with severe displacement. **B:** The soft tissue injury precluded pelvic reduction and fixation. This radiograph shows remarkable late deformity.

highest for patients who sustain these types of fractures and, in one series, about 20% of children with crushed open pelvic fractures died within hours of admission, secondary to uncontrolled hemorrhage.[60] Open fractures are more common than crush injuries, representing 13% of patients[60] with pelvic fractures, the result of motor vehicle trauma and gunshot wounds.

The principles of emergency management are similar to those applied for other unstable pelvic fractures. Surgical stabilization of the pelvic ring may be extremely challenging in the face of multiple fracture sites, comminution, and soft tissue trauma. Lacerations of the vagina and rectum, bladder injuries, and urethral disruptions complicate management and increase the risk of infection. External fixation alone may not be sufficient to manage these complex injuries, making it frequently necessary to perform internal fixation or a combination of these techniques. Stable pelvic fixation, multiple debridements, soft tissue management, and careful surveillance for infection are recommended to improve the chances of successful outcomes.[60]

Acetabular Fractures

TREATMENT OPTIONS FOR ACETABULAR FRACTURES

Acetabular fractures constitute only 2% to 17% of pediatric pelvic fractures, making them very uncommon.[23,60,86,106] Acetabular fractures associated with pelvic ring injuries tend to have less displacement and less often require operative treatment but tend to have more associated injuries.[46] Though rare, these injuries carry the potential for significant long-term morbidity. The goals of treatment for acetabular fractures in children are twofold. The first is to restore a congruent and stable joint with an anatomically reduced articular surface. The second is to preserve alignment of the triradiate cartilage in hopes of ensuring normal growth. Schlickewei et al.[74] noted that there are a variety of injury patterns and limited evidence of outcomes for any specific treatment. Thus, each fracture should be evaluated on an individual basis with the following guidelines: (i) anatomic reduction will likely result in a good long-term outcome; (ii) MRI is the best tool for identifying closure of the triradiate cartilage; and (iii) patients should be informed about the possibility of growth arrest and secondary associated problems such as joint subluxation or dysplasia.[74]

NONOPERATIVE TREATMENT OF ACETABULAR FRACTURES

In general, conservative treatment is indicated for simple, nondisplaced fracture patterns. Short-term bed rest followed by non–weight-bearing ambulation with crutches can be used for nondisplaced or minimally (≤2 mm) displaced fractures, particularly those that do not involve the superior acetabular dome. Because weight-bearing forces must not be transmitted

across the fracture, crutch ambulation is appropriate only for older children who can reliably avoid weight bearing on the injured limb. Non–weight bearing usually is continued for 6 to 8 weeks. Radiographs should be obtained frequently in the first few weeks to confirm fracture alignment. For those younger children who cannot comply with non–weight-bearing ambulation, spica cast immobilization is preferred.

Skeletal traction is an option for those rare acetabular fractures that can be reduced to less than or equal to 2 mm of displacement or those with medical contraindications to surgical treatment. To avoid injury to the physis, the traction pin is usually inserted in the distal femur under anesthesia using fluoroscopic guidance. Follow-up radiographs should confirm fracture reduction and joint congruency, and traction is generally maintained for 4 to 6 weeks until fracture healing is sufficient to allow progressive weight bearing.

There are few studies reporting the outcome of nonoperative treatment of acetabular fractures in children. Heeg et al.[34] reported on 23 patients with a variety of fracture patterns, with 18 being treated conservatively. The authors reported excellent functional and radiographic results of nonoperative treatment in those who were able to maintain congruent joints.

OPERATIVE TREATMENT OF ACETABULAR FRACTURES

Indications/Contraindications

The primary indication for operative treatment of pediatric acetabular fractures is either (1) an unstable joint or (2) an incongruent joint, regardless of fracture pattern. Instability usually results from posterior or anterior wall fractures, and, when present, must be remedied by operative reduction and fixation. Lack of congruency may result from bony fragments and/or soft tissue within the joint or from fracture displacement in the weight-bearing dome. In the former situation, open reduction is necessary to remove the offending agents and avoid premature osteoarthritis and, in the latter case, anatomic restoration of the articular surface with stable internal fixation is the operative goal. Gordon et al.[21] recommended accurate reduction and internal fixation of any displaced acetabular fracture in a child. They noted that the presence of incomplete fractures and plastic deformation may make accurate reduction difficult or impossible; they recommended that incomplete fractures be completed and that osteotomies of the pubis, ilium, or ischium be made if necessary to achieve accurate reduction of the acetabulum.[21] Improved outcomes with early (<24 hours) fixation of acetabular fractures in adults have been reported,[67] and Gordon et al.[21] noted that early fixation (before callus formation) is especially important to prevent malunion in young patients in whom healing is rapid (Fig. 23-30).

Another important indication for surgical treatment is malalignment of the triradiate cartilage, which can result in growth arrest and progressive acetabular dysplasia (Fig. 23-31). Linear growth of the acetabulum occurs by interstitial growth in the triradiate part of the cartilage complex, causing the pubis, ischium, and ilium to enlarge. The depth of the acetabulum develops in response to the presence of a spherical femoral head

Figure 23-30. A: Pelvic radiograph of a 12-year-old 1 year after an acetabular fracture. The fracture is a malunion with subluxation of the hip joint. **B:** Three-dimensional CT scan showing the malunited fragment.

and interstitial growth of the acetabular cartilage.[69] Growth derangement of all or part of the triradiate cartilage as a result of poor fracture reduction may result in a dysplastic acetabulum. Since the ilioischial limb of the triradiate contributes the most to acetabular growth, injury to the ilioischial limb of the triradiate cartilage has a greater potential for late acetabular deformity than an anterior iliopubic limb injury.[18] Due to its physeal nature and rare occurrence, triradiate cartilage injuries are often missed on initial evaluation (47% in one series).[15] Therefore a high index of suspicion and low threshold for advanced imaging is necessary when evaluating young children with acetabular fractures.

Outcomes

Sen et al.[79] reviewed a series of 38 adolescent acetabular fractures (patient ages 11–18 years) of which 37 were treated operatively. They reported generally good outcomes with 34 of 38 (89%) returning to full activity with 29 (76%) being pain free at a mean follow-up of 38.2 months. Based on these

Figure 23-31. A: AP pelvis of a 4-year-old boy who was struck by a truck demonstrates left superior and inferior pubic rami fractures and involvement of the open triradiate cartilage. **B:** AP pelvis of the same patient 8 years later demonstrates premature closure of the left triradiate cartilage and posttraumatic acetabular dysplasia. (Copyright Wudbhav N. Sankar, MD.)

results, the authors advocated a more aggressive surgical approach for any acetabular fracture with more than minimal displacement.

Open Reduction and Internal Fixation of Acetabular Fractures

Preoperative Planning

> ✔ **Open Reduction and Internal Fixation of Acetabular Fractures:**
> PREOPERATIVE PLANNING CHECKLIST

OR table	❏ Fluoroscopic table such as a Jackson table
Fluoroscopy location	❏ Contralateral side of the table (opposite the injury)
Equipment	❏ Screw set including long 3.5- to 4.5-mm and various-sized cannulated screws ❏ Threaded Kirschner wires ❏ Plate set including small fragment plates, pelvic reconstruction plates, and smaller "hook" plates ❏ Pelvic retractors, clamps, and reduction instruments ❏ Femoral distractor

The positioning and approach for ORIF of pediatric acetabular fractures varies according to the pattern of the fracture and the direction of the displacement as determined on the preoperative radiographs and CT scans (Table 23-1).[21] Fractures of the posterior wall and/or posterior column can be approached through a Kocher–Langenbeck approach with the patient in either lateral decubitus or prone position (Fig. 23-32). Anterior column injuries can be approached through an ilioinguinal approach with the patient placed supine. Some transverse fractures may require an extended iliofemoral approach. The extended lateral approaches, which include the extended iliofemoral and triradiate approaches, should be avoided as much as possible because of the risk of devascularization of the ilium and heterotopic bone formation.

TABLE 23-1. Surgical Exposure for Operative Fixation of Acetabular Fractures

Fracture Type	Exposure
Anterior column or wall	Ilioinguinal
Posterior column or wall	Kocher–Langenbeck
Transverse	Ilioinguinal (or extended lateral)
T-shaped	Ilioinguinal and Kocher–Langenbeck (or extended lateral)
Anterior column and posterior hemitransverse	Ilioinguinal
Both columns	Ilioinguinal (or extended lateral)

Reprinted from Gordon RG, et al. Techniques of operative reduction and fixation of pediatric and adolescent pelvic fractures. *Oper Tech Orthop.* 1995;5(2), 95–114. Copyright © 1995, With permission from Elsevier.

Figure 23-32. A: Radiograph of a football injury with posterior acetabular fracture and dislocation. **B, C:** Postoperative radiographs after a posterior approach and plating.

Authors' Preferred Treatment of Pelvic and Acetabular Fractures (Algorithms 23-1 and 23-2)

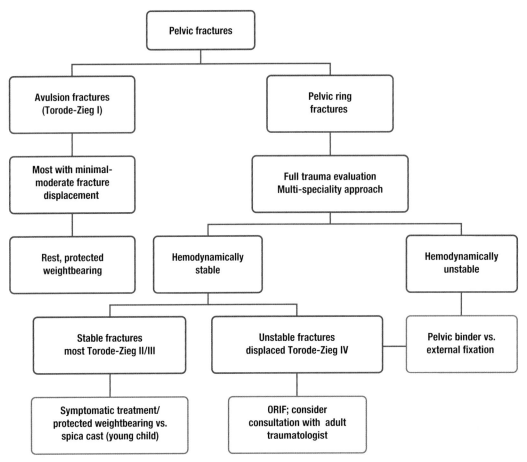

Algorithm 23-1. Authors' preferred treatment of pelvic fractures.

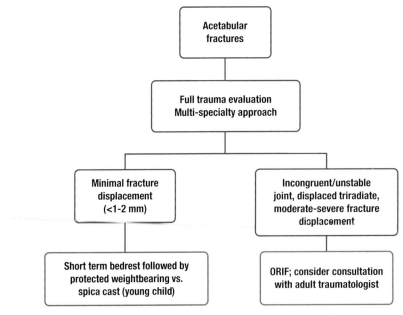

Algorithm 23-2. Authors' preferred treatment of acetabular fractures.

We almost always manage low-energy pelvic avulsion fractures (Torode and Zieg type I) conservatively with rest and partial weight bearing on crutches for 2 or more weeks, followed by gradual resumption of normal activities after about 6 weeks. For those rare fractures with significant displacement (>2 cm) or persistent disability, fragment fixation or excision may be warranted.

For higher-energy pelvic and acetabular fractures, a multispecialty approach is essential, especially at the time of initial presentation. The team should be aware of the large incidence of concomitant injuries to the head, thorax, and abdomen. The urogenital system should be carefully evaluated, specifically looking for open fractures. If there is hemodynamic instability, the trauma surgeon, orthopaedic surgeon, radiologist, and blood bank should work together to stabilize the patient. The orthopaedic surgeon can provide temporary relief with pelvic wrapping, external fixation, or pelvic packing depending on the treatment of other injuries. If needed, operative fixation can be done in the same session as surgery for associated injuries or it can be timed later when the patient is stabilized.

Definitive treatment is usually conservative for isolated iliac wing fractures (Torode and Zieg type II) and simple pubis and ischium fractures (Torode and Zieg type III) and consists of symptomatic treatment and protected weight bearing. For toddlers and younger school-aged children, this treatment may include a spica cast for immobilization and comfort. For more involved pelvic and acetabular fractures, treatment is more likely to be conservative in children with an immature pelvis and operative in children with an unstable fracture pattern and a mature pelvis or closed triradiate cartilage.[78] There is mounting evidence that unstable pelvic ring fractures and displaced acetabular fractures in children should be operatively reduced and stabilized using the same principles as in adults. Given the technically demanding nature of these operations, it is important that the surgeon has experience with these procedures and, if necessary, we recommend consultation and collaboration with an adult orthopaedic traumatologist.

Torode and Zieg class IV injuries with displacement and/or pelvic ring fractures with displacement of more than 1 cm and anterior and posterior ring fractures should undergo reduction and fixation. Open reduction of the SI joint or a posterior iliac injury can be performed with a combination of plate and/or screws. The approach can be anterior in the iliac fossa or posterior, depending on the fracture characteristics. SI screws can be used in the immature pelvis, but preoperative planning is imperative to ensure a safe corridor for screw placement. Imaging, including the use of fluoroscopy for placement of the screws, is necessary. With a widened symphysis, anterior external fixation or plating is recommended along with posterior stabilization. Similarly, we advocate ORIF for any pediatric acetabular fracture that is associated with hip instability, incongruity of the joint, or significant displacement of the triradiate cartilage. The surgical approach and technique for fixation is dictated by the fracture pattern.

MANAGEMENT OF EXPECTED ADVERSE OUTCOMES AND UNEXPECTED COMPLICATIONS RELATED TO PELVIC AND ACETABULAR FRACTURES

Pelvic and Acetabular Fractures:
ADVERSE OUTCOMES AND COMPLICATIONS

- Malunion of the pelvic ring leading to leg length discrepancy, hip and spine arthrosis, SI joint pain or fusion, and distortion of the birth canal, hindering vaginal delivery
- Premature triradiate closure after acetabular fractures leading to acetabular dysplasia and premature hip arthrosis
- Heterotopic ossification that causes pain at the site, hip impingement, and restricted hip range of motion
- Genitourinary complications including urethral and bladder injury, incontinence, chronic pelvic floor pain, and sexual dysfunction
- Disability related to associated injuries such as traumatic brain injury, thoracoabdominal trauma, and lumbosacral plexus disruption
- Venous thromboembolism from the traumatic injury, immobilization, or as a complication of surgery

The major adverse outcomes following treatment of pediatric pelvic and acetabular fractures are malunion of the pelvic ring leading to long-term morbidity and premature triradiate closure after acetabular fracture. Because of the rapid healing in young children, loss of reduction and nonunion usually are not problems. Malunion of the pelvis can lead to leg length discrepancy, SI joint arthrosis, back pain, lumbar scoliosis, incompetency of the pelvic floor, and distortion of the birth canal. Because of the possibility of dystocia during childbirth, pelvimetry is recommended before pregnancy; however, vaginal delivery is generally still safe.[104] Schwarz et al.[77] reported leg length discrepancies of 1 to 5 cm in 10 of 17 patients after nonoperative treatment of unstable pelvic fractures; 5 had low back pain at long-term follow-up. Heeg and Klasen[33] reviewed 18 children with unstable pelvic fractures and reported that 9 had a leg length discrepancy greater than 1 cm and 3 had back pain. For those patients with growth remaining, an appropriately timed epiphysiodesis may be used to manage any residual leg length discrepancy. Of course, the best way to avoid the negative effects of pelvic malunion is to achieve and maintain an adequate initial reduction.

Acetabular dysplasia, secondary to growth arrest of the triradiate cartilage, is a concerning complication after trauma to the acetabulum. Premature closure of the triradiate cartilage has an overall incidence of less than 5% (range 0%–11%) after pediatric acetabular fractures.[52,102] Heeg et al.[35] reported acetabular deformity and subluxation of the hip in two of three patients with premature fusion of the triradiate cartilage. Peterson and Robertson[66] reported formation of a physeal osseous bar in a 7-year-old boy 2 years after fracture of the lateral portion of the superior ramus

Annotated References

Reference	Annotation
Greenwald LJ, Yost MT, Sponseller PD, et al. The role of clinically significant venous thromboembolism and thromboprophylaxis in pediatric patients with pelvic or femoral fractures. *J Pediatr Orthop.* 2012;32(4):357–361.	The records of 1,782 children with pelvic or femoral fractures admitted to a single institution were reviewed. Over 90% did not receive thromboprophylaxis. Only 3 (0.17%) patients had a diagnosis of deep vein thrombosis, none were diagnosed with a pulmonary embolism, and there was no related mortality.
Holden CP, Holman J, Herman MJ. Pediatric pelvic fractures. *J Am Acad Orthop Surg.* 2007;15(3):172–177.	Pelvic and acetabular fractures are uncommon but often associated with life-threatening injuries. This article summarizes the assessment and care of these injuries in children.
McDonnell M, Schachter AK, Phillips DP, Liporace FA. Acetabular fracture through the triradiate cartilage after low-energy trauma. *J Orthop Trauma.* 2007;21(7):495–498.	This article presents an uncommon acetabular fracture through the triradiate cartilage and describes the possible long-term complications.
Shore BJ, Palmer CS, Bevin C, et al. Pediatric pelvic fracture: a modification of a preexisting classification. *J Pediatr Orthop.* 2012;32(2):162–168.	One hundred and twenty-four children with pediatric pelvic fractures were identified and classified based on a modified Torode and Zieg classification. The classification was found to be predictive of increased hospital care and blood product use.
Silber JS, Flynn JM. Changing patterns of pediatric pelvic fractures with skeletal maturation: implications for classification and management. *J Pediatr Orthop.* 2002;22(1):22–26.	One hundred and sixty-six pelvic fractures were reviewed, of which 80% had radiographs adequate to evaluate the triradiate cartilage, which was used to determine maturity. Ninety-seven were determined to be immature (mean age 5.7) and 32 mature (mean age 14). The immature more commonly had isolated stable fractures while those in the mature group were more likely to have acetabular fractures and pubic or SI diastasis, and all operative procedures were done in this group.
Smith WR, Oakley M, Morgan SJ. Pediatric pelvic fractures. *J Pediatr Orthop.* 2004;24(1):130–135.	This article reviewed 230 pediatric pelvic fractures, 23 of which were unstable. Eighteen patients were treated operatively. They noted limited remodeling of the pelvis over medium-term follow-up. Patients with greater than 1.1 cm of residual asymmetry were more likely to have nonstructural scoliosis, lumbar pain, Trendelenburg sign, and SI joint dysfunction.
Swaid F, Peleg K, Alfici R, et al. A comparison study of pelvic fractures and associated abdominal injuries between pediatric and adult blunt trauma patients. *J Pediatr Surg.* 2017;52(3):386–389.	This study is a retrospective review of 7,621 patients in a national registry. They were classified as children (0–14 years old) and adults (15–64 years old). There was a much lower incidence of these injuries in children (0.8% vs. 4.3%), and the severity of the pelvic injury was greater in adults, although in this study the morbidity was similar. The most common mechanism is pedestrian versus car in children versus motor vehicle accident in adults.
Tarman GJ, Kaplan GW, Lerman SL, et al. Lower genitourinary injury and pelvic fractures in pediatric patients. *Urology.* 2002;59(1):123–126.	Over 8,000 trauma patients presenting to a pediatric trauma center were reviewed, of which 212 patients had pelvic fractures. Seventeen percent were found to have genitourinary injuries, but of these, less than 3% had significant lower genitourinary injuries, and none were found in stable pelvic fractures or in the absence of gross hematuria.

REFERENCES

1. Abdelgawad AA, Davey S, Salmon J, et al. Ilio-sacral (IS) screw fixation for sacral and sacroiliac joint (SIJ) injuries in children. *J Pediatr Orthop.* 2016;36(2):117–121.
2. Al-Mahdi W, Ibrahim MM, Spiegel DA, et al. Is systemic inflammatory response syndrome relevant to pulmonary complications and mortality in multiply injured children? *J Pediatr Orthop.* 2020;40(1):1–7.
3. Badina A, Vialle R, Fitoussi F, Damsin JP. Case reports: treatment of traumatic triradiate cartilage epiphysiodesis. What is the role of bridge resection? *Clin Orthop Relat Res.* 2013;471(11):3701–3705.
4. Banierink H, Reininga IHF, Heineman E, et al. Long-term physical functioning and quality of life after pelvic ring injuries. *Arch Orthop Trauma Surg.* 2019;139(9):1225–1233.
5. Bent MA, Hennrikus WL, Latorre JE, et al. Role of computed tomography in the classification of pediatric pelvic fractures-revisited. *J Orthop Trauma.* 2017;31(7):e200–e204.
6. Blanchard C, Kushare I, Boyles A, et al. Traumatic, posterior pediatric hip dislocations with associated posterior labrum osteochondral avulsion: recognizing the acetabular "fleck" sign. *J Pediatr Orthop.* 2016;36(6):602–607.
7. Blasier RD, McAtee J, White R, Mitchell DT. Disruption of the pelvic ring in pediatric patients. *Clin Orthop Relat Res.* 2000;(376):87–95.
8. Brown GA, Willis MC, Firoozbakhsh K, et al. Computed tomography image-guided surgery in complex acetabular fractures. *Clin Orthop Relat Res.* 2000;(370):219–226.
9. Bucholz RW, Ezaki M, Ogden JA. Injury to the acetabular triradiate physeal cartilage. *J Bone Joint Surg Am.* 1982;64(4):600–609.
10. Burgess AR, Eastridge BJ, Young JW, et al. Pelvic ring disruptions: effective classification system and treatment protocols. *J Trauma.* 1990;30(7):848–856.
11. Chia JPY, Holland AJA, Little D, Cass DT. Pelvic fractures and associated injuries in children. *J Trauma.* 2004;56(1):83–88.
12. Clancy WG Jr, Foltz AS. Iliac apophysitis and stress fractures in adolescent runners. *Am J Sports Med.* 1976;4(5):214–218.
13. Delaney KM, Reddy SH, Dayama A, et al. Risk factors associated with bladder and urethral injuries in female children with pelvic fractures: an analysis of the National Trauma Data Bank. *J Trauma Acute Care Surg.* 2016;80(3):472–476.
14. Demetriades D, Karaiskakis M, Velmahos GC, et al. Pelvic fractures in pediatric and adult trauma patients: are they different injuries? *J Trauma.* 2003;54(6):1146–1151.
15. Dong Y, Wang J, Qin J, et al. Retrospective analysis of traumatic triradiate cartilage injury in children. *BMC Musculoskelet Disord.* 2021;22(1):674.

16. Dora C, Zurbach J, Hersche O, Ganz R. Pathomorphologic characteristics of post-traumatic acetabular dysplasia. *J Orthop Trauma*. 2000;14(7):483–489.

17. Fitze G, Dahlen C, Zwipp H. Acetabular avulsion fracture in a 13-year-old patient after a minor trauma. *J Pediatr Surg*. 2008;43(3):E13–E16.

18. Gepstein R, Weiss RE, Hallel T. Acetabular dysplasia and hip dislocation after selective premature fusion of the triradiate cartilage. An experimental study in rabbits. *J Bone Joint Surg Br*. 1984;66(3):334–336.

19. Giannoudis PV, Pape HC. Damage control orthopaedics in unstable pelvic ring injuries. *Injury*. 2004;35(7):671–677.

20. Gonzalez KW, Dalton BG, Kerisey MC, et al. Pelvic angiography for trauma in children: a rare but useful adjunct. *Eur J Pediatr Surg*. 2017;27(2):196–199.

21. Gordon RG, Karpik K, Hardy S, Mears DC. Techniques of operative reduction and fixation of the pediatric adolescent pelvic fractures. *Oper Tech Ortho*. 1995;5:95–114.

22. Greenwald LJ, Yost MT, Sponseller PD, et al. The role of clinically significant venous thromboembolism and thromboprophylaxis in pediatric patients with pelvic or femoral fractures. *J Pediatr Orthop*. 2012;32(4):357–361.

23. Grisoni N, Connor S, Marsh E, et al. Pelvic fractures in a pediatric level 1 trauma center. *J Orthop Trauma*. 2002;16(7):458–463.

24. Grosso NP, Van Dam BE. Total coccygectomy for the relief of coccygodynia: a retrospective review. *J Spinal Disord*. 1995;8(4):328–330.

25. Guillamondegui OD, Mahboubi S, Stafford PW, Nance ML. The utility of the pelvic radiograph in the assessment of pediatric pelvic fractures. *J Trauma*. 2003;55(2):236–239.

26. Guillaume JM, Pesenti S, Jouve JL, Launay F. Pelvic fractures in children (pelvic ring and acetabulum). *Orthop Traumatol Surg Res*. 2020;106(1S):S125–S133.

27. Guzman D, Sabharwal S, Zhao C, Sabharwal S. Venous thromboembolism among pediatric orthopedic trauma patients: a database analysis. *J Pediatr Orthop B*. 2018;27(2):93–98.

28. Haasz M, Simone LA, Wales PW, et al. Which pediatric blunt trauma patients do not require pelvic imaging? *J Trauma Acute Care Surg*. 2015;79(5):828–832.

29. Hamai S, Nakashima Y, Akiyama M, et al. Ischio-pubic stress fracture after periacetabular osteotomy in patients with hip dysplasia. *Int Orthop*. 2014;38(10):2051–2056.

30. Hauschild O, Strohm PC, Culemann U, et al. Mortality in patients with pelvic fractures: results from the German pelvic injury register. *J Trauma*. 2008;64(2):449–455.

31. Hearty T, Swaroop VT, Gourineni P, Robinson L. Standard radiographs and computed tomographic scan underestimating pediatric acetabular fracture after traumatic hip dislocation: report of 2 cases. *J Orthop Trauma*. 2011;25(7):e68–e73.

32. Hébert KJ, Laor T, Divine JG, et al. MRI appearance of chronic stress injury of the iliac crest apophysis in adolescent athletes. *AJR Am J Roentgenol*. 2008;190(6):1487–1491.

33. Heeg M, Klasen HJ. Long-term outcome of sacroiliac disruptions in children. *J Pediatr Orthop*. 1997;17(3):337–341.

34. Heeg M, Klasen HJ, Visser JD. Acetabular fractures in children and adolescents. *J Boint Joint Surg Br*. 1989;71(3):418–421.

35. Heeg M, Visser JD, Oostvogel HJ. Injuries of the acetabular triradiate cartilage and sacroiliac joint. *J Bone Joint Surg Br*. 1988;70(1):34–37.

36. Heinrich SD, Gallagher D, Harris M, Nadell JM. Undiagnosed fractures in severely injured children and young adults. Identification with technetium imaging. *J Bone Joint Surg Am*. 1994;76(4):561–572.

37. Holden CP, Holman J, Herman MJ. Pediatric pelvic fractures. *J Am Acad Orthop Surg*. 2007;15(3):172–177.

38. Hosalkar HS, Pennock AT, Zaps D, et al. The hip antero-superior labral tear with avulsion of rectus femoris (HALTAR)lesion: does the SLAP equivalent in the hip exist? *Hip Int*. 2012;22(4):391–396.

39. Ismail N, Bellemare JF, Mollitt DL, et al. Death from pelvic fracture: children are different. *J Pediatr Surg*. 1996;31(1):82–85.

40. Judet R, Judet J, Letournel E. Fractures of the acetabulum: classification and surgical approaches for open reduction. Preliminary report. *J Bone Joint Surg Am*. 1964;46:1615–1646.

41. Junkins EP Jr, Nelson DS, Carroll KL, et al. A prospective evaluation of the clinical presentation of pediatric pelvic fractures. *J Trauma*. 2001;51(1):64–68.

42. Karunakar MA, Goulet JA, Mueller KL, et al. Operative treatment of unstable pediatric pelvis and acetabular fractures. *J Pediatr Orthop*. 2005;25(1):34–38.

43. Keats TE, Anderson MW. *Atlas of Normal Roentgen Variants that May Stimulate Disease*. Mosby; 2001:371.

44. Keshishyan RA, Rozinov VM, Malakhov OA, et al. Pelvic polyfractures in children. Radiographic diagnosis and treatment. *Clin Orthop Relat Res*. 1995;(320):28–33.

45. Kruppa CG, Khoriaty JD, Sietsema DL, et al. Pediatric pelvic ring injuries: how benign are they? *Injury*. 2016;47(10):2228–2234.

46. Kruppa CG, Sietsema DL, Khoriaty JD, et al. Acetabular fractures in children and adolescents: comparison of isolated acetabular fractures and acetabular fractures associated with pelvic ring injuries. *J Orthop Trauma*. 2018;32(2):e39–e45.

47. Kuhn JP, Slovis TL, Haller JO. *Caffey's Pediatric Diagnostic Imaging*. 10th ed. Mosby; 2004.

48. Labuz DF, Cunningham A, Tobias J, et al. Venous thromboembolic risk stratification in pediatric trauma: a Pediatric Trauma Society Research Committee multicenter analysis. *J Trauma Acute Care Surg*. 2021;91(4):605–611.

49. Lee DH, Jeong WK, Inna P, et al. Bilateral sacroiliac joint dislocation (anterior and posterior) with triradiate cartilage injury: a case report. *J Orthop Trauma*. 2011;25(12):e111–e114.

50. Letournel E, Judet R, Elson RA. *Fractures of the Acetabulum*. 2nd ed. Springer-Verlag; 1993.

51. Lewallen LW, McIntosh AL, Sems SA. Pediatric pelvic ring injuries. *Orthopedics*. 2018;41(5):e701–e704.

52. Liporace FA, Ong B, Mohaideen A, et al. Development and injury of the triradiate cartilage with its effects on acetabular development: review of the literature. *J Trauma*. 2003;54(6):1245–1249.

53. Lynch SA, RenstrômPA. Groin injuries in sport: treatment strategies. *Sports Med*. 1999;28(2):137–144.

54. Magid D, Fishman EK, Ney DR, et al. Acetabular and pelvic fractures in the pediatric patient: value of two- and three-dimensional imaging. *J Pediatr Orthop*. 1992;12(5):621–625.

55. Marmor M, Elson J, Mikhail C, et al. Short-term pelvic fracture outcomes in adolescents differ from children and adults in the National Trauma Data Bank. *J Child Orthop*. 2015;9(1):65–75.

56. Matsuda DK, Calipusan CP. Adolescent femoroacetabular impingement from malunion of the anteroinferior iliac spine apophysis treated with arthroscopic spinoplasty. *Orthopedics*. 2012;35(3):e460–e463.

57. McDonald GA. Pelvic disruptions in children. *Clin Orthop Relate Res*. 1980;151:130–134.

58. McDonnell M, Schachter AK, Phillips DP, Liporace FA. Acetabular fracture through the triradiate cartilage after low-energy trauma. *J Orthop Trauma*. 2007;21(7):495–498.

59. Mennen AHM, Zonneveld I, Bloemers FW, van Embden D. Critical review of the classification and treatment of pediatric pelvic fractures. *Injury*. 2022;53(10):3301–3309.

60. Mosheiff R, Suchar A, Porat S, et al. The "crushed open pelvis" in children. *Injury*. 1999;30(Suppl 2):B14–B18.

61. Nierenberg G, Volpin G, Bialik V, Stein H. Pelvic fractures in children: a follow-up in 20 children treated conservatively. *J Pediatr Orthop B*. 1993;1:140–142.

62. Nieto LL, Camacho SG, Reinoso JP. [Treatment of Torode and Zieg type IV unstable pelvic fractures in children]. *Acta Ortop Mex*. 2010;24(5):338–344.

63. Ochs BG, Marintschev I, Hoyer H, et al. Changes in the treatment of acetabular fractures over 15 years: analysis of 1266 cases treated by the German Pelvic Multicentre Study Group (DAO/DGU). *Injury*. 2010;41(8):839–851.

64. Ogden JA. *Skeletal Injury in the Child*. 3rd ed. Springer-Verlag; 2000.

65. Pennal GF, Tile M, Waddell JP, Garside H. Pelvic disruption: assessment and classification. *Clin Orthop Relat Res*. 1980;(151):12–21.

66. Peterson HA, Robertson RC. Premature partial closure of the triradiate cartilage treated with excision of a physical osseous bar. Case report with a fourteen-year follow-up. *J Bone Joint Surg Am*. 1997;79(5):767–770.

67. Plaisier BR, Meldon SW, Super DM, Malangoni MA. Improved outcome after early fixation of acetabular fractures. *Injury*. 2000;31(2):81–84.

68. Pohlemann T. Pelvic ring injuries: assessment and concepts of surgical management. In: Rüedi T, Murphy W, eds. *AO Principles of Fracture Management*. Thieme; 2000.

69. Ponseti IV. Growth and development of the acetabulum in the normal child. Anatomical, histological, and roentgenographic studies. *J Bone Joint Surg Am*. 1978;60(5):575–585.

70. Reichard SA, Helikson MA, Shorter N, et al. Pelvic fractures in children—review of 120 patients with a new look at general management. *J Pediatr Surg*. 1980;15(6):727–734.

71. Rossi F, Dragoni S. Acute avulsion fractures of the pelvis in adolescent competitive athletes: prevalence, location and sports distribution of 203 cases collected. *Skeletal Radiol*. 2001;30(3):127–131.

72. Rubel IF, Kloen P, Potter HG, Helfet DL. MRI assessment of the posterior acetabular wall fracture in traumatic dislocation of the hip in children. *Pediatr Radiol*. 2002;32(6):435–439.

73. Sagi HC, Coniglione FM, Stanford JH. Examination under anesthetic for occult pelvic ring instability. *J Orthop Trauma*. 2011;25(9):529–536.

74. Schlickewei W, Keck T. Pelvic and acetabular fractures in childhood. *Injury*. 2005;36(Suppl 1):A57–A63.

75. Schlonsky J, Olix ML. Functional disability following avulsion fracture of the ischial epiphysis. Report of two cases. *J Bone Joint Surg Am*. 1972;54(3):641–644.

76. Schuett DJ, Bomar JD, Pennock AT. Pelvic apophyseal avulsion fractures: a retrospective review of 228 cases. *J Pediatr Orthop*. 2015;35(6):617–623.

77. Schwarz N, Posch E, Mayr J, et al. Long-term results of unstable pelvic ring fractures in children. *Injury*. 1998;29(6):431–433.

78. Scolaro JA, Firoozabadi R, Routt ML. Treatment of pediatric and adolescent pelvic ring injuries with percutaneous screw placement. *J Pediatr Orthop*. 2018;38(3):133–137.

79. Sen MK, Warner SJ, Sama N, et al. Treatment of acetabular fractures in adolescents. *Am J Orthop (Belle Mead NJ)*. 2015;44(10):465–470.

80. Sener M, Karapinar H, Kazimoglu C, et al. Fracture dislocation of sacroiliac joint associated with triradiate cartilage injury in a child: a case report. *J Pediatr Orthop B*. 2008;17(2):65–68.

81. Shaath MK, Koury KL, Gibson PD, et al. Analysis of pelvic fracture pattern and overall orthopaedic injury burden in children sustaining pelvic fractures based on skeletal maturity. *J Child Orthop*. 2017;11(3):195–200.

82. Shah MK, Stewart GW. Sacral stress fractures: an unusual cause of low back pain in an athlete. *Spine (Phila Pa 1976)*. 2002;27(4):E104–E108.

83. Shlamovitz GZ, Mower WR, Bergman J, et al. Lack of evidence to support routine digital rectal examination in pediatric trauma patients. *Pediatr Emerg Care*. 2007;23(8):537–543.

84. Shlamovitz GZ, Mower WR, Bergman J, et al. Poor test characteristics for the digital rectal examination in trauma patients. *Ann Emerg Med*. 2007;50(1):25–33, 33.e1.

85. Shore BJ, Palmer CS, Bevin C, et al. Pediatric pelvic fracture: a modification of a preexisting classification. *J Pediatr Orthop*. 2012;32(2):162–168.

86. Silber JS, Flynn JM. Changing patterns of pediatric pelvic fractures with skeletal maturation: implications for classification and management. *J Pediatr Orthop*. 2002;22(1):22–26.

87. Silber JS, Flynn JM, Katz MA, et al. Role of computed tomography in the classification and management of pediatric pelvic fractures. *J Pediatr Orthop.* 2001;21(2):148–151.

88. Silber JS, Flynn JM, Koffler KM, et al. Analysis of the cause, classification, and associated injuries of 166 consecutive pediatric pelvic fractures. *J Pediatr Orthop.* 2001;21(4):446–450.

89. Sinikumpu JJ, Hetsroni I, Schilders E, et al. Operative treatment of pelvic apophyseal avulsions in adolescent and young adult athletes: a follow-up study. *Eur J Ortop Surg Traumatol.* 2018;28(3):423–429.

90. Smith W, Shurnas P, Morgan S, et al. Clinical outcomes of unstable pelvic fractures in skeletally immature patients. *J Bone Joint Surg Am.* 2005;87(11):2423–2431.

91. Smith WR, Oakley M, Morgan SJ. Pediatric pelvic fractures. *J Pediatr Orthop.* 2004;24(1):130–135.

92. Sreeranga YL, Joshi PM, Bandini M, Kulkarni SB. Comprehensive analysis of paediatric pelvic fracture urethral injury: a reconstructive centre experience. *BJU Int.* 2022;130(1):114–125.

93. Stiletto RJ, Baacke M, Gotzen L. Comminuted pelvic ring disruption in toddlers: management of a rare injury. *J Trauma.* 2000;48(1):161–164.

94. Subasi M, Arslan H, Necmioglu S, et al. Long-term outcomes of conservatively treated paediatric pelvic fractures. *Injury.* 2004;35(8):771–781.

95. Sundar M, Carty H. Avulsion fractures of the pelvis in children: a report of 32 fractures and their outcome. *Skeletal Radiol.* 1994;23(2):85–90.

96. Swaid F, Peleg K, Alfici R, et al. A comparison study of pelvic fractures and associated abdominal injuries between pediatric and adult blunt trauma patients. *J Pediatr Surg.* 2017;52(3):386–389.

97. Tarman GJ, Kaplan GW, Lerman SL, et al. Lower genitourinary injury and pelvic fractures in pediatric patients. *Urology.* 2002;59(1):123–126.

98. Tile M. Pelvic fractures: operative versus nonoperative treatment. *Orthop Clin North Am.* 1980;11(3):423–464.

99. Tolo VT. Orthopaedic treatment of fractures of the long bones and pelvis in children who have multiple injuries. *Instr Course Lect.* 2000;49:415–423.

100. Tomaszewski R, Gap A. Operative treatment of pediatric pelvic fractures—our experience. *Orthop Traumatol Rehabil.* 2011;13(3):241–252.

101. Torode I, Zieg D. Pelvic fractures in children. *J Pediatr Orthop.* 1985;5(1):76–84.

102. Trousdale RT, Ganz R. Posttraumatic acetabular dysplasia. *Clin Orthop Relat Res.* 1994;(305):124–132.

103. Upperman JS, Gardner M, Gaines B, et al. Early functional outcome in children with pelvic fractures. *J Pediatr Surg.* 2000;35(6):1002–1005.

104. Vaajala M, Kuitunen I, Nyrhi L, et al. Pregnancy and delivery after pelvic fracture in fertile-aged women: a nationwide population-based cohort study in Finland. *Eur J Obstet Gynecol Reprod Biol.* 2022;270:126–132.

105. Vazquez WD, Garcia VF. Pediatric pelvic fractures combined with an additional skeletal injury is an indicator of significant injury. *Surg Gynecol Obstet.* 1993; 177(5):468–472.

106. Von Heyden J, Hauschild O, Strohm PC, et al. Paediatric acetabular fractures: data from the German Pelvic Trauma Registry Initiative. *Acta Orthop Belg.* 2012;78(5):611–618.

107. Wait A, Gaskill T, Sarwar Z, Busch M. Van neck disease: osteochondrosis of the ischiopubic synchondrosis. *J Pediatr Orthop.* 2011;31(5):520–524.

108. Watts HG. Fractures of the pelvis in children. *Orthop Clin North Am.* 1976;7(3): 615–624.

109. Whiting PS, Auston D, Avilucea FR, et al. Negative stress examination under anesthesia reliably predicts pelvic ring union without displacement. *J Orthop Trauma.* 2017;31(4):189–193.

110. Zwingmann J, Aghayev E, Südkamp NP, et al. Pelvic fractures in children results from the German pelvic trauma registry: a cohort study. *Medicine (Baltimore).* 2015; 94(51):e2325.

24

Fractures and Traumatic Dislocations of the Hip in Children

Chinmay Paranjape and Vidyadhar Upasani

Hip Fractures

INTRODUCTION TO HIP FRACTURES

While hip fractures are common in adults, they are rare in children, comprising less than 1% of all pediatric fractures.[8] In contrast with adult hip fractures which are commonly associated with osteoporosis and low-energy mechanisms, pediatric hip fractures typically result from high-energy mechanisms. This therefore warrants trauma surveys for additional extremity, visceral, or head injuries which are concurrent in 30% of patients. Occasionally, pediatric hip fractures result from minor trauma superimposed upon bone that is weakened by tumor or metabolic bone disease. These fractures can occur through the physis, but more commonly occur through the femoral neck and the intertrochanteric region.

The presence of the proximal femoral physis is an important consideration when treating pediatric hip fractures. Injury to the greater trochanter apophysis can lead to coxa valga. Damage to the proximal femoral physis from fracture or implant use can result in limb length discrepancies, coxa breva or coxa vara. The surgeon should generally place fixation across the physis in older children with poor bone quality, in adolescents who have little growth potential remaining, or if fracture location dictates that adequate fixation must cross the physis.

Pediatric hips are also at risk secondary to their limited blood supply. The physis acts as a barrier to interosseous blood supply to the femoral head. Because of this, and the fact that there is little blood supply to the femoral head from the ligamentum teres, an increased risk of osteonecrosis (ON) is present following hip fracture that may disrupt the important retinacular vessels.

Although they are less common than other pediatric fractures, pediatric hip fractures are important secondary to the high rate of complications and the potential lifetime morbidity that may result from complications. Potential complications from the fracture and its treatment include chondrolysis, ON, varus malunion, nonunion, physeal disruption, and growth abnormalities leading to leg length discrepancy or angular deformities. Because the hip is developing in the growing child, deformities can progress and change with age. However, outcomes for these complex fractures can be significantly improved by adherence to treatment principles.[8]

ASSESSMENT OF HIP FRACTURES

MECHANISMS OF INJURY FOR HIP FRACTURES

Hip fractures in children can be caused by axial loading, torsion, hyperabduction, or a direct blow to the hip. Almost all hip fractures in children are caused by severe, high-energy trauma, such as those seen with motor vehicle accidents or falls from a height.[5,23] With the exception of the physis, the proximal femur in children is extremely strong, and significant force is necessary to cause fracture. If a child suffers a fracture as a result of insignificant trauma, then one should suspect an underlying etiology such as prior injury or surgery, metabolic bone disease, or pathologic lesion of the proximal femur (Fig. 24-1).

Infants with hip fractures and without a plausible cause for fracture should be evaluated for nonaccidental trauma by a careful history and an examination of the skin, other extremities, trunk, and head. Further skeletal radiographic imaging is often indicated, and an evaluation by a child protective team is required to diagnose life-threatening head and visceral injuries that can be easily missed in this group.

INJURIES ASSOCIATED WITH HIP FRACTURES

Because these fractures are caused by high-energy trauma, they are frequently accompanied by associated injuries that can affect the patient's overall outcome. Pape et al.,[53] in a series of 28 patients with a mean follow-up of 11 years, found favorable outcomes in Delbet type II, III, and IV fractures according to Ratliff's criteria.[58] Poorer functional outcomes were attributed to associated head trauma, amputation, or peripheral neurologic damage.[53] In a series of 14 patients with hip fractures, all of which were caused by vehicular accidents or falls from height, 12 patients (86%) had associated injuries including head and facial injury, other fractures, and/or visceral injury.[43] In a series of hip fractures secondary to high-energy trauma, Bagatur and Zorer[4] similarly found associated injuries in 4 of their 17 patients.

SIGNS AND SYMPTOMS OF HIP FRACTURES

The diagnosis of hip fracture in a child is based on the history of high-energy trauma and the typical signs and symptoms of the shortened, externally rotated, and painful lower extremity.

Figure 24-1. A 10-year-old boy with a fracture through a unicameral bone cyst sustained while running for a soccer ball.

Clinical examination is usually obvious, and a patient with a complete fracture is unable to ambulate because of severe pain in the hip and has a shortened, externally rotated extremity. An infant with a hip fracture holds the extremity flexed, abducted, and externally rotated. Infants and newborns with limited ossification of the proximal femur can be challenging patients to diagnose with hip fractures as the differential diagnosis can include infection and congenital dislocation of the hip. In the absence of infection symptoms, pseudoparalysis, shortening, and a strong suspicion are the keys to a fracture diagnosis in this age group.

With an incomplete or stress fracture of the femoral neck, the patient may be able to bear weight with a limp and may demonstrate hip or knee pain only with extremes of range of motion, especially internal rotation. In a case series of six patients under the age of 10 with femoral neck stress fractures, Boyle et al. found that patients presented with a limp that worsened with activity.[12] Only half of the patients experienced pain with the terminal flexion, while the other half had no pain with hip range of motion. With these more subtle injuries, or with a chronic slipped capital femoral epiphysis (SCFE), patients may also present with primary symptoms of medial knee or thigh pain. After the knee is examined, a supine examination of bilateral hips is essential to evaluate for symmetric internal and external rotation and appropriately diagnose these children.

IMAGING AND OTHER DIAGNOSTIC STUDIES FOR HIP FRACTURES

A good-quality anteroposterior (AP) pelvic radiograph will provide a comparison view of the opposite hip if a displaced fracture is suspected. For the pelvic radiograph, the leg should be held in extension and in as much internal rotation as possible without causing extreme pain to the patient. A cross-table lateral radiograph should be considered to avoid further displacement and unnecessary discomfort to the patient from an attempt at a frog-leg lateral view.

Nondisplaced fracture or stress fractures may be difficult to detect on radiographs. Any break or offset of the bony trabeculae near Ward's triangle, the radiolucent area between the principle compressive, secondary compressive, and primary tensile trabeculae in the femoral neck, is evidence of a nondisplaced or impacted fracture (Fig. 24-2). Special studies may be required

Figure 24-2. A: Ward's triangle is the space in the center of the femoral neck formed by the intersection of the principal compressive, secondary compressive, and tensile trabeculae. B: Note the offset in this intersection in this nondisplaced femoral neck fracture. (Copyright SD PedsOrtho.)

Principle compressive group
Principle tensile group
Greater trochanter group
W = Ward's triangle
Secondary compressive group
Secondary tensile group

Figure 24-3. A: Right hip pain with nondisplaced stress fracture. **B:** The T1-weighted image shows the impacted cortex. **C:** The STIR sequence image shows surrounding bony edema.

to reveal an occult fracture as case examples of further displacement of nondisplaced fracture have been reported.[26] Adjunctive studies for stress fracture diagnosis may include a magnetic resonance imaging (MRI), computed tomography (CT) scan, or a technetium bone scan which can demonstrate increased uptake at the fracture site.

The typical MRI appearance of a fracture is a linear black line (low signal) on all sequences surrounded by a high-signal band of bone marrow edema and hemorrhage. The low signal represents the trabecular impaction (Fig. 24-3). MRI may detect an occult hip fracture within the first 24 hours after injury.[31] In addition, pathologic fractures may require special imaging to aid diagnosis or to fully appreciate bone quality which would impact implant selection. MRI is also a useful test when treating a pathologic fracture; this test will delineate soft tissues in and around the fracture, which can provide insight into diagnosis and delineate high-yield areas for biopsy.

In infants, an ultrasound can be used to detect epiphyseal separation. In addition, an ultrasound can demonstrate the presence of an effusion, which may be aspirated to aid in diagnosis. A bloody aspirate is suggestive of fracture, whereas a serous or purulent aspirate suggests synovitis or infection, respectively. If performed in the operating room, an aspiration and confirmatory arthrogram of the hip can also be useful, especially if closed reduction and cast immobilization is chosen as treatment.

In a patient with posttraumatic hip pain without evidence of a fracture, other diagnoses must be considered, including Perthes disease, synovitis, spontaneous hemarthrosis, and infection. A complete blood count, erythrocyte sedimentation rate, C-reactive protein, and vital signs are helpful to evaluate for infection. When the presentation is unclear, a perfusion MRI

to evaluate proximal femoral vascularity may be a useful test to diagnose aseptic ON as a result of Perthes disease or more remote causes of ON. In children under 5 years of age, developmental coxa vara can be confused with an old hip fracture.

CLASSIFICATION OF HIP FRACTURES

Hip Fractures: DELBET CLASSIFICATION	
Type	**Description**
IA	Transepiphyseal fracture without dislocation from the acetabulum
IB	Transepiphyseal fracture with dislocation from the acetabulum
II	Transcervical fracture
III	Cervicotrochanteric (basicervical) fracture
IV	Intertrochanteric fracture

Pediatric hip fractures generally are classified by the method of Delbet (Fig. 24-4). This classification system continues to be useful because it is not only descriptive but also has prognostic significance.[45] In general, more significant rates of ON and growth arrest are noted in fractures in the proximal end of the femoral neck (type I [38–100%] and type II [28–60%] injuries), whereas lower rates of ON are noted in type III (18–27%) and type IV (5%) injuries.[16,38,45] Conversely, the latter two groups tend to have higher rates of significant varus malunion if not treated appropriately. Subtrochanteric fractures

Figure 24-4. Delbet classification of hip fractures in children. I, transepiphyseal with (IB) or without (IA) dislocation from the acetabulum; II, transcervical; III, cervicotrochanteric; and IV, intertrochanteric.

have been included by some in the discussion of proximal femoral fractures, but they are not included in the Delbet classification and are discussed elsewhere in this book.

Type I

Transphyseal fractures occur through the proximal femoral physis, with (type IA) or without (type IB) dislocation of the femoral head from the acetabulum (Fig. 24-5). Such fractures are rare, constituting 8% of hip fractures in children.[30] Approximately half of type I fractures are associated with a dislocation of the capital femoral epiphysis. True transphyseal fractures tend to occur in young children after high-energy trauma[17] and are different from unstable SCFE, which usually follows a prodromal

period of activity-related hip or knee pain. Unstable SCFE differs from traumatic separation as it occurs following minor trauma, which is superimposed on a weakened physis while a true transphyseal fracture is secondary to a high-energy trauma.

Iatrogenic fracture of the physis in children and adolescents has been described as occurring during reduction of a hip dislocation (Fig. 24-6).[11,29] As true physeal fractures are high-energy injuries, it is possible, and perhaps more likely, that these patients had unrecognized physeal injury at the time of dislocation and the epiphysis became displaced during reduction.

Transphyseal fractures without femoral head dislocation have a better prognosis than those with dislocation. Similarly, younger children with these fractures have a better prognosis than older children. ON in younger children is unlikely, although coxa vara,

Figure 24-5. This 2-year-old boy fell from the trampoline and subsequently complained of right hip pain. **A:** AP radiographs were not grossly abnormal. **B:** Frog-leg lateral radiograph revealed a transepiphyseal fracture. **C, D:** Closed reduction in the operating room was stabilized with a percutaneous pin. **E:** At 8 months, he was asymptomatic and there was no evidence of ON.

coxa breva, and premature physeal closure can cause subsequent leg length discrepancy. In cases of femoral head dislocation in a type I fracture, the outcome is poor secondary to ON and premature physeal closure in virtually 100% of patients.[16]

Type II

Transcervical fractures are the most common fracture type (45–50% of all hip fractures).[30] These fractures occur between the proximal femoral physis and the intertrochanteric line. By definition, these fractures are considered intracapsular femoral neck fractures. Nondisplaced transcervical fractures have a better prognosis and a lower rate of ON than displaced fractures, regardless of treatment.[16,45,58] However, ON can still occur in minimally displaced fractures, and this may be secondary to the fact that it is difficult to document how much displacement and spontaneous reduction occurs at the time of trauma. Moon and Mehlman[45]

Figure 24-6. **A:** A 16-year-old with traumatic right hip dislocation. The physis appears intact and a closed reduction was attempted in the OR. **B:** Traumatic right physeal separation seen with closed reduction.

performed a meta-analysis of available literature and documented a 28% incidence of ON in type II fractures. The occurrence of ON is thought to be directly related to fracture displacement, which may lead to disruption or kinking of the blood supply to the femoral head. In addition, the meta-analysis demonstrated higher rates of ON in children older than 10 years at the time of their injury.[45] Because the pediatric hip capsule is tough and less likely to tear, some have hypothesized that a possible etiology of vascular impairment in minimally displaced fractures is intra-articular hemarthrosis leading to increased intracapsular pressure and retinacular vessel compression from tamponade.[16,30]

Type III

Cervicotrochanteric fractures are located at or slightly above the anterior intertrochanteric line and are the second most common type of hip fracture in children, representing about 34% of fractures.[30] It is conceivable that a certain portion of these fractures may be intra- and extracapsular as a result of anatomic differences in capsule insertion. Nondisplaced type III fractures also have a much lower complication rate than displaced fractures. Displaced type III fractures are similar to type II fractures in the type of complications that can occur. The incidence of ON seen with this fracture pattern is 18%, slightly less than in type II fractures.[50] Similar to type II fractures, the risk of ON is directly related to the degree of displacement at the time of injury.[11] Premature physeal closure occurs in 25% of patients, and coxa vara occurs in approximately 14% of patients.[30]

Type IV

Intertrochanteric fractures account for only 12% of hip fractures in children.[30] This fracture is completely extracapsular and has the lowest complication rate of all four types. Nonunion in this fracture is rare. Moon and Mehlman[45] documented a rate of ON of only 5%, which is much lower than in the other types of hip

fractures. Coxa vara and premature physeal closure have occasionally been reported.[17,30,58]

UNUSUAL FRACTURE PATTERNS

Rarely, proximal femoral physeal separation occurs during a difficult delivery and can be confused on radiographs with congenital dislocation of the hip. Type I fracture in a neonate deserves special attention. This injury is exceedingly rare and, because the femoral head is not visible on plain radiographs, the diagnosis can be difficult. The index of suspicion must be high in neonates, after a difficult delivery, who are not moving their leg. The differential diagnosis includes septic arthritis and developmental hip dislocation. Plain radiographs may show a high-riding proximal femoral metaphysis on the involved side, thus mimicking a developmental hip dislocation. Ultrasonography is useful in diagnosis of neonatal proximal femoral physeal fracture; with this test, the cartilaginous head remains in the acetabulum but its dissociation from the femoral shaft can be appreciated. The diagnosis can be missed if there is no history of trauma or if there is an ipsilateral fracture of the femoral shaft.[2] In the absence of a known history of significant trauma in a young child, nonaccidental trauma should be ruled out.

Stress fractures are caused by repetitive injury and result in hip or knee pain and a limp. Pain associated with long-distance running, marching, or a recent increase in physical activity is suggestive of stress fracture. Though in a recent case study of young children with femoral neck fractures, no increase in activity was noted prior to the onset of symptoms.[12] Close scrutiny of high-quality radiographs may identify sclerosis, cortical thickening, or new bone formation. Nondisplaced fractures may appear as faint radiolucencies. If radiographs are inconclusive, adjunctive tests such as MRI, CT, or bone scintigraphy may be helpful.

An unstable SCFE can be mistaken for a traumatic type I fracture; however, SCFE is caused by an underlying abnormality of the physis and occurs after trivial trauma, usually in adolescents, while type I fractures typically occur with significant high-energy trauma in younger children. Often in an SCFE, there may be signs of remodeling or callus formation in the femoral metaphysis.

Fracture after minor trauma suggests weakened bone possibly from systemic disease, tumor, cyst, or infection. If the physical examination (soft tissue bruising) and radiographic evidence of trauma is significant but the history is not consistent, non-accidental trauma must always be considered. In the multiply traumatized patient, it is easy to miss hip fractures that are overshadowed by more dramatic or painful injuries. Radiographs of the pelvis should be obtained and examined carefully in patients with femoral shaft fractures because ipsilateral hip fracture or dislocation can occur.[2] While the rate of ipsilateral femoral neck fracture is reported to be as high as 9% in adults with femoral shaft fractures, this rate is less than 1% in pediatric trauma patients.[15]

PATHOANATOMY AND APPLIED ANATOMY RELATED TO HIP FRACTURES

Ossification of the femur begins in the seventh fetal week. In early childhood, only a single proximal femoral chondroepiphysis exists. The confluence of the greater trochanteric physis with the capital femoral physis along the superior femoral neck and the unique vascular supply to the capital femoral epiphysis makes the immature hip vulnerable to growth derangement and subsequent deformity after a fracture (Fig. 24-7). During the first year of life, the medial portion of this physis grows faster than the lateral, creating an elongated femoral neck by 1 year of age. The capital femoral epiphysis begins to ossify at approximately 4 months in girls and 5 to 6 months in boys. The ossification center of the trochanteric apophysis appears at 4 years in boys and girls.[30] The proximal femoral physis is responsible for the metaphyseal growth in the femoral neck, whereas the trochanteric apophysis contributes to the appositional growth of the greater trochanter and, to a lesser extent, to the metaphyseal growth of the femur.[20] Closure of the proximal femoral and trochanteric physis occurs at about the age of 14 in girls and 16 in boys.

VASCULAR ANATOMY

The frequency and sequelae of ON of the hip in children has led to extensive study of the blood supply of the femoral head.[52] Postmortem injection and microangiographic studies have elucidated vascular changes with age. These observations are as follows:

- At birth and before age 3 to 4 months, the ligamentum teres provides a minor contribution to head perfusion along with branches of the medial and lateral femoral circumflex vessels (the metaphyseal vessels). The metaphyseal vessels traverse the neck.
- These arteries gradually diminish in size as the cartilaginous physis develops and forms a barrier, preventing transphyseal continuity of these vessels into the femoral head. As a result, the metaphyseal blood supply to the femoral head is virtually nonexistent by age 4.
- From ages 18 months to 4 years, the predominant supply shifts to the terminal retinacular branches of the medial femoral circumflex.
- These branches run along the posterior and superior aspect of the femoral neck before penetrating the lateral edge of the femoral epiphysis. The lateral epiphyseal vessels extend superiorly on the exterior of the neck, bypassing the physeal barrier, and continuing into the epiphysis.

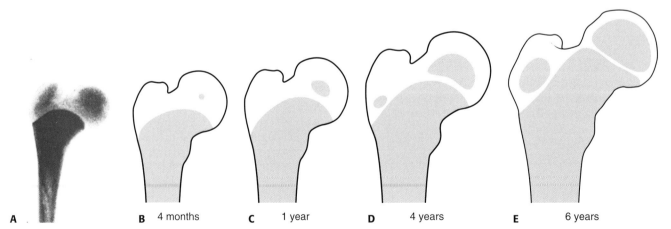

A   **B** 4 months   **C** 1 year   **D** 4 years   **E** 6 years

Figure 24-7. The transformation of the preplate to separate growth zones for the femoral head and greater trochanter. The diagram shows development of the epiphyseal nucleus. **A:** Radiograph of the proximal end of the femur of a stillborn girl, weight 325 g. **B–E:** Drawings made on the basis of radiographs. (Reprinted with permission from Edgren W. Coxa plana: a clinical and radiological investigation with particular reference to the importance of the metaphyseal changes for the final shape of the proximal part of the femur. *Acta Orthop Scand Suppl.* 1965;84:1–129.)

- Many names have been used to describe these vessels. These include the lateral cervical ascending artery, the lateral epiphyseal vessels, and the superior retinacular vessels
- Ogden[52] noted that the lateral epiphyseal vessels consist of two branches: the posterosuperior and posteroinferior branches of the medial circumflex artery. At the level of the intertrochanteric groove, the medial circumflex artery branches into a retinacular arterial system (the posterosuperior and posteroinferior arteries). These arteries penetrate the capsule and traverse proximally (covered by the retinacular folds) along the neck of the femur to supply the femoral head peripherally and proximal to the physis.
- At about 3 to 4 years of age, the lateral posterosuperior vessels appear to predominate and supply the entire anterior lateral portion of the capital femoral epiphysis. The posteroinferior and posterosuperior arteries persist and supply the femoral head throughout life.
- The vessels of the ligamentum teres are of virtually no importance. They contribute little blood supply to the femoral head until age 8, and then only about 20% as an adult.

A thorough understanding of the vascular anatomy of the femoral head is needed for understanding pediatric hip fractures (Fig. 24-8). The multiple small vessels of the young coalesce with age to a limited number of larger vessels. As a result, damage to a single vessel can have serious consequences; for example, occlusion of the posterosuperior branch of the medial circumflex artery can cause ON of the anterior lateral portion of the femoral head.

This anatomy accordingly informs the advised location for capsulotomy. To decrease iatrogenic injury to existing blood supply, anterior capsulotomy is performed. It is suspected that anterior capsulotomy does not damage the blood supply to the femoral head if the intertrochanteric notch and the superior lateral ascending cervical vessels are avoided.

SOFT TISSUE ANATOMY

The pediatric hip joint is enclosed by a thick fibrous capsule that is considered less likely to tear than in adult hip fractures. Bleeding within an intact capsule may lead to a tense hemarthrosis after intracapsular fracture which can theoretically tamponade the ascending cervical vessels and may have implications in the development of ON. The hip joint is surrounded by a protective cuff of musculature; as such, open hip fracture is rare. In the absence of associated hip dislocation, neurovascular injuries are rare.

The sciatic nerve emerges from the sciatic notch beneath the piriformis and courses superficial to the external rotators and the quadratus femoris medial to the greater trochanter. The lateral femoral cutaneous nerve lies in the interval between the tensor and sartorius muscles and supplies sensation to the lateral thigh. This nerve can be identified and preserved during an anterolateral approach to the hip. The femoral neurovascular bundle is separated from the anterior hip joint by the iliopsoas. Thus, any retractor placed on the anterior acetabular rim should be carefully placed deep to the iliopsoas to protect the femoral bundle. Inferior and medial to the hip capsule, coursing

Figure 24-8. The vascular anatomy of the proximal femur. Views sagittally with the abductors reflected and the capsule opened. The blood supply to the femoral head branches from the femoral artery as follows: the profunda femoris (PF) becomes the medial femoral circumflex (MFC) and lateral femoral circumflex (LFC). The predominant blood supply to the head emanates from the medial femoral circumflex, which gives rise to the deep branch with an ascending limb (AL) that is joined by the piriformis branch of the inferior gluteal artery (IGA). The terminal branches of this supply to the femoral upper epiphysis are the retinacular vessels that lie superiorly and posteriorly (RV).

from the deep femoral artery toward the posterior hip joint, is the medial femoral circumflex artery. Placement of a distal Hohmann retractor too deeply can tear this artery, and control of the bleeding may be difficult.

TREATMENT OPTIONS FOR HIP FRACTURES

The goal of treatment in all pediatric hip fractures is primarily anatomic union with a secondary goal of preventing late complications. The most common complications, in order of frequency, are ON, malunion leading to coxa vara, premature physeal arrest and nonunion.[65] Literature supports the concept that attempted conservative treatment can result in unacceptably high rates of coxa vara.[5] Lower rates of ON, coxa vara, and nonunion have been reported in patients who were aggressively treated with anatomic reduction (open or closed) and internal fixation (with or without supplemental casting).[4,19,24] A study that followed 36 patients until healing concluded that patients treated with open reduction had a smaller complication rate and recommended open reduction and internal fixation (ORIF) over closed reduction and internal fixation (CRIF) whenever possible.[6] Current management is directed at early anatomic reduction of these fractures with stable internal fixation and selective use of supplemental external stabilization (casting), with the goal of minimizing devastating late complications.[19,67]

NONOPERATIVE TREATMENT OF HIP FRACTURES

Indications/Contraindications

Nonoperative Treatment of Hip Fractures: INDICATIONS AND CONTRAINDICATIONS
Indications
• Infants and toddlers 0–2 years with stable minimally displaced type I fractures • Nondisplaced type II and III fractures in younger children (0–5 years) • Nondisplaced stress fractures
Relative Contraindications
• Type I fractures >2 years • Displaced fractures • Older children (>5 years with types II and III) fractures

Techniques

Nonoperative treatment in children less than 1 year may be either a Pavlik harness or abduction brace. In older children treated nonoperatively, a single-leg spica cast past the knee may be considered. There are no outcome studies on spica or brace treatment but a spica cast should only be considered in younger children up to 5 years with nondisplaced fractures. Nonoperative and spica cast treatment alone is not optimal in older children as the potential for nonunion is too great not to perform internal fixation.

OPERATIVE TREATMENT OF HIP FRACTURES

Indications/Contraindications

Internal fixation is indicated in children with displaced hip fractures. Internal fixation is also recommended for most acute nondisplaced fractures except in children where size limits the efficacy of internal fixation (0–5 years). Completely nondisplaced fractures may be treated with percutaneous screw placement with or without capsulotomy. Displaced fractures may be treated with attempted CRIF. However, if there is any residual displacement after an attempted closed reduction, an open reduction should be performed to decrease the incidence of ON and nonunion.

Watson-Jones (Anterior Lateral) Approach

Preoperative Planning

✓ **Watson-Jones (Anterior Lateral) Approach:** PREOPERATIVE PLANNING CHECKLIST	
OR table	❏ Fracture table/flattop table to allow adequate imaging
Position/ positioning aids	❏ The patient should have a bump on the back and posterior pelvis to allow access to the region posterior to the greater trochanter
Fluoroscopy location	❏ On the side opposite the operative field ❏ If percutaneous fixation is indicated, two C-arms may be helpful
Equipment	❏ Deep retractors

Surgical Approach

If open reduction is necessary, the Watson-Jones approach is a useful, direct approach to the femoral neck. A lateral incision is made over the proximal femur, slightly anterior to the greater trochanter (Fig. 24-9A). The fascia lata is incised longitudinally (Fig. 24-9B). The innervation of the tensor muscle by the superior gluteal nerve is 2 to 5 cm above the greater trochanter, and care should be taken not to damage this structure. The tensor muscle is reflected anteriorly. The interval between the gluteus medius and the tensor muscles will be used (Fig. 24-9C). The plane is developed between the muscles and the underlying hip capsule (Fig. 24-9D). If necessary, the anterior-most fibers of the gluteus medius tendon can be detached from the trochanter for wider exposure. After clearing the anterior hip capsule, longitudinal capsulotomy is made along the anterosuperior femoral neck. A transverse incision can be added superiorly for wider exposure (Fig. 24-9E). Fracture reduction can be facilitated with a Schanz pin in the proximal fragment and a pointed reduction clamp across the fracture site. Once the hip fracture is reduced, guidewires for cannulated screws can be passed perpendicular to the fracture along the femoral neck from the base of the greater trochanter.

Smith-Petersen (Anterior) Approach

Preoperative Planning

✓ **Smith-Petersen (Anterior) Approach:** PREOPERATIVE PLANNING CHECKLIST	
OR table	❏ Radiolucent
Position/ positioning aids	❏ A bump under the thoracolumbar spine to the posterosuperior iliac spine to access the greater trochanter for screw insertion
Fluoroscopy location	❏ Opposite the surgeon
Equipment	❏ Long retractors

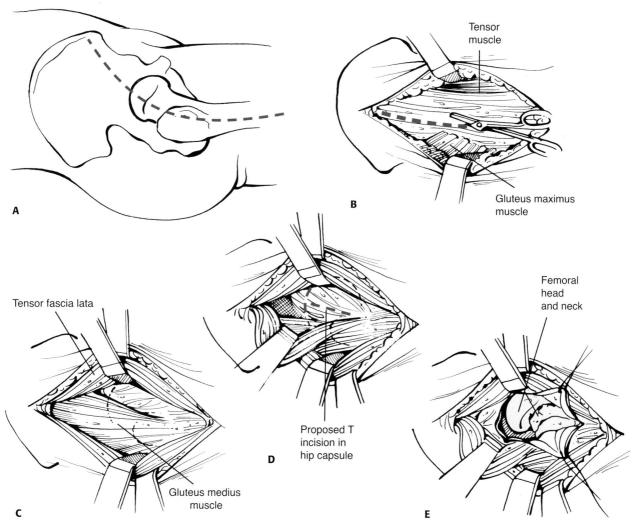

Figure 24-9. Watson-Jones lateral approach to the hip joint for open reduction of femoral neck fractures in children. **A:** Skin incision. **B:** Incision of the fascia lata between the tensor muscle (anterior) and gluteus maximus (posterior). **C:** Exposure of the interval between the gluteus medius and tensor fascia lata (retracted anteriorly). Development of the interval will reveal the underlying hip capsule. **D:** Exposure of the hip capsule. **E:** Exposure of the femoral neck after T incision of the capsule.

Surgical Approach

An oblique incision distal and lateral to the anterosuperior iliac spine can be used through the Smith-Petersen interval (Fig. 24-10). Care should be taken to identify and protect the lateral femoral cutaneous nerve. The fascia over the tensor fascia muscle is opened longitudinally. Blunt dissection is then done to expose the medial aspect of the muscle as far proximal as the iliac crest. The rectus muscle is seen and the lateral fascia of the rectus is incised and the rectus can then be retracted in a medial direction. The fascia on the floor of the rectus is incised longitudinally and the lateral iliopsoas is elevated off the hip capsule in a medial direction to expose the hip capsule. Medial and inferior retractors should be carefully placed around the femoral neck once the capsule is incised to avoid damage to the femoral neurovascular bundle and medial femoral circumflex artery, respectively. Care must be taken not to

violate the intertrochanteric notch and the lateral ascending vessels. Because the lateral aspect of the greater trochanter is not exposed, wires must be passed percutaneously or through a separate lateral incision once the hip fracture is reduced.

Lateral Approach for Decompression

In some cases, an adequate closed reduction can be obtained, thus avoiding the need to open the hip joint for reduction purposes. However, the surgeon may decide to perform a capsulotomy to decompress the hip joint. The authors prefer to do this from a lateral approach. With this method, a 4-cm incision is made distal and lateral to the greater trochanter. From this incision, the fascia lata is incised and guide pins for cannulated screws are placed and screws are inserted in the standard manner. The anterior fibers of the gluteus medius are elevated allowing incision of the anterior capsule with a

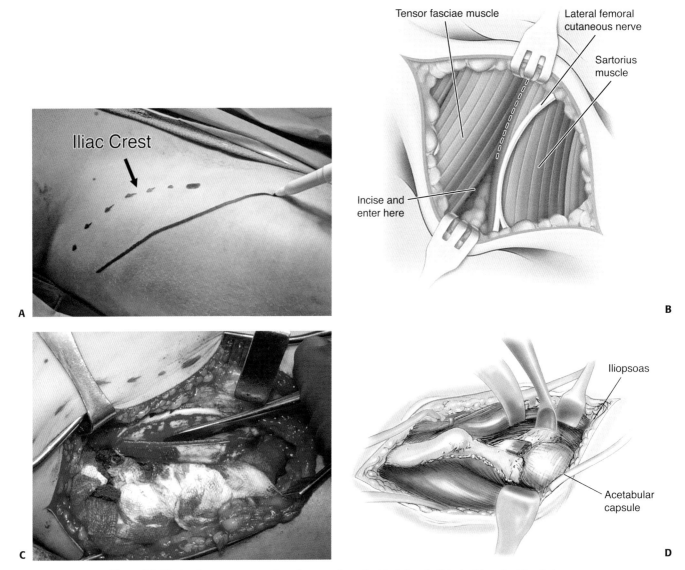

Figure 24-10. Smith-Petersen anterolateral approach to the hip joint. **A:** Skin incision. Incision is 1 cm below the iliac crest and extends just medial to the anterosuperior iliac spine. **B:** Skin is retracted, exposing the fascia overlying the anterosuperior iliac spine. The interval between the sartorius and the tensor fascia lata is identifiable by palpation. **C:** The sartorius is detached from the anterosuperior iliac spine. Splitting of the iliac crest apophysis and detachment of the rectus femoris (shown attached to anteroinferior iliac spine) will facilitate exposure of the hip capsule. **D:** The hip capsule is exposed. A T incision is made to reveal the femoral head and neck. (Reproduced from Flynn JM, et al., eds. *Operative Techniques in Pediatric Orthopaedic Surgery.* 2nd ed. Wolters Kluwer; 2016.)

Cobb elevator, knife, or osteotome. Direct visualization of the capsule is recommended instead of blunt dissection using fluoroscopic guidance.

Surgical Dislocation of the Hip

Preoperative Planning

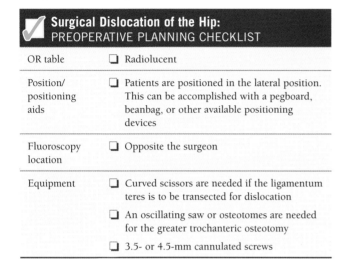

✓ Surgical Dislocation of the Hip: PREOPERATIVE PLANNING CHECKLIST	
OR table	❏ Radiolucent
Position/ positioning aids	❏ Patients are positioned in the lateral position. This can be accomplished with a pegboard, beanbag, or other available positioning devices
Fluoroscopy location	❏ Opposite the surgeon
Equipment	❏ Curved scissors are needed if the ligamentum teres is to be transected for dislocation
	❏ An oscillating saw or osteotomes are needed for the greater trochanteric osteotomy
	❏ 3.5- or 4.5-mm cannulated screws

Positioning

Patients are positioned in the lateral position on a radiolucent table. The opposite leg should be well padded so there is no pressure on the peroneal nerve. An axillary roll is needed and both upper extremities should be carefully positioned to avoid any pressure or tension on the upper extremity and brachial plexus. The complete hip and leg are draped free as high as the iliac crest.

Technique

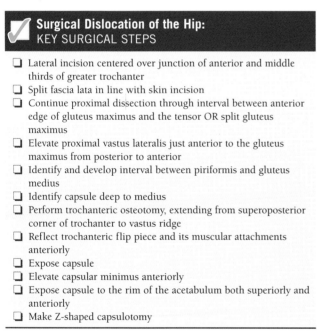

✓ Surgical Dislocation of the Hip: KEY SURGICAL STEPS
❏ Lateral incision centered over junction of anterior and middle thirds of greater trochanter
❏ Split fascia lata in line with skin incision
❏ Continue proximal dissection through interval between anterior edge of gluteus maximus and the tensor OR split gluteus maximus
❏ Elevate proximal vastus lateralis just anterior to the gluteus maximus from posterior to anterior
❏ Identify and develop interval between piriformis and gluteus medius
❏ Identify capsule deep to medius
❏ Perform trochanteric osteotomy, extending from superoposterior corner of trochanter to vastus ridge
❏ Reflect trochanteric flip piece and its muscular attachments anteriorly
❏ Expose capsule
❏ Elevate capsular minimus anteriorly
❏ Expose capsule to the rim of the acetabulum both superiorly and anteriorly
❏ Make Z-shaped capsulotomy

The technique was originally described by Ganz et al.[25] A lateral incision is created centered on the anterior third of the greater trochanter. The leg can then be abducted by placing it on a sterile, padded Mayo stand. The tensor fascia is incised longitudinally in line with the skin incision. Proximally, the dissection may be carried out between the anterior edge of the gluteus maximus and the tensor (Gibson modification[49]), or the gluteus maximus can be split bluntly. This exposes the proximal vastus lateralis, gluteus medius, and greater trochanter.

The leg is then taken off the Mayo stand and positioned with the hip in adduction and slight internal rotation to better visualize the anatomic landmarks. Identify and develop the interval between the piriformis and the gluteus medius. The piriformis is the thick, white tendon visualized deep to the posterior/distal aspect of gluteus medius. Once exposed, the tendon can be gently retracted distally to expose the inferior margin of the gluteus minimus fascia. The inferior fascia of the minimus is then opened to allow the muscle to be retracted in an anterosuperior direction off of the hip capsule. This should allow visualization of the hip capsule.

A greater trochanteric osteotomy is then performed from the posterior border of the vastus lateralis ridge to the anterior to the tip of the greater trochanter using either an oscillating saw or an osteotomy. The width of the osteotomy should be approximately 15 mm (Fig. 24-11). The piriformis and short external rotators should remain attached to the stable trochanteric bed. Maintaining the piriformis tendon intact protects the retinacular branch of the medial circumflex artery. The trochanteric flip piece with attached gluteus minimus, gluteus medius, vastus lateralis, and vastus intermedius is then reflected anteriorly.

Capsular exposure then continues anteriorly and superiorly. Gentle, progressive flexion and external rotation of the operative hip will facilitate the muscle dissection. Capsular muscular attachments are elevated anteriorly to the indirect head of the rectus tendon, superiorly to the superior rim of the acetabulum, and posteriorly to the piriformis.

The hip capsule is then opened in a Z-shaped fashion (Fig. 24-12). The longitudinal limb is along the axis of the femoral neck in line with the iliofemoral ligament. The distal aspect is proximal but in line with the intertrochanteric ridge. The posterior limb of the capsule is opened in the capsular recess of the acetabulum as far posterior as the piriformis tendon, protecting the retinaculum as it pierces the hip capsule. Once the capsule is opened, the intra-articular anatomy and fracture pattern can be visualized.

If surgical hip dislocation is indicated, temporary fixation of the fracture with a threaded Kirschner wire (K-wire) is recommended for safe dislocation. Without temporary fixation, damage may occur to the retinaculum that is easily visualized in the lateral and posterolateral regions of the femoral neck. After temporary fixation, the leg is flexed and externally rotated and the leg placed in a sterile leg bag. The hip is gently subluxated and large, curved large scissors are used to transect the ligamentum teres (Fig. 24-13).

The location and pattern of the hip fracture will dictate next steps after the capsulotomy. After fracture fixation, the hip capsule is reapproximated. The greater trochanter is reduced and

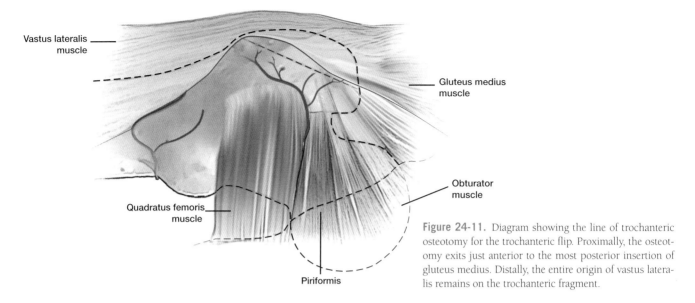

Vastus lateralis
muscle

Gluteus medius
muscle

Obturator
muscle

Quadratus femoris
muscle

Piriformis

Figure 24-11. Diagram showing the line of trochanteric osteotomy for the trochanteric flip. Proximally, the osteotomy exits just anterior to the most posterior insertion of gluteus medius. Distally, the entire origin of vastus lateralis remains on the trochanteric fragment.

fixation with two or three 3.5- or 4.5-mm screws is performed. Weight-bearing restrictions are dependent on the fracture type (Fig. 24-14).

Fracture-Specific Treatment

Type I

Fracture treatment is based on the age of the child, presence of femoral head dislocation, and fracture stability after reduction. In toddlers under 2 years of age with nondisplaced or minimally displaced fractures, simple spica cast immobilization is likely to be successful. Because the fracture tends to displace into varus and external rotation, the limb should be casted in mild abduction and neutral rotation to prevent displacement. Close follow-up in the early postinjury period is critical.

Displaced fractures in toddlers should be reduced closed by gentle traction, abduction, and internal rotation. If the fracture reduces and is stable, casting without fixation is indicated. If casting without fixation is performed, repeat radiographs should be taken in the early postoperative period to look for

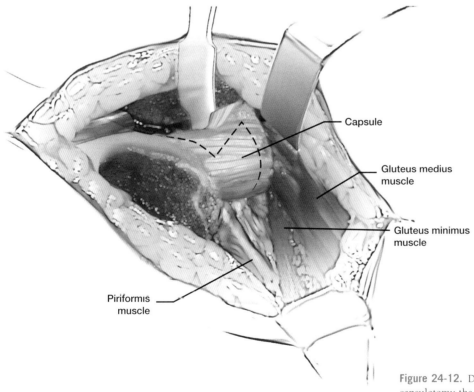

Capsule

Gluteus medius
muscle

Gluteus minimus
muscle

Piriformis
muscle

Figure 24-12. Diagram showing that for the Z-shaped capsulotomy the femur is flexed and externally rotated further (*arrows*). All external rotators are left intact.

Femoral head subluxated

Figure 24-13. Diagram showing that for subluxation and dislocation of the femoral head the hip is flexed, externally rotated and the leg brought over the front of the operating table and placed in a sterile bag.

Figure 24-14. Preoperative AP (**A**) and lateral (**B**) and postoperative AP (**C**) and lateral (**D**) demonstrating three-part Delbet 3 femoral neck fracture fixed via a surgical dislocation approach. (Copyright SD PedsOrtho.)

redisplacement. The likelihood of successful repeat reduction decreases rapidly with time and healing in a young child.

If the fracture is not stable, it should be fixed with small-diameter smooth pins that cross the femoral neck and into the epiphysis. Use of smooth pins will theoretically decrease risk of additional physeal injury in patients with a transphyseal fracture. An arthrogram *after* reduction and stabilization of the fracture may be indicated to ensure alignment is anatomic. An arthrogram *prior* to reduction and pinning may obscure bony detail and hinder assessment during reduction.

Children older than 2 years should have operative fixation, even if the fracture is nondisplaced, because the complications of late displacement are significant. Fixation must cross the physis into the capital femoral epiphysis in order to stabilize the fracture. Smooth pins can be used in young children, but cannulated screws are better for older, larger children, and adolescents. In this older group (>10 years), the effect of eventual limb length discrepancy is small and is a reasonable tradeoff for the superior fixation and stabilization needed to avoid complications in larger and older children.

Closed reduction of type IB fracture-dislocations may be attempted, but immediate open reduction is necessary if a single attempt at closed reduction is unsuccessful. Internal fixation is required to stabilize these injuries. The surgical approach should be dictated by the direction of the femoral head dislocation, most commonly posterolateral. Regardless of treatment technique chosen, parents must be advised in advance about the substantial risk of avascular necrosis (AVN) of the femoral head.

Postoperative spica cast immobilization is recommended for younger children if internal fixation stops distal to the epiphyseal physis, which makes it less stable.

Older, more reliable children may be immobilized in a hip abduction orthosis. Long-term follow-up is required in these patients to watch for growth disturbance and/or AVN. Smooth fixation should be removed shortly after fracture healing to enable further growth. Threaded fixation can be left in place or removed according to surgeon and patient preference.

Type II and Type III

Intracapsular femoral neck fractures require anatomic reduction and, in most cases, internal fixation. In rare cases, children under 5 years of age with nondisplaced, completely stable transcervical or cervicotrochanteric fractures can be managed with spica casting and close follow-up to detect varus displacement in the cast.[30] However, in almost all cases, internal fixation is recommended by most investigators for nondisplaced transcervical fractures[24,30] because the risk of late displacement in such fractures far outweighs the risk of percutaneous screw fixation, especially in young children.[14]

Displaced neck fractures should be treated with anatomic reduction and stable internal fixation to minimize the risk of late complications. Coxa vara and nonunion were frequent in several large series of displaced transcervical fractures treated with immobilization but without internal fixation.[5,16,41] However, when an anatomic closed reduction or ORIF was used, the rates of these complications were much lower.[16,17,24,47,71]

Gentle closed reduction of displaced fractures is accomplished with the use of longitudinal traction, abduction, and internal rotation. Given the findings that reduction quality significantly impacts the risk for postoperative complications, open reduction frequently is necessary for displaced fractures and should be done through a Watson-Jones lateral surgical approach or via separate bikini line anterior Smith-Petersen to assess reduction and lateral proximal femoral approaches for internal fixation.

Internal fixation with cannulated screws is performed through a small lateral incision with planned entry above the level of the lesser trochanter. Care should be taken to minimize drill holes or hardware placement in the subtrochanteric region as they create a stress riser, increasing the risk of subtrochanteric fracture. Two or three screws should be placed; if possible, the most inferior screw should skirt along the calcar with the remaining screws spaced as widely as possible.[13] Often, the small diameter of the child's femoral neck will accommodate only two screws. Alternatively, more modern implants that provide fixed-angle fixation with dynamic compression, such as the Femoral Neck System (FNS) from Synthes, are particularly useful.

In type II fractures, it may be necessary to cross the physis for fixation stability[30,47]; the sequelae of premature physeal closure and trochanteric overgrowth are much less than those of nonunion, pin breakage, and ON. Treatment of the fracture is the priority, and any subsequent growth disturbance and leg length discrepancy are secondary. Consideration may be given to simultaneous capsulotomy or aspiration of the joint to eliminate pressure from a hemarthrosis at the time of surgery.

Displaced cervicotrochanteric (type III) fractures have been shown to have a complication rate similar to that for type II fractures and should be treated similarly. Whenever possible, screws should be inserted short of the physis in type III fractures. Given the more distal anatomic location, fixation generally does not need to cross the physis in these fractures. Alternatively, a pediatric hip compression screw or a pediatric locking hip plate[32] can be used to provide more secure fixation of distal cervicotrochanteric fractures in a child over 5 years of age. These plates can be particularly useful if there is a smaller region for screw purchase distal to the fracture. Spica casting is routine in most type II and III fractures in younger children.[23] Older children, whose screws can cross the physis, may use a hip abduction orthosis as external supplementation to their internal fixation.

Type IV

Good results can be obtained after closed treatment of most intertrochanteric (type IV) fractures in younger children, regardless of displacement. Traction and spica cast immobilization are effective.[11] Instability or failure to maintain adequate reduction and polytrauma are indications for internal fixation.

Older children (>10 years) or those with significant displacement should be treated with internal fixation (Fig. 24-15). A pediatric hip screw, blade plate, or pediatric hip locking plate provide rigid internal fixation for intertrochanteric fractures.

A, B   **C**

Figure 24-15. **A:** A 14-year-old boy who fell from a tree swing sustained this nondisplaced left intertrochanteric hip fracture. **B:** Lateral radiograph shows the long spiral fracture. **C:** Three months after fixation with an adult sliding hip screw.

Smaller hip devices have made ORIF an option in children younger than 10 years. This may avoid the period of spica cast treatment and allow for a more anatomic fracture reduction.

Authors' Preferred Treatment for Hip Fractures

The choice of treatment modality for pediatric hip fractures is based on several key factors:

- The location of the fracture (i.e., Delbet classification)
- The proximity of the fracture to the physis and the need for fixation across the physis
- The age of the patient
- The amount of displacement present

The authors present their preferred techniques below based on fracture classification.

Type I

Nondisplaced or minimally displaced stable fractures in toddlers up to age 2 should be treated with a spica cast without internal fixation. The limb should be casted in a position of abduction and neutral rotation to prevent displacement into varus. If the fracture requires reduction or moves significantly during reduction or casting maneuvers, then internal fixation is mandatory. Two-millimeter smooth K-wires are inserted percutaneously to cross the physis. We recommend two or three wires. Wires should be cut off and bent below the skin for retrieval under a brief general anesthetic when the fractures healed. We do

not recommend leaving the wires outside the skin secondary to the risk for infection. Frequent radiographs are necessary to check for migration of the pins into the joint space. A spica cast is always applied in this age group and should remain in place for at least 6 weeks.[23]

Even if type I fractures in children older than 2 years are anatomically reduced, these patients should always have stabilization with internal fixation. While K-wires are appropriate for small children, 4.0- to 7.3-mm cannulated screws crossing the physis can be considered in older, larger children after closed reduction. Fluoroscopically placing a guide pin from the femoral neck, across the physis, and into the femoral head allows one to locate the proper site for a small incision overlying the lateral femur in line with the femoral neck. Two guide pins are placed into the epiphysis, and the wires are over drilled to the level of the physis (but not across to avoid growth arrest as much as possible). The hard metaphysis and lateral femoral cortex are tapped (in contrast to elderly patients with osteoporosis) to the level of the physis and stainless steel screws are placed.

If gentle closed reduction cannot be achieved, an open approach is preferred. The choice of approach is dictated by surgeon experience and position of the femoral epiphysis. For type IA fractures, an anterior approach or surgical dislocation approach is recommended. For type IB fractures, the choice of approach is dictated by the position of the femoral epiphysis. If it is anterior or inferior, a Watson-Jones approach should be used. On the other hand, most type IB fractures are displaced posteriorly, in which case a posterior approach should be selected. A surgical dislocation approach may also be used to give complete visualization of the hip and retinacular vessels.

Under direct vision, the fracture is reduced, and guidewires are passed from the lateral aspect of the proximal femur up the neck perpendicular to the fracture; predrilling is necessary before the insertion of screws. All children are immobilized. A spica cast is utilized in younger, taller patients. A hip abduction orthosis may be considered in older, larger, more compliant patients.

Older children and adolescents will usually require similar reduction methods on a fracture table, and the fracture is stabilized after closed or, if needed, open reduction. Larger 6.5- or 7.3-mm screws are needed and are placed after predrilling over the guide pins. The screws are placed through a lateral incision, and an anterior capsulotomy is performed. Such stout fixation usually obviates the need for spica casting in an adolescent but, if future patient compliance or fracture stability is in doubt, some type of external stabilization may be used. The lateral position is utilized for the surgical dislocation approach. The fracture can be reduced without the need for a traction table in the surgical dislocation approach.

Type II

Given the potential jeopardy to blood supply in type II fractures, we always desire anatomic reduction. Preoperative CT is valuable in confirming displacement, comminution, and other factors affecting the ability to obtain an anatomic reduction. For truly nondisplaced fractures, closed reduction is appropriate. However, any degree of displacement or comminution mandates open reduction to confirm adequacy of reduction. It is critical that the fracture be reduced anatomically to decrease the potential of nonunion and AVN. Our preference is an anterior Smith-Petersen bikini line incision to open the hip capsule and confirm the reduction paired with a laterally based incision to apply internal fixation. If there is experience with the surgical dislocation approach, this will give the surgeon visualization for fracture reduction and fixation. Both approaches allow the fracture to be anatomically reduced under direct vision.

Once the fracture is visualized and anatomically reduced, guidewires are then placed up the femoral neck perpendicular to the fracture. If possible, penetration of the physis should be avoided.[23] However, in most unstable type II fractures, crossing of the physis may be necessary to achieve stability and avoid the complications associated with late displacement.[11]

If the surgeon selects a surgical dislocation approach, the reduction can usually be performed without dislocation of the femoral head from the acetabulum. If femoral head dislocation is required, the fracture and femoral head should be provisionally reduced and fixed prior to subluxation and transecting the ligamentum teres to prevent traction on the retinaculum with the dislocation. Once dislocated, a guidewire can be placed retrograde through the fovea.

Type II fractures should be stabilized with 4- to 4.5-mm cannulated screws in small children up to age 8. After the age of 8, fixation with 6.5-mm or 7.3-mm cannulated screws is appropriate. Two or three appropriately sized screws should be used, depending on the size of the child's femoral neck. As in type I fractures, we recommend placing at least two guide pins. Similarly, predrilling the femoral neck is necessary to avoid displacement of the fracture while advancing the screws. Recent advances in instrumentation in the adult population, such as the Synthes Femoral Neck System (FNS) may be useful and appropriate in the adolescent population. Their relative advantage is the ability to apply a fixed-angle device without risk of rotation during application as was present in prior generations of implants such as the dynamic hip screw (DHS) (Fig. 24-16). Finally, we believe that if the physis is not crossed with implants, supplementary spica casting is needed to prevent malunion or nonunion.

Type III

Type III fractures do not pose the same risk to the blood supply of the head as type II fractures and therefore, we recommend attempted closed reduction for these fracture types. A fracture table can be useful, though potentially makes an open procedure more difficult if the reduction is unable to be obtained closed. As a result, we recommend positioning on a radiolucent flat top table. An assistant may apply a combination of longitudinal traction, adduction, and internal rotation with attempted closed reduction. If an anatomic reduction is obtained, fixation with either cannulated screws or a rigid, fixed-angle device, is therefore possible as described for type II fractures. The same open reduction maneuvers may be necessary as described in type II fractures if closed reduction is nonanatomic.

Type IV

Nondisplaced type IV fractures in children younger than 3 to 4 years are treated without internal fixation with immobilization in a spica cast for 6 to 12 weeks. Great care is needed to cast the limb in a position that best aligns the bone (Fig. 24-17A,B). Frequent radiographic examination is necessary to assess for late displacement, particularly into varus. In some cases, it may be difficult to assess reduction in a spica cast, and additional imaging like a limited CT scan may be useful (Fig. 24-17C,D).

Displaced type IV fractures in children over 3 years should be treated with internal fixation with a pediatric or juvenile compression hip screw or pediatric locking hip plate placed into femoral neck, with neck fixation stopping short of the physis. It is important to place a derotation wire prior to drilling and tapping the neck for the DHS. Closed reduction often is possible with a combination of traction and internal rotation of the limb. If open reduction is necessary, a lateral approach with anterior extension to close reduce the fracture is preferred.

Figure 24-16. Coronal (**A**) and axial (**B**) views of displaced femoral neck fracture (Delbet II) in a 13-year-old boy who fell during a ski jump. **C, D:** This was fixed using a rigid fixed-angle device, the Synthes Femoral Neck System. (Copyright SD PedsOrtho.)

Postoperative Care

In general, we believe supplementary casting or bracing should be considered for most patients with proximal femoral fractures. For instance, casting is indicated in all type I fractures except in the rare adolescents who have been treated with two to three large screws that cross the physis and who will be compliant with restricted weight bearing. For type II and III fractures, we recommend a hip spica cast to be used for at least 6 weeks in all patients whose implants do not cross the femoral physis. This recommendation makes sense when one considers

that in children younger than 10, we try to avoid crossing the physis, and these patients usually do well with these casts. On the other hand, children older than 12 years can be treated with transphyseal fixation that will be stable enough to avoid casting, which coincidently also tends to be poorly tolerated in this age group. For children 10 to 12 years, the use of a postoperative cast depends on the stability of fracture fixation and the patient's compliance; if either is in doubt, a single hip spica cast is used.

Type IV fractures treated with a hip screw and side plate do not require cast immobilization. Formal rehabilitation usually is

Figure 24-17. A: A 4-year-old boy fell from a window, causing a displaced type IV fracture. **B:** Positioning of the hip in a spica cast is usually in hip flexion and confirmed under fluoroscopy. **C:** Fluoroscopic radiographs in 90 degrees of hip flexion ensure anatomic correctness. **D:** At 1-week follow-up, radiographs were inconclusive; a CT scan assists in confirming the location.

unnecessary unless there is a severe persistent limp, which may be due to abductor weakness. Stiffness is rarely a problem in the absence of ON.

Potential Pitfalls and Preventive Measures

Hip Fracture Repair: POTENTIAL PITFALLS AND PREVENTION	
Pitfall	**Preventions**
Nonunion	• Anatomic reduction, open the fracture site if necessary • Stable internal fixation, cross the physis if necessary • Spica cast supplemental immobilization for children <10 or 10–12 years old if there is a concern for stabilization
AVN	• Urgent reduction in <24 hours • Open reduction or capsulotomy if reduction is closed • Anatomic reduction
Physeal arrest	• Stop the fixation distal to the physis but do not compromise stability. Most type III and IV fractures can achieve stable fixation without crossing the physis • If the stability of fracture fixation is not enough with implants distal to the physis, the surgeon must cross the physis • Consider removal of implants once the fracture has bony union

Management of Expected Adverse Outcomes and Unexpected Complications Related to Hip Fractures

OSTEONECROSIS

ON is the most serious and frequent complication of hip fractures in children and is the primary cause of poor results after fractures of the hip in children.[43] Its overall prevalence is approximately 30%, based on the literature.[18,30] The risk of ON is highest after displaced type IB, II, and III fractures (Fig. 24-18).[11] In the meta-analysis by Moon and Mehlman,[45] the incidences of ON in type I through type IV are 38%, 28%, 18%, and 5%, respectively. In addition to location of the fracture (as described by the Delbet classification), ON is believed to be increased with increased initial fracture displacement and older age at the time of injury.[16,39]

Several studies report lower rates of ON in their series of patients treated within 24 hours of injury with prompt reduction and internal fixation.[18,30] In contrast, other studies have

Figure 24-18. A: A 14-year-old girl with a type II fracture of the left femoral neck. **B:** After fixation with three cannulated screws. **C:** Osteonecrosis with collapse of the superolateral portion of the femoral head. **D:** After treatment with valgus osteotomy.

demonstrated no association between early treatment and risk for AVN.[72] It is hypothesized that early reduction and stabilization may decrease ON by preventing further injury to the tenuous blood supply, and alleviating the tamponade effect, as open reduction or capsulotomy may decrease intra-articular pressure caused by fracture hematoma.[33] The efficacy of alleviating the "tamponade effect" has equivocal support in the literature, with some articles reporting that aspirating the hematoma may decrease the intracapsular pressure and increase blood flow to the femoral head[19] and others suggesting that this may have little effect.[33,45]

Perhaps the most important modifiable factor in reducing ON is the quality of reduction. Schrader et al. found that better quality reduction and the use of modern cannulated implants reduced the risk of ON in their study population.[67] Timing to the operating room has remained controversial, though a 2013 systematic review suggested the odds ratio of developing ON

when definitive treatment was delayed more than 24 hours was 4.2.[76] The addition of a capsulotomy has not been previously associated with reducing ON.

ON has been classified by Ratliff as follows: type I, involvement of the whole head; type II, partial involvement of the head; and type III, an area of necrosis of the femoral neck from the fracture line to the physis[67] (Fig. 24-19). Type I is the most severe, the most common form, and has the poorest prognosis. Type I most likely results from damage to all of the retinacular epiphyseal vessels. Type II is secondary to localized damage to one or more of the lateral epiphyseal vessels near their insertion into the anterolateral aspect of the femoral head. And type III ON is from damage to the superior metaphyseal vessels. Type III is rare, but has a good prognosis provided the fracture goes on to heal.[67] Signs and symptoms of ON usually develop within the first year after injury, with a mean time to presentation of just

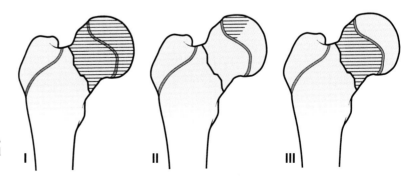

Figure 24-19. The three types of osteonecrosis. Type I, whole head; type II, partial head; and type III, femoral neck.

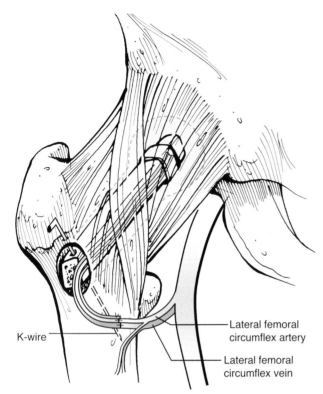

K-wire

Lateral femoral
circumflex artery

Lateral femoral
circumflex vein

Figure 24-20. Vascularized fibular grafting for osteonecrosis of the femoral head. (Redrawn with permission from Aldrich JM III, et al. Free vascularized fibular grafting for the treatment of postcollapse osteonecrosis of the femoral head. *J Bone Joint Surg Am.* 2004;86(suppl 1):87–101.)

over 11 months, but patients may not become symptomatic for up to 2 years.[15,33,66] Some authors have utilized bone scan for early detection of ON to manage family expectations and guide potential treatment. Ramachandran et al.[57] treated 28 patients with early bone scan changes of ON from SCFE or femoral neck fracture. The group was treated with an intravenous bisphosphonate (pamidronate or zoledronate) for an average of 20 months, which greatly improved the outcome at 3-year follow-up. The long-term results of established ON are likely related to age of the patient and extent and location of the necrosis within the head, and results are typically poor in over 60% of patients.[17,55] There is no clearly effective treatment for established posttraumatic ON in children.[33,66] Older children (>10 years old) tend to have worse outcomes than younger children. Treatment of ON is controversial and inconclusive and is beyond the scope of this text. Ongoing research includes the role of redirectional osteotomy,[42] distraction arthroplasty with external fixation, core decompression, vascularized fibular grafting (Fig. 24-20), injection of bone marrow concentrate, and direct bone grafting.

COXA VARA

The prevalence of postfracture coxa vara has been approximated between 20% and 30%[33]; however, it is significantly lower in

series in which internal fixation was used after reduction of displaced fractures.[17] Coxa vara may be caused by malunion, ON of the femoral neck, premature physeal closure, or a combination of these problems (Fig. 24-21). Severe coxa vara results in the greater trochanter being higher than the center of the femoral head, leading to abductor weakness and shortening of the extremity. This may result in a significant limp and functional limitation.

Remodeling of an established malunion may occur if the child is less than 8 years old, or with a neck–shaft angle greater than 110 degrees. Older patients with progressive deformity may not remodel and subtrochanteric valgus osteotomy may be considered to recreate a more normal trochanter–femoral head relationship, improve limb length inequality, and restore the abductor moment arm (Fig. 24-22).[33,40]

PREMATURE PHYSEAL CLOSURE

Premature physeal closure occurs after approximately 28% of fractures.[33] The risk of premature physeal closure increases when the physis is violated by surgical technique or when ON occurs. It is most commonly seen in patients who have type II or III ON (see Fig. 24-21).[66,67]

The capital femoral physis contributes only 13% of the growth of the entire extremity (~3 mm/year) and normally closes earlier than most of the other physes in the lower extremity. As a result, shortening secondary to premature physeal closure does not cause significant functional abnormalities except in very young children.[13,35] Treatment for leg length discrepancy is indicated only for significant discrepancy (2.5 cm or more projected at maturity).[33] If femoral growth arrest is expected because of the implant use or injury to the physis in children 8 and under, the surgeon may consider concomitant greater trochanteric epiphysiodesis to maintain a more normal articular trochanteric relationship (Fig. 24-23).

NONUNION

Nonunion occurs infrequently, with an overall incidence of 7% of hip fractures in children.[33] Nonunion is a complication seen more commonly in types II and III fractures and is rare after type I or type IV fractures. The primary cause of nonunion is failure to obtain or maintain an anatomic reduction.[13] After femoral neck fracture in a child, pain should resolve and bridging callus should be seen at the fracture site by 3 months after injury. If a delayed or nonunion is suspected, a CT scan may be helpful to look for bridging bone. If no or minimal healing is seen by 3 to 6 months, the diagnosis of nonunion is established. Nonunion should be treated operatively as soon as possible. If rigid fixation was not utilized initially, the fracture should be revised using rigid internal fixation. If stable fixation was obtained in the initial procedure, a subtrochanteric valgus osteotomy should be performed to alter the orientation of the fracture

Figure 24-21. **A:** A 12-year-old boy with a type III left hip fracture. Poor pin placement and varus malposition are evident. **B:** The fracture united in mild varus after hardware revision. **C:** Fourteen months after injury, collapse of the weight-bearing segment is evident. **D:** Six years after injury, coxa breva and trochanteric overgrowth are seen secondary to osteonecrosis, nonunion, and premature physeal closure.

Figure 24-22. **A:** A 10-year-old boy with a type III fracture treated without cast immobilization develops progressive varus deformity 4 months after surgery. Inset CT scan demonstrates delayed union. Valgus osteotomy is indicated for his progressive varus deformity and delayed healing. **B:** Three years after valgus osteotomy, the fracture is healed and the deformity corrected.

Figure 24-23. A: Greater trochanteric epiphysiodesis was performed at the time of open reduction and internal fixation of a pathologic femoral neck fracture (see Fig. 24-1) in a 10-year-old boy. Because the implant crosses the physis, growth arrest is expected and trochanteric arrest may minimize trochanteric overgrowth. **B:** Seven-year follow-up shows that growth arrest occurred and some trochanteric mismatch is present despite prior epiphysiodesis.

and allow compression across the fracture site (Fig. 24-24).[40,41] Allograft bone graft may be used to supplement in these procedures. However, given the increased morbidity required for harvest, autograft should be reserved for persistent nonunions. Internal fixation should extend across the site of the nonunion, and supplemental external forms of immobilization should be used in all but the most mature and cooperative adolescents.

LESS COMMON COMPLICATIONS

Infection is uncommon after hip fractures in children. The reported incidence of 1%[1,7] is consistent with the expected infection rate in any closed fracture treated surgically with ORIF. Chondrolysis is exceedingly rare.[4] Care must be taken to avoid persistent penetration of hardware into the joint, which can cause chondrolysis in conditions such as SCFE. Finally, SCFE has been reported as a rare complication after fixation of an ipsilateral femoral neck fracture.[34]

SUMMARY, CONTROVERSIES, AND FUTURE DIRECTIONS RELATED TO HIP FRACTURES

Pediatric femoral neck fractures have a relatively small incidence compared with other lower extremity fractures, but the potential for complications is much greater. Except for very young children, the majority of these fractures should be treated with reduction and internal fixation to assure an anatomic reduction. For closed reduction to be successful, the fracture must

be reduced nearly anatomic. Fracture reduction should be done early, but controversy persists as to whether this must be done within 24 hours. A variety of approaches exist for open reduction of pediatric hip fractures, and the chosen approach should be based on surgeon experience and fracture pattern. Surgical dislocation allows direct visualization of the fracture and the retinaculum, which may have some benefit on the incidence of AVN, but this is yet to be proven. There are a variety of fixation methods once the fracture is anatomically reduced. The goal is to avoid fixation across the physis when possible. However, if the patient is older (>10 years), or fixation would otherwise be inadequate, cross the physis. Fracture stability and union are more critical than avoiding physeal injury. Continued research is required to better understand the risk factors for AVN and to determine optimal treatment of this devastating complication.

Stress Fractures of the Femoral Neck

INTRODUCTION TO STRESS FRACTURES OF THE FEMORAL NECK

Stress fractures of the femoral neck are extremely uncommon in children, and only a few case series have been published in the English-language literature. In one study of 40 stress fractures in children, there was only one femoral neck stress fracture. Stress fractures are typically associated with strenuous activities such as repetitive running or jumping, but have also been

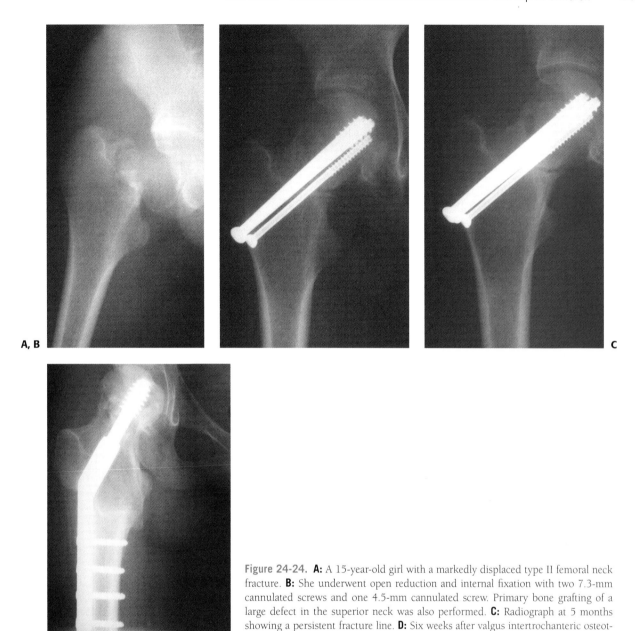

Figure 24-24. A: A 15-year-old girl with a markedly displaced type II femoral neck fracture. **B:** She underwent open reduction and internal fixation with two 7.3-mm cannulated screws and one 4.5-mm cannulated screw. Primary bone grafting of a large defect in the superior neck was also performed. **C:** Radiograph at 5 months showing a persistent fracture line. **D:** Six weeks after valgus intertrochanteric osteotomy. The fracture is healing.

described in children undertaking free play.[12] The rarity of such fractures underscores the need for a high index of suspicion when a child has unexplained hip pain. The differential can be long for hip pain in children, and early diagnosis and treatment are essential to avoid complete fracture with displacement.

ASSESSMENT OF STRESS FRACTURES OF THE FEMORAL NECK

MECHANISMS OF INJURY FOR STRESS FRACTURES OF THE FEMORAL NECK

Stress fractures of the femoral neck usually result from repetitive cyclic loading of the hip, such as that produced by a new or increased activity. A recent increase in the repetitive activity is highly suggestive of the diagnosis. An increase in intensity of soccer,[9] and an increase in distance running are examples of such activities. However, a recent case series of children under 10 with femoral neck stress fractures saw no evidence of increased activity level or elevated sporting volume before the onset of symptoms.[12]

Younger children may present with a limp or knee pain and may not have a clear history of increased activity. Underlying metabolic disorders or immobilizations that weaken the bone may predispose to stress fracture. There is an increased awareness of vitamin D deficiency in children who may predispose to a femoral neck stress fracture.[48] In adolescent female athletes, amenorrhea, anorexia nervosa, osteoporosis, and the "female athlete triad" have been implicated in the development of stress fractures of the femoral neck.

SIGNS AND SYMPTOMS OF STRESS FRACTURES OF THE FEMORAL NECK

The usual presentation is that of progressive hip or groin pain with or without a limp. The pain may be perceived in the thigh or knee and may be mild enough so that it does not significantly limit activities. In the absence of displacement, examination may reveal slight limitation of hip motion with increased pain and hip pain with terminal hip flexion.[12]

IMAGING AND OTHER DIAGNOSTIC STUDIES FOR STRESS FRACTURES OF THE FEMORAL NECK

Usually, plain radiographs reveal the fracture, but in the first 4 to 6 weeks after presentation, plain films may be negative. If there are no changes or only linear sclerosis, a bone scan or MRI will help identify the fracture. MRI has been documented as a sensitive test for nondisplaced fractures of the femoral neck. If a sclerotic lesion is seen on plain radiographs, the differential diagnosis should include osteoid osteoma, chronic sclerosing osteomyelitis, bone infarct, and osteosarcoma. The differential diagnosis of hip pain in a child is broad, but includes SCFE, Legg–Calvé–Perthes disease, infection, avulsion injuries of the pelvis, eosinophilic granuloma, and bony malignancies. Untreated stress fractures may progress with continued activity to complete fracture with displacement.[75] For this reason, prompt diagnosis and treatment are important.

CLASSIFICATION OF STRESS FRACTURES OF THE FEMORAL NECK

Femoral neck stress fractures are classified into two types: compression fractures and tension fractures. The compression type appears as reactive bone formation on the inferior cortex without cortical disruption. This type rarely becomes completely displaced but may collapse into a mild varus deformity, and compression types have been reported to progress to complete fracture without early treatment (Fig. 24-25).[75] The tension type is a transverse fracture line appearing on the superior portion of the femoral neck. This type is inherently unstable because the fracture line is perpendicular to the lines of tension. Tension stress fractures have only rarely been reported in skeletally immature children[28,37] but may occur in skeletally mature teenagers.[12,75]

TREATMENT OF STRESS FRACTURES OF THE FEMORAL NECK

Compression-type fractures generally can be treated with a period of non–weight bearing on crutches. Partial weight bearing can be allowed at 6 to 8 weeks with progression to full weight bearing at 12 to 16 weeks provided that the pain is resolved and there is radiographic evidence of healing. Close follow-up

and careful evaluation are mandatory to ensure that the fracture heals without propagation. Underlying conditions should be evaluated and addressed. In small or uncooperative children, spica casting may be necessary. Displacement into varus, however minimal, mandates internal fixation. Tension fractures are at high risk for displacement and should be treated with in situ compression fixation using cannulated screws.

Management of Expected Adverse Outcomes and Unexpected Complications Related to Stress Fractures of the Femoral Neck

Coxa vara is the most common complication of untreated compression-type fractures. Acute displacement of this type also has been described.[64] Once displaced, the stress fracture is subject to all the complications of type II and type III displaced femoral neck fractures.

Hip Dislocations

INTRODUCTION TO HIP DISLOCATIONS

Traumatic hip dislocations are uncommon injuries in children, constituting less than 5% of pediatric dislocations. In one study, the author identified only 15 cases over a 20-year period at a large trauma center.[3] The character of the injury tends to vary with age. Children under age 6 commonly suffer isolated hip dislocation from a low-energy injury, whereas older children require a high-energy mechanism to dislocate the hip, and these injuries are often associated with more severe trauma.[3,7,56,70] Most hip dislocations in children can be reduced easily, and long-term outcome is generally good with prompt and complete reduction. Delay in reduction or neglected dislocations routinely do poorly, with a high incidence of AVN of the femoral head.[6,7] Incomplete reductions can occur from interposed soft tissue or bony fragments, and postoperative imaging is mandatory to ensure complete reduction.[44] Difficult reductions or hip dislocation that occurs in adolescents (with a widened proximal femoral physis) should be performed with anesthesia, muscle relaxation, and the use of fluoroscopy to ensure that physeal separation does not occur.[31,33] Open reduction may be needed if the hip cannot be reduced, or if there is a femoral head fracture or an incarcerated fragment. Incomplete reductions may be treated open or arthroscopically. Complications, although uncommon, may occur, and these patients should be closely followed for recurrent subluxation, dislocation, and AVN.[3,70]

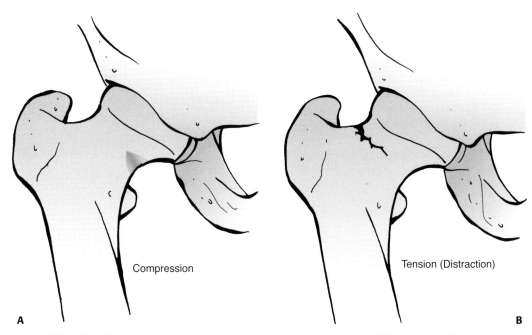

Figure 24-25. A line drawing of stress fractures, comparing compression (**A**) and tension (**B**) types.

ASSESSMENT OF HIP DISLOCATION

MECHANISMS OF INJURY FOR HIP DISLOCATIONS

The mechanism of injury in children with hip dislocation varies. Posterior hip dislocations are the most common[70] and generally occur when a force is applied to the leg with the hip flexed and slightly adducted (Fig. 24-26). Anterior dislocations comprise less than 10% of pediatric hip dislocations (Fig. 24-27).[3,70] Anterior dislocations can occur superiorly or inferiorly and result from forced abduction and external rotation. If the hip is extended while undergoing forced abduction and external rotation, it will dislocate anteriorly and superiorly;

if the hip is flexed while abducted and externally rotated, the femoral head tends to dislocate anteriorly and inferiorly. In very rare cases, the femoral head may dislocate directly inferiorly, a condition known as *luxatio erecta femoris* or infracotyloid dislocation. Although this condition is extremely rare, it tends to occur more commonly in children than in adults.[69]

In younger children, hip dislocations can occur with surprisingly little force, such as a fall while at play. The mechanism for hip dislocations in older children and adolescents is similar to that of adults in that significant trauma is needed. In a French study,[3] the authors assessed children with hip dislocations and divided them into two groups by age: those under 6 years (seven patients) and those aged 6 and older (seven patients). All of the children under age 6 had low-energy mechanisms and isolated

Figure 24-26. A typical posterior dislocation of the hip.

Figure 24-27. An anterior (inferior) dislocation of the hip.

Figure 24-30. Right hip pain after a fall. **A:** The plain film shows no significant abnormality at time of injury. **B, C:** Persistent pain prompted an MRI 2 months after injury, which showed an interposed labrum in the joint.

Pipkin Classification for Dislocations With Femoral Head/Neck Fractures

Type	Associated Fracture
1	Head fracture caudal to the fovea (small fragment)
2	Head fracture cranial to the fovea (large fragment)
3	Combined head and neck fracture
4	Combined neck and acetabular fracture

Fracture-dislocation of the hip involving the femoral head or the acetabulum is less common in children than in adults. Older adolescents generally sustain adult-type fracture-dislocations of the hip. Dislocations associated with femoral head or neck fractures are most commonly classified by the methods of Pipkin.[59] He classified the head fractures as occurring either caudal to the fovea with a resultant small fragment (type 1) (see Figs. 24-31 and 24-32), cranial to the fovea with a resultant large fragment (type 2), any combined femoral head and neck fracture (type 3), and any femoral neck fracture with an acetabular fracture (type 4). The youngest patient in his series from 1957 was 20, and most of these fractures were secondary to the relatively new phenomena of traffic accidents or other high-energy trauma such as All-Terrain Vehicle (ATV) accidents.

Habitual dislocation of the hip has been described in children. In this condition, the child can actually voluntarily dislocate the hip. Many factors may contribute to this ability, including generalized ligamentous laxity or hyperlaxity disorders, excessive anteversion of the femur and acetabulum, and coxa valga.[74] A commonly confused condition is snapping of the iliotibial band over the greater trochanter, and often the patient will describe this as "dislocating their hip." Yet, the hip remains well seated both before and after the snap, which can be quite dramatic. The more common iliotibial band snapping can usually be differentiated from a true hip dislocation by examination, or if needed, radiographs with the hip "in" versus "out." A snapping iliotibial band will demonstrate a well-seated hip on both radiographs.

PATHOANATOMY AND APPLIED ANATOMY RELATED TO HIP DISLOCATIONS

The hip joint is a synovial ball and socket joint formed by the articulation of the round head of the femur and the cup-like acetabulum of the pelvis. If this is injured early in childhood, the growth of the acetabulum can be affected and this may result in acetabular dysplasia or impingement.

TREATMENT OPTIONS FOR HIP DISLOCATIONS

The immediate goal in the treatment of a traumatic hip dislocation is to obtain concentric reduction as soon as possible. Reduction of a pediatric or adolescent hip dislocation should be

Figure 24-31. **A:** A 12-year-old boy was tackled from behind in football. The right hip was dislocated. Reduction was easily achieved, but the hip was unstable posteriorly as a result of fracture of the posterior rim of the acetabulum. This is the most common fracture, occurring with hip dislocation. **B:** The fracture and capsule were fixed via a posterior approach. **C:** Oblique view shows reconstitution of the posterior rim.

considered an orthopaedic emergency. Generally, closed reduction should be attempted initially. Successful closed reduction can be achieved with intravenous or intramuscular sedation in the emergency department in most patients. However, there is a risk of separating the femoral epiphysis from the femoral neck.

Figure 24-32. **A:** A posterior dislocation associated after reduction with a femoral head fracture caudal to the ligamentum teres (Pipkin type 2). This is uncommon in children. **B:** This was treated with open reduction and internal fixation, with follow-up radiographs taken 1 year after the injury.

Hence, complete muscle relaxation and the ability to urgently open the hip is often helpful, and this is best provided in the operating room with a general anesthetic. Open reduction is indicated if closed reduction is unsuccessful or incomplete. In children, especially in their early teenage years, cases of proximal physeal separation with attempted closed reduction have been reported, and therefore, the use of fluoroscopy to assess the stability of the proximal femoral physis is highly recommended.[31,55]

Several methods of closed reduction have been described for reduction of posterior dislocations. With any type of dislocation, traction along the axis of the thigh coupled with gentle manipulation of the hip usually results in reduction after satisfactory relaxation of the surrounding muscles.

In one method, the patient is placed supine and the surgeon stands above the patient. For this reason, either the patient must be placed on the floor or the surgeon must climb onto the bed. The knee is flexed to relax the hamstrings. While an assistant stabilizes the pelvis, the surgeon applies longitudinal traction along the axis of the femur and gently manipulates the femoral head over the rim of the acetabulum and back into the acetabulum.

The gravity method entails placing the patient prone with the lower limbs hanging over the edge of a table. An assistant stabilizes the patient while the surgeon applies gentle downward pressure with the knee and hip flexed 90 degrees, in an attempt to pull the femoral head anteriorly over the posterior rim of the acetabulum and back into the socket. Gentle internal and external rotation may assist in the reduction.

OPERATIVE TREATMENT OF HIP DISLOCATION

If satisfactory closed reduction cannot be obtained using reasonable measures or the reduction is not concentric secondary to bone fragments or soft tissue interposition, it is appropriate to proceed with open reduction and inspection of the joint. The goal of an open reduction is to remove and potentially reconstruct any obstructing soft tissues and identify and remove intra-articular osteochondral fragments. The approach for open reduction includes the approaches discussed in the prior section (anterior, posterior, or surgical dislocation). The choice of approach depends on the direction of dislocation and surgeon experience. Surgeons with extensive hip arthroscopic experience may be able to arthroscopically extract interposed soft tissue or osteochondral fragments limiting a concentric reduction.

In an irreducible hip, imaging can be performed prior to reduction to aid in surgical planning, but it should not delay treatment. As mentioned previously, in children in their early teenage years, cases of proximal physeal separation with attempted closed reduction have been reported, and therefore, the use of fluoroscopy to assess the stability of the proximal femoral physis is highly recommended.[31,55]

Surgical Technique for Open Reduction of a Posterior Hip Dislocation Through a Posterolateral Approach

Open reduction of a posterior dislocation should be performed through a posterolateral (Kocher–Langenbeck) approach or surgical dislocation approach. For the Kocher–Langenbeck approach, the patient is positioned in the lateral decubitus position with the dislocated side facing up. The incision is centered on and just posterior to the greater trochanter and extends proximally into the buttock. Generally, a straight incision can be made when the hip is flexed approximately 90 degrees. Once the fascia lata is incised, the femoral head can be palpated beneath or within the substance of the gluteus maximus muscle. The fibers of the gluteus maximus can then be divided by blunt dissection, exposing the dislocated femoral head. The path of dislocation is followed through the short external rotator muscles and capsule down to the acetabulum. The sciatic nerve lies on the short external rotators and should be identified and inspected. The piriformis may be draped across the acetabulum, obstructing the view of the reduction. It may be necessary to detach the short external rotators to see inside the joint. After the joint is inspected, repair of the fracture of the posterior acetabular rim can be performed in the standard fashion.

Surgical Technique for Open Reduction of an Anterior Hip Dislocation

Anterior dislocations should be approached through an anterior approach. This can be performed through a bikini incision that uses the interval between the sartorius and the tensor fascia lata. The deep dissection follows the defect created by the femoral head down to the level of the acetabulum. In the anterior approach, the femoral head should be dislocated and any interposed soft tissue extracted. A Schanz screw or bone hook may be needed to displace the femur enough to see inside the joint in the anterior approach. Any bony fragments displaced from the femoral head or the acetabulum should have reduction and fixation if the size is significant. In younger hips, the cartilaginous labral–chondral junction may be displaced from the bony rim. Suture anchor repair through the base of the labrum should be performed.

Surgical Technique for Open Reduction of a Hip Dislocation Through a Surgical Dislocation Approach

A surgical dislocation approach is particularly useful for hips that are reduced but are not concentric, or in hips with ongoing instability after reduction. A lateral incision is created centered on the anterior third of the greater trochanter. The leg can then be abducted by placing it on a sterile, padded Mayo stand. The tensor fascia is incised longitudinally in line with the skin incision. Proximally, the dissection may be carried out between the anterior edge of the gluteus maximus and the tensor (Gibson modification), or the gluteus maximus may be split bluntly. This exposes the proximal vastus lateralis, gluteus medius, and greater trochanter.

The leg is then taken off the Mayo and positioned with the hip in adduction and slight internal rotation to better visualize the anatomic landmarks. Identify and develop the interval between the piriformis and the gluteus medius. The piriformis is the thick, white tendon visualized deep to the posterior/distal aspect of gluteus medius. Once exposed, the tendon can be gently retracted distally to expose the inferior margin of the gluteus minimus fascia. The inferior fascia of the minimus is then opened to allow the muscle to be retracted in an anterosuperior direction off of the hip capsule. This should allow visualization of the hip capsule.

A greater trochanteric osteotomy is then performed from the posterior border of the vastus lateralis ridge to the anterior and to the tip of the greater trochanter using either an oscillating saw or an osteotomy. The width of the osteotomy should be approximately 15 mm. The piriformis and short external rotators should remain attached to the stable trochanteric bed. Maintaining the piriformis tendon intact protects the retinacular branch of the medial circumflex artery. The trochanteric flip piece with attached gluteus minimus, gluteus medius, vastus lateralis, and vastus intermedius is then reflected anteriorly.

Capsular exposure then continues anteriorly and superiorly. Gentle, progressive flexion and external rotation of the operative hip will facilitate the muscle dissection. Capsular muscular attachments are elevated anteriorly to the indirect head of the rectus tendon, superiorly to the superior rim of the acetabulum, and posteriorly to the piriformis.

The hip capsule is then opened in a Z-shaped fashion. The longitudinal limb is along the axis of the femoral neck in line with the iliofemoral ligament. The distal aspect is proximal but in line with the intertrochanteric ridge. The posterior limb of the capsule is opened in the capsular recess of the acetabulum as far posterior as the piriformis tendon, protecting the retinaculum as it pierces the hip capsule. Once the capsule is opened, the intra-articular anatomy can be visualized. The epiphysis should be provisionally pinned with a smooth K-wire if there is any concern of epiphysiolysis.

Flexion and external rotation of the leg will allow anterior dislocation of the femoral head. Complete dislocation may not be necessary if most of the soft tissue injury is located posteriorly, as is typically seen in a posterior hip dislocation. The femoral head and acetabulum should be inspected for damage. Frequently, the labrum or hip capsule is entrapped within the joint.

Surgical Technique for Treatment of Irreducible or Incomplete Hip Dislocation

Regardless of approach selected, any small intra-articular fragments should be removed. The labrum and capsule should be inspected for repairable tears. Labral fragments that cannot be securely replaced should be excised, but repair should be attempted. Any bony fragments displaced from the femoral head or the acetabulum should have reduction and fixation if the size allows. In younger hips, the cartilaginous labral–chondral junction may be displaced from the bony rim. Suture anchor repair through the base of the labrum should be performed. The hip joint is then reduced under direct vision. The capsule should be repaired and, in the case of a surgical dislocation approach, the greater trochanter should be reduced and secured with two or three 3.5- or 4.5-mm screws.

Postreduction radiographs should be taken to confirm concentric reduction. If the joint appears slightly widened, repeat investigation is indicated to rule out interposed tissue. Slight widening secondary to fluid in the hip joint or decreased muscle tone can occur, and this may improve over the next few days.

Treatment of Open Dislocations

Open injuries should be treated with immediate irrigation and debridement. The surgical incision should incorporate and enlarge the traumatic wound. Inspection should proceed as detailed above. Capsular repair should be attempted if the hip joint is not contaminated. The wound should be left open or should be well drained to prevent invasive infection. As in all open fractures, intravenous antibiotics should be administered and patients should be screened for tetanus.

Postoperative Management

After reduction, a short period of immobilization should be instituted. In younger children, a spica cast can be used for 4 to 6 weeks; older cooperative children can be treated with hip abduction orthosis. A bone scan can be obtained at 4 to 6 weeks after injury to evaluate the perfusion to the femoral head.[61] Early identification of ON allows for modification to the postoperative protocol including prolonged protected weight bearing,

medical treatment with bisphosphonates, and consideration of alternative surgical treatments including core decompression or multiple epiphyseal drilling before the femoral head has started to collapse. Range-of-motion precautions are dependent on the direction of the dislocation approach used in treatment. Patients with a posterior dislocation treated with a posterolateral approach should be restricted from excessive adduction, internal rotation, and flexion. Patients with an anterior dislocation treated with an anterior approach should be restricted from excessive extension and external rotation. And those patients treated with a surgical dislocation approach require limitations to active abduction and passive adduction past the midline. All patients may be touch-down weight bearing if developmentally appropriate.

Authors' Preferred Treatment for Hip Dislocations

Urgent closed reduction by applying traction in line with the femur and gently manipulating the femoral head back into the acetabulum should be performed. A controlled reduction with sedation or general anesthesia and muscle relaxation in the operating room is preferable, and aggressive techniques should not be attempted without muscle relaxant. The use of fluoroscopy to monitor the reduction, especially in children over 12 with open physis, is important to ensure that proximal femoral epiphysiolysis does not occur. Surgery is indicated for dislocations that are irreducible or for nonconcentric reductions. We recommend an MRI should be considered after reduction to assess for interposing fragments of bone, cartilage, or soft tissue.

Potential pitfalls and preventive measures reduce the hip urgently. The most devastating outcome is ON, and prolonged time to reduction (more than 6 hours) appears to be the greatest risk factor. In multitrauma patients, this concept needs to be expressed to the trauma team so that it can be prioritized properly.

Look for associated fractures and other injuries. In older children, it is important to evaluate the posterior rim of the acetabulum after posterior dislocation to rule out fracture. Relying on plain radiographs and CT may underestimate the extent of damage to the posterior wall of the acetabulum in children because of the incomplete ossification of the pediatric bone. MRI may be required to adequately assess the posterior wall of the acetabulum in children.[68]

Fractures at other sites in the femur must be considered. It is important to obtain radiographs that show the entire femur to rule out ipsilateral fracture. Careful evaluation of the entire patient is needed especially for high-energy injuries that result in a hip dislocation in older children and adults.

Separation of the capital femoral epiphysis and femoral neck fracture has been reported in association with dislocation of the hip and the attempted reduction. Children in their early teenage years, aged 12 to 16, should have

Figure 24-33. A: An 11-year-old boy dislocated his left hip while wrestling. **B:** The hip was easily reduced. **C:** After 5 months, hip pain led to an MRI, which shows osteonecrosis of the capital femoral epiphysis. **D:** At 10 months after injury, there are typical changes of osteonecrosis despite non–weight bearing.

reduction performed with fluoroscopy under general anesthesia when possible. This strategy may avoid the possibility of displacing the proximal femoral epiphysis (with attendant increased ON risk) during attempted closed reduction (Fig. 24-33). Spontaneous relocation of a dislocation of the hip may occur with subsequent soft tissue or osteocartilaginous interposition. Failure to appreciate the presence of hip dislocation may lead to inadequate treatment. Traumatic hip subluxation may go undetected or may be treated as a sprain or strain if the diagnosis is not considered.[51,63] After dislocation and spontaneous reduction, soft tissue may become interposed in the hip joint potentially resulting in chronic arthropathy. In a child with posttraumatic hip pain without obvious deformity, the possibility of dislocation–relocation must be considered.

Always image the hip for evaluation of interposed tissue after reduction. The incidence of widened joint space after hip reductions is as high as 26%.[44] After reduction, hemarthrosis may initially cause the hip joint to appear slightly wider on the affected side, but this should decrease after a few days. If the hip fails to appear concentric, the possibility of interposed soft tissue must be considered, and MRI or CT should be performed.

Long-term follow-up is important in children who undergo hip dislocation. Injury to the triradiate cartilage may cause acetabular dysplasia with growth. ON, although uncommon, may lead to early arthrosis, and this may not be identified radiographically for several years. If there has been a significant delay in time to reduction or the patient is otherwise at higher risk for ON, then consideration of a bone scan or MRI to evaluate for ON may be warranted, especially if early treatment with bisphosphonates is considered.

Management of Expected Adverse Outcomes and Unexpected Complications Related to Hip Dislocations in Children

ON occurs in about 10% of hip dislocations in children (Fig. 24-34).[27,47,53] Urgent reduction may decrease the incidence of this complication.[47] The risk of ON is most likely related to the severity of initial trauma. If the force of the hip dislocation is so strong as to disrupt the obturator externus muscle, the posterior ascending vessels may simultaneously be torn.[53] In the rare case of dislocation with an intact capsule, increased intracapsular pressure as a result of hemarthrosis may have a tamponade effect, resulting in ON. The type of postreduction care has not been shown to influence the rate of ON.

Early technetium bone scanning with pinhole-collimated images can be used to detect ON as an area of decreased uptake.

Findings on T2-weighted MRI images are abnormal but of variable signal intensity, and the MRI may be falsely negative if performed within a few days of injury.[62] Conversely, many perfusion defects seen on MRI spontaneously resolve after several months.[62] As treatment for early ON continues to develop, the utility of postreduction perfusion imaging may change, and early assessment may be considered for those at high risk of ON. Currently, posttraumatic hips should be followed by serial radiographs even after healing to look for signs of ON. It is

Figure 24-34. A: Anteroposterior radiograph of the pelvis, showing dislocation of the right hip. **B:** Anteroposterior radiograph of the right hip, showing the physeal separation after attempted closed reduction. Anteroposterior (**C**) and lateral (**D**) radiographs made after surgical dislocation, reduction, and fixation of the epiphysis through a trochanteric flip osteotomy.

(continues)

Figure 24-34. (*Continued*) Anteroposterior radiographs made during 4 months (**E**), 7 months (**F**), 1 year (**G**) and 2 years (**H**) after surgical reconstruction. (Reprinted with permission from Schoenecker JG, et al. Treatment of traumatic separation of the proximal femoral epiphysis without development of osteonecrosis: A report of two cases. *J Bone Joint Surg Am.* 2010;92(4):973–977.)

recommended that these studies continue for at least 2 years following a traumatic dislocation, as radiographic changes may appear late.

If ON develops, pain, loss of motion, and deformity of the femoral head may occur.[7] The course of traumatic ON in a young child resembles Legg–Calvé–Perthes disease and may be treated like Perthes disease.[7] The goals of treatment are to maintain mobility and containment of the femoral head to maximize congruity after resolution. ON in older children should be treated as in adults and may require osteotomy, reconstruction, or arthroplasty. If identified early, medical treatment with bisphosphonates or revascularization techniques, such as a vascularized fibular bone graft, may be considered.[1]

CHONDROLYSIS

Chondrolysis has been reported after hip dislocation in up to 6% of children[27,56] and probably occurs as a result of articular damage at the time of dislocation. Chondrolysis cannot be reversed by medical or surgical techniques, and treatment is symptomatic. Anti-inflammatory medication and weight-relieving devices should be used as needed. One study suggests that hip joint distraction with a hinged external fixator may

improve range of motion and decrease pain.[22] If the joint fails to reconstitute, fusion, reconstruction, or replacement should be considered.

COXA MAGNA

Coxa magna occasionally occurs after hip dislocation. The reported incidence varies widely and ranges from 0% to 47%.[27,56] It is believed to occur as a result of posttraumatic hyperemia.[56] In most children, this condition is asymptomatic and does not require any treatment.[56] There is no intervention that will prevent coxa magna.

HABITUAL DISLOCATION

Habitual or voluntary dislocation of the hip usually is unrelated to trauma. Many factors may contribute to this ability, including generalized ligamentous laxity, excessive anteversion of the femur and acetabulum, and coxa valga. Initial management should include counseling the child to cease the activity (with or without psychiatric counseling) and observation. If episodes of dislocation persist, permanent changes such as secondary capsular laxity or osteocartilaginous deformation of the hip may occur. These changes may lead to pain, residual subluxation, or degenerative joint disease. Conservative treatment should be initially attempted and may include simple observation with or without psychiatric counseling or immobilization with cast or brace.

Hip stabilization by surgical means may be indicated for persistent painful episodes of hip, despite conservative treatment or those with underlying medical conditions predisposing to habitual dislocation, such as Down syndrome.[57,74] Knight et al.[36] reported their 10-year follow-up of Down syndrome patients with habitual subluxation treated with a varus/derotation intertrochanteric osteotomy. They recommend surgery in these patients before age 7 and attempting to get the neck/shaft angle to 105 degrees to prevent later hip abnormality.[36] Therefore, corrective surgery, if considered, should be performed only to correct specific anatomic abnormality and perhaps in patients with known ligamentous laxity. Surgery may include capsular plication, although bony correction with redirectional pelvic osteotomy, or osteotomy of the proximal femur, is required to treat the underlying pathology.[74]

HETEROTOPIC OSSIFICATION

Heterotopic ossification can result after closed reduction of hip dislocations in children, but is generally asymptomatic and rarely requires intervention. In one study, three children (all under 16 years of age) developed heterotopic ossification, one of which required surgical excision.[47]

INTERPOSED SOFT TISSUE

Interposed tissues may result in a nonconcentric reduction or a complete failure of closed reduction. Muscle, bone, articular cartilage, and labrum have all been implicated.[63,73] An MRI can provide the most useful information on obstacles to complete concentric reduction.[73] Open reduction generally is necessary to clear impeding tissues from the joint.[56,63,73] Untreated, nonconcentric reduction may lead to permanent degenerative arthropathy.

LATE PRESENTATION

Not all hip dislocations in children cause severe or incapacitating symptoms. Ambulation may even be possible. As a result, treatment may be delayed or the diagnosis missed until shortening of the limb and contracture are well established, making reduction difficult. Nearly all patients with a delayed treatment of traumatic hip dislocation develop ON.[6,39] Prolonged, heavy traction has been described as a method to effect reduction. If this fails, preoperative traction, extensive soft tissue release, or

primary femoral shortening should be considered in association with an open reduction. Open reduction will likely be difficult and may not always be successful. Even if a stable, concentric reduction is achieved, progressive arthropathy may lead to a stiff and painful hip. The likelihood of a good result decreases with the duration of dislocation.

NERVE INJURY

The sciatic nerve may be directly compressed by the femoral head after a posterior dislocation of the hip in 2% to 13% of patients.[23,70] If the hip is expediently reduced, nerve function returns spontaneously in most patients.[23] If the sciatic nerve palsy is present prior to reduction, the nerve does not need to be explored unless open reduction is required for other reasons. If sciatic nerve function is shown to be intact and is lost during the reduction maneuver, the nerve should be explored to ensure that it has not displaced into the joint. Other nerves around the hip joint are rarely injured at dislocation. Treatment is generally expectant unless laceration or incarceration is suspected; if so, exploration is indicated.

RECURRENT DISLOCATION

Recurrence after traumatic hip dislocation is rare but occurs most frequently after posterior dislocation in children under 8 years of age[6] or in children with known hyperlaxity (Down syndrome, Ehlers–Danlos disease, etc.). The incidence of recurrence is estimated to be less than 3%.[56] Recurrence can be quite disabling, and in the long term may result in damage to the articular surfaces as a result of shear damage to the cartilaginous hip. Prolonged spica casting (at least 3 months) may be effective in younger chidren.[48] Surgical exploration with capsulorrhaphy can be performed if conservative treatment fails.[6,36] Prior to hip reconstruction, an MRI or arthrography is recommended to identify soft tissue defects or capsular redundancy.[6]

In older children, recurrent dislocation can occur as a result of a bony defect in the posterior rim of the acetabulum similar to that in adults and may require posterior acetabular reconstruction (Fig. 24-35). More recent literature suggests a more severe soft tissue injury associated with these fractures than had been previously appreciated.[54,60,77] These patients may have large labral tears that can contribute to ongoing issues if instability, with a near-complete or radial tear of the posterior labrum. MRI evaluation of the hip after reduction allows for evaluation of these potential findings without the risk of radiation exposure.[10]

VASCULAR INJURY

Impingement on the femoral neurovascular bundle has been described after anterior hip dislocation in children, and

Figure 24-35. An 11-year-old who had left persistent pain after closed reduction of left hip after sledding accident. **A:** Anteroposterior radiograph of reduced hip preoperatively. **B:** Preoperative CT slice clearly demonstrating entrapped fragment. **C:** Anteroposterior radiograph postoperatively.

this may occur in up to 25% of patients. The hip should be reduced as soon as possible to remove the offending pressure on the femoral vessels. If reduction of the hip fails to restore perfusion, immediate exploration of the femoral vessels is indicated.

SUMMARY, CONTROVERSIES, AND FUTURE DIRECTIONS RELATED TO HIP DISLOCATIONS

The treatment for hip disorders is evolving. We now have new surgical and medical treatment options for hip disorders such as surgical hip dislocation and hip arthroscopy. Although most do not directly apply to the urgent reduction of hip dislocations, they are applicable to the sequelae that may occur. The use of bisphosphonates and other medications that inhibit bone resorption is an active area of research and may have direct effects on limiting collapse of the femoral head if ON occurs.[1] This could soon change our paradigm for the evaluation of a hip after reduction of a dislocation, and early perfusion MRI or bone scans may be indicated.

A host of surgical methods are available to manage deformity as a result of ON or hip instability. Techniques to increase vascularity, such as vascularized bone grafting, remain a controversial method to improve the natural history. Hinged distraction across the hip may now play a role as a primary treatment for chondrolysis or as an adjunct to other techniques.[22] Hip arthroscopy is much more commonly performed and allows for a much less invasive approach for the removal of loose bodies in the hip, as well as assessing and treating chondral, labral, and capsular injuries.[13]

Together, these new techniques offer future opportunities to decrease the severity of known complications and potentially improve functional outcomes. Time and follow-up will be required to determine if these methods improve the natural history of these posttraumatic sequelae.

ACKNOWLEDGMENTS

The authors thank Rachel Y. Goldstein and Young-Jo Kim, who contributed this chapter in the previous edition, the work on which this revision was based.

Annotated References

Reference	Annotation
Mehlman CT, Hubbard GW, Crawford AH, et al. Traumatic hip dislocation in children. *Clin Orthop Relat Res.* 2000;376:68–79.	Retrospective review of 46 pediatric patients with traumatic hip dislocation with long-term follow-up. Found that functional outcomes were generally good in these patients. Time to reduction was the only studied factor predictive of the risk for avascular necrosis.
Moon ES, Mehlman CT. Risk factors for avascular necrosis after femoral neck fractures in children: 25 Cincinnati cases and meta-analysis of 360 cases. *J Orthop Trauma.* 2006;20(5):323–329.	Meta-analysis of over 300 pediatric hip fractures, which identified fracture pattern and age at injury as the two most significant risk factors for the development of avascular necrosis of the femoral head.
Schrader MW, Jacofsky DJ, Stans AA, et al. Femoral neck fractures in pediatric patients: 30 years experience at a level 1 trauma center. *Clin Orthop Relat Res.* 2007;454:169–173.	Retrospective review of 20 patients with pediatric femoral neck fractures with medium-term follow-up. Found that quality of reduction and time to reduction were associated with good outcomes.
Spence D, DiMauro JP, Miller PE, et al. Osteonecrosis after femoral neck fractures in children and adolescents: analysis of risk factors. *J Pediatr Orthop.* 2016;36(2):111–116.	Retrospective review of 70 patients with pediatric femoral neck fractures, which identified factors associated with increased risk for avascular necrosis. Risk factors identified included fracture displacement, fracture location, and time to treatment.

REFERENCES

1. Agarwala S, Jain D, Joshi VR, Sule A. Efficacy of alendronate, a bisphosphonate, in the treatment of AVN of the hip. A prospective open-label study. *Rheumatology (Oxford).* 2005;44(3):352–359.
2. Alho A. Concurrent ipsilateral fractures of the hip and femoral shaft: a meta-analysis of 659 cases. *Acta Orthop Scand.* 1996;67(1):19–28.
3. Ayadi K, Trigui M, Gdoura F, et al. [Traumatic hip dislocations in children]. *Rev Chir Orthop Reparatrice Appar Mot.* 2008;94(1):19–25.
4. Bagatur AE, Zorer G. Complications associated with surgically treated hip fractures in children. *J Pediatr Orthop B.* 2002;11(3):219–228.
5. Bali K, Sudesh P, Patel S, et al. Pediatric femoral neck fractures: our 10 years of experience. *Clin Orthop Surg.* 2011;3(4):302–308.
6. Banskota AK, Spiegel DA, Shrestha S, et al. Open reduction for neglected traumatic hip dislocation in children and adolescents. *J Pediatr Orthop.* 2007;27(2):187–191.
7. Barquet A. Natural history of avascular necrosis following traumatic hip dislocation in childhood: a review of 145 cases. *Acta Orthop Scand.* 1982;53(5):815–820.
8. Beaty JH. Fractures of the hip in children. *Orthop Clin North Am.* 2006;37(2):223–232.
9. Bettin D, Pankalla T, Böhm H, Fuchs S. Hip pain related to femoral neck stress fracture in a 12-year-old boy performing intensive soccer playing activities: a case report. *Int J Sports Med.* 2003;24(8):593–596.
10. Blanchard C, Kushare I, Boyles A, et al. Traumatic, posterior pediatric hip dislocations with associated posterior labrum osteochondral avulsion: recognizing the acetabular "fleck" sign. *J Pediatr Orthop.* 2016;36(6):602–607.
11. Boardman MJ, Herman MJ, Buck B, Pizzutillo PD. Hip fractures in children. *J Am Acad Orthop Surg.* 2009;17(3):162–173.
12. Boyle MJ, Hogue GD, Heyworth BE, et al. Femoral neck stress fractures in children younger than 10 years of age. *J Pediatr Orthop.* 2017;37(2):e96–e99.
13. Bray TJ. Femoral neck fracture fixation. Clinical decision making. *Clin Orthop Relat Res.* 1997;(339):20–31.
14. Byrd JWT, Jones KS. Traumatic rupture of the ligamentum teres as a source of hip pain. *Arthroscopy.* 2004;20(4):385–391.
15. Caldwell L, Chan CM, Sanders JO, Gorczyca JT. Detection of femoral neck fractures in pediatric patients with femoral shaft fractures. *J Pediatr Orthop.* 2017;37(3):e164–e167.
16. Canale ST, Bourland WL. Fracture of the neck and intertrochanteric region of the femur in children. *J Bone Joint Surg Am.* 1977;59(4):431–443.
17. Canale ST, Casillas M, Banta JV. Displaced femoral neck fractures at the bone-screw interface after in situ fixation of slipped capital femoral epiphysis. *J Pediatr Orthop.* 1997;17(2):212–215.
18. Cheng JC, Tang N. Decompression and stable internal fixation of femoral neck fractures in children can affect the outcome. *J Pediatr Orthop.* 1999;19(3):338–343.
19. Chun KA, Morcuende J, El-Khoury GY. Entrapment of the acetabular labrum following reduction of traumatic hip dislocation in a child. *Skeletal Radiol.* 2004;33(12):728–731.
20. Cornawall R, Radomisli TE. Nerve injury in traumatic dislocation of the hip. *Clin Orthop Relat Res.* 2000;(377):84–91.
21. Davison BL, Weinstein SL. Hip fractures in children: a long-term follow-up study. *J Pediatr Orthop.* 1992;12(3):355–358.
22. Egol KA, Koval KJ, Kummer F, Frankel VH. Stress fractures of the femoral neck. *Clin Orthop Relat Res.* 1998;(348):72–78.
23. Flynn JM, Wong KL, Yeh GL, et al. Displaced fractures of the hip in children. Management by early operation and immobilization in a hip spica cast. *J Bone Joint Surg Br.* 2002;84(1):108–112.
24. Forster NA, Ramseier LE, Exner GU. Undisplaced femoral neck fractures in children have a high risk of secondary displacement. *J Pediatr Orthop B.* 2006;15(2):131–133.
25. Ganz R, Gill TJ, Gautier E, et al. Surgical dislocation of the adult hip: a technique with full access to the femoral head and acetabulum without the risk of avascular necrosis. *J Bone Joint Surg Br.* 2001;83(8):1119–1124.
26. Ganz R, Parvizi J, Beck M, et al. Femoroacetabular impingement: a cause for early osteoarthritis of the hip. *Clin Orthop Relat Res.* 2003;(417):112–120.
27. Guevara CJ, Pietrobon R, Carothers JT, et al. Comprehensive morphologic evaluation of the hip in patients with symptomatic labral tear. *Clin Orthop Relat Res.* 2006;453:277–285.
28. Hayyun MF, Jamil S, Abd-Rashid AH, Ibrahim S. Subcapital femoral neck tension stress fracture–a rare injury in a child: a case report. *Malays Orthop J.* 2021;15(1):132–134.
29. Herrera-Soto JA, Price CT, Reuss BL, et al. Proximal femoral epiphysiolysis during reduction of hip dislocation in adolescents. *J Pediatr Orthop.* 2006;26(3):371–374.
30. Hughes LO, Beaty JH. Fractures of the head and neck of the femur in children. *J Bone Joint Surg Am.* 1994;76(2):283–292.
31. Ingari JV, Smith DK, Aufdemorte TB, Yaszemski MJ. Anatomic significance of magnetic resonance imaging findings in hip fracture. *Clin Orthop Relat Res.* 1996;(332):209–214.
32. Joeris A, Audigé L, Ziebarth K, Slongo T. The locking compression paediatric hip plate: technical guide and critical analysis. *Int Orthop.* 2012;36(11):2299–2306.
33. Joseph B, Mulpuri K. Delayed separation of the capital femoral epiphysis after an ipsilateral transcervical fracture of the femoral neck. *J Orthop Trauma.* 2000;14(6):446–448.
34. Kashiwagi N, Suzuki S, Seto Y. Arthroscopic treatment for traumatic hip dislocation with avulsion fracture of the ligamentum teres. *Arthroscopy.* 2001;17(1):67–69.
35. Kirkos JM, Papavasiliou KA, Kyrkos MJ, Kapetanos GA. Multidirectional habitual bilateral hip dislocation in a patient with Down syndrome. *Clin Orthop Relat Res.* 2005;(435):263–266.
36. Knight DMA, Alves C, Wedge JH. Femoral varus derotation osteotomy for the treatment of habitual subluxation and dislocation of the pediatric hip in trisomy 21: a 10-year experience. *J Pediatr Orthop.* 2011;31(6):638–643.
37. Lehman RA Jr, Shah SA. Tension-sided femoral neck stress fracture in a skeletally immature patient: a case report. *J Bone Joint Surg Am.* 2004;86(6):1292–1295.
38. Li Y, Sun D, Wang K, et al. Postoperative avascular necrosis of the femoral head in pediatric femoral neck fractures. *PLoS One.* 2022;17(5):e0268058.
39. Maeda S, Kita A, Fujii G, et al. Avascular necrosis associated with fractures of the femoral neck in children: histological evaluation of core biopsies of the femoral head. *Injury.* 2003;34(4):283–286.
40. Magu NK, Singh R, Sharma A, Sen R. Treatment of pathologic femoral neck fractures with modified Pauwels' osteotomy. *Clin Orthop Relat Res.* 2005;(437):229–235.
41. Magu NK, Singh R, Sharma AK, Ummat V. Modified Pauwels' intertrochanteric osteotomy in neglected femoral neck fractures in children: a report of 10 cases followed for a minimum of 5 years. *J Orthop Trauma.* 2007;21(4):237–243.
42. Mehlman CT, Hubbard GW, Crawford AH, et al. Traumatic hip dislocation in children. Long-term followup of 42 patients. *Clin Orthop Relat Res.* 2000;(376):68–79.
43. Mirdad T. Fractures of the neck of the femur in children: an experience at the Aseer Central Hospital, Abha, Saudi Arabia. *Injury.* 2002;33(9):823–827.
44. Moed BR. The modified Gibson posterior surgical approach to the acetabulum. *J Orthop Trauma.* 2010;24(5):315–322.
45. Moon ES, Mehlman CT. Risk factors for avascular necrosis after femoral neck fractures in children: 25 Cincinnati cases and meta-analysis of 360 cases. *J Orthop Trauma.* 2006;20(5):323–329.
46. Moorman CT III, Warren RF, Hershman EB, et al. Traumatic posterior hip subluxation in American football. *J Bone Joint Surg Am.* 2003;85(7):1190–1196.

47. Morsy HA. Complications of fracture of the neck of the femur in children. A long-term follow-up study. *Injury.* 2001;32(1):45–51.

48. Nagao S, Ito K, Nakamura I. Spontaneous bilateral femoral neck fractures associated with a low serum level of vitamin D in a young adult. *J Arthroplasty.* 2009;24(2):322. e1-4.

49. Nötzli HP, Siebenrock KA, Hempfing A, et al. Perfusion of the femoral head during surgical dislocation of the hip. Monitoring by laser Doppler flowmetry. *J Bone Joint Surg Br.* 2002;84(2):300–304.

50. Nötzli HP, Wyss TF, Stoecklin CH, et al. The contour of the femoral head–neck junction as a predictor for the risk of anterior impingement. *J Bone Joint Surg Br.* 2002;84(4):556–560.

51. Odent T, Glorion C, Pannier S, et al. Traumatic dislocation of the hip with separation of the capital epiphysis: 5 adolescent patients with 3 to 9 years of follow-up. *Acta Orthop Scand.* 2003;74(1):49–52.

52. Ogden JA. Changing patterns of proximal femoral vascularity. *J Bone Joint Surg Am.* 1974;56(5):941–950.

53. Pape HC, Krettek C, Friedrich A, et al. Long-term outcome in children with fractures of the proximal femur after high-energy trauma. *J Trauma.* 1999;46(1):58–64.

54. Philippon MJ, Kuppersmith DA, Wolff AB, Briggs KK. Arthroscopic findings following traumatic hip dislocation in 14 professional athletes. *Arthroscopy.* 2009;25(2):169–174.

55. Poggi JJ, Callaghan JJ, Spritzer CE, et al. Changes on magnetic resonance images after traumatic hip dislocation. *Clin Orthop Relat Res.* 1995;(319):249–259.

56. Price CT, Pyevich MT, Knapp DR, et al. Traumatic hip dislocation with spontaneous incomplete reduction: a diagnostic trap. *J Orthop Trauma.* 2002;16(10):730–735.

57. Ramachandran M, Ward K, Brown RR, et al. Intravenous bisphosphonate therapy for traumatic osteonecrosis of the femoral head in adolescents. *J Bone Joint Surg Am.* 2007;89(8):1727–1734.

58. Ratliff AH. Fractures of the neck of the femur in children. *J Bone Joint Surg Br.* 1962; 44B:528–542.

59. Rieger H, Pennig D, Klein W, Grünert J. Traumatic dislocation of the hip in young children. *Arch Orthop Trauma Surg.* 1991;110(2):114–117.

60. Riley PM Jr, Morscher MA, Gothard MD, Riley PM Sr. Earlier time to reduction did not reduce rates of femoral head osteonecrosis in pediatric hip fractures. *J Orthop Trauma.* 2015;29(5):231–238.

61. Roca I, Barber I, Fontecha CG, Soldado F. Evaluation of bone viability. *Pediatr Radiol.* 2013;43(4):393–405.

62. Rubel IF, Kloen P, Potter HG, Helfet DL. MRI assessment of the posterior acetabular wall fracture in traumatic dislocation of the hip in children. *Pediatr Radiol.* 2002;32(6):435–439.

63. Salisbury RD, Eastwood DM. Traumatic dislocation of the hip in children. *Clin Orthop Relat Res.* 2000;(377):106–111.

64. Sanders S, Egol KA. Adult periarticular locking plates for the treatment of pediatric and adolescent subtrochanteric hip fractures. *Bull NYU Hosp Jt Dis.* 2009;67(4): 370–373.

65. Sanghavi S, Patwardhan S, Shyam A, et al. Nonunion in pediatric femoral neck fractures. *J Bone Joint Surg Am.* 2020;102(11):1000–1010.

66. Schmidt GL, Sciulli R, Altman GT. Knee injury in patients experiencing a high-energy traumatic ipsilateral hip dislocation. *J Bone Joint Surg Am.* 2005;87(6): 1200–1204.

67. Schrader MW, Jacofsky DJ, Stans AA, et al. Femoral neck fractures in pediatric patients: 30 years experience at a level 1 trauma center. *Clin Orthop Relat Res.* 2007; 454:169–173.

68. Scully SP, Aaron RK, Urbaniak JR. Survival analysis of hips treated with core decompression or vascularized fibular grafting because of avascular necrosis. *J Bone Joint Surg Am.* 1998;80(9):1270–1275.

69. Sener M, Karapinar H, Kazimoglu C, et al. Fracture dislocation of sacroiliac joint associated with triradiate cartilage injury in a child: a case report. *J Pediatr Orthop B.* 2008;17(2):65–68.

70. Song KS, Choi IH, Sohn YJ, et al. Habitual dislocation of the hip in children: report of eight additional cases and literature review. *J Pediatr Orthop.* 2003;23(2):178–183.

71. Song KS, Kim YS, Sohn SW, Ogden JA. Arthrotomy and open reduction of the displaced fracture of the femoral neck in children. *J Pediatr Orthop B.* 2001;10(3): 205–210.

72. Spence D, DiMauro JP, Miller PE, et al. Osteonecrosis after femoral neck fractures in children and adolescents: analysis of risk factors. *J Pediatr Orthop.* 2016;36(2):111–116.

73. Thacker MM, Feldman DS, Madan SS, et al. Hinged distraction of the adolescent arthritic hip. *J Pediatr Orthop.* 2005;25(2):178–182.

74. Togrul E, Bayram H, Gulsen M, et al. Fractures of the femoral neck in children: long-term follow-up in 62 hip fractures. *Injury.* 2005;36:123–130.

75. Vialle R, Odent T, Pannier S, et al. Traumatic hip dislocation in childhood. *J Pediatr Orthop.* 2005;25(2):138–144.

76. Yeranosian M, Horneff JG, Baldwin K, Hosalkar HS. Factors affecting the outcome of fractures of the femoral neck in children and adolescents: a systematic review. *Bone Joint J.* 2013;95-B(1):135–142.

77. Yoo JH, Hwang JH, Chang JD, Oh JB. Management of traumatic labral tear in acetabular fractures with posterior wall component. *Orthop Traumatol Surg Res.* 2014;100(2):187–192.

25

Femoral Shaft Fractures

Keith D. Baldwin and John M. Flynn

INTRODUCTION TO FEMORAL SHAFT FRACTURES

Femur fractures are common.[55,110] When subtrochanteric and supracondylar fractures are included, femoral shaft fractures represent about 1.6% of all bony injuries in children. Fractures are more common in boys (2.6:1) and occur in a bimodal distribution with a peak occuring during the toddler years (most commonly from simple falls) and then again in early adolescence (most commonly from higher-energy injury).[69,77,101] Recent incidence studies[46,70] also showed a seasonal bimodal variation, peaks in spring and autumn. Most femur fractures (64%) are femoral shaft fractures, with 27% being distal fractures and 9% proximal fractures.[46]

Although pediatric femoral shaft fractures impart substantial short-term disability, with attention to detail and modern techniques, these major injuries can be treated successfully with few long-term sequelae. Over the past 20 years, there has been a dramatic and sustained trend toward the operative stabilization of femoral shaft fractures in school-aged children using internal fixation. These advances have decreased the substantial early disability for children as well as the family's burden of care during the recovery period.[58] This trend toward operative management of pediatric femur fractures, including much younger children than in the past, is well documented in recent studies and does not necessarily follow national guidelines.[137,145,160]

ASSESSMENT OF FEMORAL SHAFT FRACTURES

The diagnosis of pediatric femoral shaft fractures is usually not subtle: There is a clear mechanism of injury, deformity and swelling of the thigh, and obvious localized pain. The diagnosis is more difficult in patients with multiple trauma or head injury in as well as nonambulatory, severely disabled children. A physical examination is usually sufficient to document the presence of a femur fracture. In patients lacking sensation (e.g., patients with paraplegia or myelomeningocele), the swelling and redness caused by a fracture may mimic the clinical findings of an infection. Presentation may be delayed due to lack of sensation, and may be mistaken for nonaccidental trauma in some cases.[10]

In the setting of a femur fracture, a comprehensive physical examination should be performed looking for other sites of injury. Hypotension rarely results from an isolated femoral fractures. Waddell's triad of femoral fracture, intra-abdominal or intrathoracic injury, and head injury can be associated with high-velocity automobile injuries. Multiple trauma may necessitate rapid stabilization of femoral shaft fractures to facilitate overall care. This is particularly true in cases of head injury and vascular disruption.

The hemodynamic significance of femur fractures has been studied by two groups.[30,112] Hematocrit levels below 30% rarely occur without multisystem injury. A declining hematocrit should not be attributed to closed femoral fracture until other sources of blood loss have been eliminated.[30,112] Adams et al. found that in their study of 95 isolated femur fractures, only 4.2% had a preoperative hemoglobin less than 8.2 g/dL postoperatively, and none required transfusion perioperatively.[1,36] As such isolated femur fractures can largely be treated expectantly from a hemodynamic perspective.

MECHANISMS OF INJURY OF FEMORAL SHAFT FRACTURES

The etiology of femoral fractures in children varies with the age of the child. Before walking age, up to 80% of femoral fractures may be caused by nonaccidental trauma.[62,195] In a study of over 5,000 children at a trauma center, Coffey et al.[31] found that nonaccidental trauma was the cause of only 1% of lower extremity fractures in children older than 18 months, but 67% of lower extremity fractures in children younger than 18 months. Baldwin et al.[13] found three primary risk factors for abuse in young children presenting with a femur fracture: a history suspicious for abuse, physical or radiographic evidence of prior injury, and age under 18 months. Children with no risk factors had only a 4% chance of being a victim of abuse, whereas children with all three risk factors had a 92% chance that their femur fractures were the result of abuse.

Murphy et al. showed that[136] transverse fractures of the femoral shaft are a better predictor of nonaccidental trauma in young children than spiral fractures.

Older children are unlikely to have a femoral shaft fracture caused by abuse because their bone is sufficiently strong to tolerate forceful blows, and is able to resist torque without fracture. In older children, femoral fractures are most likely to be caused by high-energy injuries. Motor vehicle accidents account for up to 90% of femur fractures in this age group.[40,69] Pathologic femur fractures are relatively rare in children but may occur because of generalized osteopenia in infants or young children with osteogenesis imperfecta. Osteogenesis imperfecta should be considered when a young child, with no history suggestive of abuse or significant trauma, presents with a femoral shaft fracture and non accidental trauma has been ruled out. Radiologic evaluation is often insufficient to diagnose osteogenesis imperfecta; skin biopsy, collagen analysis, and bone biopsy may be required to make a definitive diagnosis. Generalized osteopenia also may accompany neurologic diseases, such as cerebral palsy or myelomeningocele, or metabolic diseases

such as kidney disease leading to fracture with minor trauma in osteopenic bone.[91] Pathologic fractures may occur in patients with neoplasms, most often benign lesions such as nonossifying fibroma, aneurysmal bone cyst, unicameral cyst, or eosinophilic granuloma. Although pathologic femur fractures are rare in children, it is essential that the orthopaedist and radiologists study the initial injury films closely for the subtle signs of primary lesions predisposing to fracture, particularly in cases of low-energy injury from running or tripping. Radiographic signs of a pathologic fracture may include mixed lytic–blastic areas disrupting trabecular architecture, break in the cortex, and periosteal reaction in malignant lesions such as osteosarcoma, or better-defined sclerotic borders with an intact cortex seen in benign lesions such as nonossifying fibroma (Fig. 25-1).

Stress fractures may occur in any location in the femoral shaft.[121] In this era of high-intensity, year-round youth sports, orthopaedists more commonly encouter adolescents with femoral stress fractures from running, soccer, and basketball.[22] Although uncommon (4% of all stress fractures in children), femoral shaft or femoral neck stress fractures should be considered in a child with thigh pain because an unrecognized stress fracture may progress to a displaced femoral fracture. A high index of suspicion is important, because even nontraditional sports can lead to stress fractures with extreme overuse.

IMAGING AND OTHER DIAGNOSTIC STUDIES FOR FEMORAL SHAFT FRACTURES

Radiographic evaluation should include the entire femur, including the hip and knee as injury of the adjacent joints is common. An anteroposterior (AP) pelvis x-ray is a valuable supplement to standard femoral shaft views, because there may be associated intertrochanteric fractures of the hip, fractures of the femoral neck, or physeal injuries of the proximal femur.[17] Distal femoral fractures may be associated with physeal injury about the knee, knee ligament injury, meniscal tears,[186] and tibial fractures.[105]

Plain x-rays generally are sufficient for making the diagnosis. In rare circumstances, bone scanning and magnetic resonance imaging (MRI) may be helpful in the diagnosis of small buckle fractures in limping children or stress fractures in athletes. Advanced imaging such as MRI is also indicated for mechanisms inconsistent with injury or when concern exists for a pathologic bone fracture in the setting of an otherwise healthy child to rule out malignancy. The orthopaedist should carefully evaluate radiographs for comminution or nondisplaced "butterfly" fragments, second fractures, joint dislocations, and pathologic, as these findings can substantially alter the treatment plan.

CLASSIFICATION OF FEMORAL SHAFT FRACTURES

Femoral fractures are classified as: (a) transverse (60–90 degrees relative to the long axis of the bone),[108,171] short oblique (30–60 degrees relative to the long axis of the bone), or long oblique (<30 degrees relative to the long axis of the bone), or comminuted (multifragmentary). For fixation purposes transverse and short oblique fractures are thought of as "length stable" and long oblique and comminuted are thought of as "length unstable."

Figure 25-1. **A:** Femoral fracture through a poorly demarcated, mixed, osteoblastic, osteolytic lesion—an osteosarcoma. **B:** Sclerotic borders of this lesion in the distal femur are typical of a pathologic fracture through a nonossifying fibroma.

A femur fracture can also be categorized as open or closed. Open fractures are classified according to Gustilo system.[73] The presence or absence of vascular and neurologic injury is documented and is part of the description of the fracture. The most common femoral fracture in children (>50%) is a simple transverse, closed, noncomminuted injury.

The level of the fracture (Fig. 25-2) leads to characteristic displacement of the fragments based on the attached muscles. With subtrochanteric fractures, the proximal fragment lies in abduction, flexion, and external rotation. The pull of the gastrocnemius on the distal fragment in a supracondylar fracture produces an extension deformity (posterior angulation of the femoral shaft), which may make the femur difficult to align.

PATHOANATOMY AND APPLIED ANATOMY RELATED TO FEMORAL SHAFT FRACTURES

Through remodeling during childhood, a child's bone changes from primarily weak woven bone to stronger lamellar bone. Strength also is increased by a change in geometry. The increasing diameter and area of bone result in a markedly increased area moment of inertia, leading to an increase in strength. This progressive increase in bone strength helps explain the bimodal distribution of femoral fractures. In early childhood, the femur is relatively weak and breaks under load conditions reached in normal play. In adolescence, high-velocity trauma is required to reach the stresses necessary for fracture.[46]

Figure 25-2. The relationship of fracture level and position of the proximal fragment. **A:** In the resting unfractured state, the position of the femur is relatively neutral because of balanced muscle pull. **B:** In proximal shaft fractures the proximal fragment assumes a position of flexion (iliopsoas), abduction (abductor muscle group), and lateral rotation (short external rotators). **C:** In midshaft fractures, the effect is less extreme because there is compensation by the adductors and extensor attachments on the proximal fragment. **D:** Distal shaft fractures produce little alteration in the proximal fragment position because most muscles are attached to the same fragment, providing balance. **E:** Supracondylar fractures often assume a position of hyperextension of the distal fragment because of the pull of the gastrocnemius.

TABLE 25-1. Treatment Options for Isolated Femoral Shaft Fractures in Children and Adolescents

Age	Treatments
Birth–24 months	Pavlik harness (newborn to 6 months)
	Early spica cast
	Traction → spica cast (very rare)
24 months–5 years	Early spica cast
	Traction → spica cast
	External fixation (rare)
	Flexible intramedullary nails (rare)
6–11 years	Flexible intramedullary nails
	Traction → spica cast
	Submuscular plate
	External fixation
12 years to maturity	Trochanteric entry intramedullary rod
	Flexible intramedullary nails
	Submuscular plate
	External fixation (rare)

Treatment choices are influenced by fracture pattern, the child's weight, the presence of other injuries (head, chest, abdominal, etc.) and associated soft tissue trauma.

TREATMENT OPTIONS FOR FEMORAL SHAFT FRACTURES

Treatment of femoral shaft fractures in children depends on two primary considerations: age (Table 25-1) and fracture pattern. Secondary considerations, especially in operative cases, include the child's weight, associated injuries, mechanism of injury, availability of equipment, and the experience of the surgeon. Economic concerns,[54,142,178] the family's ability to care for a child in a spica cast or external fixator, and the advantages and disadvantages of any operative procedure also are important factors.[193] Clinical practice guidelines were developed in 2009[99] and then updated in 2015. These guidelines provided the current evidence for pediatric femur fracture treatment in a clinical practice guideline summary.[87] The guidelines generated few solid recommendations, due to low-level evidence in the literature. As such a comprehensive decision-making model incorporating all of these factors has been designed based on expert consensus, and will be discussed in more detail in the authors' preferred method section.[12,193]

TREATMENT VARIATION WITH AGE

Infants

Femoral shaft fractures in infants are usually stable because their periosteum is thick. In fractures occurring in infancy, management should include evaluation for underlying metabolic bone abnormality or abuse. Once these have been ruled out, most infants with a proximal or midshaft femoral fracture are comfortably and successfully treated with simple splinting to provide some stability and comfort, with a Pavlik harness to improve the resting position of the fracture.[163,177] For the rare unstable fracture, the Pavlik harness may not offer sufficient stabilization. Morris et al.[133] reported a group of eight birth-related femoral fractures in 55,296 live births. Twin pregnancies, breech presentation, and prematurity were associated with birth-related femur fractures. The typical fracture is a spiral fracture of the proximal femur with flexion of the proximal fragment. With thick periosteum, and remarkable remodeling potential, newborns rarely need a manipulative reduction of their fracture, nor rigid external immobilization. For femoral fractures with more shortening (1–2 cm) or angulation (>30 degrees), reduction and spica casting may be used. Traction rarely is necessary in this age group.

Preschool Children

In children 6 months to 4 years of age, early spica casting (Fig. 25-3) is the treatment of choice for isolated femur fractures with less than 2 cm of initial shortening (Fig. 25-4). In low-energy fractures, the "walking spica" is ideal (Fig. 25-5). One-legged spica casts have been tested against two-legged spicas in randomized controlled trials. Both methods result in healing in acceptable alignment with one-legged spica casts being associated with less burden of care including fewer parental days of missed work and easier positioning of the child in a car seat.[52,106] Femur fractures with more than 2 cm of initial shortening or marked instability and fractures that cannot be reduced with early spica casting 3 to are recommended to recieve 10 days of

Figure 25-3. **A:** This 7-month-old sustained a low-energy spiral femoral shaft fracture. **B:** Treatment was in a spica cast. **C, D:** Excellent healing with abundant callus at only 4 weeks after injury.

Figure 25-4. **A:** This 2-year-old sustained a low-energy spiral femoral shaft fracture, ideal for walking spica treatment. **B:** Immediately after reduction, note the lateral mold at the fracture site. **C:** Six weeks after injury, there is anatomic alignment, minimal shortening, and good callus formation.

Figure 25-5. A 4-year-old with a minimally displaced midshaft femur fracture treated with a walking spica cast, shown here 4 weeks after injury.

skin or skeletal traction prior to spica casting, though it bears noting that this approach has fallen out of favor in recent years. Nevertheless, internal or external fixation should be the exception rather than the rule in children less than 4 years of age. Although internal fixation of femoral shaft fractures in toddlers can produce a very pleasing radiographic appearance, reduction, casting, and remodeling produce such consistently excellent results and recent studies have demonstrated nearly three times greater cost in treating with internal fixation compared to spica casting, with equivalent outcomes.[107,153] In rare circumstances, external fixation can be used for children with open fractures or multiple trauma. Intramedullary fixation is used in children with metabolic bone disease that predisposes to fracture or after multiple fractures, such as in osteogenesis imperfecta, or following multitrauma. Flexible nailing can be used in the normal-sized preschool child[19] but is rarely necessary. Larger children (in whom reduction cannot be maintained with a spica cast) occasionally may benefit from flexible intramedullary nailing, traction with delayed casting, or in rare cases, submuscular plating or external fixation.

Children 5 to 11 Years of Age

Femur fractures in children aged 5 to 11 years of age, may be treated successfully by several different methods, depending on the fracture type, patient characteristics, and surgeon skill and experience.[55] In rare circumstances, a nondisplaced fracture might be treated in a walking spica cast in children less than 10 years old. Although traction and casting is still a successful method of managing femur fractures in young school-aged children, the cost and the social problems related to school-aged children in casts have resulted in this technique falling out of favor. Spica cast management is generally not used for children with multiple trauma, head injury, vascular compromise, floating knee injuries, significant skin problems, or multiple fractures. Flexible intramedullary nails are the predominant treatment modality for femur fractures in 5- to 11-year-olds, although submuscular plating and external fixation have their place,[100] especially in length-unstable fractures, or in those difficult-to-manage fractures in the proximal and distal third of the femoral shaft (see Authors' Preferred Treatment section).

Age 11 to Skeletal Maturity

Lateral entry trochanteric entry, locked intramedullary nailing is the primary mode of treatment for femur fractures in the preadolescent and adolescent age groups.[38] Several studies designed to refine the indications for flexible intramedullary nailing have concluded that although most results are excellent or satisfactory in children older than 11, complications rise significantly when this popular technique is used for bigger and older children.[136] In an international multicenter, retrospective study, Moroz et al.[132] found a statistically significant relationship between age and outcome, with children older than 11 years or heavier than 49 kg faring worse. Sink et al.[171] found a much higher rate of complications in length-unstable fractures. Fortunately, surgeons can now select from several different trochanteric entry nails that allow a relatively safe, lateral entry point, with the stability of proximal and distal locking screws. With this new information and technology, locked intramedullary nailing is used commonly for obese children of ages 10 to 12, and most femoral shaft fractures in children of age 13 to skeletal maturity. In fact, recent data suggest that by and large greater trochanteric growth after the age of 8 is appositional and that cartilaginous models are largely formed by that age. As such these studies conclude that antegrade nailing through the greater trochanter is safe after age 8.[97]

TREATMENT VARIATION WITH FRACTURE PATTERN

In addition to age, the treating surgeon should consider fracture patterns, especially when choosing implants. Elastic nailing is ideal for the vast majority of length-stable midshaft femur fractures in children between the ages of 5 and 11 years old. For length-unstable fractures, the risk of shortening and malunion increases substantially when elastic nailing is used.[170] Length-unstable fractures are best treated with locked trochanteric entry nailing in older children, external fixation in younger children, or submuscular plating in either of these age cohorts.

NONOPERATIVE TREATMENT OF FEMORAL SHAFT FRACTURES

Indications/Contraindications for Nonoperative Treatment		
Age	Indications for Nonoperative Treatment	Contraindications for Nonoperative Treatment
Birth–4 years	Most fractures in this age group	The extremely rare, open, high-energy, displaced fracture, especially in the setting of multitrauma or vascular injury
5–10 years	Nondisplaced fractures	Displaced fractures (almost all fractures treated with fixation)
11 years to maturity	The very rare, nondisplaced fracture in family preferring nonoperative care Nonambulatory children, particularly those with severe medical comorbidity	Displaced fractures and most nondisplaced fractures (almost all fractures treated with fixation)

Pavlik Harness

Stannard et al.[177] popularized the use of the Pavlik harness for femur fractures in infants. This treatment is ideal for a proximal or midshaft femoral fracture that occurs as a birth-related injury. Pain can be reduced by loosely wrapping cotton cast padding around the thigh. In a newborn infant in whom a femur fracture is noted in the intensive care unit or nursery, the femur is immobilized with simple padding or a soft splint. For a stable fracture, this approach may be sufficient and will allow intravenous access to the feet if needed. The Pavlik harness can be applied with the hip in moderate flexion and abduction. This often helps align the distal fragment with the proximal fragment (Fig. 25-6). Evaluation of angulation in the coronal plane (varus–valgus) is difficult because of hyperflexion. Stannard et al.[177] reported acceptable alignment in all patients with less than 1 cm of shortening. Morris et al.[133] showed that all treatments, including traction, spica cast, and Pavlik harness, are effective and resulted in satisfactory outcomes in all patients regardless of treatment.

Podeszwa et al.[149] reported infants treated with a Pavlik had higher pain scores when compared to an immediate spica cast; however, one-third of the spica cast patients had skin problems compared with none of the Pavlik harness treated patients. Average overgrowth after Pavlik harness usage is 5 mm (1–18 mm).[113]

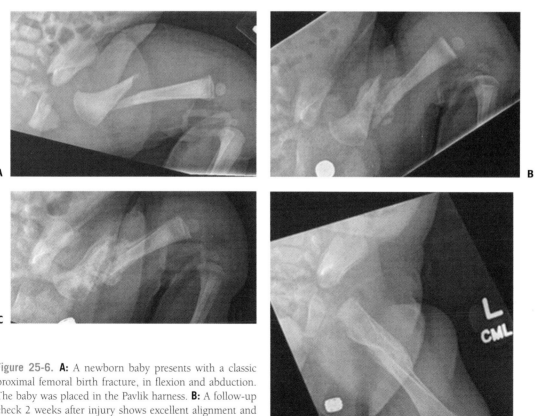

Figure 25-6. A: A newborn baby presents with a classic proximal femoral birth fracture, in flexion and abduction. The baby was placed in the Pavlik harness. **B:** A follow-up check 2 weeks after injury shows excellent alignment and early callous. **C:** A follow-up at 4 weeks shows a healed fracture. The Pavlik harness was removed. **D:** Follow-up 7 weeks after injury shows the dramatic early remodeling that is typical of these fractures.

Spica Casting

Spica casting[85,176] is usually the best treatment option for isolated femoral shaft fractures in children under 5 years of age, unless there is (a) shortening of more than 2 cm, (b) massive swelling of the thigh, or (c) an associated injury that precludes cast treatment. Several centers have adopted spica application in the emergency department as their standard treatment for infants and toddlers. Higher-energy injury, a proximal fracture location, and initial coronal angulation of greater than 8 degrees has been associated with a higher rate of suboptimal alignment at treatment conclusion, though the long-term sequelae of this malalignment appear to be minimal in this age group.[129]

Mansour et al.[115] compared spica cast placement in the emergency department versus the operating room, and concluded that the outcome and complications were similar, but the children treated in the operating room had longer hospital stays and significantly higher hospital charges. Car seating programs after spica casting are important, several studies have emphasized the need for seating evaluation following spica casting and admission is warranted if this cannot be fully assessed in an emergency room setting.[33–35,184] found that in children between 2 and 6 years old with a femur fracture treated in a spica cast, older and heavier children and those with over 2 cm of initial shortening went on to develop clinically measurable leg-length discrepancies but that none required secondary interventions as a result. Cassinelli et al.[28] treated 145 femur fractures, all in children younger than age 7, with immediate spica cast application in the emergency department. All children younger than 2 years of age, and 86.5% of children aged 2 to 5 years old, met acceptable alignment parameters on final radiographs. Re-reduction in the operating room was needed in 11 patients. The investigators concluded that initial shortening was the only independent risk factor associated with lost reduction.

The advantages of a spica cast include low cost, excellent safety profile, and a very high rate of good or excellent results, with acceptable leg-length equality, healing time, and motion.[50,84,107] Hughes et al.[80] evaluated 23 children ranging in age from 2 to 10 years who had femur fractures treated with early spica casting to determine the impact of treatment on the patients and their families. The greatest problems encountered by the family in caring for a child in a spica cast were transportation, cast intolerance by the child, and hygiene. In a similar study, Kocher[98] used a validated questionnaire for assessing the impact of medical conditions on families and demonstrated that for family, having a child in a spica cast is similar to having a child on renal dialysis. They found that the impact was greatest for children older than 5 years, and when both parents are working. Such data should inform the decisions of orthopaedic surgeons and families who are trying to choose among the many options for young school-aged children.

Illgen et al.[83] in a series of 114 isolated femoral fractures in children under 6 years of age, found that 90-degree/90-degree spica casting was successful in 86% without cast change or wedging, based on tolerance of shortening less than 1.5 cm and angulation less than 10 degrees. Similar excellent results have been reported by Czertak and Hennrikus[39] using the 90/90 spica cast.

Thompson et al.[180] described the telescope test in which patients were examined with fluoroscopy at the time of

TABLE 25-2. Acceptable Angulation			
Age	Varus/Valgus (degrees)	Anterior/Posterior (degrees)	Shortening (mm)
Birth to 2 years	30	30	15
2–5 years	15	20	20
6–10 years	10	15	15
11 years to maturity	5	10	10

reduction and casting. If more than 3 cm of shortening could be demonstrated with gentle axial compression, traction was used rather than immediate spica casting. By using the telescope test, these researchers decreased unacceptable results (>2.5 cm of shortening) from 18% to 5%. Shortening is acceptable, but should not exceed 2 cm. This is best measured on a lateral x-ray taken through the cast. If follow-up x-rays reveal significant varus (>10 degrees) or anterior angulation (>30 degrees), the cast may be wedged. However, Weiss et al.[192] noted that wedging of 90/90 spica casts can cause peroneal nerve palsy, especially during correction of valgus angulation (a problem that rarely occurs). For unacceptable position, the fracture can be manipulated and a new cast applied, or the cast can be removed and the patient placed in traction to regain or maintain length. Angular deformity of up to 15 degrees in the coronal plane and up to 30 degrees in the sagittal plane may be acceptable, depending on the patient's age (Table 25-2). Finally, if shortening exceeds 2 cm, traction or an external fixator may be considered (Fig. 25-7). A recent study showed that femur fractures

Figure 25-7. A proximal spiral femur fracture, which failed treatment with pins and plaster, and was salvaged with an external fixator.

gain an average of 5 degrees of varus and 10 degrees of procurvatum between cast application and fracture union. As such cast molding and initial alignment should be planned accordingly.[140]

The position of the hips and knees in the spica cast is controversial. Some centers prefer a spica cast with the hip and knee flexed 90 degrees each. Studies have shown that this "sitting spica" yields good clinical results.[119] The child is placed in a sitting position with the legs abducted about 30 degrees on either side. The synthetic material used for the cast gives it sufficient strength so that no bar is required between the legs. This not only allows the child to be carried on the parent's hip but also aids in toiletry needs, making bedpans unnecessary. Also, a child who can sit upright during the day can attend school in a wheelchair. More recently, with reports about compartment syndrome of the leg after using the 90/90 spica cast, several centers now cast with the hip and knee are more extended (~45 degrees each) and the bottom of the foot cut out to prevent excessive shortening. It should be noted that compartment syndrome had been thought to result from traction while first applying a short leg cast and building onto it, hence creating excessive pressure in the popliteal fossa.[102,135] Varying the amounts

of hip and knee flexion in the spica cast based on the position of the fracture also has been recommended: slightly more hip flexion is desirable with proximal fractures.[176]

Recently, there has been a resurgence of interest in the "walking spica cast" (see Fig. 25-5). Practitioners of the single-leg, or walking spica, apply the technique primarily for toddlers with very stable, low-energy fractures. The cast must be extensively reinforced at the hip. With the hip and knee much more extended, the single-leg spica not only improves function and ease of care, but also avoids a technique that has been associated with compartment syndrome in several children.[102,135] Increasingly, the walking spica is now considered the optimal treatment for low-energy femur fractures in toddlers.[52,106]

Technique

The cast is applied in the operating room or, in some centers, the sedation unit or emergency department.[115] For the sitting spica cast technique, a long leg cast is placed with the knee and ankle flexed at 90 degrees (Fig. 25-8A). Alternatively, the

Figure 25-8. Application of a 90-degree/90-degree spica cast. **A:** Generous padding is applied over the foot, and a pad is placed on the popliteal fossa to prevent injury to the peroneal nerve and popliteal vessels. **B:** A long leg cast is applied with the knee flexed 90 degrees. **C:** A mold is placed over the apex of the fracture, generally correcting a varus deformity into slight valgus. **D:** Using a standard spica table, a 1½ spica cast is applied with the hip flexed 90 degrees and abducted 30 degrees.

Figure 25-9. The dangers of pulling upward on the calf when applying a spica: This upward pull, which is used to reduce the fracture, can be dangerous, because it puts pressure on the gastrocnemius muscle and the other posterior leg structures, such as the femoral artery and femoral vein. (Reprinted with permission from Skaggs D, Flynn J. *Staying Out of Trouble in Pediatric Orthopaedics.* Lippincott Williams & Wilkins; 2006:105.)

child may be placed on a spica box initially, and the entire cast may be placed as a unit. It is important to place OR towels or a folded blanket on the abdomen during cast placement to allow for sufficient room in the cast. Waterproof linings may also be used to minimize friction, diaper rash, superficial infection, and skin damage. Casts will often need mole skin petaling to minimize discomfort and skin problems. Knee flexion greater than 60 degrees improves maintenance of length and reduction.[83] However, if one applies excessive traction to maintain length (Fig. 25-9), the risk of compartment syndrome is unacceptably high particularly when a short leg cast is applied first. Less traction, less knee flexion, and accepting slightly more shortening is a reasonable compromise. Extra padding, or a felt pad, is placed in the area of the popliteal fossa. The knee should not be flexed after the padding is placed because the lump of material in the popliteal fossa may create vascular obstruction (Fig. 25-8B). Because most diaphyseal fractures lose reduction into varus angulation while in a spica cast, a valgus mold at the fracture site is strongly recommended, and potentially even overmolding valgus (Fig. 25-8C). With more traditional placement the patient is placed on a spica table after placement of the long leg cast, supporting the weight of the legs with manual traction, and the remainder of the cast is applied with the hips in 90 degrees of flexion and 30 degrees of abduction, holding the fracture out to length (Fig. 25-8D). It is mandatory to avoid excessive traction because compartment syndromes and skin sloughs have been reported. The leg should be placed in 15 degrees of external rotation to align the distal fragment with the external rotation of the proximal fragment. After the spica cast is in place, AP and lateral x-rays are obtained to ensure that length and angular and rotational alignment are maintained.

Observation for 24 hours after spica application is recommended to be sure that the child is not at risk for neurovascular compromise or compartment syndrome.

For the single-leg spica or "walking spica" technique, the cast is applied with approximately 45 degrees of knee flexion and 45 degrees of hip flexion with 15 degrees of external rotation. The hip should be reinforced anteriorly with multiple layers of extra fiberglass. The pelvic band should be fairly wide so that the hip is controlled as well as possible. A substantial valgus mold is important to prevent varus malangulation. It is better to err on the side of mild posterior angulation, because the pull of the psoas generally leads to some procurvatum over time. We leave the foot out, stopping the distal end of the cast in the supramalleolar area, which is protected with plenty of extra padding. Seven to 10 days after injury, the child returns to clinic anticipating the need for cast wedging as fractures drift about 5 degrees varus and 10 degrees of procurvatum over the course of healing.[140] Most toddlers pull to a stand and begin walking in their walking cast about 2 to 3 weeks after injury.

If excessive angulation occurs, the cast should be changed, with manipulation in the operating room. Casts can be wedged for less than 15 degrees of angulation. If shortening of more than 2 cm is documented, the treatment strategy may be altered including cast change, traction, or conversion to external fixation. Lengthening techniques if the shortening is not detected until the fracture callus has developed. When conversion to external fixation is required, we recommend osteoclasis (either closed or open if needed) at the time of the application of the external fixator, with slow lengthening over a period of several weeks (1 mm/day) to reestablish acceptable length (see Fig. 25-7).

Generally, the spica cast is worn for 4 to 8 weeks, depending on the age of the child and the severity of the soft tissue damage accompanying the fracture. Typically, an infant's femoral shaft fracture will heal in 3 to 4 weeks; and a toddler's fracture will heal in 6 weeks. After the cast is been removed, parents are encouraged to allow their children to stand and walk whenever the child is comfortable; most children will need to be carried or pushed in a stroller for a few days until hip and knee stiffness gradually resolves. Most joint stiffness resolves spontaneously in children after a few weeks. It is unusual for a patient to require physical therapy. In fact, aggressive joint range-of-motion exercises with the therapist immediately after cast removal make children anxious, and may prolong rather than hasten recovery. Follow-up at 1-year time is helpful to assure return to baseline or expected structure and function by analyzing gait, range of motion, and leg lengths.

OPERATIVE TREATMENT OF FEMORAL SHAFT FRACTURES

Traction and Spica Casting

Since as early as the 18th century, traction has been used for management of femur fractures. Vertical overhead traction with the hip flexed 90 degrees and the knee straight was introduced by Bryant in 1873,[23] but this often resulted in vascular insufficiency,[139] and it is now rarely used for treatment of femoral fractures. Modified Bryant traction, in which the knee is flexed 45 degrees, increases the safety of overhead skin traction.[51]

Figure 25-10. This tomogram shows a bony bridge caused by a tibial traction pin that was placed for femoral fracture.

Traction prior to spica casting is indicated when the fracture is length unstable and the family and surgeon agree that nonoperative measures are preferred. In general, skeletal traction then spica casting are not currently used for children who are older than 12 years of age, because of the significant risk of shortening and angular malunion; in children older than 12 years of age, internal fixation is recommended. Children who are rapidly shortened in an early spica cast can be salvaged with cast removal and subsequent traction. The limit of skin traction is the interface between skin and tape or skin and foam traction boot. Skin complications, such as slough and blistering, usually occur when more than 5 lb of traction is applied. When more than 5 lb of traction is required or simply for ease in patient management, skeletal traction can be used to maintain alignment.[7]

The distal femur is the location of choice for a traction pin.[7,164] Although proximal tibial traction pins have been recommended by some clinicians,[81] growth arrest in the proximal tibial physis and subsequent recurvatum deformity have been associated with their use (Fig. 25-10). Also, knee ligament and meniscal injuries that sometimes accompany femoral fractures may be aggravated by the chronic pull of traction across the knee. Although traction followed by delayed spica casting results in excellent clinical and radiographic results, it has fallen out of favor because of the protracted hospital course and labor intensiveness of follow-up x-rays and nursing care.[142]

Technique

Traction and Spica Casting:
KEY SURGICAL STEPS

☐ Steinmann pin placement
☐ Traction applied and regular radiographs to monitor alignment
☐ Traction pin removed when callus seen

A large Steinmann pin is placed in the distal femur, avoiding the distal femoral physis. The insertion should be on the medial side, to have full control adjacent to the femoral artery in Hunter canal. Fluoroscopic controls are recommended, ensuring optimal pin position. The pin should be placed parallel to the joint surface. Traction is applied, initially using 5 pounds, and increasing is necessary. Traction is applied in a 90/90 position. An x-ray should be taken once or twice per week to monitor alignment. When early callus is seen on x-ray (usually about 3 weeks), the child is returned to the operating room, the traction pin is removed, the pin site is dressed, and a spica cast is applied as described above.

Unless there are extenuating circumstances, better options exist for children over 5 to 7 years of age.

Complications

Traction and Spica Casting of Femoral Shaft Fractures: PITFALLS AND PREVENTIONS	
Pitfall	**Prevention**
Compartment syndrome	• There is risk in placing an initial below-knee cast, then using that cast to apply traction while immobilizing the child in the 90/90 position. Avoid traction on a short leg cast, leave the foot out, and use less hip and knee flexion.
Malalignment and shortening	• Radiographs once or twice a week, with adjustments made based on alignment and fracture short.

Outcomes

Epps et al.[47] reported on immediate single-leg spica cast for pediatric femoral diaphyseal fracture. In a series of 45 children, 90% of the children pulled to stand and 62% of the children walked independently by the end of treatment. Fifty percent of patients were able to return to school or day care while in the cast. Only two children had unacceptable shortening, and two required repeat reduction. Flynn et al.[52] performed a prospective study of low-energy femoral shaft fractures in young children, comparing a walking spica cast to a traditional spica cast. Although the outcomes of the two treatment methods were similar, the walking spica cast resulted in substantially lower burden of care for the family. Leu et al. performed a similar randomized trial of single versus double-leg spica casting in this age group and found greater ease of care and less missed work for parents using single-leg casts.[106] Children with a walking spica are more likely to have their cast wedged in clinic to correct early loss of reduction.

In a study by Gross et al.,[61] 72 children with femoral fractures were treated with early cast brace/traction management. In this technique, a traction pin is placed in the distal femur and then incorporated into a cast brace. The traction pin is left long enough to be used for maintaining traction while the patient is in the cast brace or traction is applied directly to the cast. The patient is allowed to ambulate in the cast brace starting 3 days

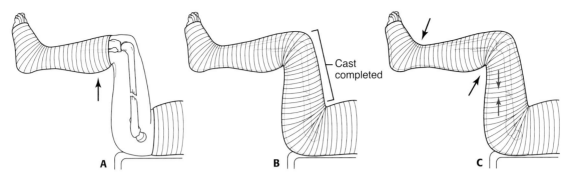

Figure 25-11. This drawing shows the pathogenesis of leg compartment syndrome caused by improper application of a spica cast. **A:** In the original description, a short leg cast was applied first, and used to pull the fracture out to length, as shown in this drawing. **B:** As the cast was completed, traction held on the short leg cast portion put pressure in the popliteal fossa. **C:** After the child awakens from general anesthesia, there is shortening of the femur from muscular contraction which causes the thigh and leg to slip somewhat back into the spica. This causes pressure to occur at the corners of the cast. (Reprinted with permission from Mubarak SJ, et al. Volkmann contracture and compartment syndromes after femur fractures in children treated with 90/90 spica casts. *J Pediatr Orthop.* 2006;26(5):570–572.)

after application. Radiographs are taken of the fracture in the cast brace to document that excessive shortening is not occurring. The patient then is returned to traction in the cast brace until satisfactory callus is present to prevent shortening or angular deformity with weight bearing. The technique was not effective in older adolescents with midshaft fractures but achieved excellent results in children 5 to 12 years of age. The average hospital stay was 17 days.

Comparative studies and retrospective reviews have demonstrated unsatisfactory results in a small, yet significant, percentage of patients treated with skeletal traction.[81,96,156] Recently, increased attention has been focused on the risk of compartment syndrome in children treated in 90/90 spica cast.[135] Mubarak et al.[135] presented a multicenter series of nine children with an average age of 3.5 years who developed compartment syndrome of the leg after treatment of a low-energy femur fracture in a 90/90 spica cast. These children had extensive muscle damage and skin loss around the ankle (Fig. 25-11). The authors emphasize the risk in placing an initial below-knee cast, and then using that cast to apply traction while immobilizing the child in the 90/90 position. The authors recommend avoiding traction on a short leg cast, leaving the foot out, and using less hip and knee flexion (Fig. 25-12).

Flexible Intramedullary Nail Fixation

In most centers, flexible intramedullary nailing is the standard treatment for midshaft femur fractures in children between the ages of 5 and 11 years old. Popularized by Metaizeau,[125] the flexible intramedullary nailing technique can be performed with either stainless steel nails[155,167,168,190] or titanium elastic nails. The popularity of flexible intramedullary nailing results from its safety, efficacy, and ease of implant removal. The flexible nailing technique offers satisfactory bridge fixation, enough stress at the fracture site to allow abundant callous formation, as well as relatively easy insertion and removal. The implants are inexpensive and the technique has a short learning curve. The primary limitation of flexible nailing is the lack of rigid fixation. Length-unstable fractures can shorten and angulate and result in prominent hardware and loss

of reduction, particularly in older and heavier children. Compared to children with rigid fixation, children who have their femur fracture treated with flexible nailing clearly have more pain and muscle spasm in the early postoperative period. The surgeon should take this into consideration in planning the early rehabilitation.

As the flexible nailing technique has become more popular, there have been many studies to refine the technique and indications,[167] and to elucidate the inherent limitations of fixation with flexible implants.[168] Analysis of these studies has been made more difficult by differences in technique, patient characteristics, implant metallurgy, as well as ability to "lock" the nail with implants such as Enders nails versus more traditional flexible intramedullary nails. Mechanical testing of femoral fracture fixation systems showed that the greatest rigidity is provided by an external fixation device and the least by flexible intramedullary rodding.[104] Stainless steel rods are stiffer than titanium in bending tests. Recognizing this flexibility, the French pioneers[103,109] of elastic nailing stressed the critical importance of proper implant technique, including prebending the nails so that the apex of the bend was at the fracture site, and so that the two implants balance one another to prevent bending and control rotation. Frick et al.[56] found there to be greater stiffness and resistance to torsional deformation when retrograde nails are contoured into a double C pattern than with the antegrade C and S configuration. Sagan et al.[165] noted that apex anterior malunion is less likely if at least one nail has its shoe tip point anteriorly, such that the nail is in procurvatum.

The prevailing technique for flexible nail insertion at most centers throughout the world has been retrograde, with small medial and lateral incisions just above the distal femoral physis. However, some prefer an antegrade technique, with entry in the subtrochanteric area. The primary advantages of a proximal insertion site are a fewer knee symptoms postoperatively.

Flexible nails are removed after fracture union at most centers. However, some surgeons choose to leave the implants permanently. There is a theoretical concern that if flexible nails are left in young children, they will come to lie in the distal diaphysis as the child grows older. This may create a stress riser in the distal diaphysis, leading to a theoretical risk of fracture (Fig. 25-13).

Figure 25-12. Authors' recommended technique of spica cast application. **A:** The patient is placed on a child's fracture table. The leg is held at about 45-degree angle of flexion at the hip and knee with traction applied to the proximal calf. **B:** The 1½ spica is then applied down to the proximal calf. Molding of the thigh is accomplished during this phase. **C:** The x-rays of the femur are obtained and any wedging of the cast that is necessary can occur at this point in time. **D:** The leg portion of the cast and the crossbar are applied. The belly portion of the spica is trimmed to the umbilicus. (Reprinted with permission from Mubarak SJ, et al. Volkmann contracture and compartment syndromes after femur fractures in children treated with 90/90 spica casts. *J Pediatr Orthop.* 2006;26(5):570–572.)

Preoperative Planning

Figure 25-13. A: A few years after titanium-lasting nailing, the nails have migrated proximally with growth, creating a stress riser and the subsequent insufficiency fracture. **B:** The refracture was treated with removal of the old nails and replacement with longer implants.

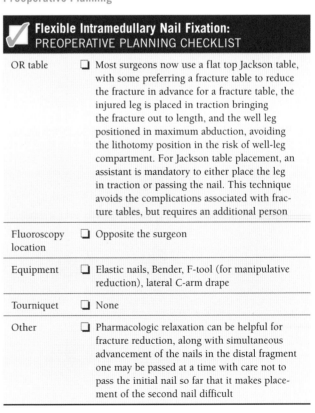

✓	**Flexible Intramedullary Nail Fixation:** PREOPERATIVE PLANNING CHECKLIST	
OR table	❑	Most surgeons now use a flat top Jackson table, with some preferring a fracture table to reduce the fracture in advance for a fracture table, the injured leg is placed in traction bringing the fracture out to length, and the well leg positioned in maximum abduction, avoiding the lithotomy position in the risk of well-leg compartment. For Jackson table placement, an assistant is mandatory to either place the leg in traction or passing the nail. This technique avoids the complications associated with fracture tables, but requires an additional person
Fluoroscopy location	❑	Opposite the surgeon
Equipment	❑	Elastic nails, Bender, F-tool (for manipulative reduction), lateral C-arm drape
Tourniquet	❑	None
Other	❑	Pharmacologic relaxation can be helpful for fracture reduction, along with simultaneous advancement of the nails in the distal fragment one may be passed at a time with care not to pass the initial nail so far that it makes placement of the second nail difficult

A

B

Figure 25-14. Titanium elastic nailing of the midshaft femur fracture through a benign lytic defect. **A:** Portable radiograph of a short oblique femur fracture through a benign lytic defect. **B:** AP radiograph taken several weeks after surgery that show the fracture well aligned with titanium elastic nail internal fixation and early callus at the fracture site.

The ideal patient for flexible intramedullary nailing is the child between the ages of 5 and 11 years old with a length-stable femur fracture, in the mid-80% of the diaphysis (Fig. 25-14), who has a body weight of less than 50 kg.[132] Unstable fracture patterns can also be treated with flexible nailing, but the risk of shortening and angular malunion may be greater,[171] though more recent data call this into question.[11]

Initial radiographs should be studied carefully for fracture lines that propagate proximally and distally and might be otherwise unnoticed (Fig. 25-15). Although it is technically difficult to obtain satisfactory fixation with a retrograde technique when the fracture is near the distal metaphysis, a recent biomechanical study[122] demonstrated that retrograde insertion provides better stability than antegrade insertion for distal femoral shaft

A, B

C

Figure 25-15. A: This high-energy, midshaft femur fracture was treated with titanium nails. **B:** A large butterfly fragment was dislodged during nail insertion. Because the fracture is now length-unstable, the surgeon wisely chose to protect the child for a few weeks in a one-leg spica cast. **C:** The fracture healed and had excellent alignment. Note how the nails have wound around each other. This can make nail removal more difficult.

fractures. Nail size is determined by measuring the minimum diameter of the diaphysis, then multiplying by 0.4 to get nail diameter. For instance, if the minimum diameter of the diaphyseal canal is 1 cm, the 4-mm nails are used. Always choose the largest possible nail size that permits two nails to fit medullary canal.

Flexible nailing can be effectively performed on a fracture table or a flat-top Jackson table, though the latter requires either thin wire traction or a surgical assistant.

Technique

Flexible Intramedullary Nail Fixation of Femoral Shaft Fractures:
KEY SURGICAL STEPS

- ❏ Fluoroscopic check of nail size
- ❏ Leg prepped and draped
- ❏ Medial and lateral incisions
- ❏ A hole is made in the cortex of the bone
- ❏ Nail is prebent and guided into the hole
- ❏ Medial and lateral rods are inserted
- ❏ Fracture reduction is optimized if necessary
- ❏ Nail deemed more difficult to pass is passed first, then the easier nail
- ❏ Nails are driven across the fracture and satisfactory reduction is confirmed fluoroscopically
- ❏ The nails are pulled back and their ends are before they are driven back securely into the femur

Fluoroscopy should be used to check the size of the nail against the canal, each nail should be the same size with the goal of filling 40% of the canal at the isthmus with each nail. Most pediatric femur fractures are fixed with 4-mm-diameter nails; in smaller children, 3.5-mm nails may be necessary. Two nails

of similar size should be used, and they should be as large as possible. With smaller diameter nails stainless steel should be considered for its increased stiffness.

After the child is placed on the fracture table and the fracture reduced as much as possible, the leg is prepared and draped with the thigh (hip to knee) exposed. The image intensifier is used to localize the placement of skin incisions by viewing the distal femur in the AP and lateral planes. If a Jackson table is used, check to make sure the fracture is reducible prior to draping. Incisions are made on the medial and lateral side distal to the insertion site in the bone. The proximal end of the 2- to 3-cm incision should be at or just distal to the level of the insertion site, which is about 2.5 to 3 cm proximal to the distal femoral physis (Fig. 25-16). A 4.5-mm drill bit or awl is used to make a hole in the cortex of the bone. The distal femoral metaphysis is opened 2.5 cm proximal to the distal femoral physis using a drill or awl. The drill or awl is then steeply angled in the frontal plane to facilitate passage of the nail through the dense pediatric metaphyseal bone. Widen the aperture of the entry point with the awl or drill on the way out of the bone to facilitate ease of entry for the elastic nail and advancement in the canal. The distance from the top of the inserted rod to the level of the fracture site is measured, and a gentle 30-degree bend is placed in the nail. A second bend is sometimes helpful near the entering tip of the nail to facilitate clearance of the opposite cortex during initial insertion. The tip of the nail can be placed just distal to the tip of the finger as it is guided into the hole in the bone to allow more simple insertion. On insertion, the rod glances off the cortex as it advances toward the fracture site. Both medial and lateral rods are inserted to the level of the fracture. At this point, the fracture reduction is optimized if necessary with a radiolucent fracture reduction tool, which holds the unstable femoral fracture in the appropriate position to allow fixation.

Figure 25-16. A: A drill bit slightly larger than the nail that will be implanted is used to broach the cortex. The drill bit can initially be placed in a perpendicular orientation. **B:** Once the cortex is broached, the drill bit is dropped to a sharply oblique angle and the medullary canal is entered. **C:** The contoured nails are inserted following the track of the drill bit. The angle insertion is sharply oblique so that the nail tip bounces off the opposite cortex and precedes up the canal. **D:** After the first nail is just across the fracture site, the second nail is inserted in a similar fashion.

The nail that is judged to be more difficult to get across the fracture site should be passed first. If the easier nail is passed first, it may stabilize the two fragments such that the second, more difficult, nail cannot be passed easily. The two nails then are driven into the proximal end of the femur, with one driven toward the femoral neck and the other toward the greater trochanter. The initial nail may be rotated to allow the second nail to pass, but care must be taken not to wind the nails on each other. After the nails are driven across the fracture and before they are seated, fluoroscopy is used to confirm satisfactory reduction of the fracture and to ensure that the nails did not comminute the fracture as they were driven into the proximal fragment. The nails are pulled back approximately 2 cm, and the end of each nail is cut, then driven back securely into the femur. The end of the nail should lie adjacent to the bone of the distal femoral metaphysis, exposed just enough to allow easy removal once the fracture is healed. Do not bend the exposed distal tip of the nail away from femoral metaphysis as this will irritate surrounding tissues. Unstable fractures of more length may require an end cap or eyelet screw if the nail design allows or a supplemental cast.

The procedure described is with titanium elastic rods, but other devices are available and can be used with slight variations in procedure. The technique of elastic fixation of femoral fractures as described by Ligier et al.[109] requires that a bend be placed in the midportion of the rod at the level of the fracture site. This produces a spring effect (Fig. 25-17), which adds to the rigidity of the fracture fixation. The spread of the rods in opposite directions provides a "prestressed" fixation, which increases resistance to bending. The opposite bends of the two rods at the level of the fracture significantly increase resistance to varus and valgus stress, as well as torsion. A second bend is sometimes helpful near the entering tip of the nail to facilitate clearance of the opposite cortex during initial insertion. Based on the report by Sagan et al.,[165] sagittal plane configuration should be considered as well. An apex-posterior bend in one of the nails, with the nail shoe pointing anteriorly in the proximal femur, resists apex-anterior malunion.

Using nails that are too small or mismatched in size increases the rate of complications.[138] It is very unusual to use nails smaller than 3.5 mm, except in the very youngest, smallest children. If smaller nails are necessary, stainless steel should be considered as this metal confers additional stiffness. On the lateral, one nail should have its tip pointing anteriorly. When passing the second nail across the fracture site and rotating it, care must be taken not to wind one rod around the other. A proximal insertion site can also be used. An insertion site through the lateral border of the trochanter avoids creating the stress riser that results from subtrochanteric entry.

Figure 25-17. A: Stability from flexible rods comes from proper technique. **B:** Torsional stability results from divergence of the rods in the metaphysis. **C:** Resistance to sagittal and coronal bending results from spreading of the prebent rods through the diaphysis, as well as the size and material properties of the rods. Elastic rods return to their predetermined alignment when loaded unless plastic deformation occurs.

Mazda et al.[118] emphasized that for insertion of titanium elastic nails, the nails have to be bent into an even curve over the entire length, and the summit of the curve must be at the level of the fracture or very close to it in comminuted fractures. The depth of curvature should be about three times the diameter of the femoral canal. Flynn et al.[53] also stressed the importance of contouring both nails with similar gentle curvatures, choosing nails that are 40% of the narrowest diaphyseal diameter and using medial and lateral starting points that are at the same level in the metaphysis. In length-unstable fractures, an endcap has been shown to confer increased stability that might lessen the risk of shortening[189] and nail backout.

Postoperative Care

A knee immobilizer is beneficial in the early postoperative course to decrease knee pain and quadriceps spasm. When the flexible nailing technique is used for length-unstable fracture, walking (or one-leg) spica is recommended, generally for about 4 to 6 weeks until callus is visible on radiographs. For length-stable fractures, touch-down weight bearing could begin as soon as the patient is comfortable. Gentle knee exercises and quadriceps strengthening can be begun, but there should be no aggressive passive motion of the knee, which increases the motion at the fracture site and increases quadriceps spasm. Postoperative knee motion does return to normal over time. Full weight bearing generally is tolerated by 6 weeks. Ozdemir et al.[147] recommended the use of postoperative functional bracing, demonstrating effectiveness in a group of patients treated with elastic rodding. Such postoperative support may occasionally be required, but in most cases, it appears not to be needed.

The nails can be removed 6 to 12 months after injury when the fracture is fully healed, usually as an outpatient procedure.

Complications

Flexible Intramedullary Nail Fixation of Femoral Shaft Fractures:
PITFALLS AND PREVENTIONS

Pitfall	Prevention
Overgrowth in preschool children[133]	• The technique should be used infrequently in preschool children.
Painful bursa and limited knee flexion[118]	• Do not leave rods too long.
Malunion	• Obtain a proper reduction of the fracture, use nails of adequate size, contour the nails so that the maximum bend is at the fracture site and there is good canal fill.
Shortening	• Use nails of adequate size, contour the nails properly, be sure that the proximal tip of the nail is embedded firmly in the strong metaphyseal bone of the proximal femur. • Consider using endcaps or eyelet screws, as well as consider casting when using the technique in length-unstable fractures.

Outcomes

A study comparing steel to titanium flexible nails found a higher complication rate in the titanium group.[190] These authors reported that a typical 3.5-mm stainless steel nail has the same strength as a 4-mm diameter titanium nail. Lee et al.[104] analyzed a group of synthetic fractured femurs instrumented with Enders rods and determined that there was sufficient axial and torsional stiffness to allow "touch-down weight bearing" despite fracture type. Gwyn et al.[64] similarly showed that 4-mm titanium rods impart satisfactory torsional stability regardless of fracture pattern.

Bourdelat[20] compared retrograde and antegrade (ascending and descending) flexible intramedullary rodding in a group of 73 femoral fractures. An antegrade transtrochanteric approach was recommended by Carey and Galpin,[26] who reported excellent results in 25 patients without growth arrest of the upper femur and no osteonecrosis. Satisfactory alignment and fracture healing were obtained in all patients.

Retrograde intramedullary nailing with Enders nails or titanium nails has been reported by Ligier et al.,[109] Mann et al.,[114] Heinrich et al.,[71] Herscovici et al.,[75] and others.[26,90,120] Heinrich et al.[71] recommended a 3.5-mm Enders nail in children 6 to 10 years of age and a 4-mm nail in children over 10 years of age. Ligier et al.[109] used titanium nails ranging from 3 to 4 mm inserted primarily in a retrograde fashion. Heinrich et al.[72] recommended flexible intramedullary nails for fixation of diaphyseal femoral fractures in children with multiple system injury, head injury, spasticity, or multiple long bone fractures. Flynn et al.[53] published the first North American experience with titanium elastic nails. In this multicenter study, 57 of 58 patients had an excellent or satisfactory result, there was no loss of rotational alignment, but four patients healed with an angular malunion of more than 10 degrees. Narayanan et al.[138] looked at one center's learning curve with titanium elastic nails, studying the complications of 79 patients over a 5-year period. Nails that were bent excessively away from the bone led to irritation at the insertion site in 41. The center also had eight malunions and two refractures. They noted that complications could be diminished by using rods with similar diameter and contour, and by avoiding bending the distal end of the nail way from the bone and out into the soft tissues. Luhmann et al.[111] reported 21 complications in 43 patients with titanium elastic nails. Most of the problems were minor, but a hypertrophic nonunion and a septic joint occurred in their cohort. They suggested that problems could be minimized by using the largest nail possible and leaving only 2.5 cm out of the femoral cortex.

Morshed et al.[134] performed a retrospective analysis of 24 children treated with titanium elastic nails and followed for an average of 3.6 years. The original plan with these children was to retain their implants. However, about 25% of the children had their nails removed for persistent discomfort.

Flynn et al.[54] compared traction and spica cast with titanium elastic nails for treatment of femoral fractures in 83 consecutive school-aged children. The three unsatisfactory results were treated with traction followed by casting. The overall complication rate was 34% in the traction group and 21% in the elastic nail group.

An international multicenter study focused on factors that predict a higher rate of complications after flexible nailing of pediatric femoral shaft fractures.[19] Analyzing 234 fractures in 229 patients from six different level 1 trauma centers, the authors found significantly more problems in older, heavier children. A poor outcome was five times more likely in patients who weigh more than 108.5 lb. A poor outcome was also almost four times more likely in patients older than 11 years old. The authors concluded that results were generally excellent for titanium elastic nailing, but poor results were more likely in children older than 11 years and heavier than 50 kg. Ho et al.[78] reported a 34% complication rate in patients 10 years and older, but only a 9% complication rate in patients younger than 10 years, emphasizing the concept that complications of flexible nailing are higher in older, heavier children. More recent data using Ender's flexible IMN suggest that complication rates are low in this group which may emphasize the importance of nail design and ability to lock the flexible nails in treating this group.[168]

Salem and Keppler[166] noted a 47% incidence of torsional malunion of 15 degrees or more in the patients they treated at one center in Germany. These authors could not determine if the torsional malunion was due to instability after fixation, or faulty surgical technique. In either case, the findings call attention to the need for rotational assessment after fixation.

Complications are relatively infrequent after flexible intramedullary nailing. In 351 fractures reported in seven studies,[15,26,49,72,109,111,118] one nonunion, one infection, and no occurrence of osteonecrosis were reported. Approximately 12% of patients had malunions, most often mild varus deformities, and approximately 3% had clinically significant leg-length discrepancies from either overgrowth or shortening. A recent study noted overgrowth of more than 1 cm in 8.2% of preschool children treated with titanium elastic nailing.[133] This is a much higher rate of overgrowth than seen in older children, suggesting the technique should be used infrequently in preschool children. Mazda et al.[118] pointed out a technique-related complication that occurred in 10 of their 34 patients: Rods were left too long and caused painful bursae and limited knee flexion. All 10 patients had the nails removed 2 to 5 months after surgery. Flexible nails inserted in a retrograde fashion may also penetrate into the knee joint, causing an acute synovitis.[161] In a multicenter study[53] that included 58 femoral fractures stabilized with titanium elastic nails, irritation of the soft tissue near the knee by the nail tip occurred in four patients (7%), leading to a deeper infection in two patients. This study also reported one refracture after premature nail removal, leading to a recommendation that nail removal be delayed until callus is solid around all cortices and the fracture line is no longer visible. Ozdemir et al.[147] measured overgrowth with a scanogram and found that the average increase in length was 1.8 mm, suggesting that significant femoral overgrowth is not seen with this method of treatment.

External Fixation

External fixation of femoral shaft fractures offers an efficient, convenient method to align and stabilize the fractured pediatric femur. Most surgeons favor internal fixation, but when severe soft tissue injury precludes nailing or submuscular plating, or in the event that a fracture shortens excessively in a spica cast or as part of a "damage-control" strategy, external fixation techniques can be invaluable.[131] In head-injured patients with vascular injuries or multiply injured patients and those with severe open fractures, external fixation offers an excellent method of rapid fracture stabilization.

Preoperative Planning

✓ External Fixation of Femoral Shaft Fractures: PREOPERATIVE PLANNING CHECKLIST	
OR table	❏ Either the fracture table or radiolucent table can be used
Fluoroscopy location	❏ Opposite surgeon
Equipment	❏ External fixator of choice
Tourniquet	❏ None

During preoperative planning, the fracture should be studied carefully for comminution, or fracture lines that propagate proximally or distally. The surgeon should assure that the fixator devices available are long enough to span the distance between the optimal proximal and distal pin insertion sites.

If the fracture is open, it should be irrigated and debrided before application of the external fixation device, if there is a vascular injury, the plan for the frame and the vascular repair are made in conjunction. With the fracture optimally aligned, fixation is begun. The minimal and maximal length constraints characteristic of all external fixation systems must be kept in mind, and the angular adjustment intrinsic to the fixation device should be determined. Rotation is constrained with uniplanar external fixation systems once the first pins are placed. That is, if parallel pins are placed with the fracture in 40 degrees of malrotation, a 40-degree malalignment will exist (Fig. 25-18). Multiplanar systems or thin wire frames can eliminate this issue.

Technique

✓ External Fixation of Femoral Shaft Fractures: KEY SURGICAL STEPS
❏ Address other surgical issues: if the fracture is open, perform irrigation and debridement; if there is a vascular injury, prep and drape in such a way that allows for vascular repair.
❏ Identify desired sites of pins
❏ Predrill the pins
❏ Place pins
❏ Reduce the fracture and place pin to bar constructs
❏ While maintaining reduction, attach bars to bars, tighten clamps
❏ Place additional bars and pins to enhance stiffness.

Technique Tips

Pin sizes vary with manufacturers, as do drill sizes. In general, the pins are placed through predrilled holes to avoid thermal

Figure 25-18. A: This proximal spiral femur fracture was deemed length unstable and a poor candidate for titanium elastic nails. The surgeon chose an external fixator, rather than a plate. **B:** Eight weeks after injury, the fracture is healing in excellent alignment and there is good early callous. Fixator removal is easier than plate removal.

necrosis of bone. Sharp drills should be used. The manufacturer's recommendation for drill and screw sizes should be checked before starting the procedure. Some self-drilling and self-tapping pins are available. At least two pins should be placed proximally and two distally. An intermediate or auxiliary pin may be beneficial, preferably out of plane.

Postoperative Care

The key to preventing pin-site irritation is avoiding tension at the skin–pin interface. We recommend that our patients clean their pin sites daily with soap and water, perhaps as part of regular bath or shower. Showering is allowed once the wound is stable and there is no communication between the pin and the fracture hematoma. Antibiotics are commonly used at some point while the fixator is in place, because pin-site infections are common and easily resolved with antibiotic treatment, usually cephalosporin.

There are two general strategies regarding fixator removal. The external fixation device can be used as "portable traction." With this strategy, the fixator is left in place until early callus stabilizes the fracture. At this point, usually 6 to 8 weeks after injury, the fixator device is removed and a walking spica cast is placed. This minimizes stress shielding from the fixator, and allows time for the pin holes to fill in while the cast is on. The alternative, classic strategy, involves using the fixator until the fracture is completely healed. Fixator dynamization, which is difficult in small, young children, is essential for this classic strategy. The surgeon should not remove the device until three or four cortices show bridging bone continuous on AP and lateral x-rays, typically 3 to 4 months after injury.

Complications

External Fixation: PITFALLS AND PREVENTIONS	
Pitfall	**Prevention**
Malalignment	• Placement of the pins perpendicular to the shaft of the femur
Pin-site infection	• Release any skin that will move against the pin when the patient begins to ambulate, perform twice daily pin care
Refracture after external fixator removal	• Be sure there are at least three cortices of bridging callus before external fixator is removed

Although joint stiffness has been noted in older patients treated with external fixation, it is relatively uncommon in children with femoral fractures unless major soft tissue injury is present.[48]

Outcomes

Aronson and Tursky[8] reported their early experience with 44 femoral fractures treated with primary external fixation and early weight bearing. Most patients returned to school by 4 weeks after fracture and had full knee motion by 6 weeks after the fixator was removed. In this early study, end-on alignment was the goal and overgrowth was minimal. Matzkin et al.[117] reported on a series of 40 pediatric femur fractures treated with external fixation. Seventy-two percent of their series were dynamized prior to external fixator removal, and their refracture rate was only 2.5%. They had no overgrowth, but one patient ended up 5 cm short.

Bar-On et al.[15] compared external fixation with flexible intramedullary rodding in a prospective randomized study. They found that the early postoperative course was similar but that the time to return to school and resume full activity was less with intramedullary fixation. Muscle strength was better in the flexible intramedullary fixation group at 14 months after fracture. Parental satisfaction was also significantly better in the flexible intramedullary rodding group. Bar-On et al.[15] recommended that external fixation be reserved for open or severely comminuted fractures.

The most common complication of external fixation is pin-track irritation/infection, which has been reported to occur in up to 72% of patients.[128] This problem generally is easily treated with oral antibiotics and local pin-site care. Sola et al.[175] reported a decreased number of pin-track infections after changing their pin care protocol from cleansing with peroxide to simply having the patient shower daily. Superficial infections should be treated aggressively with pin-track releases and antibiotics. Deep infections are rare, but if present, surgical debridement and antibiotic therapy are usually effective. Any skin tenting over the pins should be released at the time of application or at follow-up. If the external fixator is switched out for a femoral nail in a damage control setting, the secondary surgery should occur between day 5 and day 14.[143]

A comprehensive study of external fixation complications found an overall rate of refracture of 4.7%, with a pin-track infection rate of 33.1%.[27] Skaggs et al.[173] reviewed the use of external fixation devices for femoral fractures and found a 12% rate of secondary fractures in 66 patients. Fractures with fewer than three cortices with bridging callus at the time of fixator removal had a 33% risk of refracture, whereas those with three or four cortices showing bridging callus had only a 4% rate of refracture. Other reports in the literature with smaller numbers, but still substantial experience, document refracture rates as high as 21.6% with more significant complications.[42,44,60,128,152] Despite the complications, patients and treating physicians have found wound care and ability to lengthen through the fracture to be of great benefit to external fixation.

Antegrade Transtrochanteric Intramedullary Nailing

With reports by Beaty et al.[16] and others in the early 1990s alerting surgeons that antegrade intramedullary nailing can be complicated by osteonecrosis of the proximal femur, flexible nailing (either antegrade or retrograde) quickly became more popular than standard locked, antegrade rigid intramedullary nailing. Locked antegrade femoral nailing for pediatric femur fractures has enjoyed a resurgence of interest, however, with the introduction of newer-generation implants that allow a far lateral trochanteric entry point (Fig. 25-19). These newer implant systems avoid a piriformis entry site, reducing the risk of osteonecrosis.[79,93] Antegrade-locked intramedullary fixation is particularly valuable for adolescent femur fractures.

Open fractures in older adolescents can be effectively treated with intramedullary rodding, either as delayed or primary

Figure 25-19. Indication of femoral entry points relative to the proximal femoral blood supply: red, piriformis entry; blue, trochanteric entry; green, far lateral trochanteric entry. Piriformis is generally avoided, lateral entry is the preferred nail design.

treatment, including those caused by gunshot wounds and high-velocity injuries.[182] Antegrade intramedullary rod insertion maintains length, prevents angular malunion and nonunion, and allows the patient to be rapidly mobilized and discharged from the hospital. However, other techniques with fewer potential risks should be considered.

Retrograde rodding of the femur has become an accepted procedure in adults.[158] In a large patient with a bone age greater than 16 years, one may consider this method of fixation. If growth from the distal femur is predicted to be less than 1 cm, leg-length inequality should not be a problem and locking screws should be kept in the metaphysis.

Figure 25-20. AP (**A**) and lateral (**B**) radiographs immediately after internal fixation of the midshaft femur fracture in a 13-year-old child with a pediatric locking nail that permits easy lateral entry, and requires minimal reaming of the child's proximal femur.

Preoperative Planning

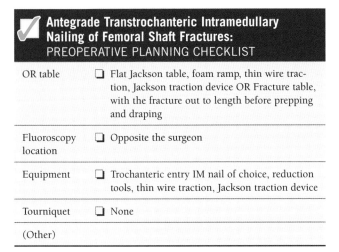

✔ **Antegrade Transtrochanteric Intramedullary Nailing of Femoral Shaft Fractures:**
PREOPERATIVE PLANNING CHECKLIST

OR table	❑ Flat Jackson table, foam ramp, thin wire traction, Jackson traction device OR Fracture table, with the fracture out to length before prepping and draping
Fluoroscopy location	❑ Opposite the surgeon
Equipment	❑ Trochanteric entry IM nail of choice, reduction tools, thin wire traction, Jackson traction device
Tourniquet	❑ None
(Other)	

The patient is placed either supine on a Jackson or fracture table. The upper end of the femur is approached through a small longitudinal proximal incision that allows access to the lateral trochanteric entry point. The skin incision can be precisely placed after localization on both the AP and lateral views, generally a guidepin may be placed to localize. Thin wire traction is placed in the distal femur prior to beginning the case if the Jackson table is used.

Technique

✔ **Antegrade Transtrochanteric Intramedullary Nailing of Femoral Shaft Fractures:**
KEY SURGICAL STEPS

❑ Dissection on lateral aspect of the greater trochanter
❑ Rod insertion through the lateral aspect of the greater trochanter
❑ Reaming and nail insertion
❑ Distal locking screws are inserted

Dissection should be limited to the lateral aspect of the greater trochanter, avoiding the piriformis fossa. This prevents dissection near the origin of the lateral ascending cervical artery medial to the piriformis fossa. The rod should be inserted through the lateral aspect of the greater trochanter, generally approximately 10 degrees off the tip of the greater trochanter, though this varies by implant. In children and adolescents, it is preferable to choose the smallest implant, with the smallest diameter opening reamer, to avoid damage to the proximal femoral insertion area. The technique for reaming and nail insertion varies according to the specifics of the implant chosen. In general, the smallest rod that maintains contact with the femoral cortices is used (generally ≤9 mm) and is locked proximally and distally (Figs. 25-20 and 25-21). Rods that have an expanded proximal cross section should be avoided, as they require excessive removal of bone

Figure 25-21. Preoperative (**A**) and postoperative (**B**) images showing the use of a newer-generation lateral entry nail to treat a proximal third femur fracture in a 14-year-old girl.

from the child's proximal femur. Only one distal locking screw is necessary, but two can be used.[92]

Technique Tips

Dissection should be limited to the lateral aspect of the greater trochanter (Fig. 25-22), without extending to the capsule or midportion of the femoral neck. Some nailing systems provide a small-diameter semiflexible tube that can be inserted up to the fracture site after initial entry-site reaming. This tube is extremely valuable in manipulating the flexed, abducted proximal fragment in proximal-third femur fractures.

Postoperative Care

Nails can be removed 9 to 18 months after radiographic union to prevent bony overgrowth over the proximal tip of the nail. We do not routinely remove locked antegrade nails from our teenage patients unless they are symptomatic or request removal for another reason. Dynamization with removal of the proximal or distal screw generally is not necessary. Distal locking screws may become symptomatic medially if the child grows away from the nail.

Complications

Antegrade Transtrochanteric Intramedullary Nailing of Femoral Shaft Fractures: PITFALLS AND PREVENTIONS	
Pitfall	**Prevention**
Avascular necrosis	• Use a far lateral, trochanteric entry point. Avoid dissection in the piriformis fossa.
Excessive reaming of a child's proximal femur	• Use the smallest diameter femoral nail possible.
Postoperative shortening or loss of reduction	• Used proximal and distal interlocks.
Irritation at the greater trochanter	• Do not leave an excessive amount of nail exposed proximally.
Rotational malreduction	• Assure proper rotational alignment before placing the distal interlocks. Beware of internal rotation deformity if using a fracture table

Outcomes

Comparative studies by Reeves et al.[156] and Kirby et al.[96] as well as retrospective reviews of traction and casting, suggest that femoral fractures in adolescents are better treated with intramedullary fixation[16,42,57,59,61,89,96,109,181,194,196] than with traditional traction and casting (Table 25-3). Keeler et al.[93] reported 80 femur fractures in patients 8 to 18 years old treated with a lateral trochanteric entry starting point. There was no osteonecrosis, no malunion, and a 2.5% infection rate.

Length-unstable adolescent femur fractures benefit from interlocking proximally and distally to maintain length and rotational alignment. Beaty et al.[16] reported the use of interlocking intramedullary nails for the treatment of 31 femoral shaft fractures in 30 patients 10 to 15 years of age. All fractures united,

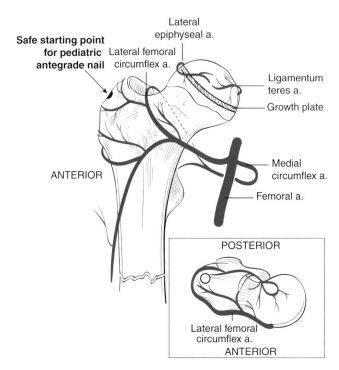

Figure 25-22. Trochanteric entry point for intramedullary nail indicated with *arrow.* Entry here with smaller diameter nails limits the risk of AVN and ensures no awl in the piriformis fossa. (Reprinted with permission from Skaggs D, Flynn J. *Staying Out of Trouble in Pediatric Orthopaedics.* Lippincott Williams & Wilkins; 2006:109.)

and the average leg-length discrepancy was 0.51 cm. No angular or rotational malunions occurred. All nails were removed at an average of 14 months after injury; no refracture or femoral neck fracture occurred after nail removal. One case of osteonecrosis of the femoral head occurred, which was thought to be secondary to injury to the ascending cervical artery during nail insertion.

Reamed antegrade nailing in children with an open proximal femoral physis must absolutely avoid the piriformis fossa, because of the risk of proximal femoral growth abnormalities,[154] the risk of osteonecrosis of the femoral head,[16,126,151,179] the size of the proximal femur, and the relative success of other treatment methods. Beaty et al.[16] reported the use of pediatric "intermediate" interlocking nails for femoral canals with diameters as small as 8 mm. Townsend and Hoffinger[183] and Momberger et al.[130] published reviews of trochanteric nailing in adolescents with very good results. The combined series includes 82 patients aged 10 to 17+ 6 years with no reported cases of osteonecrosis and no significant alteration in proximal femoral anatomy.

Ricci et al.[158] when looking at retrograde femur nailing, have shown that the complication rate with this technique compares favorably to that of antegrade nailing, with a higher rate of knee pain but a lower rate of hip pain. The malunion rate was slightly lower with retrograde rodding than with antegrade rodding of the femur.

Although good results have been reported with locked intramedullary nails and patient satisfaction is high, problems with proximal femoral growth, osteonecrosis, and leg-length discrepancy cannot be ignored. Fortunately, the osteonecrosis rate with newer lateral trochanteric entry nails is much lower.

TABLE 25-3. Results of Treatment of Femoral Shaft Fractures in Adolescents

Series	No. of Patients	Average Age (Range) in Years + Months	Treatment	Results and Complications (*n*)
Kirby et al.[96]	13	12 + 7 (10 + 11–15 + 6)	Traction + cast	Short >2.5 cm (2) Significant residual angulation (4)
	12	12 + 0 (10 + 10–15 + 7)	Intramedullary nailing	No overgrowth No significant residual angulation
Ziv et al.[196]	17	8 + 3 (6–12)	Intramedullary nailing (9 Rush pins, 9 Kuntscher nails)	No leg-length discrepancy >1 cm Change in AID 0.5–1 cm = 3 with Kuntscher nails
Reeves et al.[156]	41	12 + 4 (9 + 9–16 + 4)	Traction + cast	Delayed union (4) Malunion (5) Growth disturbance (4) Psychotic episodes (2)
	49	14 + 11 (11–16 + 10)	Intramedullary nailing	No infection, nonunion, or malunion
Beaty et al.[16]	30	12 + 3 (10–15)	Intramedullary nailing	Overgrowth >2.5 cm (2) AVN femoral head (1)
Aronson et al.[8]	42	9 + 7 (2 + 5–17 + 8)	External fixation	8.5% pin infection 10% cast or reapplication
Ligier et al.[109]	123	10 (5–16)	Flexible IM rods	1 infection 13 wound ulcerations 2 LLD >2 cm
Mazda et al.[118]	34	9.5 (6–17)	Flexible IM rods	1–1.5 cm overgrowth (3) 1–15-degree malalignment (2)

LLD, leg-length discrepancy.

In a series of intramedullary nailing of 31 fractures, Beaty et al.[16] reported one patient with segmental osteonecrosis of the femoral head (Fig. 25-23), which was not seen on x-ray until 15 months after injury. Kaweblum et al.[92] reported a patient with osteonecrosis of the proximal femoral epiphysis after a greater trochanteric fracture, suggesting that the blood supply to the proximal femur may have been compromised by vascular disruption at the level of the greater trochanter during rod insertion. Other researchers have reported single patients with osteonecrosis of the femoral head after intramedullary nailing.[126,146,179] A poll of the members of the Pediatric Orthopaedic Society disclosed 14 patients with osteonecrosis in approximately 1,600 femoral fractures. Despite the use of a "safe" transtrochanteric insertion site for antegrade femoral rodding, a case of osteonecrosis has been reported. Buford et al.[25] showed in their MRI study of hips after antegrade rodding that subclinical osteonecrosis may be present. Antegrade rodding through the trochanter or the upper end of the femur appears to be associated with a risk of osteonecrosis in children with open physes, regardless of chronologic age. Chung noted the absence of transphyseal vessels to the proximal femoral epiphysis and demonstrated that the singular lateral ascending cervical artery predominantly supplies blood to the capital femoral epiphysis[29] (Fig. 25-24). He stated that all of the epiphyseal and

metaphyseal branches of the lateral ascending cervical artery originate from a single stem that crosses the capsule at the trochanteric notch. Because the space between the trochanter and the femoral head is extremely narrow, this single artery is vulnerable to injury and appears to be so until skeletal maturity, regardless of chronologic age.

The proximal femoral physis is a continuous cartilaginous plate between the greater trochanter and the proximal femur in young children. Interference with the physis may result in abnormal growth of the femoral neck, placing the child at a small risk for subsequent femoral neck fracture. Antegrade nailing with reaming of a large defect also may result in growth disturbance in the proximal femur as well as femoral neck fracture (Fig. 25-25). Beaty et al.[16] reported no "thinning" of the femoral neck in their patients, which they attributed to an older patient group (10–15 years of age) and design changes in the femoral nail that allowed a decrease in the cross-sectional diameter of the proximal portion of the femoral rods.

Submuscular Bridge Plating

Submuscular bridge plating (Fig. 25-26)[67,88] allows for stable internal fixation with maintenance of vascularity to small fragments of bone, facilitating early healing.[108]

Figure 25-23. A: Isolated femoral shaft fracture in an 11-year-old child. **B:** After fixation with an intramedullary nail, femoral head appears normal. **C:** Eight months after injury, fracture is healed; note early signs of osteonecrosis of right femoral head. **D:** Fifteen months after injury, segmental osteonecrosis of the femoral head is evident on x-rays. **E:** MRI shows extent of osteonecrosis of right femoral head.

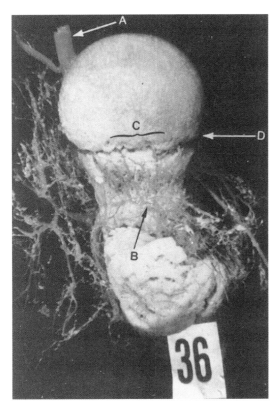

Figure 25-24. The single ascending cervical artery (B) is the predominant blood supply to the femoral head. The vessel is at risk during antegrade insertion of an intramedullary rod. (Reprinted with permission from Chung S. The arterial supply of the developing proximal end of the femur. *J Bone Joint Surg Am.* 1976;58(7):961–970.)

Figure 25-25. A 15-year-old boy 3 years after intramedullary nailing of the right femur. Articulotrochanteric distance increased by 1.5 cm; note partial trochanteric epiphysiodesis (*arrow*) with mild overgrowth of the femoral neck. (Reprinted with permission from Beaty JH, et al. Interlocking intramedullary nailing of femoral-shaft fractures in adolescents: preliminary results and complications. *J Pediatr Orthop.* 1994;14(2):178–183.)

Modern techniques of femoral plating, limiting incisions, maintaining the periosteum, and using long plates and filling only a few select screw holes, have been adopted by many pediatric orthopaedic trauma surgeons as a valuable tool to manage length-unstable femur fractures. Pathologic fractures, especially in the distal femoral metaphysis, create larger areas of bone loss that can be treated with open biopsy, plate fixation, and immediate bone grafting.

A, B   C

Figure 25-26. AP (**A**) and lateral (**B**) radiographs showing a complex spiral distal femur fracture that extends into the joint. This is a variation of Salter IV fracture. **C:** The fracture was managed with submuscular plating, and percutaneous lag screw fixation of the distal femoral condyle fractures.

In very rare situations, such as when there is limited bone for fixation between the fracture and the physes, locked plating techniques may be valuable. This technique provides greater stability by securing the plate with a fixed-angle screw in which the threads lock to the plate as well as in the bone. This effectively converts the screw plate to a fixed-angle blade plate device. In using this type of device, one should lock first, then compress, and finally lock the plate on the opposite side of the fracture. The locked plate can be used with an extensile exposure or with submuscular plating, but the latter is more difficult and should only be attempted when the technique is mastered.

We do not routinely use locking plates unless pathologic lesions, severe osteopenia, or severe comminution is present. Locking screws can "cold weld" to the plate, later turning a simple implant removal into a very difficult exercise involving large exposures, cutting of the implant, and possibly locally destructive maneuvers to remove the screws.

Technique

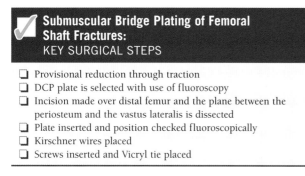

Submuscular Bridge Plating of Femoral Shaft Fractures:
KEY SURGICAL STEPS

❏ Provisional reduction through traction
❏ DCP plate is selected with use of fluoroscopy
❏ Incision made over distal femur and the plane between the periosteum and the vastus lateralis is dissected
❏ Plate inserted and position checked fluoroscopically
❏ Kirschner wires placed
❏ Screws inserted and Vicryl tie placed

The technique for submuscular bridge plating of pediatric femur fractures has been well described.[89,171,172] The patient is positioned on a fracture table or if preferred a flat-top Jackson table, and a provisional reduction is obtained with gentle traction. In most cases, a 4.5-mm narrow, low-contact DCP plate is used. A very long plate, with 10 to 16 holes, is preferred. The plate selection is finalized by obtaining an image with the plate over the anterior thigh, assuring that there are six screw holes proximal and distal to the fracture (although in some more proximal and distal fractures, only three holes will be available). The table-top plate bender is used to create a small flare proximally for the plate to accommodate the contour of the greater trochanter, or a larger flare to accommodate the distal femoral metaphysis. A 2- to 3-cm incision is made over the distal femur, just above the level of the physis. Exposure of the periosteum just below the vastus lateralis facilitates the submuscular passage of the plate. A Cobb elevator is used to dissect the plane between the periosteum and the vastus lateralis. The plate is inserted underneath the vastus lateralis and the femoral shaft is held to length by traction. The plate is advanced slowly, allowing the surgeon to feel the bone against the tip of the plate. Fluoroscopy is helpful in determining proper positioning of the plate. A bolster is placed under the thigh to help maintain sagittal alignment. Once the plate is in position and the femur is out to length, a Kirschner wire is placed in the most proximal and distal hole of the plate to maintain length (Fig. 25-27). Fluoroscopy is used to check the AP and lateral views and be sure the bone is at appropriate length at this point. A third Kirschner wire may be used to provide a more stable reduction of the femoral shaft. Although screws can be used to facilitate angular reduction to the plate, length must be achieved before the initiation of fixation. Rather than using a depth gauge directly, because the bone will be pulled to the plate, the depth gauge is placed over the thigh itself to measure appropriate length of the screw. Place one screw through the distal incision under direct visualization. At the opposite end of the femur, the next most proximal screw is placed to fix length and provisionally improve alignment. Stab holes are made centrally for drill and

A

B

Figure 25-27. A: A Kirschner wire is inserted in the end holes of the plate to maintain length. **B:** Drill holes and screws are placed with fluoroscope imaging.

screw insertion. When screws are inserted, a Vicryl tie is placed around the shank to avoid losing the screw during percutaneous placement. Self-tapping screws are required for this procedure. Six cortices are sought on either side of the fracture.

The postoperative management includes protected weight bearing on crutches with no need for cast immobilization, as long as stable fixation is achieved. At times, there is benefit to a knee immobilizer; however, in general, this is not required. Early weight bearing in some series of plate fixation has resulted in a low but significant incidence of plate breakage and non-union. These complications should be decreased by a cautious period of postoperative management.

There are occasional cases with sufficient osteopenia or comminution to require a locked plate to provide secure fixation. In using a locked plate submuscularly, a large enough incision must be used to be sure the bone is against the plate when it is locked. The articular fragment is fixed first to ensure that the angular relationship between the joint surface and the shaft is perfect.

Complications

Submuscular Bridge Plating of Femoral Shaft Fractures: PITFALLS AND PREVENTIONS	
Pitfall	**Prevention**
Refracture	• Remove the plate after satisfactory union, and about 1 year after injury.
Failure fixation/plate bending	• Restrict weight-bearing until early callus is seen.
Distal femur varus or valgus malunion	• Very carefully contour the plate distally.

Outcomes

Kanlic et al.[89] reported a series of 51 patients using submuscular bridge plating with up to 10-year follow-up. Fifty-five percent had unstable fracture patterns. There were two significant complications: one plate breakage (3.5 mm) and one fracture after plate removal. Functional outcome was excellent with 8% significant leg-length discrepancy. Hedequist et al.[66] reported on 32 patients aged 6 to 15 years old. Most fractures in their series were comminuted, pathologic, osteopenic, or in a difficult location. Rozbruch et al. described modern techniques of plate fixation popularized by the AO Association for the Study of Internal Fixation that include indirect reduction, biologic approaches to internal fixation, and greater use of blade plates and locked plates (Fig. 25-28).

Figure 25-28. A: This child with an unstable femoral fracture in osteopenic bone was managed with a submuscular locking plate providing alignment and stability. **B:** The lateral bow of the femur may be partially preserved despite a straight plate.

Sink et al.[170] reported on their center's transition to treating unstable femur fractures with submuscular plating and trochanteric entry nails, and reserving elastic nailing for stable fractures. Their complication rate declined sharply with this change in treatment philosophy.

Plate removal can be difficult after submuscular plating; in fact, the problems with plate removal keep some surgeons from using the technique routinely. Pate et al.[148] reviewed a series of 22 cases of plate removal after submuscular plating for femoral shaft fracture. In 7 of the 22 cases, the incision and surgical dissection were more extensive in the plate removal than in the initial insertion. The authors alert the reader that bone can form on the leading edge of the plate, complicating plate removal.

Quadriceps strength after plate fixation appears not to be compromised, relative to intramedullary fixation or cast immobilization. Distal femoral valgus has also been noted following plating and therefore plate removal is suggested following fixation of distal femur fractures particularly when the plate is placed 20 mm or less from the growth plate.[76,94]

Authors' Preferred Treatment for Femoral Shaft Fractures (Algorithm 25-1)

With many different treatment options, and several different factors that must be considered when choosing among the options, a comprehensive decision-making algorithm is needed; published guidelines are not being followed.[137,145,160] This method was recently evaluated based on expert consensus and by clinical outcomes.[193]

A similar classification system can be made to describe the severity, risk, and optimal treatment options for pediatric femur fractures (see Algorithm 25-1).

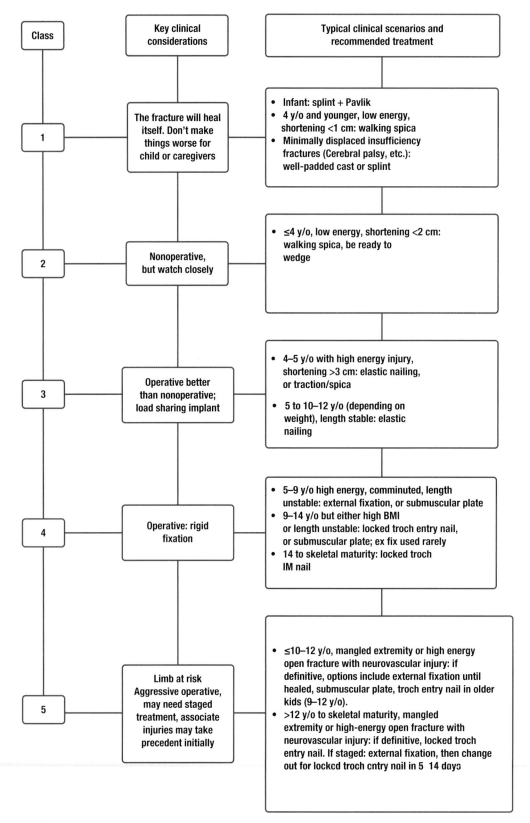

Class	Key clinical considerations	Typical clinical scenarios and recommended treatment
1	The fracture will heal itself. Don't make things worse for child or caregivers	• Infant: splint + Pavlik • 4 y/o and younger, low energy, shortening <1 cm: walking spica • Minimally displaced insufficiency fractures (Cerebral palsy, etc.): well-padded cast or splint
2	Nonoperative, but watch closely	• ≤4 y/o, low energy, shortening <2 cm: walking spica, be ready to wedge
3	Operative better than nonoperative; load sharing implant	• 4–5 y/o with high energy injury, shortening >3 cm: elastic nailing, or traction/spica • 5 to 10–12 y/o (depending on weight), length stable: elastic nailing
4	Operative: rigid fixation	• 5–9 y/o high energy, comminuted, length unstable: external fixation, or submuscular plate • 9–14 y/o but either high BMI or length unstable: locked troch entry nail, or submuscular plate; ex fix used rarely • 14 to skeletal maturity: locked troch IM nail
5	Limb at risk Aggressive operative, may need staged treatment, associate injuries may take precedent initially	• ≤10–12 y/o, mangled extremity or high energy open fracture with neurovascular injury: if definitive, options include external fixation until healed, submuscular plate, troch entry nail in older kids (9–12 y/o). • >12 y/o to skeletal maturity, mangled extremity or high-energy open fracture with neurovascular injury: if definitive, locked troch entry nail. If staged: external fixation, then change out for locked troch entry nail in 5–14 days

Algorithm 25-1. Authors' preferred treatment for femoral shaft fractures: a comprehensive decision-making system for pediatric femur fracture management.

MANAGEMENT OF EXPECTED ADVERSE OUTCOMES AND UNEXPECTED COMPLICATIONS RELATED TO FEMORAL SHAFT FRACTURES

Femoral Shaft Fractures:
COMMON ADVERSE OUTCOMES AND COMPLICATIONS

- Leg-length discrepancy
- Angular deformity
- Rotational deformity
- Delayed union
- Nonunion
- Muscle weakness
- Infection
- Neurovascular injury
- Compartment syndrome

LEG-LENGTH DISCREPANCY

The most common sequela after femoral shaft fractures in children is leg-length discrepancy. The fractured femur may be initially short from overriding of the fragments at union or conversely, growth acceleration can occur to "make up" the difference, but often this acceleration continues and the injured leg ends up being longer. The potential for growth stimulation from femoral fractures has long been recognized, but the exact cause of this phenomenon is still unknown. Growth acceleration has been attributed to age, sex, fracture type, fracture level, and the amount of overriding of the fracture fragments. Age seems to be the most constant factor, but fractures in the proximal third of the femur and oblique comminuted fractures also have been associated with relatively greater growth acceleration.

Overgrowth after femoral fracture is most common in children 2 to 10 years of age. The average overgrowth is 0.9 cm, with a range of 0.4 to 2.5 cm.[169] Overgrowth can occur with any initial length of the fractured bone. In general, overgrowth occurs most rapidly during the first 2 years after fracture and to a much lesser degree for the next year or so after. Because the average overgrowth after femoral fracture is approximately 1 cm, shortening of 2 to 3 cm in the cast is the maximal acceptable amount.

Truesdell[185] first reported the phenomenon of overgrowth in 1921, and many researchers have verified the existence of growth stimulation after fracture.[2,3,6,14,32,45,154] The relationship of the location of the fracture to growth is somewhat controversial. Staheli[176] reported that overgrowth was greatest if the fracture occurred in the proximal third of the femur, whereas Henry stated that the most overgrowth occurred in fractures in the distal third of the femur. Other investigators have found no relationship between fracture location and growth stimulation.[45,157,169] The relationship between fracture type and overgrowth also is controversial. In general, most researchers believe that no specific relationship exists between fracture type and overgrowth, but some have reported overgrowth to be more frequent after spiral, oblique, and comminuted fractures associated with greater trauma.

ANGULAR DEFORMITY

Some degree of angular deformity is frequent after femoral shaft fractures in children, but this usually remodels with growth. Angular remodeling occurs at the site of fracture, with appositional new bone formation in the concavity of the long bone. Differential physeal growth also occurs in response to diaphyseal angular deformity. Wallace and Hoffman[191] stated that 74% of the remodeling that occurs is physeal, and appositional remodeling at the fracture site occurs to a much lesser degree. However, this appears to be somewhat age dependent. It is clear that angular remodeling occurs best in the direction of motion at the adjacent joint.[191] That is, anterior and posterior remodeling in the femur occurs rapidly and with little residual deformity. In contrast, remodeling of a varus or valgus deformity occurs more slowly. The differential physeal growth in a varus or valgus direction in the distal femur causes compensatory deformity, which is usually insignificant. In severe varus bowing, however, a hypoplastic lateral condyle results, which may cause a distal femoral valgus deformity if the varus bow is corrected.

Guidelines for acceptable alignment vary widely. The range of acceptable anterior and posterior angulation varies from 30 to 40 degrees in children up to 2 years of age (Fig. 25-29), decreasing to 10 degrees in older children and adolescents. The range of acceptable varus and valgus angulation also becomes smaller with age. Varus angulation in infants and children should be limited to 10 to 15 degrees, although greater degrees of angulation may have a satisfactory outcome. Acceptable valgus angulation is 20 to 30 degrees in infants, 15 to 20 degrees in children up to 5 years of age, and 10 degrees in older children and adolescents. Compensation for deformity around the knee is limited, so guidelines for the distal femoral fractures should be stricter than proximal femoral fractures.

Late development of genu recurvatum deformity of the proximal tibia after femoral shaft fracture has been most often reported as a complication of traction pin or wire placement through or near the anterior aspect of the proximal tibial physis, excessive traction, pin-track infection, or prolonged cast immobilization. Femoral pins are preferred for traction, but if tibial pins are required, the proximal anterior tibial physis must be avoided. Femoral traction pins should be placed one or two fingerbreadths proximal to the superior pole of the patella to avoid the distal femoral physis.

If significant angular deformity is present after fracture union, corrective osteotomy should be delayed for at least a year unless the deformity is severe enough to markedly impair function. This will allow determination of remodeling potential before deciding that surgical correction is necessary. The ideal osteotomy corrects the deformity at the site of fracture. In juvenile patients, however, metaphyseal osteotomy of the proximal or distal femur may be necessary. In adolescents with midshaft deformities, diaphyseal osteotomy and fixation with an interlocking intramedullary nail are often preferable.

Distal femoral angular malunion is being recognized after submuscular plating. Care in plate contouring and postoperative monitoring is recommended.[76]

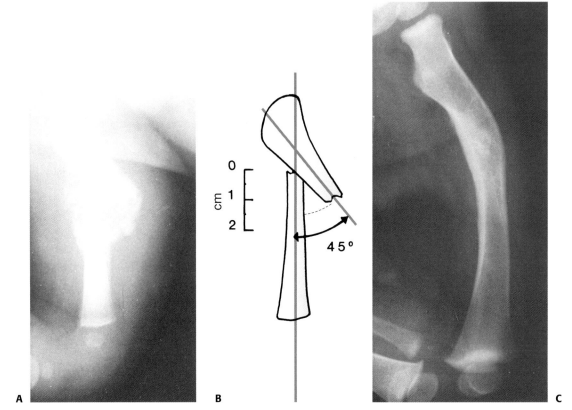

Figure 25-29. Remodeling potential of the femur during infancy. This infant sustained a femoral fracture during a breech delivery and was placed in a spica cast but with insufficient flexion of the hip. **A:** At 3 weeks, union is evident with about 45 degrees of angulation in the sagittal plane and 1.5 cm of overriding. **B:** Line drawing demonstrating true angulation. **C:** Twelve months later the anterior angulation has reduced to a level such that it was not apparent to the family, and the shortening has reduced to less than 1 cm.

ROTATIONAL DEFORMITY

According to Verbeek,[187] rotational deformities of 10 degrees to more than 30 degrees occur in one-third of children after conservative treatment of femoral shaft fractures. Salem and Keppler[166] noted a 47% incidence of torsional malunion of 15 degrees or more in the patients they treated with elastic nails at one center in Germany. Torsional deformity usually is expressed as increased femoral anteversion on the fractured side compared with the opposite side, as demonstrated by physical examination; a difference of more than 10 degrees has been the criterion of significant deformity. However, Brouwer et al.[22] challenged this criterion, citing differences of 0 to 15 degrees in a control group of 100 normal volunteers. The accuracy of measurements from plain x-rays also has been disputed, and Norbeck et al.[141] suggested the use of computed tomographic (CT) scanning for greater accuracy.

Rotational remodeling in childhood femoral fractures is another controversy in the search for criteria on which to base therapeutic judgments. According to Davids[41] and Braten et al.,[21] up to 25 degrees of rotational malalignment at the time of healing of femoral fractures appears to be well tolerated in children. In their patients with more than 25 degrees of rotational malalignment, however, deformity caused clinical complaints. Davids[41] found no spontaneous correction in his study of malunions based on CT measurements, but the length of follow-up is insufficient to state that no rotational remodeling occurs. Brouwer et al.[22] and others[65,144,187] reported slow rotational correction over time. Buchholz et al.[24] documented five children with increased femoral anteversion of 10 degrees or more after fracture healing in children between 3 and 6 years old. In three of five children, there was full correction of the rotational deformity but the oldest of the children failed to correct spontaneously.

Certainly, in older adolescents, no significant rotational remodeling will occur. In infants and juveniles, some rotational deformity can be accepted[51] because either true rotational remodeling or functional adaptation allows resumption of normal gait. Up to 30 degrees of malrotation in the femur should result in no functional impairment unless there is pre-existing rotational malalignment. The goal, however, should be to reduce a rotational deformity to 10 degrees, based on alignment of the proximal and distal femur radiographically, interpretation of skin and soft tissue envelope alignment, and correct positioning within a cast, based on the muscle pull on the proximal fragment. The distal fragment should be lined up with the position of the proximal fragment determined by the muscles inserted upon it (see Fig. 25-2).

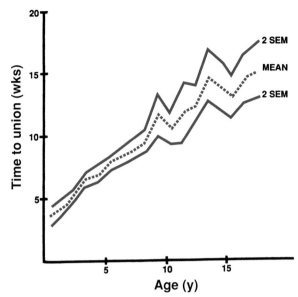

*Excludes delayed unions and pseudoarthroses.

Figure 25-30. Time required for union of femoral shaft fractures in childhood and adolescence. (Redrawn from Skak SV, Jensen TT. Femoral shaft fracture in 265 children: log-normal correlation with age of speed of healing. *Acta Orthop Scand.* 1988;59(6):704–707, with permission.)

DELAYED UNION

Delayed union of femoral shaft fractures is uncommon in children. The rate of healing also is related to soft tissue injury and type of treatment. The time to fracture union in most children is rapid and age dependent. In infants, fracture can be healed in 2 to 3 weeks. In children under 5 years of age, healing usually occurs in 4 to 6 weeks. In children 5 to 10 years of age, fracture healing is somewhat slower, requiring 8 to 10 weeks. Throughout adolescence, the time to healing continues to lengthen. By the age of 15 years, the mean time to healing is about 13 weeks, with a range from 10 to 15 weeks (Fig. 25-30). Application of an external fixation device appears to delay callus formation and slow the rate of healing. Flexible nailing allows some motion at the fracture site, promoting extensive callus formation. Bone grafting and internal fixation with either a compression plate or locked intramedullary nail is the usual treatment for delayed union in older children and adolescents. Delayed union of a femoral fracture treated with casting in a child 1 to 6 years of age is probably best treated by continuing cast immobilization until bridging callus forms or (rarely) by additional bone grafting.

NONUNION

Nonunions of pediatric femoral fractures are rare. They tend to occur in adolescents, in infected fractures, or in fractures with segmental bone loss or severe soft tissue loss. Tibial fractures are the most common source of pediatric nonunions; femoral fractures account for only 15% of nonunions in children. Even in segmental fractures with bone loss, young children may have sufficient osteogenic potential to fill in a significant fracture gap

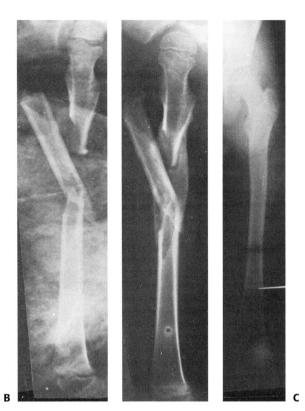

Figure 25-31. The effectiveness of remodeling of the femur in a child. **A:** Comminuted fracture in an 8-year-old child managed with a femoral pin incorporated in a spica cast. The midfragment is markedly angulated. **B:** Fracture after union 12 weeks later with filling in of the defect and early absorption of the protruding fragment. **C:** Appearance at age 12 with only a minimal degree of irregularity of the upper femur remaining.

(Fig. 25-31).[124] For the rare femoral shaft nonunion in a child 5 to 10 years of age, bone grafting and plate-and-screw fixation have been traditional treatment methods, but more recently insertion of an interlocking intramedullary nail and bone grafting have been preferred, especially in children over 10 to 12 years of age. Aksoy et al.[4] reported a small series of nonunions in malunions salvaged with titanium elastic nails. Union was achieved in 6 to 9 months in most cases.

Robertson et al. reported the use of external fixators in 11 open femoral fractures. The time to union was delayed, but a satisfactory outcome occurred without subsequent procedures. This supports the belief that the rates of delayed union and nonunion are low in pediatric femoral fractures, because open fractures would have the highest rates of delayed union.

MUSCLE WEAKNESS

Weakness after femoral fracture has been described in the hip abductor musculature, quadriceps, and hamstrings, but persistent weakness in some or all of these muscle groups seldom cause a long-term functional problem. Hennrikus et al.[74] found that quadriceps strength was decreased in 30% of his patients and 18% had a significant decrease demonstrated by a one-leg hop test. Thigh atrophy of 1 cm was present in 42% of patients.

These deficits appeared to be primarily related to the degree of initial displacement of the fracture. Finsen et al. found hamstring and quadriceps deficits in patients with femoral shaft fractures treated with either rods or plates.

Damholt and Zdravkovic documented quadriceps weakness in approximately one-third of patients with femoral fractures, and Viljanto et al.[188] reported that this weakness was present when patients were treated operatively or nonoperatively. Biyani et al. found that hip abductor weakness was related to ipsilateral fracture magnitude, long intramedullary rods, and, to a lesser degree, heterotopic ossification from intramedullary rodding. Hedin and Larsson[68] found no significant weakness in any of 31 patients treated with external fixation for femoral fractures based on either Cybex testing or a one-leg hop test. They thought that the weakness seen in other studies may be related to prolonged immobilization.

Injury to the quadriceps muscle probably occurs at the time of femoral fracture, and long-term muscle deficits may persist in some patients regardless of treatment. Severe scarring and contracture of the quadriceps occasionally require quadricepsplasty.

INFECTION

Infection may rarely complicate a closed femoral shaft fracture, with hematogenous seeding of the hematoma and subsequent osteomyelitis. Fever is commonly associated with femoral fractures during the first week after injury, but persistent fever or fever that spikes exceedingly high may be an indication of infection. One should have a high index of suspicion for infection in type III open femur fractures. A series of 44 open femur fractures[82] reported no infection in type I and II fractures, but 50% (5 of 10) of type III fractures developed osteomyelitis. Presumably this occurs because of the massive soft tissue damage accompanying this injury.

Pin-track infections occasionally occur with the use of skeletal traction, but most are superficial infections that resolve with local wound care and antibiotic therapy. Occasionally, however, the infections may lead to osteomyelitis of the femoral metaphysis or a ring sequestrum that requires surgical debridement.

NEUROVASCULAR INJURY

Nerve and vascular injuries are uncommonly associated with femoral fractures in children.[162] An estimated 1.3% of femoral fractures in children are accompanied by vascular injury[162] such as intimal tears, total disruptions, or injuries resulting in the formation of pseudoaneurysms. Vascular injury occurs most frequently with displaced Salter–Harris physeal fractures of the distal femur or distal femoral metaphyseal fractures. If arteriography indicates that vascular repair is necessary after femoral shaft fracture, open reduction with internal fixation or external fixation of the fracture is usually recommended first to stabilize the fracture and prevent injury of the repair. Secondary limb ischemia also has been reported after the use of both skin and skeletal traction. Documentation of peripheral pulses at the time of presentation, as well as throughout treatment, is necessary.

Nerve abnormalities reported with femoral fractures in children include those caused by direct trauma to the sciatic or femoral nerve at the time of fracture and injuries to the peroneal nerve during treatment. Weiss et al.[192] reported peroneal nerve palsies in 4 of 110 children with femoral fractures treated with early 90/90 hip spica casting. They recommended extending the initial short leg portion of the cast above the knee to decrease tension on the peroneal nerve.

Riew et al.[159] reported eight nerve palsies in 35 consecutive patients treated with locked intramedullary rodding. The nerve injuries were associated with delay in treatment, preoperative shortening, and boot traction. Resolution occurred in less than 1 week in six of eight patients.

Many peroneal nerve deficits after pediatric femoral shaft fractures will resolve with time. In infants, however, the development of an early contracture of the Achilles tendon is more likely. Because of the rapid growth in younger children, this contracture can develop quite early; if peroneal nerve injury is suspected, an ankle-foot orthosis should be used until the peroneal nerve recovers. If peroneal, femoral, or sciatic nerve deficit is present at initial evaluation of a closed fracture, no exploration is indicated. If a nerve deficit occurs during reduction or treatment, the nerve should be explored. Persistent nerve loss without recovery over a 4- to 6-month period is an indication for exploration.

COMPARTMENT SYNDROME

Compartment syndromes of the thigh musculature are rare, but have been reported in patients with massive thigh swelling after femoral fracture and in patients treated with intramedullary rod fixation.[127] If massive swelling of thigh musculature occurs and pain is out of proportion to that expected from a femoral fracture, compartment pressure measurements should be obtained and decompression by fasciotomy should be considered. It is probable that some patients with quadriceps fibrosis[157] and quadriceps weakness[39] after femoral fracture had intracompartmental pressure phenomenon. Mathews et al.[116] reported two cases of compartment syndrome in the "well leg" occurring when the patient was positioned for femoral nailing in the hemilithotomy position. The fracture table has recently been a source of complications.[95]

Janzing et al.[86] reported the occurrence of compartment syndrome using skin traction for treatment of femoral fractures. Skin traction has been associated with compartment syndrome in the lower leg on both the fractured and nonfractured sides. It is important to realize that in a traumatized limb, circumferential traction needs to be monitored closely and is contraindicated in the multiply injured or head-injured child. As noted in the spica cast section, several cases of leg compartment syndrome have been reported after spica cast treatment in younger children with femur fractures, typically traction and technique dependent.

SPECIAL FRACTURES OF THE FEMORAL SHAFT

SUBTROCHANTERIC FRACTURES

Subtrochanteric fractures generally heal slowly, angulate into varus, and are more prone to overgrowth. These fractures offer

Figure 25-32. A: Proximal AP view of a skeletally immature femur following flexible nailing. **B:** Distal AP view of the same patient.

a challenge, as the bone available between the fracture site and the femoral neck limits internal fixation options. In younger children, traction and casting can be successful, but are at higher risk for unacceptable alignment at conclusion of treatment.[43,129] Three weeks of traction is usually necessary, and the surgeon should place a good valgus mold at the fracture site, and monitor the fracture closely in the first 2 weeks after casting. When the patient returns for follow-up and the subtrochanteric fracture has slipped into varus malangulation, the cast can be wedged in clinic or casting can be abandoned for another method. Parents should be warned that loss of reduction in the cast is quite common, and wedging in clinic is a routine step in management. An external fixation strategy can be quite successful if there is satisfactory room proximally to place pins. Once there is satisfactory callus (about 6 weeks), the fixator can be removed and weight bearing allowed in a walking spica (long leg cast with a pelvic band—place a valgus mold to stabilize fracture in the first few weeks after external fixator removal). Flexible nailing can be used, with a proximal and distal entry strategy (Fig. 25-32). A pitfall in this fracture is thinking the proximal fragment is too short to use flexible IM nails on the AP radiograph because the proximal fragment is pulled into flexion by the unopposed psoas muscle. Pombo and Shilt[150] reported a series of 13 children, averaging 8 years old with subtrochanteric fractures, treated with flexible nailing. Results were excellent or satisfactory in all cases. Submuscular plating can also produce satisfactory results. In adolescents, there is insufficient experience with this fracture to determine at what age intramedullary fixation with a reconstruction-type nail and an angled transfixion screw into the femoral neck is indicated. Antegrade intramedullary nail systems place significant holes in the upper femoral neck and should be avoided. Unlike subtrochanteric fractures in adults, nonunions are rare in children with any treatment method. Plating can also be considered in select cases in school-aged or older children (Fig. 25-33).

Figure 25-33. This 10-year-old boy was involved in a motor vehicle accident. **A:** His left femur had a length stable transverse subtrochanteric fracture and he was treated with an anterograde lateral femoral entry nail. **B:** His right side had a more comminuted femoral shaft fracture and was treated with bridge plating.

Figure 25-34. It is difficult to treat distal femoral shaft fractures in traction. The muscle forces around the knee often result in significant flexion at the fracture site.

SUPRACONDYLAR FRACTURES

Supracondylar fractures represent as many as 12% of femoral shaft fractures[174] and are difficult to treat because the gastrocnemius muscle inserts just above the femoral condyles and pulls the distal fragment into a position of extension (Fig. 25-34),[63] making alignment difficult (see Fig. 25-2). The traditional methods of casting and single-pin traction may be satisfactory in young children (Fig. 25-35). As mentioned in the external fixation section above, supracondylar fractures through a benign lesion are safely and efficiently treated with a brief period (4–6 weeks) of external fixation (Fig. 25-36), followed by a walking cast until the callus is solid and the pin sites are healed. In other cases, internal fixation is preferable, either with submuscular plating (see Figs. 25-26 and 25-37) and fully threaded cancellous screws (if there is sufficient metaphyseal length) or with crossed smooth K-wires transfixing the fracture from the epiphysis to the metaphysis, as described for distal femoral physeal separations. If there is sufficient metaphyseal length, flexible nailing can be used, so long as fixation is satisfactory. The flexible nails can be either placed antegrade as originally described, or a retrograde if there is satisfactory distal bone for fixation near the nail entry site. Biomechanically, retrograde insertion is superior.[122] Pathologic fractures in this area are common, and an underlying lesion should always be sought.

OPEN FEMORAL FRACTURES

Open femoral fractures are uncommon in children because of the large soft tissue compartment around the femur. Proper wound care, debridement, stabilization, and antibiotic therapy are required to reduce the chance of infection.[63] In a study by Hutchins et al.,[82] 70% of children with open femoral fractures had associated injuries and 90% were automobile related. The average time to healing was 17 weeks, and 50% of the Gustilo type III injuries developed osteomyelitis.

External fixation of open femoral shaft fractures simplifies wound care and allows early mobilization. The configuration of the external fixator is determined by the child's size and the fracture pattern. Generally, monolateral half-pin frames are satisfactory, but thin-wire circular frames may be necessary if bone loss is extensive. External fixation provides good fracture control, but, as always, family cooperation is required to manage pin and fixator care.

A, B   **C, D**

Figure 25-35. A: This 6-year-old patient sustained an unstable supracondylar fracture of the femur. **B:** The fracture was managed with immediate spica casting with the knee in 90 degrees of flexion, mandatory in such a case to prevent posterior angulation. Bayonet apposition, as shown on lateral (**C**) and AP (**D**) radiographs, is acceptable in a child of this age.

Figure 25-36. AP (**A**) and lateral (**B**) radiographs showing a fracture at the junction of the distal femoral metaphysis and diaphysis. **C:** The fractures reduced into near-anatomic alignment and an external fixator was used to control the distal fragment. **D:** The fixator was removed 8 weeks after injury, and after a brief period of weight bearing is tolerated a long leg cast, the fracture has healed in anatomic alignment with no shortening.

Plate fixation also allows early mobilization as well as anatomic reduction of the femoral fracture. Wound care and treatment of other injuries are made easier in children with multiple traumas. However, this is an invasive technique with the potential for infection and additional injury to the already traumatized soft tissues in the area of the fracture. In emergency situations, plate fixation or intramedullary fixation may be used for Gustilo–Anderson type I and II fractures; type III fractures in older adolescents are better suited for external fixation or intramedullary nailing. Plate breakage can occur if bone grafting is not used for severe medial cortex comminution.

In older adolescents, submuscular plating or trochanteric entry nailing is often the optimal treatment choice. Closed nailing after irrigation and drainage of the fracture allows early mobilization and easy wound care in patients with Gustilo–Anderson type I, II, IIIA, and IIIB injuries, but the risk of osteonecrosis must be recognized.

FEMORAL FRACTURES IN PATIENTS WITH METABOLIC OR NEUROMUSCULAR DISORDERS

For patients with osteogenesis imperfecta who have potential for ambulation, surgical treatment with Rush, Bailey–Dubow, or Fassier rods or newer-generation stiff and solid rods are recommended for repeated fractures or angular deformity. Cast immobilization is minimized in patients with myelomeningocele or cerebral palsy, because of the frequency of osteoporosis and refractures in these patients. If possible, existing leg braces are modified for treatment of the femoral fracture. In nonambulatory patients, a simple pillow splint is used.

Figure 25-37. Preoperative (**A**) and postoperative (**B**) x-rays showing a fracture at the junction of the distal femoral metaphysis and diaphysis treated with plate fixation.

FLOATING KNEE INJURIES

These rare injuries occur when ipsilateral fractures of the femoral and tibial shafts leave the knee joint "floating" without distal or proximal bony attachments. They are high-velocity injuries, usually resulting from collision between a child pedestrian or cyclist and a motor vehicle. Most children with floating knee injuries have multiple-system trauma, including severe soft tissue damage, open fractures, and head, chest, or abdominal injuries.

Except in very young children, it is usually best to fix both fractures. If both fractures are open, external fixation of both the tibial and femoral fractures may be appropriate. A recent multicenter study suggested that intramedullary fixation is the preferred modality in school-age or older children for the femoral fracture employed in about 70% of cases. The same study showed that almost one-third of tibia fractures were treated successfully in a cast.[37]

Letts et al.[105] described five patterns of ipsilateral tibial and femoral fractures and made treatment recommendations based on those patterns. Because of the high prevalence of complications after closed treatment, Bohn and Durbin[18] recommended open or closed reduction and internal fixation of the femoral fracture in older children. Arslan et al.[9] evaluated the treatment of the "floating knee" in 29 consecutive cases, finding that those treated operatively had a shorter hospital stay, decreased time to weight bearing, and fewer complications than those managed with splinting casting or traction. Arslan et al.[9] demonstrated that open knee fracture rather than ligamentous injury was a risk factor for poor outcome and that angulation was a predictor of future compromise of function. The CORTICES[37] work group demonstrated that if at least the

femoral fracture was fixed outcomes were good or excellent in 93% of cases.

Bohn and Durbin[18] reported that of 19 patients with floating knee injuries, at long-term follow-up 11 had limb-length discrepancy secondary to either overgrowth of the bone after the fracture or premature closure of the ipsilateral physis (seven patients), genu valgum associated with fracture of the proximal tibial metaphysis (three patients), or physeal arrest (one patient). Four patients had late diagnosis of ligamentous laxity of the knee that required operation. Other complications included peroneal nerve palsy, infection, nonunion, malunion, and refracture.

FRACTURES IN THE MULTIPLE-SYSTEM TRAUMA PATIENT

In a study of 387 previously healthy children with femoral fractures, the authors evaluated the effect of stabilization on pulmonary function. Patients with severe head trauma or cervical spine trauma are at greatest risk for pulmonary complications. Timing of treatment of femoral fractures appears to not affect the prevalence of pulmonary complications in children. Mendelson et al.[123] similarly showed no effect of timing of femoral fixation on long-term outcome but early fracture fixation did decrease hospital stay without increasing the risk of central nervous system or pulmonary complications. Similarly. Al-Mahdi et al.[5] showed although SIRS was common among severely injured children, ARDS was rare in the multi-injured child and mortality was exclusively due to head trauma.

Annotated References

Reference	Annotation
Beaty JH, Austin SM, Warner WC, et al. Interlocking intramedullary nailing of femoral-shaft fractures in adolescents: preliminary results and complications. *J Pediatr Orthop.* 1994;14(2):178–183.	Thirty-one femoral-shaft fractures in 30 patients were treated with interlocking intramedullary nails. Two patients had overgrowth of >2.5 cm; none had angular or rotational malunions. One patient developed asymptomatic segmental avascular necrosis of the femoral head, which was not seen on radiographs until 15 months after injury. This study established that intramedullary nailing is a reasonable alternative for the treatment of isolated femoral-shaft fractures in older adolescents and in younger adolescents with multiple trauma, and noted the possible complication of AVN.
Crosby SN Jr, Kim EJ, Koehler DM, et al. Twenty-year experience with rigid intramedullary nailing of femoral shaft fractures in skeletally immature patients. *J Bone Joint Surg Am.* 2014;96(13):1080–1089.	Debate exists over the safety of rigid intramedullary nailing of femoral shaft fractures in skeletally immature patients. Among the 246 fractures, 24 complications (9.8%) occurred. At the time of the latest follow-up, 1.7% (4 of 241 patients) reported pain. The average Nonarthritic Hip Score was 92.4 points (range, 51–100 points), and 100% of patients reported satisfaction with their treatment. This large study confirmed that rigid intramedullary nailing is an effective technique for treatment of femoral shaft fractures in pediatric patients with an acceptable rate of complications.
Czertak DJ, Hennrikus WL. The treatment of pediatric femur fractures with early 90-90 spica casting. *J Pediatr Orthop.* 1999;19(2):229–232.	Twenty-three consecutive children younger than 6 years with a closed femoral shaft fracture stemming from low-energy trauma were treated with an early spica cast. Average shortening of the fracture at the time of cast removal was 1.0 cm (range, 0.1–2.1 cm). Final patient examinations were performed 18–24 months after the fracture. Overgrowth averaged 1.1 cm in the femur (range, 0.5–1.9 cm). Limb lengths in each patient were within 1 cm of the contralateral limb when measured by scanogram and by blocks. This study helped popularize "immediate spica casting" for toddlers with low-energy fractures.
Edvardsen P, Syversen SM. Overgrowth of the femur after fracture of the shaft in childhood. *J Bone Joint Surg Br.* 1976;58(3):339–342.	This study beautifully documented the expected overgrowth after femoral shaft fracture. Twenty-six children conservatively treated for fracture of the femoral shaft have been reviewed with regard to differences in limb length 7–10 years after the injury. Nearly two-thirds of the patients had overgrowth of the femur of 10 mm or more. Shortening of 15–20 mm at the fracture site was well compensated for by accelerated growth. Growth acceleration seemed to take place during the healing period and the difference at the end of healing was permanent. Overgrowth was promoted by comminuted and long oblique fractures and by overriding of the fracture ends, but was not influenced by the age at fracture, the duration of treatment, or the level of fracture of the shaft. Growth of the tibia was not affected by the femoral fracture.
Flynn JM, Garner MR, Jones KJ, et al. The treatment of low-energy femoral shaft fractures: a prospective study comparing the "Walking Spica" with the traditional spica cast. *J Bone Joint Surg Am.* 2011;93(23):2196–2202.	This prospective cohort trial comparing walking and traditional hip spica casting showed that the walking hip spica cast gave similar orthopaedic outcomes with a much lower care burden for the family, and established walking spica as the standard treatment of low-energy fractures in children 1–4 years old.
Flynn JM, Luedtke LM, Ganley TJ, et al. Comparison of titanium elastic nails with traction and a spica cast to treat femoral fractures in children. *J Bone Joint Surg Am.* 2004;86-A(4):770–777.	The results of this prospective study supported the empiric observations and published results of retrospective series indicating that a child in whom a femoral fracture is treated with titanium elastic nails achieves recovery milestones significantly faster than a child treated with traction and a spica cast. The complication rate associated with nailing compares favorably with that associated with traction and application of a spica cast. This study gave further support to TEN as centers were moving away for traction and casting in the early 21st century.

Annotated References

Reference	Annotation
Heinrich SD, Drvaric DM, Darr K, MacEwen GD. The operative stabilization of pediatric diaphyseal femur fractures with flexible intramedullary nails: a prospective analysis. *J Pediatr Orthop*. 1994;14(4):501–507.	Seventy eight diaphyseal femur fractures in 77 children were stabilized with flexible intramedullary nails. The patients ranged in age from 2 + 9 to 18 years. There were four unscheduled reoperations, but no major complications; all fractures united. The results obtained using flexible intramedullary nails for the stabilization of select pediatric diaphyseal femur fractures are comparable to nonoperative methods of treatment, but with less disruption to family life and a shorter hospitalization. This is one of the earliest and most important reports on what has become the standard of care for most femur fractures in children 5–12 years old.
Hughes BF, Sponseller PD, Thompson JD. Pediatric femur fractures: effects of spica cast treatment on family and community. *J Pediatr Orthop*. 1995;15(4):457–460.	Twenty-three consecutive children with isolated closed femur fractures treated with early spica casts were studied to determine the impact of this treatment on family, school, and other support systems. Mobility was identified by families as the major problem. In families with two working parents, a mean of 3 weeks' time off work was needed. None of the children was accepted into school in cast. Mean time to independent walking was 5 days and to running, 25 days; skills returned faster in younger children. All aspects of spica treatment were easier for preschool children. This study added to the evidence that spica casting was very challenging for families and for school-aged children, and accelerated the trend toward operative management.
Kanlic EM, Anglen JO, Smith DG, et al. Advantages of submuscular bridge plating for complex pediatric femur fractures. *Clin Orthop Relat Res*. 2004;426:244–251.	The authors investigated whether a minimally invasive submuscular bridge plating technique provides stability for early functional treatment (without protective casting or bracing) and predictable healing. They showed that the technique offered the advantage of adequate stability for early functional treatment and predictable healing with maintenance of length and alignment for all pediatric femoral shaft fractures. This was one of the earliest and best series of submuscular plating, and brought it into the list of treatment options, especially for higher-energy, length-unstable fractures.
Ligier JN, Metaizeau JP, Prévot J, Lascombes P. Elastic stable intramedullary nailing of femoral shaft fractures in children. *J Bone Joint Surg Br*. 1988; 70(1):74–77.	This is the first report from the center that popularized TEN worldwide. They showed that complications were minimal, the most common being minor skin ulceration caused by the ends of the rods. A surprising feature was the low incidence of growth changes, with a mean lengthening of only 1.2 mm after an average follow-up of 22 months. Compared with conservative treatment, Elastic Stable Intramedullary Nailing (ESIN) obviates the need for prolonged bed rest and is thus particularly advantageous for treating children.
Moroz LA, Launay F, Kocher MS, et al. Titanium elastic nailing of fractures of the femur in children. Predictors of complications and poor outcome. *J Bone Joint Surg Br*. 2006;88(10):1361–1366.	Between 1996 and 2003, six institutions in the United States and France contributed a consecutive series of 234 fractures of the femur in 229 children which were treated by titanium elastic nailing. There was a statistically significant relationship ($P = .003$) between age and outcome, and the odds ratio for poor outcome was 3.86 for children aged 11 years and older compared with those below this age. The difference between the weight of children with a poor outcome and those with an excellent or satisfactory outcome was statistically significant (54 kg vs. 39 kg; $P = .003$). A poor outcome was five times more likely in children who weighed more than 49 kg. This paper refined the age and weight indications for TEN.
Weltsch D, Baldwin KD, Talwar D, Flynn JM. Expert consensus for a principle-based classification for treatment of diaphyseal pediatric femur fractures. *J Pediatr Orthop*. 2020;40(8):e669–e675.	To determine which treatment option is best for a specific fracture type in a specific patient, pediatric femoral shaft fractures can be divided into five classes: (1) fractures that will heal with limited intervention; (2) fractures that should be treated without surgery, but must be watched closely; (3) fractures that benefit from surgical intervention with load-sharing implants; (4) fractures that may benefit from surgical intervention with rigid fixation; and (5) fractures in a patient with a limb at risk and associated injuries that require initial treatment precedence. This is currently the most useful classification for treatment of pediatric femoral shaft fractures.

REFERENCES

1. Adams AJ, Baldwin KD, Arkader A, Sankar WN. Assessing the need for common perioperative laboratory tests in pediatric patients with femoral shaft fractures. *J Pediatr Orthop.* 2019;39(6):e456–e461.
2. Aitken AP. Overgrowth of the femoral shaft following fracture in children. *Am J Surg.* 1940;49(1):147–148.
3. Aitken AP, Blackett CW, Cincotti JJ. Overgrowth of the femoral shaft following fracture in childhood. *J Bone Joint Surg Am.* 1939;21(2):334–338.
4. Aksoy MC, Caglar O, Ayvaz M, et al. Treatment of complicated pediatric femoral fractures with titanium elastic nail. *J Pediatr Orthop.* 2008;17(1):7–10.
5. Al-Mahdi W, Ibrahim MM, Spiegel DA, et al. Is systemic inflammatory response syndrome relevant to pulmonary complications and mortality in multiply injured children? *J Pediatr Orthop.* 2020;40(1):1–7.
6. Anderson M, Green WT. Lengths of the femur and the tibia: norms derived from orthoroentgenograms of children from five years of age until epiphyseal closure. *Am J Dis Child.* 1948;75(3):279–290.
7. Aronson DD, Singer RM, Higgins RF. Skeletal traction for fractures of the femoral shaft in children. A long-term study. *J Bone Joint Surg Am.* 1987;69(9):1435–1439.
8. Aronson J, Tursky EA. External fixation of femur fractures in children. *J Pediatr Orthop.* 1992;12(2):157–163.
9. Arslan H, Kapukaya A, Kesemenli C, et al. Floating knee in children. *J Pediatr Orthop.* 2003;23(4):458–463.
10. Asirdizer M, Zeyfeoglu Y. Femoral and tibial fractures in a child with myelomeningocele. *J Clin Forensic Med.* 2005;12(2):93–97.
11. Atassi O, Fontenot PB, Busel G, et al. "Unstable" pediatric femoral shaft fractures treated with flexible elastic nails have few complications. *J Orthop Trauma.* 2021;35(2):e56–e60.
12. Baldwin KD, Hosseinzadeh P, Abzug JM, et al. Femoral shaft fractures in pediatric patients: an algorithm for success. *Instr Course Lect.* 2019;68:453–462.
13. Baldwin K, Pandya N, Wolfgruber H, et al. Femur fractures in the pediatric population: abuse or accidental trauma? *Clin Orthop Relat Res.* 2011;469(3):798–804.
14. Barfod B, Christensen J. Fractures of the femoral shaft in children with special reference to subsequent overgrowth. *Acta Chir Scand.* 1959;116(3):235–250.
15. Bar-On E, Sagiv S, Porat S. External fixation or flexible intramedullary nailing for femoral shaft fractures in children. A prospective, randomised study. *J Bone Joint Surg Br.* 1997;79(6):975–978.
16. Beaty JH, Austin SM, Warner WC, et al. Interlocking intramedullary nailing of femoral-shaft fractures in adolescents: preliminary results and complications. *J Pediatr Orthop.* 1994;14(2):178–183.
17. Bennett FS, Zinar DM, Kilgus DJ. Ipsilateral hip and femoral shaft fractures. *Clin Orthop Relat Res.* 1993;296:168–177.
18. Bohn WW, Durbin RA. Ipsilateral fractures of the femur and tibia in children and adolescents. *J Bone Joint Surg Am.* 1991;73(3):429–439.
19. Bopst L, Reinberg O, Lutz N. Femur fracture in preschool children: experience with flexible intramedullary nailing in 72 children. *J Pediatr Orthop.* 2007;27(3):299–303.
20. Bourdelat D. Fracture of the femoral shaft in children: advantages of the descending medullary nailing. *J Pediatr Orthop.* 1996;5(2):110–114.
21. Braten M, Terjesen T, Rossvoll I. Torsional deformity after intramedullary nailing of femoral shaft fractures. Measurement of anteversion angles in 110 patients. *J Bone Joint Surg Br.* 1993;75(5):799–803.
22. Brouwer KJ, Molenaar JC, van Linge B. Rotational deformities after femoral shaft fractures in childhood. A retrospective study 27–32 years after the accident. *Acta Orthop Scand.* 1981;52(1):81–89.
23. Bryant T. *The Practice of Surgery.* Galaxy Publishing; 1873.
24. Buchholz IM, Bolhuis HW, Broker LH, et al. Overgrowth and correction of rotational deformity in 12 femoral shaft fractures in 3-6-year-old children treated with an external fixator. *Acta Orthop Scand.* 2002;73(2):170–174.
25. Buford D Jr, Christensen K, Weatherall P. Intramedullary nailing of femoral fractures in adolescents. *Clin Orthop Relat Res.* 1998;350:85–89.
26. Carey TP, Galpin RD. Flexible intramedullary nail fixation of pediatric femoral fractures. *Clin Orthop Relat Res.* 1996;332:110–118.
27. Carmichael KD, Bynum J, Goucher N. Rates of refracture associated with external fixation in pediatric femur fractures. *Am J Orthop (Belle Mead NJ).* 2005;34(9):439–444.
28. Cassinelli EH, Young B, Vogt M, et al. Spica cast application in the emergency room for select pediatric femur fractures. *J Orthop Trauma.* 2005;19(10):709–716.
29. Chung SM. The arterial supply of the developing proximal end of the human femur. *J Bone Joint Surg Am.* 1976;58(7):961–970.
30. Ciarallo L, Fleisher G. Femoral fractures: are children at risk for significant blood loss? *Pediatr Emerg Care.* 1996;12(5):343–346.
31. Coffey C, Haley K, Hayes J, Groner JI. The risk of child abuse in infants and toddlers with lower extremity injuries. *J Pediatr Surg.* 2005;40(1):120–123.
32. Cole WH. Compensatory lengthening of the femur in children after fracture. *Ann Surg.* 1925;82(4):609–616.
33. Collins AC, Adams N, Ostrander JD, et al. Safe transport of spica casted infants: reducing the risk of traumatic injury in side impact collisions. *Am J Surg.* 2022;223(1):164–169.
34. Collins AC, Caskey S, Peck JB, et al. Frontal crash injury metrics are below mandated limits for a spica casted child dummy in currently available restraints. *J Pediatr Orthop.* 2020;40(5):e394–e400.
35. Collins AC, McKean L, Ostrander J, et al. Crash performance of rear-facing restraints with a fracture type spica casted 1-year-old dummy. *J Pediatr Orthop.* 2022;42(1):e1–e7.
36. Compton E, Andras LM, Murgai RR, et al. Isolated femoral shaft fractures in children rarely require a blood transfusion. *Injury.* 2020;51(3):642–646.
37. CORTICES. The pediatric "floating knee" injury: a state-of-the-art multicenter study. *J Bone Joint Surg Am.* 2019;101(19):1761–1767.
38. Crosby SN Jr, Kim EJ, Koehler DM, et al. Twenty-year experience with rigid intramedullary nailing of femoral shaft fractures in skeletally immature patients. *J Bone Joint Surg Am.* 2014;96(13):1080–1089.
39. Czertak DJ, Hennrikus WL. The treatment of pediatric femur fractures with early 90-90 spica casting. *J Pediatr Orthop.* 1999;19(2):229–232.
40. Daly KE, Calvert PT. Accidental femoral fracture in infants. *Injury.* 1991;22(4):337–338.
41. Davids JR. Rotational deformity and remodeling after fracture of the femur in children. *Clin Orthop Relat Res.* 1994;302:27–35.
42. Davis TJ, Topping RE, Blanco JS. External fixation of pediatric femoral fractures. *Clin Orthop Relat Res.* 1995;318:191–198.
43. DeLee JC, Clanton TO, Rockwood CA Jr. Closed treatment of subtrochanteric fractures of the femur in a modified cast-brace. *J Bone Joint Surg Am.* 1981;63(5):773–779.
44. de Sanctis N, Gambardella A, Pempinello C, et al. The use of external fixators in femur fractures in children. *J Pediatr Orthop.* 1996;16(5):613–620.
45. Edvardsen P, Syversen SM. Overgrowth of the femur after fracture of the shaft in childhood. *J Bone Joint Surg Br.* 1976;58(3):339–342.
46. Engström Z, Wolf O, Hailer YD. Epidemiology of pediatric femur fractures in children: the Swedish Fracture Register. *BMC Musculoskelet Disord.* 2020;21(1):796.
47. Epps HR, Molenaar E, O'Connor DP. Immediate single-leg spica cast for pediatric femoral diaphysis fractures. *J Pediatr Orthop.* 2006;26(4):491–496.
48. Evanoff M, Strong ML, MacIntosh R. External fixation maintained until fracture consolidation in the skeletally immature. *J Pediatr Orthop.* 1993;13(1):98–101.
49. Fein LH, Pankovich AM, Spero CM, Baruch HM. Closed flexible intramedullary nailing of adolescent femoral shaft fractures. *J Orthop Trauma.* 1989;3(2):133–141.
50. Ferguson J, Nicol RO. Early spica treatment of pediatric femoral shaft fractures. *J Pediatr Orthop.* 2000;20(2):189–192.
51. Ferry AM, Edgar MS Jr. Modified Bryant's traction. *J Bone Joint Surg Am.* 1966;48(3):533–536.
52. Flynn JM, Garner MR, Jones KJ, et al. The treatment of low-energy femoral shaft fractures: a prospective study comparing the "Walking Spica" with the traditional spica cast. *J Bone Joint Surg Am.* 2011;93(23):2196–2202.
53. Flynn JM, Hresko T, Reynolds RA, et al. Titanium elastic nails for pediatric femur fractures: a multicenter study of early results with analysis of complications. *J Pediatr Orthop.* 2001;21(1):4–8.
54. Flynn JM, Luedtke LM, Ganley TJ, et al. Comparison of titanium elastic nails with traction and a spica cast to treat femoral fractures in children. *J Bone Joint Surg Am.* 2004;86-A(4):770–777.
55. Flynn JM, Schwend RM. Management of pediatric femoral shaft fractures. *J Am Acad Orthop Surg.* 2004;12(5):347–359.
56. Frick KB, Mahar AT, Lee SS, Newton PO. Biomechanical analysis of antegrade and retrograde flexible intramedullary nail fixation of pediatric femoral fractures using a synthetic bone model. *J Pediatr Orthop.* 2004;24(2):167–171.
57. Galpin RD, Willis RB, Sabano N. Intramedullary nailing of pediatric femoral fractures. *J Pediatr Orthop.* 1994;14(2):184–189.
58. Gordon JE, Anderson JT, Schoenecker PL, et al. Treatment of femoral fractures in children aged two to six. *Bone Joint J.* 2020;102-B(8):1056–1061.
59. Gordon JE, Swenning TA, Burd TA, et al. Proximal femoral radiographic changes after lateral transtrochanteric intramedullary nail placement in children. *J Bone Joint Surg Am.* 2003;85(7):1295–1301.
60. Gregory P, Sullivan JA, Herndon WA. Adolescent femoral shaft fractures: rigid versus flexible nails. *Orthopedics.* 1995;18(7):645–649.
61. Gross RH, Davidson R, Sullivan JA, et al. Cast brace management of the femoral shaft fracture in children and young adults. *J Pediatr Orthop.* 1983;3(5):572–582.
62. Gross RH, Stranger M. Causative factors responsible for femoral fractures in infants and young children. *J Pediatr Orthop.* 1983;3(3):341–343.
63. Gustilo RB. Current concepts in the management of open fractures. *Instr Course Lect.* 1987;36:359–366.
64. Gwyn DT, Olney BW, Dart BR, Czwala PJ. Rotational control of various pediatric femur fractures stabilized with titanium elastic intramedullary nails. *J Pediatr Orthop.* 2004;24(2):172–177.
65. Hagglund G, Hansson LI, Norman O. Correction by growth of rotational deformity after femoral fracture in children. *Acta Orthop Scand.* 1983;54(6):858–861.
66. Hedequist D, Bishop J, Hresko T. Locking plate fixation for pediatric femur fractures. *J Pediatr Orthop.* 2008;28(1):6–9.
67. Hedequist DJ, Sink E. Technical aspects of bridge plating for pediatric femur fractures. *J Orthop Trauma.* 2005;19(4):276–279.
68. Hedin H, Larsson S. Muscle strength in children treated for displaced femoral fractures by external fixation: 31 patients compared with 31 matched controls. *Acta Orthop Scand.* 2003;74(3):305–311.
69. Hedlund R, Lindgren U. The incidence of femoral shaft fractures in children and adolescents. *J Pediatr Orthop.* 1986;6(1):47–50.
70. Heideken JV, Svensson T, Blomqvist P, et al. Incidence and trends in femur shaft fractures in Swedish children between 1987 and 2005. *J Pediatr Orthop.* 2011;31(5):512–519.
71. Heinrich SD, Drvaric D, Darr K, MacEwen GD. Stabilization of pediatric diaphyseal femur fractures with flexible intramedullary nails (a technique paper). *J Orthop Trauma.* 1992;6(4):452–459.
72. Heinrich SD, Drvaric DM, Darr K, MacEwen GD. The operative stabilization of pediatric diaphyseal femur fractures with flexible intramedullary nails: a prospective analysis. *J Pediatr Orthop.* 1994;14(4):501–507.
73. Henderson J, Goldacre MJ, Fairweather JM, Marcovitch H. Conditions accounting for substantial time spent in hospital in children aged 1–14 years. *Arch Dis Child.* 1992;67(1):83–86.

74. Hennrikus WL, Kasser JR, Rand F, et al. The function of the quadriceps muscle after a fracture of the femur in patients who are less than seventeen years old. *J Bone Joint Surg Am.* 1993;75(4):508–513.

75. Herscovici D Jr, Scott DM, Behrens F, et al. The use of Ender nails in femoral shaft fractures: what are the remaining indications? *J Orthop Trauma.* 1992;6(3):314–317.

76. Heyworth BE, Hedequist DJ, Nasreddine AY, et al. Distal femoral valgus deformity following plate fixation of pediatric femoral shaft fractures. *J Bone Joint Surg Am.* 2013;95(6):526–533.

77. Hinton RY, Lincoln A, Crockett MM, et al. Fractures of the femoral shaft in children. Incidence, mechanisms, and sociodemographic risk factors. *J Bone Joint Surg Am.* 1999;81(4):500–509.

78. Ho CA, Skaggs DL, Tang CW, Kay RM. Use of flexible intramedullary nails in pediatric femur fractures. *J Pediatr Orthop.* 2006;26(4):497–504.

79. Hosalkar HS, Pandya NK, Cho RH, et al. Intramedullary nailing of pediatric femoral shaft fracture. *J Am Acad Orthop Surg.* 2011;19(8):472–481.

80. Hughes BF, Sponseller PD, Thompson JD. Pediatric femur fractures: effects of spica cast treatment on family and community. *J Pediatr Orthop.* 1995;15(4):457–460.

81. Humberger FW, Eyring EJ. Proximal tibial 90-90 traction in treatment of children with femoral-shaft fractures. *J Bone Joint Surg Am.* 1969;51(3):499–504.

82. Hutchins CM, Sponseller PD, Sturm P, Mosquero R. Open femur fractures in children: treatment, complications, and results. *J Pediatr Orthop.* 2000;20(2):183–188.

83. Illgen R III, Rodgers WB, Hresko MT, et al. Femur fractures in children: treatment with early sitting spica casting. *J Pediatr Orthop.* 1998;18(4):481–487.

84. Infante AF Jr, Albert MC, Jennings WB, Lehner JT. Immediate hip spica casting for femur fractures in pediatric patients. A review of 175 patients. *Clin Orthop Relat Res.* 2000;376:106–112.

85. Irani RN, Nicholson JT, Chung SM. Long-term results in the treatment of femoral-shaft fractures in young children by immediate spica immobilization. *J Bone Joint Surg Am.* 1976;58(7):945–951.

86. Janzing H, Broos P, Rommens P. Compartment syndrome as a complication of skin traction in children with femoral fractures. *J Trauma.* 1996;41(1):156–158.

87. Jevsevar DS, Shea KG, Murray JN, Sevarino KS. AAOS clinical practice guideline on the treatment of pediatric diaphyseal femur fractures. *J Am Acad Orthop Surg.* 2015;23(12):e101.

88. Kanlic E, Cruz M. Current concepts in pediatric femur fracture treatment. *Orthopedics.* 2007;30(12):1015–1019.

89. Kanlic EM, Anglen JO, Smith DG, et al. Advantages of submuscular bridge plating for complex pediatric femur fractures. *Clin Orthop Relat Res.* 2004;426:244–251.

90. Karaoglu S, Baktir A, Tuncel M, et al. Closed ender nailing of adolescent femoral shaft fractures. *Injury.* 1994;25(8):501–506.

91. Katz JF. Spontaneous fractures in paraplegic children. *J Bone Joint Surg Am.* 1953;35-A(1):220–226.

92. Kaweblum M, Lehman WB, Grant AD, Strongwater A. Avascular necrosis of the femoral head as sequela of fracture of the greater trochanter. A case report and review of the literature. *Clin Orthop Relat Res.* 1993;294:193–195.

93. Keeler KA, Dart B, Luhmann SJ, et al. Antegrade intramedullary nailing of pediatric femoral fractures using an interlocking pediatric femoral nail and a lateral trochanteric entry point. *J Pediatr Orthop.* 2009;29(4):345–351.

94. Kelly B, Heyworth B, Yen YM, Hedequist D. Adverse sequelae due to plate retention following submuscular plating for pediatric femur fractures. *J Orthop Trauma.* 2013;27(12):726–729.

95. Kelly BA, Naqvi M, Rademacher ES, et al. Fracture table application for pediatric femur fractures: incidence and risk factors associated with adverse outcomes. *J Pediatr Orthop.* 2017;37(6):e353–e356.

96. Kirby RM, Winquist RA, Hansen ST Jr. Femoral shaft fractures in adolescents: a comparison between traction plus cast treatment and closed intramedullary nailing. *J Pediatr Orthop.* 1981;1(2):193–197.

97. Knapik DM, McCarthy C, Liu RW. Developmental patterns of the greater trochanter in skeletally immature patients. *J Pediatr Orthop.* 2019;39(6):e412–e416.

98. Kocher M. American Academy of Orthopaedic Surgeons Specialty Day. 2004.

99. Kocher MS, Sink EL, Blasier RD, et al. Treatment of pediatric diaphyseal femur fractures. *J Am Acad Orthop Surg.* 2009;17(11):718–725.

100. Kong H, Sabharwal S. External fixation for closed pediatric femoral shaft fractures: where are we now? *Clin Orthop Relat Res.* 2014;472(12):3814–3822.

101. Landin LA. Fracture patterns in children: analysis of 8,682 fractures with special reference to incidence, etiology and secular changes in a Swedish urban population 1950–1979. *Acta Orthop Scand Supp.* 1983;202:1–109.

102. Large TM, Frick SL. Compartment syndrome of the leg after treatment of a femoral fracture with an early sitting spica cast. A report of two cases. *J Bone Joint Surg Am.* 2003;85(11):2207–2210.

103. Lascombes P, Haumont T, Journeau P. Use and abuse of flexible intramedullary nailing in children and adolescents. *J Pediatr Orthop.* 2006;26(6):827–834.

104. Lee SS, Mahar AT, Newton PO. Ender nail fixation of pediatric femur fractures: a biomechanical analysis. *J Pediatr Orthop.* 2001;21(4):442–445.

105. Letts M, Vincent N, Gouw G. The "floating knee" in children. *J Bone Joint Surg Br.* 1986;68(3):442–446.

106. Leu D, Sargent MC, Ain MC, et al. Spica casting for pediatric femoral fractures. A prospective, randomized controlled study of single-leg versus double-leg spica casts. *J Bone Joint Surg Am.* 2012;94(14):1259–1264.

107. Lewis RB, Hariri O, Elliott ME, et al. Financial analysis of closed femur fractures in 3- to 6-year-olds treated with immediate spica casting versus intramedullary fixation. *J Pediatr Orthop.* 2019;39(2):e114–e119.

108. Li Y, Hedequist DJ. Submuscular plating of pediatric femur fracture. *J Am Acad Orthop Surg.* 2012;20(9):596–603.

109. Ligier JN, Metaizeau JP, Prevot J, Lascombes P. Elastic stable intramedullary nailing of femoral shaft fractures in children. *J Bone Joint Surg Br.* 1988;70(1):74–77.

110. Loder RT, O'Donnell PW, Feinberg JR. Epidemiology and mechanisms of femur fractures in children. *J Pediatr Orthop.* 2006;26(5):561–566.

111. Luhmann SJ, Schootman M, Schoenecker PL, et al. Complications of titanium elastic nails for pediatric femoral shaft fractures. *J Pediatr Orthop.* 2003;23(4):443–447.

112. Lynch JM, Gardner MJ, Gains B. Hemodynamic significance of pediatric femur fractures. *J Pediatr Surg.* 1996;31(10):1358–1361.

113. Mahajan J1, Hennrikus W, Piazza B. Overgrowth after femoral shaft fractures in infants treated with a Pavlik harness. *J Pediatr Orthop B.* 2016;25(1):7–10.

114. Mann DC, Weddington J, Davenport K. Closed Ender nailing of femoral shaft fractures in adolescents. *J Pediatr Orthop.* 1986;6(6):651–655.

115. Mansour AA III, Wilmoth JC, Mansour AS, et al. Immediate spica casting of pediatric femoral fractures in the operating room versus the emergency department: comparison of reduction, complications, and hospital charges. *J Pediatr Orthop.* 2010;30(8):813–817.

116. Mathews PV, Perry JJ, Murray PC. Compartment syndrome of the well leg as a result of the hemilithotomy position: a report of two cases and review of literature. *J Orthop Trauma.* 2001;15(8):580–583.

117. Matzkin EG, Smith EL, Wilson A, Murray PC. External fixation of pediatric femur fractures with cortical contact. *Am J Orthop (Belle Mead NJ).* 2006;35(11):498–501.

118. Mazda K, Khairouni A, Pennecot GF, Bensahel H. Closed flexible intramedullary nailing of the femoral shaft fractures in children. *J Pediatr Orthop.* 1997;6(3):198–202.

119. McCarthy RE. A method for early spica cast application in treatment of pediatric femoral shaft fractures. *J Pediatr Orthop.* 1986;6(1):89–91.

120. McGraw JJ, Gregory SK. Ender nails: an alternative for intramedullary fixation of femoral shaft fractures in children and adolescents. *South Med J.* 1997;90(7):694–696.

121. Meaney JE, Carty H. Femoral stress fractures in children. *Skeletal Radiol.* 1992;21(3):173–176.

122. Mehlman CT, Nemeth NM, Glos DL. Antegrade versus retrograde titanium elastic nail fixation of pediatric distal-third femoral-shaft fractures: a mechanical study. *J Orthop Trauma.* 2006;20(9):608–612.

123. Mendelson SA, Dominick TS, Tyler-Kabara E, et al. Early versus late femoral fracture stabilization in multiply injured pediatric patients with closed head injury. *J Pediatr Orthop.* 2001;21(5):594–599.

124. Mesko JW, DeRosa GP, Lindseth RE. Segmental femur loss in children. *J Pediatr Orthop.* 1985;5(4):471–474.

125. Metaizeau JP. Stable elastic intramedullary nailing for fractures of the femur in children. *J Bone Joint Surg Br.* 2004;86(7):954–957.

126. Mileski RA, Garvin KL, Huurman WW. Avascular necrosis of the femoral head after closed intramedullary shortening in an adolescent. *J Pediatr Orthop.* 1995;15(1):24–26.

127. Miller DS, Markin L, Grossman E. Ischemic fibrosis of the lower extremity in children. *Am J Surg.* 1952;84(3):317–322.

128. Miner T, Carroll KL. Outcomes of external fixation of pediatric femoral shaft fractures. *J Pediatr Orthop.* 2000;20(3):405–410.

129. Misaghi A, Mahmoud MAH, Arkader A, Baldwin KD. Fracture characteristics predict suboptimal alignment in preschool femoral shaft fractures treated with spica casting: a retrospective chart review. *Curr Orthop Pract.* 2020;31(4):379–384.

130. Momberger N, Stevens P, Smith J, et al. Intramedullary nailing of femoral fractures in adolescents. *J Pediatr Orthop.* 2000;20(4):482–484.

131. Mooney JF. The use of 'damage control orthopedics' techniques in children with segmental open femur fractures. *J Pediatr Orthop.* 2012;21(5):400–403.

132. Moroz LA, Launay F, Kocher MS, et al. Titanium elastic nailing of fractures of the femur in children. Predictors of complications and poor outcome. *J Bone Joint Surg Br.* 2006;88(10):1361–1366.

133. Morris S, Cassidy N, Stephens M, et al. Birth-associated femoral fractures: incidence and outcome. *J Pediatr Orthop.* 2002;22(1):27–30.

134. Morshed S, Humphrey M, Corrales LA, et al. Retention of flexible intramedullary nails following treatment of pediatric femur fractures. *Arch Orthop Traum Surg.* 2007;127(7):509–514.

135. Mubarak SJ, Frick S, Sink E, et al. Volkmann contracture and compartment syndromes after femur fractures in children treated with 90/90 spica casts. *J Pediatr Orthop.* 2006;26(5):567–572.

136. Murphy R, Kelly DM, Moisan A, et al. Transverse fractures of the femoral shaft are a better predictor of nonaccidental trauma in young children than spiral fractures are. *J Bone Joint Surg Am.* 2015;97(2):106–111.

137. Naranje SM, Stewart MG, Kelly DM, et al. Changes in the treatment of pediatric femoral fractures: 15-year trends from United States Kids' Inpatient Database (KID) 1997 to 2012. *J Pediatr Orthop.* 2016;36(7):e81–e85.

138. Narayanan UG, Hyman JE, Wainwright AM, et al. Complications of elastic stable intramedullary nail fixation of pediatric femoral fractures, and how to avoid them. *J Pediatr Orthop.* 2004;24(4):363–369.

139. Nicholson JT, Foster RM, Heath RD. Bryant's traction; a provocative cause of circulatory complications. *JAMA.* 1955;157(5):415–418.

140. Nielsen E, Skaggs DL, Ryan D, Andras LM. Molding spica casts to maintain alignment of femur fractures. *J Pediatr Orthop.* 2018;38(5):e267–e270.

141. Norbeck DE Jr, Asselmeier M, Pinzur MS. Torsional malunion of a femur fracture: diagnosis and treatment. *Orthop Rev.* 1990;19(7):625–629.

142. Nork SE, Hoffinger SA. Skeletal traction versus external fixation for pediatric femoral shaft fractures: a comparison of hospital costs and charges. *J Orthop Trauma.* 1998;12(8):563–568.

143. Nowotarski PJ, Turen CH, Brumback RJ, Scarboro JM. Conversion of external fixation to intramedullary nailing for fractures of the shaft of the femur in multiply injured patients. *J Bone Joint Surg Am.* 2000;82(6):781–788.

144. Oberhammer J. Degree and frequency of rotational deformities after infant femoral fractures and their spontaneous correction. *Arch Orthop Traum Surg.* 1980;97(4):249–255.

145. Oetgen ME, Blatz AM, Matthews A. Impact of clinical practice guideline on the treatment of pediatric femoral fractures in a pediatric hospital. *J Bone Joint Surg Am.* 2015;97(20):1641–1646.
146. O'Malley DE, Mazur JM, Cummings RJ. Femoral head avascular necrosis associated with intramedullary nailing in an adolescent. *J Pediatr Orthop.* 1995;15(1):21–23.
147. Ozdemir HM, Yensel U, Senaran H, et al. Immediate percutaneous intramedullary fixation and functional bracing for the treatment of pediatric femoral shaft fracture. *J Pediatr Orthop.* 2003;23(4):453–457.
148. Pate O, Hedequist D, Leong N, Hresko T. Implant removal after submuscular plating for pediatric femur fractures. *J Pediatr Orthop.* 2009;29(7):709–712.
149. Podeszwa DA, Mooney JF III, Cramer KE, Mendelow MJ. Comparison of Pavlik harness application and immediate spica casting for femur fractures in infants. *J Pediatr Orthop.* 2004;24(5):460–462.
150. Pombo MW, Shilt JS. The definition and treatment of pediatric subtrochanteric femur fractures with titanium elastic nails. *J Pediatr Orthop.* 2006;26(3):364–370.
151. Pott P. *Some Few General Remarks on Fractures and Dislocations.* Howes; 1769.
152. Probe R, Lindsey RW, Hadley NA, Barnes DA. Refracture of adolescent femoral shaft fractures: a complication of external fixation. A report of two cases. *J Pediatr Orthop.* 1993;13(1):102–105.
153. Ramo BA, Martus JE, Tareen N, et al. Intramedullary nailing compared with spica casts for isolated femoral fractures in four and five-year-old children. *J Bone Joint Surg Am.* 2016;98(4):267–275.
154. Raney EM, Ogden JA, Grogan DP. Premature greater trochanteric epiphysiodesis secondary to intramedullary femoral rodding. *J Pediatr Orthop.* 1993;13(4):516–520.
155. Rathjen KE, Riccio AI, De La Garza D. Stainless steel flexible intramedullary fixation of unstable femoral shaft fractures in children. *J Pediatr Orthop.* 2007;27(4):432–441.
156. Reeves RB, Ballard RI, Hughes JL. Internal fixation versus traction and casting of adolescent femoral shaft fractures. *J Pediatr Orthop.* 1990;10(5):592–595.
157. Reynolds DA. Growth changes in fractured long-bones: a study of 126 children. *J Bone Joint Surg Br.* 1981;63-B(1):83–88.
158. Ricci WM, Bellabarba C, Evanoff B, et al. Retrograde versus antegrade nailing of femoral shaft fractures. *J Orthop Trauma.* 2001;15(3):161–169.
159. Riew KD, Sturm PF, Rosenbaum D, et al. Neurologic complications of pediatric femoral nailing. *J Pediatr Orthop.* 1996;16(5):606–612.
160. Roaten JD, Kelly DM, Yellin JL, et al. Pediatric femoral shaft fractures: a multicenter review of the AAOS Clinical Practice Guidelines before and after 2009. *J Pediatr Orthop.* 2019;39(8):394–399.
161. Rohde RS, Mendelson SA, Grudziak JS. Acute synovitis of the knee resulting from intra-articular knee penetration as a complication of flexible intramedullary nailing of pediatric femur fractures: report of two cases. *J Pediatr Orthop.* 2003;23(5):635–638.
162. Rosental JJ, Gaspar MR, Gjerdrum TC, Newman J. Vascular injuries associated with fractures of the femur. *Arch Surg.* 1975;110(5):494–499.
163. Rush JK, Kelly DM, Sawyer JR, et al. Treatment of pediatric femur fractures with the Pavlik harness: multiyear clinical and radiographic outcomes. *J Pediatr Orthop.* 2013;33(6):614–617.
164. Ryan JR. 90-90 skeletal femoral traction for femoral shaft fractures in children. *J Trauma.* 1981;21(1):46–48.
165. Sagan ML, Datta JC, Olney BW, et al. Residual deformity after treatment of pediatric femur fractures with flexible titanium nails. *J Pediatr Orthop.* 2010;30(7):638–643.
166. Salem KH, Keppler P. Limb geometry after elastic stable nailing for pediatric femoral fractures. *J Bone Joint Surg Am.* 2010;92(6):1409–1417.
167. Shaha J, Cage JM, Black S, et al. Flexible intramedullary nails for femur fractures in pediatric patients heavier than 100 pounds. *J Pediatr Orthop.* 2018;38(2):88–93.
168. Shaha JS, Cage JM, Black SR, et al. Redefining optimal nail to medullary canal diameter ratio in stainless steel flexible intramedullary nailing of pediatric femur fractures. *J Pediatr Orthop.* 2017;37(7):e398–e402.
169. Shapiro F. Fractures of the femoral shaft in children. The overgrowth phenomenon. *Acta Orthop Scand.* 1981;52(6):649–655.
170. Sink EL, Faro F, Polousky J, et al. Decreased complications of pediatric femur fractures with a change in management. *J Pediatr Orthop.* 2010;30(7):633–637.
171. Sink EL, Gralla J, Repine M. Complications of pediatric femur fractures treated with titanium elastic nails: a comparison of fracture types. *J Pediatr Orthop.* 2005;25(5):577–580.
172. Sink EL, Hedequist D, Morgan SJ, Hresko T. Results and technique of unstable pediatric femoral fractures treated with submuscular bridge plating. *J Pediatr Orthop.* 2006;26(2):177–181.
173. Skaggs DL, Leet AI, Money MD, et al. Secondary fractures associated with external fixation in pediatric femur fractures. *J Pediatr Orthop.* 1999;19(5):582–586.
174. Smith NC, Parker D, McNicol D. Supracondylar fractures of the femur in children. *J Pediatr Orthop.* 2001;21(5):600–603.
175. Sola J, Schoenecker PL, Gordon JE. External fixation of femoral shaft fractures in children: enhanced stability with the use of an auxiliary pin. *J Pediatr Orthop.* 1999;19(5):587–591.
176. Staheli LT. Femoral and tibial growth following femoral shaft fracture in childhood. *Clin Orthop Relat Res.* 1967;55:159–163.
177. Stannard JP, Christensen KP, Wilkins KE. Femur fractures in infants: a new therapeutic approach. *J Pediatr Orthop.* 1995;15(4):461–466.
178. Stans AA, Morrissy RT, Renwick SE. Femoral shaft fracture treatment in patients age 6 to 16 years. *J Pediatr Orthop.* 1999;19(2):222–228.
179. Thometz JG, Lamdan R. Osteonecrosis of the femoral head after intramedullary nailing of a fracture of the femoral shaft in an adolescent. A case report. *J Bone Joint Surg Am.* 1995;77(9):1423–1426.
180. Thompson JD, Buehler KC, Sponseller PD, et al. Shortening in femoral shaft fractures in children treated with spica cast. *Clin Orthop Relat Res.* 1997;338:74–78.
181. Timmerman LA, Rab GT. Intramedullary nailing of femoral shaft fractures in adolescents. *J Orthop Trauma.* 1993;7(4):331–337.
182. Tolo VT. External fixation in multiply injured children. *Orthop Clin North Am.* 1990;21(2):393–400.
183. Townsend DR, Hoffinger S. Intramedullary nailing of femoral shaft fractures in children via the trochanter tip. *Clin Orthop Relat Res.* 2000;376:113–118.
184. Trottier ER, Hatcher L, Feng J, et al. Incidence of secondary interventions after early spica casting for diaphyseal femur fractures in young children. *Can J Surg.* 2022;65(4):E417–E424.
185. Truesdell ED. Inequality of the lower extremities following fracture of the shaft of the femur in children. *Ann Surg.* 1921;74(4):498–500.
186. Vangsness CT Jr, DeCampos J, Merritt PO, Wiss DA. Meniscal injury associated with femoral shaft fractures. An arthroscopic evaluation of incidence. *J Bone Joint Surg Br.* 1993;75(2):207–209.
187. Verbeek HO. Does rotation deformity, following femur shaft fracture, correct during growth? *Reconstr Surg Traumatol.* 1979;17:75–81.
188. Viljanto J, Kiviluoto H, Paananen M. Remodelling after femoral shaft fracture in children. *Acta Chir Scand.* 1975;141(5):360–365.
189. Volpon JB, Perina MM, Okubo R, Maranho DA. Biomechanical performance of flexible intramedullary nails with end caps tested in distal segmental defects of pediatric femur models. *J Pediatr Orthop.* 2012;32(5):461–466.
190. Wall EJ, Jain V, Vora V, et al. Complications of titanium and stainless steel elastic nail fixation of pediatric femoral fractures. *J Bone Joint Surg Am.* 2008;90(6):1305–1313.
191. Wallace ME, Hoffman EB. Remodelling of angular deformity after femoral shaft fractures in children. *J Bone Joint Surg Br.* 1992;74(5):765–769.
192. Weiss AP, Schenck RC Jr, Sponseller PD, Thompson JD. Peroneal nerve palsy after early cast application for femoral fractures in children. *J Pediatr Orthop.* 1992;12(1):25–28.
193. Weltsch D, Baldwin KD, Talwar D, Flynn JM. Expert consensus for a principle-based classification for treatment of diaphyseal pediatric femur fractures. *J Pediatr Orthop.* 2020;40(8):e669–e675.
194. Winquist RA, Hansen ST Jr, Clawson DK. Closed intramedullary nailing of femoral fractures. A report of five hundred and twenty cases. *J Bone Joint Surg Am.* 1984;66(4):529–539.
195. Wood JN, Fakeye O, Mondestin V, et al. Prevalence of abuse among young children with femur fractures: a systematic review. *BMC Pediatr.* 2014;14:169.
196. Ziv I, Blackburn N, Rang M. Femoral intramedullary nailing in the growing child. *J Trauma.* 1984;24(5):432–434.

26

Fractures of the Distal Femoral Physis

Ying Li

INTRODUCTION TO FRACTURES OF THE DISTAL FEMORAL PHYSIS

Distal femoral physeal injuries are uncommon, accounting for fewer than 2% of all physeal injuries.[29] However, complications requiring additional surgery occur after approximately 40% to 60% of these injuries.[2,17,26,36,61] The most common complication is growth disturbance of the distal femur resulting in angular deformity and/or shortening. In one meta-analysis of the published literature from 1950 to 2007 that included 564 fractures, 52% of fractures resulted in a growth disturbance.[7] This complication has been reported in patients of all ages regardless of the mechanism of injury, type of fracture, anatomic reduction of the fracture, and the type of treatment.[1,2,9,17,26,36,61] In addition to growth complications, knee stiffness, ligamentous disruption, neurovascular injuries, and compartment syndrome may occur as a result of these injuries.[17,59,61] Although the prognosis is better for very young children and nondisplaced fractures, complications may occur after any distal femoral physeal injury. Careful clinical assessment, complete diagnostic imaging, anatomic reduction, and secure immobilization or fixation to maintain reduction are necessary to ensure the best possible outcomes. Close follow-up at regular 6-month intervals after fracture healing until skeletal maturity is recommended to allow for early detection and treatment of clinically significant growth disturbances.

ASSESSMENT OF FRACTURES OF THE DISTAL FEMORAL PHYSIS

MECHANISMS OF INJURY OF FRACTURES OF THE DISTAL FEMORAL PHYSIS

Most distal femoral physeal fractures are the result of high-energy mechanisms, such as motor vehicle- or sports-related trauma, and occur in older children and adolescents. Children between the ages of 2 and 11 years are less likely to sustain these fractures compared to adolescents or even infants.

Infants and Toddlers

Neonates are susceptible to distal femoral physeal fractures from birth trauma. Factors that predispose the newborn to this injury include breech presentation, macrosomia, difficult vaginal delivery, and rapid labor and delivery.[31] This injury has been also reported after delivery by cesarean section.[27] Child abuse should be suspected in infants and toddlers when a small peripheral metaphyseal fragment of bone, also called a "corner fracture" or the "classic metaphyseal lesion," is identified in association with widening of the distal femoral physis on radiographs of the femur or knee (Fig. 26-1).[35] This radiographic finding is pathognomonic for child abuse. If this radiographic sign is identified, regardless of the reported mechanism of injury, the child should be carefully examined for other signs of mistreatment such as skin lesions; a skeletal survey is obtained to identify other skeletal injuries and an immediate referral to your institution's child protection team and local child welfare services must be initiated.

Pathologic Fractures

Underlying conditions such as neuromuscular disorders, joint contractures, or nutritional deficiencies may predispose some

Figure 26-1. A 2-month-old girl presented with leg swelling. **A, B:** Radiographs revealed displaced Salter–Harris I fracture of the distal femur. **C, D:** Skeletal survey revealed numerous other fractures in various stages of healing consistent with nonaccidental trauma.

children, regardless of age, to separation of the distal femoral epiphysis.[3,4,37] Like other pathologic fractures, distal femoral physeal separations that occur in children with underlying conditions typically result from low-energy mechanisms, such as inadvertent twisting of the limb during transferring from a bed or stretching during physical therapy. Nonambulatory children, such as children with cerebral palsy, are particularly susceptible to pathologic metaphyseal fractures due to disuse osteopenia. Ambulatory children with spina bifida may develop epiphysiolysis, or a chronic separation of the distal femoral physis, and be unaware of it because of altered sensation. Salter–Harris fractures of the distal femur have been reported during manipulation of the knee under anesthesia in children who had developed knee contractures secondary to arthrofibrosis after treatment of displaced tibial eminence fractures.[62]

Biomechanics of Injury

In the adolescent with open growth plates about the knee, the most common mechanism of fracture of the distal femoral physis is a varus or valgus stress across the knee joint from a direct blow or buckling while landing from a jump or fall from a height. In most cases, this medially or laterally directed force is coupled with a torsional moment from direct application of force to the foot or more commonly, from twisting of the knee on the planted foot. In an animal model, the physis is least able to resist torsional forces.[10] Knee hyperextension or hyperflexion forces result in sagittal plane displacement. The combination of forces applied to the physis, however, determines the direction of displacement of the distal fragment.

Loading the limb to failure across the immature knee is more likely to lead to physeal disruption due to tensile stresses that are transmitted through the ligaments to the adjacent physis than it is to disruption of the major knee ligaments.[18] Varus or valgus forces (Fig. 26-2A) create tension on one side of the physis and compression on the opposite side. The result is the disruption of the periosteum, which may become entrapped between the epiphysis and the metaphysis (Fig. 26-2B), and the perichondrial ring on the tension side, followed by a fracture plane that begins in the hypertrophic zone and proceeds in an irregular manner through the physis.[10] In adults, a similar mechanism of injury is more likely to cause ligamentous disruption rather than bone failure because ligaments of the mature knee are less able to withstand extreme tensile forces compared to the bone of the adult distal femur and proximal tibia.

INJURIES ASSOCIATED WITH FRACTURES OF THE DISTAL FEMORAL PHYSIS

Since many of these injuries are the result of high-energy mechanisms, such as traffic accidents and motor sports, associated visceral injuries occur in approximately 5% of patients.[17] Other musculoskeletal injuries are seen in association with distal femoral physeal fractures in 10% to 15% of patients.[17,61] Other long bone fractures, as well as pelvic and spine fractures, must be ruled out, especially if the mechanism of injury is high-energy motor trauma (Fig. 26-3). Knee ligament disruption, however, is the most common concomitant musculoskeletal injury. Knee

Figure 26-2. A: In a skeletally immature patient, valgus force at the knee is more likely to cause a physeal fracture of the distal femur than a medial collateral ligament tear, an injury that occurs in adults. **B:** With correction of the valgus deformity, periosteum may become entrapped.

instability is diagnosed in 8% to 37% of patients[13,17] and is typically diagnosed after fracture healing with the initiation of rehabilitation and return to activities. Salter–Harris type III fractures of the medial femoral condyle are most frequently associated with anterior cruciate ligament injuries.[39,50] Open fractures and vascular injuries are uncommon associated injuries, occurring in about 3% of patients. Peroneal nerve injury occurs in about 2% to 7% of patients with displaced fractures.[8,17]

SIGNS AND SYMPTOMS OF FRACTURES OF THE DISTAL FEMORAL PHYSIS

Presentation

Emergency department assessment for children who are victims of high-energy trauma with a suspected distal femoral physeal separation should be initially evaluated by the trauma team to identify potential life-threatening injuries, to evaluate the ABCs, and to initiate resuscitation protocols if indicated. On the initial survey, head trauma, thoracoabdominal injuries, unstable spine and pelvic fractures, and limb-threatening extremity injuries are the priorities. After stabilization of the cardiovascular status, a thorough secondary survey should focus on the extremities. Long-bone fractures and ligamentous injuries of the extremities

Figure 26-3. A 7-year-old girl struck by a car while crossing the street sustained this closed injury. AP (**A**) and lateral (**B**) radiographs reveal an anteriorly displaced distal femoral physeal separation and a tibial shaft fracture. Upon admission, she had no pulse in the extremity. **C–E:** She underwent emergency open reduction and fixation of the distal femur and IM nail fixation of the tibia. Her pulses returned to normal after femur reduction. She did not develop a compartment syndrome.

are identified with a careful orthopaedic examination of all four extremities. Although severe injuries may occur in association with fractures of the distal femoral physis, this fracture usually occurs as an isolated injury in most patients.

For patients with displaced distal femoral physeal fractures, the diagnosis may be obvious. Patients typically describe severe pain, giving way of the limb, and obvious knee deformity after a sports injury, motor vehicle accident, or other high-energy mechanism and are unable to walk or bear weight on the injured limb. On examination, visible limb malalignment, severe swelling, and often ecchymosis at the apex of the knee deformity are identified. In fractures with severe displacement, the skin at the apex may be tented or puckered from protrusion of the metaphyseal distal femur through the periosteum and quadriceps muscle into the dermis. Hematoma may be palpable beneath the skin. Abrasions or laceration of the overlying soft tissues may be a clue to the mechanism of injury or to an open fracture. Assessment of knee range of motion and ligament stability is not possible in most cases with obvious displacement because of pain and the poor reliability of the examination in the face of fracture instability. Aggressive manipulation is also potentially harmful to the fractured physis or neurovascular structures that are already compromised.

Patients with nondisplaced fractures are more difficult to diagnose. Many children with nondisplaced distal femoral physeal fractures present with knee pain or mild knee swelling after a twisting injury or blow to the knee but are able to bear weight, albeit often with a painful limp. Point tenderness at the level of the distal femoral physis, either medially or laterally about the knee, is perhaps the most reliable way to detect this injury. Range of motion is typically painful but may not be severely restricted in all cases and fracture crepitus is absent because the periosteum is not fully disrupted. Varus/valgus stress testing of the knee ligaments is usually painful and, in some cases, may reveal subtle movement or suggest instability. The examiner, however, must be mindful that a skeletally immature patient with point tenderness at the physis is more likely to have sustained a physeal fracture of the distal femur compared to disruption of the medial or lateral collateral ligaments of the knee. Therefore, forceful or repeated stress testing of the knee in these cases should be avoided to minimize trauma to the injured physis.

Motor and Sensory Testing

Careful neurovascular examination of the lower leg and foot must be performed for all children with suspected fractures of the distal femoral physis, especially for those with obvious limb deformity. Complete motor and sensory testing of the distal limb is necessary to identify injury to the sciatic nerve and its branches, the tibial and common peroneal nerves. The peroneal nerve is injured in about 2% of patients with displaced fractures[8] and is the most commonly injured nerve related to this fracture,[17] so it is especially important that anterior (deep branch) and lateral (superficial branch) compartment muscle function and lower leg sensation be carefully documented. This nerve injury is typically a neuropraxia, the result of stretching from anterior or medial displacement of the distal femoral epiphysis.

Vascular Assessment

Although vascular injuries are rare after fractures of the distal femoral physis,[17,36,61] the vascular status must also be evaluated carefully. The distal pulses are palpated in the foot and ankle and other signs of adequate perfusion are evaluated. These other signs include assessment of capillary refill, skin temperature, and signs of venous insufficiency, such as distal swelling or cyanosis. Doppler ultrasound and measurement of ankle–brachial indices may be useful for detecting less obvious vascular injury when pulses and other signs are equivocal. Laceration, intimal tear, and thrombosis in the popliteal artery may occur by direct injury to the artery by the distal end of the metaphysis when the epiphysis is displaced anteriorly during a hyperextension injury.[8,17,55] Since anteriorly displaced fractures have an increased risk of neurovascular damage in general compared to other directions of displacement,[13,59] the examiner must be particularly suspicious for a vascular injury in patients with obvious hyperextension deformity of the knee.

Compartment syndrome after distal femoral physeal fracture is rare but in one series, occurred in 1.2% of patients.[17] Signs of compartment syndrome in the lower leg such as severe swelling, tense compartments, increasing use of analgesics or anxiety, and pain with passive motion and other examination abnormalities consistent with the diagnosis are also evaluated.[5]

Compartmental pressure recordings should be obtained if there are clinical findings of compartment syndrome of the lower leg. Compartment syndrome in association with this fracture is more likely to manifest hours after the injury rather than at the time of initial presentation. Patients at risk for developing a delayed compartment syndrome after this fracture are those with other injuries of the lower leg, such as tibial shaft fractures, and those with compromised vascularity.[17]

IMAGING AND OTHER DIAGNOSTIC STUDIES FOR FRACTURES OF THE DISTAL FEMORAL PHYSIS

Radiography

High-quality orthogonal radiographic views of the femur and knee are necessary for diagnosing distal femoral physeal separations (Table 26-1). On the AP radiograph, physeal widening and the presence of a fracture line proximally in the metaphysis or distally in the epiphysis allows the surgeon to differentiate between the four most common Salter–Harris types, types I to IV. In addition, epiphyseal varus (also called apex lateral angulation) or valgus (also called apex medial angulation) and medial or lateral translation in the coronal plane are determined on the AP view. The lateral radiograph demonstrates the amount of angulation and translation of the epiphysis in the sagittal plane. The anteriorly displaced epiphysis is usually tilted so that the distal articular surface faces anteriorly. This direction of displacement is alternatively called hyperextension of the epiphysis or apex posterior angulation. The posteriorly displaced epiphysis is tilted downward so that the distal articular surface faces the popliteal fossa, sometimes described as hyperflexion of the epiphysis or apex anterior angulation. Minor degrees

TABLE 26-1. Imaging Studies in the Evaluation of Distal Femoral Physeal Fractures

Study	Indications	Limitations
Standard radiographs	First study, often sufficient	May miss nondisplaced Salter–Harris type I or III fractures or underestimate fracture displacement
Computed tomography (CT)	Best defines fracture pattern and amount of displacement	Poor cartilage visualization Increased radiation exposure
	Useful for planning surgery, especially for metaphyseal comminution	Less useful than MRI in evaluating for occult Salter–Harris type I fractures
Magnetic resonance imaging (MRI)	Useful for evaluation of occult Salter–Harris type I fracture, especially in infants with little epiphyseal ossification	Availability, cost, duration of procedure
	Identifies associated soft tissue injuries, especially with Salter–Harris type III fractures	Fracture geometry less clear than with CT scan
Stress views	Differentiate occult Salter–Harris fracture from ligament injury	Painful, muscle spasm may not permit opening of fracture if patient awake, potentially harmful to physis
Contralateral radiographs	Useful in infants or to assess physeal width Obtain at follow-up to compare growth	Usually not helpful in acute fractures
Ultrasonography, arthrography	Helpful in infants to assess swelling and displacement of epiphysis	Not useful after infancy

of displacement may be difficult to measure on plain films unless the x-ray projection is precisely in line with the plane of the fracture. Even small amounts of displacement are significant.[26,36] Rotational malalignment of the distal fragment relative to the proximal fragment may be identified on either view and is dramatic in some cases with severe displacement.

Diagnosis of minimally displaced distal femoral physeal fractures is challenging. Because the physis is normally radiolucent, injury is typically identified because of physeal widening, epiphyseal displacement, or metaphyseal bone injury suggestive of a fracture. Without obvious radiographic abnormalities, a nondisplaced Salter–Harris type I or III fracture can be easily overlooked.[53] Oblique views of the distal femur may reveal an occult fracture through the epiphysis or metaphysis. In the past, stress views of the distal femur were recommended for patients with negative radiographs who have an effusion or tenderness localized to the physis. However, it is our practice to forego stress radiographs because they are painful to the patient and may damage the already compromised physis. Presumptive Salter–Harris I fractures are either immobilized for 1 to 2 weeks and reexamined or are further evaluated with magnetic resonance imaging (MRI).[39,60]

Magnetic Resonance Imaging

MRI is the most commonly used advanced imaging study for evaluating traumatic knee injuries in children and adolescents. The primary utility of MRI is to identify acute knee injuries when the examination and radiographs are nondiagnostic or to confirm diagnostic suspicions. In one large MRI study of 315 adolescents with acute traumatic knee injuries, physeal injuries of the distal femur were diagnosed in 7 patients with negative plain radiographs.[12] MRI also facilitates identification of knee ligament tears, meniscal pathology, and osteochondral fractures that may occur concomitantly with distal femoral physeal fractures,[39] both in the acute setting and after fracture healing. MR arteriography is one method of evaluating vascular anatomy and flow in patients with an abnormal vascular examination in association with displaced distal femoral physeal fractures.

Computed Tomography

A computed tomography (CT) scan is recommended for all patients with Salter–Harris III and IV fractures diagnosed on plain radiographs. In one study, CT identified fracture displacement and comminution that was not recognized on plain radiographs of the knee. The author encourages its use for evaluation of these fractures to identify displacement, define fracture geometry, and plan surgical fixation.[33] CT may also be useful to identify fractures and displacement in cases where the plain radiographs are negative but the examination is suspicious for a distal femoral physeal fracture.

SPECIAL SITUATIONS OF FRACTURES OF THE DISTAL FEMORAL PHYSIS

Neonate

Separation of the distal femoral epiphysis in a neonate is particularly difficult to diagnose on initial x-rays unless there is

displacement because only the center of the epiphysis is ossified at birth. This ossification center is in line with the axis of the femoral shaft on both the AP and lateral views in normal infants. Any degree of malalignment of the ossification center from the shaft should raise suspicion for this fracture. Comparison views of the opposite knee and other modalities may also be helpful to identify its presence in neonates when radiographs of the affected leg are equivocal. MRI, performed under anesthesia, is another commonly used diagnostic imaging study that may help to identify a separation of the unossified femoral epiphysis.

Unique to the neonate is the use of ultrasonography[25] to evaluate distal femoral physeal separation. Ultrasound allows visualization of the cartilaginous distal femur in a young child with incomplete ossification of the distal femoral epiphysis. Although this study is safe and readily available, it is unfamiliar to many technicians and radiologists, making its reliability questionable unless performed by an experienced team. This modality may be used not only to diagnose injuries but also to guide reduction. Knee arthrography, another option for evaluating the immature distal femoral epiphysis for possible disruption, is primarily used to facilitate reduction and fixation in the operating room.

One should remember to consider infection in a neonate with a painful or immobile limb.

Physeal Arrest

An effective method for determining the viability of the physis after healing of a traumatic injury is MRI performed with fat-suppressed three-dimensional spoiled gradient-recalled echo sequences.[15] Impending growth disturbance can be identified early with this MRI technique, and MRI can be used to map the extent of physeal bony bar formation to determine if excision is an option for treatment.[15] Although CT may also be used to map the location and area of physeal bars, it is the author's preference to use MRI because it does not expose the child to radiation and evaluates the quality of the physeal cartilage adjacent to the bar, a possible predictor of the success of bar excision.

CLASSIFICATION OF FRACTURES OF THE DISTAL FEMORAL PHYSIS

Several types of classification schemes have been used to describe fractures of the distal femoral physis, each with some merit because of the information that its use provides to the surgeon. The Salter–Harris classification[55] is the most widely used classification scheme (Fig. 26-4).

This familiar classification system, based on plain radiographs, is useful for the description of the types of physeal fractures of the distal femur. As opposed to its application to other physeal fractures, however, the Salter–Harris scheme is not as reliable in predicting the risk of growth disturbance as it relates to the fracture types.[1,9,17,36] For many physeal fractures in other anatomic sites, risk of growth disturbance is lower after type I and II fractures and higher after type III and IV fractures. Distal femoral physeal fractures, however, are at risk for significant growth disturbance regardless of type.[7,36] This classification scheme is useful for treatment planning and is also a good indicator of the mechanism of injury.[13]

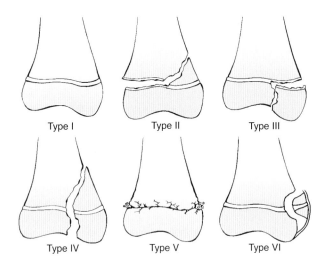

Figure 26-4. The Salter–Harris classification of fractures involving the distal femoral physis.

Salter–Harris Classification		
Salter–Harris Type	**Energy Required**	**Risk of Physeal Arrest**
I	Mild to moderate	Low
II	Moderate	Moderate
III	Significant	High
IV	Significant	High
V	Significant	High
VI	Moderate	Unknown

Direction of Displacement	**Risks**
Anterior	Vascular injury
Posterior	Nerve injury
Medial/lateral	Neurovascular injury
Magnitude of Displacement	**Risks**
More than 50% of diameter of metaphysis	Higher rate of complications

Age at Fracture	**Prognosis**
Under age 2 years	Good
2–11 years	Fair to poor
12 years and older	Fair to poor

Salter–Harris I Fractures

The Salter–Harris type I pattern is a fracture that traverses the distal femoral physis, without extension either proximally into the metaphysis or distally into the epiphysis or knee joint (Fig. 26-5). Anatomically, this fracture cleaves the physis predominantly across the physeal zones of cell hypertrophy and provisional calcification. Because of the undulation of the distal femoral physis, likely evolutionarily developed to increase the stability of the physeal plate when subjected to shear stress, most distal femoral physeal fractures do not propagate cleanly across these zones but instead also extend into the germinal zones of the physis. This encroachment of the fracture line into cartilage precursor cells is likely the explanation for increased rates of growth disturbance after Salter–Harris I and II fracture types.

Although this fracture pattern may be seen in any age group of skeletally immature patients, it occurs more frequently in infants, as the result of birth trauma or abuse, and in adolescents with sports-related trauma. Many Salter–Harris I fractures are nondisplaced and may go undetected. Sometimes, the diagnosis is made only retrospectively after subperiosteal new bone formation occurs along the adjacent metaphysis, evident on follow-up radiographs 10 to 14 days after injury, or by MRI. When displacement is present before the age of 2 years, it usually occurs in the sagittal plane. Approximately 15% of physeal fractures of the distal femur are Salter–Harris type I fractures.[7]

Salter–Harris II Fractures

The Salter–Harris type II pattern is the most common type of separation of the distal femoral epiphysis (Figs. 26-6 and 26-7). This pattern is characterized by a fracture line that extends through the physis incompletely and then exits proximally via an oblique extension of the fracture line through the metaphysis. The metaphyseal corner that remains attached to the epiphysis is called the Thurston Holland fragment. Although the direction of displacement varies, typically the direction of displacement is also the location of the metaphyseal fragment because the metaphyseal spike occurs on the side of compression forces. This fracture type may also be seen in children of all ages but is more common in adolescents. Slightly more than half (57%) of all distal femoral physeal fractures are Salter–Harris II fractures.[7]

Salter–Harris III Fractures

The Salter–Harris type III injury has a fracture line that traverses part of the physis and then exits distally, with extension of the fracture line vertically across the physis, epiphysis, and its articular surface (Fig. 26-8). Most Salter–Harris III fractures of the distal femur traverse the medial physis and extend into the joint, separating the medial condyle from the lateral condyle of the distal femur. These injuries are often produced by valgus stress across the knee, the same mechanism of injury that produces medial collateral and cruciate ligament disruption in skeletally mature patients, and may have an associated injury to the cruciate ligaments.[48] This fracture occurs most frequently in older children and adolescents and comprises about 10% of all distal femoral physeal fractures.[7]

Nondisplaced Salter–Harris III and IV fractures and other more complex patterns of distal femoral physeal fracture may not always be detectable or fully delineated on plain radiographs, requiring MRI or CT to identify.[38,39,43] It has been

Figure 26-5. Preoperative (**A, B**) and postoperative (**C, D**) radiographs of a 2.5-year-old boy with Salter–Harris I right distal femur fracture, treated with closed reduction and percutaneous pinning. Pins are separated widely at fracture site to provide more stability.

Figure 26-6. A 10-year-old boy who was hit by a car and sustained a Salter–Harris II fracture of the distal femur. Patient was petite, so the fracture was reduced and stabilized with K-wires, which were removed promptly at 4 weeks to decrease risk of infection. Follow-up radiographs 2 years later showed no evidence of growth disturbance. However, given the lateral location of the metaphyseal spike, if the patient had developed a growth arrest, a varus malalignment would have resulted.

hypothesized that the Salter–Harris type III fracture, seen mostly in older children and adolescents, may occur as a consequence of the progression of closure of the distal femoral physis. This pattern of fracture occurs near skeletal maturity when the central portion of the distal femoral physis begins to close before the medial and lateral parts of the physis, similar to a Tillaux fracture of the distal tibia.[39] Occasionally, a type III fracture may occur in the coronal plane of the distal femoral condyle, more commonly the medial femoral condyle, similar to the "Hoffa fracture" of the posterior condyle seen in adults.[43] This fracture is difficult to diagnose with standard x-rays[53] and is also challenging to reduce and fix. A triplane fracture of the distal femur, a fracture that appears as a Salter–Harris I injury in the sagittal plane and a Salter–Harris III fracture in the coronal and sagittal planes, has also been described.[38] This triplane fracture is not completely analogous to the classic triplane fracture of the ankle; however, because while the fracture line extends in three dimensions about the physis, the distal femoral physis is completely open.

Salter–Harris IV Fractures

In Salter–Harris type IV injuries of the distal femur, the fracture line extends vertically through the metaphysis, across the physis, ultimately extending through the epiphysis and its articular surface (Fig. 26-9). It is at times difficult to distinguish between Salter–Harris III and IV fractures because the metaphyseal fragment may be small and difficult to identify on plain radiographs. Salter–Harris III and IV fractures likely occur from similar mechanisms and in the same age ranges, with both presenting management challenges that require anatomic realignment of the joint line and physis to minimize risk of growth disturbance. Of fractures of the distal femoral physis, this

Figure 26-7. A 15-year-old boy with right Salter–Harris II fracture after a bike accident. **A:** Fracture was stabilized with two cannulated screws using a washer for additional compression. **B:** Patient underwent ongoing monitoring for any evidence of growth arrest. Given the fracture pattern, if this were to occur, we would expect developing valgus malalignment (in contrast to the example in Fig. 26-6).

A

B

Figure 26-8. A 15-year-old boy with left Salter–Harris III fracture shown in AP and lateral radiographs (**A**) and also on CT (**B**). Although in the AP view the screws appear to be at the level of the physis (**C**), it is clearly visualized on the lateral that they are below this level (**D**), highlighting the undulating nature of the distal femur physis.

lower extremity. The annual rate of growth is approximately three-eighths of an inch or 9 to 10 mm. The growth of the distal femur, like the physes of other long bones, ceases at a mean skeletal age of 14 years in girls and 16 years in boys, with a wide range of variability.[63]

PHYSEAL ANATOMY

At birth, the distal femoral physis is flat, or planar, making this physis in infants the least stable compared to other age groups. With maturation, the physis assumes an undulating and more convoluted shape.[34] By the age of 2 to 3 years, the physis develops an intercondylar groove, or central prominence, as well as sulci that traverse medial and lateral proximal to each condyle. This configuration effectively divides the physis into four quadrants, each with concave surfaces that match the four convex surfaces of the distal femoral metaphysis over a large surface area. The complex physeal geometry and large area of the distal femoral physis contribute to its stability by better-resisting shear and torsional forces compared to the smaller flat physes of infants. The perichondral ring also circumferentially reinforces the physis at its periphery. This structure, combined with reinforcement of the physeal periphery by the knee ligaments, provides additional resistance to disruption of the physis.[11] During adolescence, however, the perichondrial ring becomes thinner. It is hypothesized that this change contributes to relative weakening of the distal femoral physis, partially explaining the fact that fractures of this physis are more frequent in adolescents and generally occur from lower-energy mechanisms compared to children of 2 to 11 years of age.

The irregular configuration of the physis, while contributing to stability, is also an important factor in the high incidence of growth disturbance from these fractures. Fracture lines, instead of cleanly traversing the hypertrophic zone and area of provisional calcification, extend through multiple regions of the physis and damage germinal cells regardless of fracture type. In addition, during reduction of displaced fractures, epiphyseal ridges may grind against the metaphyseal projections and further damage cartilage-producing resting cells. Minimizing contact and shear across the physis during reduction is preferable to improve the chances of normal growth after injury. Reductions in the operating room with muscle-relaxing agents, use of traction during reduction, avoiding a tourniquet which can tighten muscles, and limiting the number of closed manipulation attempts before converting to open reduction are some techniques that are generally recommended.

BONY ANATOMY

Proximal to the medial border of the medial condyle, a small area of the metaphysis of the distal femur widens abruptly, forming the adductor tubercle. The lateral metaphysis, by contrast, flares only minimally at the proximal part of the lateral condyle, forming the lateral epicondyle. The distal femur is divided into two discrete condyles at the level of the knee joint, separated by the intercondylar notch. Nearly the entire distal femur is covered by hyaline cartilage for articulation with the proximal tibia. The anterior, or patellar, surface just proximal

to the intercondylar notch has a shallow midline concavity to accommodate the longitudinal convex ridge of the undersurface of the patella. Posteriorly, the distal femur contacts the tibial cartilage as the knee flexes. The posterior condyles, projections of the femoral condyles posteriorly, contain this cartilage that extends on either side of the intercondylar notch and nearly to the posterior margin of the physis.

The distal femur has well-defined normal anatomical alignment parameters. The mechanical axis of the femur is formed by a line between the centers of the hip and knee joints (Fig. 26-11). A line tangential to the distal surfaces of the two condyles (the joint line) is in approximately 3 degrees of valgus relative to the mechanical axis. The longitudinal axis of the diaphysis of the femur inclines

Figure 26-11. The mechanical and anatomic axis of the lower extremity. Note that the knee joint is in a mean of 3 degrees of valgus. The femoral shaft is inclined medially at an angle of 6 degrees relative to the mechanical axis.

medially in a distal direction at an angle of 6 degrees relative to the mechanical axis.[24]

SOFT TISSUE ANATOMY

The distal femoral physis is completely extrasynovial. Anteriorly and posteriorly, the synovial membrane and joint capsule of the knee attach to the femoral epiphysis just distal to the physis. The suprapatellar pouch, however, is a ballooning out of the synovium that extends proximally over the anterior surface of the metaphysis. On the medial and lateral surfaces of the epiphysis, the proximal attachment of the synovium and capsule is distal to the physis and separated from the physis by the insertions of the collateral ligaments. The strong posterior capsule and all of the major ligaments of the knee are attached to the epiphysis distal to the physis. Varus/valgus-directed forces that would cause collateral ligament disruption in adults often result in physeal separations in children and adolescents because the tensile strength of the ligaments is greater than that of the physis. The anterior and posterior cruciate ligaments originate in the upward-sloping roof of the intercondylar notch distal to the physis. Compression and tension forces can be transmitted across the extended knee to the epiphysis of the femur by taut ligaments. The medial and lateral heads of the gastrocnemius muscle originate from the distal femur proximal to the joint capsule and physis. Although forces generated by the gastrocnemius are probably not a major factor that contributes to fractures of the distal femoral physis, pull of the muscle may be a deforming force in metaphyseal fractures of the distal femur.

NEUROVASCULAR ANATOMY

Arterial Anatomy

The popliteal artery runs along the posterior surface of the distal femur, separated from it by only a thin layer of fat. Directly proximal to the femoral condyles, this artery sends off transverse branches medially and laterally, called the medial and lateral superior geniculate arteries, along the surface of the distal femoral metaphysis beneath the overlying muscles that they supply. The popliteal artery then continues distally, adjacent to the posterior capsule of the knee joint between the femoral condyles. At this level, the middle geniculate artery branches from it anteriorly to the posterior surface of the epiphysis, providing the primary blood supply to the distal femoral epiphysis and the physis. The distal femoral epiphysis, however, receives its blood supply from a rich anastomosis of vessels. As such, osteonecrosis of this epiphysis is exceedingly rare, occurring only in situations where the distal femoral epiphysis is completely stripped of its soft tissue attachments. Since the popliteal artery and its branches course along the posterior distal femur, it is especially vulnerable to injury because of contact with the distal femoral metaphysis from hyperextension injuries of the knee with anterior displacement of the epiphysis. While tenting of the artery causing occlusion and arterial spasm are the most common reasons for vascular abnormalities related to distal femoral physeal fractures, intimal injury and laceration may also occur.

Nerve Supply

The sciatic nerve, extending from the upper thigh, divides into the common peroneal and tibial nerves just proximal to the popliteal space. The peroneal nerve then descends posteriorly, between the biceps femoris muscle and the lateral head of the gastrocnemius muscle, to a point just distal to the head of the fibula. The peroneal nerve then changes course, wrapping around the proximal fibula to enter the anterior compartment of the lower leg, where it divides into the deep and superficial branches. The common peroneal nerve's course between muscles protects it from direct injury from fracture ends. However, because of limited excursion due to its anteriorly directed course around the fibular head, the nerve is susceptible to injury from stretch. Neuropraxia and even axonotmesis of the common peroneal nerve result most commonly from fractures with severe anterior displacement and medial translation (varus displacement).[59] The tibial nerve, coursing through the popliteal space adjacent to the popliteal artery, enters the calf along the arch of the soleus muscle. This nerve is vulnerable to injury from mechanisms that are similar to those that cause injury to the popliteal artery, although clinically, tibial nerve injury is rare.

TREATMENT OPTIONS FOR FRACTURES OF THE DISTAL FEMORAL PHYSIS

Distal femoral physeal fractures in children and adolescents are challenging fractures that require careful preoperative evaluation and assessment of the injury, including both physical and radiographic examinations, so as to devise an appropriate treatment plan (Table 26-2). The treatment principles for these injuries can be summarized as follows:

• Restore the anatomy without iatrogenically compromising the distal femoral physis.
• Stabilize the fracture in the position of anatomic reduction.

The surgeon must keep in mind that by definition, there has already been an injury to the physis and further damage to the physis by repeated or forceful manipulations may contribute to one of the complications of this injury, premature physeal closure. Closed reduction of these injuries must be done gently, preferably under either IV sedation or general anesthesia, so that the reduction is accomplished easily with minimal force. Once the reduction has been achieved, maintaining it has been shown to be vitally important for influencing outcome (as redisplaced fractures tend to have poor prognosis and higher complication rates).[7,61] Treatment is also guided by the Salter–Harris type. Salter–Harris types III and IV fractures are intra-articular and require an anatomic reduction to minimize the potential for future arthritis. Therefore, these fractures are most commonly treated with open reduction and internal fixation to restore congruency of the joint surface. The ultimate goals of treatment are to maintain anatomic alignment of the lower extremity, preserve range of motion in the knee joint, and not disturb ongoing growth of the distal femoral physis.

TABLE 26-2. Methods of Treatment for Distal Femoral Physeal Fractures

Treatment	Pros	Cons	Indications
Closed reduction and immobilization	Avoids anesthesia	High risk of loss of reduction	Nondisplaced, stable fractures
Closed reduction and screw fixation	Minimal dissection	Only in reducible fractures	Reducible Salter–Harris type II fractures, nondisplaced Salter–Harris type III and IV fractures
Closed reduction and smooth pinning	Minimal dissection	Pins may lead to joint infection, require later removal	Reducible Salter–Harris type I fractures, Salter–Harris type II fractures with small metaphyseal fragment
Open reduction and screws and/or smooth pins	Anatomic reduction	Stiffness	Irreducible Salter–Harris type I and II fractures, displaced Salter–Harris type III and IV fractures
External fixation	Allows soft tissue access	Pin site (joint) infection	Severe soft tissue injury
Rigid plate crossing physis	Rigid fixation	Can stop future growth when spans physis	Adolescents near the end of growth, severe injuries with growth disturbance inevitable
			Possible temporary fixation with extraperiosteal locked plating removed soon after union

NONOPERATIVE TREATMENT OF FRACTURES OF THE DISTAL FEMORAL PHYSIS

Nondisplaced or minimally displaced distal femoral physeal fractures, especially Salter–Harris type I or II fractures, may be treated with a gentle closed reduction and immobilization in a long-leg cast. Conceivably, even a Salter–Harris type III or IV fracture that is completely nondisplaced could also be managed in this manner. The treating surgeon must be cognizant of the fact that displacement may have been far greater at the time of injury than the injury radiographs depict. At the time of the injury, the periosteum and/or resilience of the child's bone, as well as reduction at the site of injury, may have occurred, rendering the fracture to appear non- or minimally displaced on the initial radiographs. Evidence of considerable soft tissue injury, such as swelling, ecchymosis, and/or other skin changes, may be an indication that the fracture was more displaced at the time of injury.

If minimal force is required to perform a reduction, most series indicate that these fractures can be successfully managed nonoperatively. Careful assessment of stability of the fracture by the surgeon is crucial to a successful outcome with closed reduction and casting. In a study of 82 patients immobilized in a long-leg cast, 36% had redisplacement in the first 2 weeks, including 3 patients immobilized with a hip spica cast.[17] Of the 32 patients that displaced in a cast in this series, only 8 were successfully remanipulated. Closed reduction and casting is never the best definitive treatment for displaced or unstable distal femoral physeal fractures because of the significant risk of fracture redisplacement.[2] Persistent widening after provisional reduction may reflect interposed periosteum, resulting in a less than anatomic reduction and higher risk of redisplacement. Some believe that periosteal interposition may theoretically place the physis at increased risk for

premature closure[56] but there is very little evidence to support this opinion. Anatomic reduction is always the goal with these injuries and if an adequate reduction cannot be obtained by closed means, alternative methods of treatment must be utilized. In general, with nonoperative treatment, the risk of fracture redisplacement and the risk of growth disturbance are high so only truly nondisplaced fractures should be treated nonoperatively.

OPERATIVE TREATMENT OF FRACTURES OF THE DISTAL FEMORAL PHYSIS

Distal femoral physeal fractures with more than 2 mm of displacement typically require reduction and surgical stabilization with internal fixation. The overriding principle regarding reduction maneuvers is to avoid further injury to the physis (Fig. 26-12). Most authors recommend that the reductions be done with the patient relaxed with muscle relaxants or under general anesthesia. However, the so-called gentle reduction does not preclude the possibility of a growth arrest, as has been noted by Thomson et al.[61] The technique of reduction relies on assessment of the fracture pattern. In general, the concave side of the fracture is gently manipulated to realign it with the long axis or shaft of the femur, essentially closing down the convexity of the fracture. The periosteum is typically intact on the concave side of the injury. For example, the periosteum on the side of the Thurston Holland fragment of a Salter–Harris type II fracture is usually intact but disrupted on the convex side of the fracture. Periosteal interposition at the fracture site is a frequent occurrence in these fractures and necessitates careful assessment of the postreduction imaging and anatomy.

For a Salter–Harris type II fracture that is displaced into valgus alignment such that the epiphysis is displaced laterally

Figure 26-12. Closed reduction of a Salter–Harris type I or II fracture. **A:** With medial or lateral displacement, traction is applied longitudinally along the axis of the deformity to bring the fragments back to length. **B:** For anterior displacement, the reduction can be done with the patient prone or supine. Length is gained first, then a flexion moment is added.

and there is a lateral Thurston Holland fragment, the reduction maneuver would involve gentle longitudinal traction, often with the knee flexed slightly, and counterpressure applied over the medial distal femur while the epiphyseal portion of the fracture is gently guided back in place. Reduction is 90% traction and 10% manipulation to minimize iatrogenic trauma to the physis. More challenging reductions occur in the sagittal plane when the epiphysis is displaced either anteriorly or posteriorly. Anteriorly displaced physeal fractures generally require some level of knee flexion to achieve reduction. In all reductions, longitudinal traction is the first force applied followed by the gentle manipulation of the epiphysis back into place starting with counterpressure on the proximal segment in an opposite direction. For an anteriorly displaced epiphysis, holding the fracture reduced may require a significant amount of knee flexion, which may not be advisable from a neurovascular standpoint, particularly in a really swollen knee. Fractures like these may require internal stabilization with pins simply to be able to immobilize the knee in slight flexion. Some authors recommend aspiration of the hematoma from the knee, especially in

Salter–Harris type III or IV fractures, prior to closed reduction maneuvers. Various reports indicate rates of fracture redisplacement in a cast of 30% or higher, so internal fixation for displaced fractures is advised.[61] A recent report indicated that internal fixation is the preferred method of treatment for all displaced injuries.[2]

Closed Reduction and Percutaneous Pinning

One of the most common techniques for stabilization of displaced distal femoral physeal fractures is percutaneous internal fixation with pins or screws (Fig. 26-13). These fractures can often be reduced fairly anatomically, and given their propensity to be unstable, fixation with smooth crossed pins or with one to two screws through the Thurston Holland fragment in the case of Salter–Harris type II fractures provides stable internal fixation of the fracture. Even Salter–Harris type III and IV fractures can be treated this way if there is minimal displacement on the injury films and an anatomic reduction can be achieved by closed means.

Figure 26-13. Screw fixation following closed or open reduction of Salter–Harris type II fracture with a large metaphyseal fragment. **A:** When using cannulated screws, place both guidewires before screw placement to avoid rotation of the fragment while drilling or inserting screw. Screw threads should be past the fracture site to enable compression. Washers help increase compression. Screws may be placed anterior and posterior to each other, which is particularly helpful when trying to fit multiple screws in a small metaphyseal fragment. **B:** This form of fixation is locally "rigid," but must be protected with long-leg immobilization.

Preoperative Planning

✓ Closed Reduction and Percutaneous Pinning:
PREOPERATIVE PLANNING CHECKLIST

OR table	❏ Radiolucent flat top
Position/ positioning aids	❏ Supine with soft bolster or bump under ipsilateral hip ❏ Anteriorly displaced epiphysis may require prone position
Fluoroscopy location	❏ C-arm opposite surgeon
Equipment	❏ Smooth Steinmann pins; large and small cannulated screw sets
Tourniquet	❏ Sterile tourniquet available
(Other)	❏ Doppler available to assess pedal pulses

Preoperative planning and room setup for percutaneous pinning includes the availability of a radiolucent table and C-arm. Instrumentation typically comprises of large (e.g., 6.5 mm), partially threaded cannulated screws or smooth Steinmann pins. Smaller cannulated screws may be required for some fracture patterns, such as a small Thurston Holland fragment in a Salter-Harris type II fracture or more comminuted fractures. Muscle relaxation of the patient provided by the anesthesiology team is especially helpful before initiating reduction maneuvers. Neurovascular status of the extremity should be checked routinely both before and after reduction maneuvers.

Positioning

Fracture reduction can be facilitated by placing a bump under the patient's thigh. Anteriorly displaced physeal fractures may be managed in a prone position.

Technique

✓ Closed Reduction and Percutaneous Pinning:
KEY SURGICAL STEPS

- ❏ Assure adequate positioning and setup with radiolucent table and C-arm
- ❏ Obtain closed reduction as anatomic as possible
- ❏ Verify reduction with imaging
- ❏ Stabilize reduction
- ❏ Place Steinman pins to stabilize fracture with C-arm guidance
- ❏ Place guide pins in metaphysis for cannulated screws
- ❏ Assess pin position on AP and lateral images
- ❏ For pin fixation, either bend outside skin or bury subcutaneously
- ❏ For screw fixation, measure pins to determine screw length and overdrill with cannulated drill
- ❏ Place screws over pins to stabilize fracture
- ❏ Close wounds and place long-leg cast or brace

The technique requires closed reduction to be accomplished with virtually anatomic alignment as discussed previously. For Salter–Harris type I fractures and Salter–Harris type II fractures without a significant Thurston Holland fragment or with metaphyseal comminution, two large (3.2-mm or even larger diameter) smooth Steinmann pins are typically inserted retrograde in a cross-pin configuration. With fluoroscopic guidance and the reduction held by an assistant, a small incision is made over the midpoint of the femoral condyle. The placement of the pin is not in the articular cartilage but just off the articular margin in the epiphyseal bone and directed slightly anteriorly to avoid injury to the posterior neurovascular structures. It may be helpful to insert the first pin on the side that was the concave side of the fracture pattern. Careful assessment of pin placement should be done with C-arm imaging in both the AP and lateral planes.

Fracture stability may be assessed by gently applying a varus, valgus, or flexion-extension force once pins are in place. Some authors will leave the pins external to the skin at the level of the epiphysis. Some will bend the pins slightly and cut them short under the skin, but this is falling out of favor as it requires another procedure for pin removal with no demonstrated benefit. Other authors advocate driving the pins out of the skin at the level of the metaphysis such that the pins are flush with the edge of the epiphysis at the entry site, as there is a theoretical risk that external pins at the level of the epiphysis could lead to septic knee arthritis since the pins are intra-articular. Yet another option is to start the pins proximally in the metaphysis, advancing them across the fracture in an antegrade fashion, and leaving the tips of the pins in the subchondral bone of the epiphysis to minimize pin tract infections that could communicate with the joint. It is important to note the vascular "safe zone" in the medial thigh, in which the superficial femoral artery is safely posterior to the distal femur. One study showed that the safe zone extends two times the width of the distal femoral physis proximal to the medial femoral condyle in children 6 years or older. The authors recommend avoiding retrograde pins that exit into the medial thigh in children up to 3 years old and a slightly anterior pin trajectory should be used.[21] Patients are usually immobilized in a fiberglass long-leg cast with the knee gently flexed or a brace if the pins are buried underneath the skin, there is sufficient fracture stability, good patient compliance, and a long enough femur to provide immobilization of the knee.

The technique of using transphyseal pins to stabilize distal femoral physeal fractures requires the use of smooth pins to minimize injury to the physis. A recent article looked at whether these pins could be responsible for physeal injury and subsequent growth arrest.[19] The conclusion of this study was that the potential for physeal arrest varied with increasing fracture severity based on the Salter–Harris classification and transphyseal smooth pins were not statistically associated with the growth arrest.[19]

Postoperative Care

Distal femoral physeal fractures heal readily and are healed within 4 weeks, at which point, pins may be removed. Touchdown weight-bearing in the cast may be allowed in the last week or 2 prior to pin removal. Often a splint or hinged knee brace is used for a few weeks to facilitate regaining range of motion of the knee with increasing weight-bearing, such that most patients are able to bear weight fully about 6 weeks postoperatively. Pin removal at 4 weeks may be done in the office if the pins are external or as a day surgery procedure if they were buried beneath the skin. It is important to stress that intraarticular pins should not be left in place for more than 4 weeks as this may lead to a septic joint and infection should always be considered with any increasing discomfort, fevers, drainage, etc. The patients are instructed to work on quadriceps strengthening and active range of motion of the knee often facilitated by physical therapy.

Screw Fixation

The technique for stabilizing Salter–Harris type II fractures with a significant metaphyseal fragment again involves performing a gentle closed reduction under anesthesia. A small incision is then made in the metaphysis over the Thurston Holland fragment, which typically is either on the medial or lateral aspect of the distal femur. The guide pins from the cannulated screw system are used to help stabilize the fracture (Fig. 26-14). After careful assessment of pin placement with C-arm imaging in the AP and lateral planes, the pins are measured to determine screw length, the outer cortex is drilled, and one or two 6.5 mm or larger partially threaded screws are inserted to stabilize the fracture fragment. Care must be taken to ensure that the screws do not approach or cross the physis. In general, screws are placed parallel to the distal femoral physis. The surgeon should consider use of washers as the metaphyseal bone is weak in this area. Again, assessment of fracture stability by gentle stress with the screws in place is helpful

to ensure that the internal fixation is adequate in providing optimum stability. Postoperative immobilization and care are the same as after percutaneous pinning. Screw removal is at the discretion of the family and surgeon at a convenient time in the future. Occasionally, the size of the Thurston Holland fragment permits only one screw to be placed. These fractures may be unstable enough that one screw is insufficient to provide adequate internal fixation, so supplemental fixation can be achieved with an oblique Steinmann pin inserted following the technique described for percutaneous pinning. This pin would ideally be inserted on the side opposite the screw entry site to provide improved stability to the fracture.

Closed Reduction and Screw Fixation of Salter–Harris III and IV Fractures

Minimally displaced Salter–Harris III and IV fractures may also be managed with reduction and percutaneous screw fixation. The use of bone reduction forceps or clamps may be helpful in closing down a gap or diastasis of the condyles. Again, careful and accurate assessment of intraoperative imaging is essential to ascertain whether the reduction is adequate for a percutaneous technique versus an open reduction. A large pelvic reduction forceps is helpful for obtaining and maintaining reduction during screw placement.

Screw placement in the epiphysis for both Salter–Harris III and IV fractures is performed with C-arm guidance using a cannulated screw system. Care must be taken not to place the screws too distal in the epiphysis such that they would impinge on the intercondylar notch of the femur and this should be assessed with intraoperative notch views if there is any question. Two screws are typically placed, one more anteriorly and one more posteriorly, to stabilize a Salter–Harris III fracture. A Salter–Harris IV fracture may have a metaphyseal fragment that is sufficiently large enough to be stabilized with a screw (Fig. 26-15).

Challenges with the technique of a closed reduction and internal fixation include an inadequate reduction secondary to periosteal interposition. As mentioned, the periosteum is often torn on the convex side, so an incomplete reduction with a widened physis on the convex side may need to be opened to extract the periosteum to ensure an anatomic and stable reduction. Interposed periosteum has been shown experimentally to increase the risk of growth disturbance.[49] In addition, when trying to utilize this technique for Salter–Harris type III or IV fractures, if the articular surface cannot be well aligned or if there is comminution present, an open approach is necessary.

Open Reduction and Internal Fixation

Open reduction and internal fixation is necessary for all irreducible distal femoral physeal fractures. Irreducible fractures may have interposed periosteum on the side of the widened physis or the convex side of the fracture. An incision is made over the medial or lateral aspect of the femur centered over the physis; even in sagittal plane displacements, the incision is typically still medial or lateral. The periosteum is carefully

Figure 26-14. A: Clinical photo of right knee with a Salter–Harris II fracture; note swelling compared to normal left knee. **B:** Photo of knee showing guide pin for cannulated screw in place in Thurston Holland fragment. *Vertical line* marks cephalad extent of TH fragment. *Smaller line* marks the physis. **C:** Preparing entry site for second guide pin with C-arm guidance. **D:** Using a hemostat to spread through iliotibial band and periosteum to create path to distal femur for pin placement. **E:** Placing guide pin parallel to original pin. **F:** Two pins in distal femur, parallel and verified in good position with C-arm.

Figure 26-14. (*Continued*) **G:** Measuring depth of guide pin to determine screw length. Note a third pin was added. **H:** Drilling over guide pin. Note that far cortex does not need to be drilled. **I:** Placing cannulated cancellous screw. **J:** Appearance after screws are placed. **K:** Appearance after wound closure. **L:** Dressing in place.

(*continues*)

Figure 26-14. (*Continued*) **M:** Final cast in place.

removed from the physis and care is taken to avoid causing any more injury to the physis by surgical instruments or retractors. Evacuation of organized hematoma is helpful to achieve anatomic reduction. Internal fixation may proceed accordingly with either pins or screws.

Fractures that undergo open reduction and internal fixation may be more prone to knee stiffness. Healing by 4 weeks is expected and early mobilization of the knee is recommended at that time.

Other Means of Fixation

The use of external fixators in open fractures involving the distal femoral physis may be a helpful strategy to manage severe soft tissue injuries, especially temporarily as in damage control for the multitrauma patient. Typically, one or two half pins from an external fixation set are placed in the epiphysis and two half pins are placed in the femoral shaft. Salter–Harris type III and IV fractures may be somewhat more difficult to manage with the external fixation technique and may increase the risk of a septic joint. Fixation across the knee may be necessary.

Another fixation option is a plate spanning the physis. A study from France described good outcomes with this technique.[26] Screw placement avoided the physis and the plates were removed at a relatively early timepoint after the index surgery to minimize the risk of growth disturbance. Absorbable screws have also been used in some of these patients. There is little current literature on this technique.

In Salter–Harris type III and IV fractures, arthroscopically aided reduction of the fracture may be helpful in minimally displaced fractures to ensure an anatomic reduction of the joint line and articular cartilage.[37] In addition, visualization of the knee joint, whether with arthroscopy or at the time of arthrotomy, permits assessment for other associated injuries, such as ligamentous or meniscal injuries.

Most authors recommend addressing intra-articular ligamentous injuries later after the fracture has healed and range of motion has been reestablished. Peripheral tears of the meniscus may be repaired primarily at the time of open reduction of

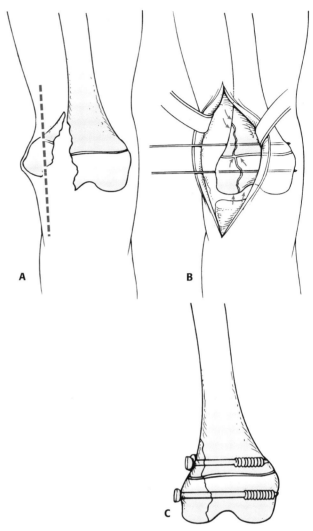

Figure 26-15. Open reduction of displaced lateral Salter–Harris type IV fracture of the distal femur. **A:** A longitudinal skin incision is made anteriorly on the knee at the location of the intra-articular fracture or in the midline if fracture severity raises concern of needing a total knee replacement in the future. **B:** Alignment of joint and physis are used to judge reduction. Guidewires for cannulated screws placed above and below physis, parallel to physis. **C:** Screws inserted in compression with washer on metaphyseal fragment. Washer is optional in epiphyseal fragment if later prominence is of more concern than need for additional compression.

the fracture. As in most current protocols for anterior cruciate ligament reconstruction, resolution of the acute phase swelling (and in this case, fracture healing and rehabilitation) should occur prior to consideration of anterior cruciate ligament reconstruction.

For fractures associated with vascular injuries, rapid and adequate reduction of the fracture and stabilization is necessary. If there is still vascular compromise to the leg, the orthopaedic team may consider compartment pressure monitoring and/or fasciotomies as warranted while the vascular team is evaluating the need for intervention for an occluded artery.

Author's Preferred Treatment of Fractures of the Distal Femoral Physis (Algorithm 26-1)

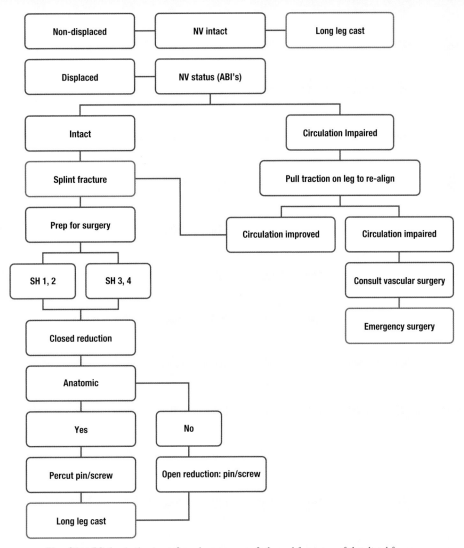

Algorithm 26-1. Author's preferred treatment of physeal fractures of the distal femur.

The management of these fractures is focused on minimizing further injury or trauma to the physis, especially with reduction maneuvers. Fracture reduction must be done gently in a relaxed patient. Often the fractures reduce with longitudinal traction and a little medial or lateral pressure; aim for 90% traction and 10% manipulation. Repeated forceful reductions must be avoided to minimize potential iatrogenic injury to the physis. Treatment principles really are based on the Salter–Harris classification, as well as the amount and degree of displacement. The author has a very low threshold for operative stabilization of these fractures with pins or screws as needed.

For truly nondisplaced fractures regardless of Salter–Harris type, the author is comfortable with a well-molded long-leg cast and careful follow-up. In children with certain body types, especially obese patients who are relatively short stature, cast immobilization may not provide fracture stability. Treatment must be individualized to the specific patient

and consideration given to the possibility that casting may not adequately stabilize a nondisplaced fracture. The treating surgeon must recall that what appears nondisplaced on radiographs in the emergency department may have displaced and returned to normal anatomic positioning at the time of injury, and not be lulled into a false sense of fracture stability for "nondisplaced" fractures. CT is generally recommended to assess for displacement.

Should cast immobilization be elected as a treatment option for nondisplaced fractures, seeing the patient back in the office and obtaining repeat radiographs within 5 to 7 days is recommended to ensure that the fracture reduction is maintained and to identify loss of anatomic position as early as possible. The literature indicates that loss of reduction and rereduction of fractures is associated with a higher incidence of physeal growth arrest, but accepting malalignment is also less than ideal for the patient's functional outcome.

Displaced Salter–Harris I and II Fractures

Many Salter–Harris type I and II fractures of the distal femoral physis that are displaced can be managed by a closed reduction in the operating room and stabilization with internal fixation. If one or two screws can be placed through the Thurston Holland fragment to stabilize a Salter–Harris type II fracture, this is the desired treatment. Washers may be helpful to increase compression. Large smooth pins (generally 2.4–3.2 mm) are also commonly used to stabilize both Salter–Harris type I fractures and type II fractures with a metaphyseal fragment that is too small to accommodate screws. Typically, these patients are managed with 4 weeks of long-leg casting. At 4 weeks, the cast is removed and pin removal is performed (if pins were used) either in the clinic or in the operating room if the pins were buried. Patients are then transitioned to a knee immobilizer or hinged knee brace to allow them to begin range of motion exercises. Weight-bearing is also initiated at that time. Therapy may be helpful to assist with regaining range of motion but the therapist must be cautioned against any forcible passive manipulation in the early postcasting phase. Most patients are weaned off crutches and ambulating by 8 weeks postinjury.

Displaced Salter–Harris III and IV Fractures

Displaced intra-articular fractures that involve the distal femoral physis require careful scrutiny of the fracture alignment and pattern preoperatively and careful assessment of the intraoperative imaging. This injury is easily missed and in some series, the diagnosis may be delayed in as many as 39% of cases.[46] Salter–Harris type III or IV fractures can on some occasions be managed with closed reduction with the use of pelvic reduction forceps but typically require either open reduction with an arthrotomy or arthroscopic assistance to ensure anatomic restoration of the articular cartilage. Once an anatomic reduction has been achieved, the fracture is stabilized with screws. These are generally epiphyseal screws placed parallel to the physis and avoiding the intercondylar notch. In some cases where the distal femoral physis is approaching closure, the physis can be crossed to achieve stronger stabilization, though typically, great care is taken to avoid screw placement near the physis to avoid any additional trauma to the already injured physis. A number of surgeons point out that imaging with the C-arm may not be the most accurate way to assess postoperative reduction in these fractures. Other options include obtaining plain radiographs intraoperatively or use of arthroscopy as a means to assess the joint alignment and integrity, though this is not a technique the author has used routinely. The postoperative regimen is the same as for type I and II fractures, with casting for 4 weeks and then transition to a knee immobilizer versus hinged knee brace to allow early initiation of motion.

The author explains to all patients and their families that all distal femoral physeal fractures may have a guarded long-term prognosis regarding growth of the physis. Follow-up should be scheduled at 3, 6, 12, and possibly 24 months postinjury to specifically assess alignment and length of the extremity and carefully assess radiographs for signs of physeal injury or arrest. Screw removal is left to the discretion of the family. Also, screws are occasionally removed if MRI is needed to assess the physis.

Potential Pitfalls and Preventive Measures

Repair of Distal Femoral Physeal Fractures: PITFALLS AND PREVENTION

Pitfall	Prevention
Missed diagnosis	• Immobilize and reexamine if uncertain or obtain an MRI • Be cognizant of nondisplaced injury in infants, pathologic conditions, polytrauma, or unresponsive patients
Inadequate reduction	• Carefully examine intraoperative radiographs • Low threshold for opening if concern for inadequate reduction, gapping from entrapped periosteum
Unrecognized vascular injury	• Thorough neurovascular examination • Prompt reduction of the fracture if concern regarding vascular status • Involvement of vascular team if perfusion does not normalize with fracture reduction
Loss of reduction	• Pin or screw fixation for all fractures that require reduction • Repeat radiographs at 5–7 days postinjury • High long-leg cast with molding proximally or spica cast
Growth disturbance	• Minimize trauma at time of reduction • Follow-up at 3, 6, 12, and possibly 24 months postinjury with full-length radiographs of both lower extremities
Knee joint instability	• Check ligaments when fracture is stabilized or healed • Consider MRI, especially for type III fractures
Stiffness	• Avoid prolonged immobilization • Remove cast at 4 weeks and apply knee immobilizer or hinged knee brace with initiation of range of motion in most cases. Avoid aggressive manipulation because of risk of additional injury to physis.

Reduction Malalignment (Poor Reduction or Loss of Reduction)

Displacement in distal femoral physeal fractures can often be significant. In an operating room with muscle relaxation, reduction can often be accomplished without significant force by simply placing traction on the leg and guiding the epiphysis back into position. Traction should be considered the most important component of this reduction, as it is imperative to avoid additional trauma to the already injured physis. Some surgeons prefer use of a fracture table for reduction though the author's preference is a standard radiolucent table. A radiolucent triangle can also be useful, particularly for anteriorly displaced physeal fractures that require some level of knee flexion to achieve reduction. Careful clinical and radiographic assessment of leg alignment and fracture reduction needs to be done to ensure that an anatomic reduction is achieved. If the fracture remains malaligned in either the coronal or sagittal plane, this may require later reconstructive surgery, as well as increase the risk for growth arrest.

It is especially critical to ensure that physeal widening, which may be subtle, is not present on imaging. Interposed periosteum may cause physeal widening and block a more anatomic reduction, as well as contribute to fracture instability that could lead to loss of reduction postoperatively. The surgeon should have a low threshold to make an incision and inspect the fracture to ensure there is no soft tissue impeding reduction in cases where the fracture may appear less than anatomically reduced.

When loss of reduction of what was thought to be a stable, nondisplaced fracture in a cast is noted, the patient should be expeditiously returned to the operating room and anatomic alignment reestablished. Once an adequate reduction has been achieved, internal fixation in the form of pins or screws is needed to maintain the alignment.

If the fracture is more than 10 days old, healing may have already occurred along the physis. Manipulation at this point may cause iatrogenic damage to the physis, so closed reduction is no longer an option.

Reduction in Cases of Vascular Injury

Distal femoral physeal injuries require significant trauma to be sustained by the extremity to cause displacement of the epiphysis, so other associated injuries may occur. Displaced fractures in particular must be carefully assessed for neurovascular damage in the emergency department. For Salter–Harris type II fractures where the epiphysis is displaced anteriorly, the popliteal artery is at risk of injury from the distal end of the metaphysis. Careful assessment of pulses and circulation to the foot are essential. In patients with documented vascular compromise or a white foot, fracture reduction is an operative emergency and careful postoperative assessment for return of vascular status is necessary. Consultation with the vascular surgical team is often required if concerns regarding vascular status remain postreduction. Vascular imaging may be needed to assess circulation if pulses are still diminished following reduction and stabilization of the distal femoral physeal fracture. In addition, some of these patients may sustain such injury to the leg that a compartment syndrome could ensue, so careful monitoring of the compartments by clinical examination or compartment pressure measurements may be necessary.

Septic Knee

There is a theoretical risk of septic knee arthritis resulting from pins placed in a retrograde manner in the epiphysis on either side of the knee joint and left externally. However, one study showed no cases of septic arthritis with retrograde percutaneous pinning of the distal femur, and pin duration of 30 days or longer was associated with an increased rate of pin tract infections.[41] Consequently, the author recommends that these pins be removed no later than 4 weeks postoperatively. In the event of a septic joint, the patient is returned to the operating room for irrigation and debridement. The pins may have to be left in place if septic arthritis occurs prior to sufficient fracture healing. Appropriate antibiotic treatment and surgical wound management are necessary in cases of an infection, especially in the first few weeks following the injury.

MANAGEMENT OF EXPECTED ADVERSE OUTCOMES AND UNEXPECTED COMPLICATIONS

Fractures of the Distal Femoral Physis: COMMON ADVERSE OUTCOMES AND COMPLICATIONS

- Loss of reduction
- Vascular injury
- Peroneal nerve injury
- Ligamentous injury
- Knee stiffness
- Growth disturbance
- Physeal arrest

In the immediate postoperative period, loss of reduction and neurovascular injuries are the most notable complications. In follow-up, the most common complications of distal femoral physeal fractures include knee ligament injury, neurovascular problems, growth disturbance of the distal femur, and persistent knee stiffness (Table 26-3).

LOSS OF REDUCTION

Redisplacement after closed reduction of distal femoral physeal separations has been reported in 30% to 70% of patients immobilized in a long-leg cast.[17,61] Placement of a hip spica cast may reduce this loss of reduction to as low as 10%.[17] Multiple attempts at initial closed reduction and late reduction are potentially damaging to the physis and may increase the risk of growth disturbance.[52] In one experimental rat model, risk of physeal injury was similar for fractures reduced after the equivalent of 7 human days. After 10 days, however, manipulation of physeal fractures led to diaphyseal fractures because of the degree of physeal healing.[16] Based on the experimental evidence and clinical experience, it is reasonable to attempt manipulation or repeat manipulation of physeal fractures up to 10 days after injury. After this time, open reduction may be required to reestablish alignment and risk of physeal arrest may be increased. For children with more than 2 years of growth remaining who have Salter–Harris I and II fractures, observation for remodeling

TABLE 26-3. Complications of Fractures of the Distal Femoral Physis

	Number of Patients	Ligamentous Injury (%)	Neurovascular Problems (%)	Angular Deformity (%)	Shortening (%)	Stiffness (%)
Lombardo and Harvey[36]	34	23	3	33	35	33
Czitrom et al.[13]	41 22	0	2.5	41	14% clinical 58% radiographic	
Riseborough et al.[7,a]	133		4	25	55	23
Thomson et al.[61]	30	Two anterior cruciate ligament injuries		18	47	18
Eid and Hafez[17]	151	8% symptomatic 14% asymptomatic	10	51	38	29
Ilharreborde et al.[26,b]	20	0		55	40	25
Arkader et al.[2]	73		1	12	12	4
Adams et al.[1]	70		3	7	26	1
Bellamy et al.[9]	101			11	24	

[a]Series contains referred patients and may not represent true incidence.
[b]Salter–Harris type II fractures only.

may be more prudent, depending on the degree of residual deformity. Osteotomy of the femur may be performed later if remodeling is incomplete. Older children with type I and II fractures are best treated with open reduction and fixation, possibly combined with epiphysiodesis of the contralateral uninjured distal femur. For patients of all ages who present late after sustaining displaced Salter–Harris type III and IV fractures, open reduction is recommended as soon as possible to restore the articular surface.[40]

NEUROVASCULAR ABNORMALITIES

Vascular Injury

Vascular injuries are possible but uncommon with this fracture, with most series reporting no vascular injuries.[17,36,61] Trauma to the popliteal artery may be caused by trauma from the distal end of the metaphysis and occurs most commonly from fractures caused by forced knee hyperextension resulting in anterior displacement of the epiphysis.[8,17,55] In the emergency department, clinical signs of vascular impairment should prompt the surgeon to perform emergency reduction of the fracture. It is our preference to perform the reduction in the operating room but in situations where a delay of treatment in the operating room is expected, reduction of the gross deformity and splinting of the fracture is a reasonable course of action. Arteriography is not indicated prior to reduction of the fracture.

In the operating room, the fracture is reduced and stabilized first. If vascular examination is normal after reduction, as evidenced by return of distal pulses, normal capillary refill, and symmetric ankle–brachial indices, the limb is splinted or casted with cutouts to allow serial evaluation of the pulses distally and the child is admitted for observation. Since intimal injuries of the artery and thrombosis may occur in a delayed fashion, the child's

vascular status is monitored closely for 24 hours after surgery for signs of worsening vascular status and compartment syndrome. Arteriography is sometimes utilized during the observation period to assess patients with distal perfusion and some abnormality of vascularity, such as diminished pulses, and for those with a worsening vascular status after reduction and pinning.

If distal perfusion does not return within 15 to 20 minutes after reduction and fixation, the time course over which vessel spasm typically recovers, immediate exploration of the vessel by a vascular surgeon is indicated. Although ischemia time may be increased when prolonged fracture stabilization is performed first, manipulation of the fracture after vascular surgery may compromise the repair. Arteriography is indicated only if the fracture has occurred in association with an ipsilateral pelvic fracture or more proximal lower extremity injury to localize the site of vascular injury. In most cases, thrombectomy and direct vessel repair or bypass of the injury with a vein graft are necessary to restore flow. If ischemia time exceeds 6 to 8 hours, four-compartment fasciotomies of the lower leg are done prophylactically in conjunction with the vascular repair to minimize the effects of reperfusion and prevent compartment syndrome of the calf.

Peroneal Nerve Injury

The peroneal nerve is the most frequently injured nerve after distal femoral physeal separations.[17] It is injured primarily from traction, most commonly when there is anteromedial displacement of the epiphysis, but may also be damaged from direct trauma. Most peroneal nerve injuries are neuropraxias that spontaneously recover within 6 to 12 weeks of injury.[17,59] Persistent neurologic deficit 3 months after fracture warrants electromyographic examination. If the conduction time is prolonged and fibrillation or denervation is present in distal muscles, exploration and microneural reanastomosis or resection of any neuroma may be indicated. Open injuries that result in peroneal nerve transection are best treated with repair or nerve grafting as early as possible after injury based on the child's condition and the status of the soft tissues adjacent to the nerve laceration. An ankle–foot orthosis is typically prescribed for patients with peroneal nerve injuries to facilitate rehabilitation and is discontinued after nerve recovery.

LIGAMENTOUS INJURIES

Symptomatic knee joint instability has been reported in 8% to 40% of patients with distal femoral physeal fractures.[17] Although these ligament injuries occur at the time of initial trauma, most are not identified until after the fracture has healed and rehabilitation has been initiated. The anterior cruciate ligament is most commonly disrupted, especially after Salter–Harris type III fractures of the medial femoral condyle.[39,50] Collateral ligament and posterior cruciate ligament disruptions and meniscal injuries may also occur after these fractures but are less common.

Difficulty with stairs, pain or swelling with activities, and episodes of giving way or knee buckling are typical presenting complaints associated with a ligamentous or meniscal injury. The physical examination may identify knee stiffness, signs of ligament instability, and joint line tenderness. Early diagnosis of injuries to the ligaments or menisci can facilitate earlier management,[13] but in many cases, the symptoms related to recovery from the fracture make identifying these other injuries challenging. A high index of suspicion is needed to diagnose associated ligamentous and meniscal injuries. When suspected, an MRI of the knee after healing of the fracture is the best way to identify these injuries. Meniscal surgery, especially repair, is ideally done soon after fracture healing to facilitate rehabilitation. Ligament reconstruction is best done after knee range of motion has been restored and other factors are taken into account, including the degree of instability, the child's age, and level of activity.

KNEE STIFFNESS

Limitation of knee motion after separation of the distal femoral epiphysis is seen in as many as one-third of patients after fracture healing. This complication is the result of several factors, including intra-articular adhesions, capsular contracture, and muscle contractures, most notably the hamstrings and quadriceps. Initial treatment consists of active and active-assistive range-of-motion exercises. Drop-out casts and dynamic bracing may be of benefit for some patients with persistent stiffness. For patients with persistent stiffness and loss of functional range of motion despite nonsurgical treatments, surgical interventions may be utilized to restore mobility. Gentle knee manipulation under anesthesia is sometimes useful but is associated with the risk of periarticular fractures of the knee.[11] Surgical release of contractures and adhesions, followed by continuous passive motion, is most reliable for regaining motion.[58]

GROWTH DISTURBANCE

The most common complication of distal femoral physeal fractures is growth disturbance. This complication is manifested clinically by the development of angular deformity in cases where the physeal injury is incomplete (Fig. 26-16), shortening of the limb after injuries that result in complete arrest, or

Figure 26-16. An 8-year-old girl struck by a car while on bicycle. Initial AP (**A**) and lateral (**B**) radiographs reveal displaced physeal fracture of the distal femur.

(continues)

Figure 26-16. *(Continued)* **C, D:** She underwent closed reduction and pinning. **E, F:** Four years later, she has angular deformity and shortening from asymmetric growth arrest.

in some cases, both angulation and limb shortening. In one meta-analysis of case series reported from 1950 to 2007 that included 564 fractures, 52% of fractures resulted in a growth disturbance.[7] Although Salter–Harris type I and II fractures in other areas of the body usually have a low risk of growth arrest, these fractures in the distal femur are at risk for premature physeal closure. Of the most common Salter–Harris types, growth abnormalities are seen in 36% of type I fractures, 58% of type

II fractures, 49% of type III fractures, and 64% of type IV fractures. Displaced distal femoral physeal fractures are four times more likely to develop growth arrest compared to nondisplaced fractures. Growth disturbance is uncommon in patients younger than 2 years of age who sustain these injuries, possibly because of the flat shape of the physis in this age group, which reduces the damage to physeal cartilage precursor cells. Older children who have more than 2 years of growth remaining are at highest risk for this complication and are most likely to have clinically significant deformities resulting from physeal arrest. One study showed that the likelihood of undergoing multiple procedures to address angular deformity or leg-length difference following surgical fixation of a distal femoral physeal fracture increased by 24.5% for each additional year of growth remaining.[9] Although adolescents frequently sustain this fracture and may develop growth complications, the clinical consequences of growth arrest are not as severe compared to patients between the ages of 2 and 12 years. Increased rate of growth arrest is also seen more commonly in patients who had surgery for these fractures, particularly if transphyseal fixation was used.[2]

Diagnosing Growth Arrest

The distal femur grows approximately 1 cm per year. Consequently, growth arrest is typically evident by 6 months after distal femoral physeal fracture healing. In some cases, however, incomplete cessation of growth and the resulting angular deformity may not be clinically evident for 12 to 18 months after injury. Subtle radiographic clues may be appreciable at 4 to 6 months postinjury in many cases. Follow-up radiographs after fracture healing should be carefully scrutinized to determine if the physeal line is reconstituted and that Park–Harris growth arrest lines are running parallel to the physis on both the AP and lateral views. Growth arrest lines develop when there is a temporary slowing of growth during periods of malnutrition, trauma, chemotherapy, or alcohol consumption, among other things.[20,44] The normal longitudinal orientation of the zone of provisional calcification becomes dense and interconnected, forming a transverse line in the metaphysis. After growth resumes, this dense layer moves away from the physis and is visible on radiographs as a radiodense line of bone in the metaphysis.[44] If the line is growing symmetrically away from the physis, then normal growth has resumed. Failure of a Park–Harris line to appear is suggestive of premature growth arrest. An oblique Park–Harris line that converges toward the physis indicates asymmetrical growth caused by a bone bridge across the physis that is preventing growth of one side of the physis and will lead to angular deformity.

Full-length standing x-rays of both lower extremities may also help determine if growth disturbance has occurred. It is the author's practice to obtain standing radiographs of the lower extremities as soon as possible following the initial injury to document baseline leg lengths and limb alignment. Imaging is then repeated at approximately 6-month intervals so that any development of a leg-length difference or change in angulation may be identified. Bilateral lower extremity scanograms and CT scanograms are also useful for measuring leg-length discrepancies but drawbacks compared to full-length radiographs include inability to assess the mechanical axis and increased radiation exposure, respectively.[54] If growth disturbance is suspected, MRI or CT is utilized to determine its extent; screw removal is typically done before imaging to improve the quality of imaging by eliminating the scatter effect of the metal. Physeal growth arrest is best detected by fat-suppressed three-dimensional spoiled gradient-recalled echo sequence MRI technique and may identify abnormalities as early as 2 months after injury.[15]

Treatment of Physeal Arrest

Early recognition and management of progressive angulation can reduce the need for osteotomy if the diagnosis is made before a clinically significant deformity develops and the physeal bar is excised to allow resumption of normal growth. After deformity has developed, however, an osteotomy is generally required whether bar excision is performed or not. The bar is typically located across the portion of the physis that was directly injured. Physeal bars may arise after any fracture type but are most common after type II, III, and IV fractures. When asymmetric growth follows a type II separation, the portion of the physis protected by the Thurston Holland fragment is usually spared, as opposed to the growth inhibition in the portion separated from the metaphyseal fragment. For fractures with a medial metaphyseal spike, the resultant deformity is more likely to be valgus because of lateral growth arrest, whereas the opposite is true for fractures with a lateral metaphyseal spike. For type III and IV fractures, the physeal bar is usually centered at the site of the physis that was traversed by the fracture line.

Excision is generally recommended for posttraumatic physeal bars that constitute less than 50% of the total cross-sectional area of the distal femoral physis in children with a mild degree of angulation and at least 2 years of growth remaining.[30,47] In one series, resumption of normal growth was seen in 80% of patients, whereas others have reported lower success rates with growth restoration seen in only 25% to 50% of patients.[22,64] Due to the unpredictable results of bar excision, it may be more prudent to perform ipsilateral distal femoral hemiepiphysiodesis combined with contralateral distal femoral epiphysiodesis for patients who have mild angulation and less than 3 to 4 cm of growth remaining in the injured physis, a scenario most commonly encountered in older children and adolescents with less than 2 years of growth potential. For children with more than 4 cm of growth remaining, physeal bar excision is attempted for those bars that encompass less than 50% of the physis because the combination of ipsilateral hemiepiphysiodesis and contralateral epiphysiodesis results in unacceptable loss of overall height. For older children and adolescents with physeal bars that already have significant angulation, distal femoral osteotomy may be done at the time of bilateral distal femoral epiphysiodesis. Physeal bar excision in combination with distal femoral osteotomy may also be considered for younger children who are candidates for bar resection and have angulation that exceeds 15 to 20 degrees.[30,47] If physeal bar excision fails to restore growth or the limb-length discrepancy is severe at the time of diagnosis of the growth disturbance, limb lengthening and other reconstructive procedures are options to consider based on the projected growth remaining and the limb-length difference.

COMPLETE PHYSEAL ARREST WITH LEG-LENGTH DISCREPANCY

Limb-length discrepancy is a frequently reported complication of distal femoral physeal fractures,[2,17,26,61] but only 22% of patients with distal femoral physeal fractures have leg-length

Figure 26-17. A 13-year-old boy fell off a wall. He sustained a comminuted fracture of the distal femur (**A**) with superficial abrasions over his leg and underwent closed reduction and fixation with smooth wires (**B, C**). Eighteen months later, he had a leg-length discrepancy of about 2 cm. **D:** After a discussion with the family, screw epiphysiodeses of the femur and tibia were done. **E:** At 1-year follow-up, he had nearly equal leg lengths.

discrepancies measuring greater than 1.5 cm (Fig. 26-17).[7] This is the case because many fractures occur in older children and adolescents with limited growth remaining at the time of injury. The treatment strategy varies depending on the projected amount of discrepancy. Since the decision for treatment must often be made at the time of diagnosis of the complete arrest, methods of predicting the ultimate leg-length discrepancy that do not require serial measurements, such as the Paley or Menelaus methods, are utilized. Immediate contralateral distal femoral epiphysiodesis is indicated for older children and adolescents with projected discrepancies greater than 2 to 2.5 cm. For children with discrepancies that are projected to be larger than 2.5 cm, planning for limb lengthening is initiated.

SUMMARY, CONTROVERSIES, AND FUTURE DIRECTIONS RELATED TO FRACTURES OF THE DISTAL FEMORAL PHYSIS

Distal femoral physeal fractures, although relatively uncommon injuries, are prone to complications and require attentive diagnostic, operative, and postoperative management. They can result from both low- and high-energy mechanisms. Acutely, patient evaluation must focus on identifying possible associated injuries and the neurovascular status of the affected limb.

Peroneal nerve and popliteal artery injuries and compartment syndrome of the leg may occur, especially in patients with high-energy mechanisms. Radiographs and CT scans are utilized to fully delineate the fracture pattern and to guide treatment. Most Salter–Harris I and II fractures may be treated with closed reduction and fixation with smooth pins or screws. Salter–Harris III and IV fractures frequently require open reduction and fixation to ensure anatomic alignment of the joint line and physis. Growth disturbances are the most common complication related to distal femoral physeal fractures and are seen in approximately half of patients, resulting in either angular deformities or leg-length discrepancies. Displaced fractures, regardless of Salter–Harris type, are prone to growth disturbances. Other complications of these injuries include ligamentous knee injuries and knee stiffness.

Some important issues regarding physeal fractures of the distal femur require clarification and warrant future study. The diagnosis of physeal separations in the face of negative radiographs by stress radiographs of the distal femur remains somewhat controversial. In a past era when open repair of medial collateral ligament injuries was performed, distinguishing nondisplaced physeal fractures from ligament tears using stress views was important for making expedient treatment decisions.[20] Iatrogenic worsening of physeal injury, however, is a concern when performing this diagnostic test. Currently, initial treatment is similar for both injuries, specifically immobilization and not surgery, and with the increasing use of MRI to evaluate acute knee injuries, stress views are no longer routinely utilized for children and adolescents with possible physeal separations with few exceptions.

The best method of advanced imaging for displaced fractures is another area of controversy. For intra-articular fractures, some[33] have recommended the routine use of CT scan as part of the preoperative evaluation to help delineate the fracture pattern and to plan fixation. Others prefer MRI for these injuries, trading some diminution of bone details for the ability to diagnose chondral, meniscal, and ligament injuries.[39,60] In the acute setting, the best choice of imaging studies is unclear. The surgeon must weigh the pros and cons of each modality, taking into consideration factors such as the availability of each of the modalities in the emergency setting, the radiation associated with a CT, and familiarity with interpretation of MRI for fracture assessment. Further study on this topic is needed to optimize decision making.

Despite advanced imaging methods for fracture evaluation and modern surgical techniques for management of displaced fractures, complications, particularly growth disturbance, affect approximately half of patients with this injury. Research on this injury must focus on the methods that diminish the incidence of growth disruption and restore growth when arrest occurs. The use of stem cells, cartilage cell regeneration, and other novel techniques are being investigated to address the problem of growth arrest after physeal injuries, including those of the distal femoral physis in children.[14,28,51,65]

ACKNOWLEDGMENTS

The author thanks Lindsay Andras and Brian G. Smith, who prepared this chapter in previous editions.

Annotated References

Reference	Annotation
Adams AJ, Mahmoud MAH, Wells L, et al. Physeal fractures of the distal femur: does a lower threshold for surgery lead to better outcomes? *J Pediatr Orthop B*. 2020;29(1):40–46.	Report of 70 patients with distal femoral physeal fractures, 63 of whom were treated surgically. Despite a lower threshold for surgery, the complication rate remained high at 36%.
Arkader A, Warner WC Jr, Horn BD, et al. Predicting the outcome of physeal fractures of the distal femur. *J Pediatr Orthop*. 2007;27(6):703–708.	Series of 73 patients that showed both presence of displacement and Salter–Harris classification to be predictive of outcome. Degree and direction of displacement did not correlate with outcomes.
Basener CJ, Mehlman CT, DiPasquale TG. Growth disturbance after distal femoral growth plate fractures in children: a meta-analysis. *J Orthop Trauma*. 2009;23(9):663–667.	Meta-analysis with more than 500 fractures and overall rate of growth disturbance of 52%.
Brone LA, Wroble RR. Salter-Harris type III fracture of the medial femoral condyle associated with an anterior cruciate ligament tear. Report of three cases and review of the literature. *Am J Sports Med*. 1998;26(4):581–586.	Report on a series of patients with Salter–Harris III fractures of the medial femoral condyle and associated anterior cruciate ligament tears which were treated in a staged fashion, with ligament reconstruction performed at a second operation.
Broughton NS, Dickens DR, Cole WG, et al. Epiphyseolysis for partial growth plate arrest. Results after four years or at maturity. *J Bone Joint Surg Br*. 1989;71(1):13–16.	Thirteen children treated with epiphysiodesis for growth arrest and there were no complications from the procedure. Eight of these had improvement or resolution of their alignment, while five underwent additional surgery.
Egol KA, Karunakar M, Phieffer L, et al. Early versus late reduction of a physeal fracture in an animal model. *J Pediatr Orthop*. 2002;22(2):208–211.	Animal model demonstrating that the smallest angular deformity developed in physeal fractures that were immediately reduced.
Garrett BR, Hoffman EB, Carrara H. The effect of percutaneous pin fixation in the treatment of distal femoral physeal fractures. *J Bone Joint Surg Br*. 2011;93(5):689–694.	Fifty-five patients showed no association between percutaneous placement of smooth pins across the physis and growth arrest.
Khoshhal KI, Kiefer GN. Physeal bridge resection. *J Am Acad Orthop Surg*. 2005;13(1):47–58.	Discuss techniques and future research directions for resection of physeal bars.
Lippert WC, Owens RF, Wall EJ. Salter-Harris type III fractures of the distal femur: plain radiographs can be deceptive. *J Pediatr Orthop*. 2010;30(6):598–605.	Demonstrated increased displacement of fracture on CT scan and MRI compared to plain radiographs.
Murgai RR, Compton E, Illingworth KD, Kay RM. The incidence of pin tract infections and septic arthritis in percutaneous distal femur pinning. *J Pediatr Orthop*. 2019;39(6):e462–e466.	Found no cases of septic arthritis in 163 patients who underwent retrograde percutaneous pinning of the distal femur. Patients with retained pins for greater than or equal to 30 days had a higher rate of pin tract infections.

REFERENCES

1. Adams AJ, Mahmoud MAH, Wells L, et al. Physeal fractures of the distal femur: does a lower threshold for surgery lead to better outcomes? *J Pediatr Orthop B*. 2020;29(1):40–46.
2. Arkader A, Warner WC Jr, Horn BD, et al. Predicting the outcome of physeal fractures of the distal femur. *J Pediatr Orthop*. 2007;27(6):703–708.
3. Aroojis AJ, Gajjar SM, Johari AN. Epiphyseal separations in spastic cerebral palsy. *J Pediatr Orthop B*. 2007;16(3):170–174.
4. Aroojis AJ, Johari AN. Epiphyseal separations after neonatal osteomyelitis and septic arthritis. *J Pediatr Orthop*. 2000;20(4):544–549.
5. Bae DS, Kadiyala RK, Waters PM. Acute compartment syndrome in children: contemporary diagnosis, treatment, and outcome. *J Pediatr Orthop*. 2001;21(5):680–688.
6. Barmada A, Gaynor T, Mubarak SJ. Premature physeal closure following distal tibia physeal fractures: a new radiographic predictor. *J Pediatr Orthop*. 2003;23(6):733–739.
7. Basener CJ, Mehlman CT, DiPasquale TG. Growth disturbance after distal femoral growth plate fractures in children: a meta-analysis. *J Orthop Trauma*. 2009;23(9):663–667.
8. Beaty JH, Kumar A. Fractures about the knee in children. *J Bone Joint Surg Am*. 1994;76(12):1870–1880.
9. Bellamy JT, Ward LA, Fletcher ND. Evaluation of pediatric distal femoral physeal fractures and the factors impacting poor outcome requiring further corrective surgery. *J Pediatr Orthop B*. 2021;30(1):6–12.
10. Bright RW, Burstein AH, Elmore SM. Epiphyseal-plate cartilage: a biomechanical and histological analysis of failure modes. *J Bone Joint Surg Am*. 1974;56(4):688–703.
11. Chung SM, Batterman SC, Brighton CT. Shear strength of the human femoral capital epiphyseal plate. *J Bone Joint Surg Am*. 1976;58(1):94–103.
12. Close BJ, Strouse PJ. MR of physeal fractures of the adolescent knee. *Pediatr Radiol*. 2000;30(11):756–762.
13. Czitrom AA, Salter RB, Willis RB. Fractures involving the distal epiphyseal plate of the femur. *Intl Orthop*. 1981;4(4):269–277.
14. Dahl WJ, Silva S, Vanderhave KL. Distal femoral physeal fixation: are smooth pins really safe? *J Pediatr Orthop*. 2014;34(2):134–138.
15. Ecklund K, Jaramillo D. Patterns of premature physeal arrest: MR imaging of 111 children. *AJR Am J Roentgenol*. 2002;178(4):967–972.
16. Egol KA, Karunakar M, Phieffer L, et al. Early versus late reduction of a physeal fracture in an animal model. *J Pediatr Orthop*. 2002;22(2):208–211.
17. Eid AM, Hafez MA. Traumatic injuries of the distal femoral physis: retrospective study on 151 cases. *Injury*. 2002;33(3):251–255.
18. El-Zawawy HB, Silva MJ, Sandell LJ, Wright RW. Ligamentous versus physeal failure in murine medial collateral ligament biomechanical testing. *J Biomech*. 2005;38(4):703–706.
19. Garrett BR, Hoffman EB, Carrara H. The effect of percutaneous pin fixation in the treatment of distal femoral physeal fractures. *J Bone Joint Surg Br*. 2011;93(5):689–694.
20. González-Reimers E, Pérez-Ramírez A, Santolaria-Fernández F, et al. Association of Harris lines and shorter stature with ethanol consumption during growth. *Alcohol*. 2007;41(7):511–515.
21. Greenhill DA, Allred G, Feldman J, Herman MJ. Vascular safe zone during percutaneous pinning of the distal femur. *J Pediatr Orthop*. 2022;42(10):608–613.
22. Hasler CC, Foster BK. Secondary tethers after physeal bar excision: a common source of failure? *Clin Orthop Relat Res*. 2002;(405):242–249.
23. Havranek P, Pesl T. Salter (Rang) type 6 physeal injury. *Eur J Pediatr Surg*. 2010;20(3):174–177.
24. Hsu RW, Himeno S, Coventry MB, Chao EY. Normal axial alignment of the lower extremity and load-bearing distribution at the knee. *Clin Orthop Relat Res*. 1990;(255):215–227.
25. Hübner U, Schlicht W, Outzen S, et al. Ultrasound in the diagnosis of fractures in children. *J Bone Joint Surg Br*. 2000;82(8):1170–1173.
26. Ilharreborde B, Raquillet C, Morel E, et al. Long-term prognosis of Salter-Harris type 2 injuries of the distal femoral physis. *J Pediatr Orthop B*. 2006;15(6):433–438.
27. Jain R, Bielski RJ. Fracture of lower femoral epiphysis in an infant at birth: a rare obstetrical injury. *J Perinatol*. 2001;21(8):550–552.
28. Jie Q, Hu Y, Yang L, et al. Prevention of growth arrest by fibrin interposition into physeal injury. *J Pediatr Orthop B*. 2010;19(2):201–206.
29. Kawamoto K, Kim WC, Tsuchida Y, et al. Incidence of physeal injuries in Japanese children. *J Pediatr Orthop B*. 2006;15(2):126–130.
30. Khoshhal KI, Kiefer GN. Physeal bridge resection. *J Am Acad Orthop Surg*. 2005;13(1):47–58.
31. Krosin MT, Lincoln TL. Traumatic distal femoral physeal fracture in a neonate treated with open reduction and pinning. *J Pediatr Orthop*. 2009;29(5):445–448.
32. Lee YS, Jung YB, Ahn JH, et al. Arthroscopic assisted reduction and internal fixation of lateral femoral epiphyseal injury in an adolescent soccer player: report of one case. *Knee Surg Sports Traumatol Arthrosc*. 2007;15(6):744–746.
33. Lippert WC, Owens RF, Wall EJ. Salter-Harris type III fractures of the distal femur: plain radiographs can be deceptive. *J Pediatr Orthop*. 2010;30(6):598–605.
34. Lippiello L, Bass R, Connolly JF. Stereological study of the developing distal femoral growth plate. *J Orthop Res*. 1989;7(6):868–875.
35. Loder RT, Bookout C. Fracture patterns in battered children. *J Orthop Trauma*. 1991;5(4):428–433.
36. Lombardo SJ, Harvey JP. Fractures of the distal femoral epiphyses. Factors influencing prognosis: a review of thirty-four cases. *J Bone Joint Surg Am*. 1977;59(6):742–751.
37. Mangurten HH, Puppala B, Knuth A. Neonatal distal femoral physeal fracture requiring closed reduction and pinning. *J Perinatol*. 2005;25(3):216–219.
38. Masquijo JJ, Allende V. Triplane fracture of the distal femur: a case report. *J Pediatr Orthop*. 2011;31(5):e60–e63.
39. Mckissick RC, Gilley JS, DeLee JC. Salter-Harris Type III fractures of the medial distal femoral physis—a fracture pattern related to the closure of the growth plate: report of 3 cases and discussion of pathogenesis. *Am J Sports Med*. 2008;36(3):572–576.
40. Meyers MC, Calvo RD, Sterling JC, Edelstein DW. Delayed treatment of a malreduced distal femoral epiphyseal plate fracture. *Med Sci Sports Exerc*. 1992;24(12):1311–1315.
41. Murgai RR, Compton E, Illingworth KD, Kay RM. The incidence of pin tract infections and septic arthritis in percutaneous distal femur pinning. *J Pediatr Orthop*. 2019;39(6):e462–e466.
42. Navascués JA, González-López JL, López-Valverde S, et al. Premature physeal closure after tibial diaphyseal fractures in adolescents. *J Pediatr Orthop*. 2000;20(2):193–196.
43. Nork SE, Segina DN, Aflatoon K, et al. The association between supracondylar-intercondylar distal femoral fractures and coronal plane fractures. *J Bone Joint Surg Am*. 2005;87(3):564–569.
44. Ogden JA. Growth slowdown and arrest lines. *J Pediatr Orthop*. 1984;4(4):409–415.
45. Ogden JA. Injury to the growth mechanisms of the immature skeleton. *Skeletal Radiol*. 1981;6(4):237–253.
46. Pennock AT, Ellis HB, Willimon SC, et al. Intra-articular physeal fractures of the distal femur: a frequently missed diagnosis in adolescent athletes. *Orthop J Sports Med*. 2017;5(10):2325967117731567.
47. Peterson HA. Partial growth plate arrest and its treatment. *J Pediatr Orthop*. 1984;4(2):246–258.
48. Petrin M, Weber E, Stauffer UG. Interposition of periosteum in joint fractures in adolescents; comparison of operative and conservative treatment (author's transl). *Z Kinderchir*. 1981;33(1):84–88.
49. Phieffer LS, Meyer RA, Gruber HE, et al. Effect of interposed periosteum in an animal physeal fracture model. *Clin Orthop Relat Res*. 2000;(376):15–25.
50. Rafee A, Kumar A, Shah SV. Salter-Harris type III fracture of the lateral femoral condyle with a ruptured posterior cruciate ligament: an uncommon injury pattern. *Arch Orthop Trauma Surg*. 2007;127(1):29–31.
51. Rajagopal K, Dutt V, Manickam AS, Madhuri V. Chondrocyte source for cartilage regeneration in an immature animal: is iliac apophysis a good alternative? *Indian J Orthop*. 2012;46(4):402–406.
52. Rang M, Wenger DR. The physis and skeletal injury. In: Wenger DR, Pring ME, eds. *Rang's Children's Fractures*. Lippincott Williams & Wilkins; 2005:11–25.
53. Sabharwal S, Henry P, Behrens F. Two cases of missed Salter-Harris III coronal plane fracture of the lateral femoral condyle. *Am J Orthop (Belle Mead NJ)*. 2008;37(2):100–103.
54. Sabharwal S, Zhao C, McKeon JJ, et al. Computed radiographic measurement of limblength discrepancy. Full-length standing anteroposterior radiograph compared with scanogram. *J Bone Joint Surg Am*. 2006;88(10):2243–2251.
55. Salter RB, Harris WR. Injuries involving the epiphyseal plate. *J Bone Joint Surg Am*. 1963;45(3):587–622.
56. Segal LS, Shrader MW. Periosteal entrapment in distal femoral physeal fractures: harbinger for premature physeal arrest? *Acta Orthop Belg*. 2011;77(5):684–690.
57. Sferopoulos NK. Type V physeal injury. *J Trauma*. 2007;63(6):E121–E123.
58. Simonian PT, Staheli LT. Periarticular fractures after manipulation for knee contractures in children. *J Pediatr Orthop*. 1995;15(3):288–291.
59. Sloboda JF, Benfanti PL, McGuigan JJ, Arrington ED. Distal femoral physeal fractures and peroneal palsy: outcome and review of the literature. *Am J Orthop (Belle Mead NJ)*. 2007;36(3):E43–E45.
60. Stanitski CL. Stress view radiographs of the skeletally immature knee: a different view. *J Pediatr Orthop*. 2002;24(3):342.
61. Thomson JD, Stricker SJ, Williams MM. Fractures of the distal femoral epiphyseal plate. *J Pediatr Orthop*. 1995;15(4):474–478.
62. Vander Have KL, Ganley TJ, Kocher MS, et al. Arthrofibrosis after surgical fixation of tibial eminence fractures in children and adolescents. *Am J Sports Med*. 2010;38(2):298–301.
63. Westh RN, Menelaus MB. A simple calculation for the timing of epiphyseal arrest: a further report. *J Bone Joint Surg Br*. 1981;63(1):117–119.
64. Williamson RV, Staheli LT. Partial physeal growth arrest: treatment by bridge resection and fat interposition. *J Pediatr Orthop*. 1990;10(6):769–776.
65. Xian C, Bruce F. Repair of injured articular and growth plate cartilage using mesenchymal stem cells and chondrogenic gene therapy. *Curr Stem Cell Res Ther*. 2006;1(2):213–229.

27

Proximal Tibial Physeal Fractures

Benjamin J. Shore and Eric W. Edmonds

INTRODUCTION TO PROXIMAL TIBIAL PHYSEAL FRACTURES

Fractures of the proximal tibia physis require a significant amount of force, and therefore these injuries account for less than 1% of all physeal injuries.[22,34] Contrasting the distal femur discussed in the previous chapter, the proximal tibial physis has intrinsic varus–valgus and side-to-side translational stability because of the collateral ligaments and the lateral fibular buttress.[7] Although potentially problematic regarding an apophyseal fracture of the tibial tubercle, the metaphyseal overhang of the tubercle can provide anteroposterior translational support.

An avulsion fracture of the tibial tuberosity is uncommon, accounting for less than 1% of all epiphyseal injuries and approximately 3% of all proximal tibial fractures.[21,22,34] Most fractures involving the proximal tibial physis result in anterior, anterolateral, and anteromedial epiphysis displacement relative to the metaphysis caused by the anatomic stability mentioned above.[39] In the rare fracture with posterior displacement, the epiphysis and tubercle apophysis are displaced as a single unit.[27] Fractures of the proximal tibial metaphysis usually occur in children aged 3 to 6 years and may be complete or greenstick. In contrast, the tibial tubercle fracture is most commonly sustained by adolescents.[24] The most critical features of proximal tibial physeal fractures are proximity to the popliteal artery and possible development of compartment syndrome associated with fracture displacement.

ASSESSMENT OF PROXIMAL TIBIAL PHYSEAL FRACTURES

MECHANISMS OF INJURY OF PROXIMAL TIBIAL PHYSEAL FRACTURES

These injuries require a significant amount of force to propagate a proximal tibial physis fracture, most often motor vehicle trauma, sports injuries, or other events such as lawn mower accidents. However, Salter–Harris type II fractures have been reported in child abuse cases and Salter–Harris I fractures have been reported in arthrogrypotic children undergoing physical therapy stretching.[42]

Despite the fact that most purely physeal fractures displace anteriorly, a hyperextension force can result in the metaphyseal portion of the tibia displacing posteriorly toward the popliteal artery, which can result in vascular compromise. Valgus stress can open the physis medially with the fibula acting as a lateral resistance force (Fig. 27-1).[46] Rarely, a flexion force can cause a

Figure 27-1. Jumping on the trampoline is a common mechanism for young children to sustain valgus and varus fractures of the proximal tibia.

Salter–Harris type II or III fracture, which has a similar injury pattern to that of tibial tubercle avulsion injuries.

Tibial tubercle apophyseal fractures are more frequently the result of jumping activities, with the two most common reported being (1) a strong quadriceps contraction during knee extension associated with jumping, and (2) rapid passive flexion of the knee against the contracting quadriceps while landing (Fig. 27-2).[9,16,23,24,27,33] Moreover, tibial tuberosity fractures are reported almost exclusively in adolescent boys who tend to have greater quadriceps strength and may overcome the stability of the apophysis with a violent contraction of the muscle.[9,16,23,24,27] Because the proximal tibial physis closes from posterior to anterior, the fracture pattern depends on the amount of physeal closure present at the time of injury, as well as the degree of knee flexion.[36] When the injury occurs with the knee in either full extension or up to 30 degrees of flexion, avulsion of the tibial tubercle without fracture of the epiphysis will result; with greater than 30 degrees of flexion, avulsion of both the tibial tubercle and proximal tibial epiphysis occur where the majority of fractures are type III.[20]

INJURIES ASSOCIATED WITH PROXIMAL TIBIAL PHYSEAL FRACTURES

Although the proximal tibial physis and the tibial tubercle apophysis are intimately associated with each other, fractures of the two locations have a unique set of associated injuries. The proximal physis fracture is at risk for ligamentous, vascular, and neurologic injury; whereas, the tubercle apophyseal fractures are at particular risk for compartment syndrome.

Ligamentous injuries and internal derangement of the knee joint may occur during Salter–Harris III and IV proximal tibial physeal injuries in 40% of patients.[35] Associated injuries such as meniscal tears, cruciate ligament laxity, patellar or quadriceps tendon avulsions, and compartment syndrome have been reported with tibial tubercle fractures.[5,13,30,45] However, in a systematic review of tibial tubercle fractures, low rates of tendon avulsion (2%), meniscal tears (2%), and cruciate ligament laxity (1%) were reported.[36]

Vascular compromise in proximal tibial physeal fractures can be devastating, but they are uncommon in isolated tubercle injuries.[7,39] The popliteal artery is tethered by its major branches near the posterior surface of the proximal tibial epiphysis. The posterior tibial branch passes under the arching fibers of the soleus. The anterior tibial artery travels anteriorly over an aperture above the proximal border of the interosseous membrane. A hyperextension injury that results in posterior displacement of the proximal tibial metaphysis may stretch and tear the tethered popliteal artery (Fig. 27-3). Even a minimally displaced fracture at presentation may have had significant displacement at the time of injury and should therefore be monitored for vascular injury.[43] Diagnostic workup of these fractures does not mandate routine angiography as long vascular status is monitored during the initial 24 to 48 hours.

Regarding vascular injuries, the tibial tubercle avulsion fractures are at risk for bleeding of the anterior tibial recurrent artery (which traverses the base of the tubercle) into the anterior compartment. Rather than resulting in direct ischemia, this vascular compromise is associated with indirect ischemia through the development of compartment syndrome.[31]

A peroneal neuropathy may also be associated with a fracture of the proximal tibial physis, but it will often undergo spontaneous resolution of symptoms.

SIGNS AND SYMPTOMS OF PROXIMAL TIBIAL PHYSEAL FRACTURES

Physical examination of children with either a proximal physis or tubercle apophysis fracture may not be dissimilar. An important and sensitive finding is an inability to actively fully extend the knee in most displaced fractures. Pain, knee effusion, and a hemarthrosis will often be present in both. Limb deformity may

Figure 27-2. The tibial tubercle is commonly fractured because of the maximum generated force of the quadriceps contracture during jumping, primarily in male adolescents.

Figure 27-3. Tethering of the popliteal artery by the more distal tibial artery creates a situation wherein posterior metaphyseal tibia displacement can damage the artery.

or may not be present in either fracture type, and hamstring spasm may limit knee extension on examination.

The physeal injuries will have pain over the tibial physis distal to the joint line, in contrast to the tubercle injuries that will hurt directly anteriorly. Sometimes, the tubercle fractures will have a freely movable osseous fragment palpated subcutaneously between the proximal tibia and the femoral condyles and may result in skin tenting; whereas, in the physeal fractures, the proximal metaphysis of the tibia is displaced posteriorly, creating a concavity that can be palpated anteriorly at the level of the tibial tubercle. A valgus deformity suggests medial displacement of the metaphysis.

Careful physical examination with special attention to the aforementioned associated injuries should be performed at the time of initial assessment. Ischemia caused by disruption of the popliteal artery or secondary to compartment syndrome should not be missed on clinical examination. Asymmetric perfusion and pallor compared to the contralateral limb and distal pain should be recognized for potential signs of vascular compromise. Pulses should be assessed and compartments should be assessed by palpation, examination of sensation, and stretch testing of the anterior compartment through passive and active toe motion.

When the proximal end of the metaphysis protrudes under the subcutaneous tissues on the medial aspect of the knee, a tear of the distal end of the medial collateral ligament (MCL)

A ©SD PedsOrtho   B

Figure 27-4. Often the only radiographic evidence of a physeal fracture may be a joint effusion, as seen in this lateral of a minimally displaced tibial tubercle fracture. **A:** Unaffected knee, right side, with *arrow* demonstrating normal crisp posterior border to the quadriceps tendon. **B:** Mild effusion with disruption of fat planes, *arrowheads* highlighting obliterated planes due to hemarthrosis.

should be suspected in association with a physeal fracture. The presence of patella alta may represent either severity of tubercle displacement or concomitant rupture of the patella tendon. With a small avulsion, the child may be able to extend the knee actively through intact retinacular tissue, but active extension is impaired with larger injuries.

IMAGING AND OTHER DIAGNOSTIC STUDIES FOR PROXIMAL TIBIAL PHYSEAL FRACTURES

In proximal tibial physeal fractures, plain radiographs are the mainstay of evaluation, but nondisplaced physeal fractures may not be visible. Associated hemarthrosis can sometimes be the only indication of fracture and is primarily recognized by identifying an obliteration of the fat planes (predominately the loss of a crisp posterior border to the quadriceps tendon in mild- to moderate-sized hemarthrosis) (Fig. 27-4) or an increased separation of the patella from the distal femur on lateral views in patients with severe hemarthrosis. Occasionally, relatively nondisplaced physeal fractures may have small Thurstan Holland fragments extending into the metaphysis. Often, fracture lines may only be visible on oblique view radiographs. At other times, the metaphyseal fragments can be quite large (Fig. 27-5). Stress views can often differentiate a proximal tibial physeal fracture from a ligament injury, but there is potential risk for physeal injury and increased pain in a clinical setting when performing these x-rays. In young children (2–5 years old), measurement of the anterior tilt angle of the proximal tibial physis on the lateral is helpful to diagnose fractures not otherwise appreciated.[41] When uncertain of the diagnosis, an MRI can distinguish between physeal fractures and ligament injuries in a safe, accurate, and more comfortable fashion than stress radiographs (Fig. 27-6).[40] Moreover, CT scans can define the bony injury better than MRI or plain film and are often helpful to define intra-articular involvement and determine treatment for Salter–Harris type III, IV, and complex tibial tubercle fractures (Fig. 27-7).

The standard method of identifying tibial tubercle fractures is via the lateral plain radiograph; however, more severe injuries should warrant advanced diagnostic imaging to help identify articular disruption and internal derangement that is often seen in these fracture patterns. Although most patients with tibial tubercle fractures are adolescents (with developed secondary ossification of the tibial tubercle), fractures may occur in the more immature child and be seen merely as a small fleck of bone on plain film (Fig. 27-8). To improve the utility of diagnostic plain film, the lateral projection view should be done with the tibia rotated slightly internal to bring the slightly lateral tubercle perpendicular to the x-ray cassette.

©SD PedsOrtho

Figure 27-5. Displaced fracture of the proximal tibial physis with a large posterior metaphyseal Thurstan Holland fragment, as well as an anterior conjoined tibial tubercle fragment.

Figure 27-6. MRI images can assist in differentiating physeal injuries from ligament ruptures. This coronal image demonstrates a proximal tibial physeal fracture with evidence of entrapped medial collateral ligament (MCL) fibers (*arrow*) limiting reduction.

Figure 27-7. Both 3D and standard CT images can help define fracture patterns that involve the joint surface to guide appropriate treatment. This 3D reconstruction demonstrates a tibial tubercle fracture with mild comminution at the joint surface (*arrow*).

With regard to the tibial tubercle, it is important to remember that normal ossification may progress from more than one secondary center of ossification. Contralateral films may be helpful to distinguish normal ossification versus minimally displaced fragments, but patella alta may be more reliable in that comparison.

CLASSIFICATION OF PROXIMAL TIBIAL PHYSEAL FRACTURES

Metaphyseal Fracture Patterns: CLASSIFICATION	
Direction of Injury	**Resultant Fracture Pattern**
Valgus	Medial-sided displacement
Varus	Lateral-sided displacement
Hyperextension	Posterior displacement

Tibial Tubercle Fracture Patterns: MODIFIED OGDEN CLASSIFICATION	
Type	**Description**
I	Apophyseal injuries at the patellar tendon insertion (displaced/nondisplaced)
II	Apophyseal/epiphyseal injuries without intra-articular extension (displaced/nondisplaced)
III	Apophyseal/epiphyseal injuries with intra-articular extension (displaced/nondisplaced)
IV	Fracture of the entire proximal tibia, with or without posterior Thurstan Holland fragment (displaced/ nondisplaced)
V	No fracture, pure avulsion injury of the patellar tendon

Proximal tibial physeal fractures are most commonly described using the Salter–Harris classification scheme that denotes the direction of fracture propagation relative to the growth plate. Age and mechanism of injury can dictate fracture location (Figs. 27-9 and 27-10).[24] Watson-Jones[44] described three types of avulsion fractures of the tibial tubercle, with subsequent modifications by Ogden and associates[27,28] who noted that the degree of displacement depends on the severity of injury to adjacent soft tissue attachments. Ryu and Debenham[37] and Inoue et al.[19] proposed a type IV fracture in which the physeal separation occurs through the tibial tuberosity and extends posteriorly into the horizontal tibial physis. Pace et al.[29] and

Figure 27-8. Young children may only have evidence of a small fleck (*arrow*) to represent an otherwise larger cartilaginous fracture of the tibial tubercle.

Figure 27-9. All proximal tibial physeal fractures can be classified based on the mechanism of injury: varus/valgus, extension, and flexion avulsion injuries.

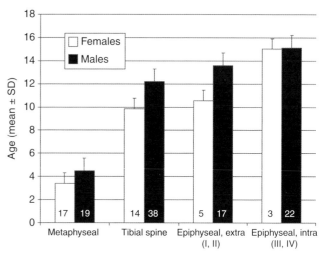

Figure 27-10. Bar graph representing the change in fracture patterns seen with increasing age.

Aerts et al.[1] have described modified surgical management techniques associated with these type IV fractures. A study delineating a three-dimensional classification of tibial tubercle fractures highlighted the risk for associated pathology when considering surgical fixation.[30] Pretell-Mazzini et al.[36] performed a systematic review of the literature surrounding tibial tubercle fractures and summarized the Ogden classification into the following five groups, where within each group, the fracture can be displaced, nondisplaced, or comminuted: type I fractures involve the tibial apophysis, where the patellar tendon inserts; type II fractures involve the apophysis and the epiphysis without intra-articular extension; type III fractures are similar to type II fracture with intra-articular extension; type IV fractures involve the entire proximal tibial physis and the fracture can exist posteroinferiorly creating an equivalent Thurstan Holland fragment; and finally type V injuries are not really fractures but pure avulsion injuries (Fig. 27-11).

OUTCOME MEASURES FOR PROXIMAL TIBIAL PHYSEAL FRACTURES

There are no specific outcome scores or tools validated for proximal tibial physeal fractures; however, most studies have used plain radiographs to determine healing and a few have utilized return to sports for functional outcomes. However, some studies have reported high rates of return to sport after these injuries ranging from 60% to 100%.[8,36]

PATHOANATOMY AND APPLIED ANATOMY RELATING TO PROXIMAL TIBIAL PHYSEAL FRACTURES

Present at birth, the ossific nucleus of the proximal tibial epiphysis lies central in the cartilaginous anlage. Usually singular, it can occasionally have two ossification centers, not including the universal secondary center of ossification of the tubercle that appears between 9 and 14 years of age. Closure of the proximal tibial physis and union between the epiphysis and tubercle centers occurs commonly in girls between 10 and 15 years and in boys between 11 and 17 years of age.

The development of the tibial tubercle was further defined by Ehrenborg.[12] After birth is the cartilaginous stage that exists prior to development of the secondary ossification center and persists until the age of 9 years in girls and age of 10 years in boys. This is followed by the apophyseal stage, in which the ossification center appears in the tongue of cartilage that

Figure 27-11. Modified Ogden classification of tibial tubercle fractures.

A, B   C

Figure 27-12. Example case with open reduction of the tibial tubercle fracture. **A:** Lateral radiograph demonstrating displaced tibial tubercle that does not extend into the joint (modified Ogden type II). **B:** Sagittal CT scan that highlights that although this fracture does not involve the joint (*solid arrow*), it does involve the proximal tibial physis (*broken arrow*). **C:** Intraoperative photograph demonstrating that patella tendon fibers (*broken arrow*) extend greater than 2 cm distal to the fracture fragment (*solid arrow*), highlighting the soft tissue disruption that occurs. (Used with permission of the Children's Orthopaedic Center, Los Angeles.)

drapes over the anterior tibial metaphysis. The epiphyseal stage is marked by the tubercle and epiphyseal bony union, and this is followed by the final bony stage, wherein the proximal tibia becomes fully ossified. There is evidence that closure of the physis follows a predictable pattern.[4,27,30] In the sagittal plane, the proximal tibial physis has been shown to close in a posterior-to-anterior direction, with subsequent progression of closure toward the tubercle apophysis which is closing in a proximal-to-distal direction, simultaneously. In the coronal planes, the proximal tibial physis is closing in a medial-to-lateral direction; whereas, in the axial plane, the tibia is closing in a posteromedial-to-anterolateral direction.

The anatomy of the collateral ligaments provides some protection from epiphyseal disruption. The superficial portion of the MCL extends distal to the physis inserting into the medial metaphysis, therefore acting as a medial buttress. The lateral collateral ligament inserts on the proximal pole of the fibula, and this entire lateral construct acts like a lateral buttress. Anteriorly, the patellar ligament attaches to the secondary ossification center of the tibial tuberosity that is draped over the metaphysis, serving as a constraint to posterior displacement. The terminal insertion of the powerful quadriceps at the boundary between the secondary ossification centers of the tubercle and the proximal tibial epiphysis places the tubercle at risk for isolated or combined avulsion fractures. This risk is minimal until adolescence when the quadriceps mechanism is matured because some fibers of the patella tendon extend distal to the apophysis into the anterior aspect of the upper tibial diaphysis. Therefore, it is important to recognize that these adolescent avulsions often have extensive soft tissue damage that extends down the anterior diaphysis of the tibia (Fig. 27-12). The distal portion of the popliteal artery lies close to the posterior aspect of the proximal tibia. Firm connective tissue septa hold the vessel against the knee capsule, placing it at risk for injury during proximal tibia physeal fractures (Fig. 27-13). The lateral inferior geniculate artery crosses the surface of the popliteus muscle, anterior to the lateral head of the gastrocnemius, and turns forward underneath the

lateral collateral ligament. The medial inferior geniculate artery passes along the proximal border of the popliteus muscle, anterior to the medial head of the gastrocnemius, and extends anterior along the medial aspect of the proximal tibia. The popliteal artery divides into the anterior tibial and posterior tibial branches beneath the arch of the soleus muscle. Much of the blood supply to the proximal tibial epiphysis is derived from an anastomosis

Figure 27-13. Arteriogram after a proximal tibial physeal fracture. Even with minimal displacement, note the construction of the popliteal artery (*arrow*).

between these geniculate arteries.[10,17] The tibial tubercle receives its main blood supply from a plexus of arteries behind the patellar ligament at the level of the attachment to the tibial tubercle.[10] This vascular anastomosis arises from the anterior tibial recurrent artery and may be torn with this fracture.[31,45] Several small branches extend down into the secondary ossification center. A smaller part of the blood supply enters the superficial surface of the tubercle from adjacent periosteal vessels.

TREATMENT OPTIONS FOR PROXIMAL TIBIAL PHYSEAL FRACTURES

NONOPERATIVE TREATMENT OF PROXIMAL TIBIAL PHYSEAL FRACTURES

Non- or minimally displaced fractures can often be treated with closed reduction. If there is any displacement requiring manipulation for closed reduction, this is best done under anesthesia. One should have a low threshold for operative fixation; however, recent studies have demonstrated that closed reduction can be safely achieved in displaced Ogden type IV fractures.[8,21]

Regarding tubercle reductions, a persistent gap between the distal end of the tubercle and the adjacent metaphysis may indicate an interposed flap of periosteum.[9,16] Minimally displaced, small avulsion fragments have been treated successfully with immobilization in a cylinder cast or long-leg cast with the knee fully extended.[8,9,23,27]

Indications/Contraindications

Nonoperative Treatment of Proximal Tibial Physeal Fractures:
INDICATIONS AND CONTRAINDICATIONS

Indications

• No to minimal displacement

Relative Contraindications

• Displacement
• Joint involvement
• Compartment syndrome
• Open fracture
• Displaced floating knee fractures

Closed Reduction of Proximal Tibial Tubercle and Physeal Fractures

Traction during the reduction maneuver will reduce the risk of physeal damage. There is little reason to recreate the deformity during reduction, and doing so may injure the physis. Prior to closed reduction, a tense knee effusion may be aspirated using sterile technique followed by an injection of 2 to 5 mL of either 0.5% bupivacaine or 0.2% ropivacaine to relieve pain and augment the reduction attempt. However, many children will not tolerate this method of anesthesia and either moderate conscious sedation or general anesthesia should be employed, to

ensure adequate muscle relaxation and protection of the physis with closed reduction.

Patients with a nondisplaced (≤2 mm) and stable proximal tibial epiphyseal fractures can be simply placed in a long-leg cast generally in full extension if that best reduces the fracture. Appropriate padding is important and thick (0.5-inch) foam may be placed either along the popliteal fossa or on the bony prominences to protect the skin. The cast may be either univalved or bivalved to permit swelling. Almost universally, the child is then admitted to the hospital for observation and gentle elevation to monitor for the possibility of vascular injury and compartment syndrome, even in seemingly minimally displaced fractures.

Radiographs should be obtained at the time of reduction and cast placement to confirm appropriate alignment of the fracture. Future films should include both the AP and lateral x-rays at 1 week after reduction to confirm maintenance of reduction. The cast may be removed 4 to 6 weeks after injury if the fracture demonstrates radiographic and clinical union. Return to normal activities can be permitted about 4 to 8 weeks following cast removal.

OPERATIVE TREATMENT OF PROXIMAL TIBIAL PHYSEAL FRACTURES

Indications/Contraindications

Fractures that are reducible via closed methods, but unstable, may be stabilized with crossing percutaneous smooth pins or screws. Fractures that cannot be anatomically reduced require open reduction for removal of soft tissue interposition (entrapped pes anserinus and periosteum have been reported).[42,46] Another relative indication for open reduction and internal fixation (ORIF) is to facilitate wound management when a vascular repair is necessary.

Open reduction is also indicated for all type III displaced injuries with intra-articular extension.[9,16,23,26,28] Residual displacement greater than 2 to 3 mm may lead to an extensor lag and quadriceps weakness.

Closed Reduction and Percutaneous Fixation

Preoperative Planning

Closed Reduction and Percutaneous Pinning of Proximal Tibial Physeal Fractures:
PREOPERATIVE PLANNING CHECKLIST

OR table	❏ Radiolucent, preferably without metallic sidebars
Position/positioning aids	❏ Assistant for countertraction, bump under operative leg to facilitate easy cross-table lateral fluoroscopy
Fluoroscopy location	❏ Opposite to surgeon and back table
Equipment	❏ C-arm, smooth pins, unopened trays for open reduction
Tourniquet	❏ Nonsterile ❏ May not need to inflate, unless surgery converted to open reduction, can tether quadriceps inhibiting anatomic reduction

Figure 27-14. A modified Ogden type IV tibial tubercle fracture or Salter–Harris type II (with posterior metaphyseal fragment and tibial tubercle fracture). **A:** AP radiograph demonstrating cross-pin technique. **B:** Lateral radiograph demonstrating anatomic reduction with fixation.

If the reduction is performed in the emergency department but the fracture is deemed unstable, then a temporary splint should be placed and plans to move to the operating room should be made. However, if the initial attempt was undertaken in the operating room and the fracture was deemed unstable, then percutaneous pinning could be done immediately.

Positioning

The patient should be placed supine on a radiolucent table. A bolster under the ipsilateral buttocks helps keep the patella facing anteriorly and can be helpful for imaging during the procedure. A bump under the ankle makes lateral imaging easier and can aid in reduction, or an assistant can elevate the leg for lateral imaging. The surgeon stands on the ipsilateral side of the table. The C-arm comes in from the contralateral side, the image screen is positioned so that the surgeon does not have to turn their head away from the field to see the screen, and the back table should be positioned behind the surgeon.

Surgical Approach

If an anatomic reduction is achieved, smooth K-wires are usually sufficient for fixation of the epiphyseal fragment and minimize the risk of iatrogenic growth plate injury. One can use K-wires for the tibial tuberosity but screws are stronger and closing the apophyseal growth plate near the end of growth is not a concern. Pin size choice will depend on the size of the tibia but usually ranges from a 0.062-inch pin to a 2.5-mm pin in bigger

children. One should consider leaving the pins extra-articular, coming out distally, to help mitigate the risk of a septic joint from a pin tract infection (Fig. 27-14).

Technique

 Closed Reduction and Percutaneous Pinning of Proximal Tibial Physeal Fractures:
KEY SURGICAL STEPS

- ❑ Closed reduction of the fracture with C-arm guidance
  - Pin placement (with relaxing incision on the skin if any excessive pressure)
- ❑ For smooth pin placement, bend and cut pins to be pulled at 4 weeks postoperatively and apply a relaxing skin incision if there is any pressure caused by the pins
- ❑ For cannulated screws, close stab incisions with suture
- ❑ Place dressing and apply long-leg cast in full extension

Occasionally, for large Thurstan Holland fragments, a percutaneous compression screw may be placed to secure the fracture. Rather than using the cross-pin technique, or in conjunction with that technique, a small stab incision can be made directly over the fragment after reduction. Fluoroscopy guidance is then utilized to place the guide pin from a cannulated screw system, being sure not to violate the physis or the apophysis anteriorly. Length is measured, the proximal cortex drilled, and the screw is inserted and secured into place with fluoroscopy. If a bicortical purchase can be achieved, then that is optimal. Yet, cancellous screws can be utilized if the width of the tibial metaphysis exceeds the screw options (Fig. 27-15).

Figure 27-15. Salter–Harris type II proximal tibial physis fracture with two cannulated, partially threaded cancellous screws in the Thurstan Holland fragment. **A:** AP radiograph. **B:** Lateral radiograph.

For the extra-articular tibial tubercle fragments, a choice between the smooth pin (Fig. 27-16) and the screw (Fig. 27-17) can be made but the technique is the same. These fractures will often have soft tissue interposition and conversion to open reduction is common.

Fluoroscopy can confirm the reduction is anatomic. Even with open reduction, an anatomically reduced fragment has some space between the osseous tubercle and the tibia, so a lateral image of the contralateral leg may help evaluate the reduction. While smooth K-wires may be preferable if there is lots of growth expected, cannulated screws provide more strength. There is no need to violate the posterior cortex of the tibia, which could harm neurovascular structures.

Figure 27-16. Intraoperative lateral fluoroscopy image demonstrating multiple smooth pin fixation of a tubercle fracture.

Open Reduction and Internal Fixation

Preoperative Planning

✓ ORIF of Proximal Tibial Physeal Fractures: PREOPERATIVE PLANNING CHECKLIST

OR table	❏ Radiolucent, preferably without metallic sidebars
Position/ positioning aids	❏ Assistant for countertraction, bump under operative leg to facilitate easy cross-table lateral fluoroscopy
Fluoroscopy location	❏ Opposite to operative limb, surgeon, and back table
Equipment	❏ C-arm, smooth pins, trays for open reduction including a cannulated compression screw system (4.0–6.5-mm sizes available)
Tourniquet	❏ Nonsterile ❏ May not need to inflate, unless surgery converted to open reduction, can tether quadriceps inhibiting anatomic reduction
Other	❏ Confirm vascular status prior to surgery and have sterile Doppler available

A CT scan can help define if there is intra-articular involvement. If there is, one should plan for either open or arthroscopic visualization of the joint surface. Have cannulated screws available, 4.0 to 6.5 mm for most cases.

Positioning

The patient should be placed supine on a radiolucent table. A bolster under the ipsilateral buttocks helps keep the patella facing anteriorly and can be helpful for imaging during the procedure. A bump under the knee or ankle makes lateral imaging easier, or an assistant can elevate the leg for lateral imaging. The surgeon stands on the ipsilateral side of the table. The C-arm

Figure 27-17. Postoperative lateral radiograph with single compression screw and washer fixation of an extra-articular tibial tubercle fracture.

comes in from the contralateral side, the image screen is positioned so the surgeon does not have to turn their head away from the field to see the screen, and the back table should be positioned behind the surgeon.

Surgical Approach

A longitudinal incision just lateral to the tibial tubercle (rather than directly over it) to minimize the potential for scar discomfort over the prominent bone. It may extend proximally into the joint if the articular surface is to be evaluated open and may extend distally a bit for an anterior compartment release and replace avulsed extensor mechanism tissue. Care should be taken not to score or further damage the physis at the perichondral ring of LaCroix during the approach (Fig. 27-18). Often the extent of soft tissue

disruption extends past the middle of the tibial diaphysis and an adequate incision is necessary to facilitate appropriate exposure. There are no vascular or neurologic structures at risk during this approach. A tourniquet is usually not needed and may need to be released if it is hindering reduction of a displaced fracture caused by constriction of the quadriceps muscle.

Technique

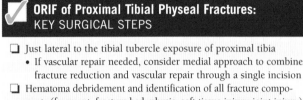

ORIF of Proximal Tibial Physeal Fractures:
KEY SURGICAL STEPS

- ☐ Just lateral to the tibial tubercle exposure of proximal tibia
  - If vascular repair needed, consider medial approach to combine fracture reduction and vascular repair through a single incision
- ☐ Hematoma debridement and identification of all fracture components (fragment, fracture bed, physis, soft tissue injury, joint injury)
- ☐ Isolated tibial tubercle fractures are directly reduced with straight knee. Type IV fractures involving the entire physis may require traction and some leverage (90% traction, 10% leverage)
- ☐ Utilize C-arm fluoroscopy and place tentative smooth wire fixation or guidewires for cannulated screws
- ☐ Consider release of fascia off lateral tibia to release anterior compartment
- ☐ Closure of incision
- ☐ Cast application (long-leg or cylinder) in near full extension, or a hinged knee brace locked in extension

After performing the anterior approach, the fracture bed is carefully cleared of debris such as fracture hematoma and an assessment is taken of the entire fracture personality. For example, a periosteal flap (from the diaphysis) is frequently entrapped in the fracture, blocking an anatomic reduction.[9,16] Isolated tibial tubercle fractures are directly reduced with straight knee. Type IV fractures involving the entire physis may require traction and some leverage (90% traction, 10% leverage). For type II and III fractures, screws should not violate the epiphysis (Fig. 27-19). For

Figure 27-18. Intraoperative photograph of a C fracture. The patella is to the upper right foot and the lower left, with the physis (*curved arrow*) and fracture bed (*double-headed arrow*). There is evidence of a large periosteal avulsion attached to the tubercle fragment (*arrowhead*).

Figure 27-19. Lateral radiograph demonstrating multiple compression screw fixation of a Salter–Harris type IV proximal tibial physeal fracture.

should be done between 4 and 6 months postoperatively via plain radiographs.

Potential Pitfalls and Preventive Measures for Proximal Tibial Physeal Fractures

Proximal Tibial Physeal Fracture Repair:
PITFALLS AND PREVENTIONS

Pitfall	Prevention
Unrecognized physeal or apophyseal fracture	• Scrutinize radiographs for signs of nondisplaced fractures • Obtain stress radiographs or MRI to confirm diagnosis • MCL injuries are unusual in the very young
Unrecognized arterial injury	• Understand that maximal displacement at the time of injury can be far greater than that seen on static resting radiograph • Thorough physical examination particularly concerning the circulatory system • Repeat examination during in-hospital observation
Compartment syndrome	• Vigilance during the first 24 hours to assess compartment status • Be aware that a neurologic injury may confound physical examination results • Univalve, bivalve, or place foam in cast to allow for swelling postreduction
Growth disruption of the affected physis	• Metaphyseal fractures (Cozen injuries) may autocorrect the valgus deformity and observation is warranted • Recurvatum is the most common (especially following tubercle injuries) and may require surgical intervention
Intra-articular pin placement	• May result in septic arthritis and should be avoided, try to place pins in a retrograde fashion from metaphysis to epiphysis
Tourniquet utilization in tubercle fractures can hinder reduction	• Releasing the tourniquet, and thereby the quadriceps muscle, will assist in the reduction of tubercle fractures

With open physes, children with knee trauma or those with polytrauma should have their radiographs scrutinized for nondisplaced proximal tibial fractures.[14,38] Overnight observation in the hospital is recommended for all fractures of the proximal tibia because of the risk of vascular injury or development of compartment syndrome. All casts should be at least univalved during early immobilization, and repeated compartment assessments must be performed and documented (Fig. 27-21). However, several recent large series have not identified compartment syndrome after tibial tubercle fractures,[6,8,21] suggesting that perhaps the increased concern with compartment syndrome is not well substantiated. Arterial injuries can go unrecognized, especially in "minimally" displaced fractures, since the full displacement at time of injury is not known. Nondisplaced fractures can

Figure 27-21. Physical examination findings in the setting of compartment syndrome.

be misdiagnosed as MCL injuries. Stress radiographs, or preferably an MRI, can assist in correct diagnosis. Be aware of the Cozen fracture and the proximal tibial growth disturbance that can occur following metaphyseal fractures; however, the true incidence of this phenomenon may actually be much lower than previously thought.[25,47] Recurvatum is the most common deformity following a physeal injury and should be carefully followed radiographically, with comparisons of the contralateral side. Osteotomies may be necessary for correction.[32] An intra-articular placement of the smooth pins may result in a septic joint and should be avoided. There is an association of anterior cruciate ligament injuries with these proximal fractures that may result in late instability if untreated.

Tibial tubercle fractures have an increased risk of compartment syndrome caused by bleeding of the recurrent anterior tibial artery into the anterior compartment. Use of a tourniquet may bind the quadriceps and hinder reduction of a displaced fracture.

Outcomes

Functional outcomes have not been consistently reported in the management of proximal tibial fractures. A systematic review showed that most (88%) proximal tibial fractures were treated operatively, and return to preinjury activity was reported in 79% of patients.[2,5,9,13,15,18,20,23,26,28] Ninety-four percent of patients were able to return to preinjury activities in a mean of 28.9 weeks, and 98% achieved full range of knee motion in a mean of 22.3 weeks.[13,18,20,48] Fracture union was successful in 99% of fractures, with the painful nonunion fragments treated with delayed excision.[20,45]

In reviewing the literature, the overall complication rate in the management of tibial tubercle fractures is 28% (95/336 fractures). However, the most common complication is related to hardware irritation and bursitis (56%), followed by tenderness or prominence of tibial tubercle (18%).[36]

MANAGEMENT OF EXPECTED ADVERSE OUTCOMES AND UNEXPECTED COMPLICATIONS FOR PROXIMAL TIBIAL PHYSEAL FRACTURES

Proximal Tibial Physeal Fractures:
COMMON ADVERSE OUTCOMES AND COMPLICATIONS[36]

- Hardware irritation (56%)
- Tenderness over tibial tubercle (18%)
- Refracture (6%)
- Leg-length inequality (5%)
- Recurvatum (4%)
- Wound infection (3%)
- Stiffness (3%)
- Vascular injury (1%)
- Deep vein thrombosis (DVT)/Pulmonary embolus (PE) (1%)
- Instability (1%)
- Hardware failure (1%)
- Compartment syndrome (0%)

Injuries to the proximal tibia physis are subject to limb shortening or angulation from subsequent growth arrest (Fig. 27-22A). Any of the fracture patterns mentioned above can result in this

particular complication; and, as with any physeal (or apophyseal) fracture, an anatomic reduction with fixation reduces but does not eliminate the risk of growth disturbance. If a partial or complete growth arrest is diagnosed, there is limited recourse. Surgery can be done to limit deformity progression via epiphysiodesis or excision of an epiphyseal bar depending on estimations of remaining growth and location of the arrest within the physis (Fig. 27-22B–D). Therefore, frequent radiographic follow-up is important to achieve early recognition of the growth arrest and thereby limit the extent of disturbance through early intervention. As a reminder, the proximal tibia grows longitudinally at a mean rate of 6 mm/year. And the mean age of physeal closure at the proximal tibia is 14 years old in girls and 16 years old in boys. If angular growth disturbances are identified late, then an osteotomy can be done to correct the deformity. Even recurvatum following a tibial tubercle fracture can be corrected with an osteotomy.[32]

Compartment syndrome may occur following any proximal tibial physeal fracture caused by either a mechanical blockage of the vascular structures by a displaced fracture, damage to the popliteal artery, or tearing of the anterior tibial recurrent vessels that bleed into the anterior compartment.[31,45] It is important to recognize that even a minimally displaced fracture at the time of presentation may have injured one of these vessels at the moment of fracturing. Furthermore, even minimal posterior displacement of the metaphysis can obstruct popliteal blood flow since that vessel is tethered against the bone by soft tissues and the distal anterior tibial artery.[7] Vigilant monitoring is recommended for all patients with proximal tibial physis or displaced tibial tuberosity avulsion fractures. Prophylactic anterior compartment fasciotomy has been described at the time of open reduction to help mitigate the risk of compartment syndrome associated with these fractures, but recent literature suggests

Figure 27-22. A: Sagittal CT scan 1 year after reduction and smooth wire fixation of a 12-year-old tibial tubercle fracture with subsequent physeal bar formation (*arrow*) and developing genu recurvatum. **B:** Initial lateral radiograph after physeal bar excision and fat graft placement to correct deformity showing initial postcorrective surgery.

(continues)

Figure 27-22. *(Continued)* Three years after corrective surgery, the operated limb had 7 degrees of persistent recurvatum (**C**) compared to contralateral limb (**D**) but also more than 2.5 cm of uninhibited longitudinal growth.

that this practice may actually be unnecessary and should only be indicated in Odgen type IV or V fractures where the posterior cortex has been disrupted.[6]

Bursitis over prominent implants is common, especially for tibial tubercle fractures.[2,36,45] Countersinking the screw heads may not always be possible without risking fracture of the tuberosity fragment; however, 4.0 or 4.5 screw heads without washers can usually sink below the level of the patella tendon fibers without complication. Fixation with small screws or use of a tension band construct may be good alternatives, but fixation of these fractures should not be sacrificed for a potential risk of bursitis since the pull of the quadriceps muscle can displace fixed fractures. Families should be consulted that approximately 50% of patients may require a secondary procedure for implant removal after successful union of the fracture.

Less frequently, there have been reports of symptomatic knee instability, primarily in children sustaining Salter–Harris type III and IV proximal tibial injuries.[3,35] Refracture has also been reported for tibial tubercle fractures.[45] This was seen in two children, one after a rapid return to sports (4 weeks after injury) and one wherein a transverse proximal tibial fracture occurred 7 months postoperatively at the level of the retained screws. There is one report of arthrofibrosis and persistent loss of motion of 25 degrees in a Salter–Harris type III fracture at almost 2 years postinjury.[9] Finally, even a thrombophlebitis has been reported in the literature.[25]

SUMMARY OF PROXIMAL TIBIAL PHYSEAL FRACTURES

Fractures of the proximal tibial physis may be relatively uncommon, but they can result in deleterious consequences if poorly managed. Unrecognized compartment syndrome or arterial injury would be devastating to a young limb.

Annotated References

Reference	Annotation
Brown C, Kelly BA, Brouillet K, Luhmann SJ. Ogden Type I to III tibial tubercle fractures in skeletally immature patients: is routine anterior compartment fasciotomy of the leg indicated? *J Child Orthop*. 2021 Dec 1; 15(6):515–524.	Retrospective study over 12 years of 49 Ogden I–III fractures. Thirteen patients had a prophylactic fasciotomy and 8 of those had traumatic fascial disruptions. No instances of compartment syndrome, growth arrest, or recurvatum.
Checa Betegón P, Arvinius C, Cabadas González MI, et al. Management of pediatric tibial tubercle fractures: Is surgical treatment really necessary? *Eur J Orthop Surg Traumatol*. 2019;29(5):1073–1079.	Retrospective study of 10 patients with 11 acute avulsions. Fifty percent of the cases were treated successfully with closed reduction and casting. No compartment syndrome and 100% return to sport by 25 weeks.
Koivisto ST, Laaksonen T, Ahola JA, et al. Epidemiology and management of proximal tibia fractures in children and adolescents: a population-based study based on the Kids' Fracture Tool. *Acta Orthop*. 2022;93:826–830.	This retrospective study over 6 years involved 241 children who received care in the city of Helsinki. The overall incidence of vascular compromise was 0% and compartment syndrome was 1 of 241 or 0.4%. The annual incidence for proximal tibial fractures in children 13–16 years of age was 21 of 100,000.

Annotated References

Reference	Annotation
Mubarak SJ, Kim JR, Edmonds EW, et al. Classification of proximal tibial fractures in children. *J Child Orthop*. 2009;3(3):191–197.	Retrospective study of 135 proximal tibia fractures over an 8-year period. The authors developed a new classification system that reflects the direction of force and fracture pattern.
Ogden JA, Tross RB, Murphy MJ. Fractures of the tibial tuberosity in adolescents. *J Bone Joint Surg Am*. 1980;62(2):205–215.	This retrospective review reports 15 adolescent physeal fractures. In this paper, the authors modified the existing Watson-Jones classification into the Ogden classification, creating fracture subtypes based on displacement and comminution.
Pace L, McCulloch, Momoh E, et al. Operatively treated type IV tibial tubercle apophyseal fractures. *J Pediatr Orthop*. 2013;33(8):791–796.	Twenty-four operatively treated Ogden type IV tibial tubercle fractures were reviewed in 23 patients. This retrospective review discusses the management and complications associated with type IV variant injuries. In this article, the authors advocate for plate and screw fixation for the type IV B tibial tubercle fractures.
Pandya N, Edmonds EW, Roocroft JH, et al. Tibial tubercle fractures: complications, classification, and the need for intra-articular assessment. *J Pediatr Orthop*. 2012;32(8):749–759.	This retrospective review of 41 operatively treated tibial tubercle fractures introduces a four-part classification system that helps guide physicians regarding surgical management. The authors advocate preoperative CT or MRI to help identify intra-articular pathology that is often missed on plain radiographs.
Pretell-Mazzini J, Kelly DM, Sawyer JR, et al. Outcomes and complications of tibial tubercle fractures in pediatric patients: a systematic review of the literature. *J Pediatr Orthop*. 2016;36(5):440–446.	This systematic review reports on 23 eligible articles reporting on the management of tibial tubercle fractures for a review of 336 fractures. This is the most comprehensive review in the literature. This paper reviews the functional outcome, complications, and methods of treatment for tibial tubercle fractures. In addition, this paper attempts to synthesize the classification systems which have been previously published and reported on.
Ryu RK, Debenham JO. An unusual avulsion fracture of the proximal tibial epiphysis. Case report and proposed addition to the Watson-Jones classification. *Clin Orthop Relat Res*. 1985;(194):181–184.	A case report which makes modification to the Watson-Jones/Ogden tibial tubercle classification by adding type IV, which are tubercle fractures that extend into the posterior cortex of the tibia.
Yang BW, Shore BJ, Rademacher E, et al. Prevalence of Cozen's Phenomenon of the Proximal Tibia. *J Pediatr Orthop*. 2019;39(6):e417–e421.	This single-center retrospective study over 3 years identified 181 proximal tibia fractures with a mean age of 4.5 years. A total of four patients (4/181, 2%) developed valgus greater than 5 degrees at clinical follow-up, indicating that Cozen phenomenon is an uncommon complication of proximal tibia fractures.

REFERENCES

1. Aerts BRJ, Ten Brinke B, Jakma TSC, Punt BJ. Classification of proximal tibial epiphysis fractures in children: four clinical cases. *Injury*. 2015;46(8):1680–1683.
2. Ares-Rodriguez O, Seijas R, Nunez-Pereira S, et al. Type III fracture of the anterior tibial tuberosity in adolescents: two case reports. *Eur J Orthop Surg Traumatol*. 2008;18(5):399–403.
3. Bertin KC, Goble EM. Ligament injuries associated with physeal fractures about the knee. *Clin Orthop Relat Res*. 1983;(177):188–195.
4. Blanks RH, Lester DK, Shaw BA. Flexion-type Salter II fracture of the proximal tibia. Proposed mechanism of injury and two case studies. *Clin Orthop Relat Res*. 1994;(301):256–259.
5. Brey JM, Conoley J, Canale ST, et al. Tibial tuberosity fractures in adolescents: is a posterior metaphyseal fracture component a predictor of complications? *J Pediatr Orthop*. 2012;32(6):561–566.
6. Brown C, Kelly BA, Brouillet K, Luhmann SJ. Ogden type I to III tibial tubercle fractures in skeletally immature patients: is routine anterior compartment fasciotomy of the leg indicated? *J Child Orthop*. 2021;15(6):515–524.
7. Burkhart SS, Peterson HA. Fractures of the proximal tibial epiphysis. *J Bone Joint Surg Am*. 1979;61(7):996–1002.
8. Checa Betegón P, Arvinius C, Cabadas González MI, et al. Management of pediatric tibial tubercle fractures: is surgical treatment really necessary? *Eur J Orthop Surg Traumatol*. 2019;29(5):1073–1079.
9. Christie MJ, Dvonch VM. Tibial tuberosity avulsion fracture in adolescents. *J Pediatr Orthop*. 1981;1(4):391–394.
10. Crock H. *An Atlas of Vascular Anatomy of the Skeleton and Spinal Cord*. Martin Dunitz; 1996.
11. Davidson D, Letts M. Partial sleeve fractures of the tibia in children: an unusual fracture pattern. *J Pediatr Orthop*. 2002;22(1):36–40.
12. Ehrenborg G. The Osgood-Schlatter lesion: a clinical study of 170 cases. *Acta Chir Scand*. 1962;124:89–105.
13. Frey S, Hosalkar H, Cameron DB, et al. Tibial tuberosity fractures in adolescents. *J Child Orthop*. 2008;2(6):469–474.
14. Gupta SP, Agarwal A. Concomitant double epiphyseal injuries of the tibia with vascular compromise: a case report. *J Orthop Sci*. 2004;9(5):526–528.
15. Hajdu S, Kaltenecker G, Schwendenwein E, Vécsei V. Apophyseal injuries of the proximal tibial tubercle. *Int Orthop*. 2000;24(5):279–281.
16. Hand WL, Hand CR, Dunn AW. Avulsion fractures of the tibial tubercle. *J Bone Joint Surg Am*. 1971;53(8):1579–1583.
17. Hannouche D, Duparc F, Beaufils P. The arterial vascularization of the lateral tibial condyle: anatomy and surgical applications. *Surg Radiol Anat*. 2006;28(1):38–45.
18. Howarth WR, Gottschalk HP, Hosalkar HS. Tibial tubercle fractures in children with intra-articular involvement: surgical tips for technical ease. *J Child Orthop*. 2011;5(6):465–470.
19. Inoue G, Kuboyama K, Shido T. Avulsion fractures of the proximal tibial epiphysis. *Br J Sports Med*. 1991;25(1):52–56.
20. Jakoi A, Freidl M, Old A, et al. Tibial tubercle avulsion fractures in adolescent basketball players. *Orthopedics*. 2012;35(8):692–696.
21. Koivisto ST, Laaksonen T, Ahola JA, et al. Epidemiology and management of proximal tibia fractures in children and adolescents: a population-based study based on the Kids' Fracture Tool. *Acta Orthop*. 2022;93:826–830.
22. Mann DC, Rajmaira S. Distribution of physeal and nonphyseal fractures in 2,650 long-bone fractures in children aged 0–16 years. *J Pediatr Orthop*. 1990;10(6):713–716.
23. Mosier SM, Stanitski CL. Acute tibial tubercle avulsion fractures. *J Pediatr Orthop*. 2004;24(2):181–184.

24. Mubarak SJ, Kim JR, Edmonds EW, et al. Classification of proximal tibial fractures in children. *J Child Orthop.* 2009;3(3):191–197.
25. Navascués JA, González-López JL, López-Valverde S, et al. Premature physeal closure after tibial diaphyseal fractures in adolescents. *J Pediatr Orthop.* 2000;20(2):193–196.
26. Nikiforidis PA, Babis GC, Triantafillopoulos IK, et al. Avulsion fractures of the tibial tuberosity in adolescent athletes treated by internal fixation and tension band wiring. *Knee Surg Sports Traumatol Arthrosc.* 2004;12(4):271–276.
27. Ogden JA, Southwick WO. Osgood-Schlatter's disease and tibial tuberosity development. *Clin Orthop Relat Res.* 1976;(116):180–189.
28. Ogden JA, Tross RB, Murphy MJ. Fractures of the tibial tuberosity in adolescents. *J Bone Joint Surg Am.* 1980;62(2):205–215.
29. Pace JL, McCulloch PC, Momoh EO, et al. Operatively treated type IV tibial tubercle apophyseal fractures. *J Pediatr Orthop.* 2013;33(8):791–796.
30. Pandya NK, Edmonds EW, Roocroft JH, Mubarak SJ. Tibial tubercle fractures: complications, classification, and the need for intra-articular assessment. *J Pediatr Orthop.* 2012;32(8):749–759.
31. Pape JM, Goulet JA, Hensinger RN. Compartment syndrome complicating tibial tubercle avulsion. *Clin Orthop Relat Res.* 1993;(295):201–204.
32. Pappas AM, Anas P, Toczylowski HM Jr. Asymmetrical arrest of the proximal tibial physis and genu recurvatum deformity. *J Bone Joint Surg Am.* 1984;66(4):575–581.
33. Pesl T, Havranek P. Acute tibial tubercle avulsion fractures in children: selective use of the closed reduction and internal fixation method. *J Child Orthop.* 2008;2(5):353–356.
34. Peterson HA, Madhok R, Benson JT, et al. Physeal fractures: Part 1. Epidemiology in Olmsted County, Minnesota, 1979–1988. *J Pediatr Orthop.* 1994;14(4):423–430.
35. Poulsen TD, Skak SV, Jensen TT. Epiphyseal fractures of the proximal tibia. *Injury.* 1989;20(2):111–113.
36. Pretell-Mazzini J, Kelly DM, Sawyer JR, et al. Outcomes and complications of tibial tubercle fractures in pediatric patients: a systematic review of the literature. *J Pediatr Orthop.* 2016;36(5):440–446.
37. Ryu RK, Debenham JO. An unusual avulsion fracture of the proximal tibial epiphysis. Case report and proposed addition to the Watson-Jones classification. *Clin Orthop Relat Res.* 1985;(194):181–184.
38. Sferopoulos NK, Rafailidis D, Traios S, Christoforides J. Avulsion fractures of the lateral tibial condyle in children. *Injury.* 2006;37(1):57–60.
39. Shelton WR, Canale ST. Fractures of the tibia through the proximal tibial epiphyseal cartilage. *J Bone Joint Surg Am.* 1979;61(2):167–173.
40. Stanitski CL. Stress view radiographs of the skeletally immature knee: a different view. *J Pediatr Orthop.* 2004;24(3):342.
41. Stranzinger E, Leidolt L, Eich G, Klimek PM. The anterior tilt angle of the proximal tibia epiphysial plate: a significant radiological finding in young children with trampoline fractures. *Eur J Radiol.* 2014;83(8):1433–1436.
42. Thompson GH, Gesler JW. Proximal tibial epiphyseal fracture in an infant. *J Pediatr Orthop.* 1984;4(1):114–117.
43. Tjoumakaris FP, Wells L. Popliteal artery transection complicating a non-displaced proximal tibial epiphysis fracture. *Orthopedics.* 2007;30(10):876–877.
44. Watson-Jones R, Wilson JN, eds. *Fractures and Joint Injuries.* Churchill Livingstone; 1976.
45. Wiss DA, Schilz JL, Zionts L. Type III fractures of the tibial tubercle in adolescents. *J Orthop Trauma.* 1991;5(4):475–479.
46. Wood KB, Bradley JP, Ward WT. Pes anserinus interposition in a proximal tibial physeal fracture. A case report. *Clin Orthop Relat Res.* 1991;(264):239–242.
47. Yang BW, Shore BJ, Rademacher E, et al. Prevalence of Cozen's phenomenon of the proximal tibia. *J Pediatr Orthop.* 2019;39(6):e417–e421.
48. Zrig M, Annabi H, Ammari T, et al. Acute tibial tubercle avulsion fractures in the sporting adolescent. *Arch Orthop Trauma Surg.* 2008;128(12):1437–1442.

28

Intra-Articular Injuries of the Knee

Dennis E. Kramer and Mininder S. Kocher

Fractures of the Tibial Spine (Intercondylar Eminence)

INTRODUCTION TO FRACTURES OF THE TIBIAL SPINE

Fractures of the tibial spine occur because of a chondroepiphyseal avulsion of the anterior cruciate ligament (ACL) insertion on the anteromedial tibial spine.[141,199] Tibial spine fractures were once thought to be the pediatric equivalent of midsubstance ACL tears in adults,[89,197] though recent evidence suggests that the relative incidence of ACL tears in children may be increasing,[170] and that tibial spine fractures in some adult populations may be more common than previously appreciated.[49,88]

Avulsion fracture of the tibial spine is a relatively uncommon injury in children, occurring in 3 per 100,000 children each year. Most common age is 11 to 12 years, and it accounts for 2% to 5% of traumatic knee effusions in adolescents.[44]

Historically, a variety of treatment options have been reported; however, modern treatment is based specifically on fracture type. Nondisplaced fractures and hinged fractures which are able to be closed reduced can be treated without surgery. Displaced fractures that are not able to be reduced require open or arthroscopic reduction with internal fixation.

The prognosis for closed treatment of nondisplaced and reduced tibial spine fractures and for operative treatment of displaced fractures is good. Most series report healing with an excellent functional outcome despite some residual knee laxity.[90,112,175,197] Potential complications include nonunion, malunion, arthrofibrosis, residual knee laxity, and growth disturbance.[90,175,188,197]

ASSESSMENT OF FRACTURES OF THE TIBIAL SPINE

MECHANISMS OF INJURY FOR FRACTURES OF THE TIBIAL SPINE

The most common mechanism of tibial spine fracture in children was once a fall from a bicycle, but increased participation in youth sports at earlier ages at higher competitive levels has led to tibial spine fractures resulting from sporting activities being seen with increased frequency. The most common biomechanical scenario leading to tibial spine fracture is forced valgus and external rotation of the tibia, although tibial spine avulsion fractures can also occur from hyperflexion, hyperextension, or tibial internal rotation.

A tibial spine fracture represents a chondroepiphyseal avulsion of a fragment of the anteromedial tibial spine from the rest of the central proximal tibial epiphysis. In a cadaver study, fracture of the anterior intercondylar spine was simulated by oblique osteotomy beneath the spine and traction on the ACL. In each specimen, the displaced fragment could be reduced into its bed by extension of the knee. In adults, the same stress might cause an isolated tear of the ACL, but in children, the incompletely ossified tibial spine is generally weaker to tensile stress than the ligament, so failure occurs through the cancellous bone beneath the subchondral bone of the tibial spine. In addition, loading conditions may result in differential injury patterns. In experimental models, midsubstance ACL injuries tend to occur under rapid loading rates, whereas tibial spine avulsion fractures tend to occur under slower loading rates.[141,199]

A narrow intercondylar notch may predispose to tibial spine fracture versus midsubstance ACL tears as shown by Kocher et al.[94] in a retrospective case-control study.

INJURIES ASSOCIATED WITH FRACTURES OF THE TIBIAL SPINE

Associated intra-articular injuries are uncommon. Although Shea et al.[169] identified bone bruises in 18 of 20 MRI studies in children with tibial spine fractures, in a series of 80 skeletally immature patients who underwent surgical fixation of tibial spine fractures, Kocher et al. found no intra-articular chondral injuries. Associated meniscal tears (Fig. 28-1) have been reported in 0%[83] to 40% of MRI studies. A recent prospective study reported meniscal injuries in 20 of 54, 37% of consecutive patients who underwent surgical treatment for tibial spine fractures.[63] Higher age, advanced tanner stage, and pubescence

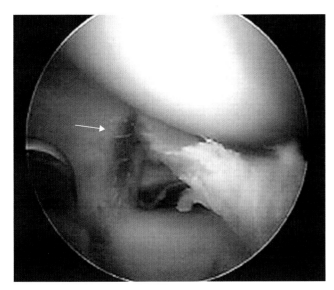

Figure 28-1. Longitudinal meniscus tear (*white arrow*) associated with tibial spine fracture.

Figure 28-2. Sagittal CT cut showing a minimally displaced tibial spine fracture (*white arrow*) that can be treated conservatively without surgery as the majority of the ACL insertion on the tibia is reduced. (From Kramer et al. In: Skaggs DL, Kocher MS, eds. *Master Techniques in Orthopaedic Surgery: Pediatrics.* 2nd ed. Wolters Kluwer; 2016:449–461, with permission.)

were significantly associated with an accompanying meniscal injury and 90% of these injuries involved the lateral meniscus.[63] Associated collateral ligament injury or proximal ACL avulsion is uncommon but has been described in case reports.

SIGNS AND SYMPTOMS OF FRACTURES OF THE TIBIAL SPINE

Patients typically present with a painful, swollen knee and difficulty weight bearing after an acute traumatic event. On physical examination, there is often a large hemarthrosis due to the intra-articular fracture and limited motion due to pain, and swelling. Sagittal plane laxity is often present, but the contralateral knee should be assessed for physiologic laxity. Gentle stress testing should be performed to rule out other ligamentous injuries.

Patients with late malunion of a displaced tibial spine fracture may lack full extension because of a mechanical bony block, and/or have increased knee laxity, with a positive Lachman and pivot-shift examination.

IMAGING AND OTHER DIAGNOSTIC STUDIES FOR FRACTURES OF THE TIBIAL SPINE

Anteroposterior (AP) and lateral knee radiographs typically demonstrate the fracture, which is often seen best on the lateral view. The lateral radiograph is most useful in fracture classification (see below). Radiographs should be carefully scrutinized, as the avulsed fragment may be mostly nonossified cartilage with only a small, thin ossified portion visible on the lateral view.

Bone age radiographs may be obtained for patients around the time of skeletal maturity if transphyseal screw fixation is being considered. In cases where displacement is unclear, a computerized tomography (CT) scan can be obtained (Fig. 28-2). If

most of the ACL insertion on the tibia is reduced, the fracture can be treated without surgery.

MRI can be helpful to confirm the diagnosis in cases with a very thin ossified portion of the avulsed fragment or evaluate for suspected associated injuries (Fig. 28-3).[83,105,169]

Figure 28-3. Sagittal T2 MRI showing a displaced McKeever type III tibial spine fracture (*white arrow*) that requires surgical reduction and fixation. (From Kramer et al. In: Skaggs DL, Kocher MS, eds. *Master Techniques in Orthopaedic Surgery: Pediatrics.* 2nd ed. Wolters Kluwer; 2016:449–461, with permission.)

CLASSIFICATION OF FRACTURES OF THE TIBIAL SPINE

Fractures of the Tibial Spine: MEYERS AND MCKEEVER CLASSIFICATION	
Type	**Description**
I	Minimal displacement of the fragment from the rest of the proximal tibial epiphysis
II	Displacement of the anterior third to half of the avulsed fragment, which is lifted upward but remains hinged on its posterior border in contact with the proximal tibial epiphysis
III	Complete separation of the avulsed fragment from the proximal tibial epiphysis, with upward displacement and rotation

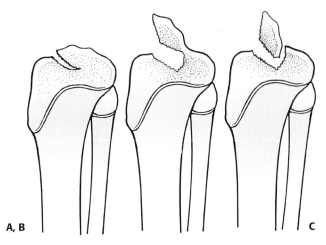

Figure 28-4. Classification of tibial spine fractures. **A:** Type I—minimal displacement. **B:** Type II—hinged posteriorly. **C:** Type III—complete separation.

The classification system of Meyers and McKeever, which is based on the degree of displacement of the tibial spine fragment, continues to be widely used to classify fractures and guide treatment (Fig. 28-4). Radiographs of these fracture types are shown in Figure 28-5. The interobserver reliability between type I and type II/III fractures is good; however, differentiation between type II and III fractures may be difficult.[94]

Zaricznyj[202] further classified a type IV fracture to describe comminution of the tibial spine fragment.

OUTCOME MEASURES FOR FRACTURES OF THE TIBIAL SPINE

Although healing of the fracture on radiographs is important in determining timing for return to activities, the most important

long-term outcome measures used to assess the results of tibial spine fracture fixation include functional knee scores, such as the Pedi-IKDC[100] and Lysholm[174] knee scores, and a patient's ability to make a full return to activities of daily life and sports activities, which can be assessed using the Marx or Tegner activity scores.[122] Asymmetry in the Lachman examination is not uncommon,[195] even after anatomic fixation of fractures, but has not been shown to correlate with symptomatic instability or long-term clinic results.

Figure 28-5. Stages of displacement of tibial spine fractures. **A:** Type I fracture (*white arrow*), minimal displacement (*open arrow*). **B:** Type II fracture (*white arrow*), posterior hinge intact.

Figure 28-5. *(Continued)* **C:** Type III fracture (*white arrow*), complete displacement and proximal migration.

PATHOANATOMY AND APPLIED ANATOMY RELATING TO FRACTURE OF THE TIBIAL SPINE

The intercondylar spine lies between the anterior poles of the menisci. It is triangular shaped with its base along the anterior border of the proximal tibia. In the immature skeleton, the proximal surface of the spine is covered entirely with cartilage. The ACL attaches in the interspinous region of the spine and just anteriorly to the tibial spines, with separate slips anteriorly and laterally as well (Fig. 28-6). The ACL originates off the posterior margin of the lateral aspect of the intercondylar notch. The anterior horn of the lateral meniscus is typically attached in the region of the tibial intercondylar spine just adjacent to the ACL insertion. In 12 patients with displaced tibial spine fractures that did not reduce closed, Lowe et al.[113] reported that

Figure 28-6. Anterior cruciate ligament insertion on the tibial spine (*white arrow*).

Figure 28-7. Meniscal entrapment under a tibial spine fracture (*black arrow*).

the anterior horn of the lateral meniscus consistently remained attached to the tibial spine fracture fragment.

Meniscal or intermeniscal ligament entrapment under the displaced tibial spine fragment has been reported and may be a rationale for considering arthroscopic or open reduction in displaced tibial spine fractures (Fig. 28-7).[95] Meniscal entrapment prevents anatomic reduction of the tibial spine fragment, which may result in a block to extension and/or anterior laxity.[84,195] Furthermore, meniscal entrapment itself may cause knee pain after fracture healing. Meniscal incarceration-blocking reduction of type II or III tibial spine fractures has occurred in children. The prevalence of meniscal entrapment in tibial spine fractures may be common for displaced fractures. Although the anterior horn of the lateral meniscus may remain attached to the tibial spine fracture fragment, it may instead remain attached to the intermeniscal ligament, generating a soft tissue complex that can become incarcerated between the elevated bony or cartilaginous fracture fragment and its underlying bony bed. In a consecutive series of 80 skeletally immature patients who underwent surgical fixation of hinged or displaced tibial spine fractures which did not reduce in extension, Kocher et al.[95] found entrapment of the anterior horn medial meniscus (*n* = 36), intermeniscal ligament (*n* = 6), or anterior horn lateral meniscus (*n* = 1) in 26% (6/23) of hinged (type II) fractures and 65% (37/57) of displaced (type III) fractures. The entrapped meniscus can typically be extracted with an arthroscopic probe and retracted with a retaining suture (Fig. 28-8).

TREATMENT OPTIONS OF FRACTURES OF THE TIBIAL SPINE

Treatment options include brace or cast immobilization with or without closed reduction,[196,197] open reduction with immobilization,[131] open reduction with internal fixation,[133]

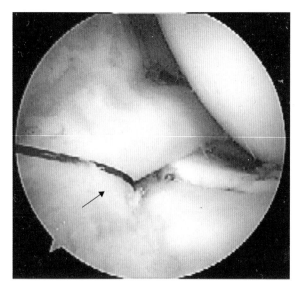

Figure 28-8. Retraction of an entrapped anterior horn medial meniscus using a retaining suture (*black arrow*).

arthroscopic reduction with immobilization,[125] arthroscopic reduction with suture fixation,[80] or suture mattress technique,[119] and arthroscopic reduction with wire,[19] screw fixation,[25] percutaneous K-wire fixation,[68,79] anchor fixation,[189] suture button fixation,[10] and bioabsorbable implant fixation.[132,166] Studies of the biomechanical strength of internal fixation suggest similar fixation strength between bioabsorbable and metallic internal fixation and[117] nonabsorbable and absorbable suture fixation,[110] inconsistent strength with suture anchor fixation,[10] and increased fixation strength of suture fixation over screw fixation,[30,53] with advocates of both bioabsorbable implant fixation and suture techniques emphasizing the advantage of avoiding subsequent hardware removal procedures.[119,201]

NONOPERATIVE TREATMENT OF FRACTURE OF THE TIBIAL SPINE

Indications/Contraindications

Nonoperative Treatment of Fractures of the Tibial Spine: INDICATIONS AND CONTRAINDICATIONS	
Indications	**Relative Contraindications**
• Type I (nondisplaced) fractures	• Type III fractures
• Anatomic reduction of type II (hinged) fractures	• Persistent/recurrent displacement of type II fractures

Closed treatment is typically utilized for type I fractures and for type II fractures that successfully reduce with closed reduction.

Techniques

Closed reduction is usually performed with placement of the knee in full extension or 20 to 30 degrees of flexion. Aspiration

Figure 28-9. Reduction of type II tibial fracture with knee in 10 to 20 degrees of flexion.

of the intra-articular fracture hematoma, with or without the intra-articular injection of a short-acting local anesthetic, has historically been utilized prior to reduction but is not required. Radiographs, most importantly the lateral view, are obtained to assess adequacy of reduction. If the proximal fracture fragment includes bony segments of the medial or lateral tibial plateau, extension may affect a reduction through pressure applied by medial femoral condyle or lateral femoral condyle (LFC) congruence (Fig. 28-9). Fractures confined within the intercondylar notch, however, are unlikely to reduce in this manner. Portions of the ACL are tight in all knee flexion positions; therefore, there may not be any one position that eliminates the traction effect of the ACL on the fragment. Interposition of the anterior horn medial meniscus or intermeniscal ligament may further block reduction.

Outcomes

Closed reduction can be successful for some type II fractures but is not typically attempted in type III fractures. While Bakalim and Wilppula[16] reported successful closed reduction in 10 patients, and Meyers and McKeever[127] recommended cast immobilization with the knee in 20 degrees of flexion for all type I and II fractures, Kocher et al.[95] reported successful closed reduction in only 50% of type II fractures (26/49). However, no type III fractures were closed reduced (0/57), in their series, and Meyers and McKeever[127] similarly recommended open reduction or arthroscopic treatment for all type III fractures. Smillie[173] suggested that closed reduction by hyperextension can be accomplished only with a large fragment.

OPERATIVE TREATMENT OF FRACTURE OF THE TIBIAL SPINE

Indications/Contraindications

Arthroscopic or open reduction with internal fixation of all type III fractures and type II fractures which do not reduce has been advocated for a variety of reasons, including concern over meniscal entrapment, the potential for instability and loss of extension associated with closed reduction,[84] the ability to evaluate and treat associated intra-articular pathology (meniscal tears or entrapment), and the opportunity for earlier mobilization following fixation. For displaced fractures, Wiley and Baxter[195] found a correlation between fracture displacement at healing with knee laxity and functional outcome.

Arthroscopic Reduction and Internal Fixation With Epiphyseal Cannulated Screws

Preoperative Planning

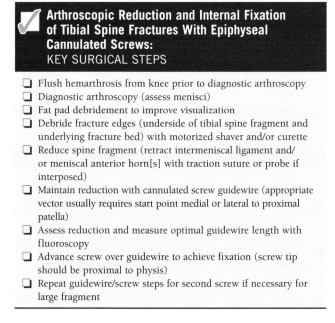

Arthroscopic Reduction and Internal Fixation of Tibial Spine Fractures With Epiphyseal Cannulated Screws:
PREOPERATIVE PLANNING CHECKLIST

OR table	❏ Standard table with lateral thigh post
Position/positioning aids	❏ Supine
Fluoroscopy location	❏ From operative side, perpendicular to table
Equipment	❏ Knee arthroscopy setup, 3.5- or 4-mm cannulated screw system (partially threaded)
Tourniquet	❏ Nonsterile

Technique

Arthroscopic Reduction and Internal Fixation of Tibial Spine Fractures With Epiphyseal Cannulated Screws:
KEY SURGICAL STEPS

- ❏ Flush hemarthrosis from knee prior to diagnostic arthroscopy
- ❏ Diagnostic arthroscopy (assess menisci)
- ❏ Fat pad debridement to improve visualization
- ❏ Debride fracture edges (underside of tibial spine fragment and underlying fracture bed) with motorized shaver and/or curette
- ❏ Reduce spine fragment (retract intermeniscal ligament and/or meniscal anterior horn[s] with traction suture or probe if interposed)
- ❏ Maintain reduction with cannulated screw guidewire (appropriate vector usually requires start point medial or lateral to proximal patella)
- ❏ Assess reduction and measure optimal guidewire length with fluoroscopy
- ❏ Advance screw over guidewire to achieve fixation (screw tip should be proximal to physis)
- ❏ Repeat guidewire/screw steps for second screw if necessary for large fragment

The patient is positioned supine on the operating room table. A thigh high tourniquet and standard arthroscope is used in most patients with small joint scope reserved for only the smallest knees. Standard anteromedial and anterolateral portals are used. Prior to insertion of the arthroscope through the arthroscopic cannula in the anterolateral portal, the large hemarthrosis should be evacuated to optimize arthroscopic visualization. An accessory superomedial or superolateral portal can be later developed for guidewire and screw insertion.

A thorough diagnostic arthroscopic examination is essential to evaluate for concomitant injuries. Anterior fat pad is then excised with a shaver for complete visualization of the intercondylar spine fragment. Entrapped medial meniscus or intermeniscal ligament is extracted with an arthroscopic probe and retracted with a retention suture (see Fig. 28-7). The base of the tibial spine fragment is elevated (Fig. 28-10A) and the fracture bed debrided with an arthroscopic shaver or hand curette (Fig. 28-10B). Anatomic reduction is obtained using an arthroscopic probe or microfracture pick with the knee in 30 to 90 degrees of flexion (Fig. 28-10C). Cannulated guidewires can be placed through portals just off the superomedial or superolateral border of the patella, using a spinal needle to determine the optimal inferiorly directed vector for fracture fixation and taking care to avoid injury to the chondral surfaces adjacent to the intercondylar notch. The guidewires are placed into the intercondylar spine at the base of the ACL. Fluoroscopic assistance is utilized to confirm anatomic reduction and to guide correct wire orientation. A cannulated drill is used over the guidewires, taking care to drill the entire depth of the proximal fragment but avoiding plunging through the proximal tibial physis. One or two screws are placed, based on the size of the tibial spine fragment (Fig. 28-10D). Partially threaded 3.5-mm diameter screws (Fig. 28-10E) are used in children and either 4- or 4.5-mm diameter screws are used in adolescents. For patients near skeletal maturity, the screw can cross the proximal tibial physis to get better fixation. The knee is brought through a range of motion (ROM) to ensure rigid fixation without fracture displacement and to evaluate for impingement of the screw head(s) in extension.

Arthroscopic Reduction and Internal Fixation With Sutures

Preoperative Planning

Arthroscopic Reduction and Suture Fixation of Fractures of the Tibial Spine:
PREOPERATIVE PLANNING CHECKLIST

OR table	❏ Standard table with lateral thigh post
Position/positioning aids	❏ Supine
Fluoroscopy location	❏ Optional
Equipment	❏ Knee arthroscopy setup, ACL tibial guide with <3-mm guidewire (but not reamer), suture passing devices (to advance through ACL at level of footprint and to retrieve through <3-mm tibial tunnels), repair suture (no. 2 size or greater)
Tourniquet	❏ Nonsterile

Figure 28-10. Arthroscopic reduction and cannulated screw internal fixation of a displaced tibial spine fracture. **A:** Elevation of the tibial spine fragment. **B:** Debridement of the fracture bed **C:** Reduction of the tibial spine. **D:** Drilling over the cannulated screw guidewire. **E:** Cannulated screw fixation.

Technique

> ### Arthroscopic Reduction and Suture Fixation of Fractures of the Tibial Spine:
> KEY SURGICAL STEPS
>
> ❏ Flush hemarthrosis from knee prior to diagnostic arthroscopy
> ❏ Diagnostic arthroscopy (assess menisci)
> ❏ Debride fat pad
> ❏ Debride fracture edges (underside of spine fragment and underlying fracture bed) with motorized shaver and/or curette. Consider removing excess bone from tibial side of fragment to allow for slight overreduction of spine fragment and account for ligamentous stretch of ACL fibers
> ❏ Reduce spine fragment (retract intermeniscal ligament and/or meniscal anterior horn[s] if interposed with tagging suture or probe through accessory transpatellar portal)
> ❏ Pass repair sutures through base of ACL at level of tibial footprint (one anterior, one posterior to maximize fixation/repair stability)
> ❏ Through a new proximal tibial incision, create two tibial tunnels (<3 mm) with ACL guide/guidewire on either side of fragment with 1-cm cortical bone bridge between tunnel starting points
> ❏ Pull trans-ACL sutures through tunnels using suture passer device
> ❏ Optimize reduction, tie sutures over bone bridge on maximum tension

Arthroscopic setup and examination is similar to the technique described for epiphyseal screw fixation. Accessory superomedial and superolateral portals are not used, though an accessory transpatellar working portal may be considered to facilitate fracture reduction and suture management. The fracture is elevated and the fracture base debrided (Fig. 28-11A) using tiny curettes. The authors typically remove some excess bone from the tibial side of the fracture site to allow for slight overreduction of the

tibial spine fragment which may account for the intrinsic ACL fiber stretch injury which can occur at the time of tibial spine fracture. The fracture is reduced, or slightly overreduced, and an optimal reduction may be provisionally maintained with a small K-wire directed inferiorly, though reduction of a previously entrapped intermeniscal ligament or anterior meniscal horn over the anterior aspect of the fragment often maintains the reduction adequately and the K-wire can interfere with suture passage through the base of the ACL. Two proximally directed guide pins, approximately 2.7 mm in size, are then placed using the tibial ACL guide system from a small incision made just medial to the tibial tubercle and distal to the proximal tibial physis (Fig. 28-11B). Care is taken to create separate starting points for the two guidewires, to ensure a 1-cm cortical bone bridge between the tibial tunnels for later suture tying, and to place the intra-articular exit points through either side of the base of the intercondylar spine fragment (Fig. 28-11C) right along the fracture line. Either suture passing devices or small wire loops (<2.7 mm in diameter) are then placed up the tibial tunnels, toward the medial and lateral sides of the base of the tibial spine fragment (Fig. 28-11D). At this point, a is used to pass a suture through the medial wire loop, across the posterior aspect of the base of the ACL/tibial spine fragment and back out through the lateral wire loop. This process can be facilitated with the use of a transpatellar tendon portal to retrieve the suture. A second suture is then typically placed in the same direction through the medial wire loop, across the anterior base of the ACL/tibial spine fragment and out through the lateral wire loop (Fig. 28-11E). Once both sutures have been passed, these transtibial wire loops then pull the suture ends out through the inferior incision, and the sutures are tied down onto the tibia over the bony bridge, using arthroscopic

A   B

Figure 28-11. A: Preparation of the tibial spine fracture site with debridement of fibrinous clot using a curette. **B:** An ACL drill guide is used to plan tunnel placement.

(continues)

Figure 28-11. (*Continued*) **C:** The medial guide pin is drilled retrograde into the medial aspects of the tibial fracture site. **D:** Suture retrievers are passed separately through the medial and lateral tunnel. **E:** A curved suture passer is used to pass a suture through the retrievers and the base of the ACL. **F:** The suture retrievers are pulled distally to pull each end of the suture through the corresponding tibial tunnel and the fracture is slightly overreduced following suture fixation. (From Kramer et al. In: Skaggs DL, Kocher MS, eds. *Master Techniques in Orthopaedic Surgery: Pediatrics.* 2nd ed. Wolters Kluwer; 2016:449–461, with permission.)

assessment to confirm maintenance of the optimal reduction (Fig. 28-11F). Alternatively, the sutures can be secured into an anchor distal to the tunnel drilled to achieve fixation. Two or more ACL repair sutures are typically utilized to space the position of the "suture bridge" over a large segment of the ACL footprint and improve rotational stability of the fragment. Both absorbable and nonabsorbable braided sutures may be utilized for the ACL repair sutures as studies have not shown a difference,[162] and there are no published reports of complications

associated with growth disturbance secondary to the bony bridging or prolonged nonabsorbable suture retention through the small transtibial guidewire tracts. If following fixation there is slight residual elevation of the anterior-most portion of the tibial spine fragment which does not contain ACL insertion fibers, this portion of the fragment can be excised with a basket or burr. The knee is brought to full extension following fixation to ensure there is no residual bony impingement or block to extension.

Authors' Preferred Treatment of Fractures of the Tibial Spine (Algorithm 28-1)

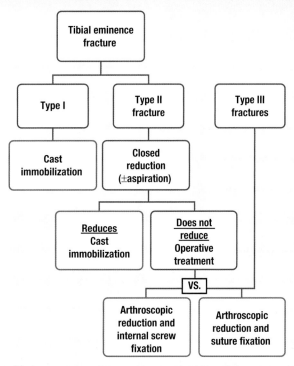

Algorithm 28-1. Authors' preferred treatment of tibial spine fractures in children.

Type I fractures are treated with a locked hinged knee brace in an older child or adolescent or long-leg cast immobilization in a younger child, applied in full extension (0 degrees), to prevent loss of reduction and a flexion contracture, which is generally harder to treat than loss of extension. Radiographs are repeated in 1 to 2 weeks to ensure that the fragment has not displaced. The cast/brace is removed at 6 weeks after injury once bony healing is evident on radiographs. A hinged knee brace is then used and physical therapy initiated to regain motion and strength. Patients are typically allowed to return to sports 3 to 4 months after injury if they demonstrate fracture healing and adequate motion and strength.

Type II fractures may be treated with a gentle attempt at closed reduction with simple knee extension. Radiographs are taken to assess reduction. If the fragment is reduced,

closed management then can be initiated, and follow-up radiographs are performed at 1 and 2 weeks postreduction to ensure maintenance of reduction. Length of casting and postcasting management is similar to type I fractures. If the fracture does not reduce or later displaces, operative treatment as below be performed to optimize outcomes.

Type III fractures: We favor primary operative management in the absence of significant medical comorbidities with arthroscopic reduction and internal fixation. However, open reduction through a medial parapatellar incision can also be performed per surgeon preference/experience, or if arthroscopic visualization is difficult. The authors' preferred fixation is epiphyseal cannulated screws if the fragment is large and the patient is near skeletal maturity or suture fixation for smaller fragments, comminuted fragments and younger patients.

Postoperative Care

Following arthroscopic reduction and internal fixation, patients are placed in a postoperative hinged knee brace and maintained touch-down weight bearing for 6 weeks postoperatively. Motion is generally restricted to 0 to 30 degrees for 6 weeks. The brace is kept locked in extension at night to prevent a flexion contracture. Radiographs are obtained at 2 and 6 weeks to evaluate for maintenance of reduction and fracture healing (Fig. 28-12).

Cast immobilization for 4 to 6 weeks postoperatively may be considered in younger children. Initiation of physical therapy at 6 weeks postoperatively is routinely utilized to optimize motion, strength, and sports-specific training. Patients are typically allowed to return to sports at 12 to 16 weeks postoperatively, depending on knee function. Screws are not routinely removed. Functional ACL bracing is utilized if there is residual knee laxity.

Figure 28-12. Type III tibial spine fracture in an 11-year-old male child treated with arthroscopic reduction and 3.5-mm cannulated screw fixation. Preoperative AP (**A**) and lateral (**B**) radiographs showing fracture (*white arrow*). Postoperative AP (**C**) and lateral (**D**) radiographs.

Potential Pitfalls and Preventive Measures

Repair of Fractures of the Tibial Spine:
POTENTIAL PITFALLS AND PREVENTIONS

Pitfall	Prevention
Failure/loss of reduction of type II	• Ensure cast is in full extension • Obtain MRI or consider surgical intervention if meniscal interposition is suspected • Follow x-rays closely (5–7 days and 12–14 days postreduction) • Consider surgical intervention
Inadequate visualization during arthroscopy	• Before starting arthroscopy, flush hemarthrosis until arthroscopy fluid clear • Make sure fat pad debridement is adequate
Comminution of spine fragments during attempted screw fixation (or upon initial assessment)	• Use suture fixation instead of screw fixation
Growth disturbance with screw fixation	• Multiple fluoroscopic views to ensure no physeal screw penetration
Postoperative arthrofibrosis	• Ensure adequate fixation to allow early ROM • Immobilize in extension at night to avoid loss of extension

For closed management of tibial spine fractures, follow-up radiographs must be obtained at 1 to 2 weeks postinjury to verify maintenance of reduction. Late displacement and malunion can occur, particularly for type II fractures.

During arthroscopic reduction, visualization can be difficult unless the large hematoma is evacuated and flushed and the large inflamed fat pad is adequately debrided. Careful attention to preparation of the fracture bed is important to provide optimal conditions for bony healing. Attempted epiphyseal cannulated screw fixation of small or comminuted tibial spine fragments can fail as the screw may further comminute the fragment. In many cases, suture fixation is preferred for this reason. If epiphyseal cannulated screw fixation is used, fluoroscopy is necessary to ensure that the drill or screw does not traverse the proximal tibial physis (in skeletally immature patients), which may result in a proximal tibial physeal growth arrest.

Early mobilization and nighttime bracing in full extension is helpful to avoid arthrofibrosis which can occur with immobilization. However, in younger children, compliance with protected weight bearing and brace use can be problematic.

Outcomes

The prognosis for closed treatment of nondisplaced and reduced tibial spine fractures and for operative treatment of displaced fractures is good. Most series report healing with an excellent functional outcome despite some residual knee laxity.[90,183,195,197] Potential complications include nonunion, malunion, arthrofibrosis, residual knee laxity, and growth disturbance.[90,187,195,197] Type I fractures may not be completely benign, however. A 2022 report by Shimberg et al. found that in 48 patients with type I tibial spine fractures, 25% had concomitant injuries and 4 (8%) required subsequent ACL-R while another 4 (8%) required later surgery for meniscal issues.[172]

Mild residual knee laxity is seen frequently, even after anatomic reduction and healing of tibial spine fractures. Baxter and Wiley[20,195] found excellent functional results without symptomatic instability in 17 pediatric knees with displaced tibial spine fractures, despite a positive Lachman examination in 51% of patients and increased mean instrumented knee laxity of 3.5 mm. After open reduction and internal fixation (ORIF) of type III fractures in 13 pediatric knees, Smith[175] identified patient-reported instability in only two patients, despite a positive Lachman examination in 87% of patients. In a group of 50 children after closed or open treatment, Willis et al.[197] found excellent clinical results despite a positive Lachman examination in 64% of patients and instrumented knee laxity of 3.5 mm for type II fractures and 4.5 mm for type III fractures. Similarly, Janarv et al.[84] and Kocher et al.[90] found excellent functional results despite persistent laxity even in anatomically healed fractures. More recent long-term follow-up studies have replicated these findings.[37,183] Despite four patients demonstrating signs, but no symptoms, of instability, Tudisco et al.[183] recently reported good results in 13 of 14 knees followed for a mean of 29 years postinjury, with the one suboptimal result reported in a type III fracture treated nonoperatively.

Persistent laxity despite anatomic reduction and healing of tibial spine fractures in children is likely related to plastic deformation of the collagenous fibers of the ACL occurring

in association with tibial spine fracture. At the time of tibial spine fixation, the ACL often appears hemorrhagic within its sheath, but grossly intact and in continuity. In a primate animal model, Noyes et al.[141] found frequent elongation and disruption of ligament architecture despite gross ligament continuity in experimentally produced tibial spine fractures at both slow and fast loading rates. This persistent AP laxity despite anatomic reduction may be avoided by countersinking the tibial spine fragment within the epiphysis at the time of reduction and fixation. Later ACL injury after previous tibial spine fracture may be more common than previously thought. One case series of 101 patients over a 20-year period reported a 19% rate of delayed ACL reconstruction (ACL-R) in patients who had a prior tibial spine fracture.[130] Quinlan et al. recently reported a 10% rate of ipsilateral ACL rupture and 21% rate of requiring an additional knee procedure in 66 patients treated with arthroscopic tibial spine repair at a mean follow-up of 5.8 years.[151]

> ### MANAGEMENT OF EXPECTED ADVERSE OUTCOMES AND UNEXPECTED COMPLICATIONS IN FRACTURE OF THE TIBIAL SPINE
>
> **Fractures of the Tibial Spine:**
> COMMON ADVERSE OUTCOMES AND COMPLICATIONS
>
> - Arthrofibrosis
> - Nonunion
> - Malunion
> - ACL laxity

Poor results may occur after tibial spine fractures associated with unrecognized injuries of the collateral ligaments or complications from associated physeal fracture.[175] In addition, hardware across the proximal tibial physis may result in growth disturbance with recurvatum deformity or shortening.

Malunion of type II and III fractures may cause mechanical impingement of the knee during full extension (Fig. 28-13). For symptomatic patients, this can be corrected by either osteotomy of the fragment and fixation in a more recessed, anatomic position or excision of the manumitted fragment with anatomic suture repair of the ACL to its bony footprint. Alternatively, excision of the fragment and ACL-R can be considered in adults and older adolescents.

Nonunion of type II and III tibial spine fractures treated closed can usually be managed by arthroscopic or open reduction with internal fixation.[188] Debridement of the fracture bed and the fracture fragment to fresh, bleeding bone is essential to optimize bony healing. Similarly to management of malunions described above, excision of the fragment and ACL-R can be considered in adults and older adolescents, and may be preferable, given the increasingly favorable reports of outcomes of pediatric ACL-R techniques.

Arthrofibrosis is the most common complication following tibial spine injury.[44] Stiffness and arthrofibrosis can be a challenging problem after both nonoperative and operative

Figure 28-13. Lateral radiograph of a malunited displaced fracture of the intercondylar spine of the tibia (*white arrow*) with an extension block.

management of tibial spine fractures. The milieu of a major traumatic intra-articular injury, a large hemarthrosis, and immobilization can predispose to arthrofibrosis. Vander Have et al. reported on 20 cases of arthrofibrosis out of 205 patients (10%) from four institutions over a 10-year period who had undergone surgical intervention for tibial spine fracture, as well as 12 additional cases referred from other institutions. Of the 32 total cases, 25 (78%) had been immobilized for 4 to 6 weeks postoperatively without motion, and 24 (75%) required additional operative treatment within 6 months to address debilitating loss of knee motion.[187] The authors concluded that for fractures that undergo fixation, early mobilization utilizing physical therapy can minimize the risk of arthrofibrosis, an approach supported by subsequent analyses.[147] If stiffness is detected, dynamic splinting and aggressive physical therapy can be employed during the first 3 months from fracture.[143] If significant stiffness remains, patients should be managed with arthroscopy, lysis of adhesions. and manipulation under anesthesia.[187] Overly vigorous manipulation should be avoided to avert iatrogenic proximal tibial or distal femoral physeal fracture, which may lead to growth arrest or deformity requiring further treatment.[187]

Patellar Sleeve Fractures

INTRODUCTION TO PATELLAR SLEEVE FRACTURES

Patellar sleeve fractures occur in adolescents with growth remaining following sudden quadriceps contraction in a flexed knee position. They represent the most common patellar fracture

Figure 28-14. Lateral radiograph of the knee showing a patellar sleeve avulsion injury to the distal patella in association with patella alta.

pattern in adolescents. These fractures occur from a shear-type mechanism where the thick adolescent periosteum of the patella remains attached to the patellar tendon/extensor mechanism and shears away from its weaker attachment to the underlying bony patella.[176] This causes the patella to displace proximally.

ASSESSMENT OF PATELLAR SLEEVE FRACTURES

Patellar sleeve fractures are typically diagnosed on lateral radiographs which show patella alta possibly in association with distal ossification at the intact periosteal attachment to the patellar tendon (Fig. 28-14). Patients typically present with a large swollen knee, often held in flexion. On physical examination, patients are unable to straight-leg raise and often have pain with any knee ROM. If lateral radiographs are equivocal, MRI can be considered to better assess bony displacement and integrity of the extensor mechanism.

TREATMENT OPTIONS FOR PATELLAR SLEEVE FRACTURES

NONOPERATIVE TREATMENT FOR PATELLAR SLEEVE FRACTURES

Conservative management with immobilization in full knee extension with either a cast or locked brace can be considered for nondisplaced or minimally displaced fractures with an intact extensor mechanism as evidenced by the ability to do a straight-leg raise.[176]

OPERATIVE TREATMENT FOR PATELLAR SLEEVE FRACTURES

Surgical repair is indicated for periosteal sleeve fractures with significant displacement especially if the patient is unable to do a straight-leg raise.

Technique

Operative Repair of Patellar Sleeve Fractures:
KEY SURGICAL STEPS

☐ Anatomic reduction of the patellar sleeve fracture to restore congruency to the underlying patellar cartilage and restore the extensor mechanism at proper tension.
☐ Identify and repair associated injuries such as retinacular tears or loose fragments in the joint
☐ Achieve satisfactory fixation in the distal fragment, which has limited bone for purchase and allows for earlier motion following a period of immobilization

Following induction of general anesthesia, a midline vertical incision is made directly over the patella. The patella, patellar tendon, and medial and lateral retinaculum are exposed to identify the zone of injury. The distal patellar sleeve fracture fragment is identified and is typically larger than it appears on radiographs due to a large cartilaginous component. The fracture is often seen in combination with horizontal medial and lateral retinacular tears.

The knee hemarthrosis is then lavaged and the joint assessed for loose chondral fragments. The patellar sleeve fracture site is identified. Nonabsorbable sutures are placed across the retinacular tear sites but not tied. A suture-through bone technique is then employed to repair the patellar sleeve fracture. Three vertical holes are drilled retrograde through the proximal patellar fragment—one medial, one central, and one lateral using a small drill bit. Two no. 2 braided nonabsorbable stitches are placed into the patellar tendon/distal patellar fragment in a locking-stitch Krakow technique so that four free suture ends (one medial strand, two central strands, one lateral strand) are present at the proximal portion of the distal fragment.

The fracture site is then reapproximated and the medial-most suture is passed retrograde through the medial tunnel in the proximal fragment using a suture passing device. Similarly, the two middle sutures were passed through the middle tunnel and the most lateral suture is passed through the lateral tunnel. Sutures are then retrieved out the proximal aspect of the patellar tunnels. Tension is held on the sutures which reduces the distal fragment. The sutures are then tied to each other for secure stabilization. Finger palpation confirms anatomic reduction of the patellar joint surface. A fluoroscopic lateral view is obtained to confirm anatomic reduction.

The medial and lateral retinacular sutures are tied to repair the retinacular tears. The knee incision was closed in layers with absorbable sutures. The patient is then placed into a cylinder cast or a hinged knee brace locked in extension. Radiographs are obtained at the 2- and 6-week postoperative visits (Fig. 28-15). Progressive weight bearing, knee ROM, and physical therapy is typically initiated as adequate healing is seen on radiographs.

Figure 28-15. A: Two-week postoperative lateral radiograph of the knee in cast after reduction and fixation of a patellar sleeve fracture. **B:** Six-month postoperative lateral radiograph of the knee showing a healed patellar sleeve fracture.

Patellar Sleeve Fractures:
SURGICAL PITFALLS AND PREVENTIONS

Pitfall	Prevention
Small distal patellar bony fragment makes screw fixation challenging and prone to further comminution	• Suture fixation of the distal fragment that includes the patellar tendon provides a more secure method of fixation and does not rely on the limited bone of the distal patellar pole. • Incorporating the periosteum of the patella in the repair provides strong reinforcement for fixation
Anatomic reduction of the cartilagenous surface of the patella is of primary importance though visualization can be challenging	• Use direct visualization (when possible), fluoroscopic imaging, and finger palpation to confirm anatomic reduction of the underlying intra-articular patellar cartilage • Retinacular tears can be used to facilitate visualization of the underlying patellar cartilage if necessary
Loose chondral fragments are common and may require fixation if large or cause mechanical loose body symptoms if not identified and removed	• Look for intra-articular chondral fragments that may be present; large osteochondral fragments should be reduced and fixated separately or incorporated into the repair

MANAGEMENT OF EXPECTED ADVERSE OUTCOMES AND UNEXPECTED COMPLICATIONS RELATED TO PATELLAR SLEEVE FRACTURES

Patellar Sleeve Fractures:
COMMON ADVERSE OUTCOMES AND COMPLICATIONS

Arthrofibrosis
Extensor lag
Delayed diagnosis resulting in chronic knee pain and weakness

ARTHROFIBROSIS

While younger patients can be placed into cylinder casts for immobilization for up to 4 to 6 weeks without significant risk of arthrofibrosis, older adolescents with secure fixation should be placed into a hinged knee brace with gradual increase in knee ROM over a 6-week period to lower the risk of arthrofibrosis. Physical therapy is necessary to regain strength and ROM and prevent arthrofibrosis following discontinuation of immobilization. In severe cases of arthrofibrosis refractory to physical therapy, surgical intervention in the form of arthroscopic lysis of adhesions may be necessary.

EXTENSOR LAG

Extensor lag may occur following improper tensioning of the repair, especially in cases of persistent patella alta. Often this will respond to physical therapy, though failure to respond may require revision surgical repair.

MISSED DIAGNOSIS

In certain cases, the diagnosis may be missed because the distal bony fragment is not readily discernible on radiographs—patella alta may be indicative of this injury. Close attention should be directed to this injury in the appropriate clinical scenario involving a direct blow to the patella with the knee in flexion in a younger patient who is unable to extend the knee, and MRI may be useful for diagnosing a sleeve fracture when the diagnosis is not clear from the clinical and plain radiographic findings.

Osteochondral Fractures

INTRODUCTION TO OSTEOCHONDRAL FRACTURES

Osteochondral fractures in skeletally immature patients are more common than once thought. They are typically associated with acute lateral patellar dislocations. The most common locations for these fractures are the inferior aspect of the patellar median ridge, the inferior medial patellar facet, or the lateral aspect of the LFC (Fig. 28-16). The osteochondral fracture fragments may range from small incidental loose bodies to large portions of the articular surface.

Diagnosis can be difficult to make by plain radiographs as even a large osteochondral fragment may contain no ossified bone or

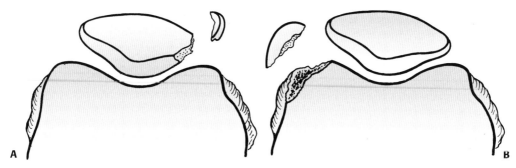

Figure 28-16. Osteochondral fractures associated with dislocation of the right patella. **A:** Medial facet. **B:** Lateral femoral condyle.

only a minimal ossified portion that is visible. MRI has therefore emerged as having a critical role in identifying associated osteochondral fractures or chondral-only fractures in cases of large knee hemarthroses. Acute osteochondral fractures must be differentiated from acute chondral injuries, which do not involve subchondral bone, and osteochondritis dissecans (OCD),[65,96] which is most often a repetitive overuse lesion of the subchondral bone, which may result in a nonhealing stress fracture that can progress to separation of the overlying chondral fragment.

Treatment of acute osteochondral fractures includes removal of small loose bodies or reduction and fixation of larger osteochondral fragments. In cases associated with an acute lateral patellar dislocation, patellar stabilization procedures such as medial retinacular repair or medial patellofemoral ligament reconstruction (MPFLR) may be performed adjunctively.

ASSESSMENT OF OSTEOCHONDRAL FRACTURES

MECHANISMS OF INJURY FOR OSTEOCHONDRAL FRACTURES

There are two primary mechanisms that produce an osteochondral fracture.[5,27] First, a direct blow to the knee with a shearing force applied to either the medial femoral condyle or LFC can create an osteochondral fracture. The second mechanism involves a flexion-rotation injury of the knee in which an internal rotation force is placed on a fixed foot, usually coupled with a strong quadriceps contraction. The subsequent contact between the tibia and femur or patella and LFC causes the fracture. This latter contact mechanism occurs during an acute patellar dislocation. When the patella dislocates laterally, the medial retinaculum and the associated medial patellofemoral ligament (MPFL) tears, while the extensor mechanism still applies significant compressive forces as the patella shears laterally across the LFC. The medial border of the patella then temporarily becomes impacted on the

prominent edge of the LFC before it slides back tangentially over the surface of the LFC because of pull of the quadriceps. Either the dislocation or the relocation phase of this injury can cause an osteochondral fracture to the LFC, the medial facet of the patella, or both (Fig. 28-17). Interestingly, osteochondral fractures are relatively uncommon in the setting of chronic, recurrent patellar subluxations or dislocations. In these situations, the laxity of the medial knee tissues and decreased compressive forces between the patella and the LFC prevent development of excessive shear forces. With more acute or traumatic dislocations, even if a frank osteochondral fracture does not occur, bone bruising is generally seen on MRI on both the patella and LFC, and chondral injuries, such as fissuring of the articular surface of the medial facet and median ridge, are also common.[87,140]

Most patients give a history of a twisting injury consistent with acute patellar dislocation, but a few report a direct blow to the lateral or medial femoral condyle, accounting for a shear injury. The prevalence of osteochondral fractures associated with acute patella dislocation ranges from 19% to 50% in the literature.[5,27,140]

INJURIES ASSOCIATED WITH OSTEOCHONDRAL FRACTURES

As described above, common injuries associated with osteochondral fractures caused by an acute patellar dislocation include MPFL tear and bone bruises or impaction injuries to the LFC and medial aspect of the patella. Occasionally the MCL is injured in these patients due to valgus knee moments.[102] Other osteochondral fractures may occur in association with severe cruciate or collateral ligament tears, especially in the setting of a knee dislocation.

SIGNS AND SYMPTOMS OF OSTEOCHONDRAL FRACTURES

Acutely, osteochondral fractures present with severe pain, swelling, and difficulty in weight bearing.[173,198] The swelling typically

Figure 28-17. Osteochondral fractures associated with dislocation of the patella. **A:** Medial facet of patella (*black arrow*). **B:** Lateral femoral condyle (*black arrow*).

Figure 28-18. Osteochondral fracture of lateral femoral condyle after patellar dislocation. **A:** Fragment seen in lateral joint space (*black arrow*). **B:** Lateral view (*black arrow*).

represents a hemarthrosis from the fracture. If the osteochondral fracture is associated with an acute patellar dislocation, there is often tenderness to palpation over the medial patella and lateral aspect of the LFC, though medial femoral condylar tenderness may also be exhibited, either from a femoral-sided tear of the MPFL or because of a partial MCL sprain. The patient will usually resist attempts to flex or extend the knee significantly due to the hemarthrosis. The large hemarthrosis is due to an intra-articular fracture of the highly vascular subchondral bone. Joint aspiration may reveal fatty globules or a supernatant layer of fat indicating an intra-articular fracture. Similarly, fluid–fluid levels may be seen on MRI, from the separation of fat and blood. Patients who present in a delayed fashion after injury may complain of mechanical loose-body–type symptoms such as intermittent locking or catching of the knee associated with a knee effusion.

IMAGING AND OTHER DIAGNOSTIC STUDIES FOR OSTEOCHONDRAL FRACTURES

Radiographic assessment of a possible osteochondral fracture should begin with AP, lateral, and skyline plain radiographs. A tunnel view may help locate a fragment in the region of the intercondylar notch. Because the osteochondral fragment may be difficult to see on plain radiographs, radiographs should be carefully assessed for even the smallest ossified fragment (Fig. 28-18).

Matelic et al.[123] report that standard radiographs failed to identify the osteochondral fracture in 36% of children who had an osteochondral fracture found during arthroscopy. For this reason, MRI is recommended in most patients who present with a large knee effusion that could potentially be a hemarthrosis, due to the importance of identifying a possible osteochondral

fracture despite negative radiographs.[29,164,194] A high-riding patella may also have a protective effect against associated intra-articular osteochondral fractures. Patients with an Insall index greater than 1.3 have a decreased chance of sustaining an osteochondral fracture compared with patients who have an Insall index within normal limits.[29]

CLASSIFICATION OF OSTEOCHONDRAL FRACTURES

The classification of osteochondral fractures of the knee is based on the site, the type, and the mechanism of injury. The classification outlined in Table 28-1 is based on the descriptions of osteochondral fractures by Kennedy[86] and Smillie.[173]

OUTCOME MEASURES FOR OSTEOCHONDRAL FRACTURES

Healing of osteochondral fractures must be followed closely with radiographs, where applicable, as healing is the most important predictor of outcome. For fixation of osteochondral fractures with minimal subchondral bone or purely chondral fractures,

TABLE 28-1. Mechanism of Osteochondral Fractures	
Site	**Mechanism**
Medial femoral condyle	Direct blow (fall)
	Compression and rotation (tibiofemoral)
Lateral condyle	Direct blow (kick)
	Compression and rotation (tibiofemoral)
	Acute patellar dislocation
Patella (medial margin)	Acute patellar dislocation

follow-up MRI may be necessary to determine healing. Once healed, standard outcome measures, such as functional knee metrics (the Pedi-IKDC[100] and Lysholm[174] knee scores), can be used to assess the results and, paired with the Marx or Tegner activity scores,[122] ascertain a patient's ability to make a full return to activities of daily life and sports activities.

PATHOANATOMY AND APPLIED ANATOMY RELATING TO OSTEOCHONDRAL FRACTURES

The patella tracks in the trochlear groove between the medial femoral condyle and LFC during flexion and extension of the knee. With increasing knee flexion, the contact area on the articular surface of the patella moves from the distal to the proximal aspect of the articular surface of the patella. Between 90 and 135 degrees of flexion, the patella glides into the intercondylar notch between the femoral condyles. The two primary areas of contact are the medial patellar facet with the medial femoral condyle and the superolateral quadrant of the lateral patellar facet with the LFC. Soft tissue support for the patellofemoral joint includes the quadriceps muscle, the MPFL, the patellar tendon, and the vastus medialis and lateralis muscles.

Dislocation of the patella may tear the medial retinaculum and MPFL, but the rest of the quadriceps muscle–patellar ligament complex continues to apply significant compression forces as the patella dislocates laterally. These forces are believed to cause fracture of the medial patellar facet, the LFC articular rim, or both (see Fig. 28-16).[85,86,141,155] Osteochondral fractures are uncommon with chronic recurrent subluxation or dislocation of the patella because of relative laxity of the medial retinaculum.

A histopathologic study by Flachsmann et al.[64] helps to explain the occurrence of osteochondral fractures in the skeletally immature at an ultrastructural level. They noted that in young patients, interdigitating fingers of uncalcified cartilage penetrate deep into the subchondral bone, providing a relatively strong bond between the articular cartilage and the subchondral bone. In the adult, the articular cartilage is bonded to the subchondral bone by the well-defined calcified cartilage layer, the cement line. When shear stress is applied to the juvenile joint, the forces are transmitted into the subchondral bone by the interdigitating cartilage with the resultant bending forces causing the open pore structure of the trabecular bone to fail. In mature tissue, the plane of failure occurs between the deep and calcified layers of the cartilage, the tidemark, leaving the osteochondral junction undisturbed.

As the tissue transitions from the juvenile to the adult pattern during adolescence, fracture toughness to the osteochondral region diminishes. The calcified cartilage layer is only partially formed and the interdigitating cartilage fingers are progressively replaced with calcified matrix. Consequently, the interface between the articular cartilage and the subchondral bone becomes a zone of potential weakness. This may explain why osteochondral fractures are seen frequently in adolescents.

TREATMENT OPTIONS FOR OSTEOCHONDRAL FRACTURES

NONOPERATIVE TREATMENT OF OSTEOCHONDRAL FRACTURES

Nonoperative management of osteochondral fractures is reserved for small fragments, 5 mm or less, that have failed to cause or are unlikely to cause mechanical symptoms typically associated with a loose body. Each osteochondral fracture is unique, so treatment should be individualized, based on a patient's age and activity level, the size, donor site location and chondral status of the injured osteochondral fragment, time to diagnosis, and the degree of surrounding injury. The larger the osteochondral fragment, the more bone attached to the fragment, and the more central the weight-bearing zone from which the fragment detached, the more the surgeon should consider an attempt at refixation.

OPERATIVE TREATMENT OF OSTEOCHONDRAL FRACTURES

Indications/Contraindications

The recommended management of acute osteochondral fractures of the knee is either surgical removal of the fragment or reduction and fixation of the fragment, depending on fragment size and the quality.[95] In patients with an osteochondral fracture after acute patellar dislocation, concomitant repair of the medial retinaculum or MPFL reconstruction at the time of fragment excision or fixation may decrease the risk of recurrent patellar instability,[2,36,156] though if repair is chosen, there is conflicting evidence whether this improves the redislocation rate.[42,138,144]

Fixation

If the lesion is large (≥5 mm), easily accessible, involves a weight-bearing area, and has adequate subchondral bone attached to the chondral surface, then fixation should be considered.[86,173,198] It also should be noted that large chondral-only fragments can also be successfully repaired, especially in the patellofemoral joint.[59]

Preoperative Planning

Fixation of Osteochondral Fractures: PREOPERATIVE PLANNING CHECKLIST

OR table	❏ If fluoroscopy planned, radiolucent table
Position/positioning aids	❏ Supine
Fluoroscopy location	❏ Nonoperative side, perpendicular to table
Equipment	❏ Small K-wires, bioabsorbable pins/tacks/screws, headless compression screws ❏ Instruments to assist with potential need for arthrotomy: Z-retractors, etc.
Tourniquet	❏ Nonsterile

Technique

Fixation of Osteochondral Fractures:
KEY SURGICAL STEPS

- ❏ Diagnostic arthroscopy to retrieve loose body, assess viability, and assess fracture bed and feasibility of fixation
- ❏ If optimal fixation is achievable through arthroscopic means (rare), skip below arthrotomy step
- ❏ Arthrotomy (medial parapatellar or lateral parapatellar or directly over the donor site) to optimize access to fracture bed; if donor site on patella, make arthrotomy long enough to ensure adequate eversion of patella. If donor site on femoral condyles, consider knee flexion on a triangle to center donor site at level of incision. Take care during arthrotomy to avoid injury to the anterior horn of the meniscus
- ❏ Debride/prepare fracture bed and fragment
- ❏ Reduce fragment, provisionally fix with small K-wire
- ❏ Fixation with bioabsorbable pins, tacks, or screws or headless metal compression screws (reserved for larger fragments with adequate bone)
- ❏ Repair arthrotomy (For medial peripatellar arthrotomy, take care not to overtension during closure to avoid increasing patellofemoral contact forces)

Fixation can be performed via arthroscopy or arthrotomy. Fixation options include K-wires, cannulated or solid metal screws, variable pitch headless screws, or bioabsorbable pins,[40,69,192] tacks, or screws, which have recently increased in popularity and have the advantage of not requiring implant removal.[51] For metal implants, hardware removal is typically performed after fracture healing, though headless compression screws may be buried beneath the superficial level of the cartilage and may be retained. Traditionally, purely chondral fragments with no subchondral bone attached were previously not considered amenable to refixation because of concerns regarding poor healing capacity. However, new reports have suggested that large chondral-only fragments may be able to heal in children or adolescents if early refixation is pursued.[58,59,134,184] Fixation can also be successful in the setting of a chronic osteochondral fracture fragment and should be considered in chronic cases if tissue quality is good.[56] In these cases, there is often overgrowth of the osteochondral fragment that may require careful trimming by the surgeon in order to get an anatomic reduction.

Removal of Fragments

If the osteochondral fracture fragment is small (<5 mm), damaged, has minimal subchondral bone, or has fractured from a non–weight-bearing or minimally weight-bearing region of the knee, removal of loose bodies is typically recommended.[107] The fragment's crater should be debrided to stable edges and the underlying subchondral bone should be perforated through marrow stimulation techniques to encourage fibrocartilage formation.[107]

Larger defects may be treated either concurrently or in a delayed fashion with more advanced cartilage restoration techniques including osteochondral grafting (mosaicplasty), or autologous chondrocyte implantation (MACI).

Authors' Preferred Treatment of Osteochondral Fractures (Algorithm 28-2)

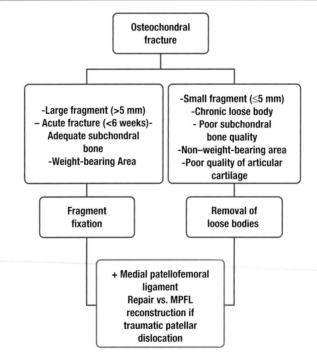

Algorithm 28-2. Authors' preferred treatment of osteochondral fracture in children.

In patients with an acute, traumatic patellar dislocation with a large hemarthrosis, MRI is performed, even if initial radiographs do not clearly show any associated osteochondral fracture.

Patients with small (≤5 mm) osteochondral fractures, damaged fragments, and fractures involving non–weight-bearing areas are treated with either observation (less likely) or arthroscopic removal of loose bodies. For patients seen more than 4 weeks following the initial injury with imaging evidence of a small loose body but no symptoms, arthroscopy may be deferred unless the patient develops mechanical symptoms. If arthroscopy is pursued for a small osteochondral fracture, the fragment's crater is debrided to stable edges to prevent further loose bodies from developing and the underlying subchondral bone should be perforated with marrow stimulation techniques, such as microfracture, to encourage fibrocartilage formation. MPFL reconstruction (more commonly) or medial retinacular/patellofemoral ligament repair at the site of injury is typically performed adjunctively in cases of acute patellar dislocation to decrease the risk of recurrent patellofemoral instability.

Patients with large (>5 mm) osteochondral fractures where the chondral surface remains in good condition and the osteochondral fragment can be anatomically reduced back to the native donor site, or purely chondral fragments with intact chondral surfaces that involve large weight-bearing areas, are treated with fragment fixation. At times, these fragments can be very large, involving nearly the entire weight-bearing surface of the medial patellar facet (Fig. 28-19) or LFC (Fig. 28-20). Medial patellar facet osteochondral fractures can be fixed through an open lateral retinacular release by manually tilting the patella (see Fig. 28-19) or more commonly via an arthroscopic lateral release combined with a medial parapatellar arthrotomy, from which the patella can be completely everted with the aid of two K-wires temporarily placed into the patella and held by needle drivers. This approach also allows for tensioning of the medial retinacular repair or assists with MPFL reconstruction following fixation. LFC osteochondral fractures typically require a lateral parapatellar arthrotomy for fragment fixation (see Fig. 28-20). Z-shaped knee retractors are helpful for exposure and the knee is flexed or extended to optimize visualization of the fracture bed. The osteochondral fracture fragment and the fracture bed are debrided of fibrous tissue to healthy bone. The donor site edges should be cleared of all fibrinous debris and tested for stability using a tiny curette. The subchondral bone of the donor site may be perforated at this step to initiate bleeding prior to fragment reduction. The fragment is then reduced anatomically. At times, the osteochondral fragment will have swelled and be larger than the donor site and may require trimming with a sharp knife or overcuretting of the donor site to achieve an anatomic reduction. For osteochondral fragments with large thick areas of subchondral bone, headless compression screws are often preferable for fixation, compared to bioabsorbable tacks or screws, as stronger fixation allows for fragment compression and early mobilization. For osteochondral fragments with thin layers of subchondral bone, bioabsorbable tacks or screws are routinely employed for fixation which obviates the need for later implant removal (Fig. 28-21).[103] Because chondral-only fragments will have no subchondral bone upon which to compress metal screws, bioabsorbable tacks or a suture-based repair are preferred techniques.[58]

Figure 28-19. Fixation of a medial patellar facet osteochondral fracture in an adolescent male athlete. **A:** Skyline radiograph demonstrating a fracture of the medial patellar facet with the fragment in the lateral recess (*white arrow*). **B:** Axial MRI demonstrating medial facet fracture and loose fragment (*black arrow*).

(continues)

Figure 28-19. *(Continued)* **C:** Arthroscopic view of osteochondral fragment in the lateral recess. **D:** Open view of patella. **E:** Open view of osteochondral fragment. **F:** Open view of reduction and cannulated screw fixation of medial patellar facet. **G:** Intraoperative lateral radiograph after fracture fixation. **H:** Lateral radiograph 3 months after fracture fixation and 6 weeks after screw removal demonstrating healing.

Postoperative Care

Postoperatively, patients treated with fragment excision can begin ROM exercises immediately. Crutches may be necessary in the immediate postoperative period, but patients can progress to weight bearing as tolerated. For weight-bearing lesions of the femoral condyles in which a microfracture/marrow stimulation technique was employed, weight bearing may be delayed and continuous passive motion (CPM) of the knee may be employed to aid formation of fibrocartilage.

Following osteochondral or chondral fragment fixation, patients are treated with protected weight bearing in a postoperative brace until fracture healing. ROM, when not weight bearing, is allowed from 0 to 30 degrees for the first 2 weeks, followed by gradual progression until fracture healing. Healing typically occurs between 6 and 12 weeks postoperatively. Confirmation with follow-up MRI may be utilized though is not routinely employed (Fig. 28-22).[104] For metal screw fixation cases, second look arthroscopy is performed at a later date to confirm fragment healing, remove hardware, and assess the integrity of the articular surface. Return to athletic activities is permitted when knee ROM and strength recover fully.

Figure 28-20. Fixation of a lateral femoral condyle osteochondral fracture in an adolescent female athlete. **A:** Arthroscopic view of the lateral femoral condyle. **B:** Open view of the fracture fragment. **C:** Open view of fracture fixation using cannulated screws through a limited lateral arthrotomy. **D:** Six weeks postoperative lateral radiograph demonstrating fracture healing. **E:** Arthroscopic appearance at the time of screw removal 6 weeks postoperatively.

Potential Pitfalls and Preventative Measures of Osteochondral Fractures

Repair of Osteochondral Fractures: POTENTIAL PITFALLS AND PREVENTIONS	
Pitfall	**Prevention**
Missed osteochondral injury/delayed diagnosis	• Low threshold to obtain an MRI in cases of traumatic knee hemarthrosis/acute patellar dislocation even if radiographs do not show a loose body
Injury to anterior horn meniscus during arthrotomy	• Take care when excising fat pad during arthrotomy not to damage anterior horn of meniscus • If damaged, can perform suture repair via arthrotomy
Further fragmentation of fracture fragment	• Extend portal incisions adequately for removal • Be careful using arthroscopic graspers not to damage the cartilage during removal • Arthroscopically position fragment in gutter/anterior recess near arthrotomy site; retrieve only after full arthrotomy
Fragment does not fit in bed	• Plan surgery acutely/urgently to prevent excessive swelling of fragment • Trim fragment cartilage with sharp knife to fit bed. Protect the most important weight-bearing areas of the fragment and trim the least important • Remove more bone from the donor site as needed to achieve anatomic reduction
Inadequate fixation	• When possible, achieve at least two points of fixation for rotational stability
Growth disruption	• In skeletally immature patients, implants should be short enough to avoid physeal trauma during fixation

Figure 28-21. Arthroscopic knee images following a patellar dislocation. **A:** A loose body is identified and removed (note the subchondral bone on the loose fragment). **B:** The donor site on the lateral femoral condyle is identified (it is weight bearing) and prepared. **C:** The loose fragment is reduced and fixed into the donor site with bioabsorbable implants. (Reprinted from Kramer DE, Pace JL. Acute traumatic and sports-related osteochondral injury of the pediatric knee. *Orthop Clin North Am.* 2012;43(2):227–236. Copyright © 2012, with permission from Elsevier.)

In cases of osteochondral fracture fixation, adequate fixation should be obtained to allow for early motion. Screw heads must be countersunk or headless, variable pitch screws may be used to avoid scuffing of articular surfaces. When chondral-only fixation is pursued with bioabsorbable tacks or screws, care must be taken to partially countersink the implant heads below the articular surface without fissuring through the cartilage completely. Suture repair or fibrin glue can be added to the edges of the reduced chondral-only fragment if more fixation is desired. Moreover, close postoperative clinical monitoring of crepitus, swelling, or new pain must be maintained, and advanced imaging obtained when necessary due to the risk of potential back out of the implants not seen on radiographs. In children or adolescents with growth remaining, care must also be taken to prevent crossing the distal femoral physis with hardware.

Figure 28-22. A: Postoperative T1 sagittal MRI. **B:** Postoperative proton density axial MRI. Both showing the bioabsorbable implant across an osteochondral fracture of the lateral trochlea (*white arrows*). (Reprinted by permission from Kramer DE, et al. Surgical management of osteochondritis dissecans lesions of the patella and trochlea in the pediatric and adolescent population. *Am J Sports Med.* 2015; 43(3):654–662. Copyright © 2015 SAGE Publications.)

Outcomes

Osteochondral fractures with small fragments not involving the weight-bearing portion of the joint usually have a good prognosis following loose body removal. The prognosis for larger osteochondral fractures involving the weight-bearing surfaces is more variable.[69,161] Excision of large fragments involving the weight-bearing articular surfaces predictably leads to the development of degenerative changes.[9] Fracture fixation resulting in fragment healing with a congruous articular surface offers the best long-term prognosis; however, even these cases may develop crepitus, stiffness, and degenerative changes. In a recent series of patients with osteochondral fractures in association with acute patellar dislocations, patients with osteochondral fractures of the weight-bearing femoral condyles had lower IKDC scores at final follow-up compared to those patients with non–weight-bearing lesions or patellar lesions.[164] Recently reported results of chondral-only fragment fixation have been favorable, but only small series or case reports with short-term follow-up have emerged.[58,59,82,134,184]

MANAGEMENT OF EXPECTED ADVERSE OUTCOMES AND UNEXPECTED COMPLICATIONS OF OSTEOCHONDRAL FRACTURES

Osteochondral Fractures:
COMMON ADVERSE OUTCOMES AND COMPLICATIONS

- Arthrofibrosis
- Loss of fixation/nonunion
- Osteoarthritis/focal chondral degeneration

Among the most common complications following an acute patellar dislocation with an osteochondral fracture treated with either excision or repair is recurrent patellar instability. Although studies have suggested that concomitant MPFL repair decreases the risk of recurrent instability,[156] this concept remains controversial.[36,42,138,144] Recent data suggest MPFL reconstruction can be safely combined with osteochondral fracture repair or loose body removal and minimize risk of recurrent patellar instability in the short term.[73,152] Gurusamy et al. in a prospective analysis of 76 adolescents with an acute patellar dislocation with loose body treated with MPFL reconstruction, MPFL repair, or no treatment found that MPFL reconstruction was associated with less recurrent instability (10.0% vs. 58.7%; $P < .001$), fewer secondary procedures (6.7% vs. 47.8%; $P < .001$), and more frequent return to sports (66.7% vs. 39.1%; $P = .003$).[73]

Stiffness is also a common complication following patellofemoral dislocation, particularly after fracture fixation. Adequate internal fixation is necessary to allow for early motion, which decreases the risk of arthrofibrosis. Stiffness may be treated with aggressive therapy and dynamic splinting during the first 3 to 4 months after injury.[143] Beyond this time frame, arthroscopic lysis of adhesions and manipulation under anesthesia is typically required, with care taken to avoid distal femoral physeal injury through excessive manipulation in skeletally immature patients. Nonunion after fragment fixation may also occur, necessitating further attempts at fracture fixation or fracture excision. Excision of larger osteochondral fractures involving the weight-bearing articular surfaces requires associated chondral resurfacing, such as marrow stimulation procedures (microfracture), osteochondral grafting (mosaicplasty), or autologous chondrocyte implantation,[24,148,178] which are technically challenging, and have less optimal outcomes, in the patellofemoral joint, compared with the tibiofemoral articular surfaces.[60,70,76,118] Complications related to implants for fracture fixation may also occur. Proud screw heads may scuff articular surfaces. Prior to reabsorption, bioabsorbable implants may also scuff the cartilage, and over time may be associated with reactive synovitis, sterile effusions, or fragmentation. In addition, bioabsorbable implants can loosen and break off over time, causing a large effusion and mechanical loose-body–type symptoms.[34,82]

Patellar Dislocation

INTRODUCTION TO PATELLAR DISLOCATION

Patellar instability events are relatively common in adolescents. These episodes can range from an acute, traumatic patellar dislocation to chronic, recurrent patellar subluxations in patients with ligamentous laxity. The age- and sex-adjusted annual incidence of first-time lateral patellar dislocation has been estimated at 23.2 per 100,000 person-years with a mean age at dislocation of 21.4 ± 9.9 years and 55% occurring in females.[160] For high school athletes, a recent study noted an overall injury rate of 1.95 per 100,000 athletic exposures (AEs). The highest injury rates were noted for girls' gymnastics (6.19 per 100,000 AEs), boys' football (4.10), and boys' wrestling (3.45) with the rate of injury higher in competition (3.72) than practice (1.34).[129]

Acute, traumatic patellar dislocation occurs more commonly in adolescents. In younger children, these usually occur in the context of underlying patellofemoral dysplasia. Chronic, atraumatic, recurrent patellofemoral instability occurs most frequently in adolescent females, often with underlying laxity and risk factors related to abnormal coronal and rotational lower extremity alignment, such as genu valgum, femoral anteversion, and external tibial torsion.

First-time acute, traumatic patellar dislocations without associated osteochondral loose bodies are often treated with a short period of immobilization followed by patellofemoral bracing and rehabilitation. Acute, traumatic patellar dislocations with osteochondral fractures were discussed above. Chronic, recurrent, atraumatic patellofemoral instability is typically treated with patellofemoral bracing and rehabilitation, with surgery reserved for symptomatic failures of above management. Recurrent patellofemoral instability can be surgically managed with a variety of proximal and distal realignment procedures.

Figure 28-24. The Q angle. Normal valgus alignment of the quadriceps mechanism: Line drawn from the anterosuperior iliac spine to center of the patella, line drawn from center of the patella to tibial spine.

TT/LTR (lateral trochlear ridge) which attempt to predict recurrent instability based on patient-specific anatomy.[35,193]

TREATMENT OPTIONS FOR PATELLAR DISLOCATION

NONOPERATIVE TREATMENT OF PATELLAR DISLOCATION

Indications/Contraindications

Nonoperative Treatment of Patellar Dislocations:
INDICATIONS AND CONTRAINDICATIONS

Indications

- Primary patellar dislocation
- Second patellar dislocation with few/no risk factors for recurrence

Relative Contraindications

- Osteochondral fracture/loose body >5 mm seen on x-ray or MRI
- Recurrent patellar dislocation with underlying/anatomic risk factors for recurrence

---

Most acute patellar dislocations in children reduce spontaneously; if they do not, reduction usually can be easily performed. Surgery is typically not initially recommended for primary acute patellar dislocations in children without associated loose bodies or osteochondral injuries unless they remain symptomatic following nonoperative management. Most patellar dislocations are treated nonoperatively with immobilization in extension, followed by patellofemoral bracing and rehabilitation focused on regaining normal ROM and strengthening of the quadriceps, particularly the VMO.

Technique

After appropriate sedation, reduction is achieved by flexing the hip to relax the quadriceps muscle, gradually extending the knee, and gently pushing the patella medially back into its normal position. Gentle reduction should be emphasized to avoid the risk of osteochondral fracture associated with patellar relocation.

Outcomes

The prognosis following patellar dislocations in children, when not associated with osteochondral injury, is generally good with success rates (no recurrent instability) of 60% to 70%. Patients with a younger age at first dislocation and trochlear dysplasia are at higher risk for recurrent instability.[108,109] Cash and Hughston[38] noted 75% satisfactory results after nonoperative treatment in carefully selected patients.

Recurrent patellar dislocations with associated osteochondral injuries can lead to osteoarthritis of the patellofemoral joint. A recent study found patellar dislocation increases the likelihood of development of patellofemoral arthritis, with an adjusted odds ratio of 3.2.[43]

OPERATIVE TREATMENT OF PATELLAR DISLOCATION

Indications/Contraindications

For acute first-time patellar dislocations without an osteochondral fracture, surgical intervention may be considered for complete MPFL avulsions with severely lateralized patella or for cases with persistent symptoms of patellar apprehension despite adequate conservative management.

If a displaced osteochondral fracture has occurred in association with an acute first-time patellar dislocation, surgical intervention is recommended to treat the loose osteochondral fracture with either removal or repair and stabilize the patella. The patellar stabilization procedure typically involves either an MPFL reconstruction[73] or MPFL repair/medial reefing with or without lateral retinacular release or lengthening.[36,42,115,138,144] Distal bony realignment in the form of tibial tubercle osteotomy might also be considered although is less likely to be employed in the acute setting following a single patellar instability event.

Surgical intervention is also indicated in cases of recurrent patellar instability despite prior proper conservative management. In these cases, patellar stabilization can involve one of various proximal and/or distal patellofemoral realignment procedures. Proximal realignment options include isolated or combination procedures, including lateral retinacular release or lateral retinacular z-lengthening, medial retinacular plication, reefing, or MPFL reconstruction using hamstring autograft, or, more commonly, allograft.[1,21,26,32,33,41,45,46,126,139,155] Distal realignment can be bony in the form of tibial tubercle osteotomy or soft tissue in the form of medial partial (Roux–Goldthwait procedure)/full patellar tendon transfers.

Preoperative Planning

Operative Realignment of Patellar Dislocation:
PREOPERATIVE PLANNING CHECKLIST

OR table	❏ If fluoroscopy planned, radiolucent table
Position/positioning aids	❏ Supine
Fluoroscopy location	❏ Nonoperative side, perpendicular to table
Equipment	❏ If osteochondral fragment fixation planned), small K-wires, bioabsorbable pins/tacks/ screws, headless compression screws
Tourniquet	❏ Nonsterile

Positioning

A standard arthroscopy setup should be used. For both arthroscopic and open techniques, most of the surgery is performed with the knee in full extension. If osteochondral fragment fixation is planned, a bump for both the knee and ankle are helpful to elevate the entire leg and facilitate true lateral x-rays, if necessary.

Operative Realignment of Patellar Dislocation

Surgical Approach and Technique

Operative Realignment of Patellar Dislocation:
KEY SURGICAL STEPS

❏ Perform diagnostic arthroscopy to assess status of patellar and lateral condylar cartilage, assess patellofemoral alignment/tracking, rule out intra-articular loose bodies, consider arthroscopic lateral release, if indicated by lateral patellar tilt or severe patellar lateralization
❏ Distal patellar realignment (tibial tubercle osteotomy [TTO] if skeletally mature, Roux–Goldthwait or patellar tendon transfer if skeletally immature) and indicated by significantly elevated TT-TG
❏ Proximal patellar realignment: medial reefing versus MPFL reconstruction

The most common distal realignment approach in skeletally mature patients is the TTO, which may involve straight medialization of the tubercle (the Elmslie–Trillat procedure),[182] straight anteriorization (the Maquet procedure),[120] or a combination anteromedialization (an "AMZ," or the Fulkerson osteotomy).[66] However, these are contraindicated in patients with an open tibial tubercle apophysis because of the risk of a growth arrest, which can result in recurvatum deformity. In cases of significant patella alta, some authors have additionally proposed distalization of the tibial tubercle, with and without patellar tendon tenodesis, designed to shorten the tendon.[47,124] In skeletally immature patients, Galeazzi semitendinosus tenodesis[14,71] or the Roux–Goldthwait reconstruction[121,137] are distal realignment soft tissue procedures that have been traditionally utilized, though more recent studies have suggested that outcomes of these procedures may be less favorable than historically reported.[14,71,137]

These perspectives have further stimulated interest in MPFL reconstruction techniques in skeletally immature children. Prior studies reported conflicting data on the true anatomic MPFL attachment relative to the distal femoral physis and how this relationship changes over time.[52,87,167] In addition, past literature detailed complications associated with MPFL reconstruction often related to femoral fixation points.[126,137,181] However, many recent studies have reported MPFL reconstruction in skeletally immature patients with attention to proper technique as a safe and effective procedure in adolescents with an open distal femoral physis.[31,135,165,185] In the skeletally immature patient, using an epiphyseal type MPFL reconstruction with the femoral attachment site distal to the physis results in a more isometric graft compared with techniques with attachment sites proximal to the physis and can avoid injury to the distal femoral physis.[28] Shamrock et al. in a recent systemic review on 132 MPFL reconstructions in skeletally immature patients identified only 5 redislocations (3.8%) and no cases of premature physeal closure at nearly 5-year follow-up.[165]

Authors' Preferred Treatment of Patellar Dislocation (Algorithm 28-3)

Most acute patellar dislocations in children without osteochondral fracture are treated by closed methods with satisfactory results. Patients are allowed to weight-bear in a knee immobilizer for approximately 2 weeks. The patient is then placed in a patellofemoral brace with a lateral bolster and physical therapy is initiated, emphasizing straight-leg raises, progressive resistance exercises, patellar mobilization, and vastus medialis strengthening. Patients are allowed to return to sports 6 to 12 weeks after injury, depending on their progress with rehabilitation.

Acute surgical intervention for first-time patellar dislocations is indicated most commonly for an associated osteochondral fracture as described above. Following treatment of the osteochondral loose body, we typically perform a patellar

stabilization procedure in the form of an MPFL reconstruction or less commonly a medial retinacular/MPFL reefing with or without lateral retinacular release to reduce the risk of recurrent patellar instability.

Recurrent patellar instability is most common in adolescents, especially females. Risk factors have been identified and include age 16 years or less, abnormal Q angle, genu valgum, patella or trochlea dysplasia, LFC hypoplasia, femoral anteversion or external tibial torsion, VMO weakness, connective tissue disorders predisposing to patellar hypermobility (e.g., Ehlers–Danlos syndrome), elevated TT-TG distance, and multiple previous dislocations (Fig. 28-25).[6] Initial treatment is bracing followed by aggressive physical therapy for rehabilitation of the VMO/quadriceps muscles.

Algorithm 28-3. Authors' preferred treatment of patellar dislocations in children and adolescents. *Can be achieved with closure of medial parapatellar arthrotomy if used for open fixation of osteochondral fracture. **Consider guided growth if significant knee valgus. MPFL, medial patellofemoral ligament; MQTFL, medial quadriceps tendon–femoral ligament; ROM, range of motion; TT-TG, tibial tuberosity to trochlear groove distance.

Surgical intervention is indicated in children who continue to have subluxation or dislocation episodes. For the rare patient with minimal risk factors for recurrence or only minor, but recurrent symptomatic subluxation episodes, an isolated proximal soft tissue realignment procedure, consisting of medial retinaculum/MPFL reefing with lateral retinacular release or lengthening, may be considered (Fig. 28-26A).

More commonly, patients have multiple underlying risk factors (such as young age, trochlear dysplasia, elevated Q angles, hypermobility, and lateralized TT-TG distances), and an MPFL reconstruction with or without a distal realignment procedure is indicated. MPFL reconstruction allows for reconstitution of a robust medial patellar checkrein.[21,32,46] In our practice, a folded hamstring allograft (gracilis or semitendinosus) is generally used to reconstruct the MPFL with the folded portion used for femoral fixation.

It is important for the surgeon to ensure MPFL graft isometry and appropriate tension prior to establishing the insertion points during MPFL reconstruction. The goal of the reconstructed MPFL is to act as a checkrein from lateral patellar translation at knee ROM 0 to 30 degrees without increasing medial patellofemoral forces and to not tighten with knee flexion. Placing the MPFL insertion point proximal to the distal femoral physis will cause tightening of the graft with knee flexion and block knee flexion as the patient grows. Before securing the graft, isometry is checked by passing and securing a suture to the intended MPFL graft positions on the femur through the medial retinaculum and to the patella and then taking the knee through full ROM and ensuring the suture does night tighten in flexion but rather remains isometric or loosens slightly in knee flexion (where the MPFL is less important for patellar stability).

For skeletally immature patients, femoral fixation is achieved with a suture anchor or suture to periosteum at Schottle point[61] identified with intraoperative fluoroscopy ensuring a perfect lateral fluoroscopic image is obtained. Care is taken to ensure the femoral fixation point is distal to the distal medial femoral physis. For adolescents closer to skeletal maturity, femoral fixation of the folded portion of the hamstring autograft can also be achieved with a short and small bone tunnel and biocomposite interference screw fixation.

For patellar fixation, we prefer to utilize a single anchor into the patella at the third of the patella for the larger limb of the folded hamstring allograft. Fluoroscopy is utilized to confirm patellar insertion position. For the second limb, we prefer to pass this through the quadriceps tendon at the superior pole of the patella to replicate the medial quadriceps tendon–femoral ligament (MQTFL) as has been described by Fulkerson and Edgar,[67] although dual anchor patellar fixation is also well described.

A guided growth procedure such as medial hemiepiphysiodesis may be added in skeletally immature patients with significant genu valgum and patellar instability.

In skeletally *mature* patients with a significantly abnormal Q angle or elevated TT-TG distance (>16–20 mm), TTO in conjunction with medial plication or, more commonly, MPFL reconstruction is preferred. Tubercle medialization with the Elmslie–Trillat procedure (Fig. 28-26C) is effective in improving patellofemoral kinematics in the coronal plane, though a Fulkerson osteotomy incorporating anteriorization of the patella is preferred in cases with pre-existing patellar chondrosis or significant osteochondral injury which has undergone fixation or microfracture.

Postoperative Care

Following an MPFL reconstruction or medial reefing, patients are placed into a hinged knee brace with ROM limited to 0 to 30 degrees and protected weight bearing for the first 2 weeks. Patients start physical therapy and progress toward full weight bearing and increased ROM in the larger brace between weeks 3 and 6 postoperatively. They are then transitioned to a smaller knee brace and physical therapy advanced to full ROM at 6 weeks postoperatively. Patients who underwent a TTO procedure are kept at knee ROM 0 to 30 degrees and protected weight bearing until 6 weeks postoperatively. If there is radiographic evidence of healing, at 6 weeks, a smaller brace is used when ambulating. For both groups, straight-ahead running is allowed at 3 months postop, with advancement to agility and sports-specific exercises as indicated. Return to athletic activities is permitted at approximately 4 to 6 months postoperatively when full ROM is recovered and strength is symmetric.

Figure 28-25. Chronic lateral patellar subluxation in a 13-year-old girl.

A, B   **C**

Figure 28-26. Surgical technique for the treatment of chronic patellar subluxation or dislocation. **A:** Lateral retinacular release and medial imbrication. **B:** Semitendinosus tenodesis. **C:** Elmslie–Trillat procedure.

Potential Pitfalls and Preventive Measures

Repair of Patellar Dislocation: POTENTIAL PITFALLS AND PREVENTIONS	
Pitfall	**Prevention**
Unrecognized osteochondral fractures or chondral injuries	• Careful and detailed diagnostic arthroscopy to assess for chondral injuries in expected locations at start of patellar stabilization procedure
Overconstraint of the knee blocking flexion following MPFL reconstruction	• Ensure graft isometry and appropriate tension prior to establishing insertion points during MPFL reconstruction so MPFL acts as a medial "checkrein" at knee ROM 0–30 degrees without increasing medial patellofemoral forces and does not tighten with knee flexion
Patellar fracture from patellar fixation of MPFL graft	• Avoid using long tunnels (>20 mm), large-diameter tunnels (>5 mm), oblique tunnels, complete transpatellar tunnels, or multiple tunnels

Unrecognized osteochondral fractures may present later as loose bodies. Overzealous and injudicious use of lateral retinacular release may result in iatrogenic medial patellar instability. For MPFL reconstruction procedures, while there are conflicting reports about the appropriate degrees of knee flexion at which MPFL tensioning and fixation should be pursued, ranging from 30 to 90 degrees,[1,2,7,22,33,41,45,111,126,136,155,203] graft isometry and assessment of tension through a wide ROM is indicated to avoid increasing patellar contact forces.[22,126] Fluoroscopy is indicated to identify and confirm MPFL graft insertion points. We recommend against long tunnels (>20 mm), complete transpatellar tunnels, or multiple patellar tunnels to avoid subsequent patellar fracture.

Outcomes

A variety of surgical approaches are associated with relatively low rates of redislocation and good short-term knee scores in both adults and children.[1,15,36,142,203] Studies on MPFL reconstruction in pediatric and adolescent patients show promising results.[165] Allahabadi and Pandya[4] recently reported on 24 MPFL reconstructions in adolescents of mean age 15.7 (range 11–19). At a minimum of 2 years postoperatively, three (12.5%) had recurrent instability and there were no cases of growth disturbance.[4] Bremond et al.[31] reported a 9% redislocation rate and no cases of growth disturbance following MPFLR with soft tissue femoral fixation in 54 skeletally immature knees. Nelitz et al.[135] reported on anatomic MPFL reconstruction in 21 consecutive children of mean age 12.2 years (range 10.3–13.9 years). At mean 2.8-year follow-up, no recurrent dislocations occurred.

MANAGEMENT OF EXPECTED ADVERSE OUTCOMES AND UNEXPECTED COMPLICATION OF PATELLAR DISLOCATION

Patellar Dislocation:
COMMON ADVERSE OUTCOMES AND COMPLICATIONS

- Arthrofibrosis
- Patellar subluxation/instability
- Patellar redislocation

Recurrent patellar instability may occur, especially after lateral release alone without medial retinaculum repair.[154] Arthrofibrosis, with lack of knee flexion, may occur after MPFL reconstruction or Galeazzi tenodesis, if the graft is overly tensioned or positioned proximal to the distal femoral physis.[54] A recent report noted at 16% rate of complications following MPFL reconstruction in 179 knees in a young patient population.[146] Complications included recurrent lateral patellar instability (eight patients), knee motion stiffness with flexion deficits (eight patients), patellar fractures (six patients), and patellofemoral arthrosis/pain (five patients). Eighteen of 38 (47%) complications were secondary to technical factors and were considered preventable and female sex and bilateral MPFL reconstructions were risk factors associated with postoperative complications.[146] It is also possible to overconstrain the patellofemoral joint with an MPFL reconstruction if the MPFL graft is overtensioned which may increase contact pressure to the medial patellar cartilage leading to patellofemoral arthritis.[54,55,179] After TTO, nonunion, painful hardware requiring second surgery for screw removal, neurovascular injury, and compartment syndrome have been reported.

Ligament Injuries and Knee Dislocations

INTRODUCTION TO LIGAMENT INJURIES

Ligamentous injuries of the knee in children and adolescents were once considered rare. Tibial spine avulsion fractures were considered the pediatric ACL injury equivalent.[90,94,95] However, major ligamentous injuries are being seen with increased frequency and have received increased attention.[3,8,12,23,57,74,78,97,98,114,171,190] The increased frequency of diagnosis of knee ligament injuries in children is likely related to increased participation in youth sports at higher competitive levels and an increased awareness of injuries in this age group.

ACL injury has been reported in 10% to 65% of pediatric knees with acute traumatic hemarthroses in series ranging from 35 to 138 patients.[114,186] Stanitski[177] reported 70 children and adolescents with acute traumatic knee hemarthroses;

arthroscopic examination revealed ACL injuries in 47% of those 7 to 12 years of age and in 65% of those 13 to 18 years of age.

Injury patterns in the skeletally immature knee are dependent on the loading conditions and the developmental anatomy. Isolated knee ligament injury in children younger than 14 years of age was once believed to be rare because of the relative strength of the ligaments compared to the physes, but a report investigating rates of pediatric knee injuries presenting to a large children's hospital emergency room suggested that over a 12-year period, the rate of tibial spine fractures increased by 1%, whereas cases of ACL tears had increased by 11%.[159] The inherent ligamentous laxity in children also may offer some protection against ligament injury. Faster loading conditions favor ligamentous injuries, whereas slower loading conditions favor fracture. Narrowing of the intercondylar notch during skeletal development may also predispose to ligamentous injury.[94] Fractures and ligamentous injuries may also occur concurrently.

ASSESSMENT OF LIGAMENT INJURIES

MECHANISMS OF INJURY FOR LIGAMENT INJURIES

The mechanism of ligamentous injury varies with the child's age. In younger children, ligamentous injury is often associated with significant polytrauma. In contrast, adolescents are more likely to sustain ligamentous injury during contact sports or sports that require "cutting" maneuvers while running. Older adolescents may describe the knee as buckling or moving out of place and can usually relate the location and severity of their pain. Rapid intra-articular effusion within 2 hours of injury suggests hemarthrosis, most commonly from injury to the ACL. The most common mechanism in adolescents is abduction, flexion, and internal rotation of the femur on the tibia occurring during athletic competition when the weight-bearing extremity is struck from the lateral side.

Isolated injury of the LCL is rare in children, but a direct blow to the medial aspect of the knee may tear the LCL, usually with avulsion from the fibula or a physeal injury through the distal femur. MCL injuries are very common in young athletic adults but do also occur in children and adolescents and typically result from a direct lateral blow to the knee or a pivoting activity that produces a valgus moment across the joint.[102,153,168] They are most commonly purely ligamentous injuries although bony avulsions do occur. Isolated injuries of the ACL or PCL are more common. Disruption of the ACL with minimal injury to other supporting structures may be caused by hyperextension, marked internal rotation of the tibia on the femur, and pure deceleration. In contrast, isolated injury of the PCL most often is caused by a direct blow to the front of the tibia with the knee in flexion. The most extensive description of PCL injuries in children to date recently demonstrated that most of these injuries are sustained during sports, with less common causes including falls from height, trampoline injuries, and motor vehicle accidents.[99]

Figure 28-27. Valgus stress test of medial collateral ligament. Extremity is abducted off table, knee is flexed to 20 degrees, and valgus stress is applied. **A:** Frontal view. **B:** Lateral view.

INJURIES ASSOCIATED WITH LIGAMENT INJURIES

Common injuries associated with ACL tear include meniscus injuries (lateral more commonly than medial, in the acute setting) and MCL tears. MCL injuries are commonly seen with patellar dislocation events, both of which may be caused by a valgus moment across the knee.[102,150] Posterolateral corner and PCL injuries frequently occur in conjunction with each other. Complete and partial knee dislocations may have a variety of patterns of associated injuries.

SIGNS AND SYMPTOMS OF LIGAMENT INJURIES

In general, acute knee hemarthrosis suggests rupture of a cruciate ligament, an osteochondral fracture often associated with a patellar dislocation, a peripheral tear in the vascular portion of a meniscus, or a tear in the deep portion of the joint capsule. The absence of hemarthrosis is not, however, an indication of a less severe ligament injury, because with complete disruption, the blood in the knee joint may escape into the soft tissues.

Palpation of the collateral ligaments and their bony origins and insertions should locate tenderness at the site of the ligament injury. A defect in the collateral ligaments may be felt if the MCL is avulsed from its insertion on the tibia or if the LCL is avulsed from the fibular head. If the neurovascular status is normal, stability should be evaluated by varus/valgus stress testing, which may be done immediately after injury in cooperative adolescents but can be more difficult in younger ages or those with significant pain. Beginning the examination by testing the uninjured knee often calms patients and makes them more cooperative; it also establishes a baseline for assessing the ligamentous stability of the injured knee as knee laxity varies during childhood.[77] Valgus and varus stress testing of the MCL and LCL should be done at both 20 degrees of flexion and full extension, which may demonstrate gross instability if there is cruciate ligament rupture as well (Fig. 28-27).

The anterior drawer test, as described by Slocum, is the classic maneuver for testing the stability of the ACL (Fig. 28-28). The Lachman and pivot-shift tests, however, are considered

Figure 28-28. Anterior drawer test of anterior cruciate ligament. Foot is positioned in internal, external, and neutral rotation during examination. With anterior cruciate insufficiency, an anterior force (**A**) displaces the tibia forward (**B**).

Figure 28-29. Posterior cruciate ligament injury. Note posterior sagging of the tibia with posterior cruciate injury.

more sensitive for evaluating ACL injury when the examination can be done in a relaxed, cooperative adolescent, but may be confounded if there is significant guarding. The posterior drawer test (Fig. 28-29), quad active test, and assessment of the posterior sag sign are the key maneuvers for evaluation of the integrity of the PCL.

IMAGING AND OTHER DIAGNOSTIC STUDIES FOR LIGAMENT INJURIES

AP and lateral radiographs are obtained when any ligament injury of the knee is suspected in children. The radiographs are carefully inspected for evidence of occult epiphyseal or physeal fractures or bony avulsions. The intercondylar notch, especially, is inspected to detect a tibial spine fracture. Occasionally, a small fragment of bone avulsed from the medial femur or proximal tibia indicates injury to the MCL. Similarly, avulsion of a small fragment of bone from the proximal fibular epiphysis or the lateral aspect of the distal femur may indicate LCL injury.

MRI is frequently used to further delineate ligamentous injuries in the knee. MRI should be used to confirm an uncertain diagnosis or to gain further information that may affect treatment. Conventional MRI can give information regarding MCL injury, LCL injury, ACL injury, PCL injury, posterolateral corner injury, bone bruising, chondral injury, and meniscal injury.

CLASSIFICATION OF LIGAMENT INJURIES

Classification of knee ligament injuries is based on the severity of the injury, the specific anatomic location of the injury, and the direction of the subsequent instability caused by an isolated ligament injury or combination of ligament injuries.

A grade 1 ligament sprain is a tear of a minimal number of fibers of the ligament with localized tenderness but no instability. A grade 2 sprain is disruption of more ligamentous fibers, causing asymmetry with stress testing, compared with the contralateral knee, but minimal or minor instability. A grade 3 sprain is complete disruption of the ligament, resulting in gross instability. Although difficult to assess clinically, the degree of sprain also is determined with collateral ligaments during stress testing by the amount of separation of the joint surfaces: Grade 1 sprain, 5 mm or less (normal/baseline); grade 2 sprain, 5 to 10 mm; and grade 3 sprain, more than 10 mm.

The anatomic classification of knee ligament injuries (femoral attachment avulsion, midsubstance/interstitial tear, or tibial attachment avulsion) describes the exact location of the disruption, whether in the MCL (Fig. 28-30), ACL, LCL (Fig. 28-31), or PCL. Finally, the instability of the knee joint caused by the ligament disruption may be classified as having one-plane instability (simple or straight), rotary instability (anteromedial, anterolateral, posterolateral, or posteromedial), or combined instability (anterolateral–posterolateral, anterolateral–anteromedial, or anteromedial–posteromedial), which may be helpful in planning treatment.

Authors' Preferred Treatment of Ligament Injuries

Isolated Medial Collateral Ligament and Combined ACL/MCL Injuries (Algorithm 28-4)

Isolated grade I or II sprains of the MCL are treated with a hinged knee brace for 1 to 3 weeks. Return to sports is allowed when full ROM is achieved and the patient can run

and cut without pain. Isolated complete (grade III) disruption of the MCL can be treated with 6 weeks of immobilization in a hinged knee brace followed by formal physical therapy focused on rehabilitation of the quadriceps muscles and knee motion. Grade III disruptions of the MCL associated with an

Figure 28-30. Medial collateral ligament injury. **A:** Femoral origin. **B:** Middle portion. **C:** Tibial insertion.

Figure 28-31. Lateral collateral ligament injury. **A:** Femoral origin. **B:** Middle portion. **C:** Fibular insertion.

Algorithm 28-4. Authors' preferred treatment of medial cruciate ligament injuries.

ACL injury are usually treated with ACL-R without formal MCL repair, but medial stability must be confirmed under anesthesia prior to ACL-R, and ACL-R should be delayed at least 4 to 6 weeks to ensure adequate time for MCL healing. While some authors do not routinely employ hinged knee bracing following ACL-R, in the presence of an MCL tear, we recommend a hinged knee brace in the early postoperative period. Surgical treatment of isolated MCL injuries is rarely, if ever necessary. Acute repair could be considered in the setting of a large, widely displaced bony avulsion with significant associated knee instability or chronic reconstruction may be considered in the setting of symptomatic chronic valgus instability.

Isolated Anterior Cruciate Ligament (Algorithm 28-5)

When treating a skeletally immature athlete with an ACL injury, we divide patients into three groups: preadolescents, adolescents with significant growth remaining, and older adolescents with closing physes. Patients are classified based on skeletal age and physiologic age via Tanner staging. Skeletal age can be determined from an AP radiograph of the left hand and wrist as per the atlas of Greulich et al.[72] Alternatively, skeletal age can be estimated from knee radiographs as per the atlas of Pyle and Hoerr.[149] Physiologic age is established using the Tanner staging system (Table 28-3).

For preadolescent patients, who have the most growth remaining, we perform a physeal-sparing, combined intra-articular and extra-articular reconstruction utilizing autogenous iliotibial band (Fig. 28-32).[91,92] This procedure is a modification of the combined intra-articular and extra-articular reconstruction described by MacIntosh and Darby.[116] This procedure provides knee stability while avoiding the risk of iatrogenic growth disturbance by violating the distal femoral and/or proximal tibial physes. In our opinion, the consequences of potential iatrogenic growth disturbance caused by transphyseal reconstruction in these young patients are prohibitive, and the outcomes of this physeal-sparing technique[91,93] are comparable or superior to many series of adult-type reconstructions. Moreover, in a recent 3D motion analysis study, Sugimoto et al.[180] showed that ITB ACL-R appears to restore normal, symmetric, physiologic kinetic. and kinematic function in the growing knee by 1 year after reconstruction, with maintenance of normal parameters for up to 20 years. In a cadaveric study, Kennedy et al.[85] demonstrated better—AP and rotational stability than the all-epiphyseal and transphyseal over-the-top reconstruction techniques.

In adolescent patients with significant growth remaining, we perform a "physeal respecting" transphyseal ACL-R with autogenous hamstrings tendons with smaller centralized

Algorithm 28-5. Authors' preferred treatment for ACL reconstruction in skeletally immature patients.

TABLE 28-3. Tanner Staging Classification of Secondary Sexual Characteristics

Tanner Stage		Male	Female
Stage 1 (Prepubertal)	Growth Development	5–6 cm/year Testes <4 mL or <2.5 cm No pubic hair	5–6 cm/year No breast development No pubic hair
Stage 2	Growth Development	5–6 cm/year Testes 4 mL or 2.5–3.2 cm Minimal pubic hair at base of penis	7–8 cm/year Breast buds Minimal pubic hair on labia
Stage 3	Growth Development	7–8 cm/year Testes 12 mL or 3.6 cm Pubic hair over pubis Voice changes Muscle mass increases	8 cm/year Elevation of breast; areolae enlarge Pubic hair of mons pubis Axillary hair Acne
Stage 4	Growth Development	10 cm/year Testes 4.1–4.5 cm Pubic hair as adult Axillary hair Acne	7 cm/year Areolae enlarge Pubic hair as adult
Stage 5	Growth Development	No growth Testes as adult Pubic hair as adult Facial hair as adult Mature physique	No growth Adult breast contour Pubic hair as adult
Other		Peak height velocity: 13.5 years	Adrenarche: 6–8 years Menarche: 12.7 years Peak height velocity: 11.5 years

Figure 28-32. Physeal-sparing, combined intra- and extra-articular reconstruction utilizing autogenous iliotibial band for prepubescents. **A:** The iliotibial band graft is harvested free proximally and left attached to Gerdy tubercle distally. **B:** The graft is brought through the knee in the over-the-top position posteriorly. **C:** The graft is brought through the knee and under the intermeniscal ligament anteriorly. **D:** Resulting intra-articular and extra-articular reconstruction.

tunnels and suspensory fixation on the femur while avoiding bone plugs or fixation across physes.[101] Caution should be taken in these patients if new femoral tunnel drilling techniques are used to avoid significant obliquity of the distal femoral tunnel which would violate more of the distal femoral physis. In older adolescent patients approaching skeletal maturity, we perform conventional adult ACL-R with interference screw fixation using either autogenous central third patellar tendon or autogenous purely soft tissue graft (quadriceps or hamstrings).

In skeletally immature patients as in adult patients, acute ACL-R is not performed within the first 3 weeks after injury to minimize the risk of arthrofibrosis. Rehabilitation is instituted to regain ROM, decrease swelling, and resolve the reflex inhibition of the quadriceps. Skeletally immature patients must be emotionally mature enough to actively participate in the extensive rehabilitation required after ACL-R. Treatment of multiligamentous injuries that involve the ACL are discussed in the MCL, LCL, PCL, and knee dislocation sections.

Isolated Lateral Collateral Ligament and Combined ACL/LCL Injuries (Algorithm 28-6)

Grade III injuries of the LCL are extremely rare in children. Occasionally, the lateral capsular sign[200] is seen on radiographs obtained for evaluation of knee injury. Most often, the LCL is avulsed from the proximal fibular epiphysis, with or without a cortical fleck fragment, as proximal and midsubstance tears are uncommon. This injury is treated in the same manner as injury to the MCL. For isolated grade III injuries, a 6-week period of immobilization in a hinged knee brace is recommended. For the rare case of a large displaced LCL bony avulsion or combined LCL/posterolateral corner injury associated with a displaced bony avulsion in an unstable knee, acute repair may be considered.[191] If ACL injury is associated with a grade 1 or 2 LCL injury, treatment is ACL-R without formal LCL repair, but lateral stability must be confirmed under anesthesia prior to ACL-R, and ACL-R should be delayed at least 4 to 6 weeks to ensure adequate time for LCL healing. In the setting of a complete LCL avulsion with

Algorithm 28-6. Authors' preferred treatment of lateral cruciate ligament injuries.

complete ACL tear, repair of the LCL, in conjunction with ACL-R is pursued, usually between 2 and 4 weeks, so as to optimize the healing potential of the collateral ligament without undue risk of arthrofibrosis. If the surgery is delayed and tissue is suboptimal, ACL-R is combined with a posterolateral corner/LCL reconstruction with allograft as has been previously described.[106]

Isolated Posterior Cruciate Ligament and Combined ACL/PCL (Algorithm 28-7)

In general, PCL injuries have traditionally been considered rare in children, with most case reports describing a bony avulsion injury.[157] Kocher et al.[99] reported a series of 26 knees in patients aged 18 years or younger with PCL injuries, 15 of which underwent surgery for gross instability secondary to either a partial tear ($n = 1$, 7%), a complete ligamentous tear ($n = 4$, 27%), or an osteochondral avulsion fragment from either the tibial or femoral footprint ($n = 10$, 67%). Of note, 53% of the operative cohort had an additional ligamentous injury, and 60% had a meniscal tear.

For skeletally immature patients with isolated, purely ligamentous injuries, we treat nonoperatively with bracing and physical therapy focusing on quadriceps strengthening. For displaced bony avulsions similar to tibial spine fractures, we prefer acute repair. Bony avulsions of the femoral insertion can be treated with arthroscopic repair using bone tunnels and suture fixation, similar to tibial spine techniques, being careful to avoid the distal femoral physis. Bony avulsions of the tibia can be challenging to access and treat arthroscopically. If desired, an arthroscopic-assisted repair of avulsions through small bony tunnels, with the limbs of suture tied over a cortical bone bridge, similar to the technique described above for tibial spine fractures can be attempted. We prefer a formal open posteromedial approach for these injuries with direct repair of the avulsed tibial fragment back to its donor bed, with suture or screw fixation, being cautious to avoid implants across the proximal tibial physis. For skeletally mature adolescents with symptomatic chronic PCL insufficiency, we will perform a PCL reconstruction with adult-based techniques, generally with an Achilles allograft.

For combined ACL/PCL injuries, we typically treat the PCL injury nonoperatively with bracing for 6 weeks prior to ACL-R. We then assess the stability of the PCL intraoperatively during ACL-R and simultaneously reconstruct the PCL

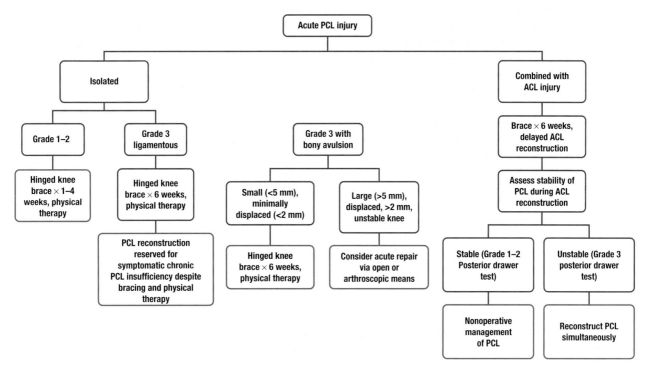

Algorithm 28-7. Authors' preferred treatment of posterior cruciate ligament injuries.

in the setting of chronic grade 3 laxity to posterior drawer testing.

Knee Dislocation (Algorithm 28-8)

Acute dislocations of the knee are uncommon in children because the forces required to produce dislocation are more likely to fracture the distal femoral or proximal tibial physis. Acute knee dislocation usually involves major injuries of associated soft tissues and ligaments and often neurovascular injuries. Injuries typically occur in older skeletally mature adolescents from high-energy trauma, such as motor vehicle injuries, pedestrian versus motor vehicle injury, bicycle versus motor vehicle injury, trampoline injuries, and high-energy contact sports.

Adequate follow-up studies of acute knee dislocations in children younger than 10 years of age are few, and most information has been obtained from reports of knee dislocations in adults. Because of the potential for associated vascular injury, acute knee dislocations in children may be emergent situations. The dislocation causes obvious deformity about the knee. With anterior dislocation, the tibia is prominent in an abnormal anterior position (Fig. 28-33). With posterior dislocation, the femoral condyles are abnormally prominent anteriorly.

After the dislocation is reduced, the stability of the knee should be evaluated with gentle stress testing. For isolated anterior or posterior dislocations, the integrity of the collateral ligaments should be carefully evaluated. Some knees

may spontaneously reduce after dislocation or reduce with manipulation of the leg for transport.

The neurovascular status of the extremity should be carefully evaluated both before and after reduction, especially the dorsalis pedis and posterior tibial pulses and peroneal nerve function. There is increasing evidence supporting the diagnostic and prognostic value of the ankle–brachial index,[128] which may be positive (<0.9) because of significant vascular injury, despite normal pulses and Doppler. Any abnormal vascular findings, either before or after reduction, require arteriography, which may be done in the operating room to facilitate rapid transition to repair. Popliteal artery laceration or intimal tear may occur in a fifth to a third of cases. Abnormalities in the sensory or motor function of the foot and distribution of the peroneal nerve function should be noted. Peroneal nerve injury has been reported in up to 40% of cases. MRI is usually performed to assess the integrity of the cruciate and collateral ligaments, the posterolateral and posteromedial corners, the menisci, and the articular surfaces.

Knee dislocation usually occurs with disruption of both cruciate ligaments. With direct anterior or posterior dislocation, the collateral ligaments and the soft tissues may be retained because the femoral condyles are stripped out of their capsular and collateral ligament attachments, and when reduced slip back inside them. Associated medial displacement is often accompanied by LCL disruption. Associated lateral displacement is often accompanied by MCL disruption. Knee dislocations in adolescents have been associated with tibial spine fractures, osteochondral fractures

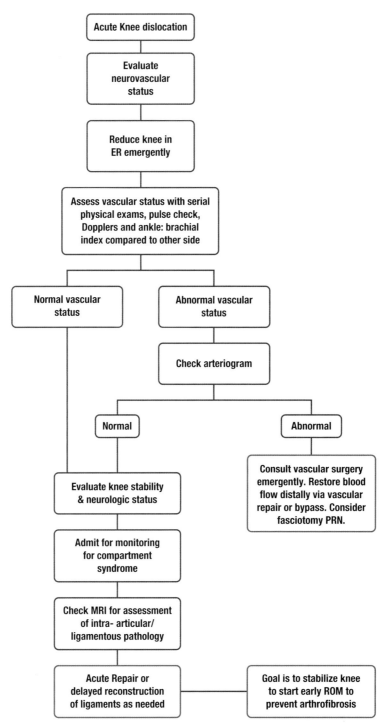

Algorithm 28-8. Authors' preferred treatment of knee dislocation.

of the femur or tibia, meniscal injuries, and peroneal nerve injuries.

Treatment of knee dislocations includes both acute and delayed reconstructive management. Acutely, the knee is reduced under anesthesia. If emergent vascular surgery is necessary, fasciotomies are usually also performed. However, ligamentous reconstruction is typically delayed. The knee is braced with protected weight bearing and limited motion, or occasionally application of external fixation is warranted to protect the vascular repair.

Figure 28-33. Anteromedial dislocation of the knee in a 14-year-old girl. **A:** AP x-ray. **B:** Lateral x-ray.

Multiligamentous reconstruction may be delayed approximately 2 to 4 weeks after injury, depending on the injury pattern. Primary ligament repairs become more difficult after this period of time because of scarring and lack of definition of tissues. Reconstructions may be staged or performed in a single multiligamentous knee procedure. Surgery often combines arthroscopic and open techniques. General principles include ligament repair or reconstruction for collateral ligament injuries, ligament reconstruction for midsubstance cruciate ligament injuries, and meniscal repair. Allograft tissue is often used for the PCL/ MCL or LCL when necessary because of the multiligamentous nature of the injury and the need to minimize tourniquet time and any additional knee trauma that would come from graft harvesting. Postoperatively, prolonged immobilization should be avoided because of the substantial risk of arthrofibrosis after knee dislocation surgery. Limited motion in a hinged knee brace and protected weight bearing are prescribed, followed by increasing mobilization and strengthening.

Annotated References

Reference	Annotation
Cruz AI Jr, Lee RJ, Kushare I, et al. Tibial spine fractures in young athletes. *Clin Sports Med.* 2022;41(4):653–670.	The Tibial Spine Research Group reports on current management of tibial spine fractures in young athletes
Fabricant PD, Yen YM, Kramer DE, et al. Fixation of traumatic chondral-only fragments of the knee in pediatric and adolescent athletes: a retrospective multicenter report. *Orthop J Sports Med.* 2018;6(2):2325967117753140.	This study reports on successful treatment of fixation of chondral-only loose bodies in the pediatric and adolescent knee
Featherall J, Metz AK, Froerer DL, et al. The Schöttle point is consistently located distal to the medial femoral physis in pediatric patients: a digitally reconstructed radiographic study. *Am J Sports Med.* 2022;50(13):3565–3570.	This study describes the location of Schottle point in pediatric patients as distal to the medial femoral physis
Flachsmann R, Broom ND, Hardy AE, Moltschaniwskyj G. Why is the adolescent joint particularly susceptible to osteochondral shear fracture? *Clin Orthop Relat Res.* 2000;381:212–221.	A histopathologic study that helps to explain the occurrence of osteochondral fractures in the skeletally immature at an ultrastructural level

Annotated References

Reference	Annotation
Gurusamy P, Pedowitz JM, Carroll AN, et al. Medial patellofemoral ligament reconstruction for adolescents with acute first-time patellar dislocation with an associated loose body. *Am J Sports Med*. 2021;49(8):2159–2164.	This study reports on the success of treating acute first-time patellar dislocations in adolescents with an associated loose body with loose body excision versus repair and concomitant MPFL reconstruction
Lewallen LW, McIntosh AL, Dahm DL. Predictors of recurrent instability after acute patellofemoral dislocation in pediatric and adolescent patients. *Am J Sports Med*. 2013;41(3):575–581.	This article reports on the importance of young age and trochlear dysplasia as risk factors for recurrent instability following patellar dislocations in young patients
Meyers MH, McKeever FM. Fracture of the intercondylar eminence of the tibia. *J Bone Joint Surg Am*. 1970;52:1677–1684.	Origin of classification system for tibial spine fractures
Mills WJ, Barei DP, McNair P. The value of the ankle-brachial index for diagnosing arterial injury after knee dislocation: a prospective study. *J Trauma*. 2004;56(6):1261–1265.	The authors report on a prospective study of 38 patients that supports the ABI as a rapid, reliable, noninvasive tool for diagnosing vascular injury associated with knee dislocation
Sousa PL, Stuart MJ, Prince MR, Dahm DL. Nonoperative management of minimally displaced patellar sleeve fractures. *J Knee Surg*. 2021;34(3):242–246.	The authors report on a case series of minimally displaced patellar sleeve fractures that were successfully managed nonoperatively with excellent clinical outcomes

REFERENCES

1. Ahmad CS, Brown GD, Stein BES. The docking technique for medial patellofemoral ligament reconstruction: surgical technique and clinical outcome. *Am J Sports Med*. 2009;37(10):2021–2027.
2. Ahmad CS, Stein BE, Matuz D, Henry JH. Immediate surgical repair of the medial patellar stabilizers for acute patellar dislocation: a review of eight cases. *Am J Sports Med*. 2000;28(6):804–810.
3. Aichroth PM, Patel DV, Zorrilla P. The natural history and treatment of rupture of the anterior cruciate ligament in children and adolescents. A prospective review. *J Bone Joint Surg Br*. 2002;84(1):38–41.
4. Allahabadi S, Pandya NK. Allograft medial patellofemoral ligament reconstruction in adolescent patients results in a low recurrence rate of patellar dislocation or subluxation at midterm follow-up. *Arthroscopy*. 2022;38(1):128–138.
5. Alleyne KR, Galloway MT. Management of osteochondral injuries of the knee. *Clin Sports Med*. 2001;20(2):343–364.
6. Amis AA. Current concepts on anatomy and biomechanics of patellar stability. *Sports Med Arthrosc Rev*. 2007;15:48–56.
7. Amis AA, Firer P, Mountney J, et al. Anatomy and biomechanics of the medial patellofemoral ligament. *Knee*. 2003;10(3):215–220.
8. Anderson AF. Transepiphyseal replacement of the anterior cruciate ligament in skeletally immature patients. A preliminary report. *J Bone Joint Surg Am*. 2003;85-A(7):1255–1263.
9. Anderson AF, Pagnani MJ. Osteochondritis dissecans of the femoral condyles. Long-term results of excision of the fragment. *Am J Sports Med*. 1997;25(6):830–834.
10. Anderson CN, Nyman JS, McCullough KA, et al. Biomechanical evaluation of physeal-sparing fixation methods in tibial eminence fractures. *Am J Sports Med*. 2013;41(7):1586–1594.
11. Arendt EA, Dejour D. Patella instability: building bridges across the ocean a historic review. *Knee Surg Sports Traumatol Arthrosc*. 2013;21(2):279–293.
12. Aronowitz ER, Ganley TJ, Goode JR, et al. Anterior cruciate ligament reconstruction in adolescents with open physes. *Am J Sports Med*. 2000;28(2):168–175.
13. Askenberger M, Arendt EA, Ekström W, et al. Medial patellofemoral ligament injuries in children with first-time lateral patellar dislocations: a magnetic resonance imaging and arthroscopic study. *Am J Sports Med*. 2016;44(1):152–158.
14. Aulisa AG, Falciglia F, Giordano M, et al. Galeazzi's modified technique for recurrent patella dislocation in skeletally immature patients. *J Orthop Sci*. 2012;17(2):148–155.
15. Baier C, Springorum HR, Beckmann J, et al. Treatment of patellar instability in children and adolescents. *Orthopade*. 2011;40(10):868–876.
16. Bakalim G, Wilppula E. Closed treatment of fracture of the tibial spines. *Injury*. 1974;5(3):210–212.
17. Balcarek P, Jung K, Frosch KH, Stürmer KM. Value of the tibial tuberosity-trochlear groove distance in patellar instability in the young athlete. *Am J Sports Med*. 2011;39(8):1756–1761.
18. Balcarek P, Walde TA, Frosch S, et al. Patellar dislocations in children, adolescents and adults: a comparative MRI study of medial patellofemoral ligament injury patterns and trochlear groove anatomy. *Eur J Radiol*. 2011;79(3):415–420.
19. Bale RS, Banks AJ. Arthroscopically guided Kirschner wire fixation for fractures of the intercondylar eminence of the tibia. *J R Coll Surg Edinb*. 1995;40(4):260–262.
20. Baxter MP, Wiley JJ. Fractures of the tibial spine in children. An evaluation of knee stability. *J Bone Joint Surg Br*. 1988;70(2):228–230.
21. Beasley LS, Vidal AF. Traumatic patellar dislocation in children and adolescents: treatment update and literature review. *Curr Opin Pediatr*. 2004;16(1):29–36.
22. Beck P, Brown NAT, Greis PE, Burks RT. Patellofemoral contact pressures and lateral patellar translation after medial patellofemoral ligament reconstruction. *Am J Sports Med*. 2007;35(9):1557–1563.
23. Behr CT, Potter HG, Paletta GA Jr. The relationship of the femoral origin of the anterior cruciate ligament and the distal femoral physeal plate in the skeletally immature knee. An anatomic study. *Am J Sports Med*. 2001;29(6):781–787.
24. Bentley G, Biant LC, Carrington RWJ, et al. A prospective, randomised comparison of autologous chondrocyte implantation versus mosaicplasty for osteochondral defects in the knee. *J Bone Joint Surg Br*. 2003;85(2):223–230.
25. Berg EE. Pediatric tibial eminence fractures: arthroscopic cannulated screw fixation. *Arthroscopy*. 1995;11(3):328–331.
26. Bicos J, Fulkerson JP, Amis A. Current concepts review: the medial patellofemoral ligament. *Am J Sports Med*. 2007;35(3):484–492.
27. Birk GT, DeLee JC. Osteochondral injuries. Clinical findings. *Clin Sports Med*. 2001;20(2):279–286.
28. Black SR, Meyers KN, Nguyen JT, et al. Comparison of ligament isometry and patellofemoral contact pressures for medial patellofemoral ligament reconstruction techniques in skeletally immature patients. *Am J Sports Med*. 2020;48(14):3557–3565.
29. Bohndorf K. Imaging of acute injuries of the articular surfaces (chondral, osteochondral and subchondral fractures). *Skeletal Radiol*. 1999;28(10):545–560.
30. Bong MR, Romero A, Kubiak E, et al. Suture versus screw fixation of displaced tibial eminence fractures: a biomechanical comparison. *Arthroscopy*. 2005;21(10):1172–1176.
31. Bremond N, Prima R, Rabattu PY, et al. Isolated MPFL reconstruction with soft tissue femoral fixation technique in 54 skeletally immature patients: Clinical outcomes at 2 years follow-up: a French multicenter retrospective study. *Orthop Traumatol Surg Res*. 2022;103530.
32. Brown GD, Ahmad CS. Combined medial patellofemoral ligament and medial patellotibial ligament reconstruction in skeletally immature patients. *J Knee Surg*. 2008;21(4):328–332.
33. Buckens CFM, Saris DB. Reconstruction of the medial patellofemoral ligament for treatment of patellofemoral instability: a systematic review. *Am J Sports Med*. 2010;38(1):181–188.
34. Camathias C, Gögüs U, Hirschmann MT, et al. Implant failure after biodegradable screw fixation in osteochondritis dissecans of the knee in skeletally immature patients. *Arthroscopy*. 2015;31(3):410–415.
35. Camp CL, Heidenreich MJ, Dahm DL, et al. Individualizing the tibial tubercle-trochlear groove distance: patellar instability ratios that predict recurrent instability. *Am J Sports Med*. 2016;44(2):393–399.
36. Camp CL, Krych AJ, Dahm DL, et al. Medial patellofemoral ligament repair for recurrent patellar dislocation. *Am J Sports Med*. 2010;38(11):2248–2254.
37. Casalonga A, Bourelle S, Chalencon F, et al. Tibial intercondylar eminence fractures in children: the long-term perspective. *Orthop Traumatol Surg Res*. 2010;96(5):525–530.
38. Cash JD, Hughston JC. Treatment of acute patellar dislocation. *Am J Sports Med*. 1988;16(3):244–249.
39. Chotel F, Bérard J, Raux S. Patellar instability in children and adolescents. *Orthop Traumatol Surg Res*. 2014;100(1 Suppl):S125–S137.

40. Chotel F, Knorr G, Simian E, et al; French Arthroscopy Society. Knee osteochondral fractures in skeletally immature patients: French multicenter study. *Orthop Traumatol Surg Res.* 2011;97(8 Suppl):S154–S159.
41. Christiansen SE, Jacobsen BW, Lund B, Lind M. Reconstruction of the medial patellofemoral ligament with gracilis tendon autograft in transverse patellar drill holes. *Arthroscopy.* 2008;24(1):82–87.
42. Christiansen SE, Jakobsen BW, Lund B, Lind M. Isolated repair of the medial patellofemoral ligament in primary dislocation of the patella: a prospective randomized study. *Arthroscopy.* 2008;24(8):881–887.
43. Conchie H, Clark D, Metcalfe A, et al. Adolescent knee pain and patellar dislocations are associated with patellofemoral osteoarthritis in adulthood: a case control study. *Knee.* 2016;23(4):708–711.
44. Cruz AI Jr, Lee RJ, Kushare I, et al; PRiSM, Tibial Spine Research Interest Group. Tibial spine fractures in young athletes. *Clin Sports Med.* 2022;41(4):653–670.
45. Davis DK, Fithian DC. Techniques of medial retinacular repair and reconstruction. *Clin Orthop Relat Res.* 2002;(402):38–52.
46. Deie M, Ochi M, Sumen Y, et al. Reconstruction of the medial patellofemoral ligament for the treatment of habitual or recurrent dislocation of the patella in children. *J Bone Joint Surg Br.* 2003;85(6):887–890.
47. Dejour H, Walch G, Nove-Josserand L, Guier C. Factors of patellar instability: an anatomic radiographic study. *Knee Surg Sports Traumatol Arthrosc.* 1994;2(1):19–26.
48. Desio SM, Burks RT, Bachus KN. Soft tissue restraints to lateral patellar translation in the human knee. *Am J Sports Med.* 1998;26(1):59–65.
49. Di Caprio F, Buda R, Ghermandi R, et al. Combined arthroscopic treatment of tibial plateau and intercondylar eminence avulsion fractures. *J Bone Joint Surg Am.* 2010;92(Suppl 2):161–169.
50. Dickens AJ, Morrell NT, Doering A, et al. Tibial tubercle-trochlear groove distance: defining normal in a pediatric population. *J Bone Joint Surg Am.* 2014;96(4):318–324.
51. Dines JS, Fealy S, Potter HG, Warren RF. Outcomes of osteochondral lesions of the knee repaired with a bioabsorbable device. *Arthroscopy.* 2008;24(1):62–68.
52. Düppe K, Gustavsson N, Edmonds EW. Developmental morphology in childhood patellar instability: age-dependent differences on magnetic resonance imaging. *J Pediatr Orthop.* 2016;36(8):870–876.
53. Eggers AK, Becker C, Weimann A, et al. Biomechanical evaluation of different fixation methods for tibial eminence fractures. *Am J Sports Med.* 2007;35(3):404–410.
54. Elias JJ, Cosgarea AJ. Technical errors during medial patellofemoral ligament reconstruction could overload medial patellofemoral cartilage: a computational analysis. *Am J Sports Med.* 2006;34(9):1478–1485.
55. Elias JJ, Jones KC, Lalonde MK, et al. Allowing one quadrant of patellar lateral translation during medial patellofemoral ligament reconstruction successfully limits maltracking without overconstraining the patella. *Knee Surg Sports Traumatol Arthrosc.* 2018;26(10):2883–2890.
56. Enea D, Busilacchi A, Cecconi S, Gigante A. Late-diagnosed large osteochondral fracture of the lateral femoral condyle in an adolescent: a case report. *J Pediatr Orthop B.* 2013;22(4):344–349.
57. Engebretsen L, Steffen K, Bahr R, et al. The International Olympic Committee Consensus statement on age determination in high-level young athletes. *Br J Sports Med.* 2010;44(7):476–484.
58. Fabricant PD, Yen YM, Kramer DE, et al. Fixation of chondral-only shear fractures of the knee in pediatric and adolescent athletes. *J Pediatr Orthop.* 2017;37(2):156.
59. Fabricant PD, Yen YM, Kramer DE, et al. Fixation of traumatic chondral-only fragments of the knee in pediatric and adolescent athletes: a retrospective multicenter report. *Orthop J Sports Med.* 2018;6(2):2325967117753140.
60. Farr J. Autologous chondrocyte implantation improves patellofemoral cartilage treatment outcomes. *Clin Orthop Relat Res.* 2007;463:187–194.
61. Featherall J, Metz AK, Froerer DL, et al. The Schöttle point is consistently located distal to the medial femoral physis in pediatric patients: a digitally reconstructed radiographic study. *Am J Sports Med.* 2022;50(13):3565–3570.
62. Felus J, Kowalczyk B. Age-related differences in medial patellofemoral ligament injury patterns in traumatic patellar dislocation: case series of 50 surgically treated children and adolescents. *Am J Sports Med.* 2012;40(10):2357–2364.
63. Feucht MJ, Brucker PU, Camathias C, et al. Meniscal injuries in children and adolescents undergoing surgical treatment for tibial eminence fractures. *Knee Surg Sports Traumatol Arthrosc.* 2017;25(2):445–453.
64. Flachsmann R, Broom ND, Hardy AE, Moltschaniwskyj G. Why is the adolescent joint particularly susceptible to osteochondral shear fracture? *Clin Orthop Relat Res.* 2000;381:212–221.
65. Flynn JM, Kocher MS, Ganley TJ. Osteochondritis dissecans of the knee. *J Pediatr Orthop.* 2004;24(4):434–443.
66. Fulkerson JP, Becker GJ, Meaney JA, et al. Anteromedial tibial tubercle transfer without bone graft. *Am J Sports Med.* 1990;18(5):490–496.
67. Fulkerson JP, Edgar C. Medial quadriceps tendon-femoral ligament: surgical anatomy and reconstruction technique to prevent patella instability. *Arthrosc Tech.* 2013;2(2):e125–e128.
68. Furlan D, Pogorelić Z, Biočić M, et al. Pediatric tibial eminence fractures: arthroscopic treatment using K-wire. *Scand J Surg.* 2010;99(1):38–44.
69. Gkiokas A, Morassi LG, Kohl S, et al. Bioabsorbable pins for treatment of osteochondral fractures of the knee after acute patella dislocation in children and young adolescents. *Adv Orthop.* 2012;2012:249687.
70. Gobbi A, Kon E, Berruto M, et al. Patellofemoral full-thickness chondral defects treated with second-generation autologous chondrocyte implantation: results at 5 years' follow-up. *Am J Sports Med.* 2009;37(6):1083–1092.
71. Grannatt K, Heyworth BE, Ogunwole O, et al. Galeazzi semitendinosus tenodesis for patellofemoral instability in skeletally immature patients. *J Pediatr Orthop.* 2012;32(6):621–625.
72. Greulich WW, Pyle SI, Todd TW. *Radiographic Atlas of Skeletal Development of the Hand and Wrist.* Stanford University Press; 1959.
73. Gurusamy P, Pedowitz JM, Carroll AN, et al. Medial patellofemoral ligament reconstruction for adolescents with acute first-time patellar dislocation with an associated loose body. *Am J Sports Med.* 2021;49(8):2159–2164.
74. Guzzanti V, Falciglia F, Stanitski CL. Preoperative evaluation and anterior cruciate ligament reconstruction technique for skeletally immature patients in Tanner stages 2 and 3. *Am J Sports Med.* 2003;31(6):941–948.
75. Haas JP, Collins MS, Stuart MJ. The "sliver sign": a specific radiographic sign of acute lateral patellar dislocation. *Skeletal Radiol.* 2012;41(5):595–601.
76. Henderson IJ, Lavigne P. Periosteal autologous chondrocyte implantation for patellar chondral defect in patients with normal and abnormal patellar tracking. *Knee.* 2006;13(4):274–279.
77. Hinton RY, Rivera VR, Pautz MJ, Sponseller PD. Ligamentous laxity of the knee during childhood and adolescence. *J Pediatr Orthop.* 2008;28(2):184–187.
78. Houle JB, Letts M, Yang J. Effects of a tensioned tendon graft in a bone tunnel across the rabbit physis. *Clin Orthop Relat Res.* 2001;391:275–281.
79. Hua GJ, Liu YP, Xu PR, Luo YC. Arthroscopic minimally invasive treatment of tibial intercondylar eminence fractures in children. *Zhongguo Gu Shang.* 2011;24(9):723–725.
80. Huang TW, Hsu KY, Cheng CY, et al. Arthroscopic suture fixation of tibial eminence avulsion fractures. *Arthroscopy.* 2008;24(11):1232–1238.
81. Hughston JC, Deese M. Medial subluxation of the patella as a complication of lateral retinacular release. *Am J Sports Med.* 1988;16(4):383–388.
82. Husen M, Krych AJ, Stuart MJ, et al. Successful fixation of traumatic articular cartilage-only fragments in the juvenile and adolescent knee: a case series. *Orthop J Sports Med.* 2022;10(11):23259671221138074.
83. Ishibashi Y, Tsuda E, Sasaki T, Toh S. Magnetic resonance imaging AIDS in detecting concomitant injuries in patients with tibial spine fractures. *Clin Orthop Relat Res.* 2005;(434):207–212.
84. Janarv PM, Westblad P, Johansson C, Hirsch G. Long-term follow-up of anterior tibial spine fractures in children. *J Pediatr Orthop.* 1995;15(1):63–68.
85. Kennedy A, Coughlin DG, Metzger MF, et al. Biomechanical evaluation of pediatric anterior cruciate ligament reconstruction techniques. *Am J Sports Med.* 2011;39(5):964–971.
86. Kennedy JC. *The Injured Adolescent Knee.* Williams & Wilkins; 1979.
87. Kepler CK, Bogner EA, Hammoud S, et al. Zone of injury of the medial patellofemoral ligament after acute patellar dislocation in children and adolescents. *Am J Sports Med.* 2011;39(7):1444–1449.
88. Kieser DC, Gwynne-Jones D, Dreyer S. Displaced tibial intercondylar eminence fractures. *J Orthop Surg (Hong Kong).* 2011;19(3):292–296.
89. Kocher M, Micheli LJ. The pediatric knee: evaluation and treatment. In: Insall JN, Scott WN, eds. *Surgery of the Knee.* 3rd ed. Churchill-Livingstone; 2001:1356–1397.
90. Kocher MS, Foreman ES, Micheli LJ. Laxity and functional outcome after arthroscopic reduction and internal fixation of displaced tibial spine fractures in children. *Arthroscopy.* 2003;19(10):1085–1090.
91. Kocher MS, Garg S, Micheli LJ. Physeal sparing reconstruction of the anterior cruciate ligament in skeletally immature prepubescent children and adolescents. *J Bone Joint Surg Am.* 2005;87(11):2371–2379.
92. Kocher MS, Garg S, Micheli LJ. Physeal sparing reconstruction of the anterior cruciate ligament in skeletally immature prepubescent children and adolescents. Surgical technique. *J Bone Joint Surg Am.* 2006;88(suppl 1 pt 2):283–293.
93. Kocher MS, Heyworth BE, Fabricant PD, et al. Outcomes of physeal-sparing ACL reconstruction with iliotibial band autograft in skeletally immature prepubescent children. *J Bone Joint Surg Am.* 2018;100(13):1087–1094.
94. Kocher MS, Mandiga R, Klingele K, et al. Anterior cruciate ligament injury versus tibial spine fracture in the skeletally immature knee: a comparison of skeletal maturation and notch width index. *J Pediatr Orthop.* 2004;24(2):185–188.
95. Kocher MS, Micheli LJ, Gerbino P, Hresko MT. Tibial eminence fractures in children: prevalence of meniscal entrapment. *Am J Sports Med.* 2003;31(3):404–407.
96. Kocher MS, Micheli LJ, Yaniv M, et al. Functional and radiographic outcome of juvenile osteochondritis dissecans of the knee treated with transarticular arthroscopic drilling. *Am J Sports Med.* 2001;29(5):562–566.
97. Kocher MS, Micheli LJ, Zurakowski D, Luke A. Partial tears of the anterior cruciate ligament in children and adolescents. *Am J Sports Med.* 2002;30(5):697–703.
98. Kocher MS, Saxon HS, Hovis WD, Hawkins RJ. Management and complications of anterior cruciate ligament injuries in skeletally immature patients: survey of the Herodicus Society and The ACL Study Group. *J Pediatr Orthop.* 2002;22(4):452–457.
99. Kocher MS, Shore B, Nasreddine AY, Heyworth BE. Treatment of posterior cruciate ligament injuries in pediatric and adolescent patients. *J Pediatr Orthop.* 2012;32(6):553–560.
100. Kocher MS, Smith JT, Iversen MD, et al. Reliability, validity, and responsiveness of a modified International Knee Documentation Committee Subjective Knee Form (Pedi-IKDC) in children with knee disorders. *Am J Sports Med.* 2011;39(5):933–939.
101. Kocher MS, Smith JT, Zoric BJ, et al. Transphyseal anterior cruciate ligament reconstruction in skeletally immature pubescent adolescents. *J Bone Joint Surg Am.* 2007;89(12):2632–2639.
102. Kramer DE, Miller PE, Berrahou IK, et al. Collateral ligament knee injuries in pediatric and adolescent athletes. *J Pediatr Orthop.* 2020;40(2):71–77.
103. Kramer DE, Pace JL. Acute traumatic and sports-related osteochondral injury of the pediatric knee. *Orthop Clin North Am.* 2012;43(2):227–236.
104. Kramer DE, Yen YM, Simoni MK, et al. Surgical management of osteochondritis dissecans lesions of the patella and trochlea in the pediatric and adolescent population. *Am J Sports Med.* 2015;43(3):654–662.
105. Lafrance RM, Giordano B, Goldblatt J, et al. Pediatric tibial eminence fractures: evaluation and management. *J Am Acad Orthop Surg.* 2010;18(7):395–405.

106. Larsen MW, Moinfar AR, Moorman CT III. Posterolateral corner reconstruction: fibular-based technique. *J Knee Surg.* 2005;18(2):163–166.

107. Lee BJ, Christino MA, Daniels AH, et al. Adolescent patellar osteochondral fracture following patellar dislocation. *Knee Surg Sports Traumatol Arthrosc.* 2013;21(8):1856–1861.

108. Lewallen L, McIntosh A, Dahm D. First-time patellofemoral dislocation: risk factors for recurrent instability. *J Knee Surg.* 2015;28(4):303–309.

109. Lewallen LW, McIntosh AL, Dahm DL. Predictors of recurrent instability after acute patellofemoral dislocation in pediatric and adolescent patients. *Am J Sports Med.* 2013;41(3):575–581.

110. Liao W, Li Z, Zhang H, et al. Arthroscopic fixation of tibial eminence fractures: a clinical comparative study of nonabsorbable sutures versus absorbable suture anchors. *Arthroscopy.* 2016;32(8):1639–1650.

111. Lind M, Jakobsen BW, Lund B, Christiansen SE. Reconstruction of the medial patellofemoral ligament for treatment of patellar instability. *Acta Orthop.* 2008;79(3):354–360.

112. Louis ML, Guillaume JM, Launay F, et al. Surgical management of type II tibial intercondylar eminence fractures in children. *J Pediatr Orthop B.* 2008;17(5):231–235.

113. Lowe J, Chaimsky G, Freedman A, et al. The anatomy of tibial eminence fractures: arthroscopic observations following failed closed reduction. *J Bone Joint Surg Am.* 2002;84-A(11):1933–1938.

114. Luhmann SJ. Acute traumatic knee effusions in children and adolescents. *J Pediatr Orthop.* 2003;23(2):199–202.

115. Ma LF, Wang CH, Chen BC, et al. Medial patellar retinaculum plasty versus medial capsule reefing for patellar dislocation in children and adolescents. *Arch Orthop Trauma Surg.* 2012;132(12):1773–1780.

116. MacIntosh DL, Darby DT. Lateral substitution reconstruction in proceedings and reports of universities, colleges, councils, and associations. *J Bone Joint Surg Br.* 1976;58:142.

117. Mahar AT, Duncan D, Oka R, et al. Biomechanical comparison of four different fixation techniques for pediatric tibial eminence avulsion fractures. *J Pediatr Orthop.* 2008;28(2):159–162.

118. Mandelbaum BR, Browne JE, Fu F, et al. Articular cartilage lesions of the knee. *Am J Sports Med.* 1998;26(6):853–861.

119. Mann MA, Desy NM, Martineau PA. A new procedure for tibial spine avulsion fracture fixation. *Knee Surg Sports Traumatol Arthrosc.* 2012;20(12):2395–2398.

120. Maquet P. Advancement of the tibial tuberosity. *Clin Orthop Relat Res.* 1976;(115):225–230.

121. Marsh JS, Daigneault JP, Sethi P, Polzhofer GK. Treatment of recurrent patellar instability with a modification of the Roux-Goldthwait Technique. *J Pediatr Orthop.* 2006;26(4):461–465.

122. Marx RG, Jones EC, Allen AA, et al. Reliability, validity, and responsiveness of four knee outcome scales for athletic patients. *J Bone Joint Surg Am.* 2001;83-A(10):1459–1469.

123. Matelic TM, Aronsson DD, Boyd DW Jr, LaMont RL. Acute hemarthrosis of the knee in children. *Am J Sports Med.* 1995;23(6):668–671.

124. Mayer C, Magnussen RA, Servien E, et al. Patellar tendon tenodesis in association with tibial tubercle distalization for the treatment of episodic patellar dislocation with patella alta. *Am J Sports Med.* 2012;40(2):346–351.

125. McLennan JG. The role of arthroscopic surgery in the treatment of fractures of the intercondylar eminence of the tibia. *J Bone Joint Surg Br.* 1982;64(4):477–480.

126. Melegari TM, Parks BG, Matthews LS. Patellofemoral contact area and pressure after medial patellofemoral ligament reconstruction. *Am J Sports Med.* 2008;36(4):747–752.

127. Meyers MH, McKeever FM. Fracture of the intercondylar eminence of the tibia. *J Bone Joint Surg Am.* 1970;52:1677–1684.

128. Mills WJ, Barei DP, McNair P. The value of the ankle-brachial index for diagnosing arterial injury after knee dislocation: a prospective study. *J Trauma.* 2004;56(6):1261–1265.

129. Mitchell J, Magnussen RA, Collins CL, et al. Epidemiology of patellofemoral instability injuries among high school athletes in the United States. *Am J Sports Med.* 2015;43(7):1676–1682.

130. Mitchell JJ, Mayo MH, Axibal DP, et al. Delayed anterior cruciate ligament reconstruction in young patients with previous anterior tibial spine fractures. *Am J Sports Med.* 2016;44(8):2047–2056.

131. Molander ML, Wallin G, Wikstad I. Fracture of the intercondylar eminence of the tibia: a review of 35 patients. *J Bone Joint Surg Br.* 1981;63-B(1):89–91.

132. Momaya AM, Read C, Steirer R, Estes R. Outcomes after arthroscopic fixation of tibial eminence fractures with bioabsorbable nails in skeletally immature patients. *J Pediatr Orthop B.* 2018;27:8–12.

133. Mulhall KJ, Dowdall J, Grannell M, McCabe JP. Tibial spine fractures: an analysis of outcome in surgically treated type III injuries. *Injury.* 1999;30(4):289–292.

134. Nakamura N, Horibe S, Iwahashi T, et al. Healing of a chondral fragment of the knee in an adolescent after internal fixation. A case report. *J Bone Joint Surg Am.* 2004;86-A(12):2711–2716.

135. Nelitz M, Dreyhaupt J, Reichel H, et al. Anatomic reconstruction of the medial patellofemoral ligament in children and adolescents with open growth plates: surgical technique and clinical outcome. *Am J Sports Med.* 2013;41(1):58–63.

136. Nelitz M, Reichel H, Dornacher D, Lippacher S. Anatomical reconstruction of the medial patellofemoral ligament in children with open growth-plates. *Arch Orthop Trauma Surg.* 2012;132(11):1647–1651.

137. Nelitz M, Theile M, Dornacher D, et al. Analysis of failed surgery for patellar instability in children with open growth plates. *Knee Surg Sports Traumatol Arthrosc.* 2012;20(5):822–828.

138. Nikku R, Nietosvaara Y, Aalto K, Kallio PE. Operative treatment of primary patellar dislocation does not improve medium-term outcome: a 7-year follow-up report and risk analysis of 127 randomized patients. *Acta Orthop.* 2005;76(5):699–704.

139. Nomura E, Inoue M, Kobayashi S. Long-term follow-up and knee osteoarthritis change after medial patellofemoral ligament reconstruction for recurrent patellar dislocation. *Am J Sports Med.* 2007;35(11):1851–1858.

140. Nomura E, Inoue M, Kurimura M. Chondral and osteochondral injuries associated with acute patellar dislocation. *Arthroscopy.* 2003;19(7):717–721.

141. Noyes FR, DeLucas JL, Torvik PJ. Biomechanics of anterior cruciate ligament failure: an analysis of strain-rate sensitivity and mechanisms of failure in primates. *J Bone Joint Surg Am.* 1974;56(2):236–253.

142. Oliva F, Ronga M, Longo UG, et al. The 3-in-1 procedure for recurrent dislocation of the patella in skeletally immature children and adolescents. *Am J Sports Med.* 2009;37(9):1814–1820.

143. Pace JL, Nasreddine AY, Simoni M, et al. Dynamic splinting in children and adolescents with stiffness after knee surgery. *J Pediatr Orthop.* 2018;38:38–43.

144. Palmu S, Kallio PE, Donell ST, et al. Acute patellar dislocation in children and adolescents: a randomized clinical trial. *J Bone Joint Surg Am.* 2008;90(3):463–470.

145. Parikh SN, Lykissas MG. Classification of lateral patellar instability in children and adolescents. *Orthop Clin North Am.* 2016;47(1):145–152.

146. Parikh SN, Nathan ST, Wall EJ, Eismann EA. Complications of medial patellofemoral ligament reconstruction in young patients. *Am J Sports Med.* 2013;41(5):1030–1038.

147. Patel NM, Park MJ, Sampson NR, Ganley TJ. Tibial eminence fractures in children: earlier posttreatment mobilization results in improved outcomes. *J Pediatr Orthop.* 2012;32(2):139–144.

148. Peterson L, Minas T, Brittberg M, Lindahl A. Treatment of osteochondritis dissecans of the knee with autologous chondrocyte transplantation: results at two to ten years. *J Bone Joint Surg Am.* 2003;85-A(suppl 2):17–24.

149. Pyle SI, Hoerr NL. *A Radiographic Standard of Reference the Growing Knee.* Charles Thomas; 1969.

150. Quinlan JF, Farrelly C, Kelly G, Eustace S. Co-existent medial collateral ligament injury seen following transient patellar dislocation: observations at magnetic resonance imaging. *Br J Sports Med.* 2010;44(6):411–414.

151. Quinlan NJ, Hobson TE, Mortensen AJ, et al. Tibial spine repair in the pediatric population: outcomes and subsequent injury rates. *Arthrosc Sports Med Rehabil.* 2021;3(4):e1011–e1023.

152. Repo JP, Uimonen MM, Nevalainen MT, et al. Outcomes following the operative treatment of intra-articular fracture combined with medial patellofemoral ligament reconstruction after patellar dislocation. *Knee Surg Relat Res.* 2022;34(1):21.

153. Roach CJ, Haley CA, Cameron KL, et al. The epidemiology of medial collateral ligament sprains in young athletes. *Am J Sports Med.* 2014;42(5):1103–1109.

154. Robles E, Michelin RM, Schlechter JA. Use of an accessory anteromedial portal to facilitate repair of mid-body radial tears of the lateral meniscus in children and adolescents. *Arthrosc Tech.* 2021;10(12):e2675–e2681.

155. Ronga M, Oliva F, Giuseppe Longo U, et al. Isolated medial patellofemoral ligament reconstruction for recurrent patellar dislocation. *Am J Sports Med.* 2009;37(9):1735–1742.

156. Rorabeck CH, Bobechko WP. Acute dislocation of the patella with osteochondral fracture: a review of eighteen cases. *J Bone Joint Surg Br.* 1976;58(2):237–240.

157. Ross AC, Chesterman PJ. Isolated avulsion of the tibial attachment of the posterior cruciate ligament in childhood. *J Bone Joint Surg Br.* 1986;68(5):747.

158. Rothermich MA, Nepple JJ, Raup VT, et al. A Comparative analysis of international knee documentation committee scores for common pediatric and adolescent knee injuries. *J Pediatr Orthop.* 2016;36(3):274–277.

159. Sampson NR, Beck NA, Baldwin KD, et al. Knee injuries in children and adolescents: has there been an increase in ACL and meniscus tears in recent years?. In: Presented at the 2011 American Academy of Pediatrics National Conference and Exhibition. 15–18(Abstract 14815).

160. Sanders TL, Pareek A, Hewett TE, et al. Incidence of first-time lateral patellar dislocation: a 21-year population-based study. *Sports Health.* 2018;10:146–151.

161. Schmal H, Strohm PC, Niemeyer P, et al. Fractures of the patella in children and adolescents. *Acta Orthop Belg.* 2010;76(5):644–650.

162. Schneppendahl J, Thelen S, Twehues S, et al. The use of biodegradable sutures for the fixation of tibial eminence fractures in children: a comparison using PDS II, Vicryl and FiberWire. *J Pediatr Orthop.* 2013;33(4):409–414.

163. Seeley M, Bowman KF, Walsh C, et al. Magnetic resonance imaging of acute patellar dislocation in children: patterns of injury and risk factors for recurrence. *J Pediatr Orthop.* 2012;32(2):145–155.

164. Seeley MA, Knesek M, Vanderhave KL. Osteochondral injury after acute patellar dislocation in children and adolescents. *J Pediatr Orthop.* 2013;33(5):511–518.

165. Shamrock AG, Day MA, Duchman KR, et al. Medial patellofemoral ligament reconstruction in skeletally immature patients: a systematic review and meta-analysis. *Orthop J Sports Med.* 2019;7(7):2325967119855023.

166. Sharma A, Lakshmanan P, Peehal J, David H. An analysis of different types of surgical fixation for avulsion fractures of the anterior tibial spine. *Acta Orthop Belg.* 2008;74(1):90–97.

167. Shea KG, Grimm NL, Belzer J, et al. The relation of the femoral physis and the medial patellofemoral ligament. *Arthroscopy.* 2010;26(8):1083–1087.

168. Shea KG, Grimm NL, Ewing CK, Aoki SK. Youth sports anterior cruciate ligament and knee injury epidemiology: who is getting injured? In what sports? When?. *Clin Sports Med.* 2011;30(4):691–706.

169. Shea KG, Grimm NL, Laor T, Wall E. Bone bruises and meniscal tears on MRI in skeletally immature children with tibial eminence fractures. *J Pediatr Orthop.* 2011;31(2):150–152.

170. Shea KG, Pfeiffer R, Wang JH, et al. Anterior cruciate ligament injury in pediatric and adolescent soccer players: an analysis of insurance data. *J Pediatr Orthop.* 2004;24(6):623–628.

171. Shelbourne KD, Gray T, Wiley BV. Results of transphyseal anterior cruciate ligament reconstruction using patellar tendon autograft in tanner stage 3 or 4 adolescents with clearly open growth plates. *Am J Sports Med.* 2004;32(5):1218–1222.

172. Shimberg JL, Leska TM, Cruz AI Jr, et al. Is nonoperative treatment appropriate for all patients with type 1 tibial spine fractures? A multicenter study of the Tibial Spine Research Interest Group. *Orthop J Sports Med.* 2022;10(6):23259671221099572.
173. Smillie I. *Injuries of the Knee Joint.* Churchill-Livingstone; 1978.
174. Smith HJ, Richardson JB, Tennant A. Modification and validation of the Lysholm Knee Scale to assess articular cartilage damage. *Osteoarthritis Cartilage.* 2009;17(1):53–58.
175. Smith JB. Knee instability after fractures of the intercondylar eminence of the tibia. *J Pediatr Orthop.* 1984;4(4):462–464.
176. Sousa PL, Stuart MJ, Prince MR, Dahm DL. Nonoperative management of minimally displaced patellar sleeve fractures. *J Knee Surg.* 2021;34(3):242–246.
177. Stanitski CL. Correlation of arthroscopic and clinical examinations with magnetic resonance imaging findings of injured knees in children and adolescents. *Am J Sports Med.* 1998;26(1):2–6.
178. Steadman JR, Briggs KK, Rodrigo JJ, et al. Outcomes of microfracture for traumatic chondral defects of the knee: average 11-year follow-up. *Arthroscopy.* 2003;19(5):477–484.
179. Stephen JM, Kittl C, Williams A, et al. Effect of medial patellofemoral ligament reconstruction method on patellofemoral contact pressures and kinematics. *Am J Sports Med.* 2016;44(5):1186–1194.
180. Sugimoto D, Whited AJ, Brodeur JJ, et al. Long-term follow-up of skeletally immature patients with physeal-sparing combined extra-/intra-articular iliotibial band anterior cruciate ligament reconstruction: a 3-dimensional motion analysis. *Am J Sports Med.* 2020;48(8):1900–1906.
181. Thaunat M, Erasmus PJ. Recurrent patellar dislocation after medial patellofemoral ligament reconstruction. *Knee Surg Sports Traumatol Arthrosc.* 2008;16(1):40–43.
182. Trillat A, Dejour H, Couette A. Diagnosis and treatment of recurrent dislocations of the patella. *Rev Chir Orthop Reparatrice Appar Mot.* 1964;50:813–824.
183. Tudisco C, Giovarruscio R, Febo A, et al. Intercondylar eminence avulsion fracture in children: long-term follow-up of 14 cases at the end of skeletal growth. *J Pediatr Orthop B.* 2010;19(5):403–408.
184. Uchida R, Toritsuka Y, Yoneda K, et al. Chondral fragment of the lateral femoral trochlea of the knee in adolescents. *Knee.* 2012;19(5):719–723.
185. Uppstrom TJ, Price M, Black S, et al. Medial patellofemoral ligament (MPFL) reconstruction technique using an epiphyseal femoral socket with fluoroscopic guidance helps avoid physeal injury in skeletally immature patients. *Knee Surg Sports Traumatol Arthrosc.* 2019;27(11):3536–3542.
186. Vahasarja V, Kinnuen P, Serlo W. Arthroscopy of the acute traumatic knee in children. Prospective study of 138 cases. *Acta Orthop Scand.* 1993;64(5):580–582.
187. Vander Have KL, Ganley TJ, Kocher MS, et al. Arthrofibrosis after surgical fixation of tibial eminence fractures in children and adolescents. *Am J Sports Med.* 2010;38(2):298–301.
188. Vargas B, Lutz N, Dutoit M, Zambelli PY. Nonunion after fracture of the anterior tibial spine: case report and review of the literature. *J Pediatr Orthop B.* 2009;18(2):90–92.
189. Vega JR, Irribarra LA, Baar AK, et al. Arthroscopic fixation of displaced tibial eminence fractures: a new growth plate-sparing method. *Arthroscopy.* 2008;24(11):1239–1243.
190. Volpi P, Galli M, Bait C, Pozzoni R. Surgical treatment of anterior cruciate ligament injuries in adolescents using double-looped semitendinosus and gracilis tendons: supraepiphysary femoral and tibial fixation. *Arthroscopy.* 2004;20(4):447–449.
191. von Heideken J, Mikkelsson C, Boström Windhamre H, Janarv PM. Acute injuries to the posterolateral corner of the knee in children: a case series of 6 patients. *Am J Sports Med.* 2011;39(10):2199–2205.
192. Walsh SJ, Boyle MJ, Morganti V. Large osteochondral fractures of the lateral femoral condyle in the adolescent: outcome of bioabsorbable pin fixation. *J Bone Joint Surg Am.* 2008;90(7):1473–1478.
193. Weltsch D, Chan CT, Mistovich RJ, et al. Predicting risk of recurrent patellofemoral instability with measurements of extensor mechanism containment. *Am J Sports Med.* 2021;49(3):706–712.
194. Wessel LM, Scholz S, Rüsch M, et al. Hemarthrosis after trauma to the pediatric knee joint: what is the value of magnetic resonance imaging in the diagnostic algorithm? *J Pediatr Orthop.* 2001;21(3):338–342.
195. Wiley JJ, Baxter MP. Tibial spine fractures in children. *Clin Orthop Relat Res.* 1990;(255):54–60.
196. Wilfinger C, Castellani C, Raith J, et al. Nonoperative treatment of tibial spine fractures in children-38 patients with a minimum follow-up of 1 year. *J Orthop Trauma.* 2009;23(7):519–524.
197. Willis RB, Blokker C, Stoll TM, et al. Long-term follow-up of anterior tibial eminence fractures. *J Pediatr Orthop.* 1993;13(3):361–364.
198. Woo R, Busch MT. Management of patellar instability in children. *Oper Tech Sports Med.* 1998;6:247–258.
199. Woo SL, Hollis JM, Adams DJ, et al. Tensile properties of the human femur-anterior cruciate ligament-tibia complex. The effects of specimen age and orientation. *Am J Sports Med.* 1991;19(3):217–225.
200. Woods GW, Stanley RF, Tullos HS. Lateral capsular sign: x-ray clue to a significant knee instability. *Am J Sports Med.* 1979;7(1):27–33.
201. Wouters DB, De Graaf JS, Hemmer PH, et al. The arthroscopic treatment of displaced tibial spine fractures in children and adolescents using Meniscus Arrows®. *Knee Surg Sports Traumatol Arthrosc.* 2011;19(5):736–739.
202. Zaricznyj B. Avulsion fracture of the tibial eminence: treatment by open reduction and pinning. *J Bone Joint Surg Am.* 1977;59(8):1111–1114.
203. Zhao J, Huangfu X, He Y, Liu W. Recurrent patellar dislocation in adolescents: medial retinaculum plication versus vastus medialis plasty. *Am J Sports Med.* 2012;40(1):123–132.

29

Fractures of the Shaft of the Tibia and Fibula

Brendan A. Williams and Christine Ann Ho

Fractures of the Shaft of the Tibia and Fibula

INTRODUCTION TO FRACTURES OF THE SHAFT OF THE TIBIA AND FIBULA

The true incidence of tibia/fibula fractures in pediatric patients is unknown. The most recent North American data are derived from a review of a national U.S. injury database reported by Naranje et al. in 2016.[96] The authors found that fractures of the tibial/fibular shaft are the second most common long bone fractures in children, after forearm fractures, with an annual occurrence of 11 per 1,000 children over the course of childhood.[96] In addition, fractures of tibia and fibula are the second most frequent injuries among pediatric orthopaedic trauma admissions (21.5%), after femur fractures.[40] The peak incidence occurs in children between the ages of 10 and 14 years[96] with an approximate 2:1 ratio of males to females injured.[40,65]

Seventy percent of pediatric tibial fractures are isolated injuries; ipsilateral fibular fractures occur with 30% of tibial fractures.[21,139] These fractures can be incomplete (torus, greenstick) or complete. Shannak reviewed 117 pediatric tibia fractures in 1988 and found that 51% occurred in the distal third, and 39% in the middle third.[121] In that study, 35% of pediatric tibial fractures were oblique, 32% comminuted, 20% transverse, and 13% spiral.[121] Isolated spiral or short oblique tibia fractures (often minimally or nondisplaced) in children less than 3 to 4 years of age constitute a unique fracture type often termed a "toddler's fracture."

ASSESSMENT OF FRACTURES OF THE SHAFT OF THE TIBIA AND FIBULA

MECHANISMS OF INJURY FOR FRACTURES OF THE SHAFT OF THE TIBIA AND FIBULA

Rotational forces result in oblique or spiral fractures and are responsible for approximately 80% of all tibial fractures that present without an associated fibular fracture.[21,87,121] Most tibial fractures in children of 4 to 14 years of age are the result of sporting or traffic accidents.[21,87,121] In addition, the tibia is one of the most commonly fractured long bones in abused children.[70] Approximately 11% to 26% of all abused children with a long bone injury have a fractured tibia.[81,108] The vast majority of tibia fracture in children and adolescents, regardless of mechanism, are closed injuries.

INJURIES ASSOCIATED WITH FRACTURES OF THE SHAFT OF THE TIBIA AND FIBULA

Concomitant fractures of the ankle and foot are the most common injuries associated with fractures of the tibia and fibula, followed by humeral, femoral, and radial/ulnar fractures.[18] In a 1994 report, the average Injury Severity Score of a child with a tibial fracture was 10 (range 0–45) with an average hospital stay of 6.5 days (range 1–50 days).[18] There have been no updates of this information in the recent English literature. Isolated fibular fractures are fairly uncommon in children, and in the majority of cases are the results of a direct blow to the area of the fracture.[53,130]

CLASSIFICATION OF FRACTURES OF THE SHAFT OF THE TIBIA AND FIBULA

Nonphyseal injuries of the tibia and the fibula can be classified into three major categories based on the combination of bones fractured and the location of the injuries. These include fractures of the proximal or distal tibial metaphysis, and those involving the diaphyseal region.

PATHOANATOMY AND APPLIED ANATOMY OF FRACTURES OF THE SHAFT OF THE TIBIA AND FIBULA

BONY STRUCTURE OF THE TIBIA AND FIBULA

The tibia ("flute") is the second largest bone in the body. There are two concave condyles at the proximal aspect of the tibia. The medial condyle is larger, deeper, and narrower than the lateral condyle. An elevated process, the tibial tubercle, located anteriorly between the two condyles, is the site of attachment of the patellar tendon. The shaft of the tibia is the shape of a prism, with a broad proximal extent that decreases in size until the distal third, where it gradually increases again in size. The tibial crest is prominent anteromedially from the tibial tubercle to the tibial plafond and is subcutaneous without overlying musculature.

The tibia develops from three ossification centers: one in the shaft and one each in the proximal and distal epiphysis. The tibial diaphysis begins to ossify at 7 weeks of gestation and ossification expands proximally and distally. The proximal epiphyseal center appears shortly after birth and unites with the shaft as the growth plate closes between 14 and 16 years of age. The distal epiphyseal ossification center appears in the second year of life, and the distal tibial physis closes between 14 and 15 years of age. Average age of growth plate closure varies between males and females. Additional ossification centers are found occasionally in the medial malleolus and in the tibial tubercle. The tibia articulates with the condyles of the femur proximally, with the fibula at the knee and the ankle, and with the talus distally.[46] Twelve muscles have either their origin or insertion on the tibia (Table 29-1).

The fibula articulates with the tibia and the talus. The fibular diaphysis ossifies at approximately 8 weeks of gestation. The distal fibular ossification center becomes visible at approximately 2 years of age, in most patients, and the proximal secondary ossification center generally appears at 4 years. The distal fibular physis closes completely by approximately 16 years; the proximal physis closes later, between the ages of 15 and 18 years. Nine muscles have either their origin or insertion on the fibula (Table 29-2).

TABLE 29-1. Muscle Origins and Insertions on the Tibia

Muscle	Origin or Insertion
Semimembranosus	Inserts on the inner tuberosity of the proximal tibia
Tibialis anterior, extensor digitorum longus, biceps femoris	Insert into lateral condyle of the tibia
Sartorius, gracilis, semitendinosus	Insert into the proximal medial surface of the tibial metaphysis
Popliteus	Inserts into posterior metadiaphysis of the tibia
Tibialis anterior	Arises from the lateral surface of the tibial diaphysis
Soleus, flexor digitorum longus, tibialis posterior	Arise from to the posterior diaphysis of the tibia
Patellar tendon	Inserts into the tibial tubercle
Tensor fascia lata	Inserts to Gerdy tubercle, the lateral aspect of the proximal tibial metaphysis
Secondary slip of the tensor fascia lata	Occasionally inserts into the tibial tubercle

VASCULAR ANATOMY OF THE TIBIA AND FIBULA

The popliteal artery descends vertically and posteriorly between the condyles of the femur and passes between the medial and lateral heads of the gastrocnemius muscle. It ends at the distal border of the popliteus muscle, where it divides into the anterior and posterior tibial arteries. The anterior tibial artery passes between the tibia and the fibula over the proximal aspect of the intraosseous membrane, enters the anterior compartment of the lower leg, and divides into a series of smaller branches. The posterior tibial artery divides several centimeters distal to this point, giving rise to the peroneal artery that travels in the deep posterior compartment of the leg (Fig. 29-1).

TABLE 29-2. Muscle Origins and Insertions on the Fibula

Muscle	Origin or Insertion
Biceps femoris	Inserts into head of fibula
Soleus, flexor hallucis longus, tibialis posterior	Arise from the posterior aspect of the fibular diaphysis
Peroneus longus, peroneus brevis	Arise from the lateral aspect of the fibular diaphysis
Extensor digitorum longus, peroneus tertius, extensor hallucis longus	Arise from the anterior surface of the fibular shaft

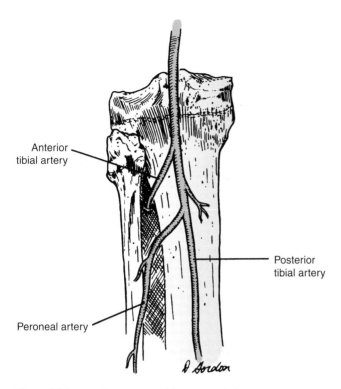

Figure 29-1. Vascular anatomy of the proximal tibia.

NEURAL ANATOMY OF THE TIBIA AND FIBULA

The posterior tibial nerve runs adjacent and posterior to the popliteal artery in the popliteal fossa and then enters the deep posterior compartment of the leg after it gives off a branch as the medial sural cutaneous nerve. The posterior tibial nerve provides innervation to the muscles of the deep posterior compartment and sensation to the plantar aspect of the foot. The common peroneal nerve passes laterally around the proximal neck of the fibula. It divides into deep and superficial branches and then passes into the anterior and the lateral compartments of the lower leg, respectively. Each branch innervates the muscles within its compartment. The deep peroneal nerve provides sensation to the first web space. The superficial branch is responsible for sensation across the dorsal and lateral aspects of the foot. The lateral sural cutaneous nerve arises from the common peroneal nerve proximal to the knee.

FASCIAL COMPARTMENTS

The lower leg has four fascial compartments (Fig. 29-2). The anterior compartment contains the extensor digitorum longus, the extensor hallucis longus, and the tibialis anterior muscles as well as the anterior tibial artery and deep peroneal nerve. The lateral compartment contains the peroneus longus and brevis muscles and the superficial peroneal nerve. The superficial posterior compartment contains the soleus and gastrocnemius muscles. The deep posterior compartment contains the flexor digitorum longus, the flexor hallucis longus, and the tibialis posterior muscles as well as the posterior tibial artery, peroneal artery, and posterior tibial nerves.

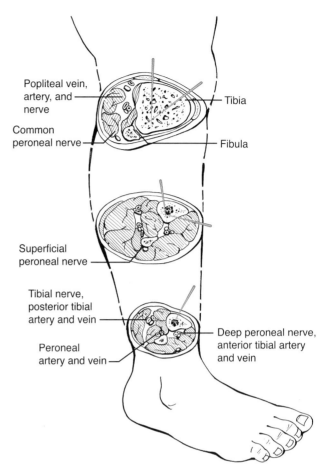

Figure 29-2. Fibroosseous compartments of the leg.

Fractures of the Proximal Tibial Metaphysis

INTRODUCTION TO FRACTURES OF THE PROXIMAL TIBIAL METAPHYSIS

Proximal tibial fractures are the least common nonphyseal tibial fractures in children.[4] Greater attention is given to the sequelae of pediatric proximal tibial metaphyseal fractures than to the management of the acute injury itself. The peak incidence for proximal tibia metaphyseal fractures is between the ages of 3 and 6 years.[71,92] The most common mechanism of injury is a low-energy force applied to the lateral aspect of the extended knee either directly or indirectly through axial loading. The cortex of the medial tibial metaphysis fails in tension, often resulting in an incomplete greenstick fracture. Compression (torus) and complete fractures can occur in this area but are less common. The fibula generally escapes injury, although plastic deformation may occur.[26] As a child matures, physeal fractures are seen more commonly in the proximal tibia due to the relative weakness of the physis compared to maturing cortical bone.[71]

ASSESSMENT OF FRACTURES OF THE PROXIMAL TIBIAL METAPHYSIS

MECHANISM OF INJURY OF PROXIMAL TIBIAL METAPHYSIS FRACTURES

Pediatric proximal tibial metaphyseal fractures most commonly occur secondary to valgus force, followed by varus, then extension, and finally flexion. An axial load on an extended knee, such as during trampoline-related activities, is a common mechanism for the valgus fractures. Varus metaphyseal fractures are rarer; it is hypothesized that the proximal fibula may act as a protective buttress on the lateral tibial metaphysis.[92]

INJURIES ASSOCIATED WITH FRACTURES OF THE PROXIMAL TIBIAL METAPHYSIS

Unlike physeal proximal tibial fractures, there are few associated injuries that occur in conjunction with proximal tibial metaphyseal fractures. Completely displaced metaphyseal fractures may be associated with injury to the popliteal artery, but this is an uncommon scenario in this younger age group.

SIGNS AND SYMPTOMS OF FRACTURES OF THE PROXIMAL TIBIAL METAPHYSIS

Children with proximal tibia metaphyseal fractures present with pain, swelling, and tenderness in the region of the fracture. Motion of the knee causes moderate pain, and in most cases, the child will not walk. Crepitance is seldom identified on physical examination, particularly if the fracture is incomplete.

IMAGING AND OTHER DIAGNOSTIC STUDIES FOR FRACTURES OF THE PROXIMAL TIBIAL METAPHYSIS

Orthogonal plain radiographs of the affected tibia are sufficient to diagnose proximal tibial metaphyseal fractures in most cases.

Radiographs usually demonstrate a complete or greenstick fracture of the proximal tibial metaphysis. The medial aspect of the fracture often is widened, producing a valgus deformity of the proximal tibia. Subtle fractures from a purely axial load may not be visualized on radiographs, but an increase in the anterior tilt angle of the proximal tibial physis (an anterior slope of the tibial plateau) may be detected on the lateral radiograph and may serve as indirect evidence of a fracture (Fig. 29-3).[131]

CLASSIFICATION OF FRACTURES OF THE PROXIMAL TIBIAL METAPHYSIS

There is no commonly accepted comprehensive classification system specifically for pediatric proximal tibial metaphyseal fractures; however, Mubarak et al.[92] provided a more global descriptive system of proximal tibial fractures dividing injuries based on the direction of force (valgus, varus, extension, and flexion/avulsion; Fig. 29-4). Varus and valgus injuries typically result in metaphyseal or physeal proximal tibial injuries, while extension and flexion avulsion injuries are more commonly associated with epiphyseal and apophyseal injuries, respectively, and typically occur in older pediatric age groups.

OUTCOME MEASURES FOR FRACTURES OF THE PROXIMAL TIBIAL METAPHYSIS

There are no commonly used outcome measures for fractures of the proximal tibial metaphysis.

PATHOANATOMY AND APPLIED ANATOMY RELATED TO PROXIMAL TIBIAL METAPHYSIS FRACTURES

The popliteal artery, popliteal vein, and tibial nerve vein lie close to the posterior proximal tibia. As the popliteal artery exits the

Figure 29-3. Anteroposterior (**A**) and lateral (**B**) radiographs of the proximal tibial metaphyseal fracture with an intact fibula in a 3-year-old child. Note the subtle increased anterior angle of the proximal tibial physis.

Figure 29-4. Classification schemes for pediatric proximal tibial fractures. (Adapted from Mubarak SJ, et al. Classification of proximal tibial fractures in children. *J Child Orthop.* 2009;3:191–197.)

distal popliteus muscle, it divides into the anterior and posterior tibial arteries. The anterior tibial artery pierces the interosseous membrane at the level of the fibular neck and joins the deep peroneal nerve in the anterior compartment of the leg. The tibial nerve lies adjacent to the posterior tibial artery in the deep posterior compartment of the leg. The common peroneal nerve lies just posterior and deep to the inserting tendon of the biceps femoris and courses anteriorly at the level of the fibular neck, where it divides into the deep and superficial peroneal nerves. Open approaches to the proximal tibia are rarely needed to remove interposed tissue, but when required, they are most safely performed from the medial side to avoid the neurovascular structures and to access the pes anserinus if repair is needed.

TREATMENT OPTIONS FOR FRACTURES OF THE PROXIMAL TIBIAL METAPHYSIS

NONOPERATIVE TREATMENT OF FRACTURES OF THE PROXIMAL TIBIAL METAPHYSIS

Indications/Contraindications

Nonoperative Treatment of Fractures of the Proximal Tibial Metaphysis:
INDICATIONS AND CONTRAINDICATIONS

Indications

- Nondisplaced closed fractures
- Displaced closed fractures amenable to closed reduction

Contraindications

- Open fractures
- Body habitus unamenable to long-leg cast treatment
- Failure to attain or maintain adequate closed reduction in a cast

Casting

Nondisplaced proximal tibial metaphyseal fractures can be treated with an appropriately padded long-leg cast for 4 to 6 weeks until there is radiographic healing, the fracture is nontender, and the patient can bear weight comfortably. As many of these fractures occur in younger children who may have limited verbal skills, care must be taken to place sufficient cast padding in areas of bony prominence and to mold the cast so as to minimize the risk of slippage. This level of attention to detail will aid in limiting skin breakdown and irritation, such as over the calcaneal tuberosity. A pillow under the calf with the heel free floating also helps to prevent cast-related pressure injuries of the heel. In a standard medial metaphyseal fracture, a varus mold should be applied as the fracture tends to go into valgus over time, one of the rare situations in orthopaedics when initial varus may be of benefit.

Displaced proximal tibial metaphyseal fractures are treated with closed manipulation under sedation or general anesthesia. Fluoroscopy is useful to verify reduction. A slight varus mold in the cast is preferred to anticipate the postfracture tibial valgus that may occur. While a long-leg cast in flexion may help to prevent weight bearing, it is often easier to mold, manipulate, and radiographically visualize the fracture with a long-leg cast in a position closer to full extension. Most of these transverse fractures are stable enough to permit weight bearing as tolerated (Fig. 29-5).

Figure 29-5. Anteroposterior and lateral radiographs of the proximal tibia and distal femur in a child who sustained a nondisplaced fracture of the proximal tibial and fibular metaphysis. The knee is casted in extension which facilitates accurate measurements of fracture alignment.

OPERATIVE TREATMENT OF PROXIMAL TIBIAL METAPHYSIS FRACTURES

Indications/Contraindications

In rare cases, an acceptable closed reduction cannot be attained or maintained, and an open reduction is required. This may be secondary to interposition of soft tissue in the fracture site, usually on the medial side. In such a situation, a standard approach to the anteromedial proximal tibia may be required to facilitate removal and fracture reduction. The pes anserinus insertion may also be repaired through this approach if necessary. Occasionally, a larger adolescent child may have a body habitus that precludes successful cast treatment, or severe swelling may also exclude circumferential casting as a safe treatment option.

Percutaneous fixation with smooth pins or an external fixator may be required in rare circumstances. Pin placement should avoid physeal violation and knee joint penetration if possible. Retrograde insertion of smooth crossed pins may be technically easier than an antegrade approach, and careful dissection should be used to avoid injury to the deep peroneal nerve and anterior tibial artery on the lateral entry point. Stabilization with pins or external fixation is often useful in polytrauma patients or those with extensive associated soft tissue injuries (Fig. 29-6).

Figure 29-6. Clinical photo of a 3-year-old girl 4 months after right proximal tibia fracture demonstrating Cozen phenomenon. (Courtesy of Keith Baldwin, MD.)

Authors' Preferred Treatment of Fractures of the Proximal Tibial Metaphysis (Algorithm 29-1)

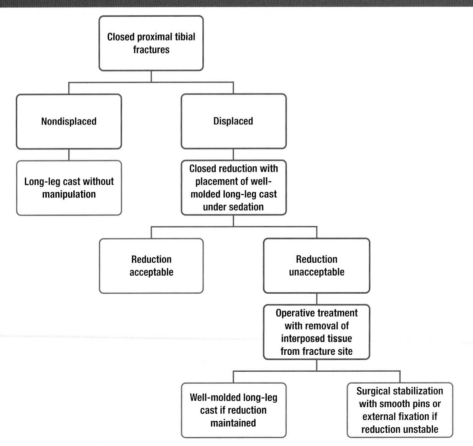

Algorithm 29-1. Authors' preferred treatment of fractures of the proximal tibial metaphysis.

Postoperative Care

After surgical intervention, a period of limited weight bearing is recommended for most patients without stable fixation. These fractures may have slightly prolonged healing due to soft tissue stripping and may require lengthier immobilization. Smooth pins may be protected under a sterile dressing and cast until removal. External fixator pins should be cleansed with dilute saline/hydrogen peroxide solution twice a day, or as per the treating surgeon's external fixator care protocol. Fractures stabilized with isolated cast treatment require regular weekly follow-up visits and radiographs to verify maintenance of the reduction. If there is loss of reduction, cast wedging or repeat reduction efforts may be indicated. In most cases, immobilization is required for approximately 4 to 6 weeks after injury. Weight bearing and discontinuation of cast treatment or pins may occur when there is visible callus and the fracture is nontender to palpation. The child may return to regular activities after recovery of normal knee and ankle range of motion. Long-term follow-up with forewarning to the family of the possibility of progressive tibial deformity is mandatory.

MANAGEMENT OF EXPECTED ADVERSE OUTCOMES AND UNEXPECTED COMPLICATIONS RELATED TO FRACTURES OF THE PROXIMAL TIBIAL METAPHYSIS

The most recognized late sequela of a proximal tibial metaphyseal fracture is development of a progressive valgus deformity (Figs. 29-7 and 29-8A,B). When the child initially presents for treatment of a tibia fracture at risk of developing genu valgum, it is crucial that the possibility of this unpredictable postfracture problem is discussed with the family. Parents should be counseled at the time of initial treatment about this possibility

Figure 29-7. Anteroposterior radiograph of a 3-year-old girl with a severe closed head injury, ipsilateral femur, and proximal tibia metaphyseal fractures. The tibia fracture was stabilized with a modified uniplanar external fixator.

and the need for clinical monitoring and follow-up radiographs if dictated by physical examination after the fracture is healed.

In 1953, Cozen[26] was the first to report valgus deformity following a proximal tibial metaphyseal fracture. He described four patients with valgus deformities after fractures in this area. In two cases, the valgus was present at the time of cast removal, suggesting loss of reduction as a potential cause of the deformity. In the other two patients, the tibia valga developed gradually during subsequent growth of the patient. Other investigators have reported development of tibia valga, even in fractures without any significant malalignment at the time of initial treatment. Nenopoulos reported a 90% incidence of progressive tibial valgus deformity in patients with minimally or nondisplaced proximal tibia metaphyseal fractures.[99] Robert et al.[116] analyzed 25 patients with proximal tibial fractures. Twelve children with a greenstick or a complete fracture developed valgus deformities, whereas no child with a torus fracture developed a deformity. Altered growth at the distal tibial physis appeared to compensate for the proximal tibia valga in three children. Corrective osteotomies were performed in four children. The valgus deformity recurred in two of these four children, and two had iatrogenic compartment syndromes. More recent work has suggested that a Cozen phenomenon of any clinical significance may be a less common occurrence. Yang et al.[141] reviewed 181 proximal tibia injuries occurring in pediatric patients with only a small proportion developing clinically significant angulation and no patients requiring surgical correction of valgus deformity. This brings into question the necessity of serial imaging for these children, but preemptive counseling and clinical monitoring for this phenomenon remain tenets of pediatric fracture management regardless.

Many theories have been proposed to explain the development of a valgus deformity after a proximal tibial metaphyseal fracture (Table 29-3).

While even appropriate operative and nonoperative treatment may still result in development of posttraumatic tibial valgus, several preventive measures have been proposed. Exploration of the fracture, followed by removal and repair of any in-folded periosteum that forms the foundation of the pes anserinus tendon plate, has been suggested as an approach that may decrease the risk of a developmental valgus deformity, but there is little data to support this approach. Houghton and Rooker demonstrated that division of the periosteum around the medial half of the proximal tibia in rabbits induced a valgus deformity and hypothesized that the increasing valgus angulation was due to a mechanical release of the restraints that the periosteum imposes on activity of the physis.[61]

Development of tibia valga has been reported to occur after simple excision of a bone graft from the proximal tibial metaphysis, proximal tibial osteotomy, and osteomyelitis of the proximal tibial metaphysis. Tibia valga deformity can occur after healing of a nondisplaced fracture and can recur after corrective tibial osteotomy, further supporting the premise that asymmetric physeal growth is the cause of most posttraumatic tibia valga deformities.

The natural history of postfracture proximal tibia valga is one of slow progression of the deformity, followed by gradual

Figure 29-8. **A:** Anteroposterior radiographs demonstrating anatomic alignment of proximal tibia metaphyseal fracture after reduction. **B:** One year after fracture union, postfracture tibia valgus is present. **C:** Spontaneous correction of postfracture tibial valgus 2 years after fracture union.

restoration of normal alignment over time. The deformity usually is apparent by 6 months postinjury and may progress for up to 18 to 24 months. Zionts and MacEwen[144] followed seven children with progressive valgus deformities of the tibia for an average of 39 months after metaphyseal fractures. Most of the deformity developed during the first year after injury, but angulation continued at a slower rate for up to 17 months after injury. Six of their seven patients had spontaneous clinical corrections. At an average of 39 months follow-up, all children had less than a 10-degree deformity. Long-term follow-up (average, 15 years) of these same seven patients revealed spontaneous correction of metaphyseal–diaphyseal and mechanical tibiofemoral angles with the mechanical axis remaining lateral to the center of the knee joint.[135] A child with a posttraumatic valgus deformity should be followed until adequate spontaneous correction occurs. This may take 18 to 36 months (Fig. 29-8C).

Bracing does not alter the natural history of posttraumatic tibia valga and is not recommended. Surgical intervention may be indicated in patients more than 18 months postinjury with a mechanical axis deviation greater than 10 degrees as a result of tibial valgus. Tibial osteotomies are not recommended in patients with postfracture valgus if they have significant growth remaining because of the possibility of recurrent valgus or other potential complications (Fig. 29-9). Instead, guided growth with temporary mechanical tethering (hemiepiphysiodesis) of the proximal medial tibial physis can restore alignment gradually without the risks of osteotomy. Hemiepiphysiodesis may be accomplished through a variety of methods utilizing staples, screws, or tension band plate and screw devices (Fig. 29-10).[88] Because the valgus deformity is often associated with some element of overgrowth, a contralateral shoe lift of appropriate size may make the deformity appear less apparent.[116]

TABLE 29-3. Proposed Etiologies of Postfracture Tibia Valga in Proximal Tibial Metaphyseal Fractures

Overgrowth of medial proximal tibial callus or medial physis

- Entrapped medial periosteum leads to increase in physeal growth
- Increased vascular flow to medial proximal physis with asymmetric physeal response
  - Bone scans demonstrating increased tracer uptake in medial physis months after fracture
  - Increase in medial collateral geniculate vascularity

Growth arrest of the lateral proximal tibial physis

Inadequate reduction or loss of reduction

Interposed soft tissue (medial collateral ligament/pes anserinus/periosteum) leading to medial gapping and a valgus deformity

Loss of tethering effect of pes anserinus tendon plate on medial physis leading to medial physeal overgrowth and hemichonrodiastasis

Tethering effect of fibula

Early weight bearing producing developmental valgus

Diaphyseal Fractures of the Tibia and Fibula

INTRODUCTION TO DIAPHYSEAL FRACTURES OF THE TIBIA AND FIBULA

Fractures of the tibial/fibular shaft may occur in children of any age and may be caused by a variety of mechanisms, ranging from a low-energy fall to a high-energy motor vehicle accident. While most closed pediatric diaphyseal tibia fractures are treated successfully with nonoperative methods, fractures with significant displacement, soft tissue injury, or open injuries may be more commonly treated with surgical management.

ASSESSMENT OF DIAPHYSEAL FRACTURES OF THE TIBIA AND FIBULA

MECHANISMS OF INJURY FOR DIAPHYSEAL FRACTURES OF THE TIBIA AND FIBULA

Most tibial fractures in children under 11 years of age are caused by torsional forces and occur in the distal third of the tibial diaphysis.

A, B   **C, D**

Figure 29-9. Developmental valgus after a proximal tibial metaphyseal fracture and subsequent corrective osteotomy. **A:** Radiograph taken 6 months after a fracture of the proximal tibia. The injury was nondisplaced. The scar from the initial proximal metaphyseal fracture is still seen (*arrow*). This child developed a moderate valgus deformity of the tibia within 6 months of fracture. **B:** A proximal tibial corrective osteotomy was performed. **C:** Two months postoperatively, the osteotomy was healed and the deformity corrected. **D:** Five months later, there was a recurrent valgus deformity of 13 degrees. (Courtesy of John J.J. Gugenheim, MD.)

A, B   **C, D**

Figure 29-10. A: Anteroposterior image of a Salter–Harris type II fracture of the proximal tibia. Notice the valgus alignment. **B:** This fracture was treated with percutaneous pin fixation after reduction. **C:** This patient developed tibia valga over a period of approximately 2 years following the injury. **D:** A medial proximal tibial hemiepiphysiodesis using a staple was performed.

These oblique and spiral fractures occur when the body rotates above a foot that is in a fixed position on the ground. The fracture line generally initiates in the distal anteromedial aspect of the bone and propagates proximally in a posterolateral direction.

If there is not an associated fibula fracture, the intact fibula prevents significant shortening of the tibia; however, varus angulation develops in approximately 60% of isolated tibial fractures within the first 2 weeks after injury (Fig. 29-11).[142] In such cases, forces generated by contraction of the long flexor muscles of the lower leg are converted into an angular moment by the intact fibula, increasing the risk of varus malalignment (see Fig. 29-11C). Isolated transverse and comminuted fractures of the tibia are caused

A, B   **C**

Figure 29-11. Anteroposterior radiograph of a distal one-third tibial fracture without concomitant fibular fracture in a 10-year-old child. **A:** The alignment in the coronal plane is acceptable (note that the proximal and distal tibial growth physes are parallel). **B:** A varus angulation developed within the first 2 weeks after injury. **C:** A 10-degree varus angulation was present after union.

most commonly by direct trauma. Transverse fractures of the tibia with an intact fibula generally are stable and seldom displace significantly.[17] Comminuted or segmental tibial fractures with an intact fibula tend to drift into varus alignment similar to oblique and spiral fractures.[17,142]

INJURIES ASSOCIATED WITH DIAPHYSEAL FRACTURES OF THE TIBIA AND FIBULA

Approximately 30% of pediatric tibial diaphyseal fractures have an associated fibular fracture.[139,142] The fibular fracture may be either complete or incomplete with some element of plastic deformation. A diaphyseal tibia fracture with an associated displaced fracture of the fibula often tends toward valgus angulation because of the action of the muscles in the anterolateral aspect of the leg and the lack of an intact lateral strut (Fig. 29-12). Any fibular injury must be identified and corrected to minimize the risk of recurrence of angulation after reduction (Fig. 29-13).

An isolated fracture of the fibular shaft is rare in children and results most commonly from a direct blow to the lateral aspect of the leg. Most isolated fractures of the fibular shaft

A
B

Anterior
tibialis muscle

Extensor digitorum
longus muscle

Extensor hallucis
longus muscle

Figure 29-12. A: Fractures involving the middle third of the tibia and fibula may shift into a valgus alignment because of the activity of the muscles in the anterior and the lateral compartments of the lower leg. **B:** Fracture of the middle tibia without an associated fibular fracture tends to shift into varus because of the force created by the anterior compartment musculature of the lower leg and the tethering effect of the intact fibula.

are nondisplaced and heal quickly with symptomatic care and immobilization (Fig. 29-14). As with any fracture, the joints above and below must be examined to evaluate for any ipsilateral injuries, such as a subtle concomitant transitional ankle fracture, which a recent series reported identified in 33% of pediatric patients with distal third shaft fractures.[86]

SIGNS AND SYMPTOMS OF DIAPHYSEAL FRACTURES OF THE TIBIA AND FIBULA

The signs and symptoms associated with tibial and fibular diaphyseal fractures vary with the severity of the injury and the mechanism by which the fractures were produced. Pain is the most common symptom. Children with fractures of the tibia or fibula have swelling at the fracture site, and the area is tender to palpation. Almost all children with any type of tibia fracture will refuse to bear weight on the injured limb. If there is significant fracture displacement, a bony defect or prominence may be palpable. Immediate neurologic impairment is rare except with fibular neck fractures, which may cause symptoms due to the adjacent common peroneal nerve.

Although arterial disruption is uncommon in pediatric tibial and fibular diaphyseal fractures, both dorsalis pedis and the posterior tibial pulses should be assessed, and a Doppler examination should be performed if the pulses are not palpable or are asymmetric with the contralateral limb. Capillary refill, sensation, and pain response patterns, particularly pain with passive motion, should be monitored. Concomitant soft tissue injuries must be evaluated carefully. Bone and soft tissue injuries associated with open fractures should be treated in an urgent manner to reduce the risk of late complications.

IMAGING AND OTHER DIAGNOSTIC STUDIES OF DIAPHYSEAL FRACTURES OF THE TIBIA AND FIBULA

Anteroposterior (AP) and lateral radiographs that include the knee and ankle joints should be obtained whenever a tibial and/or fibular shaft fracture is/are suspected. Though uncommon, tibial shaft fractures may occur in combination with transitional fractures involving the distal tibial metaphysis, and as such, close evaluation of the ankle radiographs is essential (Fig. 29-15). Comparison views of the uninvolved leg are rarely indicated. Children with suspected fractures not apparent on the initial radiographs may need treatment with supportive splinting or casting to control symptoms associated with the injuries. Periosteal new bone formation evident on plain radiographs obtained 10 to 14 days after injury confirms the diagnosis in most cases.

CLASSIFICATION OF DIAPHYSEAL FRACTURES OF THE TIBIA AND FIBULA

There is no commonly used pediatric classification system for tibia/fibular shaft fractures. Fractures are generally described based on location, fracture pattern, the direction of displacement, whether the fibula is intact, and the presence of an open injury.

A

B

C

Figure 29-13. A: Anteroposterior and lateral radiograph of the lower leg in a 12-year-old child showing a comminuted tibial fracture with a concomitant plastic deformation of the fibula. Note the valgus alignment of the tibia. **B:** This patient had a closed manipulation and casting correcting the valgus alignment in the tibia and partially correcting the plastic deformation of the fibula. **C:** At union, there is an anatomic alignment of the tibia with a mild residual plastic deformation of the fibula.

OUTCOME MEASURES FOR DIAPHYSEAL FRACTURES OF THE TIBIA AND FIBULA

While there are no specific outcome measures for pediatric diaphyseal tibia and fibula fractures, the titanium elastic nail (TEN) outcome scoring system (Table 29-4), initially proposed for use in pediatric femur fractures treated with TENs,[36] may be used to assess results after treatment of pediatric tibia fractures with flexible intramedullary fixation.[55,105,120] In addition, the Pediatric Outcome Data Collection Instrument (PODCI) or Patient-Reported Outcomes Measurement Information System (PROMIS) may be used to assess functional recovery after pediatric injuries.[118]

Figure 29-14. Distal one-third fibular fracture in an 8 year old who was struck on the lateral side of the leg (**right**). There is moderate new bone formation 6 weeks after injury (**left**).

TREATMENT OPTIONS FOR DIAPHYSEAL FRACTURES OF THE TIBIA AND FIBULA

NONOPERATIVE TREATMENT OF DIAPHYSEAL FRACTURES OF THE TIBIA AND FIBULA

Indications/Contraindications

Nonoperative Treatment of Diaphyseal Fractures of Tibia and Fibula: INDICATIONS AND CONTRAINDICATIONS[57]
Indications
• Nondisplaced closed fractures • Displaced closed fractures amenable to closed reduction
Contraindications
Relative
• Open fractures • Body habitus unamenable to long-leg cast treatment • Severe swelling with concern for compartment syndrome • Segmental fractures • Polytrauma
Absolute
• Failure to attain or maintain adequate closed reduction in a cast

Figure 29-15. A, B: Anteroposterior and lateral radiographs of an adolescent patient with a tibial shaft fracture.

(continues)

C   D

Figure 29-15. *(Continued)* **C, D:** Dedicated anteroposterior and lateral views of the ankle demonstrate an associated Salter–Harris II distal tibia fracture.

Cast Immobilization

Most uncomplicated pediatric diaphyseal tibial shaft factures, with/or without associated fibular shaft fractures, can be managed with closed manipulation and casting. Displaced fractures should be managed with reduction under appropriate sedation, using fluoroscopic assistance when available. This can be done in the emergency room or in the operating room depending on the availability of sedation and fluoroscopy. An experienced assistant is extremely helpful. A reduction plan should be made before manipulation based on review of the deforming forces

TABLE 29-4. TEN Outcome Scoring

	Excellent Result	Satisfactory Result	Poor Result
Leg-length inequality	<1 cm	<2 cm	>2 cm
Malalignment	<5 degrees	5–10 degrees	>10 degrees
Pain	None	None	Present
Complication	None	Minor and resolved	Major/lasting morbidity

Reprinted with permission from Flynn JM, et al. Titanium elastic nails for pediatric femur fractures: a multicenter study of early results with analysis of complications. *J Pediatr Orthop.* 2001;21(1):4–8.

associated with the specific fracture pattern. In most cases, a short-leg cast is applied with the foot in the appropriate position and either a varus or valgus mold at the fracture site, depending on the fracture pattern and alignment. The cast material is taken to the inferior aspect of the patella anteriorly and to a point 2 cm distal to the popliteal flexion crease posteriorly. It may be beneficial to use plaster for the initial cast because of its ability to conform to the contour of the leg and the ease with which it can be manipulated while setting. The alignment of the fracture is reassessed after the short-leg cast has been applied, and the cast is then extended to the midthigh with the knee partially flexed. Some believe it is safer to apply a long-leg cast all at once to avoid the proximal edges of the short cast causing skin problems, but maintaining fracture reduction with this approach can be difficult. Most children with complete, unstable diaphyseal tibial fractures are placed into a bent-knee (45-degree) long-leg cast to control rotation at the fracture site and to assist in maintaining non–weight-bearing status during the initial healing phase. The child's ankle initially may be left in a partially plantarflexed position to prevent generation of apex posterior angulation (recurvatum) at the fracture site. There is little risk of developing a permanent equinus contracture as any initial plantarflexion can be corrected at a cast change once the fracture becomes more stable. In the face of any significant swelling, regardless of the cast material used, consideration should be given to a univalved or bivalved cast splitting so as to minimize the risk of cast-induced compartment syndrome. Alternatively, foam may be placed under the Webril to allow for swelling. After casting, hospital admission for elevation and neurovascular monitoring should be considered, especially in higher-energy injuries with significant fracture displacement and/or initial swelling. Note that it is not critical to have anatomic alignment at this time, as the cast may be wedged at 7 to 14 days after some healing and decreased swelling has taken place.

It is important to have a discussion with the family at the initiation of care that cast treatment of tibial fractures, especially in adolescent patients, may be lengthy. They require frequent clinical and radiographic follow-up and may need further intervention to maintain alignment. The radiographic position of the fracture should be checked weekly during the first 2 or 3 weeks after the cast has been applied. Muscle atrophy and a reduction in soft tissue swelling may cause the fracture to drift into unacceptable alignment. Cast wedging may be performed in an attempt to improve alignment, and in some cases, a second cast application with remanipulation of the fracture under sedation or anesthesia may be necessary to obtain acceptable alignment. Acceptable position is somewhat controversial and varies based on patient age as well as location and direction of the deformity.[33] Remodeling of angular deformity is more limited in the tibia than other long bones with more active regional physes. No absolute criteria exist, but the following general alignment guidelines may be beneficial in decision making (Table 29-5):

- Varus and valgus deformity in the upper and midshaft tibia remodel slowly, if at all. Up to 10 degrees of deformity can be accepted in patients less than 8 years old, while less than 5 degrees of angulation is recommended in those over 8 years of age.
- Moderate translation of the shaft of the tibia in a young child is acceptable, whereas in an adolescent, at least 50% apposition is recommended.
- Up to 10 degrees of apex anterior angulation may be tolerated, although remodeling is slow.
- Minimal apex posterior angulation (recurvatum) may be accepted.
- Up to 1 cm of shortening is acceptable.

TABLE 29-5. Acceptable Alignment of a Pediatric Diaphyseal Tibial Fracture

Parameter	Patient Age	
	<8 Years	≥8 Years
Valgus	5 degrees	5 degrees
Varus	10 degrees	5 degrees
Angulation anterior	10 degrees	5 degrees
Posterior angulation	5 degrees	0 degrees
Shortening	10 mm	5 mm
Rotation	5 degrees	5 degrees

Cast Wedging

Patients with a loss of fracture reduction and unacceptable angulation may benefit from repeated manipulation of the fracture. This can be attempted in the clinic setting through the use of cast "wedging." Fracture alignment in the cast can be altered with this method obviating the need for repeated sedation. For tibia fractures, correction is most commonly performed using an opening wedge technique to permit restoration of length and alignment correction. Closing wedge technique is generally not recommended as it shortens the fracture and can pinch soft tissues.

The location for wedge placement is determined by evaluating the child's leg radiographically and marking the midpoint of the tibial fracture on the outside of the cast. One should approach wedging similar to using the center of rotation of angulation (CORA) in lower extremity deformity correction. If fluoroscopy is not available, a series of paper clips can be placed at 2-cm intervals on the surface of the cast and AP and lateral radiographs are then taken. The radiographic position of the paper clips will help define the location of the fracture and the site most suitable for placement of the wedge. Alternatively, the distance from contours of the cast from known bony prominences (e.g., medial malleolus) may be measured radiographically and an appropriate position on the cast to place a wedge can be referenced.

Author's Recommended Cast Wedging Technique

The side of the cast opposite the apex of the fracture is cut perpendicular to the long axis of the bone. A small segment of the cast is left intact directly over the apex of the malaligned fracture (~25%). A cast spreader is used to spread the cast open in a controlled manner. Premade and measured plastic shims (Fig. 29-16) or a stack of tongue depressors of the appropriate size are placed into the open segment to maintain the distraction of the site, and the cast is wrapped with new casting material after the alignment has been assessed radiographically (Fig. 29-17). It is imperative that the edges of any shims or wedging material added do not protrude into the cast padding or cause pressure on the underlying skin. This wedging technique effectively lengthens the tibia while correcting the malalignment (Fig. 29-18). Providers can estimate approximately 1 cm wedging for every 10 degrees of desired angular correction.

After any cast wedging, especially early after injury when there may be residual leg swelling, it is recommended to observe the patient for a period of time to be certain that signs and symptoms of compartment syndrome do not develop. Cast wedging may be somewhat painful, but any discomfort should subside quickly. The family should be alerted that if increasing pain develops after cast wedging, the patient should return urgently for evaluation.

Outcomes of Nonoperative Treatment of Diaphyseal Fractures of the Tibia and Fibula

The length of immobilization varies with the child's age and the type of fracture. Hoaglund and States[59] reported that in

Figure 29-16. A, B: Blocks used to hold casts open after wedge corrections of malaligned fractures. The wings on the blocks prevent the blocks from migrating toward the skin.

Figure 29-17. Comminuted fracture of the tibia and fibula in a 12-year-old boy struck by a car (**left**). Notice the extension of the fracture into the metaphysis from the diaphyseal injury. The fracture is in a valgus alignment. The fracture could not be maintained in an acceptable alignment. The cast was wedged with excellent result (**right**).

43 closed fractures in children, the average time in a cast was 2.5 months (range 1.5–5.5 months). Prolonged immobilization (>3 months) may be necessary for some fractures, especially in the adolescent population.[58]

Rates of success of cast treatment of pediatric tibial fractures range from 60% to 96%.[58,68] The wide variation in success may be related to the level of experience in the art of casting and resources available in clinic to mold and wedge casts as well as providers' willingness and dedication to serial clinical monitoring with closed treatment. The need for a cast wedge or cast change to maintain alignment occurred in 21% of a series of adolescent patients, but nonoperative management has been found to be safe and effective in treating 96% of closed pediatric tibial fractures.[58,67]

Few children with a tibial fracture require extensive rehabilitation beyond basic crutch or walker training. Most children limp with an out-toeing rotation gait on the involved extremity for several weeks to a month after the cast is removed. This is secondary to muscle weakness, joint stiffness, and a tendency to circumduct the limb during swing phase rather than malalignment or malrotation of the fracture. As the muscle atrophy and weakness resolve, the limp improves. Knee range-of-motion exercises and quadriceps strengthening may be useful in an older child progressing from a bent-knee cast to weight bearing on a short-leg cast. The child may return to sports when the fracture is healed and the patient has regained strength and function comparable to that of the uninjured leg.

OPERATIVE TREATMENT OF DIAPHYSEAL FRACTURES OF THE TIBIA AND FIBULA

Indications/Contraindications

Surgical Stabilization of Diaphyseal Tibia Fractures: INDICATIONS
Indications
Absolute
• Failure to attain or maintain adequate closed reduction
Relative

• Open fracture
  • Fracture associated with significant soft tissue injury
  • Fracture associated with compartment syndrome
  • Floating knee
• Segmental fracture
  • Fracture associated with closed head injury and/or polytrauma
• Fractures in large, obese children that may be difficult to control in a cast
• Patients for whom external circumferential immobilization may be contraindicated

Historically, operative treatment has been recommended infrequently for tibial shaft fractures in children. In 1980, Weber et al.[139] reported that only 29 (4.5%) of 638 pediatric tibial fractures in their study required surgical intervention. However, there has been increasing use of surgical stabilization in recent years,[128] particularly for unstable closed tibial shaft fractures as well as open fractures or those with associated soft tissue injuries. The current relative indications for operative treatment include open fractures, most fractures with an associated compartment syndrome, some fractures in children with spasticity (head injury or cerebral palsy), fractures in

which open treatment facilitates nursing care (floating knee, multiple long bone fractures, multiple system injuries), and unstable fractures in which adequate alignment cannot be either attained or maintained (see Table 29-3).[14,28] Common methods of fixation for tibial fractures undergoing operative treatment include percutaneous metallic pins, bioabsorbable pins,[12] external fixation,[1,30,94] and plates with screws; the use of flexible intramedullary titanium or stainless steel nails or, in some cases, intramedullary Steinmann pins, is becoming increasingly common.[41,45,47,75,94,101,113,119,137]

Flexible Intramedullary Nails

Preoperative Planning

Flexible Intramedullary Nailing of Diaphyseal Tibial Fractures: PREOPERATIVE PLANNING CHECKLIST	
OR table	❑ Radiolucent
Position/ positioning aids	❑ Supine ❑ Bump under the ipsilateral hip to rotate leg to neutral ❑ Folded blankets or foam positioner (ramp or wedge) to permit lateral imaging
Fluoroscopy location	❑ Contralateral side of operative extremity
Equipment	❑ Flexible nail implants and instrumentation (commercially available) ❑ Pin distractor available or adequate assistance for intraoperative traction
Tourniquet	❑ Nonsterile at thigh level but do not elevate unless necessary
Other	❑ Preoperative antibiotics ❑ General anesthesia with adequate muscle relaxation

A, B

C

Figure 29-18. A: Anteroposterior and lateral tibial radiographs of an 11-year-old boy who was struck by an automobile, sustaining a markedly comminuted tibial fracture without concomitant fibular fracture. **B:** Despite the comminution, length and alignment were maintained in a cast. **C:** The patient's fracture shifted into a varus malalignment that measured 10 degrees (**right**). The cast was wedged, resulting in the reestablishment of an acceptable coronal alignment (**left**).

(continues)

Figure 29-18. *(Continued)* **D:** The patient's fracture healed without malunion.

Positioning

The patient is positioned supine on a radiolucent table with a bump under the ipsilateral hip to maintain the leg in neutral rotation. Additional soft tissue bumps or commercially available foam ramps or triangles are also helpful to elevate and stabilize the operative leg above the nonoperative leg and to assist in obtaining lateral fluoroscopy images. Fluoroscopy is positioned perpendicular to the limb adjacent to the contralateral extremity.

Surgical Approach

Intramedullary fixation is performed most commonly in children using stainless steel or TENs. In most cases, the implants are placed in a proximal to distal fashion from medial and lateral proximal insertion points, although there are reports of successful management with insertion of two implants through a single insertion site.[25] Retrograde fixation through the medial malleolus may be used in rare instances because of soft tissue injuries about the planned proximal insertion sites or very proximal shaft fractures that preclude proximal entry points, but there is minimal soft tissue coverage of the nail at this insertion site. When performing flexible nail fixation, fluoroscopy is used to localize the medial and lateral entry points for the elastic nails at the level of the tibial tubercle (Fig. 29-19). The skin incision must extend proximally 2 to 3 cm to prevent skin injury during insertion of nails. Medially, the bony entry point is easily found due to its subcutaneous nature. Laterally, dissection proceeds through the anterolateral musculature down to bone. Dissection should be limited distally and posteriorly so as to avoid the branches of the peroneal nerve. Care must be taken to avoid injury to the proximal tibial physes, including the tibial tubercle apophysis.

Figure 29-19. Fluoroscopy is used to localize the entry point for placement of medial and lateral elastic nails.

Technique

 Flexible Intramedullary Nail Placement for Diaphyseal Tibia Fractures:
KEY SURGICAL STEPS

- ❏ Preselect size of flexible nails based on canal size at isthmus
- ❏ Supine position with ipsilateral bump on a radiolucent table
- ❏ Prep extremity toes-to-thigh tourniquet
- ❏ Have adequate soft blanket bumps or knee triangle available
- ❏ Medial and lateral proximal tibial incisions—do not violate perichondrial ring
- ❏ Distal aspect of incision at the point of proposed nail insertion sites
  - Starting holes medially and laterally at, or just proximal to, the level of tibial tubercle. Use drill or awl and confirm trajectory in AP and lateral planes
- ❏ Contour flexible nails to allow maximum balanced spread at the level of the fracture site
- ❏ Pass nails to fracture site. Reduce fracture with traction and manipulation
- ❏ Pass nails into distal metaphysis. Ensure fracture does not distract during insertion
  - Check lateral view on C-arm. Rotate nails as necessary to minimize possible recurvatum deformity

Selection of nail diameter should be based on a target of 60% to 80% total canal fill at the isthmus. Two nails of equal diameter and identical material should be selected; placement of differently sized nails or nails of different metallurgy will lead to unbalanced fixation. Care should be taken to ensure that

Figure 29-20. After entering the cortex, the awl is directed distally in the metaphysis.

Figure 29-21. The medial nail is being inserted with the "ski tip" end rotated so that perpendicular to the entry site. The already inserted lateral nail has been rotated 180 degrees so that the rounded portion can glide along the far cortex during advancement.

the entry points are distal enough to avoid the physes. Either an awl or a power drill may be used to enter the intramedullary canal. The drill should be at least 1 mm larger than the selected nail. Begin the drill or awl perpendicular to the long axis of the tibia until the cortex is engaged. The drill or awl should then be directed distally bevel the starting site so as to facilitate insertion of the nail into the canal (Fig. 29-20). The opposite cortex should not be violated with the drill or awl and the trajectory should be in line with the shaft on lateral imaging.

Many commercially available nails have a "ski tip" or spatulated end. Keeping the rounded portion of the end against the far cortex prevents perforation during nail insertion (Fig. 29-21). Twisting the nail inserter during insertion can also help to avoid cortical perforation. Once the nails are advanced to the level of the fracture site, the fracture is reduced, and one nail is advanced just past the fracture. The second nail is then advanced across the fracture site before both nails are driven farther into the distal fragment (Fig. 29-22). Alternatively, one nail may be advanced all the way, then the surgeon may start placing the second nail. Each nail is then advanced to a point approximately 1 cm proximal to the desired final distal position (Fig. 29-23). The nails are cut as close to the bone as possible, then a tamp is used to advance the nails to their final position, taking care to stay proximal to the distal tibia physis (Fig. 29-24). If removal of the nails is anticipated after healing, leave enough length of flexible nail to simplify future retrieval. External splinting or short-leg casting is commonly used to supplement stability.

External Fixation

Preoperative Planning

✔	**External Fixation of Diaphyseal Tibia Fractures:** PREOPERATIVE PLANNING CHECKLIST	
OR table	❑ Radiolucent	
Position/ positioning aids	❑ Supine ❑ Bump under the ipsilateral hip to rotate leg to neutral ❑ Folded blankets or foam positioner (ramp or wedge) to allow slight knee flexion	
Fluoroscopy location	❑ Ipsilateral side of operative extremity	
Equipment	❑ Large external fixator set	
Tourniquet	❑ Nonsterile at thigh level but do not inflate unless necessary	
(Other)	❑ Preoperative antibiotics ❑ General anesthesia with adequate muscle relaxation	

Positioning

Positioning is identical to positioning for flexible nail placement, but the fluoroscopy unit should be positioned on the ipsilateral side of the injured extremity. This is done so as to

A   B

Figure 29-22. A: The medial nail is carefully inserted across the fracture site. **B:** The lateral nail is rotated to allow passage across the fracture site, then will be derotated to direct the tip laterally into the distal fragment.

Figure 29-23. Both nails are inserted, leaving 1 cm proximal to the physis.

Figure 29-24. Nails have been cut close to the skin at the proximal entry point, then a tamp used to seat the distal end, taking care to not violate to the physis.

A, B

C

Figure 29-25. A, B: Type II open fracture of the tibia in a 5-year-old boy treated with debridement, unilateral external fixation, and split-thickness skin graft. **C:** Four months after removal of the external fixation.

allow placement of the external fixation pins with a minimum of obstruction by the unit itself.

Surgical Approach

Knowledge of cross-sectional anatomy is crucial for safe placement of external fixation devices. The anteromedial subcutaneous border of the tibia is safest for placement of unilateral fixation pins. In addition, the lack of soft tissue coverage minimizes soft tissue movement around the pins and thereby limits the risk of pin-tract infections.

Safe zones for half-pin fixation (see Fig. 29-2):

- Proximal tibia—distal to the tibial tuberosity, over the oblique medial subcutaneous tibia shaft
- Middle tibia—medial subcutaneous tibia shaft. The anterior tibial artery/vein and deep peroneal nerve lie along the posterolateral border of the tibia, and care should be taken that pin insertion does not violate the neurovascular bundle
- Distal tibia—medial subcutaneous tibia. Anterior placement will jeopardize the anterior tibial artery and vein

A, B

C

Figure 29-26. A: Anteroposterior and lateral radiographs of the tibia of a 12-year-old boy who was struck by a car. This child sustained a grade IIIB open middle one-third tibial fracture, a Salter–Harris type II fracture of the distal tibial physis with associated distal fibular fracture (*closed arrows*), and a tibial eminence fracture (*open arrow*). **B:** Irrigation and debridement and application of an external fixation device were performed. **C:** The fracture of distal tibial physis was stabilized with a supplemental pin attached to the external fixation device. Open reduction and internal fixation of the fibula was performed to enhance the stability of the external fixator in the distal tibia.

(continues)

Figure 29-26. *(Continued)* **D:** Anteroposterior and lateral radiographs of the tibia approximately 9 months after injury demonstrate healing of the tibial eminence fracture, the comminuted middle one-third tibial fracture, and the distal tibial physeal fracture. The distal tibial physis remains open at this time.

Technique

> ### ✓ Unilateral External Fixator for Diaphyseal Tibia Fractures:
> ### KEY SURGICAL STEPS
>
> - ❏ Planned pin insertion sites marked at the level of the skin in the safe zones
> - ❏ Two pins inserted in each of the proximal and distal fragments
> - ❏ Conventional pins
>   - Predrill both cortices through a trocar
>   - Insert pins through a drill sleeve by hand, engage both cortices so that the pin is threaded into the far cortex but not protruding excessively
> - ❏ Self-drilling pins/Schanz screws
>   - Insert pins through a drill sleeve, advance until pin reaches the far cortex
>   - Advance by hand until tip of the pin engages the inside of the far cortex
> - ❏ Connect the two pins of each main fragment to a rod via pin-to-rod clamps
> - ❏ Loosely connect the two rods with a third rod using rod-to-rod clamps
> - ❏ Manually reduce the fracture and verify under fluoroscopy
> - ❏ Tighten the rod-to-rod clamps and reconfirm reduction with fluoroscopy
> - ❏ Add additional rods if extra stability is needed
> - ❏ Note: In cases without use of rod-to-rod clamps, the proximal and distal-most pins are placed first to establish fracture length and then attached to a single longitudinal rod. Intermediate pins are then placed and attached to the rod. A second bar can be added to form a more rigid "double-stack" construct if desired

The most versatile and most widely available external fixation device for pediatric tibial fractures is a unilateral frame. The technique is identical to placement of a monolateral external fixator for adult tibia fractures, except for the care taken to not violate the physes, and pins are rarely placed proximal to the tibial tubercle. The unilateral frame is easy to apply and allows minor corrections in angular alignment and length. Secondary

Figure 29-27. An anterior frame allows for rubber bands to prevent equinus, but care must be taken to ensure ankle dorsiflexion is not limited by the frame. (Used with permission by the Children's Orthopaedic Center, Los Angeles.)

pins can be used for added support (Fig. 29-25); these are connected to the standard pins or the body of the external fixation device. This allows control of segmental fragments as needed. Fracture reduction tools can be applied to the pin clamps to assist in manipulating the fracture. A small-pin or thin-wire circular frame may be indicated for complicated fractures adjacent to the joint. Unilateral frames may be placed to span an adjacent joint so as to use ligamentotaxis as an indirect reduction method to establish and maintain alignment (Fig. 29-26). An anterior frame allows for rubber bands rather than second metatarsal half-pins to prevent equinus (Fig. 29-27). While medial frames are sometimes easiest for the surgeon to apply, they may lead to months of discomfort for the patients when they hit the frame against the other leg when walking or sleeping. If frames are placed in two parts, with the proximal and distal part connected by a separate bar (Fig. 29-28), later minor adjustments are much easier than when all pins are connected by straight bars.

Unusual fracture patterns, such as periphyseal fractures, fractures with significant bone or soft tissue loss, or fractures with delayed presentation, are appropriate candidates for multiplanar or circular external fixation.[62]

Figure 29-28. An external fixator with pins in the proximal and distal fragment independently mobile makes later adjustments much easier than if all pins are connected to a straight rod. (Used with permission by the Children's Orthopaedic Center, Los Angeles.)

Authors' Preferred Treatment of Closed Diaphyseal Fractures (Algorithm 29-2)

Algorithm 29-2. Authors' preferred treatment of closed diaphyseal fractures.

Simple pediatric diaphyseal tibial fractures unite quickly in most cases, and cast immobilization can be used without affecting the long-term range of motion of the knee and the ankle. A bent-knee, long-leg cast provides maximal comfort to the patient and controls rotation of the fracture fragments. The cast should be bivalved initially to limit the effect of any swelling. Children with nondisplaced or minimally displaced fractures that do not require manipulation generally are not admitted to the hospital. Children with more extensive injuries should be admitted for neurovascular observation and instruction in wheelchair, crutch, or walker use.

Significantly displaced fractures disrupt the surrounding soft tissues and produce a large hematoma in the fascial compartments of the lower leg. Circulation, sensation, and both active and passive movement of the toes should be monitored carefully after injury. The child should be admitted to the hospital, and reduction should be performed with adequate sedation and fluoroscopy if available. Most fractures are casted after reduction, and the cast may be bivalved or split to allow room for swelling. The limb should be kept elevated for 48 to 72 hours after injury to minimize swelling. The fracture should be evaluated clinically and radiographically within a week of initial manipulation to verify maintenance of the reduction. The cast can be wedged to correct minor

alignment problems. Significant loss of alignment requires repeat reduction with adequate anesthesia and/or utilization of a more rigid fixation method. The long-leg cast may be changed to a short-leg, weight-bearing cast or a removable boot at 4 to 6 weeks after injury. In some cases, children over 11 years of age may transition to a patellar tendon-bearing cast after removal of the long-leg cast in an effort to maintain immobilization of the fracture, while limiting the potential for significant knee stiffness. Weight-bearing immobilization is maintained until sufficient callus is evident and the fracture is nontender to palpation.

Fractures in patients with complicating factors—including spasticity, a floating knee, multiple long bone fractures, an associated transitional ankle fracture, concern for current or future compartment syndrome, extensive soft tissue damage, multiple system injuries, or an inability to obtain or maintain an acceptable reduction—should be stabilized with a more rigid fixation method, such as external fixation or flexible intramedullary nails (Figs. 29-29 and 29-30.). It is the authors' preference to use either stainless steel or titanium flexible intramedullary nails, if at all possible, in these situations. In closed fractures, external fixation is reserved for comminuted or highly unstable fracture patterns or damage control in multitrauma.

A, B

C

Figure 29-29. **A:** Anteroposterior and lateral radiographs of a 12-year-old who was involved in a motor vehicle accident sustaining a grade I open middle one-third tibial and fibular fractures. **B:** This injury was treated with intramedullary nail fixation. **C:** At union, the patient has an anatomic alignment and no evidence of a growth disturbance.

Postoperative Care

Despite surgical stabilization, many pediatric tibia fractures still require some level of external stabilization such as a cast.[44,120] Weight bearing is dependent on the pattern of fracture and stability of fixation. In general, weight bearing is allowed by 6 weeks postinjury if adequate callus is observed and the fracture is nontender.

For patients treated with external fixation, a posterior splint may be applied to help prevent the patient from developing an equinus contracture. This splint should be easy to remove for pin care and dressing changes of any associated soft tissue injury. Splinting to maintain position of the ankle and foot can be avoided by external fixation, be it unilateral or circular, to the forefoot. Routine pin care with dilute saline/hydrogen peroxide solution once or twice daily is instituted postoperative day 1.

Potential Pitfalls and Preventive Measures

Diaphyseal Fractures of the Tibia/Fibula: SURGICAL PITFALLS AND PREVENTIONS

Pitfall	Prevention
Flexible Intramedullary Nails	
Inability to pass nails	• Prebend gentle curve (10 degrees) at leading end of nail • Decrease nail diameter
Penetration of opposite cortex	• Orient smooth curved end of "ski tip" to bounce off opposite cortex. Rotating the nail back and forth slightly during insertion can also assist with preventing impaction into the opposite cortex
Inability to reduce fracture	• Femoral distractor or qualified assistant to maintain traction • Open reduction • Anesthetic muscle relaxation
Inability to maintain alignment after nails passed	• Contour nails for maximum spread at level of fracture • Balanced fixation with nails of similar size and material
External Fixation	
Lack of stability after fixation	• Add more pins or bars • Plate the fibula
Early loosening of pins	• Careful insertion technique to avoid heat necrosis
Pin-tract infections	• Small skin incisions to release tension around pins and wires • Daily pin cleaning • Insert pins in subcutaneous areas with minimal surrounding soft tissue movement
Development of delayed or pending nonunion	• Dynamize the fixator frame, increase weight bearing

Figure 29-30. Anteroposterior radiograph of a 14-year-old who was involved in a motor vehicle accident sustaining a distal one-third tibial fracture and comminuted distal fibular fracture. This was stabilized with titanium elastic nails.

Outcomes

Treatment of closed diaphyseal pediatric tibial shaft fractures remains controversial. Operative treatment with flexible elastic nailing has been compared with nonoperative management for displaced tibia fractures with similar maintenance of reduction with both techniques.[20,115] A systematic review of the topic examining 1,083 patients across 10 studies identified a higher rate of complications with operative treatment as compared to nonoperative management (24% vs. 9%; $p < .05$)[129]; however, surgically managed patients were notably older and had a higher proportion of associated fibula fractures indicative of greater instability. Among all patients treated primarily with closed management, the risk of reduction loss requiring surgical management is approximately 5%.[29,129] Cast index greater than 1.02 and postreduction angulation of more than 3.4 degrees and translation (>24.3%) were found to be risk factors for redisplacement after closed reduction in one series of 196 pediatric tibia fractures.[76]

Canavese et al. retrospectively compared these treatment options in 80 closed, displaced tibial shaft fractures at two institutions.[20] While the surgically treated fractures had greater initial displacement than those treated closed, valgus and procurvatum deformities were statistically significantly improved from injury radiographs in the flexible nailing group. In addition, the small numerical differences between the surgical and casting groups were not clinically significant; however, the immobilization time was significantly shorter in the surgical group. Rivera et al.[115] more recently compared these treatment modalities in 141 adolescents at a single center. While the elastic nail group was older and had a greater proportion of comminuted fractures and fractures also involving the fibula, the authors identified faster healing in the casted treatment group. Reduction maintenance and complication rates were similar between groups, but delayed and nonunion occurred only among patients treated with elastic nails. Ultimately, these studies indicate both methods to be safe and effective means of treatment but support initial attempts of closed management with casting whenever possible as this modality has overall low rates of failure and conversion to surgical management always remains possible.[29,129]

Numerous studies have reported on the outcomes of flexible elastic nails in the management of pediatric tibia fractures. In the most current systematic review of this topic, Fanelli et al.[34] identified 28 studies with 835 patients with a mean age of 11 years old treated for tibia fractures with elastic nailing. The overall complication rate was 28.1%, but this was greatest among open fractures (13.6% vs. 5.1%; $p = .007$). The authors found high rates of union (97.5%) at a mean of roughly 12 weeks. Infection and compartment syndrome were uncommon (1%–3%). Nearly all patients returned to unrestricted activities. A more recent work not included in this review by Pogorelić et al.[112] retrospectively examined a cohort of 132 patients with displaced tibia fractures treated with TENs over a 20-year period with a mean age of 12 years old. The authors reported no use of postoperative immobilization in their series and early mobilization with weight bearing gradually permitted after 3 to 4 weeks. The authors reported a mean healing time of 7 weeks, although their definition of healing was not clearly defined, with an overall complication rate of 11.4%. Six patients (4.5%) required reoperation due to loss of reduction or refracture. Open fractures ($n = 32$) in this cohort had prolonged healing times (mean of 10 weeks) and a higher rate of complications (21.9%).

In contrast to femoral shaft fractures, studies have failed to find poorer outcomes in regard to malunion rate or time to union in use of intramedullary flexible nails in the older, heavier pediatric patient population,[44,84] although severity of injury for these patients may be higher.[5] Pandya et al. reported a 20% rate of compartment syndrome after flexible nailing of 31 pediatric closed and open tibia fractures.[110] In this series, 83% of children who were 50 kg or greater developed compartment syndrome. Overall, the authors found that pediatric patients who developed compartment syndrome after intramedullary nailing were heavier (53 kg vs. 39 kg), more likely to present with a neurologic injury, and more likely to have comminuted tibia fractures.[110] Despite the rising popularity of surgical stabilization, the advantages of flexible nailing over casting of pediatric tibia fractures are still unclear.[57]

In regard to implant material, both titanium and stainless steel alloy flexible elastic nails exist as available treatment options. While titanium nails have theoretical biomechanical features of benefit, the majority of prior work comparing these implant options (performed largely in the management of femoral shaft fractures) has found no reproducible difference in the rate of union, infection, or skin irritation as evidenced by a 2017 systematic review of the topic.[89] Examining implant comparisons in tibial shaft fractures specifically, Marengo et al.[83] compared these implants in a series of 34 patients (21 tibia, 14 femur) and found no differences in bone healing, mechanical stability, return to activity, and complication rate. They concluded that while titanium is a superior option for patients with metal allergy, stainless steel implants are a cheaper and equally effective alternative. Implant selection is thus left to the discretion of the treating surgeon.

Open reduction and internal fixation (ORIF) of pediatric tibial fractures has been demonstrated to have statistically significantly increased rates of anatomic reduction, lower rates of subsequent surgery, but longer surgical times and higher rates of wound complications when compared to flexible nailing.[111] However, both methods have high rates of union and return to activity.

Although monolateral and multiplanar external fixator constructs have been shown to safely achieve union and maintain alignment without cost or complication differences between these fixator constructs, there is limited data comparing external fixation with ORIF or flexible nailing. Kubiak et al.[75] retrospectively compared the use of titanium flexible nails with external fixation in a mixed group of patients with open and closed tibial fractures. Although the groups were not matched and were reviewed retrospectively, the authors reported a clinically significant decrease in time to union and improved functional outcome scores with titanium nails compared to external fixation. Therefore, in most circumstances, elastic nailing is the preferred operative treatment method for the majority of diaphyseal tibia fractures requiring operative stabilization.

There are some older pediatric patients who may be best managed with reamed or unreamed rigid tibial nails, as one would a skeletally mature adult patient as this permits earlier weight bearing and may more adequately stabilize certain fracture patterns (metadiaphyseal). Maturation-related indications for transition to this technique are uncertain, but Court-Brown et al.[24] reported on 36 adolescents with open physes (13–16 years old) treated with rigid nailing with no reported cases of premature physeal arrest. Some authors have even proposed physeal-sparing approaches for rigid intramedullary nailing in this age cohort, but existing cohorts are small and outcome data for this technique are limited.[19,140] Until more robust evidence is available, authors generally advise avoiding implants that cross the physis in patients with greater than 2 years of growth remaining and utilization of established fixation strategies (i.e., flexible nailing or ORIF) especially given that these techniques have well-established outcomes and rigid nailing possesses its own array of surgical risks including knee pain.[78,134,136]

Open Tibial Fractures

INTRODUCTION TO OPEN TIBIAL FRACTURES

Most open tibial fractures in children involve the diaphyseal region and are treated similarly to comparable injuries in adults. In addition, these fractures and associated soft tissue injuries are classified utilizing the Gustilo–Anderson system.[50] Most open fractures of the tibia result from high-velocity/high-energy injuries.[117]

TREATMENT OPTIONS FOR OPEN TIBIAL FRACTURES

Management principles for open tibial fractures include the following:

- Initiation of appropriate antibiotic therapy immediately.
- Timely debridement and irrigation.
  - Consideration may be given to nonoperative treatment with irrigation and debridement in the emergency room and administration of antibiotics in select, noncontaminated, low-energy grade I open fractures,[10,43] although studies supporting this practice are underpowered.
- Fracture reduction followed by stabilization with either internal or external devices.
- Intraoperative angiography (after rapid fracture stabilization) and management of possible elevation of compartment pressures when sufficiency of the vascular perfusion is unclear.
- Open wound treatment with loose gauze packing or negative pressure dressing.[30,91]
- Staged debridement of necrotic soft tissue and bone in the operating room as needed until the wounds are ready for closure or coverage.

- Delayed closure, application of a split-thickness skin graft, or use of delayed local or free vascularized flaps as needed.[125]
- Acute shortening when soft tissues and vascular status allow in fractures with segmental bone loss.[77]
- Cancellous bone grafting (autologous or allograft) for bone defects or delayed union after maturation of soft tissue coverage.
- Bone transport or limb lengthening in patients with segmental loss after definitive soft tissue coverage achieved.[77]

These principles are similar to those used in adult patients. However, there is evidence that differences exist between pediatric and adult fracture patients. As such, the principles of treatment for open tibial fractures in adults are altered somewhat by the unique characteristics of the pediatric skeleton. These differences include the following[28,45,49,126]:

- Comparable soft tissue and bony injuries heal more reliably in children than in adults, particularly in patients less than 11 years of age.[66]
- Devitalized uncontaminated bone that can be covered with soft tissue can incorporate into the fracture callus, and in some cases may be left within the wound.
- External fixation can be maintained, when necessary, until fracture consolidation with fewer concerns about delayed or nonunion than in adults.
- Retained periosteum can regenerate bone, even after segmental bone loss in younger children.
- After thorough irrigation and debridement, many uncontaminated grade I open wounds may be closed primarily without an increased risk of infection.[60,95]
- Casts may be used for definitive stabilization in select stable open tibia fractures.[60,95]

OPERATIVE TREATMENT OF OPEN TIBIAL FRACTURES

Preoperative Planning

When surgical stabilization is planned, preoperative planning for open tibia fractures is similar to the previously described techniques for flexible intramedullary nailing or external fixation of closed tibia fractures. As with all open fractures, a thorough debridement of devitalized tissue and copious irrigation with sterile saline is necessary. Adequate soft tissue coverage is a mandatory part of operative treatment of these injuries, and early involvement with appropriate teams, such as plastic surgery or microsurgery specialists, is crucial to the management strategy.

Technique

Open tibial fractures of any grade should have a thorough and expedient irrigation and debridement of the wound, although there is evidence that infection rate is similar in injuries managed at less than 6 hours after injury and those treated later.[124] The patient's tetanus status must be determined, and prophylaxis should be administered as indicated. Appropriate intravenous (IV) antibiotic treatment is initiated as soon as possible and maintained as required based on the severity of the open fracture. There is a growing body of evidence to suggest that emergency department irrigation and debridement with administration of antibiotics alone may be appropriate for some simple, uncontaminated grade I open fractures.[10,43,107] In a retrospective comparative study of grade I open tibia fractures specifically, Padgett et al.[107] identified no infections in patients treated with bedside debridement and antibiotics (12 patients) and no difference in noninfectious complications when compared with those operatively debrided (21 patients). However, the remaining literature on this topic is limited in its inclusion of lower extremity injuries, and thus widespread adoption of this approach is not recommended at this time.

In those fractures requiring formal operative debridement, the soft tissue wounds should be extended to be certain that the area is cleansed and debrided of all nonviable tissue and foreign material. If in doubt of tissue viability, especially in younger children, leave the tissue in place and reevaluate later. Children heal more reliably than adults. Devitalized bone may be left in place if it is clean and can be covered by soft tissue, and this is determined on a case-by-case basis. The operative wound extension may be closed along with the open segment in clean grade I injuries. The traumatic wound should be allowed to heal by secondary intention if there is moderate contamination after irrigation and debridement. Patients with uncomplicated grade I fractures can be placed in a splint or a cast, or simple smooth pin fixation will prevent displacement of the fracture (Fig. 29-31). Use of this limited fixation does not preclude supplemental splinting or casting. Wounds associated with grade II and III fractures are debrided of devitalized tissue and foreign material. Most children with grade II and all children with grade III wounds require more rigid fracture stabilization to facilitate timely soft tissue coverage (Fig. 29-32). External fixation or intramedullary nails may be used at the surgeon's discretion based on fracture stability and personal experience. More rigid fixation limits the need for significant external splinting, thereby allowing better access for wound care and sequential compartment evaluation as needed.

Delayed primary closure can be performed if the wound is clean and does not involve significant skin and muscle loss. In such cases, it is imperative that closure under tension is avoided. Negative pressure dressings have been widely adopted in many trauma centers, are convenient to use, and some evidence suggests they have beneficial effects on soft tissues such as less need for flap coverage[30] and decreased infection rate.[52] Flap coverage was associated with a decreased rate of infection in a review of the literature of 54 grade IIIB tibial shaft fractures in children.[42] Definitive options include a wide variety of local rotational or pedicled myocutaneous flaps. Vascularized free flaps are viable options in cases for which no other method of closure is appropriate. In cases with segmental bone loss as well as significant soft tissue injury, acute shortening with plans for subsequent lengthening has been successful.[77]

Outcomes of Open Tibial Fractures

A number of notable differences exist when comparing the outcomes of open and closed tibia fractures in pediatric patients. Chiefly, an increased risk of complications (13.6% for open fracture vs. 5.1% for closed fracture) is evident across the existing literature base.[34,133] In addition, studies indicate open

Figure 29-31. A: Anteroposterior radiograph of a grade I open distal one-third tibial fracture in a 7-year-old child. **B:** Two percutaneous pins were used to stabilize this fracture after irrigation and debridement. **C:** Good fracture callus was present and the pins were removed 4 weeks after injury. **A, B**   **C**

Figure 29-32. A, B: Anteroposterior and lateral radiographs of a grade IIIB open tibia/fibula fractures sustained by a 9-year-old male in an agricultural accident. **C–E:** Anteroposterior/lateral radiographs and clinical image of a patient 8 weeks after placement of spanning monolateral external fixator with additional percutaneous pin fixation and delayed coverage with anterior thigh free flap. **F, G:** Anteroposterior and lateral radiographs of a patient 9 months after injury. Patient had excellent clinical result.

injuries may have slower time to union; however, patient age and selected fixation strategy may play a major role in these differences as comparative studies on open fractures are unable to control appropriately for these factors.[34,49,55,95,112] Neverthe-less, while historic outcomes for these injuries suggested higher rates of infection and more frequent delayed/nonunion, more recent evidence has suggested a more favorable outlook even for

high-grade injuries with high rates of eventual union and low rates of infection.[34,125]

Kreder and Armstrong[74] found an average time to union of 5.4 months (range 1.5–24.8 months) in a series of 56 open tib-ial fractures in 55 children with union time most impacted by patient age. Grimard et al.[49] reported that the age of the patient and the grade of the fracture were significantly associated with union time. Blasier and Barnes[13] found that children under 12 years of age required less aggressive surgical treatment and healed more rapidly than older children. They also found that younger children were more resistant to infection and had fewer complications than older children.

Hope and Cole[60] reported the results of open tibial fractures in 92 children (22 grade I, 51 grade II, and 19 grade III). Irrigation and debridement were performed on admission, IV antibiotics were given for 48 hours, and tetanus prophylaxis was administered when necessary. Primary closure was performed in 51 children, and 41 traumatic wounds were left open. Eighteen soft tissue injuries healed secondarily, and 23 required either a split-thickness skin graft or a tissue flap. Sixty-five (71%) of the 92 fractures were reduced and immobilized in an above-the-knee plaster cast. External fixation was used for unstable fractures, injuries with significant soft tissue loss, and fractures in patients with multiple system injuries. Early complications of open tibial fractures in these children were comparable with those in adults. Primary closure did not increase the risk of infection if the wound was small and uncontaminated. At reevaluation 1.5 to 9.8 years after injury, the authors found that 50% of the patients complained of pain at the fracture site; 23% reported decreased abilities to participate in sports, joint stiffness, and cosmetic defects; and 64% had leg-length inequalities. Levy et al.[79] found comparable late sequelae after open tibial fractures in children, including a 25% prevalence of nightmares surrounding the events of the accident. Blasier and Barnes[13] and Song et al.[126] found that most late complications associated with pediatric open tibial fractures occurred in children over the age of 12 and 11 years, respectively.

Most recently, in a 2017 report of pediatric open tibia fractures, Nandra et al. reported on 61 pediatric open tibial fractures with a mean age of 9 years, who were treated with a variety of fixation and wound management methods.[95] Increasing Gustilo–Anderson classification and age greater than 12 years were statistically associated with longer union time. Two of the three deep infections occurred in patients who underwent open plate fixation. Nine patients required revision of their monolateral external fixator to a multiplanar fixator due to delayed union or unacceptable alignment.

Some published reports highlight concerns about the use of external fixators in open tibia fractures in pediatric patients. Myers et al.[94] reviewed 31 consecutive high-energy tibia fractures in children treated with external fixation. Nineteen of the fractures were open, with mean follow-up of 15 months. The authors found a high rate of complications in this patient population, including delayed union (particularly in patients of at least 12 years of age), malunion, leg-length discrepancy, and pin-tract infections. However, Monsell et al. reported no nonunions and no complications in a group of 10 pediatric patients with open diaphyseal tibia fractures managed with a programmable circular external fixator. In addition, they had no patients with deep infection, nor were there any cases of refracture after fixator removal.[90]

While used infrequently, plating of pediatric tibia fractures has been reported. One series of 14 open pediatric tibial fractures treated with limited-contact places in minimally invasive

percutaneous osteosynthesis reported mean union time of 18 weeks (range 11–32 weeks) and no infections.[106] Supracutaneous plates with locking screws in lieu of traditional external fixation have also been described.[114]

Most of the literature addressing the subject of soft tissue coverage for open tibia fractures involves adult patients, and they may be relevant to the skeletally mature but less relevant to young children with better healing potential. However, combined orthoplastic management as traditionally utilized in adults, has shown favorable outcomes in pediatric patients. Smith et al.[125] reported on a series of 44 open tibia fractures in 43 patients with a majority of Gustilo–Anderson grade IIIB injuries treated with a high proportion (75%) of free flaps and demonstrated 100% union rates at a median of 12 weeks. They observed no cases of deep infection or flap failures.

Multiple authors have reported on the use of negative pressure dressings in the management of soft tissue injuries in pediatric patients. Dedmond et al.[30] reviewed the Wake Forest experience with negative pressure dressings in pediatric patients with type III open tibia fractures. They found that use of this device decreased the need for free tissue transfer to obtain coverage in this patient population. When focusing on the rate of infection, Halvorson et al.[52] found that use of negative pressure dressings in the management of open fractures, including open tibia fractures, appeared to be safe and effective when compared to historical controls. A recent literature review of adults with open tibial fractures concluded negative pressure dressings applied immediately after the first debridement seem to be an optimal bridge to the final reconstruction up to 7 days.[22] It has been our experience that negative pressure dressings have little downside other than skin irritation and may be used to speed up healing by secondary intention.

MANAGEMENT OF EXPECTED ADVERSE OUTCOMES AND UNEXPECTED COMPLICATIONS RELATED TO DIAPHYSEAL FRACTURES OF THE TIBIA AND FIBULA

It is uncommon to have poor outcomes or complications related to nonoperative treatment of closed tibial shaft fractures, as long as the appropriate radiographic follow-up and need for subsequent cast adjustment is respected. The majority of complications in pediatric tibial shaft fractures are most related to open fractures.

Diaphyseal Fractures of the Tibia and Fibula: COMMON ADVERSE OUTCOMES AND COMPLICATIONS

- Compartment syndrome
- Vascular injuries
- Infection
- Angular deformity
- Malrotation
- Leg-length discrepancy
- Anterior tibial physeal closure
- Delayed union and nonunion

COMPARTMENT SYNDROME

Compartment syndrome may occur after any type of tibia fracture, ranging from a seemingly minor closed injury to a severe, comminuted fracture. Using the Healthcare Cost and Utilization Project (HCUP) database, Obey et al.[102] identified 309 cases of compartment syndrome among 50,640 tibia fractures in pediatric patients over a 10-year period (0.6%) with older patients, motor vehicle accident and open fractures carrying an increased risk of occurrence. However, this database did not permit the review of radiographic or clinical characteristics and likely included a large proportion of lower-risk fracture types (e.g., low-energy mechanisms or toddler's fractures).

Among operatively treated patients, the pooled rate of compartment syndrome following after flexible nailing of pediatric tibial fractures across the available literature was 1.4% in the 2022 meta-analysis by Fanelli et al.[34] but has been reported as high as in the range from 2% to 20% in individual cohorts and may be associated with larger, obese children.[44,110] However, these cohorts included open tibia fractures, which sustained higher-energy injuries that were potentially more displaced with more soft tissue injury and therefore more biased toward complications. It is important to remember that compartment syndrome may occur in the face of significant soft tissue injury associated with extensively open fractures, as well as with closed injuries and after tibia fracture stabilization. In fact, Pandya and Edmonds[109] found no difference in the rate of compartment syndrome (14% open, 17% closed) following flexible nailing of pediatric tibial shaft fractures. Shore et al. reported an 11.6% incidence of compartment syndrome in 216 tibial shaft fractures with age of 14 years and older and motor vehicle accidents identified as predictors of occurrence.[123]

Diagnosis

Close observation and elevation of these affected limbs, whether the fracture was treated with casting or surgical stabilization, is necessary in all patients with displaced tibia fractures. It is crucial to monitor soft tissue swelling, pain escalation, and neurovascular examinations. In pediatric patients, this should be carefully scrutinized for the first 24 to 48 hours after treatment. Patients with a compartment syndrome often complain of pain out of proportion to the apparent severity of the injury. Increasing pain, often noted as continually increasing analgesic requirements, is the most important early sign of potential compartment syndrome in children.[6] In addition, pain with passive range of motion appears to be an early and strong clinical finding. Hyperesthesia, motor deficits, and decreased pulses are late changes and denote significant tissue injury. These signs occur only after the ischemia has been well established and the injury is permanent. Late complications of untreated lower extremity compartment syndrome include clawed toes, dorsal bunion, and limited subtalar motion secondary to necrosis and subsequent fibrous contracture of the muscles originating in the deep posterior compartment.

Treatment

Any cast or splint should be bivalved, split or otherwise loosened, and the cast padding divided, in a patient with increased or increasing pain associated with treatment of a tibia fracture. If, after removal of all encircling wraps, there is no relief, compartment syndrome should be considered. Compartment pressures may be obtained, but in most cases, pediatric patients with clinical findings consistent with elevated pressures should undergo surgical release. Any child who has objective or subjective evidence of a compartment syndrome should undergo an emergent fasciotomy. Although there is some controversy in the literature, if compartmental pressure monitoring is utilized, symptomatic patients with compartment pressures greater than 30 mm Hg may benefit from fasciotomy.[63,127]

The two-incision technique is used most widely for fasciotomies, although a single-incision, perifibular release is favored at some centers (Fig. 29-33). The fascia surrounding each

A

1 - Anterior compartment
2 - Lateral compartment
3 - Deep posterior compartment
4 - Superficial posterior compartment

B

Figure 29-33. *Arrows* show the trajectories of the decompressive fasciotomies. **A:** Decompressive fasciotomies through a two-incision approach. The anterolateral incision allows decompression of the anterior and lateral compartments. The medial incision allows decompression of the superficial posterior and the deep posterior compartments. **B:** A one-incision decompression fasciotomy can be performed through a lateral approach that allows a dissection of all four compartments.

compartment of concern should be opened widely. The wounds are left open and delayed primary closure is performed when possible. Negative pressure wound dressings may be of benefit in the management of fasciotomy wounds before closure or coverage. Split-thickness skin grafting of the wounds may be necessary in some cases. Fibulectomy has been recommended by some authors as a method by which all compartments can be released through a single approach. Most literature does not support its use, and this procedure should not be performed in skeletally immature patients due to the risk of potential proximal migration of the distal fibular remnant and resulting ankle valgus. Long-term ankle valgus may result in ankle instability, gait impairment, and potentially problematic limb length discrepancy.

In a long-term review of patients from the Children's Hospital of Philadelphia, Flynn et al. found that most children with lower extremity compartment syndrome, including those associated with tibia fractures, had good or excellent clinical results. This appeared to be true even in those patients with long time periods from injury to fasciotomy.[35] Shore et al. reported that full functional recovery was achieved in 92% of patients with tibial compartment syndrome; however, one below-knee amputation was necessary in their cohort of 25 cases.[123]

VASCULAR INJURIES

Vascular injuries associated with tibial fractures are uncommon in children; however, when they do occur, the sequelae can be devastating. In an evaluation of 14 patients with lower extremity fractures and concomitant vascular injuries, Allen et al.[2] noted that only three children returned to normal function. One factor leading to a poor outcome was a delay in diagnosis. Evaluation for vascular compromise is imperative in all children with tibial fractures.

The displaced proximal tibial metaphyseal fracture is the pattern of injury most frequently associated with vascular injury and often involves the anterior tibial artery as it passes between the fibula and the tibia into the anterior compartment. The anterior tibial artery may be injured with distal tibial fractures, as the vessel may be injured if the distal fragment translates posteriorly. Posterior tibial artery injuries are rare, except in fractures associated with crushing or shearing caused by accidents involving heavy machinery, or those secondary to gunshot wounds involving the lower leg and ankle region.

Vascular injuries have been reported in approximately 5% of children with open tibial fractures. Arterial injuries associated with open tibial fractures include those to the popliteal artery, the posterior tibial artery, the anterior tibial artery, and the peroneal artery. Amputation rates as high as 79% have been reported with grade IIIC fractures. Isolated anterior tibial and peroneal artery injuries generally have a good prognosis, whereas injuries of the posterior tibial and popliteal arteries have much less satisfactory prognoses and more commonly require vascular repairs or reconstructions.[2] Patients with open tibial fractures and vascular disruption may benefit from temporary arterial, and possibly venous, shunting before the bony reconstruction is performed. This approach allows meticulous debridement and

repair of the fracture, while maintaining limb perfusion until the primary vascular repair is performed. However, in most cases, rapid fracture stabilization, usually using external fixation, can be performed before vascular reconstruction without the need for temporary shunts.

INFECTION

The risk of infection in treatment of pediatric tibial diaphyseal fractures is mainly isolated to open tibial shaft fractures and is at highest risk in those with grade III injuries.[124] The best treatment is prevention with timely IV antibiotic administration, timely irrigation and debridement, repeated debridement as needed, and early soft tissue coverage. Surgical stabilization of the fracture protects that soft tissue and can reduce infection risk.

Prolonged wound healing, continued drainage, delayed fracture union, and hardware failure may all be signs of infection. Laboratory values may be normal in low-grade, chronic infections, and intraoperative bone biopsy and culture are sometimes needed to establish the diagnosis of osteomyelitis. As in any treatment of osteomyelitis, initial surgical treatment includes debridement of involved bone and nonviable soft tissue as well as removal of any loose or broken retained implants. A spanning external fixator device placed through noninfected areas maintains bony stabilization to allow fracture healing in cases of nonunion. Antibiotics are tailored to intraoperative bony culture results, and soft tissue coverage options include local wound care, negative pressure dressings, skin grafts, or local or free soft tissue flaps.

Ostermann et al. reported 115 grade II and 239 grade III tibial fractures in a series of 1,085 open fractures. All patients were treated with early broad-spectrum antibiotics, serial debridements, and the application of an external fixation device. Tobramycin-impregnated polymethylmethacrylate (PMMA) was placed into the wounds, and dressings were changed every 48 to 72 hours until the wounds spontaneously closed, underwent delayed primary closure, or received flap coverage. No infections occurred in grade I fractures; approximately 3% of grade II fractures and 8% of grade III fractures developed infections. No infections occurred in patients who had the wound closed within 8 days of injury. On the basis of these and other analyses, it is now recommended that wounds associated with open tibial fractures be covered within 7 days of injury whenever possible.[103]

ANGULAR DEFORMITY

Spontaneous correction of significant axial displacement after a diaphyseal fracture of a child's forearm or femur is common. Remodeling of an angulated tibial shaft fracture, however, is often incomplete (Fig. 29-34).[15] As such, the goal of treatment should be to obtain as close to anatomic alignment as possible. Swaan and Oppers[132] evaluated 86 children treated for fractures of the tibia. The original angulation of the fracture was measured on radiographs in the sagittal and frontal projections. Girls 1 to 8 years of age and boys 1 to 10 years of age demonstrated moderate spontaneous correction of residual angulation after union. In girls 9 to 12 years of age and boys 11 to 12 years

Figure 29-34. A 4-year 2-month-old child with a middle one-third transverse tibial fracture and a plastically deformed fibular fracture. **A:** Lateral view shows 20-degree posterior angulation. **B:** The deformity is still 15 degrees 4 years after the injury.

of age, approximately 50% of the angulation was corrected. No more than 25% of the deformity was corrected in children over 13 years of age.

Bennek and Steinert[11] found that recurvatum malunion of more than 10 degrees did not correct completely. In this study, 26 of 28 children with varus or valgus deformities at union had significant residual angular deformities at follow-up. Valgus deformities had a worse outcome because the tibiotalar joint was left in a relatively unstable position. Weber et al.[139] demonstrated that a fracture with varus malalignment of 5 to 13 degrees completely corrected at the level of the physis. Most children with valgus deformities of 5 to 7 degrees did not have a full correction.

Hansen et al.[53] reported on 102 pediatric tibial fractures, 25 of which had malunions of 4 to 19 degrees. Residual angular malunions ranged from 3 to 19 degrees at final follow-up, without a single patient having complete remodeling and correction. The spontaneous correction was approximately 13.5% of the total deformity. Shannak[121] reviewed the results of treatment of 117 children with tibial shaft fractures treated with closed reduction and long-leg casts. Multiplanar deformities did not remodel as completely as those in a single plane. The least correction occurred in apex posterior angulated fractures, followed by fractures with valgus malalignment (Fig. 29-35). Spontaneous remodeling of malunited tibial fractures in children appears to be limited to the first 18 months after fracture.[31,53]

MALROTATION

Rotational malalignment of the tibia does not correct spontaneously with remodeling and should be avoided.[53] A computerized tomographic (CT) evaluation of tibial rotation can be performed if there is any question about the rotational alignment of the fracture that is not evident on clinical examination.

Figure 29-35. A: Anteroposterior and lateral radiographs 2 months after injury in a 6-year-old boy reveal a valgus and anterior malunion at the fracture. **B:** One year later, the child still has a moderate valgus and anterior malalignment of the distal fractured segment. This malalignment produced painful hyperextension of the knee at heel strike during ambulation.

Rotational malunion of more than 20 to 30 degrees may produce functional impairment and may necessitate a subsequent derotational osteotomy of the tibia, though this is quite rare. Most commonly, derotational osteotomy of the tibia is performed in the supramalleolar aspect of the distal tibia. The fibula may be left intact, particularly for planned derotation of less than 30 degrees. Maintaining continuity of the fibula adds stability and limits the possibility of introducing an iatrogenic angular deformity to the distal tibia.

LEG-LENGTH DISCREPANCY

Hyperemia associated with fracture repair may stimulate the physes in the involved leg, producing growth acceleration, particularly in younger children. Tibial growth acceleration after fracture is less than that seen after femoral fractures in children of comparable ages. Shannak[121] showed that the average growth acceleration of a child's tibia after fracture is approximately 4.5 mm. Comminuted fractures appear to have the greatest risk of accelerated growth and overgrowth.

Swaan and Oppers[132] reported that young children have a greater chance for overgrowth than older children. Accelerated growth after tibial fracture generally occurs in children under 10 years of age, whereas older children may have a mild growth inhibition associated with the fracture.[53] The amount of fracture shortening also has an effect on growth stimulation. Fractures with significant shortening have more physeal growth after fracture union than injuries without shortening at union.[87] The presence of angulation at union does not appear to affect the amount of overgrowth.

Anterior Tibial Physeal Closure

Patients have demonstrated apparently iatrogenic closure after placement of a proximal tibial traction pin, the application of pins and plaster, and after application of an external fixation device. Some children may have an undiagnosed injury of the tibial physis at the time of the ipsilateral tibial diaphyseal fracture.[69] Regardless of etiology, premature closure of the physis produces a progressive recurvatum deformity and loss of the normal anterior to posterior slope of the proximal tibia as the child grows. Management may require surgical intervention including proximal tibial osteotomy with all the inherent risks and potential complications of that procedure.

NONUNION/DELAYED UNION

Nonunions and delayed unions are rare in pediatric patients with lower-energy, closed fractures. Achieving adequate fracture stability is of utmost importance in prevention of delayed healing, regardless of method employed. Inadequate immobilization or noncompliance with weight-bearing restrictions that allows patterned micro- or macromotion may slow the rate of healing and lead to delayed or nonunion. Fractures treated with flexible nailing must have some compression and motion at the fracture site. As such, use of stiffer and larger diameter nails may limit necessary micromotion or may introduce distraction at the fracture site which may slow fracture healing. However, even among operatively treated injuries with flexible nailing, the pooled rate of nonunion and delayed union across the available literature base is approximately 5%, with fewer than 2% requiring further surgical treatment.[34] The rate of nonunion is not affected by open reduction of a closed fracture.[82] The use of an external fixation device may be associated with increased time to union in some patients, particularly those with open fractures resulting from high-energy injury.[47,80,94] In patients treated with external fixation, care must be taken to advance weight bearing appropriately and to dynamize the fixator frame as soon as possible to maximize bone healing. In patients with a suspected delayed union or nonunion, a 1-cm fibulectomy will allow increased compression at the delayed union or nonunion site with weight bearing and often will induce healing (Fig. 29-36).

A, B   **C, D**

Figure 29-36. A: Anteroposterior radiograph of the distal tibia and fibula in a 5-year-old boy with an open fracture. **B:** Early callus formation is seen 1 month after injury. **C:** The tibia has failed to unite 10 months after injury. **D:** The patient underwent a fibulectomy 4 cm proximal to the tibial nonunion. The tibial fracture united 8 weeks after surgery.

Figure 29-37. A: Nonunion of an open tibial fracture. **B:** After posterolateral tibial bone graft.

In any pediatric long bone fracture that exhibits delayed healing, infection must be ruled out. With a proven aseptic nonunion, treatment is targeted to the type of nonunion, hypertrophic or atrophic. Hypertrophic nonunions have a failure of stability, and callus debridements, additional fixation or revision of existing fixation, and protected weight bearing help to achieve union. Atrophic nonunions are uncommon in pediatric patients unless there is severe soft tissue and bony loss at the time of injury. Posterolateral bone grafting is an excellent technique to produce union in children (Fig. 29-37). Avascular bone may require resection, bone grafting (autograft or vascularized bone graft), or even bone transport. Adolescents near skeletal maturity with a delayed or nonunion of the tibia can be managed with a reamed intramedullary nail, concomitant fibular osteotomy, and correction of any angulation at the nonunion site as necessary (Fig. 29-38). Addressing soft tissue coverage with vascularized tissue flaps can improve vascular perfusion to the area of the delayed or nonunion.

Fractures of the Distal Tibial Metaphysis

INTRODUCTION TO FRACTURES OF THE DISTAL TIBIAL METAPHYSIS

Fractures of the distal tibial metaphysis are uncommon injuries in children, with an incidence between 0.35% and 0.45% of all pediatric fractures.[31]

MECHANISM OF INJURY FOR DISTAL TIBIAL METAPHYSIS FRACTURES

Distal tibial metaphyseal fractures are often greenstick injuries resulting from increased compressive forces along the anterior

Figure 29-38. A: Anteroposterior and lateral radiographs of a 14-year-old adolescent who was struck by a car, sustaining a grade IIIB open fracture of the tibia. **B:** Anteroposterior and lateral radiographs of the tibia after irrigation and debridement and application of an external fixation device. **C:** The patient developed a nonunion at the tibia, which progressively deformed into an unacceptable varus alignment. **D:** The nonunion was treated with a fibular osteotomy followed by a closed angular correction of the deformity and internal fixation with a reamed intramedullary nail.

tibial cortex. This fracture often occurs secondary to an axial load on a dorsiflexed foot. The anterior cortex is impacted while the posterior cortex is displaced under tension, with a tear of the overlying periosteum. A combined valgus and recurvatum deformity may occur, which can be corrected by reducing the fracture with the ankle in plantarflexion (Fig. 29-39).

TREATMENT OPTIONS FOR FRACTURES OF THE DISTAL TIBIAL METAPHYSIS

NONOPERATIVE TREATMENT OF FRACTURES OF THE DISTAL TIBIAL METAPHYSIS

Reduction of these injuries should be performed with adequate sedation and maintained with a long-leg cast. In cases in which the fracture has displaced or angulated into recurvatum, the ankle can be left in moderate plantarflexion to minimize the risk of apex

A, B   **C**

Figure 29-39. **A:** Fracture of the distal tibia in a 7-year-old child. The lateral radiograph demonstrates a mild recurvatum deformity. **B:** The ankle was initially immobilized in an ankle neutral position, producing an increased recurvatum deformity. The cast was removed and the ankle remanipulated into plantarflexion to reduce the deformity. **C:** The ankle was then immobilized in plantarflexion, which is the proper position for this type of fracture.

posterior angulation at the fracture site. The ankle can then be brought up to neutral after 3 to 4 weeks, and a short-leg walking cast is applied. Nondisplaced fractures can be immobilized in either a short- or long-leg cast at the surgeon's discretion; a recent study reported earlier time to weight bearing and shorter time to fracture union for distal tibial fractures treated in short-leg casts.[7]

OPERATIVE TREATMENT OF FRACTURES OF THE DISTAL TIBIAL METAPHYSIS

Unstable, displaced fractures can be treated with closed reduction and percutaneous pins[16] (Fig. 29-40), antegrade flexible nails,[8,27,122] ORIF, or percutaneous plating[85] (Fig. 29-41), with good reported results for all techniques. ORIF of an associated distal fibula fracture may limit the risk of malalignment in an unstable distal tibia fracture. The surgical technique for management of these fractures with flexible nails is essentially identical to that described previously for diaphyseal tibia fractures although the location of the metaphyseal fracture typically is where the nails cross distally and the lack of canal fill may make the distal segment difficult to control. Because of this, alternate constructs such as quadruple stacked flexible nails or divergent intramedullary nailing, where the nails are not curved and only cross in the proximal tibia, have been proposed.[54,145]

A, B   **C**

Figure 29-40. **A, B:** Unstable distal metadiaphyseal fractures of the tibia and fibula in a 15-year-old girl. **C:** This fracture was stabilized with percutaneous pins because of marked swelling and fracture instability.

Figure 29-41. A: Anteroposterior radiograph of a distal one-third tibial and fibular fractures in a 9-year-old girl with a closed head injury and severe spasticity. The initial reduction in a cast could not be maintained. **B:** Open reduction and internal fixation with a medial plate was used to achieve and maintain the alignment.

Special Fractures

TODDLER'S FRACTURES

INTRODUCTION TO TODDLER'S FRACTURES

Seemingly minor episodes involving preschool-aged children that result in external rotation of the foot with the knee in a fixed position may produce a spiral fracture of the tibia without a concomitant fibular fracture. This entity is most frequently termed a "toddler's fracture" (Fig. 29-42). This fracture pattern was first reported by Dunbar et al., with 83% (63/76) of these fractures occurring in children under 2.5 years of age[32] in 1964. The traumatic episode may be unwitnessed by the parent or adult caretaker.[104] Common examples of this include injuries occurring when a child sustains a low-energy fall or attempts to extricate their foot from between the uprights of a playpen or crib, although toddler's fractures can also commonly occur while going down a playground slide on an adult's lap.[39,64] Oudjhane et al.[104] analyzed the radiographs of 500 acutely limping toddlers and identified 100 in whom a fracture was the etiology of the gait disturbance. Although this low-energy injury is presumed to be low risk for child abuse, a recent series found low-risk fractures (buckle, clavicle, supracondylar, and toddler's fractures) have a similar rate of concomitant suspicious injuries for child abuse as moderate-risk fractures (defined as all other fractures excluding spine, rib, scapula, and sternal fractures).[93]

ASSESSMENT OF TODDLER'S FRACTURES

The physical findings in a patient with a possible toddler's fracture are often subtle. The child typically presents with a history of a new-onset limp or refusal to bear weight on the limb. The

Figure 29-42. A: Anteroposterior and lateral radiographs of an 18-month-old child who presented with refusal to bear weight on her leg. Note the spiral middle one-third "toddler's" fracture (*arrowheads*). **B:** This fracture healed uneventfully after 4 weeks of immobilization in a cast.

examination should begin with an evaluation of the uninvolved side, as this serves as a control for the symptomatic extremity. The examination begins at the hip and proceeds to the thigh, knee, lower leg, ankle, and foot. It is important to note areas of point tenderness, any increase in local or systemic temperature, and any swelling or bruising of the leg. In those patients in whom the examination appears to point to the leg as the source of the problem, plain AP, lateral, and internal oblique radiographic views should be obtained of the tibia and fibula. The internally rotated oblique view may be the only view that will demonstrate an acute nondisplaced toddler's fracture. In cases in which initial radiographs are negative, but the history and examination are consistent with diagnosis of a toddler's fracture, treatment immobilization is indicated.[51,53] In these cases, follow-up radiographs will often demonstrate periosteal new bone formation approximately 10 to 14 days after injury (Fig. 29-43). Osteomyelitis may also present as a limp in the absence of trauma; laboratory markers (complete blood count, C-reactive protein, erythrocyte sedimentation rate) may need to be obtained if the diagnosis is in doubt. Magnetic resonance imaging (MRI) is rarely used due to the need for sedation or anesthesia at this young age.

TREATMENT OF TODDLER'S FRACTURES

As these fractures are inherently stable, a child with a toddler's fracture may be immobilized in a long-leg cast, short-leg cast, a walking boot, or even no immobilization for approximately 3 to 4 weeks at the discretion of the treating physician. The fracture is stable, and the patient may bear weight on the cast, splint, or boot when comfortable. Bauer and Lovejoy reported a statistically significant earlier return to weight bearing for patients in

Figure 29-43. A, B: Anteroposterior and lateral radiographs of a 27-month-old refusing to bear weight at presentation are negative. **C:** Three weeks later, an anteroposterior radiograph demonstrates the fracture line (*black arrow*) and periosteal bone formation (*white arrows*), confirming the diagnosis of a toddler's fracture. (Used with permission by the Children's Orthopaedic Center, Los Angeles.)

a boot compared to a short-leg cast (2.5 weeks vs. 2.8 weeks), but found that nearly all patients in their cohort of 192 toddlers resumed full weight bearing by 4 weeks, regardless of immobilization type.[9] Simple observation without immobilization has been compared to long-leg casting, and authors found that observation alone had equivalent clinical and radiographic outcomes with high family satisfaction, fewer minor complications (wet casts), and slightly earlier return to walking.[38]

FLOATING KNEE

INTRODUCTION TO FLOATING KNEE

Although uncommon in children, significant trauma can cause ipsilateral fractures involving both the tibia and the femur. The term "floating knee" describes the flail knee joint resulting from fractures of the shaft or metaphyseal region of the ipsilateral femur and tibia.[3] A recent series of 25 pediatric floating knee injuries found 96% of cases were caused by traffic accidents with 60% (15/25) of the injuries being open fractures.[98]

TREATMENT OF FLOATING KNEE

Historically, these injuries often were treated with traction and casting. The extent of the injuries often left permanent

functional deficits, including malunion, limb-length discrepancy, and knee stiffness when not managed aggressively.[15,23]

Today, children with ipsilateral tibia and femoral fractures are most often treated with operative stabilization of the femur and either cast immobilization after closed reduction or operative fixation of the tibia,[143] especially given the high percentage of open fractures with loss of inherent periosteal stability. In pediatric patients, multiple treatment combinations can safely be utilized to care for a patient with floating knee injury as was demonstrated in CORTICES'[23] multicenter cohort of 130 pediatric floating knee injuries. In this study, 91.5% of femur fractures and 72.3% of tibia fractures were treated operatively with a variety of constructs dictated by fracture pattern and patient age. Femur fractures were most commonly treated with flexible or rigid nailing, while flexible nailing was the most commonly utilized fixation method for tibia fractures. Good to excellent outcomes were observed in over 90% of patients according to Karlstrom criteria and no differences in outcomes were noted when comparing treatment strategies. Therefore, closed management for both injuries may represent an acceptable strategy for select patients.

In most cases, the tibial fracture is addressed after the femoral fracture has been stabilized. Closed tibial fractures in these situations may be treated with cast immobilization or operative fixation. Open tibial fractures associated with an ipsilateral femoral fracture should be stabilized with an external

A, B   **C, D**

Figure 29-44. **A, B:** Floating knee injury in a 7-year-old boy. **C:** Femoral fracture was fixed with flexible intramedullary nails. **D:** Tibial fracture was stabilized with external fixation.

fixator, flexible intramedullary nails, or plate and screw construct (Fig. 29-44). Stable fixation of both fractures allows early range of motion of the knee, earlier weight bearing, and improves overall function.[143] Despite surgical management, limb discrepancy and loss of motion may still occur given the high severity of these injuries.[98]

STRESS FRACTURES OF THE TIBIA AND FIBULA

INTRODUCTION TO STRESS FRACTURES OF THE TIBIA AND FIBULA

The pattern of stress fractures of the tibia and fibula in children differs from that in adults. In adults, the fibula is involved in stress fractures twice as often as the tibia; in pediatric patients, the tibia is affected more often than the fibula (Fig. 29-45). The prevalence of stress fractures in boys and girls appears to be equal, although stress fractures have been reported to be increasingly common in females with eating disorders.[97] These injuries typically occur in pediatric and adolescent athletes older than 10 years of age and have a history of insidious onset of pain that worsens with sporting activities.[48,138]

ASSESSMENT AND TREATMENT OF STRESS FRACTURES OF THE TIBIA AND FIBULA

Stress fractures occur when the repetitive force applied to a bone is exceeded by the bone's capacity to withstand it. Initially, osteoclastic tunnel formation increases. These tunnels

normally fill with mature bone. With continued force, cortical reabsorption accelerates. Woven bone is produced to splint the weakened cortex. However, this bone is disorganized and does not have the strength of the bone it replaces. A fracture occurs when bone reabsorption outstrips bone production.

Figure 29-45. Bilateral midtibial stress fractures in an adolescent with genu varus.

When the offending force is reduced or eliminated, bone production exceeds bone reabsorption. This produces cortical and endosteal widening with dense repair bone that later remodels to mature bone.[104]

A child with a tibial stress fracture usually has an insidious onset of symptoms. There is evidence of local tenderness that worsens with activity. The pain tends to be worse in the day, particularly during activities, and improves at night and with rest. The knee and the ankle have full range of motion. Usually, there is minimal, if any, swelling at the fracture site.[72]

Initial radiographs may be normal. Radiographic changes consistent with a stress fracture generally become evident approximately 2 weeks after the onset of symptoms. Radiographic findings consistent with fracture repair can manifest in one of three ways: localized periosteal new bone formation, endosteal thickening, or, rarely, a radiolucent cortical fracture line (Fig. 29-46).[72]

The differential diagnosis includes sarcoma of bone, osteomyelitis, and a soft tissue injury without accompanying bony injury. A careful history, physical examination, laboratory workup, and use of necessary radiographic imaging can usually allow differentiation of a stress fracture from infection or neoplasm.[138]

In cases in which the plain radiographs are normal, MRI may be helpful. MRI[72] shows a localized band of very low signal intensity continuous with the cortex. These MR findings can be diagnostic for a stress fracture and will differentiate such lesions from malignancy, thereby obviating the need for biopsy. CT rarely demonstrates the fracture line, but often delineates increased marrow density, endosteal and periosteal new bone formation, and may show soft tissue edema within the area of concern.

Tibia Stress Fractures

The most common location for a tibial stress fracture is in the proximal third.[37] The child normally has a limp of gradual onset with no history of a specific injury. The pain is described as dull, occurring in the calf near the upper end of the tibia on its medial aspect, and occasionally is bilateral. Physical findings include local tenderness on one or both sides of the tibial crest with a varying degree of swelling.

The treatment of a child with a stress fracture of the tibia begins with activity modification. An active child can rest in a prefabricated walking boot for 4 to 6 weeks followed by gradual increase in activity.[100] Nonunions of stress fractures of the tibia have been described. Green et al.[48] reported six nonunions, each in the middle third of the tibia. Three of these nonunions were in children. Two required excision of the nonunion site with iliac crest bone grafting. The third was treated by electromagnetic stimulation. In cases of stress fractures involving female athletes with dietary, nutritional, and menstrual irregularities, collaboration between pediatric orthopaedists, primary care physicians, endocrinologists, and nutritionist is recommended.[56]

Fibula Stress Fractures

Pediatric fibular stress fractures normally occur between the ages of 2 and 8 years.[73] The fractures are normally localized to the distal third of the fibula. The child presents with a limp and may complain of pain. Swelling normally is not present. The obvious bony mass commonly seen in a stress fracture of the fibula in an adult is rarely seen in a comparable fracture in a child.

Often the earliest plain radiographic sign of a stress fracture of the fibula is the presence of "eggshell" callus along the shaft of the fibula. The fracture itself cannot always be seen because the periosteal callus may obscure the changes in the narrow canal. MRI can help to identify stress fractures before the presence of radiographic changes.

SUMMARY, CONTROVERSIES, AND FUTURE DIRECTIONS RELATED TO PEDIATRIC TIBIAL SHAFT FRACTURES

Tibia fractures are extremely common injuries in all pediatric age groups. While the risk of potential complications does exist, most tibia fractures, regardless of anatomic location within the bone, heal without difficulty and cause few long-term functional deficits. Tibia fractures that pose particular concerns, either due to potential problems with management of the acute fracture or secondary to secondary to delayed complications, include proximal tibial metaphyseal fractures and open fractures of the diaphyseal region.

The management of tibial shaft fractures has demonstrated the greatest change in recent years. While an initial attempt at closed management remains appropriate for most injuries, there has been increasing use of flexible nails, with or without external immobilization, in the care of diaphyseal and metadiaphyseal

Figure 29-46. Anteroposterior and lateral radiographs of the knee of a 15-year-old with adolescent-onset tibia vara. Note the posteromedial stress fracture.

fractures while the use of closed cast treatment for the same fractures has diminished. Especially for diaphyseal fractures in older pediatric patients, the long-leg cast is being replaced by flexible intramedullary nails due to the relative conveniences that they offer to the patient, family, and physician.

Changes in the management of pediatric tibia fractures in the future seem inevitable, and it will most likely mirror approaches to care for other pediatric fractures. An increasing number of diaphyseal tibia fractures will receive surgical treatment if closed methods fail, most likely with some form of "growth plate friendly" intramedullary fixation, particularly in older children and adolescents. However, closed treatment with cast immobilization remains the primary method of care for most tibia fractures, particularly in younger children.

Annotated References

Reference	Annotation
Buckley SL, Smith G, Sponseller PD, et al. Open fractures of the tibia in children. *J Bone Joint Surg Am.* 1990;72(10):1462–1469.	Report of single-center experience with operative management of open tibia fractures in children. The incidences of compartment syndrome, vascular injury, infection, and delayed unions were similar when compared to the adult literature with open injuries.
Fanelli D, Perrotta G, Stocco F, et al. Outcomes and complications following flexible intramedullary nailing for the treatment of tibial fractures in children: a meta-analysis. *Arch Orthop Trauma Surg.* 2022;142:1469–1482.	2022 systematic review and meta-analysis of flexible intramedullary nailing in the treatment of tibial fracture in children providing pooled rates of complications across 835 patients from 28 studies with a mean age of 11 years old.
Flynn JM, Bashyal RK, Yeger-McKeever M, et al. Acute compartment syndrome of the leg in children: Diagnosis and outcome. *J Bone Joint Surg Am.* 2011;93:937–941.	Large two-center study that reviewed a 17-year experience with acute compartment of the leg in children. Despite often lengthy delays in time to treatment, most children with compartment syndrome had acceptable results after surgical management.
Gordon JE, Gregush RV, Schoenecker PL, et al. Complications after titanium elastic nailing of pediatric tibial fractures. *J Pediatr Orthop.* 2007;27(4):442–446.	Single-center, retrospective review of 60 diaphyseal tibia fractures in children treated with intramedullary fixation. While complications were low, 11% of patients demonstrated delayed or nonunions.
Kinney MC, Nagle D, Bastrom T, et al. Operative versus conservative management of displaced tibial shaft fractures in adolescents. *J Pediatr Orthop.* 2016;36(7):661–666.	Outcomes were similar in patients treated originally with both closed and operative treatments. Predictors of failure of closed reduction included initial fracture displacement and presence of a fibula fracture.
Rinker B, Valerio IL, Stewart DH, et al. Microvascular free flap reconstruction in pediatric lower extremity trauma: a 10-year review. *Plat Reconstr Surg.* 2005;115(6):1618–1624.	Review of 28 flaps placed due to lower extremity trauma in 26 patients over a 10-year period. Patients receiving free-flap coverage within 7 days of injury had a statistically lower rate of complications than those having a longer time period to soft tissue coverage.
Shore BJ, Glotzbecker MP, Zurakowski D, et al. Acute compartment syndrome in children and teenagers with tibial shaft fractures; incidence and multivariate risk factors. *J Orthop Trauma.* 2013;27(11):616–621.	Single-center review of the incidence of acute compartment syndrome in pediatric patients with tibia fractures. The incidence was much higher than previously reported in the literature and associated with patient age more than 14 years old and when the injury was secondary to an motor vehicle accident.
Smith JRA, Fox CE, Wright TC, et al. Orthoplastic management of open tibial fractures in children: a consecutive five-year series from a paediatric major trauma centre. *Bone Joint J.* 2021;103-B:1160–1167.	Single-center review of 44 open tibia fractures in 43 pediatric patients (mean 9.9 years old) with minimum 1 year treated with combined orthoplastic approach with 75% of patients undergoing free flap. No cases of flap failure or deep infection. All fractures united at median 12 weeks.
Tuten HR, Keeler KA, Gabos PG, et al. Posttraumatic tibia valga in children. A long-term follow-up note. *J Bone Joint Surg Am.* 1999;81(6):799–810.	A small case series with long-term mean follow-up of 15 years that documents spontaneous resolution of the post–Cozen fracture deformity and provides the basis for a period of watchful observation in these patients.

REFERENCES

1. Al-Sayyad MJ. Taylor Spatial Frame in the treatment of pediatric and adolescent tibial shaft fractures. *J Pediatr Orthop.* 2006;26(2):164–170.
2. Allen MJ, Nash JR, Ioannidies TT, Bell PR. Major vascular injuries associated with orthopaedic injuries to the lower limb. *Ann R Coll Surg Engl.* 1984;66(2):101–104.
3. Arslan H, Kapukaya A, Kesemenli C, et al. Floating knee in children. *J Pediatr Orthop.* 2003;23(4):458–463.
4. Aslani H, Tabrizi A, Sadighi A, Mirblok AR. Treatment of open pediatric tibial fractures by external fixation versus flexible intramedullary nailing: a comparative study. *Arch Trauma Res.* 2013;2(3):108–112.
5. Backstrom IC, MacLennan PA, Sawyer JR, et al. Pediatric obesity and traumatic lower-extremity long-bone fracture outcomes. *J Trauma Acute Care Surg.* 2012;73(4):966–971.
6. Bae DS, Kadiyala RK, Waters PM. Acute compartment syndrome in children: contemporary diagnosis, treatment, and outcome. *J Pediatr Orthop.* 2001;21(5):680–688.
7. Barnett SA, Fontenot B, Leonardi C, et al. Comparison of short-leg and long-leg casts for the treatment of distal third tibial shaft fractures in children. *J Pediatr Orthop.* 2021;41(3):e259–e265.
8. Bauer J, Hirzinger C, Metzger R. Quadruple ESIN (elastic stable intramedullary nailing): modified treatment in pediatric distal tibial fractures. *J Pediatr Orthop.* 2017;37(2):e100–e103.

9. Bauer JM, Lovejoy SA. Toddler's fractures: time to weight-bear with regard to immobilization type and radiographic monitoring. *J Pediatr Orthop.* 2019;39(6): 314–317.

10. Bazzi AA, Brooks JT, Jain A, et al. Is nonoperative treatment of pediatric type I open fractures safe and effective? *J Child Orthop.* 2014;8(6):467–471.

11. Bennek J, Steinert V. [Bone development after abnormal healing of lower leg shaft fractures in children]. *Zentralbl Chir.* 1966;91(17):633–639.

12. Benz G, Kallieris D, Seeböck T, et al. Bioresorbable pins and screws in paediatric traumatology. *Eur J Pediatr Surg.* 1994;4(2):103–107.

13. Blasier RD, Barnes CL. Age as a prognostic factor in open tibial fractures in children. *Clin Orthop Relat Res.* 1996;(331):261–264.

14. Blick SS, Brumback RJ, Poka A, et al. Compartment syndrome in open tibial fractures. *J Bone Joint Surg Am.* 1986;68(9):1348–1353.

15. Bohn WW, Durbin RA. Ipsilateral fractures of the femur and tibia in children and adolescents. *J Bone Joint Surg Am.* 1991;73(3):429–439.

16. Brantley J, Majumdar A, Jobe JT, et al. A biomechanical comparison of pin configurations used for percutaneous pinning of distal tibia fractures in children. *Iowa Orthop J.* 2016;36:133–137.

17. Briggs TW, Orr MM, Lightowler CD. Isolated tibial fractures in children. *Injury.* 1992;23(5):308–310.

18. Buckley SL, Gotschall C, Robertson W Jr, et al. The relationships of skeletal injuries with trauma score, injury severity score, length of hospital stay, hospital charges, and mortality in children admitted to a regional pediatric trauma center. *J Pediatr Orthop.* 1994;14(4):449–453.

19. Burkus M, Tömböl F, Wiegand N, Kretzer A. Physeal-sparing unreamed locked intramedullary nailing for adolescent tibial fractures. *Injury.* 2021;52(Suppl 1): S67–S73.

20. Canavese F, Botnari A, Andreacchio A, et al. Displaced tibial shaft fractures with intact fibula in children: nonoperative management versus operative treatment with elastic stable intramedullary nailing. *J Pediatr Orthop.* 2016;36(7):667–672.

21. Cheng JC, Shen WY. Limb fracture pattern in different pediatric age groups: a study of 3,350 children. *J Orthop Trauma.* 1993;7(1):15–22.

22. Cherubino M, Valdatta L, Tos P, et al. Role of negative pressure therapy as damage control in soft tissue reconstruction for open tibial fractures. *J Reconstr Microsurg.* 2017;33(Suppl 1):S08–S13.

23. CORTICES. The pediatric "floating knee" injury: a state-of-the-art multicenter study. *J Bone Joint Surg Am.* 2019;101(19):1761–1767.

24. Court-Brown CM, Byrnes T, McLaughlin G. Intramedullary nailing of tibial diaphyseal fractures in adolescents with open physes. *Injury.* 2003;34(10):781–785.

25. Coury JG, Lum ZC, O'Neill NP, Gerardi JA. Single incision pediatric flexible intramedullary tibial nailing. *J Orthop.* 2017;14(3):394–397.

26. Cozen L. Fracture of the proximal portion of the tibia in children followed by valgus deformity. *Surg Gynecol Obstet.* 1953;97(2):183–188.

27. Cravino M, Canavese F, De Rosa V, et al. Outcome of displaced distal tibial metaphyseal fractures in children between 6 and 15 years of age treated by elastic stable intramedullary nails. *Eur J Orthop Surg Traumatol.* 2014;24(8):1603–1608.

28. Cullen MC, Roy DR, Crawford AH, et al. Open fracture of the tibia in children. *J Bone Joint Surg Am.* 1996;78(7):1039–1047.

29. Cummings JL, Rivera AE, Pereira DE, et al. Nonoperative management of closed displaced tibia shaft fractures in patients under 18 years of age: low failure rate. *J Pediatr Orthop.* 2022;42(8):421–426.

30. Dedmond BT, Kortesis B, Punger K, et al. Subatmospheric pressure dressings in the temporary treatment of soft tissue injuries associated with type III open tibial shaft fractures in children. *J Pediatr Orthop.* 2006;26(6):728–732.

31. Domzalski ME, Lipton GE, Lee D, Guille JT. Fractures of the distal tibial metaphysis in children: patterns of injury and results of treatment. *J Pediatr Orthop.* 2006;26(2):171–176.

32. Dunbar JS, Owen HF, Nogrady MB, Mcleese R. Obscure tibial fracture of infants—the toddler's fracture. *J Can Assoc Radiol.* 1964;15:136–144.

33. Dwyer AJ, John B, Krishen M, Hora R. Remodeling of tibial fractures in children younger than 12 years. *Orthopedics.* 2007;30(5):393–396.

34. Fanelli D, Perrotta G, Stocco F, et al. Outcomes and complications following flexible intramedullary nailing for the treatment of tibial fractures in children: a meta-analysis. *Arch Orthop Trauma Surg.* 2022;142(7):1469–1482.

35. Flynn JM, Bashyal RK, Yeger-McKeever M, et al. Acute traumatic compartment syndrome of the leg in children: diagnosis and outcome. *J Bone Joint Surg Am.* 2011;93(10):937–941.

36. Flynn JM, Hresko T, Reynolds RA, et al. Titanium elastic nails for pediatric femur fractures: a multicenter study of early results with analysis of complications. *J Pediatr Orthop.* 2001;21(1):4–8.

37. Fottner A, Baur-Melnyk A, Birkenmaier C, et al. Stress fractures presenting as tumours: a retrospective analysis of 22 cases. *Int Orthop.* 2009;33(2):489–492.

38. Fox J, Enriquez B, Bompadre V, et al. Observation versus cast treatment of toddler's fractures. *J Pediatr Orthop.* 2022;42(5):e480–e485.

39. Gaffney JT. Tibia fractures in children sustained on a playground slide. *J Pediatr Orthop.* 2009;29(6):606–608.

40. Galano GJ, Vitale MA, Kessler MW, et al. The most frequent traumatic orthopaedic injuries from a national pediatric inpatient population. *J Pediatr Orthop.* 2005;25(1):39–44.

41. Gicquel P, Giacomelli MC, Basic B, et al. Problems of operative and non-operative treatment and healing in tibial fractures. *Injury.* 2005;36(Suppl 1):A44–A50.

42. Glass GE, Pearse M, Nanchahal J. The ortho-plastic management of Gustilo grade IIIB fractures of the tibia in children: a systematic review of the literature. *Injury.* 2009;40(8):876–879.

43. Godfrey J, Choi PD, Shabtai L, et al. Management of pediatric type I open fractures in the emergency department or operating room: a multicenter perspective. *J Pediatr Orthop.* 2019;39(7):372–376.

44. Goodbody CM, Lee RJ, Flynn JM, Sankar WN. Titanium elastic nailing for pediatric tibia fractures: do older, heavier kids do worse? *J Pediatr Orthop.* 2016;36(5): 472–477.

45. Goodwin RC, Gaynor T, Mahar A, et al. Intramedullary flexible nail fixation of unstable pediatric tibial diaphyseal fractures. *J Pediatr Orthop.* 2005;25(5): 570–576.

46. Gordon JE, Gregush RV, Schoenecker PL, et al. Complications after titanium elastic nailing of pediatric tibial fractures. *J Pediatr Orthop.* 2007;27(4):442–446.

47. Gordon JE, Schoenecker PL, Oda JE, et al. A comparison of monolateral and circular external fixation of unstable diaphyseal tibial fractures in children. *J Pediatr Orthop B.* 2003;12(5):338–345.

48. Green NE, Rogers RA, Lipscomb AB. Nonunions of stress fractures of the tibia. *Am J Sports Med.* 1985;13(3):171–176.

49. Grimard G, Naudie D, Laberge LC, Hamdy RC. Open fractures of the tibia in children. *Clinical Orthop Relat Res.* 1996;(332):62–70.

50. Gustilo RB, Anderson JT. Prevention of infection in the treatment of one thousand and twenty-five open fractures of long bones: retrospective and prospective analyses. *J Bone Joint Surg Am.* 1976;58(4):453–458.

51. Halsey MF, Finzel KC, Carrion WV, et al. Toddler's fracture: presumptive diagnosis and treatment. *J Pediatr Orthop.* 2001;21(2):152–156.

52. Halvorson J, Jinnah R, Kulp B, Frino J. Use of vacuum-assisted closure in pediatric open fractures with a focus on the rate of infection. *Orthopedics.* 2011;34(7): e256–e260.

53. Hansen BA, Greiff J, Bergmann F. Fractures of the tibia in children. *Acta Orthop Scand.* 1976;47(4):448–453.

54. Harly E, Angelliaume A, Lalioui A, et al. Divergent intramedullary nailing (DIN): a modified intramedullary nailing technique to treat paediatric distal tibial fractures. *J Pediatr Orthop.* 2019;39(10):e773–e776.

55. Heo J, Oh CW, Park KH, et al. Elastic nailing of tibia shaft fractures in young children up to 10 years of age. *Injury.* 2016;47(4):832–836.

56. Heyworth BE, Green DW. Lower extremity stress fractures in pediatric and adolescent athletes. *Curr Opin Pediatr.* 2008;20(1):58–61.

57. Ho CA. Tibia shaft fractures in adolescents: how and when can they be managed successfully with cast treatment? *J Pediatr Orthop.* 2016;36(Suppl 1):S15–S18.

58. Ho CA, Dammann G, Podeszwa DA, Levy J. Tibial shaft fractures in adolescents: analysis of cast treatment successes and failures. *J Pediatr Orthop B.* 2015;24(2):114–117.

59. Hoaglund FT, States JD. Factors influencing the rate of healing in tibial shaft fractures. *Surg Gynecol Obstet.* 1967;124(1):71–76.

60. Hope PG, Cole WG. Open fractures of the tibia in children. *J Bone Joint Surg Br.* 1992;74(4):546–553.

61. Houghton GR, Rooker GD. The role of the periosteum in the growth of long bones. An experimental study in the rabbit. *J Bone Joint Surg Br.* 1979;61-B(2):218–220.

62. Iobst CA. Hexapod external fixation of Tibia fractures in children. *J Pediatr Orthop.* 2016;36(Suppl 1):S24–S28.

63. Janzing HM, Broos PL. Routine monitoring of compartment pressure in patients with tibial fractures: beware of overtreatment! *Injury.* 2001;32(5):415–421.

64. Jennissen CA, Koos M, Denning G. Playground slide-related injuries in preschool children: increased risk of lower extremity injuries when riding on laps. *Inj Epidemiol.* 2018;5(Suppl 1):13.

65. Joeris A, Lutz N, Wicki B, et al. An epidemiological evaluation of pediatric long bone fractures—a retrospective cohort study of 2716 patients from two Swiss tertiary pediatric hospitals. *BMC pediatr.* 2014;14:314.

66. Jones G, Duncan RDD. Open tibial fractures in children under 13 years of age—10 years experience. *Injury.* 2003;34(10):776–780.

67. Kattan JM, Leathers MP, Barad JH, Silva M. The effectiveness of cast wedging for the treatment of pediatric fractures. *J Pediatr Orthop B.* 2014;23(6):566–571.

68. Kinney MC, Nagle D, Bastrom T, et al. Operative versus conservative management of displaced tibial shaft fracture in adolescents. *J Pediatr Orthop.* 2016;36(7): 661–666.

69. Knight JL. Genu recurvatum deformity secondary to partial proximal tibial epiphyseal arrest: case report. *Am J Knee Surg.* 1998;11(2):111–115.

70. Kocher MS, Kasser JR. Orthopaedic aspects of child abuse. *J Am Acad Orthop Surg.* 2000;8(1):10–20.

71. Koivisto ST, Laaksonen T, Ahola JA, et al. Epidemiology and management of proximal tibia fractures in children and adolescents: a population-based study based on the Kids' Fracture Tool. *Acta Orthop.* 2022;93:826–830.

72. Kozlowski K, Azouz M, Barrett IR, et al. Midshaft tibial stress fractures in children (report of four cases). *Australas Radiol.* 1992;36(2):131–134.

73. Kozlowski K, Urbonaviciene A. Stress fractures of the fibula in the first few years of life (report of six cases). *Australas Radiol.* 1996;40(3):261–263.

74. Kreder HJ, Armstrong P. A review of open tibia fractures in children. *J Pediatr Orthop.* 1995;15(4):482–488.

75. Kubiak EN, Egol KA, Scher D, et al. Operative treatment of tibial fractures in children: are elastic stable intramedullary nails an improvement over external fixation? *J Bone Joint Surg Am.* 2005;87(8):1761–1768.

76. Kumbaracı M, Hancıoğlu S, Turgut A. Analysis of risk factors for re-displacement of pediatric tibia fractures: a retrospective study of 196 cases. *Acta Orthop Traumatol Turc.* 2022;56(1):36–41.

77. Laine JC, Cherkashin A, Samchukov M, et al. The management of soft tissue and bone loss in type IIIB and IIIC pediatric open tibia fractures. *J Pediatr Orthop.* 2016;36(5):453–458.

78. Lefaivre KA, Guy P, Chan H, Blachut PA. Long-term follow-up of tibial shaft fractures treated with intramedullary nailing. *J Orthop Trauma.* 2008;22(8):525–529.

79. Levy AS, Wetzler M, Lewars M, et al. The orthopedic and social outcome of open tibia fractures in children. *Orthopedics.* 1997;20(7):593–598.

80. Liow RYL, Montgomery RJ. Treatment of established and anticipated nonunion of the tibia in childhood. *J Pediatr Orthop.* 2002;22(6):754–760.

81. Loder RT, Bookout C. Fracture patterns in battered children. *J Orthop Trauma.* 1991;5(4):428–433.

82. Magnusson EA, Weltsch D, Baldwin KD, Blumberg TJ. Open reduction of closed pediatric tibial shaft fractures treated with intramedullary stabilization does not increase risk of postoperative complications. *J Orthop Trauma.* 2020;34(9):482–487.

83. Marengo L, Nasto LA, Michelis MB, Boero S. Elastic stable intramedullary nailing (ESIN) in paediatric femur and tibia shaft fractures: comparison between titanium and stainless steel nails. *Injury.* 2018;49(Suppl 3):S8–S11.

84. Marengo L, Paonessa M, Andreacchio A, et al. Displaced tibia shaft fractures in children treated by elastic stable intramedullary nailing: results and complications in children weighing 50 kg (110 lb) or more. *Eur J Orthop Surg Traumatol.* 2016;26(3):311–317.

85. Masquijo JJ. Percutaneous plating of distal tibial fractures in children and adolescents. *J Pediatr Orthop B.* 2014;23(3):207–211.

86. McGraw-Heinrich JA, Ezeokoli EU, Mitchell P, et al. Pediatric distal third tibial shaft fractures: a comparison of surgical fixation methods and incidence of concomitant physeal fractures. *J Pediatr Orthop B.* 2023;32(4):393–400.

87. Mellick LB, Reesor K, Demers D, Reinker KA. Tibial fractures of young children. *Pediatr Emerg Care.* 1988;4(2):97–101.

88. Métaizeau JP, Wong-Chung J, Bertrand H, Pasquier P. Percutaneous epiphysiodesis using transphyseal screws (PETS). *J Pediatr Orthop.* 1998;18(3):363–369.

89. Mohamed A, Rajeev AS. Clinical outcomes and complications of titanium versus stainless steel elastic nail in management of paediatric femoral fractures-a systematic review. *Eur J Orthop Surg Traumatol.* 2017;27(2):157–167.

90. Monsell FP, Howells NR, Lawniczak D, et al. High-energy open tibial fractures in children: treatment with a programmable circular external fixator. *J Bone Joint Surg Br.* 2012;94(7):989–993.

91. Mooney JF III, Argenta LC, Marks MW, et al. Treatment of soft tissue defects in pediatric patients using the V.A.C. system. *Clin Orthop Relat Res.* 2000;(376):26–31.

92. Mubarak SJ, Kim JR, Edmonds EW, et al. Classification of proximal tibial fractures in children. *J Child Orthop.* 2009;3(3):191–197.

93. Murray L, Fickenscher K, Moffatt M, et al. Fractures presumed to be low risk for abuse in young mobile children: association with concomitant suspicious injuries. *Pediatr Emerg Care.* 2022;38(1):e5–e11.

94. Myers SH, Spiegel D, Flynn JM. External fixation of high-energy tibia fractures. *J Pediatr Orthop.* 2007;27(5):537–539.

95. Nandra RS, Wu F, Gaffey A, Bache CE. The management of open tibial fractures in children: a retrospective case series of eight years' experience of 61 cases at a paediatric specialist centre. *Bone Joint J.* 2017;99-B(4):544–553.

96. Naranje SM, Erali RA, Warner WC Jr, et al. Epidemiology of pediatric fractures presenting to emergency departments in the United States. *J Pediatr Orthop.* 2016;36(4):e45–e48.

97. Nattiv A. Stress fractures and bone health in track and field athletes. *J Sci Med Sport.* 2000;3(3):268–279.

98. Navarro Vergara AD, Fretes AN. The floating knee in pediatric patients: a single-center retrospective study from a referral center. *Cureus.* 2022;14(9):e29517.

99. Nenopoulos S, Vrettakos A, Chaftikis N, et al. The effect of proximal tibial fractures on the limb axis in children. *Acta Orthop Belg.* 2007;73(3):345–353.

100. Niemeyer P, Weinberg A, Schmitt H, et al. Stress fractures in adolescent competitive athletes with open physis. *Knee Surg Sports Traumatol Arthrosc.* 2006;14(8):771–777.

101. O'Brien T, Weisman DS, Ronchetti P, et al. Flexible titanium nailing for the treatment of the unstable pediatric tibial fracture. *J Pediatr Orthop.* 2004;24(6):601–609.

102. Obey MR, Shlykov MA, Nickel KB, et al. Incidence and risk factors for acute compartment syndrome in pediatric tibia fractures. *J Pediatr Orthop B.* 2023;32(4):401–404.

103. Ostermann PA, Henry SL, Seligson D. Timing of wound closure in severe compound fractures. *Orthopedics.* 1994;17(5):397–399.

104. Oudjhane K, Newman B, Oh KS, et al. Occult fractures in preschool children. *J Trauma.* 1988;28(6):858–860.

105. Ozkul E, Gem M, Arslan H, et al. How safe is titanium elastic nail application in the surgical treatment of tibia fractures in children? *Acta Orthop Belg.* 2014;80(1):76–81.

106. Ozkul E, Gem M, Arslan H, et al. Minimally invasive plate osteosynthesis in open pediatric tibial fractures. *J Pediatr Orthop.* 2016;36(4):416–422.

107. Padgett AM, Torrez TW, Kothari EA, et al. Comparison of nonoperative versus operative management in pediatric Gustilo-Anderson type I open tibia fractures. *Injury.* 2023;54(2):552–556.

108. Pandya NK, Baldwin K, Wolfgruber H, et al. Child abuse and orthopaedic injury patterns: analysis at a level I pediatric trauma center. *J Pediatr Orthop.* 2009;29(6):618–625.

109. Pandya NK, Edmonds EW. Response to letter to the editor re: Immediate intramedullary flexible nailing of open pediatric tibial shaft fractures. *J Pediatr Orthop.* 2015;35(2):e19.

110. Pandya NK, Edmonds EW, Mubarak SJ. The incidence of compartment syndrome after flexible nailing of pediatric tibial shaft fractures. *J Child Orthop.* 2011;5(6):439–447.

111. Pennock AT, Bastrom TP, Upasani VV. Elastic intramedullary nailing versus open reduction internal fixation of pediatric tibial shaft fractures. *J Pediatr Orthop.* 2017;37(7):e403–e408.

112. Pogorelić Z, Vegan V, Jukić M, et al. Elastic stable intramedullary nailing for treatment of pediatric tibial fractures: a 20-year single center experience of 132 cases. *Children (Basel).* 2022;9(6):845.

113. Qidwai SA. Intramedullary Kirschner wiring for tibia fractures in children. *J Pediatr Orthop.* 2001;21(3):294–297.

114. Radhakrishna VN, Madhuri V. Management of pediatric open tibia fractures with supracutaneous locked plates. *J Pediatr Orthop B.* 2017;27(1):13–16.

115. Rivera AE, Cummings JL, Pereira DE, et al. Displaced tibia fractures in adolescents: closed reduction and casting versus flexible intramedullary nails. *J Pediatr Orthop.* 2023;43(1):7–12.

116. Robert M, Khouri N, Carlioz H, Alain JL. Fractures of the proximal tibial metaphysis in children: review of a series of 25 cases. *J Pediatr Orthop.* 1987;7(4):444–449.

117. Robertson P, Karol LA, Rab GT. Open fractures of the tibia and femur in children. *J Pediatr Orthop.* 1996;16(5):621–626.

118. Sabatini CS, Curtis TA, Mahan ST. Patient-based outcomes after tibia fracture in children and adolescents. *Open Orthop J.* 2014;8:41–48.

119. Salem KH, Lindemann I, Keppler P. Flexible intramedullary nailing in pediatric lower limb fractures. *J Pediatr Orthop.* 2006;26(4):505–509.

120. Sankar WN, Jones KJ, David Horn B, Wells L. Titanium elastic nails for pediatric tibial shaft fractures. *J Child Orthop.* 2007;1(5):281–286.

121. Shannak AO. Tibial fractures in children: follow-up study. *J Pediatr Orthop.* 1988;8(3):306–310.

122. Shen K, Cai H, Wang Z, Xu Y. Elastic stable intramedullary nailing for severely displaced distal tibial fractures in children. *Medicine (Baltimore).* 2016;95(39):e4980.

123. Shore BJ, Glotzbecker MP, Zurakowski D, et al. Acute compartment syndrome in children and teenagers with tibial shaft fractures: Incidence and multivariable risk factors. *J Orthop Trauma.* 2013;27(11):616–621.

124. Skaggs DL, Friend L, Alman B, et al. The effect of surgical delay on acute infection following 554 open fractures in children. *J Bone Joint Surg Am.* 2005;87(1):8–12.

125. Smith JRA, Fox CE, Wright TC, et al. Orthoplastic management of open tibial fractures in children: a consecutive five-year series from a paediatric major trauma centre. *Bone Joint J.* 2021;103-B(6):1160–1167.

126. Song KM, Sangeorzan B, Benirschke S, Browne R. Open fractures of the tibia in children. *J Pediatr Orthop.* 1996;16(5):635–639.

127. Staudt JM, Smeulders MJC, van der Horst CMAM. Normal compartment pressures of the lower leg in children. *J Bone Joint Surg Br.* 2008;90(2):215–219.

128. Stenroos A, Laaksonen T, Nietosvaara N, et al. One in three of pediatric tibia shaft fractures is currently treated operatively: a 6-year epidemiological study in two university hospitals in Finland treatment of pediatric tibia shaft fractures. *Scand J Surg.* 2018;107(3):269–274.

129. Stenroos A, Puhakka J, Nietosvaara Y, Kosola J. Treatment of closed tibia shaft fractures in children: a systematic review and meta-analysis. *Eur J Pediatr Surg.* 2020;30(6):483–489.

130. Stevens PM. Guided growth for angular correction: a preliminary series using a tension band plate. *J Pediatr Orthop.* 2007;27(3):253–259.

131. Stranzinger E, Leidolt L, Eich G, Klimek PM. The anterior tilt angle of the proximal tibia epiphyseal plate: a significant radiological finding in young children with trampoline fractures. *Eur J Radiol.* 2014;83(8):1433–1436.

132. Swaan JW, Oppers VM. Crural fractures in children. A study of the incidence of changes of the axial position and of enhanced longitudinal growth of the tibia after the healing of crural fractures. *Arch Chir Neerl.* 1971;23(4):259–272.

133. Thabet AM, Craft M, Pisquiy J, et al. Tibial shaft fractures in the adolescents: treatment outcomes and the risk factors for complications. *Injury.* 2022;53(2):706–712.

134. Toivanen JAK, Väistö O, Kannus P, et al. Anterior knee pain after intramedullary nailing of fractures of the tibial shaft. A prospective, randomized study comparing two different nail-insertion techniques. *J Bone Joint Surg Am.* 2002;84(4):580–585.

135. Tuten HR, Keeler KA, Gabos PG, et al. Posttraumatic tibia valga in children. A long-term follow-up note. *J Bone Joint Surg Am.* 1999;81(6):799–810.

136. Väistö O, Toivanen J, Kannus P, Järvinen M. Anterior knee pain after intramedullary nailing of fractures of the tibial shaft: an eight-year follow-up of a prospective, randomized study comparing two different nail-insertion techniques. *J Trauma.* 2008;64(6):1511–1516.

137. Vallamshetla VRP, De Silva U, Bache CE, Gibbons PJ. Flexible intramedullary nails for unstable fractures of the tibia in children. An eight-year experience. *J Bone Joint Surg Br.* 2006;88(4):536–540.

138. Walker RN, Green NE, Spindler KP. Stress fractures in skeletally immature patients. *J Pediatr Orthop.* 1996;16(5):578–584.

139. Weber BG, Brunner C, Freuner F. *Treatment of Fractures in Children and Adolescents.* Springer-Verlag; 1980.

140. Williams KA, Thier ZT, Mathews CG, Locke MD. Physeal-sparing rigid intramedullary nailing in adolescent tibial shaft fractures: a pilot study. *Cureus.* 2021;13(3):e13893.

141. Yang BW, Shore BJ, Rademacher E, et al. Prevalence of Cozen's phenomenon of the proximal tibia. *J Pediatr Orthop.* 2019;39(6):e417–e421.

142. Yang JP, Letts RM. Isolated fractures of the tibia with intact fibula in children: a review of 95 patients. *J Pediatr Orthop.* 1997;17(3):347–351.

143. Yue JJ, Churchill RS, Cooperman DR, et al. The floating knee in the pediatric patient. Nonoperative versus operative stabilization. *Clin Orthop Relat Res.* 2000;(376):124–136.

144. Zionts LE, MacEwen GD. Spontaneous improvement of post-traumatic tibia valga. *J Bone Joint Surg Am.* 1986;68(5):680–687.

145. Zubair A, Samuelson EM, Morris RP, et al. Quadruple versus double flexible intramedullary nails to treat pediatric distal-third tibial shaft fractures: a biomechanical comparison. *J Pediatr Orthop.* 2020;40(9):487–491.

30

Ankle Fractures

Jaime R. Denning

INTRODUCTION TO ANKLE FRACTURES

Injuries to the distal tibial and fibular physes are generally reported to account for 25% to 38% of all physeal fractures,[81,161] second in frequency only to distal radial physeal fractures[146]; however, Peterson et al.[148] reported that phalangeal physeal fractures were most common, followed by physeal injuries of the radius and ankle. In skeletally immature individuals, physeal ankle fractures are slightly more common than fractures of the tibial or fibular diaphysis,[125] and these fractures are a common cause of hospital admission in children.[47]

Participation in sports is associated with a significant number of ankle injuries, including sprains and fractures. Up to 58% of physeal ankle fractures occur during sports activities[70,205] and account for 10% to 40% of all injuries to skeletally immature athletes.[137,165] Physeal ankle fractures are more common in males than in females in some studies.[187] Other studies have demonstrated that ankle injuries may be more likely in young female soccer athletes compared with males.[109] Fractures of the ankle are associated with the following sports activities: trampolines,[175] scooters,[124] soccer,[109] basketball,[51] skating,[136] and downhill skiing.[15] Increased body mass index (BMI) is also a risk factor for ankle injury in the skeletally immature.[206,4,98] Obese children tend to sustain fractures in the distal portions of long bones and are twice as likely as nonobese children to sustain physeal fractures.[4] In a recent population study, Kessler et al. found that fractures of the foot and ankle had the strongest correlation with obesity.[98]

In addition to sports, higher-energy trauma is associated with a significant number of distal tibia and fibular fractures in children. These fractures occur in approximately 10% to 20% of trauma patients presenting to the emergency room (ER).[15] Tibial physeal fractures are most common between the ages of 8 and 15 years, and fibular fractures are most common between 8 and 14 years of age.[187]

Figure 30-1. Salter–Harris anatomic classification as applied to injuries of the distal tibial epiphysis. This can also be applied to the distal fibula. This system has the highest interobserver reproducibility and is recommended for communication among care providers who have not seen radiographs.

ASSESSMENT OF ANKLE FRACTURES

CLASSIFICATIONS AND MECHANISMS OF INJURY FOR ANKLE FRACTURE

There is no generally accepted fracture classification for ankle fractures in children that predicts outcome and directs treatment. Fracture classifications are usually based on anatomy,[140,147,187] or mechanism of injury[3,11,106] descriptions. Anatomical classifications distinguish fractures based on the regions of the metaphysis, physis, and epiphysis. Mechanism of injury classifications incorporate the forces, which produce the fracture and the anatomic position of the foot and ankle that existed at the time of the injury.

Since its description, the Salter–Harris classification system has been widely used to describe the anatomic features of fractures associated with open physes. This straightforward anatomic classification (Fig. 30-1) has five distinct categories, which can be applied to most periarticular regions.

Injury classifications based on the mechanism of injury may have some advantages. The description of the injury includes the anatomic deformity and the forces that produced the injury. An understanding of these forces can facilitate reduction of a displaced fracture. Advanced imaging techniques that allow for comprehensive three-dimensional visualization of the fracture anatomy also facilitate surgical planning and reduction techniques.

Both anatomical and mechanism of injury classifications can provide useful information for determining appropriate treatment. The prognoses for growth and deformity have been predicted on the basis of both types of classification.[91,90,187] A theoretical advantage of mechanism-of-injury classifications is that identification of the force producing the injury might give even more information about the possible development of growth arrest than anatomical classifications.

Ideally, classification systems should have high inter- and intraobserver agreement. Thomsen et al.[191] studied the reproducibility of the Lauge-Hansen (mechanism of injury) and Weber (anatomical) classifications in a series of adult ankle fractures. After all investigators in the study had received a tutorial on both systems and their application, they were asked to classify 94 fractures. On the first attempt, only the Weber classification produced an acceptable level of interobserver agreement. On a second attempt, the Weber classification and most of

the Lauge-Hansen classification achieved an acceptable level of interobserver agreement. These authors concluded that all fracture classification systems should have demonstrably acceptable interobserver agreement rates before they are adopted, an argument made even more forcefully in an editorial by Burstein.[32] Vahvanen and Aalto[196] compared their ability to classify 310 ankle fractures in children with the Weber, Lauge-Hansen, and Salter–Harris classifications. They found that they were "largely unsuccessful" using the Weber and Lauge-Hansen classifications, but they could easily classify the fractures using the Salter–Harris system. We thus recommend using the Salter–Harris classification when assessing ankle fractures, and especially when communicating to others who have not seen x-rays (Fig. 30-2).

Dias and Tachdjian[56] modified the Lauge-Hansen classification based on their review of 71 fractures (Fig. 30-3). Their

Figure 30-2. Comminuted Salter–Harris type IV fracture of the distal tibia and displaced Salter–Harris type I fracture of the distal fibula produced by an inversion (shearing) mechanism in a 10-year-old girl.

| A. Supination–inversion | B. Pronation–eversion external rotation | C. Supination–plantarflexion | D. Supination–external rotation |

Figure 30-3. Dias–Tachdjian classification of physeal injuries of the distal tibia and fibula.

original classification (1978) consisted of four types in which the first word refers to the position of the foot at the time of injury and the second word refers to the force that produces the injury.

Other fracture types were subsequently added, including axial compression, juvenile Tillaux, triplane, and other physeal injuries. Syndesmosis injuries have also been described.[49] "Axial compression injury" describes the mechanism of injury but not the position of the foot. Juvenile Tillaux and triplane fractures are called transitional fractures as they occur when the physis is transitioning from open to closed and are believed to be caused by external rotation.[164] The final category, "other physeal injuries," includes diverse injuries, many of which have no specific mechanism of injury.

Dias–Tachdjian Classification of Ankle Fracture in Children

Supination–Inversion

- Grade I: The adduction or inversion force avulses the distal fibular epiphysis (Salter–Harris type I or II fracture). Occasionally, the fracture is transepiphyseal; rarely, the lateral ligaments fail (see Fig. 30-3).
- Grade II (Fig. 30-4): Further inversion produces a tibial fracture, usually a Salter–Harris type III or IV and rarely a Salter–Harris type I or II injury, or the fracture passes through the medial malleolus below the physis (see Fig. 30-2).

Figure 30-4. Variants of grade II supination–inversion injuries (Dias–Tachdjian classification). **A:** Salter–Harris type I fracture of the distal tibia and fibula. **B:** Salter–Harris type I fracture of the fibula, Salter–Harris type II tibial fracture. **C:** Salter–Harris type I fibular fracture, Salter–Harris type III tibial fracture. **D:** Salter–Harris type I fibular fracture, Salter–Harris type IV tibial fracture.

Figure 30-5. Lateral view of a supination–plantarflexion injury.

Figure 30-6. Stage I supination–external rotation injury in a 10-year-old child; the Salter–Harris type II fracture begins laterally.

Supination–Plantarflexion

The plantarflexion force displaces the epiphysis directly posteriorly, resulting in a Salter–Harris type I or II fracture. Fibular fractures were not reported with this mechanism. The tibial fracture may be difficult to see on anteroposterior (AP) radiographs (Fig. 30-5).

Supination–External Rotation

• Grade I: The external rotation force results in a Salter–Harris type II fracture of the distal tibia (Fig. 30-6). The distal fragment is displaced posteriorly, as in a supination–plantarflexion injury, but the Thurstan-Holland fragment is visible on the AP radiographs, with the fracture line extending proximally and medially.
• Grade II: With further external rotation, a spiral fracture of the fibula is produced, running from anteroinferior to posterosuperior (Fig. 30-7).

Pronation–Eversion–External Rotation

A Salter–Harris type I or II fracture of the distal tibia occurs simultaneously with a transverse fibular fracture. The distal tibial fragment is displaced laterally and the Thurstan-Holland fragment, when present, is lateral or posterolateral (Fig. 30-8). Less frequently, a transepiphyseal fracture occurs through the medial malleolus (Salter–Harris type II).

Axial Compression

This results in a Salter–Harris type V injury of the distal tibial physis. Initial radiographs usually show no abnormality, and the diagnosis is established when growth arrest is demonstrated on follow-up radiographs.

Transitional Fractures of the Distal Tibia and Fibula

Because the distal tibial physis closes in an asymmetric pattern over a period of about 18 months, injuries sustained during this period can produce fracture patterns that are not seen in younger children with completely open physes.[120] This group of fractures has been labeled "transitional" fractures because they occur during the transition from a skeletally immature ankle to a skeletally mature ankle. Such fractures, which include juvenile Tillaux and "triplane" fractures with two to four fracture fragments, have been described by Kleiger and Mankin,[102] Marmor,[126] Cooperman et al.,[44] Kärrholm et al.,[89] and Denton and Fischer.[54] The adolescent pilon fracture has been described by Letts et al.[112] The incisural fracture has been described by Cummings and Hahn.[50] Syndesmosis injuries have been described by Cummings.[49]

Classification of these fractures is even more confusing than that of other distal tibial fractures. Advocates of mechanism-of-injury systems agree that most juvenile Tillaux and triplane fractures are caused by external rotation, but they disagree as to the position of the foot at the time of the injury.[55,56,154] Some authors[55] classify juvenile Tillaux fractures as stage I injuries,

Figure 30-7. Stage II supination–external rotation injury. **A:** Oblique fibular fracture also is visible on anteroposterior view. **B:** Lateral view shows the posterior metaphyseal fragment and posterior displacement.

Figure 30-8. A: According to the Dias–Tachdjian classification, this injury in a 12-year-old boy would be considered a pronation–eversion–external rotation injury resulting in a Salter–Harris type II fracture of the distal tibia and a transverse fibular fracture. **B:** The anterior displacement of the epiphysis, visible on the lateral view, however, makes external rotation an unlikely component of the mechanism of injury; the mechanism is more likely pronation–dorsiflexion.

A   B

Figure 30-9. A: Anteroposterior radiograph of Salter–Harris type III/juvenile Tillaux fracture. **B:** Lateral radiograph of Salter–Harris type III/juvenile Tillaux fracture.

with further external rotation causing triplane fractures, and still further external rotation causing stage II injuries with fibular fracture. Others emphasize the extent of physeal closure as the only determinant of fracture pattern.[43]

Advocates of anatomical classifications are handicapped by the different anatomical configurations triplane fractures may exhibit on different radiograph projections, making computed tomography (CT) scanning or examination at open reduction necessary to determine fracture anatomy and number of fragments. In one study, the addition of CT scan review when classifying triplane fractures improved the inter- and intrarater reliability. The intra-articular displacement (>/<2 mm) and decision for nonoperative versus operative treatment were changed by 39% and 27%, respectively, by the addition of CT to plain films alone in this study as well.[61] Because these fractures occur near the end of growth, growth disturbance is rare. Anatomical classification is, therefore, more useful for descriptive purposes than for prognosis.

Juvenile Tillaux Fracture of the Distal Tibia and Fibula

The juvenile Tillaux fracture is a Salter–Harris type III fracture involving the anterolateral distal tibia. The portion of the physis not involved in the fracture is closed (Fig. 30-9).

Triplane Fracture of the Distal Tibia and Fibula

A group of fractures that have in common the appearance of a Salter–Harris type III fracture on the AP radiographs and of a Salter–Harris type II fracture on the lateral radiographs (Fig. 30-10A,B). CT scans can be very helpful to understand the complex anatomy of these fractures (Fig. 30-10C–E).[12,47,61,101] Ipsilateral triplane and diaphyseal fractures have been reported, and one of the fractures can be missed if adequate images are not obtained.[12,47,84,176] In a study of 517 pediatric tibia shaft fractures in 515 patients, 4.3% had concurrent ipsilateral distal tibial fractures, and half of those distal tibia fractures were classified as triplanes. The tibia shaft fractures with highest rate of distal tibia fractures were in older patients (12.7 years vs. 11 years in isolated fractures), were located at the junction between middle and distal third of the tibia, and were oblique or spiral pattern. Thirty-six percentage of concurrent distal tibia fractures were missed until the time of chart review for this study.[176]

Adolescent Pilon Fractures of the Distal Tibia and Fibula

The pediatric/adolescent pilon fracture[112] is defined as a fracture of the "tibial plafond with articular and physeal involvement, variable talar and fibular involvement, variable comminution, and greater than 5 mm of displacement" (Fig. 30-11). Based on a small number of cases, Letts et al. developed a three-part classification system. Type I fractures have minimal comminution and no physeal displacement. Type II fractures have marked comminution and less than 5 mm of physeal displacement. Type III fractures have marked comminution and more than 5 mm of physeal displacement.

Incisura Fractures of the Distal Tibia and Fibula

Incisural fractures are fractures that resemble Tillaux on standard radiographs, but the size of the fragment is smaller than

Figure 30-10. **A:** Anteroposterior view of a fibula fracture and triplane fracture. Note that the involvement of the joint (*arrow*) does not appear significant on plain radiographs. **B:** Lateral radiograph suggests physeal involvement (*arrow*). **C:** Coronal CT demonstrates significant displacement of the joint surface (*arrow*) that requires surgery. **D:** Sagittal CT demonstrates complex fracture fragments at the joint. **E:** 3D reconstruction can aid in surgical planning. (Used with permission of the Children's Orthopaedic Center, Los Angeles.)

that typically seen with the Tillaux fractures (Fig. 30-12).[50] On the CT scan, this fracture does not extend to the anterior cortex of the distal tibia (Fig. 30-13). The mechanism of injury may be an avulsion of the fragment by the interosseous ligament. This may be a variant of an adult tibiofibular diastasis injury.

SYNDESMOSIS INJURIES OF THE DISTAL TIBIAL AND FIBULAR FRACTURES

Syndesmosis injuries in young patients are rare and have been associated with fractures of the distal fibula, Tillaux injuries, Salter–Harris I fractures, and proximal fibula fractures

Figure 30-11. Anteroposterior (**A**) and lateral (**B**) radiographs of a pilon fracture in an adolescent.

Figure 30-12. Anteroposterior (**A**), lateral (**B**), and oblique (**C**) views of the ankle demonstrating an apparent small juvenile Tillaux fracture in a 14-year-old girl.

Figure 30-13. Incisural fracture: CT scan at the level of the tibiotalar joint demonstrates that the fracture fragment does not include the attachment of the anteroinferior tibiofibular ligament.

(Figs. 30-14 and 30-15). There was previously very limited literature on this injury, but recent publications indicate that adolescents with closed distal tibia physis and a concomitant fibula fracture are at risk for these injuries.[145,179] In a study of 77 adolescents with syndesmotic fractures, treatment with screws or suture buttons was compared and found that both modes of fixation maintained syndesmotic reduction, had functional outcomes that were equivalent at mean follow-up of

4 years, and suture button fixation had lower rates of implant removal.[119]

STRESS FRACTURES OF THE DISTAL TIBIA AND FIBULA

Stress fractures around the ankle can occur in the distal tibial metaphyseal area (Fig. 30-16) or through the distal fibular physis (Fig. 30-17). These patients (often gymnasts, ice skaters, or running/endurance athletes) may present with warmth, swelling, and pain around the metaphyseal or physeal regions. These fractures are typically diagnosed on plain radiographs if symptoms have been present long enough for endosteal sclerosis or new periosteal bone formation to appear. Magnetic resonance imaging (MRI) can also be used if more recent symptoms occur or if more urgent diagnosis is needed.[178] In general, treatment for these low-risk stress fractures in this area is treated nonoperatively with rest, immobilization, activity modification, and possibly evaluation by a metabolic bone disease specialist. Patients with stress fractures in the setting of female athlete triad (disordered eating, osteoporosis, amenorrhea) should also receive multidisciplinary treatment in addition to orthopaedic treatment of their fractures.[178]

SIGNS AND SYMPTOMS OF DISTAL TIBIAL AND FIBULAR FRACTURES

Patients with significantly displaced fractures have severe pain and obvious deformity. The position of the foot relative to the leg may provide important information about the mechanism of injury (Fig. 30-18) and should be considered in planning reduction. The status of the skin, pulses, and sensory and motor function should be determined and recorded. Tenderness, swelling, and deformity in the ipsilateral leg and foot should be noted. In patients with tibial shaft fractures, the ankle should be carefully evaluated clinically and radiographically.

Figure 30-14. A: Syndesmosis injury with distal fibula fracture. Radiographs with comparison of right and left sides. Note the widening of the medial clear space and the syndesmosis. **B:** Use of two percutaneously placed cannulated screws to reduce the syndesmosis.

A

B

Figure 30-15. Deltoid and possible syndesmosis injury associated with triplane fracture pattern.

A

B

Although compartment syndromes are rare, they do occur in these locations.[45,131] If patients are admitted to the hospital, discussion with the nursing staff about signs and symptoms of compartment syndrome is important. If patients are treated as outpatients, the patient and family should be informed about the possibility of compartment syndrome and instructed to return to the hospital for evaluation if problems with pain control develop.

EVALUATION FOR OTHER INJURIES

In low-energy ankle fractures, or those that occur during sports and play activity, other injuries are uncommon. In cases of higher-energy trauma such as motor vehicle/pedestrian accidents, the possibility of other injuries needs to be considered. A thorough physical evaluation to identify occult injuries is important. Some injuries can be missed, and ongoing awareness of this possibility is important during the hospitalization for more significant injuries.

Figure 30-16. Distal tibia stress fracture. A 15-year-old boy with 6 weeks of pain while running cross-country. Anteroposterior radiograph shows callus formation in the distal tibia metaphysis.

Figure 30-17. Stress fracture of distal fibula. A 16-year-old boy with 6 weeks of pain while running track. Anteroposterior radiograph shows widened physis. The clinical examination shows point tenderness over the fibular physis.

Figure 30-18. Severe clinical deformity in a 14-year-old boy with an ankle fracture. It is obvious without radiographs that internal rotation will be needed to reduce this fracture.

IMAGING AND OTHER DIAGNOSTIC STUDIES FOR DISTAL TIBIAL AND FIBULAR FRACTURES

Patients with nondisplaced or minimally displaced ankle fractures often have no deformity, minimal swelling, and moderate pain. Because of their benign clinical appearance, such fractures may be easily missed if radiographs are not obtained. Petit et al.[150] reviewed 2,470 radiographs from pediatric ERs, demonstrating abnormal radiographic findings in 9%. Guidelines known as the Ottawa Ankle Rules have been established for adults to determine which injuries require radiographs.[190] The Ottawa Ankle Rules have also been evaluated in children over the age of 5. These rules appear to be a reliable tool to exclude fractures in children greater than 5 years of age presenting with ankle and midfoot injuries and may significantly decrease x-ray use with a low likelihood of missing a fracture.[58] The indications for radiographs according to the guidelines are complaints of pain near a malleolus with either inability to bear weight or tenderness to palpation at the malleolus. Chande[41] prospectively studied 71 children with acute ankle injuries to determine if these guidelines could be applied to pediatric patients with ankle injuries. It was determined that if radiographs were obtained only in children with tenderness over the malleoli, and inability to bear weight, a 25% reduction in radiographic examinations could be achieved without missing any fractures. Boutis later studied 607 children between ages 3 to 16 with ankle injuries (of which 381 had low-risk examinations where signs were limited to the distal fibula) to determine if even further reduction in radiographic examinations could be achieved without missing any high-risk

fractures (defined as any fracture except for avulsion, buckle, or nondisplaced Salter–Harris I/II). None of the low-risk examination patients had a high-risk fracture, which allowed for 62.8% reduction in radiographs (even more than applying Ottawa Ankle Rules).[22] The physical examination should focus on physeal areas of the tibia and fibula, when evaluating ankle injuries, to determine if radiographs are necessary. The low-risk ankle examination is defined as isolated pain and/or tenderness with or without edema or ecchymosis of the distal fibula below the level of the joint line of the ankle or over the adjacent lateral ligaments.[22] Interpretation of radiographs (if necessary) should focus on signs of physeal injury, including soft tissue swelling in these regions.

For patients with obvious deformities, AP, mortise, and lateral radiographs centered over the ankle may provide sufficient information to plan treatment. Although obtaining views of the joint above and below is recommended for most fractures, obtaining a film centered over the midtibia to include the knee and ankle joints on the radiographs significantly decreases the quality of ankle views and is not recommended.

For patients without obvious deformities, a high-quality mortise view of the ankle is essential in addition to AP and lateral views. On a standard AP view, the lateral portion of the distal tibial physis is usually partially obscured by the distal fibula. The vertical component of a triplane or Tillaux fracture can be hidden behind the overlying fibular cortical shadow.[111] A study by Vangsness et al.[198] found that diagnostic accuracy was essentially equal when using anteroposterior, lateral, and mortise views compared with using only mortise and lateral views. Therefore, if only two views are to be obtained, the AP view may be omitted and lateral and mortise views obtained.

Haraguchi et al.[75] described two special views designed to detect avulsion fractures from the lateral malleolus that are not visible on routine views and to distinguish whether they represent avulsions of the anterior tibiofibular ligament or the calcaneofibular ligament attachments. The anterior tibiofibular ligament view is made by positioning the foot in 45 degrees of plantarflexion and elevating the medial border of the foot 15 degrees. The calcaneofibular ligament view is obtained by rotating the leg 45 degrees inward.

Stress views are occasionally recommended historically to rule out ligamentous instability, but the authors see only rare indications for stress radiography in skeletally immature patients. The discomfort of stress views in an acute injury can be avoided by using other imaging options, such as MRI. Stress views under anesthesia (regional and/or general) may be appropriate in some cases. This approach can allow for painless evaluation of the injured ankle with intraoperative comparison to the uninjured ankle.

Bozic et al.[27] studied the age at which the radiographic appearance of the incisura fibularis, tibiofibular clear space, and tibiofibular overlap develop in children. The purpose of their study was to facilitate the diagnosis of distal tibiofibular syndesmotic injury in children. They found that the incisura became detectable at a mean age of 8.2 years for girls and 11.2 years for boys. The mean age at which tibiofibular overlap appeared on the AP view was 5 years for both sexes; on the mortise view, it

Figure 30-19. Coronal and sagittal CT images of Tillaux fracture. **A:** CT scan sagittal image of juvenile Tillaux fracture. Note the degree of intra-articular displacement. **B:** CT scan coronal image of juvenile Tillaux fracture. **C:** CT scan can facilitate screw placement/ orientation. **D:** Reduction with intraepiphyseal screws.

was 10 years for girls and 16 years for boys. The range of clear space measurements in normal children was 2 to 8 mm, with 23% of children having a clear space greater than 6 mm—a distance considered abnormal in adults.

CT is useful in the evaluation of intra-articular fractures, especially juvenile Tillaux and triplane fractures (Fig. 30-19).[6,12,30,47,61,87,101] Transverse images are obtained with thin cuts localized to the joint, and high-quality reconstructions can be produced in the coronal and sagittal planes without repositioning the ankle. Three-dimensional CT reconstructions may add further useful information, and readily available software packages allow easy production of such images (Fig. 30-20). These images can assist with minimally invasive approaches, the use of percutaneous reduction clamps, and positioning of fixation screws.

MRI may be useful in the evaluation of complex fractures of the distal tibia and ankle in patients with open physes. Smith et al.[185] found that of four patients with acute (3–10 days) physeal injuries, MRI showed that three had more severe fractures than indicated on plain films (Fig. 30-21). Early MRI studies (3–17 weeks after injury) not only added information about the pattern of physeal disruption but also supplied early information about the possibility of growth abnormality. MRI has been reported to be occasionally helpful in the identification of osteochondral injuries to the joint surfaces in children with ankle fractures.[100] Although these injuries may be more common in adult fractures, we believe that these types of injuries are rare in younger patients.

Carey et al.[35] obtained MRI studies on 14 patients with known or suspected growth plate injury. The MRI detected 5 radiographically occult fractures in the 14 patients, changed the Salter–Harris classification in 2 cases, and resulted in a change in treatment plan in 5 of the 14 patients studied. These studies would seem to contradict an earlier study by Petit et al.[149] that showed only 1 patient in a series of 29 patients in whom MRI revealed a diagnosis different from that made on plain films. Iwinska-Zelder et al.[83] found that the MRI changed the management in 4 of 10 patients with ankle fractures seen on plain radiographs. Siffert et al.[181] found the MRI identified physeal injuries that were not identified by plain radiographs. At this time, the indications for MRI in the evaluation of ankle fractures in skeletally immature patients are still being defined, but this imaging modality may be a more sensitive tool for identification of minimally displaced or more complex injuries.[12] In a prospective study of skeletally immature patients with clinically diagnosed Salter I fractures of the distal fibula, none of the 18 patients imaged by MRI had evidence of physeal injury. The patients had a mean age of 8 years, and over 70% had evidence of ligamentous sprain on MRI. This questions the principle that the physis is the weak link in the musculoskeletal system in this age group.[23] If physeal arrest occurs, MRI scans are useful for mapping physeal bars.[67,77]

The use of ultrasound to detect radiographically occult fractures may be used for pediatric ankle fractures.[182]

Figure 30-20. Three-dimensional CT reconstruction of juvenile Tillaux fracture. **A:** Coronal CT image of minimally displaced juvenile Tillaux fracture. **B:** Sagittal CT image of minimally displaced juvenile Tillaux fracture. **C, D:** Three-dimensional reconstruction of juvenile Tillaux fracture.

Pitfalls in Diagnosis

A number of accessory ossification centers and normal anatomical variations may cause confusion in the interpretation of plain films of the ankle (Fig. 30-22). In a group of 100 children between the ages of 6 and 12 years, Powell found accessory ossification centers on the medial side (os subtibiale) in 20% and on the lateral side (os subfibulare) in 1%. If they are asymptomatic on clinical examination, these ossification centers are of little concern, but tenderness localized to them may indicate an injury. Stress views to determine motion of the fragments or MRI scanning may occasionally be considered if an injury to an accessory ossification center is suspected.

Clefts in the lateral side of the tibial epiphysis may simulate juvenile Tillaux fractures, and clefts in the medial side may simulate Salter–Harris type III fractures.[96] The presence of these clefts on radiographs of a child with an ankle injury may result in overtreatment if they are misdiagnosed as a fracture. Conversely, attributing a painful irregularity in these areas to anatomical variation may lead to undertreatment (Fig. 30-23).

Figure 30-21. A: Follow-up radiograph of a 7-year-old boy 1 week after an initially non-displaced Salter–Harris type III fracture from a supination–inversion injury of the distal tibia. **B:** Because of the incomplete ossification of this area and concern that the fracture might have displaced, MRI was performed. Note that the distance between the medial malleolus and the talus is greater than the distance between the talus and the distal tibia or lateral malleolus, confirming displacement of the fracture.

Figure 30-22. A: Secondary ossification center in the lateral malleolus (*arrow*) of a 7-year-old girl. Note the smooth border of the fibula and the ossification center. She also has a secondary ossification center in the medial malleolus. **B:** The same girl at age 9 after several repeat injuries and lateral instability of her ankle. She went on to have resection of the os subfibulare (*arrow*) and modified Brostrom with excellent relief of pain and instability. Notice the maturity/fusion of the medial malleolus 2 years later.

Figure 30-23. A: Mortise view of the ankle of a 10-year-old girl who had slight swelling and tenderness at the medial malleolus after an "ankle sprain." The ossicle at the tip of the medial malleolus was correctly identified as an os subtibiale. A subtle line extending from the medial physis to just distal to the medial tibial plafond (*arrow*) was also believed to be an anatomic variant. **B:** Four weeks after injury, soreness persisted and radiographs clearly demonstrated a displaced Salter–Harris type III fracture.

Figure 30-24. Posterior view of the distal tibia and fibula and the ligaments making up the ankle mortise.

Other anatomical variations include a bump on the distal fibula that simulates a torus fracture and an apparent offset of the distal fibular epiphysis that simulates a fracture. These radiographic findings should be correlated with physical examination findings of focal swelling and point tenderness that correspond with the imaging in the diagnosis of skeletal injury.

PATHOANATOMY AND APPLIED ANATOMY RELATING TO ANKLE FRACTURES

The ankle joint closely approximates a hinge joint. It is the articulation between the talus and the ankle mortise, which is a syndesmosis consisting of the distal tibial articular surface, the medial malleolus, and the distal fibula or lateral malleolus.

Four ligamentous structures bind the distal tibia and fibula into the ankle mortise (Fig. 30-24). The anterior and posteroinferior tibiofibular ligaments course inferiorly from the anterior and posterior surfaces of the distal lateral tibia to the anterior and posterior surfaces of the lateral malleolus. The anterior ligament is important in the pathomechanics of "transitional" ankle fractures. Just anterior to the posteroinferior tibiofibular ligament is the broad, thick inferior transverse ligament, which extends down from the lateral malleolus along the posterior border of the articular surface of the tibia, almost to the medial malleolus. This ligament serves as a part of the articular surface for the talus. Between the anterior and posteroinferior tibiofibular ligaments, the tibia and fibula are bound by the interosseous ligament, which is continuous with the interosseous membrane above. This ligament may be important in the pathomechanics of what we have termed incisural fractures.

On the medial side of the ankle, the talus is bound to the ankle mortise by the deltoid ligament (Fig. 30-25). This ligament arises from the medial malleolus and divides into superficial and deep layers. Three parts of the superficial layer are identified by their attachments: tibionavicular, calcaneotibial, and posterior talotibial ligaments. The deep layer is known as the anterior talotibial ligament, again reflecting its insertion and origin. On the lateral side, the anterior and posterior talofibular ligament, with the calcaneofibular ligaments, make up the lateral collateral ligament (Fig. 30-26).

In children, all medial and lateral ligaments originate distal to the tibial or fibular physis. Because the ligaments are often stronger than the physes, physeal fractures have generally been viewed as more common than ligamentous injuries in children. Advanced imaging studies have shown that the rate of ankle fractures compared to ligamentous injuries is variable,[64] and this is likely dependent on multiple factors such as the mechanism of injury, rate of force application, relative strength of the physis, and age of the patient. When distal tibia and fibular

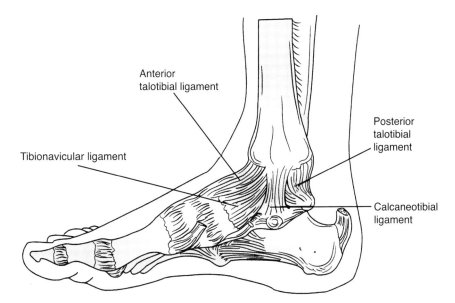

Figure 30-25. Medial view of the ankle demonstrating the components of the deltoid ligament.

Figure 30-26. Lateral view of the ankle demonstrating the anterior and posterior talofibular ligaments and the calcaneofibular ligament.

fragments are displaced together, the syndesmosis at the level of the fracture is usually intact (Fig. 30-27).

The distal tibial ossification center generally appears at 6 to 24 months of age. Its malleolar extension begins to form around the age of 7 or 8 years and is mature or complete at the age of 10 years. The medial malleolus develops as an elongation of the distal tibia ossific nucleus, although in 20% of cases, this may originate from a separate ossification center, the os tibial. This can be mistaken as a fracture.[94] The physis usually closes around the age of 15 years in girls and 17 years in boys. This process takes approximately 18 months and occurs first in the central part of the physis, extending next to the medial side, and finally ending laterally. This asymmetric closure sequence is an important anatomical feature of the growing ankle and is responsible for certain fracture patterns in adolescents, especially transitional fractures (Fig. 30-28).

The distal fibular ossification center appears around the ages of 9 to 24 months. This physis is located at the level of the ankle joint initially and moves distally with growth.[92,203] Closure of this physis generally follows closure of the distal tibial physis by 12 to 24 months.

The locations of the sensory nerves are important anatomic landmarks, as surgical exposures should aim to protect these structures. The superficial peroneal nerve branches may be most vulnerable around the ankle, especially during arthroscopic and arthrotomy approaches for triplane and Tillaux fractures.[13] This is important when arthroscopic and percutaneous reduction techniques are employed for fracture treatment.

A, B   C

Figure 30-27. **A:** Pronation–external rotation injury resulting in a Salter–Harris type I fracture of the distal tibial physis. Note that despite this severe displacement, the relationship between the distal epiphysis of the tibia and distal fibula is preserved, and widening of the syndesmosis between the tibia and fibula is not present in this region. **B, C:** Anteroposterior and lateral radiographs demonstrate satisfactory closed reduction.

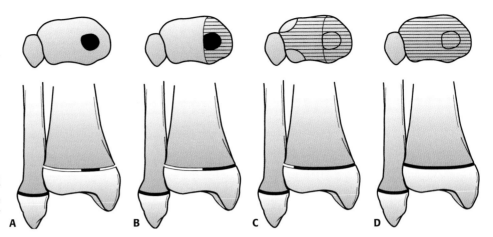

Figure 30-28. Closure of the distal tibial physis begins centrally (**A**), extends medially (**B**), and then laterally (**C**) before final closure (**D**).

TREATMENT OPTIONS FOR ANKLE FRACTURES

NONOPERATIVE TREATMENT OF ANKLE FRACTURES

Indications/Contraindications

Nonoperative Treatment of Ankle Fractures:
INDICATIONS AND CONTRAINDICATIONS

Indications

- Nondisplaced, stable fracture patterns
- Stable, minimally displaced fracture patterns

Contraindications

- Significant intra-articular displacement or step-off of articular surface, >2 mm
- Unstable fracture patterns
- Significant fracture displacement

Appropriate treatment of ankle fractures in children depends on the location of the fracture, the degree of displacement, and the age of the child (Table 30-1). Nondisplaced fractures may be simply immobilized. A randomized clinical trial of minimally displaced low-risk ankle fractures compared a fiberglass posterior splint to a removable ankle stirrup brace. This study demonstrated good outcomes in both groups.[7] Closed reduction and cast immobilization may be appropriate for displaced fractures; if the closed reduction cannot be maintained with casting, skeletal fixation may be necessary. If closed reduction is not possible, open reduction may be indicated, followed by internal fixation or cast immobilization.

The anatomic type of the fracture (usually defined by the Salter–Harris classification), the mechanism of injury, and the amount of displacement of the fragments are important considerations. When the articular surface is disrupted, the amount of articular step-off or separation must be measured. The neurologic and vascular status of the limb or the status of the skin may require emergency treatment of the fracture and associated problems. The general health of the patient and the time since injury must also be considered.

OPERATIVE TREATMENT OF ANKLE FRACTURES

Preoperative Planning

Operative treatment is indicated for open fractures or injuries with severe soft tissue injury, when there is displacement of the articular surface, or when acceptable position and alignment cannot be maintained with closed methods.

Operative Repair of Ankle Fractures:
PREOPERATIVE PLANNING CHECKLIST

OR table	☐ Radiolucent component can be valuable. Confirm that the fracture can be easily seen prior to prepping and draping the patient's fracture site.
Position/ positioning aids	☐ Allowing the ankle to be moved off the table to the side can allow easy access for C-arm evaluation. Alternatively, a bump can be placed behind the hip on the injured side, to allow for the ankle to be positioned with more inward rotation and the leg can be elevated on a stack of blankets or commercial ramp to allow easy lateral fluoroscopic imaging.
Fluoroscopy location	☐ Best location may be just off to the side of the patient, as they are positioned on the table. This allows the ankle to be moved off the side of the table, to allow easy visualization with the C-arm. We find that use of the mini C-arm has many advantages over the larger C-arm, including lower radiation dose, easy maneuverability, and it does not require additional OR staff to operate, but not all operative rooms have access to the mini C-arm.
Equipment	☐ Appropriate orthopaedic reduction tools, including large and medium bone reduction clamps, dental picks, excellent lighting source, cannulated screw systems, Kirschner wires (K-wires), or any anticipated implants. Headlights or lighted suction tips may be valuable in some cases. Local anesthetic and casting and splinting material should also be available.
Tourniquet	☐ Use may be optional, depending on surgeon preference. Clear visualization of the fracture planes may be enhanced by use of the tourniquet.

TABLE 30-1. Current Treatment Options

Fracture	Options	Pros	Cons
Distal tibia physis	Above-knee vs. below-knee cast	Below-knee casts may allow for less knee stiffness and muscle atrophy of the thigh	For fractures with potential for displacement, the below-knee cast may increase the risk of displacement and pain from lack of rotational control
	Local anesthesia with sedation vs. general anesthesia (closed reduction of fractures)	Local anesthesia techniques combined with sedation in the emergency room (ER) may be less expensive and allow for early reduction	Guidelines for sedation techniques must follow guidelines established by the American Society of Anesthesiologists, and adequate facilities and personnel may not be available in all ERs
	Minimally invasive approaches (including arthroscopic assistance) vs. traditional open surgical exposures	Arthroscopic-assisted procedures may allow for smaller incisions, and better assessment of articular reductions than open exposures	Additional equipment and OR staffing requirements for arthroscopy are necessary. Surgeon experience with arthroscopy may be more limited
	Bioabsorbable vs. metal implants	Bioabsorbable devices do not require removal, and subsequent imaging studies (CT, MRI) are not affected by these implants	First-generation implants have a higher risk of local inflammation, and the quality of fixation may be less secure

CT, computed tomography; MRI, magnetic resonance imaging; OR, operating room.

Advanced Imaging Studies

CT gives better bone resolution than MRI for intra-articular fractures. For intra-articular and multifragmented fracture patterns, CT can help plan reduction and fixation techniques. High-resolution scans with three-dimensional reconstructions provide excellent anatomic detail. For minimally invasive approaches using percutaneous screw fixation, these images can be used to plan small incisions and for precise screw placement during surgery. The CT scan can also facilitate percutaneous placement of clamps, to allow for compression perpendicular to the plane of the fracture. A clear preoperative evaluation should determine optimal screw position and orientation, and these images should also be available during the procedure to assist with screw placement.

OPEN REDUCTION AND INTERNAL FIXATION (ORIF) OF ANKLE FRACTURES

Technique

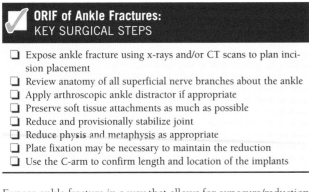

ORIF of Ankle Fractures:
KEY SURGICAL STEPS

- [ ] Expose ankle fracture using x-rays and/or CT scans to plan incision placement
- [ ] Review anatomy of all superficial nerve branches about the ankle
- [ ] Apply arthroscopic ankle distractor if appropriate
- [ ] Preserve soft tissue attachments as much as possible
- [ ] Reduce and provisionally stabilize joint
- [ ] Reduce physis and metaphysis as appropriate
- [ ] Plate fixation may be necessary to maintain the reduction
- [ ] Use the C-arm to confirm length and location of the implants

Expose ankle fracture in a way that allows for exposure/reduction of the metaphyseal, epiphyseal, and intra-articular portion as necessary. Use of CT and x-rays is invaluable for planning incision placement. Also avoid any skin compromise or fracture blisters if possible. Review the anatomy of all superficial nerve branches about the ankle, to avoid inadvertent nerve injury and secondary neuroma formation. Apply arthroscopic ankle distractor across ankle joint if traction may facilitate reduction and visualization of the fracture. In many cases, minimal fracture exposure is necessary. In some cases, more extensive exposure is valuable, to help with reduction. Preserve soft tissue attachments as much as possible, to avoid injury to bone vascularity. In some cases, contralateral ankle x-rays may be obtained of the opposite ankle from the C-arm, to help guide reduction of the injured side. Keep these images readily available to help with reduction. Because of the importance of intra-articular surface reduction, prioritize reduction of joint surface. Joint reduction may be obtained and enhanced with strategic bone clamp placement. Provisional stabilization may be obtained with K-wires. K-wires from cannulated screw systems may be placed, and some of these K-wires may be used for placement of cannulated screws over the wires. In some cases, cannulated screws can be placed over washers, to enhance compression across the fracture planes and minimize the penetration of screws into the relatively soft epiphyseal and metaphyseal bone.

Reduce physis and metaphysis as appropriate. Use of K-wires and cannulated screws can facilitate and maintain reduction. In some cases, placement of K-wires may be used as a "joystick" and a reduction tool to help with anatomic reduction of a displaced fragment. When possible, use of smooth K-wires across the physis may be necessary to maintain reduction. Smooth wires may be less likely to cause physeal arrest. In some cases, screws may be placed across the physis that is approaching closure, including juvenile plafond fractures and transitional fracture patterns. Plate fixation may be necessary in some cases, to help the reduction on the fibula, and in some cases, on the tibial side as well. Use the C-arm to confirm length and location of the implants. A preoperative CT scan can be used to help plan placement of all screws, as well as allow the surgeon to plan for the appropriate screw and thread length. Optimized screw and thread length can improve compression of fractures. During screw, K-wire placement, be vigilant about surrounding neurovascular structures. If these devices penetrate too deeply, they can injure these structures. Remain vigilant for the possibility

Figure 30-29. Ankle arthroscopy. **A:** Arthroscopic view of fracture gap in distal tibia articular surface. **B:** Arthroscopic view of fracture gap in distal tibial articular surface after reduction.

A   B

of compartment syndrome, as this may rarely occur after ankle fracture in children.

Arthroscopy

The use of arthroscopy can facilitate minimally invasive procedures, and also be a tool to help guide reduction during open procedures using larger incisions. Several clinical series document the effectiveness of arthroscopic assistance for Tillaux fractures[85,143] and triplane fractures.[82,85] The joint surfaces can be readily visualized through small incisions, avoiding the need for a larger arthrotomy. Even in cases where an arthrotomy is used, the scope can be utilized either with or without fluid to visualize the reduction of the fragments (Fig. 30-29). The fluid of the arthroscopy pump can also be used to wash out the fracture site, increasing visualization during reduction. Avoidance of high pump pressure will minimize the risks of soft tissue infiltration.

Different size scopes are available, including 2.8 and 4.5 mm. We prefer to use smaller-diameter scopes, especially in younger patients. The smaller scope has a smaller field of view, but this does not seem to be much of a disadvantage for viewing the displaced cartilage surfaces. The smaller scope also delivers less fluid to the joint, which may require additional time to clean the hematoma from the joint and fracture but has a lower risk of causing soft tissue infiltration around the joint.

Fluoroscopy

The small C-arm unit will also assist with minimally invasive approaches. This can be easily rotated to allow for AP, oblique, or lateral views. If the ankle distractor is used, position the foot and distractor to allow easy access by the C-arm (Fig. 30-30).

Ankle Distraction

Use of the ankle distractor (normally used for arthroscopy procedures) can assist with reduction of displaced extra-articular fractures, such as Salter–Harris type I or II patterns. When combined with the relaxation of general anesthesia, a few minutes of distraction across the physis can facilitate reduction. The distraction across the fracture may increase the likelihood that the first attempt at reduction will be successful; this may reduce the trauma to the physis during the reduction, perhaps reducing the risk of physeal arrest. Juvenile Tillaux and triplane fracture reduction can also be facilitated with ankle distraction, and this will also facilitate arthroscopic ankle visualization. The ankle distractor obviates the need to have the surgeon pull manually for several minutes. The surgeon can then focus on the application of other forces, such as rotation or varus/valgus to facilitate fracture reduction. Although skeletal traction using a calcaneal pin is an option,[38] we prefer to use an ankle strap and special distractor routinely used

A   B

Figure 30-30. Use of ankle distractor. **A:** Thigh positioner to allow for ankle distractor. **B:** Sterile ankle distractor in place.

(continues)

C

D

Figure 30-30. *(Continued)* **C:** Distractor can remain in place during reduction maneuvers. **D:** C-arm can be brought into the field to evaluate the reduction.

for arthroscopy (Arthrex, Naples, Florida). The ankle distractor can be positioned to allow for AP and lateral mini C-arm images (see Fig. 30-30).

Percutaneous Clamps

Precise placement of clamps can facilitate the reduction of fractures. Careful study of imaging studies, especially CT scans, can guide precise placement of clamps to provide maximal compression across fracture planes. Forces normal or near normal to the fracture planes are ideal. Care should be taken during placement, to prevent injury to neurologic and vascular structures, including sensory nerves. The skin can be divided, and then deeper dissection through the subcutaneous tissues can be performed with a hemostat. The hemostat is used to bluntly distract the tissues away from the skin portal and then advanced

A, B

C

D, E

F

Figure 30-31. **A:** Anteroposterior view of displaced Salter–Harris type I fibula fracture and Salter–Harris type IV intra-articular medial malleolus fracture. **B:** Use of percutaneous clamps to facilitate reduction of medial malleolus fracture. **C:** Use of percutaneous clamps to facilitate reduction. **D:** Use of two pins as "joysticks" to guide reduction of the displaced medial malleolus fracture. **E:** Use of percutaneous clamps to facilitate reduction and compression across the epiphyseal fracture. **F:** Use of percutaneous epiphyseal screws to gain compression across the fracture and to facilitate reduction.

Figure 30-32. Anteroposterior (**A**) and lateral (**B**) radiograph of triplane fracture with involvement of medial malleolus. Use of percutaneous clamps for reduction, viewed in the anteroposterior plane (**C**) and in the lateral plane (**D**). **E, F:** Use of percutaneous clamps for reduction, followed by placement of guidewires to hold reduction. Anteroposterior (**G**) and lateral (**H**) views of percutaneous and miniopen placement of cannulated screws.

to the bone surface. The tips of the clamp can now be placed with minimal risk to neurovascular structures. The clamp can be compressed, to facilitate reduction of triplane and Tillaux fractures (Figs. 30-31 and 30-32).

Implants

Different implants are available for fixation of ankle fractures. Smooth pins have the advantage that they do not place a threaded tip across the physis, therefore reducing the risk of iatrogenic physeal arrest. The main disadvantage of smooth pins is that they do not allow for compression. These pins can also migrate through bone and into soft tissues. Bending the ends at the surface of the skin to prevent migration is important. These pins should be removed early, as soon as the fracture stability is adequate. In most cases, we remove the pins between 14 and 21 days after surgery. Careful management of the pin–skin interface with dressings that limit motion is believed to lower the risk of pin inflammation and infection.

In most physeal injuries, the use of screws or threaded devices across the physis should be avoided when possible. In

some cases, a screw implant may be necessary to cross a physis, to maintain an articular reduction. The adequacy of reduction of the joint surface is probably more important than the physis. In patients approaching skeletal maturity, the use of screw implants across a physis that is approaching closure is probably a reasonable choice, especially in case where compression and/or stability are important, such as juvenile Tillaux fractures (Fig. 30-33).

Distal Tibial Fractures

Salter–Harris Type I and II Fractures

Cast immobilization or leg/ankle walking boot is sufficient treatment for nondisplaced Salter–Harris type I fractures of the distal tibia. The immobilization should be worn for 3 to 4 weeks, with the first 1 to 2 weeks limited to non–weight bearing. After cast or boot removal, a therapy program may be recommended in older patients or those trying to return to competitive sports at an earlier time. In our experience, formal supervised therapy is not necessary in younger patients. The normal activity of these children is usually sufficient therapy.

Figure 30-33. A, B: Displaced juvenile Tillaux fracture. Closed reduction was not successful. **C:** After open reduction with internal fixation with a small fragment screw.

Most displaced fractures can be treated with closed reduction and cast immobilization. Though an above-knee non–weight-bearing cast has often been recommended initially, as this should reduce the risk of rotational displacement after reduction, there is new literature to support the safety of using below-knee casting for these injuries. In a study of 120 patients with distal tibia physeal injuries treated with below-knee casting, only 2 of the 120 patients had displacement of the fracture in the below-knee cast.[186] These fractures can displace in the first 1 to 2 weeks after reduction, and close follow-up with radiographic surveillance for this is necessary. One or two K-wires can be placed at the time of closed reduction (if it is performed in an operating room setting), to prevent displacement after reduction under anesthesia (Fig. 30-34). These pins can be removed 2 to 3 weeks after placement.

Salter–Harris Type II Fractures

Salter–Harris type II fractures can be caused by any of the four mechanisms of injury described by Dias and Giegerich.[55] In the series of Spiegel et al.,[187] Salter–Harris type II fractures were the most common injuries (44.8%). In addition to the direction of displacement of the distal tibial epiphysis and the nature of any associated fibular fracture, the location of the Thurstan-Holland fragment is helpful in determining the mechanism of injury; for example, a lateral fragment indicates a pronation–eversion–external rotation injury; a posteromedial fragment, a supination–external rotation injury; and a posterior fragment, a supination–plantarflexion injury (Fig. 30-35).

Nondisplaced fractures can be treated with cast immobilization for 3 to 4 weeks, followed by a removable cast/walking boot for another 3 to 4 weeks.

Although most authors agree that closed reduction of significantly displaced Salter–Harris type II ankle fracture should be attempted, opinions differ as to what degree of residual displacement or angulation is unacceptable and requires open reduction. Based on follow-up of 33 Salter–Harris type II ankle fractures, Carothers and Crenshaw[36] concluded that "accurate reposition of the displaced epiphysis at the expense of forced or repeated manipulation or operative intervention is not indicated since spontaneous realignment of the ankle occurs even late in the growing period." They found no residual angulation at follow-up in patients who had up to 12 degrees of tilt after reduction, even in patients as old as 13 years of age at the time of injury. Spiegel et al.,[187] however, reported complications at

Figure 30-34. A, B: Displaced distal tibial Salter–Harris type II fracture, with distal diaphyseal fibula fracture. **C, D:** Fracture treated with closed reduction and internal fixation.

Figure 30-35. **A:** Severe plantarflexion injury with severe swelling of the ankle and foot; the reduction obtained was unstable. **B:** The reduction was stabilized by two transmetaphyseal screws placed percutaneously. **C:** Anteroposterior view confirms an anatomic reduction.

follow-up in 11 of 16 patients with Salter–Harris type II ankle fractures. Because 6 of these 11 patients had angular deformities that were attributed to lack of adequate reduction of the fracture, Spiegel et al. recommend "precise anatomical reduction."

Barmada et al.[6] reviewed a series of Salter–Harris type I and II fractures. In patients with more than 3 mm of physeal widening, the risk of premature physeal closure was 60%, compared with 17% in patients with less than 3 mm of physeal widening. Although they were unable to demonstrate a significant decrease in partial physeal arrest in those treated with surgery, they recommended open reduction and removal of the entrapped periosteal flap. A subsequent study at the same institution recommended avoiding open reduction if gross deformity was not present, as patients treated with open reduction for entrapped periosteum did not have lower rates of premature physeal closure. Leary et al.[107] studied 15 distal tibia fractures with premature physeal closure and found residual gap and number of reduction attempts did not predict early closure, but initial

displacement did. The literature on the value of open reduction and removal of interposed periosteum to lower the incidence of premature physeal closure is conflicted in these fractures, and it is likely that multiple variables are involved (energy of initial injury, amount of displacement, number of reduction attempts, age of patient).

Incomplete reduction is frequently caused by interposition of soft tissue between the fracture fragments. Grace[72] reported three patients in whom the interposed soft tissue included the neurovascular bundle, resulting in circulatory embarrassment when closed reduction was attempted. In this situation, open reduction and extraction of the soft tissue obviously is required. As noted above, a less definitive indication for open reduction is interposition of the periosteum, which causes physeal widening with no or minimal angulation. Good results have been reported after open reduction and extraction of the periosteal flap (Fig. 30-36).[97] It is not clear that failure to extract the periosteum in such cases results in physeal arrest sufficient to

Figure 30-36. **A:** Severely displaced pronation–eversion–external rotation injury. **B:** Closed reduction was unsuccessful, and a valgus tilt of the ankle mortise was noted. At surgery, soft tissue was interposed laterally (*arrows*). **C:** Reduction completed and stabilized with two cancellous screws placed above the physis.

warrant operative treatment. Wattenbarger et al.[201] and Phieffer et al.[153] have attempted to determine the relationship between physeal bar formation and interposed periosteum, although at this time it is unclear if the periosteal flap increases the risk of physeal arrest.

Because of risk of iatrogenic damage to the distal tibial physis during closed reduction, many authors recommend the use of general anesthesia with adequate muscle relaxation for children with Salter–Harris type II distal tibial fractures. However, no study has compared the frequency of growth abnormalities in patients with these fractures reduced under sedation and local analgesia to those with fractures reduced with the use of general anesthesia. Using general anesthesia and an arthroscopic ankle distractor to distract the fracture before reduction has the theoretical advantage of reducing the risk of physeal damage during the reduction maneuver (see Fig. 30-30).

When closed reductions are not performed under general anesthesia, they are usually done under IV sedation. Alioto et al.[1] demonstrated significantly improved pain relief with hematoma block for ankle fractures in a study comparing patients treated with IV sedation to patients receiving hematoma block.[54] Intravenous (IV) regional anesthesia or Bier block has also been reported to be effective for pain relief in lower extremity injuries.[108]

One advantage of reduction in the operating room with general anesthesia is the ease with which percutaneous pins can be placed to maintain reduction of the fractures. If there is any concern about redisplacement or stability after closed reduction under general anesthesia, smooth pins can be placed.

Surgeons using regional block anesthesia within the first 2 to 3 days after the fracture should consider the potential for compartment syndrome. In fractures that have a higher risk of compartment syndrome, regional anesthesia, especially peripheral nerve blocks with longer-acting agents, might delay the recognition of a compartment syndrome.[133]

Salter–Harris Type III and IV Fractures

Salter–Harris type III and IV fractures are discussed together because the mechanism of injury is the same (supination–inversion) and their treatment and prognosis are similar. Juvenile Tillaux and triplane fractures are considered separately. In the series of Spiegel et al.,[187] 24.1% of the fractures were Salter–Harris type III injuries and 1.4% were type IV. These injuries are usually produced by the medial corner of the talus being driven into the junction of the distal tibial articular surface and the medial malleolus. As the talus shears off the medial malleolus, the physis may also be damaged (Fig. 30-37).

Nondisplaced Salter–Harris types III and IV fractures can be treated with below-knee or above-knee cast immobilization, but care must be taken to be sure that the significant intra-articular displacement is not present. Salter–Harris III and IV fractures were included in the Souder study and were found to be safely immobilized by below-knee casts.[186] Radiographs frequently underestimate the degree of intra-articular involvement and step-off of the articular surfaces. CT imaging may be necessary to fully appreciate the degree of displacement. We

recommend any time there is a question of joint involvement of an ankle fracture that a CT, preferably with 3D reconstructions is obtained. Follow-up radiographs and/or CT scans in the first 2 weeks may also be necessary to confirm that no displacement occurs after casting.

Salter–Harris type III fractures of the medial malleolus have a high risk of physeal arrest. One study suggested that the rate of physeal arrest could be reduced by the use of open reduction and internal fixation.[94,104] Luhmann et al.[117] studied a series of medial malleolar fractures with growth disturbance following treatment and recommended anatomic reduction as fractures with as little as 2 mm of step-off went on to premature physeal closure. Others have also emphasized the importance of anatomic reduction and early treatment to reduce the risk of physeal arrest.[151]

Based on principles of fracture treatment in adults, displaced intra-articular fractures are treated with as anatomical a reduction as possible. Studies in children confirming the importance of articular reduction to within 2 mm are few, although most recommend anatomic articular reduction in displaced fractures involving the articular surface. Failure to obtain anatomical reduction may result in articular incongruity and posttraumatic arthritis, which often becomes symptomatic 5 to 8 years after skeletal maturity.[39] The risk of growth arrest has also been linked to the adequacy of reduction, although the literature is still unclear if anatomic reduction reduces the risk of physeal arrest (Fig. 30-38).[174] Some series suggest early anatomic reduction is associated with a lower risk of physeal arrest.[174] Closed reduction may be attempted but is likely to succeed only in minimally displaced fractures. If closed reduction is obtained, it can be maintained with a cast or with percutaneous pins or screws supplemented by a cast.

If anatomical reduction cannot be obtained by closed methods, open reduction and internal fixation or miniopen arthroscopic reduction should be carried out. Lintecum and Blasier[114] described a technique of open reduction achieved through a limited exposure of the fracture with the incision centered over the fracture site combined with percutaneous cannulated screw fixation. This technique was performed on 13 patients—8 Salter–Harris IV fractures, 4 Salter–Harris III fractures, and 1 triplane fracture. The authors reported one growth arrest at follow-up averaging 12 months. Beaty and Linton[8] reported a Salter–Harris type III fracture with an intra-articular fragment; these fractures require open reduction for inspection of the joint to ensure that no osteochondral fragments are impeding reduction. Arthroscopic evaluation of the joint may also be an option. Internal fixation devices should be inserted within the epiphysis, parallel to the physis in patients with more than 2 years of growth remaining, and should avoid entering ankle joint (Fig. 30-39; see Fig. 30-19).

Arthroscopic-assisted fixation of fractures with intra-articular involvement has been described by several centers. Jennings et al.[85] presented a series of five triplane and one Tillaux fractures treated with arthroscopic assistance. The outcome was excellent for fracture reduction and ankle function. Kaya et al.[95] review 10 patients with juvenile Tillaux fractures treated with arthroscopic assistance, demonstrating excellent

Figure 30-37. **A:** Severe ankle injury sustained by an 8-year-old involved in a car accident. The anteroposterior view in the splint does not clearly show the Salter–Harris type IV fracture of the tibia. The dome of the talus appears abnormal. **B:** CT scan shows the displaced Salter–Harris type IV fracture of the medial malleolus and a severe displaced intra-articular fracture of the body of the talus. **C, D:** Open reduction of both fractures was performed, and Herbert screws were used for internal fixation. (Courtesy of Armen Kelikian, MD.)

reduction and clinical outcomes.[143] One of the primary advantages of arthroscopic fixation is that it allows for visualization of the articular surfaces, although the need for open reduction of the metaphyseal and epiphyseal regions may still require open incisions.

Options for internal fixation include smooth K-wires, small fragment cortical and cancellous screws, and 3- and 4-mm cannulated screws (Fig. 30-40). Several reports[17,18,31] have advocated the use of absorbable pins for internal fixation of ankle fractures. Benz et al.[10] reported no complications or growth abnormalities after the use of absorbable pins with metal

screw supplementation for fixation of five ankle fractures in patients between the ages of 5 and 13 years. In reports of the use of absorbable pins without supplemental metal fixation in adults,[19,55] complications have included displacement (14.5%), sterile fluid accumulation requiring incision and drainage (8.1%), pseudarthrosis (8%), distal tibiofibular synostosis (3.8%), and infection (1.6%). Bucholz et al.[31] reported few complications in a series of fractures in adults fixed with absorbable screws made of polylactide and suggested that complications in earlier series might be related to the fact that those pins were made of polyglycolide. A report in 1993 by Böstman et al.,[18]

Figure 30-38. **A:** Anteroposterior view of a patient with a pronation–eversion–external rotation fracture. **B:** Postreduction view shows residual gapping of physis suggesting periosteal interposition. **C:** Anteroposterior view obtained for a new injury (medial malleolar fracture) shows premature closure of the physis.

however, included few complications in a series of fractures in children fixed with polyglycolide pins. A follow-up report by Rokkanen et al.[163] in 1996 reported 3.6% infection and 3.7% failure of fixation.

The main advantage of absorbable pins and screws is that hardware removal is avoided. Böstman compared the cost-effectiveness of absorbable implants in 994 patients treated with absorbable implants to 1,173 patients treated with metallic implants. To be cost-effective, the hardware removal rates required were calculated to range from 19% for metacarpal

fractures to 54% for trimalleolar fractures.[20] At this time, the indications for absorbable pins remain unclear.

Studies in the adult literature suggest second-generation bioabsorbable screws have lower complication rates, and their use may be increasing.[155,184] Additional studies in adult patients using ultrasound and MRI have not detected deleterious effects on healing with newer screw designs.[74,126] The presence of the physis, and the low-grade inflammation that may accompany the dissolution of these implants, however, may increase the risk of physeal arrest, and additional studies in adult and

Figure 30-39. **A:** Grade II supination–inversion injury in a 12-year-old girl, resulting in a displaced Salter–Harris type IV fracture of the distal tibia and a nondisplaced Salter–Harris type I fracture of the distal fibula. **B:** After anatomic open reduction and stable internal fixation.

Figure 30-40. A: Supination–inversion injury with a Salter–Harris type III fracture of the medial malleolus. **B:** Six months after open reduction and internal fixation with two transepiphyseal cannulated screws. **C:** Eighteen months after injury, the fracture has healed with no evidence of growth arrest or angular deformity. (*Arrows* show normal, symmetric Park–Harris growth arrest line.)

pediatric patients will be necessary to confirm the effectiveness and safety of these devices.[93]

Open Reduction and Internal Fixation of Salter–Harris Type III or IV Fracture of the Distal Tibia

The patient is placed supine on an operating table that is radiolucent at the lower extremity. For a minimally displaced Salter III fracture of the medial malleolus, closed reduction with percutaneous screws may be sufficient, but we have a low threshold for a small incision over the anteromedial joint to verify joint congruity after reduction (Fig. 30-41).

Periosteum often flips into this fracture, preventing an anatomic reduction. This can usually be removed with a very small incision and a skin hook (Fig. 30-42).

The incision should allow visualization of the joint surface at the fracture site and can be vertical or diagonal, depending on the nature of the fracture. The saphenous vein may be identified, dissected free, and retracted depending on the size of the incision. The fracture site is identified, and an anteromedial capsulotomy of the ankle joint is performed. The fracture surfaces are exposed and gently cleaned with irrigation and forceps (curettage is not used).

For Salter–Harris type IV fractures, the periosteum may be elevated several millimeters from the metaphyseal fracture edges. The epiphyseal edges and joint surfaces are examined through the arthrotomy. The perichondral ring should not be elevated from the physis. For Salter–Harris type III fractures, the reduction is evaluated by checking the joint surface and epiphyseal fracture edges through the arthrotomy. The epiphyseal fragment

Figure 30-41. **A:** Medial malleolus fracture. **B:** Two parallel threaded pins from a cannulated screw system are placed across the fracture site. **C:** As the screws are compressed, the fracture is reduced. An arthrogram, arthroscope, or direct visualization can confirm anatomic joint reduction. Washers help prevent the screw heads from entering the bone and maximize compressive force. **D:** Lateral view confirms good position of screws. Note that particular care must be taken with screw placement. **E:** In a different patient, the screws look acceptable in the AP plane. **F:** In the lateral plane, however, it is evident that one screw is in the joint. This is unacceptable and must be revised. Because of the curve of the distal tibia in the sagittal plane, this view is essential before the patient leaves the operating room. (Used with permission of the Children's Orthopaedic Center, Los Angeles.)

Figure 30-42. Displaced medial malleolus fracture. *Dashed arrow* shows the distal tibial metaphysis. *Solid arrow* shows the interposed periosteum. Usually a smaller incision is adequate for removal of periosteum and fracture reduction. (Used with permission of the Children's Orthopaedic Center, Los Angeles.)

Figure 30-43. Compression-type injury of the tibial physis. Early physeal arrest can cause leg-length discrepancy.

is grasped with a small towel clip or reduction forceps, and the fracture is reduced. Internal fixation is performed under direct vision and fluoroscopic control. It is important to view both the lateral and AP projections because of the curved shape of the distal tibial articular surface. If the fragment is large enough, 4-mm cannulated lag screws are inserted through the epiphyseal fragment; if the fragment is too small for screws, smooth K-wires are used. The reduction and the position of the internal fixation are checked through the arthrotomy. In fractures with a significant Thurstan-Holland fragment, a metaphyseal screw may be used if a gap exists after the epiphyseal screws are inserted. After reduction of the tibial fracture, an associated Salter–Harris type I or II fibular fracture usually reduces and is stable. If it is not, closed reduction and fixation with percutaneous oblique smooth K-wires are performed.

The patient is kept non–weight bearing in a cast for 3 weeks, and then the cast is changed to a below-knee walking cast, which is worn for an additional 3 weeks. Frequent follow-up evaluations (every 3–6 months for the first year and yearly thereafter until normal growth resumes) are necessary to detect growth abnormalities.

Salter–Harris Type V Fractures

Salter–Harris type V fractures of the ankle are believed to be caused by severe axial compression and crushing of the physis (Fig. 30-43). As originally described, these injuries are not usually associated with significant displacement of the epiphysis relative to the metaphysis, which make diagnosis of acute injury impossible from plain radiographs; the diagnosis can only be made on follow-up radiographs when premature physeal closure is evident (Fig. 30-44).

Spiegel et al.[187] have designated comminuted fractures that are otherwise unclassifiable as Salter–Harris type V injuries.

The incidence of Salter–Harris type V ankle fractures is difficult to establish because of the difficulty of diagnosing acute injuries. Spiegel et al.[187] included two type V fractures in their series, but both were comminuted fractures rather than the classic crush injury without initial radiographic abnormality.

Because of the uncertain nature of this injury, no specific treatment recommendations have been formulated. Treatment is usually directed primarily toward the sequelae of growth arrest that invariably follows Salter–Harris type V fractures. Perhaps more sophisticated scanning techniques will eventually allow identification and localization of areas of physeal injury so that irreparably damaged cells can be removed and replaced with interposition materials to prevent growth problems, but at present, this diagnosis is made only several months after injury (see Fig. 30-71, later).

Other Fractures of the Distal Tibia

Accessory ossification centers of the distal tibia (os subtibiale) and distal fibula (os fibulare) are common and may be injured. Treatment usually consists of cast immobilization for 3 to 4 weeks. Ogden and Lee[141] reported good results after cast immobilization in 26 of 27 patients with injuries involving the medial side of the tibia; only one patient required surgery. In contrast, 5 to 11 patients with injuries involving the lateral side had persistent symptoms that required excision.

Injuries to the perichondral ring of the distal tibial and fibular physes, with physeal disruption, have been described.[78] Most of these injuries are caused by skiving of the bone by machinery such as lawn mowers. They may result in growth arrest or angular deformities.

Juvenile Tillaux Fractures

This fracture is the adolescent counterpart of the fracture in adults described by the French surgeon Tillaux. It occurs when the foot externally rotates, causing the anteroinferior tibiofibular ligament to avulse a fragment of bone through its attachments to the anterolateral tibia. The avulsed fragment of bone corresponds to the portion of the distal tibial physis that is still

Figure 30-44. A: An 8-year-old girl had a minimally displaced fracture of the distal fibula; this is her standing x-ray from about 4 weeks after the injury. This was a Salter II fracture as there is a very small metaphyseal piece present. Note the normal relative lengths of the lateral malleolus, more distal than the medial malleolus. *Solid arrow* shows distal fibular physis in normal position at level of ankle joint. **B:** Two years later, at age 10, a complete growth arrest is noted. The tips of the lateral malleolus and medial malleolus (*dashed arrow* indicates that her distal tibia and fibula physes are at the same level) are at the same level and she has relative ankle valgus and pain. **C:** Intraoperative fluoroscopic images show a lengthening osteotomy of the distal fibula and a completion epiphysiodesis of the distal tibia. **D:** Postoperative AP x-ray of the ankle in the corrected position. **E:** X-ray 6 years postoperatively shows complete healing, maintenance of correction.

open (Fig. 30-45). In the series of Spiegel et al.,[187] these fractures occurred in 2.9% of patients.

Tillaux fractures may be isolated injuries or may be associated with ipsilateral tibial shaft fractures.[46] The fibula usually prevents marked displacement of the fracture and clinical deformity is generally absent. Swelling is usually slight, and local tenderness is at the anterolateral joint line, in contrast to ankle sprains where the tenderness tends to be below the level of the ankle joint.

A mortise view is essential to see the distal tibial epiphysis unobstructed by the fibula (Fig. 30-46). Steinlauf et al.[188] reported a patient in whom the Tillaux fragment became

Figure 30-45. Juvenile Tillaux fracture. Mechanism of injury: The anteroinferior tibiofibular ligament avulses a fragment of the lateral epiphysis (**A**) corresponding to the portion of the physis that is still open (**B**).

Figure 30-46. Mortise view of a 14-year-old who sustained a juvenile Tillaux fracture.

Figure 30-47. Anatomy of a three-part triplane fracture (left ankle). Note the large epiphyseal fragment (which usually has the metaphyseal component attached) and the smaller anterolateral epiphyseal fragment.

entrapped between the distal tibia and fibula, producing apparent diastasis of the ankle joint. To allow measurement of displacement from plain films, the radiograph beam would have to be directly in line with the fracture site, which makes CT confirmation of reduction desired after all closed reductions of these fractures.

Both below-knee and above-knee casts have been used for immobilization of nondisplaced juvenile Tillaux and triplane fractures. Fractures with more than 2 mm of displacement, especially those associated with articular incongruity, may be best treated with closed or open reduction.[47,95] Closed reduction is attempted by internally rotating the foot and applying direct pressure over the anterolateral tibia. If necessary, percutaneous pins can be used for stabilization of the reduction. If closed reduction is not successful, open reduction or percutaneous reduction with arthroscopic assistance may be needed. Occasionally, percutaneously inserted pins can be used to manipulate the displaced fragment into anatomical position and then advanced to fix the fragment in place.[172] Screw fixation within the epiphysis is usually the preferred fixation method (see Figs. 30-19, 30-30, and 30-31).

Triplane Fracture

Kärrholm notes that Gerner-Smidt in 1963 described triplane and Tillaux fractures as different stages of the same injury.[88] In 1957, Johnson and Fahl[86] described a triplane fracture in their report of 27 physeal ankle injuries and reported that they had seen 10 such fractures. Despite these earlier reports, the nature of triplane fractures was not appreciated until Marmor's[126] report in 1970 of an irreducible ankle fracture that at surgery was found to consist of three parts (Fig. 30-47). Two years after Marmor's report, Lynn[120] reported two additional such fractures and coined the term triplane fracture. He described the fracture as consisting of three major fragments: (1) the anterolateral

quadrant of the distal tibial epiphysis, (2) the medial and posterior portions of the epiphysis in addition to a posterior metaphyseal spike, and (3) the tibial metaphysis. Cooperman et al.,[44] however, in their 1978 report of 15 such fractures concluded that, based on tomographic studies, most were two-part fractures produced by external rotation (Fig. 30-48). Variations in fracture patterns were attributed to the extent of physeal closure at the time of injury. Kärrholm et al.[89] reported that CT evaluation of four adolescents with triplane fractures confirmed the existence of two-part and three-part fractures and also revealed four-part fractures (Fig. 30-49).

El-Karef et al.[62] studied 21 triplane fractures, identifying 19 as lateral triplane variants, and 2 as medial variants. A lateral triplane looks like a Tillaux fracture on AP radiograph because the epiphyseal fracture occurs in the sagittal plane and the metaphyseal fracture occurs in the coronal plane (more simply, the lateral part of the epiphysis has broken off). By contrast, a medial triplane has the epiphyseal fracture in the coronal plane and the metaphyseal fracture in the sagittal plane (the medial part of the epiphysis has broken off).[54,62] In the El-Karef study, 12 were two-part fractures, 6 were three-part fractures, and 3 were four-part fractures.[62]

Figure 30-48. Anatomy of a two-part lateral triplane fracture (left ankle). Note the large posterolateral epiphyseal fragment with its posterior metaphyseal fragment. The anterior portion of the medial malleolus remains intact.

C   **D**

Figure 30-52. *(Continued)* **C, D:** After open reduction with internal fixation. Note anterior-to-posterior and medial-to-lateral screw placement that avoids the physis.

surgical approach depends on the fracture anatomy as determined by the preoperative CT scan and can vary greatly. A two-part medial triplane fracture can be approached through a hockey-stick anteromedial incision. The fracture fragments are irrigated to remove debris, and any interposed periosteum is removed. The fracture is reduced, and reduction is confirmed by direct observation through an anteromedial arthrotomy and by image intensification. Two 4-mm cancellous screws are inserted from medial to lateral or from anterior to posterior or both, depending on the fracture pattern (Fig. 30-52). Anterior-to-posterior screw placement may require an additional anterolateral incision or the screws may be inserted percutaneously. Arthroscopic-assisted techniques, with the use of percutaneous clamps and screws, may also be used (see Fig. 30-32).

Fractures with three or more parts may occasionally require more exposure for reduction and internal fixation. If the fibula is fractured, posterior exposure of the tibial fracture can be readily obtained by detaching the anterior and posteroinferior tibiofibular ligaments and turning down the distal fibula on the lateral collateral ligament (Fig. 30-53). If the fibula is not fractured, a fibular osteotomy may be needed in very rare circumstances for adequate visualization of the articular surface. Careful dissection is necessary to avoid iatrogenic fractures through the physis of the fibula. Medial exposure is obtained through an anteromedial or posteromedial incision. Reduction and internal fixation are carried out in a stepwise fashion. For typical three-part fractures, the Salter–Harris type II fracture may be reduced first by provisional fixation to the distal tibia through the metaphyseal fragment. Usually, the Salter–Harris type III fragment can then be reduced and provisionally fixed to the stabilized type II fragment (Fig. 30-54). Occasionally, the order of reduction and fixation should be reversed. Fractures with four or more fragments

require additional steps, but fixation of the Salter–Harris type II or IV fragment through the metaphysis to the distal tibia is usually best performed first. This step can be followed by fixation of the Salter–Harris type III fragment or fragments (Fig. 30-55). After reduction, reliable patients may be treated with immobilization in a short-leg, non–weight-bearing cast for 3 to 4 weeks. At 3 to 4 weeks, they may be converted to a weight-bearing cast or walking boot for an additional 3 to 4 weeks.

Pilon Fractures

Although these fractures are relatively rare in young patients, they can be associated with severe soft tissue

Figure 30-53. Transfibular approach to a complex triplane fracture.

Figure 30-54. Open reduction with internal fixation of a three-part lateral triplane fracture. **A, B:** Reduction and fixation of the Salter–Harris type II fragment to the metaphysis. **C, D:** Reduction and internal fixation of the Salter–Harris type III fragment to the Salter–Harris type II fragment.

Figure 30-55. A, B: Irreducible three-part lateral triplane fracture in a 14-year-old boy. **C, D:** After open reduction through a transfibular approach and internal fixation with anterior-to-posterior and lateral-to-medial screws.

swelling. Similar to the treatment in adults with these injuries, management of the soft tissues is critical to prevent complications of skin loss, infection, wound healing problems, etc.[59,192] Initial approaches may consist of application of external fixation, or dressings to address swelling and edema, with delay in surgical intervention for 5 to 15 days (Figs. 30-56 and 30-57).[59]

Letts et al.[112] have described a small series of pilon fractures in the skeletally immature. The patients in this series did not have wound/skin complications, and only two of eight had postoperative osteoarthritis at short-term follow-up. As these fractures may be at higher risk for complications, we believe that treatment principles used in adult patients should be applied to this patient population as well.[5,14,110,112,144,160]

Figure 30-56. Preoperative CT scan views (**A, B**) and postoperative (**C, D**) anteroposterior and lateral views of a pilon fracture in an adolescent.

Figure 30-57. Pilon fracture treated with spatial frame. **A, B:** Preoperative antero-posterior and lateral view of adolescent pilon fracture with depressed articular region. **C:** Axial CT scan showing comminution of articular surface. **D, E:** Sagittal CT scan and coronal CT scan showing comminution of metaphysic and involvement of articular surface. **F, G:** Reduction of fracture with Taylor Spatial Frame and placement of percutaneous screws to reduce the articular surface.

Syndesmosis Injuries

Syndesmosis injuries have been associated with the following fracture patterns: distal fibula, Salter I and II, triplane, and Til-laux.[49,105,119,179] Medial joint space widening may be an important anatomic factor to evaluate during treatment of external rotation mechanism injuries, and this should improve after surgical treatment.[71] During surgical treatment of pediatric/ adolescent ankle fractures, evaluation for syndesmosis injuries should be performed in a manner similar to the treatment of adult fractures since the predictive factor most associated with improved functional outcome is anatomic reduction of the syndesmosis.[179] Syndesmosis reduction and fixation may be necessary (see Fig. 30-14), in some cases. Screws and suture buttons are both safe options for fixation of the reduced syndesmosis.[119]

Figure 30-58. A: Severe lawn mower injury in a 5-year-old boy. **B:** One year after initial treatment with debridement, free flap, and skin graft coverage.

Open Fractures and Lawn Mower Injuries

Severe open ankle fractures are often produced by high-velocity motor vehicular accidents or lawn mower injuries (Fig. 30-58).[78] Approximately 25,000 lawn mower injuries occur each year, 20% of which are in children. Ride-on mowers produce the most severe injuries, requiring more surgical procedures and resulting in more functional limitations.[2,57,99,200] In 1997, Loder et al.[115] reviewed 144 children injured by lawn mowers. The average age at the time of injury was 7 years. The child was a bystander in 84 cases. Sixty-seven children required amputation. Soft tissue infection occurred in 8 of 118 and osteomyelitis in 6 of 117. In an updated study 25 years later, Khansa et al. reviewed 142 children injured by lawn mowers. The average age at the time of injury was 7.5 years, 38% required amputation, and riding mowers resulted in more operative procedures, longer length of stay, and more soft tissue reconstructive procedures. The incidence of lawn mower injuries to children has not decreased despite recommendations for lawn mower safety.[99]

Principles of treatment are the same as in adults: copious irrigation and debridement, tetanus toxoid, and IV antibiotics. Gaglani et al.[68] reported the bacteriologic findings in three children with infections secondary to lawn mower injuries. They found that organisms infecting the wounds were frequently different than those found on initial debridement, calling into question the value of intraoperative cultures. Gram-negative organisms were common, and all three patients were infected with fungi as well. In children with lawn mower injuries, grass, dirt, and debris are pushed and blown into the wound under pressure, and removal of these embedded foreign objects requires meticulous mechanical debridement.

In most patients, the articular surface and physis should be aligned and fixed with smooth pins that do not cross the physis at the time of initial treatment. Exposed physeal surfaces can be covered with local fat to help prevent union of the metaphysis to the epiphysis. An external fixator may be used if neurovascular structures are injured, but small pins should be used through the metaphysis and epiphysis, avoiding the physis.[158,166] Wound closure may be a problem in cases with significant soft tissue injury and exposed bone. Skin coverage with local tissue is ideal; but if local coverage is not possible, split-thickness skin grafting is generally the next choice. Free vascular flaps and rotational flaps may be required for adequate coverage, although the necessity for flap coverage has decreased with the widespread use of vacuum-assisted closure techniques. Klein et al.[103] reported two cases that had associated vascular injury precluding such flaps that were covered successfully with local advancement flaps made possible by multiple relaxing incisions. Mooney et al.[130] reported cross-extremity flaps for such cases. They found external fixation for linkage of the lower extremities during the procedure to be valuable. After fixation removal, range of motion (ROM) returned readily.

Vosburgh et al.[200] reported 33 patients with lawn mower injuries to the foot and ankle. They found that the most severe injuries were to the posterior plantar aspect of the foot and ankle. Of their patients, five required split-thickness skin grafts and one vascularized flap for soft tissue coverage. Two ultimately required Syme amputation. Four of the patients had complete disruption of the Achilles tendon. Three had no repair or reconstruction of the triceps surae tendon, and one had delayed reconstruction 3 months after injury. Vosburgh et al.[200] speculate that dense scarring in the posterior ankle results in a "physiologic tendon" and that extensive reconstructive surgery is not always necessary for satisfactory function. Boyer et al.[26] reported a patient with deltoid ligament loss because of a severe grinding injury that was reconstructed with a free plantaris tendon graft. Soft tissue coverage was achieved using a free muscle transfer. Rinker et al.[159] have also described the use of soft tissue transfer to assist pediatric patients with severe soft tissue loss.

The development of vacuum-assisted closure devices has been a dramatic improvement in the treatment of these injuries and may reduce the need for tissue transfers.[80] Referral to centers with experience with these treatment protocols may be necessary for these severe injuries. Our experience with the use of vacuum-assisted closure devices in high-energy trauma with severe soft tissue injury has shown very good results for limb salvage.

Distal Fibula Fractures

Fractures involving the fibular physis are most commonly Salter–Harris type I or II fractures that are caused by a supination–inversion injury. Isolated fibular fractures are usually minimally displaced and can be treated with immobilization in a brace or walking boot for 3 to 4 weeks. A randomized, controlled trial comparing removable brace versus casting in children with low-risk ankle fractures showed that removable ankle brace is a cost-effective choice that allows better recovery of physical function compared to cast immobilization, faster return to baseline activities, and patients prefer the brace over the cast.[9,25]

Significantly displaced fibular fractures often accompany Salter–Harris types III and IV tibial fractures and usually reduce when the tibial fracture is reduced. Internal fixation of the tibial fracture generally results in stability of the fibular fracture such that cast immobilization is sufficient. If the fibular fracture is unstable after reduction and fixation of the tibial fracture, fixation with a smooth intramedullary or obliquely inserted K-wire is recommended (see Fig. 30-31). In older adolescents in whom growth is not a consideration, an intramedullary rod, screw, plate and screw, or lag screws only may be used as in adults (Fig. 30-59). Paez et al. recently studied 83 adolescents with unstable distal fibula fractures treated with either plate and screw construct or lag screws only, all of whom achieved fracture union without loss of reduction and had similar Foot and Ankle Ability Measure (FAAM) outcome scores. The lag screw group had shorter operative time and less symptomatic hardware, so this may be a good alternative to the traditional plate and screw constructs.[142]

Avulsion fractures from the lateral malleolus are seen in children with inversion "sprain" type injuries to the ankle. These may fail to unite with cast immobilization. Patients with such nonunions may have pain without associated instability. In such patients, simple excision of the ununited fragment usually relieves their pain.[54,76] When the nonunions are associated with instability, reconstruction of one or more of the lateral ankle ligaments is needed (see next section).[28,29]

Avulsion fracture of the accessory ossification centers of the distal fibula (os subfibulare) is also common. These will frequently heal with immobilization but are prone to reinjury through the synchondrosis between the ossicle and the fibula. In the series report by Ogden and Lee,[141] 5 of 11 patients with injuries treated with casting had persistent symptoms and required excision.

Figure 30-59. **A:** Salter–Harris type II fracture of the distal fibula in a 15-year-old. **B:** Lateral view shows the fibular metaphyseal fragment (*arrow*). Considerable soft tissue swelling was noted in the medial aspect of the ankle.

(continues)

A

B

C

D

Figure 30-59. *(Continued)* **C:** Stress films showed complete disruption of the deltoid ligament. **D:** The fibular fracture was fixed with a cannulated screw; the deltoid ligament was not repaired.

Lateral Ankle Sprains

In 2020, Beck et al. performed a systematic review of low-energy lateral ankle injuries in children and adolescents.[9] In most of the studies included in the systematic review, lateral ankle ligamentous injuries outnumber Salter–Harris I distal fibula fractures. The sports associated with highest rate of lateral ankle sprains in the adolescent population are dance, basketball, football, volleyball, gymnastics, and soccer. Other risk factors for pediatric lateral ankle sprains were high BMI, increased height, history of a prior lateral ankle injury, and poor balance. Balance training can help prevent lateral ankle sprains, and wearing a rigid brace during athletic activity can prevent repeat injury after a previous sprain.[9]

In 1984, Vahvanen[197] published a prospective study of 559 children who presented with severe supination injuries or sprains of the ankle.[202] Forty patients, 28 boys and 12 girls, with an average age of 12 years (range 5–14 years) were surgically explored. The indications for surgery included swelling, pain over the anterior talofibular ligament, limp, clinical instability, and when visible, a displaced avulsion fracture. Such fractures were visible radiographically in only 8 patients but were found at surgery in 19. Thirty-six ankles were found to have injury of the anterior talofibular ligament at surgery. Only 16 of these had either a positive lateral or anterior drawer stress test. At follow-up, all patients were pain free and none complained of instability. Based on the incidence of residual disability after such injuries in adults reported in the literature (21%–58%), these authors suggested primary surgical repair may be indicated in some cases. In our clinical experience, acute surgical repair of ankle sprains is very rarely indicated in the skeletally immature.

In cases with residual laxity and associated symptoms, delayed surgical repair may be necessary in older patients. Busconi and Pappas[34] reported 60 skeletally immature children with chronic ankle pain and instability. Fifty of these children responded to rehabilitation, but 10 had persistent symptoms. Although three of these patients' initial radiographs were within normal limits, all patients with persistent symptoms eventually were found to have ununited osteochondral fractures of the fibular epiphysis. All 10 patients with persistent symptoms were treated with excision of the ununited osteochondral fracture and a Broström reconstruction of the lateral collateral ligament. All were able to return to activities and none reported further pain or instability.

Ankle Dislocations

Nusem et al.[138] reported a 12-year-old girl who was seen with a posterior dislocation of the ankle without associated fracture. This was a closed injury and resulted from forced inversion of a maximally plantarflexed foot. The dislocation was reduced under IV sedation and the ankle immobilized in a short-leg cast for 5 weeks. The patient was asymptomatic at follow-up 4 years after injury. The inversion stress views at that time revealed only a three-degree increase in laxity compared to the uninjured side. The anterior drawer sign was negative. There was no evidence of avascular necrosis of the talus on follow-up radiographs. Mazur et al.[127] have also reported ankle dislocation without a fracture in a pediatric patient.

Author's Preferred Treatment of Distal Tibial and Fibular Fractures (Algorithm 30-1)

Algorithm 30-1. Treatment of distal tibial and fibular fractures.

Salter–Harris Type I and II Fractures of the Distal Tibia

We prefer to treat nondisplaced Salter–Harris type I and II fractures initially with immobilization using a below-knee cast. Non–weight bearing is continued until 3 to 4 weeks after injury, when the cast is changed to a walking boot which is worn for an additional 2 to 3 weeks. Follow-up radiographs are obtained every 6 months for 1 to 2 years or until a Park–Harris growth arrest line parallel to the physis is visible and there is no evidence of physeal deformity.

For displaced fractures in children with at least 3 years of growth remaining, our objective is to obtain no more than 10 to 15 degrees of plantar tilt for posteriorly displaced fractures, 5 to 10 degrees of valgus for laterally displaced fractures, and 0 degrees of varus for medially displaced fractures (Fig. 30-60). Studies in the adult literature suggest that minor alteration in alignment of the ankle joint may have significant effect on tibiotalar contact pressures.[94,193,195] If there is a question about the ability to remodel the fracture, it is probably best to perform a reduction. For children with 2 years or less of growth

remaining, the amount of acceptable angulation is reduced to 5 degrees or less. We recognize that all of the recommendations about acceptable alignment are based on clinical experience and judgment, and none have been rigorously studied.

If resources are available, we may attempt reduction of markedly displaced fractures with the use of general anesthesia with good muscle relaxation and image intensifier control. The use of an ankle distractor can facilitate distraction across the fracture and may facilitate reduction (see Fig. 30-30). In children with mildly displaced fractures, especially if anesthesia is not going to be available for many hours, an attempt at gentle closed reduction under a hematoma block supplemented as needed by well-monitored IV sedation is a good option. Many ERs are well equipped and have adequate staff to perform appropriate and safe sedation for treatment of fractures and dislocation. This approach may allow for more timely treatment, especially if operating room access is limited. Once adequately reduced, the fractures are usually stable, and a short- or long-leg cast can be used for

A, B   C

Figure 30-60. A: Displaced pronation–eversion–external rotation fracture of the distal tibia in a 12-year-old boy was treated with closed reduction and cast immobilization. **B:** After cast removal, a 10-degree valgus tilt was present. **C:** At maturity, the deformity has completely resolved.

immobilization. Rarely, for markedly unstable fractures or severe soft tissue injuries that require multiple debridements, percutaneous screws are used when the Thurstan-Holland fragment is large enough to accept screw fixation. When the fragment is too small, smooth wire fixation across the physis is the only alternative. Repeated attempts at closed manipulation of these fractures may increase the risk of growth abnormality and should be avoided. In patients with fractures that are not seen until 7 to 10 days after injury, residual displacement is probably best accepted, unless significant deformity or angulation is present. If growth does not sufficiently correct malunion, corrective osteotomy can be performed later.

Open reduction of these fractures is occasionally indicated. The exception usually has been pronation–eversion–external rotation fractures with interposed soft tissue, which may include lateral and posterior displacement. For cases that have undergone an attempt at closed reduction, close inspection of the medial physis should be performed with image intensification. In some cases, the medial physeal space will appear abnormally widened, which may suggest incarceration of a large flap of periosteum in the physis. If alignment is satisfactory, these can be treated nonoperatively. For malaligned fractures, a small anteromedial incision is made and any interposed soft tissues, such as periosteum or tendons, are extracted. Even though reduction is usually stable, we generally use internal fixation. Fixation options include screw fixation through both the metaphyseal and epiphyseal fragments, avoiding fixation across the physis if possible (Fig. 30-61). Percutaneous smooth pins can also be placed from the medial malleolus, oriented proximally to engage the metaphysis (Fig. 30-62; see Fig. 30-29).

A, B   C, D

Figure 30-61. Salter–Harris type II distal tibial fracture with fibular fracture. **A:** Lateral view. **B:** Anteroposterior view. **C, D:** After percutaneous placement of tibial screws and plating of fibular fracture.

A, B   **C, D**

Figure 30-62. Salter–Harris type II distal tibial fracture with fibular fracture. **A:** Anteroposterior view. **B:** Lateral view. **C, D:** Percutaneous placement of K-wires.

Salter–Harris Types III and IV Fractures of the Distal Tibia

Treatment of nondisplaced Salter–Harris type III and IV fractures is the same as for nondisplaced type I and II fractures with three modifications. First, after casting, the alignment is confirmed with a CT scan and/or radiographs. Second, these patients are examined more frequently (once a week) for the first 2 to 3 weeks after cast application to ensure that the fragments do not become displaced. Third, these patients are examined every 6 to 12 months after cast removal for 24 to 36 months to detect any growth abnormality.

Fractures with 2 mm or more of displacement after the best possible closed reduction may be treated with open reduction and internal fixation with anatomical alignment of the physis and intra-articular fracture fragments.

For minimally displaced fractures, closed reduction is attempted in the ER or the operating room, depending on local resources and practices. Reduction may be attempted by applying longitudinal traction to the foot, followed by eversion of the foot and direct digital pressure over the medial malleolus. If image intensification confirms anatomical reduction, but the fracture is unstable, the fracture may be fixed with two percutaneous smooth wires placed in the epiphysis parallel to the physis. Reduction is confirmed by a short, continuous fluoroscopic examination. Percutaneous clamp placement may also facilitate reduction in some of these cases. Cannulated screws can be inserted if the epiphysis is large enough. For fractures that are seen more than 7 to 14 days after injury, we may accept up to 2 mm of displacement without attempting closed or open reduction. Patients whose fractures are fixed with pins and/or screws may be immobilized in below-knee casts.

In cases where arthroscopic assistance is used, the visualization of the ankle joint can also assist with the evaluation of reduction. In some cases, the fractures may still have a small gap present with the articular surface, but the presence of step-off or intra-articular incongruity can be clearly evaluated with the scope visualization of the articular surface. It has been our experience that the C-arm views may show excellent reduction of the subchondral bone of the articular surface, and the arthroscopic or open views may show that the cartilage surfaces are not as well reduced as one would expect based on these radiographic images. Arthrogram is helpful if open or arthroscopic visualization is not done.

Fractures with more than 2 mm of displacement or step-off should be reduced, regardless of whether the fracture is acute or not. Closed reduction can be attempted, but these fractures typically require open or arthroscopic-assisted reduction. Occasionally, primary debridement of callus and soft tissue back to normal-appearing physis and fat grafting has been successful for fractures that are more than 2 weeks old.

For fractures stabilized with internal fixation, below-knee casts may be used.

Salter–Harris Type V Fractures of the Distal Tibia

These injuries are quite rare. The risk of physeal arrest is thought to be quite high for this injury pattern, because of direct damage of the germinal layer of the physis.[94] A pure Salter–Harris V fracture is not identified until months after the injury.

The prognosis for this injury is poor, and treatment is usually focused on treating the complications of angular deformity and/or physeal arrest (see Fig. 30-71, later).[94]

Juvenile Tillaux Fractures

For nondisplaced fractures and fractures displaced less than 2 mm, we prefer immobilization in an above-knee cast with the knee flexed 30 degrees and the foot neutral or internally rotated. If the position appears acceptable on plain films, CT scanning in the transverse plane with coronal and sagittal reconstructions may be used to confirm acceptable reduction. For fractures with more than 2 mm of initial displacement, manipulation may be attempted by internal rotation of the foot and application of direct pressure over the anterolateral joint line. If reduction is not obtained with this maneuver, reduction can be attempted by dorsiflexing the pronated foot and then internally rotating the foot.[123] If successful reduction is obtained, percutaneous fixation (screws or pins) can be placed with C-arm guidance. Percutaneous clamps can be used to obtain and hold reduction during screw placement. If there are questions about the adequacy of reduction, this can be confirmed by use of an arthrotomy or ankle arthroscope.

In cases in which the reduction is not ideal, there are several options. Schlesinger and Wedge[172] have described a technique using percutaneous manipulation of a Tillaux fragment with a Steinmann pin.[94] Small K-wires or the threaded tip wires from a cannulated screw set can be inserted into the Tillaux fragment under fluoroscopic control, to act as a "joystick" to reduce the fracture (Fig. 30-63). Ideally, one or both of these pins can then be passed across the fracture site after reduction has been obtained if the guidewire is carefully placed initially, and the cannulated screw can then be placed over the pins (Figs. 30-64 and 30-65). As there is no meaningful growth present in most patients who get Tillaux fractures, crossing the growth plate with a screw is acceptable, and may help in fracture reduction (see Fig. 30-33).

If reduction is not successful, open reduction is performed. The patient is placed in a supine position, and a vertical incision is placed over the fracture. A small incision is made, perhaps 2 to 3 cm, to allow for visualization. The fracture plane is identified, and direct pressure or clamps can be applied to maintain the reduction. A guidewire from the cannulated screw system (a 4-mm cannulated system usually works well in this age group) is placed, followed by placement of the screw.

A short-leg, non–weight-bearing cast or boot is worn for 3 weeks, followed by a weight-bearing cast or walking boot for another 3 weeks.

Triplane Fractures

For nondisplaced or minimally displaced (<2 mm) fractures, we prefer immobilization in a long-leg cast with the knee flexed 30 to 40 degrees. The position of the foot is determined by whether the fracture is lateral (internal rotation) or medial (eversion). A CT scan may be obtained after reduction and casting to document adequate reduction. Plain films or CT scans are obtained approximately 7 days after cast application to verify that displacement has not recurred. At 3 to 4 weeks, the cast is changed to a below-knee walking cast or walking boot, which is worn for another 3 to 4 weeks.

The ability to reduce fractures in the ER with appropriate conscious sedation varies among institutions. For institutions that have such capabilities, fracture reduction can be attempted in the ER. For fractures with more than 2 mm of displacement, an attempt at closed reduction with sedation in the emergency department is warranted. An above-knee cast is applied. If plain radiographs show satisfactory reduction, a CT scan is obtained. If reduction is acceptable, treatment is the same as for nondisplaced fractures.

If the reduction is unacceptable, closed reduction is attempted in the operating room with the use of general anesthesia. If fluoroscopy shows an acceptable reduction, percutaneous screws are inserted, avoiding the physis, and a short-leg cast is applied. If closed reduction is unacceptable, open reduction or miniopen reduction with the use of percutaneous clamps is performed. Preoperative CT scanning may be helpful for evaluating the position of the fracture fragments in the AP and lateral planes and for determining the appropriate skin incisions, percutaneous clamp placements, and screw length, location, and trajectory.

Figure 30-63. Technique for reduction of a Salter–Harris type IV fracture of the distal tibia.

Figure 30-64. Advancement of pin after reduction of juvenile Tillaux fracture.

Figure 30-65. Percutaneous insertion of 4-mm cannulated screw over pin that has been advanced into the medial distal tibia after reduction of the juvenile Tillaux fracture fragment.

Fractures Involving the Distal Fibula

It is at times difficult to differentiate between a nondisplaced Salter fracture of the distal fibula and a sprain of the talofibular ligaments, but a series of recent studies summarized in a systematic review shows evidence that all low-risk ankle injuries (whether they are a nondisplaced distal fibula fracture or a sprain) can be treated similarly with good outcomes).[9] A study of children with ankle injuries evaluated with MRI suggests the incidence of a Salter fracture of the distal fibula is 3%.[24] A careful physical examination can help differentiate between a fracture and a sprain. A sprain should have maximal tenderness over the ligaments, anterior to the distal fibula, while a fracture should have maximal tenderness on the bone, which is often best palpated from a posterior approach to avoid overlap with the anterior ligament pain and help differentiate the two. However, a few days after the injury, generalized swelling and pain can make localization more challenging. When an examination is carried out by an orthopaedic surgeon who feels there is bony tenderness, it has been shown that almost 20% of the time, a physeal fracture is present as evidenced by periosteal new bone formation weeks later.[169] Putting the patient in a functional ankle splint or cast boot will treat either a physeal fracture or sprain. Although follow-up x-rays and examination 10 to 14 days after injury might help to differentiate the two, follow-up x-rays are likely not necessary when symptoms improve in the expected time course. An MRI or ultrasound at the time of injury could also help differentiate a physeal fracture from a sprain, but this is not clinically necessary as both injury types are likely a spectrum of the same inversion injury and can be treated similarly.

We usually treat radiologically confirmed nondisplaced fibular physeal fractures with immobilization in a below-knee walking boot for 3 to 4 weeks. Studies have found use of a removable ankle brace to be as effective and to be preferable from a patient satisfaction and economic standpoint when compared to fiberglass posterior splints.[7,24,25] Closed reduction of displaced Salter–Harris types I and II fibular fractures is usually successful. In cases where reduction is unsuccessful, one may accept up to 50% displacement without problems at long-term follow-up, especially in those with 3 to 4 years of growth remaining. Acceptance of this displacement may be more reasonable in young patients with significant remodeling potential, although in older patients, displaced fractures may have more effect on ankle function, and more anatomic reduction may be advantageous. Dias and Giegerich,[55] however, reported a patient with a symptomatic spike that required excision after incomplete reduction.

Lateral Ankle Sprains and Lateral Ligament Avulsion Injuries

Diagnosis of ankle sprain in younger patients used to be thought of as rare, but in most of the recent studies of low-energy lateral ankle injuries in pediatric and adolescent patients, lateral ankle ligamentous injuries significantly outnumber Salter–Harris I distal fibula fractures.[9] If the pain can be localized to the ligaments, and there is no pain over the distal fibular physis, then ankle sprain is the likely diagnosis. The author prefer functional treatment for ankle sprains, allowing weight bearing as tolerated in a supportive device such as a walking boot or lace-up ankle brace until the patient is pain free (typically 3 weeks), and then progressive return to activities. Very severe ankle sprains are offered casting for 1 week which seems to significantly relieve pain. Elevation is also very important for pain relief over the first few days. Surgical treatment is reserved for those patients who develop late symptoms. Chronic pain and instability can occur in young patients, especially adolescents. In these cases, a Broström-type reconstruction[29] may be appropriate, although Letts et al.[113] have described nonanatomic reconstruction in younger patients such as Evans, Watson–Jones, Chrisman and Snook procedures.

Avulsion fractures can be identified that originate from the distal fibula, and special radiographic views may facilitate diagnosis (Fig. 30-66).[75] These avulsion-type injuries can lead to symptoms, and a high index of suspicion is important in younger patients. Haraguchi et al.[75] evaluated a series of severe ankle sprains and found that 26% had evidence of distal fibular avulsion injury. Children and adults over 40 years of age had the highest incidence of this injury. Patients were treated with weight-bearing casts for 3 to 4 weeks. Nonoperative treatment yielded satisfactory results in this series.

Postoperative Care and Rehabilitation

Usually a below-knee cast is worn during the last 2 to 3 weeks of immobilization, and weight bearing to tolerance is allowed during this time. After immobilization is discontinued, ankle range-of-motion exercises and strengthening exercises are begun. Protective splinting or bracing is usually not required after cast removal. Running is restricted until the patient demonstrates an essentially full, painless range of ankle and foot motion and can walk without a limp. Running progresses from jogging to more strenuous running and jumping as soreness and endurance dictate. For athletes, unrestricted running and jumping ability should be achieved before returning to sports. Protective measures such as taping or functional bracing may be beneficial for returning to sports.

Younger patients with physeal ankle fractures recover quickly and require little or no formal physical therapy. For this reason, and because of compliance considerations, fractures treated with internal fixation are usually protected with below-knee casting instead of starting an early range-of-motion program in a removable splint. In older patients who may have a higher risk of arthrofibrosis, we may start early motion in a removable boot and have them start a formal supervised physical therapy program.

Potential Pitfalls and Preventive Measures

Ankle Fractures:
SURGICAL PITFALLS AND PREVENTIONS

Pitfall	Prevention
Arthrofibrosis	• Prevention—early ROM. Fractures heal more rapidly in young patients, and early ROM and weight bearing is usually possible
Nonunion, malunion	• This is very rare in younger patients, and anatomic reduction will reduce this risk, particularly in intra-articular fractures
Physeal arrest	• This complication is rarely related to surgical technique—it is usually a direct complication from the severe trauma to the physis which occurs at the time of the fracture. Counsel patients and families about this ahead of time and let them know that close follow-up and even surgery may be necessary to address growth plate arrests
Weakness, delayed recovery	• In more severe injuries, physical therapy may be a valuable tool to help with weakness and delayed recovery. Many of these patients recover well without formal physical therapy programs, especially low-energy, minimally displaced injuries

Figure 30-66. Fibula avulsion fracture in a 7-year-old. (Used with permission of the Children's Orthopaedic Center, Los Angeles.)

MANAGEMENT OF EXPECTED ADVERSE OUTCOMES AND UNEXPECTED COMPLICATIONS OF DISTAL TIBIAL AND FIBULAR FRACTURES

Ankle Fractures:
ADVERSE OUTCOMES AND COMPLICATIONS

• Delayed union and nonunion
• Deformity secondary to malunion
• Physeal arrest or growth disturbance
• Medial malleolus overgrowth
• Arthritis
• Chondrolysis
• Osteonecrosis of the distal tibial epiphysis
• Compartment syndrome
• Osteochondral defects
• Synostosis
• Complex regional pain syndrome (CRPS)
• Osteopenia

DELAYED UNION AND NONUNION

Delayed union and nonunion are extremely rare after distal tibial physeal fractures (Fig. 30-67). Dias and Giegerich[55] reported one patient with a delayed union and one patient with a previous physeal bar excision who had a nonunion that healed after open reduction, internal fixation, and bone grafting. Siffert and Arkin[181] reported nonunion in a patient with avascular necrosis of the distal tibial epiphysis. We have seen two younger patients with Salter–Harris type III fractures that appeared to be progressing to nonunion. Because neither patient had any complaints of pain nor any evidence of progressive displacement of

Figure 30-67. Complex nonunion of a Salter–Harris type III fracture of the medial malleolus in an 8-year-old boy. Note that the distal tibial epiphysis is in valgus, whereas the talus is in varus. (Courtesy of Brent Broztman, MD.)

the fracture and stress views showed no instability, no treatment was undertaken. Both fractures eventually united. We have seen one patient with a nonunion after open reduction and internal fixation in whom pin fixation and cast immobilization were discontinued prematurely. The fracture healed after repeat open reduction and internal fixation.

Nonunion of a fracture of the fibular epiphysis has been reported by Mirmiran and Schuberth.[129] This was treated successfully with open reduction and internal fixation.

DEFORMITY SECONDARY TO MALUNION

Malunion usually occurs after triplane fractures that are either incompletely reduced or are initially immobilized in below-knee casts. It has also been reported after Salter–Harris type I and II injuries. Phan et al.[152] reported an increase in the outward foot progression angle in children following transitional fractures, but it is not known if perhaps an outwardly rotated foot predisposes one to these fractures. Derotational osteotomy may be performed for extra-articular fractures if discomfort and stiffness occur. Guille et al.[73] reported a rotational malunion of lateral malleolar fracture that led to a stress fracture of the distal fibula that went on to delayed union. Their patient improved after correction of the malrotated distal fibula and bone grafting of the delayed union site.

Takakura et al.[191] described successful open wedge osteotomy for varus deformity in nine patients. Scheffer and Peterson[170] recommend opening wedge osteotomy when the angular deformity is 25 degrees or less and the limb length discrepancy is or will be 25 mm or less at maturity. Preoperative planning should include templating the various types of osteotomies to determine which technique will maintain the proper mechanical alignment of the tibia and ankle joint and will not make the malleoli unduly prominent. Osteotomy is rarely recommended for malunion of intra-articular fractures because it is challenging to correct the joint incongruity that results from malunion (Fig. 30-68).

The use of the three-dimensional frames continues to evolve. Its use for correction of complex deformities can allow for multiplanar corrections, including rotation, length, and angular deformity.[65,180] Another option to treat secondary deformity is the use of "guided growth," the use of medial malleolar screws or medial stapling devices.[189]

A, B   C

Figure 30-68. A: This apparently nondisplaced medial malleolar fracture in an 11-year-old boy was treated with immobilization in a long-leg cast. **B:** Fourteen months after injury, there is a clear medial osseous bridge and asymmetric growth of the Park–Harris growth arrest lines (*black arrows*). Note the early inhibition of growth on the subchondral surface of the fracture (*open arrow*). **C:** Five years after injury, the varus deformity has increased significantly and fibular overgrowth is apparent.

(continues)

D   E

Figure 30-68. *(Continued)* **D:** The deformity was treated with a medial opening-wedge osteotomy of the tibia, an osteotomy of the fibula, and epiphysiodesis of the most lateral portion of the tibial physis and fibula. **E:** Three months after surgery, the osteotomies are healed and the varus deformity is corrected; the joint surface remains irregular. (Courtesy of Earl A. Stanley Jr, MD.)

PHYSEAL ARREST OR GROWTH DISTURBANCE

Deformity caused by growth arrest usually occurs after Salter–Harris types III and IV fractures in which a physeal bar develops at the fracture site, leading to varus deformity that progresses with continued growth. Spiegel et al.[187] reported growth problems in 9 of 66 patients with Salter–Harris type II fractures.

Earlier reports[36,48,69] attributed the development of physeal bars to crushing of the physis at the time of injury, but more recent reports[86,104] discount this explanation and claim that with anatomical reduction (open reduction and internal fixation if needed), the incidence of physeal bar formation can be decreased. The validity of this claim is difficult to determine from published reports. One problem is the small numbers of patients in all series, and the even smaller numbers within each group in each series. Another problem is the age of the patients in operative and nonoperative groups in the various series; for example, many children reported to do well with a particular treatment method and have so little growth remaining that treatment may have had little or no effect on growth.

A study by Rohmiller et al.[162] analyzed the outcome of 91 Salter–Harris I and II fractures of the distal tibia. They identified premature physeal closure in 40%. This series identified a trend toward increased premature physeal closure in fractures that had worse displacement after reduction. They recommended operative reduction to restore anatomic alignment, to reduce the risk of premature physeal closure.

Kling et al.[104] reported physeal bars in two of five patients treated nonoperatively and in none of three patients treated operatively in children 10 years of age and younger. In another series of 65 physeal ankle fractures, Kling[104] concluded that the frequency of growth-related deformities could be reduced by open reduction and internal fixation of Salter–Harris III and IV fractures.

However, the conclusion of Cass and Peterson,[37] Ogden,[140] and others is that growth problems after these injuries may not always be prevented by open reduction and internal fixation. Open reduction of displaced Salter–Harris type III and IV ankle fractures would seem advisable to restore joint congruity, regardless of whether growth potential can be preserved.

Harris growth lines have been reported to be reliable predictors of growth abnormality.[81] The use of MRI and/or CT scan may assist with evaluation of physeal bars. Spontaneous resolution of physeal bars has been reported[21,40] but is rare. Excision of small bony bars (~25%–40% of the surface area of the affected physis) in a patient who is expected to have greater than 2 years of growth remaining can help prevent an angular or length deformity. The location of the bar determines the best surgical technique to use; those on the periphery can usually be approached by a direct open physeal bar resection with interposition and a central bar can be done in a hybrid room or with interventional radiology assistance to perform CT-guided physeal bar resection with interposition (Fig. 30-69).[53] Large bars may require osteotomy.

Kårrholm et al.[92] reported on eight children with growth arrest of the distal tibial and/or fibular physis. Distal fibular physeal arrest could lead to either progressive ankle valgus (Fig. 30-70; see Fig. 30-44) or an otherwise normal ankle.

They found that continued fibular growth with complete arrest of tibial growth was usually compensated by proximal migration of the fibula so that varus deformity did not occur.

Because the amount of growth remaining in the distal tibial physis is small (approximately 0.25 in per year) in most older patients with these injuries, the amount of leg-length discrepancy resulting from complete growth arrest tends to be relatively small. Treatment may be required if the anticipated discrepancy is projected to be clinically significant.

A   **B**

Figure 30-69. A: One year after open reduction and internal fixation of a Salter–Harris type III fracture of the distal tibia in a 7-year-old boy, varus deformity has been caused by a physeal bar. **B:** Two years after excision of the physeal bar and insertion of cranioplast, satisfactory growth has resumed and the deformity has resolved.

Imaging techniques to identify physeal arrest and bars include radiographs, CT, and MRI. Radiographs can identify interrupted or nonparallel Park–Harris growth stimulation lines. CT scans can be useful for clear delineation of the bony anatomy, especially in cases in which surgical intervention is necessary. Studies have also used MRI scans to quantify the percentage of a physis affected by a bony bar.[67,116,168] Although the resolution capability is more limited, the avoidance of ionizing radiation is a theoretical advantage of MRI scans over CT scans, in some areas of the body, but a limited cut CT scan of a distal tibia should not have a dangerous dose of radiation.

Figure 30-70. Valgus deformity of the ankle, lateral displacement of the talus with widening of the joint medially, and severe shortening of the fibula after early physeal arrest in a child who sustained an ankle injury at 6 years of age. (Courtesy of James Roach, MD.)

Physeal injuries of the distal tibia should be followed with clinical examination and radiographs every 4 to 6 months until skeletal maturity or at least 12 months postinjury with clear evidence of symmetric physeal growth by parallel Park–Harris line (Fig. 30-71).[107] A standing bilateral hip-to-ankle radiograph is also useful to compare leg lengths and comparative angles of both lower extremities (ankle varus or valgus). If there is an asymmetric Park–Harris line seen at any point during these physeal growth checks, an MRI can be performed, specifically a fat-suppressed three-dimensional spoiled gradient echo-weight sequence to quantify what percentage of the physis is affected by the physeal bar (Fig. 30-72).[60] Animal studies have shown that physeal bars greater than 7% of the cross-sectional area of the physis can be expected to result in angular or length deformity of a bone with further growth.[121]

It is okay to continue serial exams and radiographs every 4 to 6 months without intervening surgically if the physeal bar is less than 7% to 10% of cross-sectional area of the physis (regardless of growth remaining) or if the patient has less than 2 years of growth remaining (and patient has a >7%–10% physeal bar).

Surgical intervention should include osteotomy for any angular deformity correction that occurs due to a physeal bar. If the physeal bar is 25% to 40% surface area of physis (sometimes up to 50% surface area) and the patient has more than 2 years of growth remaining, physeal bar resection is the intervention of choice. Central bars and peripheral bars can be resected using different methods and interposition of fat or polymethylmethacrylate to prevent reformation of a bony bar should also be done. The author prefers to get a preoperative planning CT.

If the physeal bar affects over 50% surface area of the physis and the patient has less than 2 years of growth remaining, ipsilateral completion epiphysiodesis can be performed. This can also be done if length deformity alone without angular

Figure 30-71. Diagnosing and treating clinically significant physeal bar arrest or disturbance.

deformity will be easier to treat (and subsequent contralateral epiphysiodesis or ipsilateral lengthening can be done concurrently depending on the expected leg length difference).

MEDIAL MALLEOLUS OVERGROWTH

Overgrowth of the medial malleolus has been reported after fractures of the distal tibia metaphysis and epiphysis. A series of 83 patients with fractures in this region demonstrated 2 patients with medial malleolus overgrowth. In both cases, there was no evidence of functional impairment.[135]

ARTHRITIS

Epiphyseal ankle fractures that do not extend into the joint have a low risk of posttraumatic arthritis, but injuries that extend into

the joint may produce this complication. Caterini et al.[39] found that 8 of 68 (12%) patients had pain and stiffness that began from 5 to 8 years after skeletal maturity. Ertl et al.[63] found that at 36 months to 13 years after injury, only 8 of 15 patients evaluated were asymptomatic. Lurie et al. retrospectively reviewed 34 patients with triplane fractures and 23 with Tillaux fractures (average 4.5-year follow-up). The factors that predicted negative functional outcome after these fractures were larger gap after closed reduction, nonoperative treatment, and complications of the fracture or treatment.[118]

Ramsey and Hamilton[156] demonstrated in a cadaver study that 1 mm of lateral talar displacement decreases tibiotalar contact area by 42%, which greatly increases the stress on this weight-bearing joint. More recently, Michelson et al.[128] reported that a cadaver study using unconstrained specimens suggested

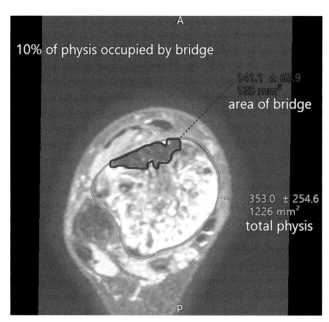

Figure 30-72. MRI of a distal tibial physis that has a small physeal bar (quantified as 10% of the surface area of the physis) that resulted from a nonoperatively treated, initially minimally displaced triplane fracture in a 13-year-old girl.

that some lateral talar displacement occurs with normal weight bearing. Because of their findings, they questioned the current criterion of 2 mm of displacement for unstable ankle fractures. However, the results of Ramsey and Hamilton's study correlate well with other studies that have shown increased symptoms in patients in whom more than 2 mm of displacement was accepted.[39,110]

Implant removal after fracture surgery remains controversial, and the indications for removal are not well defined in the literature.[33] Charlton et al.[42] have demonstrated that the periepiphyseal or subchondral screws may alter the joint contact pressures about the ankle. After removal of the screws from the subchondral bone, the contact pressure is normalized. For hardware in the subchondral bone, Charlton's study suggests that implant removal of transepiphyseal screws may be appropriate, but since this was a cadaver study, there is not clinical data to support or refute this.

CHONDROLYSIS

Chondrolysis is a rare complication of adolescent ankle fractures.[16,167] Treatment options include therapy, nonsteroidal anti-inflammatories, and activity modification. Clinical studies have evaluated the effects of joint distraction for posttraumatic chondrolysis, although experience with this technique in young patients is very limited.[167]

COMPARTMENT SYNDROME

This complication is discussed in detail in Chapter 6. Fractures of the distal tibia and ankle joint are infrequently associated with compartment syndromes.[45,131] A similar clinical picture to compartment syndrome can present with severe pain, decreased

sensation in the first web space, and weakness of extensor hallucis longus (EHL) and extensor digitorum longus (EDL). These symptoms, especially in the setting of an unreduced triplane fracture or Salter–Harris II distal tibia fracture with anterior metaphyseal fragment, can represent extensor retinaculum syndrome and treatment with immediate reduction of the fracture and release of the superior retinaculum.[53,131,132]

OSTEOCHONDRAL DEFECTS

Osteochondral injuries, primarily of the talus, are increasingly recognized after ankle injury in adults and the skeletally immature.[122,139,171] MRI may play a role in identification of treatment of these injuries.[12]

SYNOSTOSIS

Posttraumatic tibiofibular synostosis is a rare complication of fractures in this region. This can lead to growth disturbance, including angular deformity and lower extremity length discrepancy.[134,203] Synostosis in this area alters the normal pattern of movement between the tibia and fibula and has been associated with pain in some patients. In a small clinical series, Frick et al.[66] demonstrated symptoms of pain, prominence of the fibula, and ankle deformity in five of eight patients with this synostosis. In this series, the normal growth pattern of distal migration of the fibula was altered, resulting in decreased distances between the proximal physes of the tibia and fibula, and proximal positioning of the distal fibula with respect to the distal tibia. Munjal et al.[134] demonstrated successful synostosis excision in a 7-year-old patient, which led to normalization of the ankle joint at 16 months after surgery.

COMPLEX REGIONAL PAIN SYNDROME

CRPS occasionally develops after ankle injuries and is treated initially with an intensive formal physical therapy regimen that encourages desensitization of the painful area, ROM and weight bearing.[94] For patients who do not respond quickly to such a program, multimodal treatment with pain specialist, psychologist, and physical therapist in association with regional anesthesia interventions may be considered. Girls are more commonly affected by CRPS than boys (84%); the average age of onset of CRPS symptoms is 12.5 years, and the signs/symptoms in addition to pain out of proportion to injury are edema, sensory, vasomotor, sweating, motor, or temperature changes in a non-nerve distribution area.[52]

SUMMARY, CONTROVERSIES, AND FUTURE DIRECTIONS RELATED TO ANKLE FRACTURES

Many questions remain unanswered about the optimal treatment of ankle fractures in skeletally immature patients and will have to be answered with clinical trials. The relationship between physeal displacement and the development of subsequent physeal arrest is still unclear. Interposition of periosteum in the fracture may play a role in physeal arrest, although this has not been clarified in animal models or clinical trials. Studies in the adult literature have suggested that minimally angular deformities about the distal tibia can have pronounced effects on the tibiotalar contact pressures.[94,193,195] The limits of fracture remodeling and the magnitude of acceptable deformity in growing children are still not well defined in the literature.

Advanced imaging techniques have improved our understanding of these fractures and may play an increasing role in the use of computer-aided reduction techniques and other forms of minimally invasive surgery. CT scanning requires ionizing radiation but provides high-resolution model reconstruction. In addition, studies using advanced imaging have cast doubt on the commonly accepted principle that the physis is always weaker than ankle ligaments. It appears that ankle sprain injuries are more common than previously believed and are often misdiagnosed as Salter I fractures of the distal fibula.

The use of cultured chondrocytes and gene therapy may eventually play a role in the treatment of these fractures, either to prevent or treat a physeal arrest.[100] The surgical treatment of physeal bars to restore normal growth remains unsuccessful in a substantial percentage of cases, and further understanding of the basic mechanisms controlling physeal growth may help us develop more successful strategies.

ACKNOWLEDGMENTS

The author and editors wish to acknowledge Drs. Kevin G. Shea and Steven L. Frick for their past contributions to this chapter.

Annotated References

Reference	Annotation
Boutis K, Komar L, Jaramillo D, et al. Sensitivity of a clinical examination to predict need for radiography in children with ankle injuries: a prospective study. *Lancet*. 2001;358(9299):2118–2121.	None of the 381 children with low-risk ankle examinations after acute injury (fibula-only signs) had a high-risk fracture. Therefore, radiographs could be eliminated in 62.8% of children with low-risk examinations (even further reduction of radiographs/radiation exposure than Ottawa Ankle Rules). Level of evidence: I
Boutis K, Willan AR, Babyn P, et al. A randomized, controlled trial of a removable brace versus casting in children with low-risk ankle fractures. *Pediatrics*. 2007;119(6):e1256–e1263.	A randomized, controlled trial comparing removable brace versus casting in children with low-risk ankle fractures showed that removable ankle brace is a cost-effective choice that allows better recovery of physical function compared to cast immobilization, faster return to baseline activities, and patients prefer the brace over the cast. Level of evidence: I
Ertl JP, Barrack RL, Alexander AH, VanBuecken K. Triplane fracture of the distal tibial epiphysis. Long-term follow-up. *J Bone Joint Surg Am*. 1988;70:967–976.	Twenty-three patients with triplane fracture were followed for a minimum of 18 months. Residual displacement of the fracture of more than 2 mm predicted a suboptimal result; however, some patients with anatomic reduction had early degenerative arthritis and ankle symptoms. CT was helpful in delineating the fracture pattern and degree of displacement. Level of evidence: IV
Khansa I, Pearson GD, Bjorklund K, et al. Pediatric lawnmower injuries: a 25-year review. *JPRAS Open*. 2021;29:135–143.	Reviewed 142 children injured by lawn mowers. The average age at the time of injury was 7.5 years, 38% required amputation. Riding mowers resulted in more operative procedures, longer length of stay, and more soft tissue reconstructive procedures. Incidence of lawn mower injuries to children has not decreased despite recommendations for lawn mower safety. Level of evidence: IV
Kling TF Jr, Bright RW, Hensinger RN. Distal tibial physeal fractures in children that may require open reduction. *J Bone Joint Surg Am*. 1984; 66:647–657.	Case series demonstrating that growth disturbances are common following Salter–Harris type III and type IV fractures of the distal tibia, and that anatomic reduction of the physis decreases the incidence of growth disturbance. Level of evidence: III
Lurie B, Van Rysselberghe N, Pennock AT, Upasani VV. Functional outcomes of Tillaux and triplane fractures with 2 to 5 millimeters of intra-articular gap. *J Bone Joint Surg Am*. 2020;102(8):679–686.	Retrospective review of 34 patients with triplane fractures and 23 with Tillaux fractures (average 4.5-year follow-up). Factors that predicted negative functional outcome were larger gap after closed reduction, nonoperative treatment, and complications of the fracture or treatment. Level of evidence: III

Annotated References

Reference	Annotation
Lurie BM, Paez CJ, Howitt SR, Pennock AT. Suture-button versus screw fixation in adolescent syndesmotic injuries: functional outcomes and maintenance of reduction. *J Pediatr Orthop*. 2021;41(6):e427–e432.	A study of 77 adolescents with syndesmotic injuries, treatment with screws or suture buttons both maintained syndesmotic reduction, had functional outcomes that were equivalent at mean follow-up of 4 years, and suture button fixation had lower rates of implant removal. Level of evidence: III
Mubarak SJ. Extensor retinaculum syndrome of the ankle after injury to the distal tibial physis. *J Bone Joint Surg Br*. 2002;84:11–14.	Six patients presented after distal tibial physeal injury with severe pain and swelling, anesthesia in the web space of the great toe, and weakness of the toe extensors. Pain with passive flexion was present. Compartment syndrome was diagnosed and can exist beneath the superior extensor retinaculum of the ankle and is treated by release of the superior extensor retinaculum with fracture fixation. Level of evidence: IV
Ogden JA, Lee J. Accessory ossification patterns and injuries of the malleoli. *J Pediatr Orthop*. 1990;10:306–316.	This article reviews the normal growth and development of the ossification centers of the distal tibia and distal fibula. Differentiation between normal accessory ossification centers and avulsion fractures can be difficult. Radiographic and histologic samples are presented. Level of evidence: IV
Phieffer LS, Meyer RA Jr, Gruber HE, et al. Effect of interposed periosteum in an animal physeal fracture model. *Clin Orthop Relat Res*. 2000;15–25.	This animal model studies the effect of interposed periosteum on physeal fracture healing. Interposition of periosteum in a physeal fracture model resulted in small histologic bar formation and a small increase in leg-length discrepancy compared to fracture alone.
Spiegel PG, Cooperman DR, Laros GS. Epiphyseal fractures of the distal ends of the tibia and fibula: A retrospective study of two hundred and thirty-seven cases in children. *J Bone Joint Surg Am*. 1978;60:1046–1050.	Classic article evaluating 237 fractures of the distal end of the tibia and or fibula. Thirty-two percent complication rate, highest in patients with Salter–Harris type III and IV tibial fractures with more than 2 mm of displacement. Complications correlated with type of fracture, severity of displacement/comminution, and adequacy of reduction. Level of evidence: IV
Sheffer BW, Villarreal ED, Ochsner MG III, et al. Concurrent ipsilateral tibial shaft and distal tibial fractures in pediatric patients: risk factors, frequency, and risk of missed diagnosis. *J Pediatr Orthop*. 2020;40(1):e1–e5.	Study of 517 tibia shaft fractures where 4.3% had ipsilateral distal tibia fractures. Half of those distal tibia fractures were triplanes. Thirty-six percent of the distal tibia fractures were not diagnosed until chart review for the study. Level of evidence: III

REFERENCES

1. Alioto RJ, Furia JP, Marquardt JD. Hematoma block for ankle fractures: a safe and efficacious technique for manipulations. *J Orthop Trauma*. 1995;9(2):113–116.
2. Alonso JE, Sanchez FL. Lawn mower injuries in children: a preventable impairment. *J Pediatr Orthop*. 1995;15:83–89.
3. Ashhurst APC, Bromer RS. Classification and mechanism of fractures of the leg bones involving the ankle. *Arch Surg*. 1992;4:51–129.
4. Ashley P, Gilbert SR. Obesity in pediatric trauma. *Orthop Clin North Am*. 2018;49(3):335–343.
5. Assal M, Ray A, Stern R. The extensile approach for the operative treatment of high-energy pilon fractures: surgical technique and soft-tissue healing. *J Orthop Trauma*. 2007;21:198–206.
6. Barmada A, Gaynor T, Mubarak SJ. Premature physeal closure following distal tibia physeal fractures: a new radiographic predictor. *J Pediatr Orthop*. 2003;23:733–739.
7. Barnett PLJ, Lee MH, Oh L, et al. Functional outcome after air-stirrup ankle brace or fiberglass backslab for pediatric low-risk ankle fractures: a randomized observer-blinded controlled trial. *Pediatr Emerg Care*. 2012;28:745–749.
8. Beaty JH, Linton RC. Medial malleolar fracture in a child. A case report. *J Bone Joint Surg Am*. 1988;70:1254–1255.
9. Beck JJ, VandenBerg C, Cruz AI, Ellis HB Jr. Low energy, lateral ankle injuries in pediatric and adolescent patients: a systematic review of ankle sprains and nondisplaced distal fibula fractures. *J Pediatr Orthop*. 2020;40(6):283–287.
10. Benz G, Kallieris D, Seeböck T, et al. Bioresorbable pins and screws in paediatric traumatology. *Eur J Pediatr Surg*. 1994;4:103–107.
11. Bishop PA. Fractures and epiphyseal separation fractures of the ankle: classification of 332 cases according to mechanism of their production. *AJR Am J Roentgenol*. 1932;28:49–67.
12. Blackburn EW, Aronsson DD, Rubright JH, Lisle JW. Ankle fractures in children. *J Bone Joint Surg Am*. 2012;94:1234–1244.
13. Blair JM, Botte MJ. Surgical anatomy of the superficial peroneal nerve in the ankle and foot. *Clin Orthop Relat Res*. 1994;305:229–238.
14. Blauth M, Bastian L, Krettek C, et al. Surgical options for the treatment of severe tibial pilon fractures: a study of three techniques. *J Orthop Trauma*. 2001;15:153–160.
15. Blitzer CM, Johnson RJ, Ettlinger CF, Aggeborn K. Downhill skiing injuries in children. *Am J Sports Med*. 1984;12:142–147.
16. Bojescul JA, Wilson G, Taylor DC. Idiopathic chondrolysis of the ankle. *Arthroscopy*. 2005;21:224–227.
17. Böstman O, Hirvensalo E, Vainionpää S, et al. Degradable polyglycolide rods for the internal fixation of displaced bimalleolar fractures. *Int Orthop*. 1990;14:1–8.
18. Böstman O, Mäkelä EA, Södergård J, et al. Absorbable polyglycolide pins in internal fixation of fractures in children. *J Pediatr Orthop*. 1993;13:242–245.
19. Böstman OM. Distal tibiofibular synostosis after malleolar fractures treated using absorbable implants. *Foot Ankle*. 1993;14:38–43.
20. Böstman OM. Metallic or absorbable fracture fixation devices. A cost minimization analysis. *Clin Orthop Relat Res*. 1996;329:233–239.
21. Bostock SH, Peach BG. Spontaneous resolution of an osseous bridge affecting the distal tibial epiphysis. *J Bone Joint Surg Br*. 1996;78:662–663.
22. Boutis K, Komar L, Jaramillo D, et al. Sensitivity of a clinical examination to predict need for radiography in children with ankle injuries: a prospective study. *Lancet*. 2001;358(9299):2118–2121.

23. Boutis K, Narayanan UG, Dong FFT, et al. Magnetic resonance imaging of clinically suspected Salter-Harris I fracture of the distal fibula. *Injury.* 2010;41:852–856.
24. Boutis K, Plint A, Stimec J, et al. Radiograph-negative lateral ankle injuries in children: occult growth plate fracture or sprain? *JAMA Pediatr.* 2016;170(1):e154114.
25. Boutis K, Willan AR, Babyn P, et al. A randomized, controlled trial of a removable brace versus casting in children with low-risk ankle fractures. *Pediatrics.* 2007;119(6):e1256–e1263.
26. Boyer MI, Bowen V, Weiler P. Reconstruction of a severe grinding injury to the medial malleolus and the deltoid ligament of the ankle using a free plantaris tendon graft and vascularized gracilis free muscle transfer: case report. *J Trauma.* 1994;36:454–457.
27. Bozic KJ, Jaramillo D, DiCanzio J, et al. Radiographic appearance of the normal distal tibiofibular syndesmosis in children. *J Pediatr Orthop.* 1999;19:14–21.
28. Broström L. Sprained ankles. V. Treatment and prognosis in recent ligament ruptures. *Acta Chir Scand.* 1966;132:537–550.
29. Broström L. Sprained ankles. VI. Surgical treatment of "chronic" ligament ruptures. *Acta Chir Scand.* 1966;132:551–565.
30. Brown SD, Kasser JR, Zurakowski D, Jaramillo D. Analysis of 51 tibial triplane fractures using CT with multiplanar reconstruction. *AJR Am J Roentgenol.* 2004;183:1489–1495.
31. Bucholz RW, Henry S, Henley MB. Fixation with bioabsorbable screws for the treatment of fractures of the ankle. *J Bone Joint Surg Am.* 1994;76:319–324.
32. Burstein AH. Fracture classification systems: do they work and are they useful? *J Bone Joint Surg Am.* 1993;75:1743–1744.
33. Busam ML, Esther RJ, Obremskey WT. Hardware removal: indications and expectations. *J Am Acad Orthop Surg.* 2006;14:113–120.
34. Busconi BD, Pappas AM. Chronic, painful ankle instability in skeletally immature athletes. Ununited osteochondral fractures of the distal fibula. *Am J Sports Med.* 1996;24:647–651.
35. Carey J, Spence L, Blickman H, Eustace S. MRI of pediatric growth plate injury: correlation with plain film radiographs and clinical outcome. *Skeletal Radiol.* 1998;27:250–255.
36. Carothers CO, Crenshaw AH. Clinical significance of a classification of epiphyseal injuries at the ankle. *Am J Surg.* 1955;89:879–889.
37. Cass JR, Peterson HA. Salter-Harris Type-IV injuries of the distal tibial epiphyseal growth plate, with emphasis on those involving the medial malleolus. *J Bone Joint Surg Am.* 1983;65:1059–1070.
38. Castelyen PP, Handelberg F. Distraction for ankle arthroscopy. *Arthroscopy.* 1995;11:633–634.
39. Caterini R, Farsetti P, Ippolito E. Long-term followup of physeal injury to the ankle. *Foot Ankle.* 1991;11:372–383.
40. Chadwick CJ. Spontaneous resolution of varus deformity at the ankle following adduction injury of the distal tibial epiphysis. A case report. *J Bone Joint Surg Am.* 1982;64:774–776.
41. Chande VT. Decision rules for roentgenography of children with acute ankle injuries. *Arch Pediatr Adolesc Med.* 1995;149:255–258.
42. Charlton M, Costello R, Mooney JF III, Podeszwa DA. Ankle joint biomechanics following transepiphyseal screw fixation of the distal tibia. *J Pediatr Orthop.* 2005;25:635–640.
43. Clement DA, Worlock PH. Triplane fracture of the distal tibia. A variant in cases with an open growth plate. *J Bone Joint Surg Br.* 1987;69:412–415.
44. Cooperman DR, Spiegel PG, Laros GS. Epiphyseal fractures of the distal ends of the tibia and fibula. A retrospective study of two hundred and thirty-seven cases in children. *J Bone Joint Surg Am.* 1978;60:1046–1050.
45. Cox G, Thambapillay S, Templeton PA. Compartment syndrome with an isolated Salter Harris II fracture of the distal tibia. *J Orthop Trauma.* 2008;22:148–150.
46. Cox PJ, Clarke NM. Juvenile Tillaux fracture of the ankle associated with a tibial shaft fracture: a unique combination. *Injury.* 1996;27:221–222.
47. Crawford AH. Triplane and Tillaux fractures: is a 2 mm residual gap acceptable? *J Pediatr Orthop.* 2012;32(Suppl 1):S69–S73.
48. Crenshaw AH. Injuries of the distal tibial epiphysis. *Clin Orthop Relat Res.* 1965;41:98–107.
49. Cummings RJ. Triplane ankle fracture with deltoid ligament tear and syndesmotic disruption. *J Child Orthop.* 2008;2:11–14.
50. Cummings RJ, Hahn GA Jr. The incisural fracture. *Foot Ankle Int.* 2004;25:132–135.
51. Damore DT, Metzl JD, Ramundo M, et al. Patterns in childhood sports injury. *Pediatr Emerg Care.* 2003;19:65–67.
52. Denning JR. Complications of pediatric foot and ankle fractures. *Orthop Clin North Am.* 2017;48(1):59–70.
53. Denning JR. Lower extremity physeal bar resection. *Oper Techn Orthop.* 2021;31(2):1–6.
54. Denton JR, Fischer SJ. The medial triplane fracture: report of an unusual injury. *J Trauma.* 1981;21:991–995.
55. Dias LS, Giegerich CR. Fractures of the distal tibial epiphysis in adolescence. *J Bone Joint Surg Am.* 1983;65:438–444.
56. Dias LS, Tachdjian MO. Physeal injuries of the ankle in children: classification. *Clin Orthop Relat Res.* 1978;136:230–233.
57. Dormans JP, Azzoni M, Davidson RS, Drummond DS. Major lower extremity lawn mower injuries in children. *J Pediatr Orthop.* 1995;15:78–82.
58. Dowling S, Spooner CH, Liang Y, et al. Accuracy of Ottawa Ankle Rules to exclude fractures of the ankle and midfoot in children: a meta-analysis. *Acad Emerg Med.* 2009;16:277–287.
59. Dunbar RP, Barei DP, Kubiak EN, et al. Early limited internal fixation of diaphyseal extensions in select pilon fractures: upgrading AO/OTA type C fractures to AO/OTA type B. *J Orthop Trauma.* 2008;22:426–429.
60. Ecklund K, Jaramillo D. Patterns of premature physeal arrest: MR imaging of 111 children. *AJR Am J Roentgenol.* 2002;178:967–972.
61. Eismann EA, Stephan ZA, Mehlman CT, et al. Pediatric triplane ankle fractures: impact of radiographs and computed tomography on fracture classification and treatment planning. *J Bone Joint Surg Am.* 2015;97:995–1002
62. El-Karef E, Sadek HI, Nairn DS, et al. Triplane fracture of the distal tibia. *Injury.* 2000;31:729–736.
63. Ertl JP, Barrack RL, Alexander AH, VanBuecken K. Triplane fracture of the distal tibial epiphysis. Long-term follow-up. *J Bone Joint Surg Am.* 1988;70:967–976.
64. Farley FA, Kuhns L, Jacobson JA, DiPietro M. Ultrasound examination of ankle injuries in children. *J Pediatr Orthop.* 2001;21:604–607.
65. Feldman DS, Shin SS, Madan S, Koval KJ. Correction of tibial malunion and non-union with six-axis analysis deformity correction using the Taylor Spatial Frame. *J Orthop Trauma.* 2003;17:549–554.
66. Frick SL, Shoemaker S, Mubarak SJ. Altered fibular growth patterns after tibiofibular synostosis in children. *J Bone Joint Surg Am.* 2001;83(2):247–254.
67. Gabel GT, Peterson HA, Berquist TH. Premature partial physeal arrest. Diagnosis by magnetic resonance imaging in two cases. *Clin Orthop Relat Res.* 1991;272:242–247.
68. Gaglani MJ, Friedman J, Hawkins EP, Campbell JR. Infections complicating lawn mower injuries in children. *Pediatr Infect Dis J.* 1996;15:452–455.
69. Gill GG, Abott LO. Varus deformity of ankle following injury to distal epiphyseal cartilage of tibia in growing children. *Surg Gynecol Obstet.* 1941;72:659–666.
70. Goldberg VM, Aadalen R. Distal tibial epiphyseal injuries: the role of athletics in 53 cases. *Am J Sports Med.* 1978;6:263–268.
71. Gourineni P, Gupta A. Medial joint space widening of the ankle in displaced Tillaux and Triplane fractures in children. *J Orthop Trauma.* 2011;25:608–611.
72. Grace DL. Irreducible fracture-separations of the distal tibial epiphysis. *J Bone Joint Surg Br.* 1983;65:160–162.
73. Guille JT, Lipton GE, Bowen JR, Uthaman U. Delayed union following stress fracture of the distal fibula secondary to rotational malunion of lateral malleolar fracture. *Am J Orthop (Belle Mead NJ).* 1997;26:442–445.
74. Handolin L, Kiljunen V, Arnala I, et al. Effect of ultrasound therapy on bone healing of lateral malleolar fractures of the ankle joint fixed with bioabsorbable screws. *J Orthop Sci.* 2005;10:391–395.
75. Haraguchi N, Kato F, Hayashi H. New radiographic projections for avulsion fractures of the lateral malleolus. *J Bone Joint Surg Br.* 1998;80:684–688.
76. Haramati N, Roye DP, Adler PA, Ruzal-Shapiro C. Non-union of pediatric fibula fractures: easy to overlook, painful to ignore. *Pediatr Radiol.* 1994;24:248–250.
77. Havránek P, Lízler J. Magnetic resonance imaging in the evaluation of partial growth arrest after physeal injuries in children. *J Bone Joint Surg Am.* 1991;73:1234–1241.
78. Havranek P, Pesl T. Salter (Rang) type 6 physeal injury. *Eur J Pediatr Surg.* 2010;20:174–177.
79. Healy WA III, Starkweather KD, Meyer J, Teplitz GA. Triplane fracture associated with a proximal third fibula fracture. *Am J Orthop (Belle Mead NJ).* 1996;25:449–451.
80. Herscovici D Jr, Sanders RW, Scaduto JM, et al. Vacuum-assisted wound closure (VAC therapy) for the management of patients with high-energy soft tissue injuries. *J Orthop Trauma.* 2003;17:683–688.
81. Hynes D, O'Brien T. Growth disturbance lines after injury of the distal tibial physis. Their significance in prognosis. *J Bone Joint Surg Br.* 1988;70:231–233.
82. Imade S, Takao M, Nishi H, Uchio Y. Arthroscopy-assisted reduction and percutaneous fixation for triplane fracture of the distal tibia. *Arthroscopy.* 2004;20:e123–e128.
83. Iwinska-Zelder J, Schmidt S, Ishaque N, et al. Epiphyseal injuries of the distal tibia: Does MRI provide useful additional information? *Radiologe.* 1999;39:25–29.
84. Jarvis JG, Miyanji F. The complex triplane fracture: ipsilateral tibial shaft and distal triplane fracture. *J Trauma.* 2001;51:714–716.
85. Jennings MM, Lagaay P, Schuberth JM. Arthroscopic assisted fixation of juvenile intra-articular epiphyseal ankle fractures. *J Foot Ankle Surg.* 2007;46:376–386.
86. Johnson EW Jr, Fahl JC. Fractures involving the distal epiphysis of the tibia and fibula in children. *Am J Surg.* 1957;93:778–781.
87. Jones S, Phillips N, Ali F, et al. Triplane fractures of the distal tibia requiring open reduction and internal fixation. Pre-operative planning using computed tomography. *Injury.* 2003;34:293–298.
88. Kärrholm J. The triplane fracture: four years of follow-up of 21 cases and review of the literature. *J Pediatr Orthop B.* 1997;6:91–102.
89. Kärrholm J, Hansson LI, Laurin S. Computed tomography of intraarticular supination–eversion fractures of the ankle in adolescents. *J Pediatr Orthop.* 1981;1:181–187.
90. Kärrholm J, Hansson LI, Laurin S. Pronation injuries of the ankle in children. Retrospective study of radiographical classification and treatment. *Acta Orthop Scand.* 1983;54:1–17.
91. Kärrholm J, Hansson LI, Laurin S. Supination–eversion injuries of the ankle in children: a retrospective study of radiographic classification and treatment. *J Pediatr Orthop.* 1982;2:147–159.
92. Kärrholm J, Hansson LI, Selvik G. Changes in tibiofibular relationships due to growth disturbances after ankle fractures in children. *J Bone Joint Surg Am.* 1984;66:1198–1210.
93. Kaukonen JP, Lamberg T, Korkala O, Pajarinen J. Fixation of syndesmotic ruptures in 38 patients with a malleolar fracture: a randomized study comparing a metallic and a bioabsorbable screw. *J Orthop Trauma.* 2005;19:392–395.
94. Kay RM, Matthys GA. Pediatric ankle fractures: evaluation and treatment. *J Am Acad Orthop Surg.* 2001;9:268–278.
95. Kaya A, Altay T, Ozturk H, Karapinar L. Open reduction and internal fixation in displaced juvenile Tillaux fractures. *Injury.* 2007;38:201–205.
96. Keats TE. *Atlas of Normal Roentgen Variants That May Simulate Disease.* 5th ed. Year Book; 1992.

97. Keats TE. Fractures of the ankle and foot. In: Drennan JC, ed. *The Child's Foot and Ankle*. Raven Press; 1992.

98. Kessler J, Koebnick C, Smith N, Adams A. Childhood obesity is associated with increased risk of most lower extremity fractures. *Clin Orthop Relat Res*. 2013; 471(4):1199–1207.

99. Khansa I, Pearson GD, Bjorklund K, et al. Pediatric lawnmower injuries: a 25-year review. *JPRAS Open*. 2021;29:135–143.

100. Khoshhal KI, Kiefer GN. Physeal bridge resection. *J Am Acad Orthop Surg*. 2005; 13:47–58.

101. Kim JR, Song KH, Song KJ, Lee HS. Treatment outcomes of triplane and Tillaux fractures of the ankle in adolescence. *Clin Orthop Surg*. 2010;2:34–38.

102. Kleiger B, Mankin HJ. Fracture of the lateral portion of the distal tibial epiphysis. *J Bone Joint Surg Am*. 1964;46:25–32.

103. Klein DM, Caligiuri DA, Katzman BM. Local-advancement soft-tissue coverage in a child with ipsilateral grade IIIB open tibial and ankle fractures. *J Orthop Trauma*. 1996;10:577–580.

104. Kling TF Jr, Bright RW, Hensinger RN. Distal tibial physeal fractures in children that may require open reduction. *J Bone Joint Surg Am*. 1984;66:647–657.

105. Kramer DE, Cleary MX, Miller PE, et al. Syndesmosis injuries in the pediatric and adolescent athlete: an analysis of risk factors related to operative intervention. *J Child Orthop*. 2017;11(1):57–63.

106. Lange-Hansen N. Fractures of the ankle. II. Combined experimental-surgical and experimental-roetgenologic investigations. *Arch Surg (1920)*. 1950;60;957–985.

107. Leary JT, Handling M, Talerico M, et al. Physeal fractures of the distal tibia: predictive factors of premature physeal closure and growth arrest. *J Pediatr Orthop*. 2009;29:356–361.

108. Lehman WL, Jones WW. Intravenous lidocaine for anesthesia in the lower extremity: a prospective study. *J Bone Joint Surg Am*. 1984;66:1056–1060.

109. Leininger RE, Knox CL, Comstock RD. Epidemiology of 1.6 million pediatric soccer-related injuries presenting to US emergency departments from 1990 to 2003. *Am J Sports Med*. 2007;35:288–293.

110. Lerner A, Stein H. Hybrid thin wire external fixation: an effective, minimally invasive, modular surgical tool for the stabilization of periarticular fractures. *Orthopedics*. 2004;27:59–62.

111. Letts RM. The hidden adolescent ankle fracture. *J Pediatr Orthop*. 1982;2:161–164.

112. Letts M, Davidson D, McCaffrey M. The adolescent pilon fracture: management and outcome. *J Pediatr Orthop*. 2001;21:20–26.

113. Letts M, Davidson D, Mukhtar I. Surgical management of chronic lateral ankle instability in adolescents. *J Pediatr Orthop*. 2003;23:392–397.

114. Lintecum N, Blasier RD. Direct reduction with indirect fixation of distal tibial physeal fractures: a report of a technique. *J Pediatr Orthop*. 1996;16:107–112.

115. Loder RT, Brown KL, Zaleske DJ, Jones ET. Extremity lawn-mower injuries in children: report by the Research Committee of the Pediatric Orthopaedic Society of North America. *J Pediatr Orthop*. 1997;17:360–369.

116. Lohman M, Kivisaari A, Vehmas T, et al. MRI in the assessment of growth arrest. *Pediatr Radiol*. 2002;32:41–45.

117. Luhmann SJ, Oda JE, O'Donnell J, et al. An analysis of suboptimal outcomes of medial malleolus fractures in skeletally immature children. *Am J Orthop (Belle Mead NJ)*. 2012;41:113–116.

118. Lurie BM, Van Rysselberghe N, Pennock AT, Upasani VV. Functional outcomes of Tillaux and triplane fractures with 2 to 5 millimeters of intra-articular gap. *J Bone Joint Surg Am*. 2020;102(8):679–686.

119. Lurie BM, Paez CJ, Howitt SR, Pennock AT. Suture-button versus screw fixation in adolescent syndesmotic injuries: functional outcomes and maintenance of reduction. *J Pediatr Orthop*. 2021;41(6):e427–e432.

120. Lynn MD. The triplane distal tibial epiphyseal fracture. *Clin Orthop Relat Res*. 1972;86:187–190.

121. Mäkelä EA, Vainionpää S, Vihtonen K, et al. The effect of trauma to the lower femoral epiphyseal plate: an experimental study in rabbits. *J Bone Joint Surg Br*. 1988;70:187–191.

122. Malanga GA, Ramirez-Del Toro JA. Common injuries of the foot and ankle in the child and adolescent athlete. *Phys Med Rehabil Clin N Am*. 2008;19:347–371, ix.

123. Manderson EL, Ollivierre CO. Closed anatomic reduction of a juvenile Tillaux fracture by dorsiflexion of the ankle. A case report. *Clin Orthop Relat Res*. 1992:262–266.

124. Mankovsky AB, Mendoza-Sagaon M, Cardinaux C, et al. Evaluation of scooter-related injuries in children. *J Pediatr Surg*. 2002;37:755–759.

125. Mann DC, Rajmaira S. Distribution of physeal and nonphyseal fractures in 2,650 long-bone fractures in children aged 0–16 years. *J Pediatr Orthop*. 1990;10:713–716.

126. Marmor L. An unusual fracture of the tibial epiphysis. *Clin Orthop Relat Res*. 1970;73:132–135.

127. Mazur JM, Loveless EA, Cummings RJ. Ankle dislocation without fracture in a child. *Am J Orthop (Belle Mead NJ)*. 2007;36:E138–E140.

128. Michelson JD, Clarke HJ, Jinnah RH. The effect of loading on tibiotalar alignment in cadaver ankles. *Foot Ankle*. 1990;10:280–284.

129. Mirmiran R, Schuberth JM. Nonunion of an epiphyseal fibular fracture in a pediatric patient. *J Foot Ankle Surg*. 2006;45:410–412.

130. Mooney JF III, DeFranzo A, Marks MW. Use of cross-extremity flaps stabilized with external fixation in severe pediatric foot and ankle trauma: an alternative to free tissue transfer. *J Pediatr Orthop*. 1998;18:26–30.

131. Mubarak SJ. Extensor retinaculum syndrome of the ankle after injury to the distal tibial physis. *J Bone Joint Surg Br*. 2002;84:11–14.

132. Mubarak SJ. Extensor retinaculum syndrome of the ankle after injury to the distal tibial physis. *J Bone Joint Surg Br* 2002;84B(1):11–14.

133. Mubarak SJ, Wilton NC. Compartment syndromes and epidural analgesia. *J Pediatr Orthop*. 1997;17:282–284.

134. Munjal K, Kishan S, Sabharwal S. Posttraumatic pediatric distal tibiofibular synostosis: a case report. *Foot Ankle Int*. 2004;25:429–433.

135. Nenopoulos SP, Papavasiliou VA, Papavasiliou AV. Outcome of physeal and epiphyseal injuries of the distal tibia with intra-articular involvement. *J Pediatr Orthop*. 2005;25:518–522.

136. Nguyen D, Letts M. In-line skating injuries in children: a 10-year review. *J Pediatr Orthop*. 2001;21:613–618.

137. Nilsson S, Roaas A. Soccer injuries in adolescents. *Am J Sports Med*. 1978;6:358–361.

138. Nusem I, Ezra E, Wientroub S. Closed posterior dislocation of the ankle without associated fracture in a child. *J Trauma*. 1999;46:350–351.

139. O'Loughlin PF, Heyworth BE, Kennedy JG. Current concepts in the diagnosis and treatment of osteochondral lesions of the ankle. *Am J Sports Med*. 2010;38:392–404.

140. Ogden JA. *Skeletal Injury in the Child*. Lea & Febiger; 1982.

141. Ogden JA, Lee J. Accessory ossification patterns and injuries of the malleoli. *J Pediatr Orthop*. 1990;10:306–316.

142. Paez CJ, Lurie BM, Bomar JD, et al. plate versus lag screw only fixation of unstable ankle fractures involving the fibula in adolescent patients. *J Pediatr Orthop*. 2021;41(2):e161–e166.

143. Panagopoulos A, van Niekerk L. Arthroscopic assisted reduction and fixation of a juvenile Tillaux fracture. *Knee Surg Sports Traumatol Arthrosc*. 2007;15:415–417.

144. Papadokostakis G, Kontakis G, Giannoudis P, Hadjipavlou A. External fixation devices in the treatment of fractures of the tibial plafond: a systematic review of the literature. *J Bone Joint Surg Br*. 2008;90:1–6.

145. Pesl T, Havranek P. Rare injuries to the distal tibiofibular joint in children. *Eur J Pediatr Surg*. 2006;16:255–259.

146. Peterson CA, Peterson HA. Analysis of the incidence of injuries to the epiphyseal growth plate. *J Trauma*. 1972;12:275–281.

147. Peterson HA. Physeal fractures: part 3. Classification. *J Pediatr Orthop*. 1994;14:439–448.

148. Peterson HA, Madhok R, Benson JT, et al. Physeal fractures: part 1. Epidemiology in Olmsted County, Minnesota, 1979–1988. *J Pediatr Orthop*. 1994;14:423–430.

149. Petit P, Panuel M, Faure F, et al. Acute fracture of the distal tibial physis: role of gradient-echo MR imaging versus plain film examination. *AJR Am J Roentgenol*. 1996;166:1203–1206.

150. Petit P, Sapin C, Henry G, et al. Rate of abnormal osteoarticular radiographic findings in pediatric patients. *AJR Am J Roentgenol*. 2001;176:987–990.

151. Petratos DV, Kokkinakis M, Ballas EG, Anastasopoulos JN. Prognostic factors for premature growth plate arrest as a complication of the surgical treatment of fractures of the medial malleolus in children. *Bone Joint J*. 2013;95-B:419–423.

152. Phan VC, Wroten E, Yngve DA. Foot progression angle after distal tibial physeal fractures. *J Pediatr Orthop*. 2002;22(1):31–35.

153. Phieffer LS, Meyer RA Jr, Gruber HE, et al. Effect of interposed periosteum in an animal physeal fracture model. *Clin Orthop Relat Res*. 2000;376:15–25.

154. Pollen AG. Fractures involving the epiphyseal plate. *Reconstr Surg Traumatol*. 1979;17:25–39.

155. Raikin SM, Ching AC. Bioabsorbable fixation in foot and ankle. *Foot Ankle Clin*. 2005;10:667–684, ix.

156. Ramsey PL, Hamilton W. Changes in tibiotalar area of contact caused by lateral talar shift. *J Bone Joint Surg Am*. 1976;58:356–357.

157. Rapariz JM, Ocete G, González-Herranz P, et al. Distal tibial triplane fractures: long-term follow-up. *J Pediatr Orthop*. 1996;16:113–118.

158. Reff RB. The use of external fixation devices in the management of severe lower-extremity trauma and pelvic injuries in children. *Clin Orthop Relat Res*. 1984;188:21–33.

159. Rinker B, Amspacher JC, Wilson PC, Vasconez HC. Subatmospheric pressure dressing as a bridge to free tissue transfer in the treatment of open tibia fractures. *Plast Reconstr Surg*. 2008;121:1664–1673.

160. Ristiniemi J. External fixation of tibial pilon fractures and fracture healing. *Acta Orthop Suppl*. 2007;78(3):5–34.

161. Rogers LF. The radiography of epiphyseal injuries. *Radiology*. 1970;96:289–299.

162. Rohmiller MT, Gaynor TP, Pawelek J, Mubarak SJ. Salter-Harris I and II fractures of the distal tibia: does mechanism of injury relate to premature physeal closure? *J Pediatr Orthop*. 2006;26:322–328.

163. Rokkanen P, Böstman O, Vainionpää S, et al. Absorbable devices in the fixation of fractures. *J Trauma*. 1996;40:S123–S127.

164. Rosenbaum AJ, DiPreta JA, Uhl RL. Review of distal tibial epiphyseal transitional fractures. *Orthopedics*. 2012;35:1046–1049.

165. Roser LA, Clawson DK. Football injuries in the very young athlete. *Clin Orthop Relat Res*. 1970;69:219–223.

166. Ross PM, Schwentker EP, Bryan H. Mutilating lawn mower injuries in children. *JAMA*. 1976;236:480–481.

167. Sabharwal S, Schwechter EM. Five-year followup of ankle joint distraction for post-traumatic chondrolysis in an adolescent: a case report. *Foot Ankle Int*. 2007;28:942–948.

168. Sailhan F, Chotel F, Guibal AL, et al. Three-dimensional MR imaging in the assessment of physeal growth arrest. *Eur Radiol*. 2004;14:1600–1608.

169. Sankar WN, Chen J, Kay R, Skaggs DL. Incidence of occult fracture in children with acute ankle injuries. *J Pediatr Orthop*. 2008;28:500–501.

170. Scheffer MM, Peterson HA. Opening-wedge osteotomy for angular deformities of long bones in children. *J Bone Joint Surg Am*. 1994;76:325–334.

171. Schenck RC Jr, Goodnight JM. Osteochondritis dissecans. *J Bone Joint Surg Am*. 1996;78:439–456.

172. Schlesinger I, Wedge JH. Percutaneous reduction and fixation of displaced juvenile Tillaux fractures: a new surgical technique. *J Pediatr Orthop*. 1993;13:389–391.

173. Schnetzler KA, Hoernschemeyer D. The pediatric triplane ankle fracture. *J Am Acad Orthop Surg*. 2007;15:738–747.

174. Schurz M, Binder H, Platzer P, et al. Physeal injuries of the distal tibia: long-term results in 376 patients. *Int Orthop*. 2010;34:547–552.

175. Shankar A, Williams K, Ryan M. Trampoline-related injury in children. *Pediatr Emerg Care*. 2006;22:644–646.

176. Sheffer BW, Villarreal ED, Ochsner MG III, et al. Concurrent ipsilateral tibial shaft and distal tibial fractures in pediatric patients: risk factors, frequency, and risk of missed diagnosis. *J Pediatr Orthop*. 2020;40(1):e1–e5.

177. Shin AY, Moran ME, Wenger DR. Intramalleolar triplane fractures of the distal tibial epiphysis. *J Pediatr Orthop*. 1997;17:352–355.

178. Shindle MK, Endo Y, Warren RF, et al. Stress fractures about the tibia, foot, and ankle. *J Am Acad Orthop Surg*. 2012;20(3):167–176.

179. Shore BJ, Kramer DE. Management of syndesmotic ankle injuries in children and adolescents. *J Pediatr Orthop*. 2016;36(Suppl 1):S11–S14.

180. Siapkara A, Nordin L, Hill RA. Spatial frame correction of anterior growth arrest of the proximal tibia: report of three cases. *J Pediatr Orthop B*. 2008;17:61–64.

181. Siffert RS, Arkin AM. Post-traumatic aseptic necrosis of the distal tibial epiphysis; report of a case. *J Bone Joint Surg Am*. 1950;32-A:691–694.

182. Simanovsky N, Lamdan R, Hiller N, Simanovsky N. Sonographic detection of radiographically occult fractures in pediatric ankle and wrist injuries. *J Pediatr Orthop*. 2009;29:142–145.

183. Singleton TJ, Cobb M. High fibular fracture in association with triplane fracture: reexamining this unique pediatric fracture pattern. *J Foot Ankle Surg*. 2010;49:491–494.

184. Sinisaari IP, Luthje PMJ, Mikkonen RHM. Ruptured tibio-fibular syndesmosis: comparison study of metallic to bioabsorbable fixation. *Foot Ankle Int*. 2002;23:744–748.

185. Smith BG, Rand F, Jaramillo D, Shapiro F. Early MR imaging of lower-extremity physeal fracture-separations: a preliminary report. *J Pediatr Orthop*. 1994;14:526–533.

186. Souder CD, Vaughan CT. Below-knee cast immobilization for distal tibial physeal fractures. *J Foot Ankle Surg*. 2021;60(3):529–534.

187. Spiegel PG, Cooperman DR, Laros GS. Epiphyseal fractures of the distal ends of the tibia and fibula: a retrospective study of two hundred and thirty-seven cases in children. *J Bone Joint Surg Am*. 1978;60:1046–1050.

188. Steinlauf SD, Stricker SJ, Hulen CA. Juvenile Tillaux fracture simulating syndesmosis separation: a case report. *Foot Ankle Int*. 1998;19:332–335.

189. Stevens PM, Kennedy JM, Hung M. Guided growth for ankle valgus. *J Pediatr Orthop*. 2011;31:878–883.

190. Stiell IG, Greenberg GH, McKnight RD, et al. A study to develop clinical decision rules for the use of radiography in acute ankle injuries. *Ann Emerg Med*. 1992;21:384–390.

191. Takakura Y, Takaoka T, Tanaka Y, et al. Results of opening-wedge osteotomy for the treatment of a post-traumatic varus deformity of the ankle. *J Bone Joint Surg Am*. 1998;80:213–218.

192. Tarkin IS, Clare MP, Marcantonio A, Pape HC. An update on the management of high-energy pilon fractures. *Injury*. 2008;39:142–154.

193. Tarr RR, Resnick CT, Wagner KS, Sarmiento A. Changes in tibiotalar joint contact areas following experimentally induced tibial angular deformities. *Clin Orthop Relat Res*. 1985;199:72–80.

194. Thomsen NO, Overgaard S, Olsen LH, et al. Observer variation in the radiographic classification of ankle fractures. *J Bone Joint Surg Br*. 1991;73:676–678.

195. Ting AJ, Tarr RR, Sarmiento A, et al. The role of subtalar motion and ankle contact pressure changes from angular deformities of the tibia. *Foot Ankle*. 1987;7:290–299.

196. Vahvanen V, Aalto K. Classification of ankle fractures in children. *Arch Orthop Trauma Surg (1978)*. 1980;97:1–5.

197. Vahvanen V, Westerlund M, Nikku R. Lateral ligament injury of the ankle in children. Follow-up results of primary surgical treatment. *Acta Orthop Scand*. 1984;55(1):21–25.

198. Vangsness CT Jr, Carter V, Hunt T, et al. Radiographic diagnosis of ankle fractures: are three views necessary? *Foot Ankle Int*. 1994;15:172–174.

199. von Laer L. Classification, diagnosis, and treatment of transitional fractures of the distal part of the tibia. *J Bone Joint Surg Am*. 1985;67:687–698.

200. Vosburgh CL, Gruel CR, Herndon WA, Sullivan JA. Lawn mower injuries of the pediatric foot and ankle: observations on prevention and management. *J Pediatr Orthop*. 1995;15:504–509.

201. Wattenbarger JM, Gruber HE, Phieffer LS. Physeal fractures, part I: histologic features of bone, cartilage, and bar formation in a small animal model. *J Pediatr Orthop*. 2002;22:703–709.

202. Whipple TL, Martin DR, McIntyre LF, Meyers JF. Arthroscopic treatment of triplane fractures of the ankle. *Arthroscopy*. 1993;9:456–463.

203. Wuerz TH, Gurd DP. Pediatric physeal ankle fracture. *J Am Acad Orthop Surg*. 2013;21:234–244.

204. Yung CS, Kuong EE, Chow W. A previously unreported type of extra-articular triplane fracture: a revised classification system. *J Orthop Surg (Hong Kong)*. 2019;27(1):2309499019828500.

205. Zaricznyj B, Shattuck LJ, Mast TA, et al. Sports-related injuries in school-aged children. *Am J Sports Med*. 1980;8:318–324.

206. Zonfrillo MR, Seiden JA, House EM, et al. The association of overweight and ankle injuries in children. *Ambul Pediatr*. 2008;8:66–69.

31

Fractures, Dislocations, and Other Injuries of the Foot

Amy L. McIntosh

Fractures and Dislocations of the Foot

INTRODUCTION TO FRACTURES AND DISLOCATIONS OF THE FOOT

Trauma to the pediatric foot has been traditionally treated nonoperatively by orthopaedic surgeons. The dogma existed that the bones of the foot were predominantly cartilaginous and would remodel as the child matures. Few, if any, long-term studies exist to measure the outcomes of these treatments.

Children are now involved in sports and activities of greater physical intensity, leading to more complex fractures and dislocations.[2,26,101] It is not uncommon for young children to be competing in motocross, extreme skiing, go-karting, and rock climbing.[2,56,123] Professional sport has brought about more intense training and greater expectations from the child, the parent, and the coach. Physicians may feel pressure that injuries need to be treated "quicker" and rehabilitation time decreased. These expectations should not get in the way of treating the child's foot injury in the best possible way.

As the child grows into a young adult, the largely cartilaginous foot becomes ossified and fracture and dislocation patterns change. Ogden[92] showed that the cartilaginous bones were elastic, absorbing, and dissipating the energy from the trauma differently than the adult foot, which resulted in different fracture patterns. The management algorithms for the adolescent foot are therefore quite different from the infant's foot; however, the exact age at which this occurs needs to be individualized for each patient. The amount of fracture angulation and joint line displacement to accept is one of the real challenges in treating the skeletally immature foot. Some complex fractures of the talus and calcaneus in adolescents are best internally fixed according to the principles used to treat adult trauma.

An in-depth knowledge of the anatomy of the growing foot is helpful as the variable ossification centers, apophyses, and physes make fracture recognition difficult. Most of the papers quoted in this chapter are level IV (uncontrolled case series) or level V (expert consensus). One of the problems with pediatric foot and ankle research is that long follow-up intervals are necessary to validate treatments. The Oxford Ankle Foot Questionnaire for Children (OxAFQ-C) is a validated functional outcome tool used to measure subjective well-being for child patients (aged 5–16) affected by foot and ankle conditions.[83] However, there are no pediatric outcome scores for children's foot and ankle trauma, so prediction of outcome is dependent on orthopaedic-first principles of anatomic reduction, union, and effective rehabilitation. Long-term retrospective studies also have the difficulty of locating children treated decades earlier and, therefore, the follow-up rate is low.

ANATOMY OF THE GROWING FOOT

The child's foot is different from the adult foot in that the bones are largely cartilaginous until adolescence. Although the mechanisms of injury are similar, the resulting fracture is usually less severe in the child as the energy of the injury is dissipated by the elasticity of the cartilage. The cartilage also makes interpretation of imaging more difficult, and fractures may not be appreciated on plain radiograph. Computed tomography (CT) and magnetic resonance imaging (MRI) scans assist in clarification of anatomy and identification of fractures. The remodeling potential of cartilage allows some displacement and angulation of fractures to be accepted in children, whereas in adults it may be unacceptable.

Secondary areas of ossification, accessory bones, and growth plates also make fracture recognition more difficult. The appearance of the ossification centers is summarized in Figure 31-1. The calcaneus and talus are usually ossified at birth and the cuboid ossification center usually becomes evident shortly after. The navicular does not develop its primary ossification center until the child is around 3 years of age. Figure 31-2 shows the

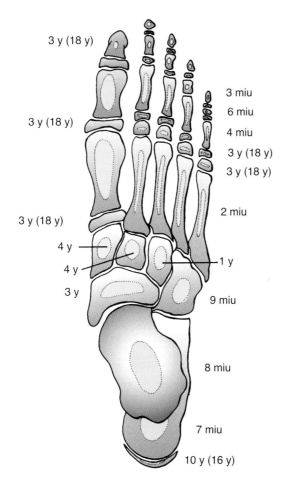

Figure 31-1. Appearance and fusion times of foot ossification centers, with figures in parentheses indicating the time of fusion of the primary and secondary ossification centers (y, years; miu, months in utero).

accessory ossicles and sesamoid bones in the foot which can also be confused with fractures especially if they are bipartite or if the accessory bones are closely adhered. It is useful clinically to radiograph the opposite foot if any doubt exists as to what may be normal or pathologic.

MECHANISMS OF INJURY AND ASSESSMENT OF FRACTURES AND DISLOCATIONS OF THE FOOT

The history provided by the patient is not always accurate in childhood trauma. Often, other children or adults who witnessed the accident can give a more accurate account than the patient. The degree of force, the speed and height of the fall, and the way the foot is twisted all help predict the degree of displacement or severity of the injury. Additionally, the ability to weight bear, degree of instability, and the location of the pain are important to ascertain.

Careful examination of the foot often will guide the surgeon to the site of injury. The child frequently complains of the whole foot "hurting"; however, systematic palpation helps localize the most painful site. Appropriate radiographs can then be obtained. Bruising and swelling will also help predict the injury pattern. Isolated bruising on the sole of the midfoot often overlies a subtle Lisfranc injury, whereas excessive dorsal swelling may predict a more severe fracture-dislocation.[107] In a crush injury, the possibility of increased compartment pressures should be considered.

Multiple injuries must also be ruled out via a complete secondary survey. For example, bilateral calcaneus fractures following a fall may be associated with a tibial fracture or spinal column injury.

Talar Fractures

INTRODUCTION TO TALAR FRACTURES

Fractures of the talus are rare in children and adolescents. Talus fractures most commonly occur through the neck and occasionally the body. Although rare, talus fractures are important to recognize because of the possible complication of avascular necrosis (AVN), which can occur because of the precarious blood supply. Most talus fractures in children can be treated with cast immobilization, whereas displaced fractures in adolescents need to be treated operatively similar to an adult fracture.[131]

ASSESSMENT OF TALAR FRACTURES

MECHANISMS OF INJURY FOR TALAR FRACTURES

A fall from a height is a common mechanism of injury causing talar fractures.[55] The foot is forcibly dorsiflexed and the neck of

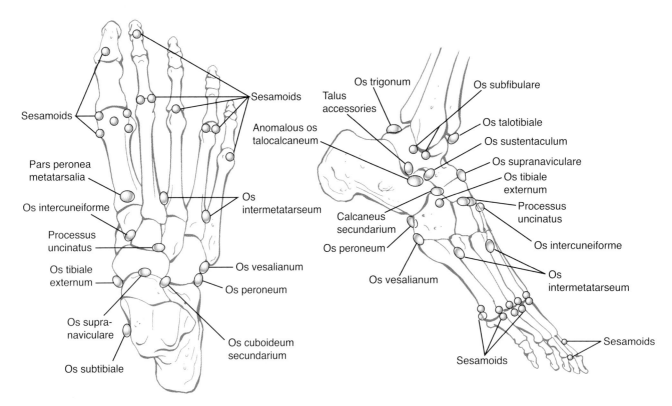

Figure 31-2. Diagrammatic representation of accessory ossicles and sesamoid bones about the foot and ankle. Note that the sesamoid bones can be bipartite and that accessory ossicles can be multicentric. (From Traughber PD. Imaging of the foot and ankle. In: Coughlin MJ, Mann RA. *Surgery of the Foot and Ankle.* 7th ed. Mosby; 1999.)

the talus impinges against the anterior lip of the distal tibia. This shear force usually results in a vertical or slightly oblique fracture line at the junction of the body and neck of the talus. When dorsiflexion is combined with supination of the foot, impingement occurs more medially and the medial malleolus may be fractured as well. With displaced fractures, the subtalar joint may become subluxed. The talus can also be fractured with crushing injuries, and open fractures are well described in lawnmower accidents.[92] Fractures of the lateral process of the talus have been described in snowboarding accidents, for which the mechanism appears to be forced dorsiflexion and inversion of the ankle.[78]

INJURIES ASSOCIATED WITH TALAR FRACTURES

The force required to fracture a child's talus is almost twice that required to fracture the other ankle and tarsal bones.[96] Therefore, other injuries often coexist with talus fractures. Fractures of the calcaneus, malleoli, tibia, and lumbar spine may be seen in the presence of a talus fracture. Hawkins,[43] in his study of adult talus fractures, found 64% of the patients had an associated musculoskeletal injury.

SIGNS AND SYMPTOMS OF TALAR FRACTURES

Other foot fractures and dislocations can present similarly to talus fractures. The ankle and foot are swollen and the foot is usually held plantarflexed. Because of this soft tissue swelling, the foot

needs to be examined closely for increased compartment pressure. As with all fractures, the soft tissues need to be inspected for any puncture wounds, abrasions, or fracture blisters as these are important in determining the management of the patient.

There may be less swelling so careful palpation around the talus is needed to detect the source of the pain. Once the foot has been clinically assessed, the appropriate radiographic investigations can be performed.

IMAGING AND OTHER DIAGNOSTIC STUDIES FOR TALAR FRACTURES

The routine radiographs for a fractured talus include an anteroposterior (AP), lateral, and oblique views. Canale and Kelly[17] have described a pronated oblique view of the talus which may demonstrate the fracture more clearly. The fractures are not always easy to see in young children, as the talus is largely cartilaginous until the second decade.[77] The cartilage anlage often leads to an underestimation of fracture displacement. MRI may show the morphology better in children less than 10 years old.

Once the fracture is identified, a CT scan can be useful in assessing the fracture plane, comminution, degree of displacement, and any other associated foot or ankle fractures. This study is particularly useful when pain prohibits the full range of radiographs mentioned above to be taken. If an open reduction is planned, the CT scan will also aid in the preoperative planning.

Figure 31-3. Hawkins classification of talar neck fractures (see text for details). **A:** Type I, nondisplaced fracture of the talar neck. **B:** Type II, displaced talar neck fracture with subluxation or dislocation of the subtalar joint. **C:** Type III, displaced talar neck fracture with associated dislocation of the talar body from both the subtalar and tibiotalar joints. **D:** Type IV, as suggested by Canale and Kelly, displaced talar neck fracture with associated dislocation of the talar body from subtalar and tibiotalar joints and dislocation of the head and neck fragment from the talonavicular joint. (Reprinted with permission from Canale ST, Kelly FB Jr. Fractures of the neck of the talus: Long-term evaluation of seventy-one cases. *J Bone Joint Surg Am.* 1978;60(2):143–156.)

CLASSIFICATION OF TALAR FRACTURES

Fractures of the talus can be classified as occurring either in the body or the neck. Some authors suggest classifying talar fractures based on the age of the patient as children less than 6 years of age generally have a better prognosis.[77] Hawkins[42] described an x-ray classification to define the different types of fractures of the talar neck and used it to predict the risk of AVN (Fig. 31-3).

Hawkins Classification of Talar Fractures	
Type	**Description**
I	Undisplaced talar neck fracture
II	Displaced talar neck fracture with subtalar subluxation or dislocation
III	Displaced fracture of the talar neck with dislocation of both the subtalar and ankle joints
IV	Displaced fracture of the talar neck with dislocation of both the subtalar, ankle, and talonavicular joints

FRACTURES OF THE TALAR NECK

Most talar fractures in children are of the talar neck. The Hawkins classification (see Fig. 31-3) was developed so it could be used to predict if the talus would become avascular because of

the disruption of the tenuous blood supply. Canale and Kelly[17] later modified the classification (see Fig. 31-3) to include a type IV injury in which there is subluxation or dislocation of the ankle, subtalar, and talonavicular joints. Most talar fractures in adults are type II or III. This classification has been used to help predict the type of treatment required and the outcome one can expect (Table 31-1).

PATHOANATOMY AND APPLIED ANATOMY RELATED TO TALAR NECK FRACTURES

The talus is composed of three parts: the body, neck, and head. Ossification starts from one center that appears in the sixth intrauterine month. The talus ossification process starts in the head and neck and proceeds in a retrograde direction toward the subchondral bone of the body. Approximately two-thirds of the talar body is articular cartilage with just a small area of bare bone on the neck where the bone receives its nutrient blood supply. There are no tendon insertions into the talus. The stability is provided by the capsular and ligamentous attachments to the surrounding bones.

The superior articular surface of the talus is wider anteriorly than it is posteriorly. Traditional teaching suggests the ankle should generally be immobilized in neutral dorsiflexion so this widest part of the talus is engaged in the ankle mortise to help prevent an equinus contracture. This technique is of less importance in younger children who are less likely to develop equinus contractures. The lateral wall of the superior articular surface curves posteriorly whereas the medial wall is straight. The two walls converge posteriorly to form the posterior tubercle of the

TABLE 31-1. Hawkins Classification of Talar Neck Fractures

Type	Description	Treatment	Affect on Blood Supply[a]	Osteonecrosis Rate (%)
Type I	Stable, undisplaced vertical fracture through talar neck.	8 weeks in cast, 4 weeks in CAM cast.	Theoretical damage to only one vessel entering talar neck.	0–10
Type II	Displaced fracture with subtalar joint subluxation or dislocation; normal ankle joint.	Immediate closed reduction.[b] A near anatomic reduction delays surgical treatment.	Two of three blood supply vessels lost: Neck vessel and one entering the tarsal canal.	20–50
Type III	Same as type II but with subluxation or dislocation of both the ankle and subtalar joint.	Direct to operating room for combined anteromedial and anterolateral surgical approach (see text).	All three sources of blood affected.	80–100
Type IV	Very rare; basically a type III with talonavicular joint displacement.	Same as type III.	Not related to blood supply.	100

CAM, controlled active motion.

[a]See text for further details of blood supply to the talus.

[b]Reduction maneuver: Maximal plantarflexion and foot traction to realign head and body in sagittal plane. Varus/valgus with or without supination/pronation stress realigns neck in coronal plane.

talus. Often, there is a separate ossification center (os trigonum) that appears here on radiographs at 11 to 13 years of age in boys and 8 to 10 years of age in girls. It usually fuses to the talus a year after it appears (Fig. 31-4).

The short neck of the talus is medially deviated approximately 10 to 44 degrees and plantarflexed between 5 and 50 degrees in relation to the axis of the body.[36] Beneath the talar

neck is the tarsal canal, a funnel-shaped area that contains the anastomotic ring formed between the artery of the tarsal canal and the artery of the tarsal sinus.[84] The broad interosseous ligament joining the calcaneus and talus is also within the canal.

The tarsal canal is conical in shape and runs from posteromedial (apex) to anterolateral where the base of the cone is known as the sinus tarsi (Fig. 31-5).

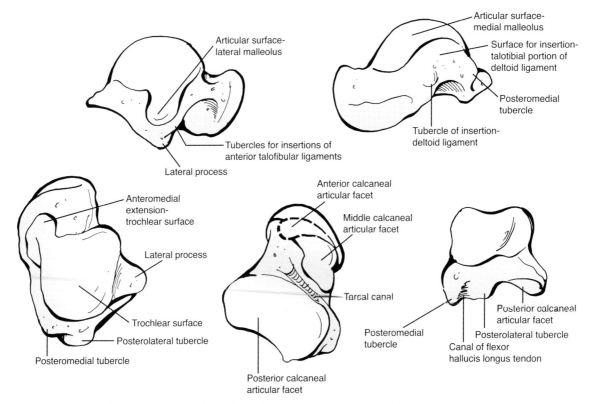

Figure 31-4. Anatomic details of the talus are important when correlating high-definition imaging, such as CT scans, with normal anatomy for the purposes of fracture management decision making.

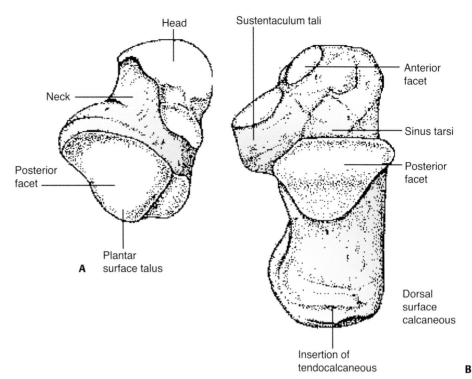

Figure 31-5. Subtalar joint opened such that the medial borders of the joint face each other. **A:** Plantar surface of the talus, which articulates with the dorsal surface of the calcaneus. Note the extensive area of the talus that is articular cartilage. **B:** Dorsal surface of the calcaneus with the articular facets occupying the anterior half of the calcaneus. (Reprinted with permission from Sammarco GJ. Anatomy. In: Helal B, et al., eds. *Surgery of Disorders of the Foot and Ankle*. Lippincott-Raven; 1996.)

The lateral process of the talus is a large wedge-shaped process that is covered in articular cartilage. It articulates with the fibula superiorly and laterally and with the subtalar joint inferiorly. The lateral talocalcaneal ligament is attached to the most distal part of the process.

The head of the talus is entirely cartilaginous, convex, and articulates with the concave surface of the navicular. The undersurface of the talus is comprised of three articulating surfaces for the calcaneus: the posterior, middle, and anterior facet. Between the posterior and middle facets is a transverse groove which forms the roof of the tarsal canal.

Blood Supply

The blood supply of the talus has been extensively studied.[5,84] The nutrient arteries are derived from the three major vessels that cross the ankle joint: posterior tibial artery, anterior tibial artery, and peroneal artery (Fig. 31-6). Branches of these three vessels perforate circumferentially the short talar neck, which is the only part of the talus denude of articular cartilage. A fracture in this area can disrupt this intricate anastomosis of vessels and leads to AVN of the body of the talus.

The main blood supply to the talus is through the artery of the tarsal canal, which branches off the posterior tibial artery approximately 1 cm proximal to the origin of the medial and lateral plantar arteries. It passes between flexor digitorum longus and flexor hallucis longus before entering the tarsal canal where it anastomoses with the artery of the tarsal sinus. Before entering the canal, the artery of the tarsal canal gives off a deltoid branch that penetrates the deltoid ligament and supplies the medial third of the talar body.[40] A dorsal vessel of the deltoid branch anastomoses with the medial branch of the dorsalis pedis artery to enter the talar neck.

The second source of blood supply is from the anterior tibial artery and its terminal extension, the dorsalis pedis artery. Multiple vessels from these arteries penetrate the dorsal neck of the talus. The third source of blood supply is from the peroneal artery. Small branches supply the posterior process of the talus and a larger branch forms the artery of the sinus tarsi to supply the lateral aspect of the talus.

Within the capsular and ligamentous attachments to the talus there are small vessels that also contribute to the blood supply.

TREATMENT OPTIONS FOR FRACTURES OF THE TALAR NECK

The treatment of talar fractures is based on the severity of the fracture and the age of the child. The Hawkins classification system is useful in directing the treatment. In a child less than 8 years of age, a less than perfect reduction of the fracture can be accepted because of the remodeling potential,[55,69,77] and the outcome in patients less than 12 years old is favorable in most cases.[32] Adolescent fractures should be treated the same way as an adult injury. Complications following pediatric talus fracture treatment are correlated with high-energy mechanism of injury and displacement requiring reduction.[121]

Nonoperative Treatment

Hawkins Type I Fractures

Undisplaced fractures of the talar neck can be treated for 6 to 8 weeks of non–weight bearing in a below-knee cast. The child can then start taking full weight if the fracture has healed radiographically. Canale and Kelly[17] accepted 5 mm of displacement and 5 degrees of angulation of the talar neck in their series.

A. Medial

1 - Anterior tibial artery
2 - Medial recurrent
    tarsal artery
3 - Medial talar artery
4 - Posterior tibial artery
5 - Posterior tubercle artery
6 - Deltoid branches
7 - Artery of tarsal canal
8 - Medial plantar artery
9 - Lateral plantar artery

B. Lateral

1 - Anterior tibial artery
2 - Lateral talar artery
3 - Lateral tarsal artery
4 - Posterior recurrent branch
    of lateral tarsal
6 - Perforating peroneal artery
7 - Anterior lateral malleolar artery

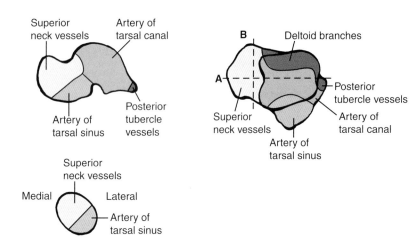

Figure 31-6. Arterial blood supply to the talus. Medial blood supply (**A**) and lateral blood supply (**B**). Dorsal view with sagittal cut through length (*a*) of talus and transverse cut through neck of talus (*b*). (Reprinted by permission from Gelberman RH, Mortensen WW. The arterial anatomy of the talus. *Foot Ankle*. 1983;4(2):64–72. Copyright © 1983 SAGE Publications.)

Hawkins Type II Fractures

A displaced or severely angulated talar neck fracture usually presents with significant soft tissue swelling and pain. This makes management more difficult than type I injuries. Achieving adequate radiographs to assess the degree of displacement is difficult without sedation. The distal fragment of the neck is usually displaced dorsally and medially.

The fracture and subluxation of the subtalar joint should be reduced under general anesthesia, most often by gentle plantarflexion and pronation of the foot. If a stable reduction is achieved, a well-molded below-knee cast can be applied with the foot in plantarflexion. This initial cast is changed to a more neutral position at 4 weeks and then removed 8 weeks following fracture reduction. Postoperative serial radiographs or a CT scan should be performed as the fracture position may be lost when the soft tissue swelling subsides. If the fracture is unstable after reduction, percutaneous Kirschner wire (K-wire) fixation is useful to hold the fracture. Two K-wires can be passed through a small dorsomedial incision and across the fracture. The incision should be on the medial side of extensor hallucis longus to avoid damage to the tibial vessels. Although the amount of residual displacement or angulation acceptable is not clearly defined, it may be better to accept a few millimeters of offset and up to 10 degrees of angulation rather than perform an open reduction and risk devascularizing the talus further.

Hawkins Type III and IV Fractures

These fractures are a result of a serious injury and require urgent surgery to openly reduce and internally fix the talus.

Operative Treatment of Talar Fractures

Surgical Approaches

There are three surgical approaches to the fractured talar neck: posterolateral, anteromedial, and anterolateral. The decision on the approach depends on the condition of the soft tissues and the familiarity of the approach by the surgeon. Occasionally, more than one approach is required if adequate reduction cannot be achieved. It is preferable to use the posterolateral approach as this causes less potential disruption to the blood supply; however, direct visualization of the talar neck is not possible. The timing of the open reduction of these fractures is somewhat controversial. With such a tenuous blood supply, one would think that urgent reduction and internal fixation is indicated. Lindvall et al.[72] compared the results of surgery within 6 hours to delayed surgery in 26 fractures of the talus in adult patients and found no significant difference in outcome. One can conclude that the severity of the injury, the quality of the reduction, and the surgical outcomes had a bigger influence on long-term outcome than if the surgery was fixed emergently or delayed (>12 hours).

Posterolateral Approach

This approach is commonly used to internally fixate fractures of the talar neck once it has been reduced. The patient is positioned supine so the other approaches can be utilized if necessary. The incision is made just lateral to the Achilles tendon. Blunt dissection is then carried out down to the joint capsule avoiding damage to the sural nerve. The posterior joint capsule can then be opened if not already torn by the injury and the posterior process of the talus can be identified. If possible, two partially threaded cannulated 4.5- or 6.5-mm screws can be used to provide compression across the fracture. It is preferable to use titanium screws which are MRI compatible to allow investigation of AVN during fracture healing if necessary. If only one screw is used, a separate K-wire should also be passed across the fracture for rotational stability. These posterior screws are more stable biomechanically than anterior screws (Fig. 31-7).[125]

Anteromedial Approach

This approach is useful to visualize the talar neck and directly reduce the fracture. Often, there is comminution of the medial wall of the neck which makes restoring length difficult. With the patient supine, the incision is made from just anterior to the medial malleolus and directly distally down the midfoot. Deeper dissection is carried out medial to the tibialis anterior and the extensor hallucis longus tendons. The dissection down to the capsule is in the interval between the tibialis anterior and tibialis posterior tendons. This approach avoids damage to the deltoid branch of the posterior tibial artery and the medial branches of the anterior tibial artery. This approach is potentially less harmful to the blood supply of the talus when compared to the anterolateral approach.[1]

Figure 31-7. Posterolateral approach to the talus. Incision is based lateral to the Achilles tendon. The Achilles tendon and flexor hallucis longus are reflected medially. The posterolateral talar tubercle is the starting point for the guide pin. **Right:** Screws are directed in line with the long axis of the neck of the talus in a plantar–medial direction such that the distal threads of the screw are all in the distal fragment (talar head), beyond the fracture line to allow for compression. Combinations of two screws or one screw and one smooth pin are determined by size and anatomy. (From Adelaar RS. Complex fractures of the talus. *Instr Course Lect.* 1997;46:323–338, with permission.)

Anterolateral Approach

One advantage of this approach is that it permits excellent exposure of the lateral talar neck, which is not usually comminuted allowing anatomic reduction. The approach also gives good access to the subtalar joint. The disadvantage to this approach is that it may disrupt the blood supply more than the other approaches. The incision starts at the tip of the lateral malleolus and extends to the base of the fourth metatarsal. Care must be taken to avoid damaging the sural nerve with deeper dissection. In the base of the incision is the artery of the sinus tarsi which should be visualized if possible.

Following open reduction and internal fixation (ORIF) of talar neck fractures, the foot is placed in a non–weight-bearing below-knee cast for 6 to 8 weeks. Radiographs are then taken to assess fracture healing and the presence or absence of the Hawkins sign. If the subchondral lucent line is present, one can assume there is adequate blood supply to the body of the talus and osteonecrosis is unlikely to occur. If the fracture has also healed, the child can start progressive weight bearing as tolerated. The absence of a subchondral lucency during healing should alert the surgeon to the possible development of osteonecrosis (Fig. 31-8). The patient should continue to be non–weight bearing until the lucency is present. If it is still not present 3 months postinjury, an MRI scan should be performed to assess the vascularity more accurately.[45] The use of titanium screws in the open reduction makes this possible. The

Figure 31-8. A 14-year-old girl with a talar neck fracture and a positive Hawkins sign (*arrow*). Disuse osteoporosis leads to halo-like image of the talus on the AP view denoting adequate talar dome vascularization; if there had been no blood supply, there would be no blood flow to lose calcium. If this happens, the dome of the talus would become denser and more radio-opaque than the surrounding bones that are undergoing diffuse osteoporosis.

decision on the amount of weight bearing in the presence of altered blood supply to the talus is not clear. AVN of the talus often takes 18 months to 2 years to revascularize so it would be impractical, if not impossible, to keep a child non—weight bearing for this period in the hope it will prevent premature collapse of the body.

FRACTURES OF THE TALAR BODY AND DOME

Fractures of the talar body are less common than of the neck, representing 29% and 45% of pediatric talus fractures in two series.[55,122] In 1977, Sneppen et al.[122] described a classification system based on the anatomic position of the fracture in the talus, which was later modified into a five-part classification.

Sneppen Classification of Talar Body Fractures	
Grade	**Fracture Type**
1	Transchondral/osteochondral
2	Coronal, sagittal, or horizontal shear
3	Posterior tubercle
4	Lateral process
5	Crush fracture

Undisplaced fractures can be treated in a non–weight-bearing below-knee cast for 6 to 8 weeks until the fracture is healed and the outcome is excellent. Undisplaced intra-articular fractures can be treated in the same way; however, serial radiographs must be taken to confirm displacement does not occur. Anatomic reduction of displaced fractures has been recommended because residual displacement of the articular surfaces leads to degenerative osteoarthritis.[68]

FRACTURES OF THE LATERAL PROCESS OF THE TALAR BODY

Fractures of the lateral process of the talus are uncommon in adults and children, and a high level of suspicion is required if the diagnosis is to be made. The lateral process is a wedge-shaped prominence that forms almost the whole lateral wall of the talus. The mechanism of injury is a forced dorsiflexion injury with inversion of the foot.[42] The talocalcaneal ligament may avulse the lateral process.

Isolated fractures of the lateral process of the talus are often not recognized on the initial radiographs.[42,44,78] Wu et al.[139] found that 42% of fractures were missed initially in their series of lateral process fractures. The lateral process is best visualized on the mortise view so the fibula is not overlying it. On the lateral radiograph, the lateral process is seen just superior to the angle of Gissane.[44] This is the angle between a line drawn along the lateral border of posterior facet and a line drawn along the anterior process (Fig. 31-9). If there is persistent pain laterally around the ankle following an inversion ankle injury, one should have a high suspicion for a lateral process fracture or an osteochondral injury. If injury not clearly seen on the plain films, a CT scan should be performed to assess the talus and rule out any other coexisting fractures.[59,90]

The incidence of this once-rare injury increased with the rising popularity of snowboarding.[59,78,89] Kirkpatrick et al.[59] reviewed 3,213 snowboarding injuries and found an unusually high incidence of lateral process fractures, representing 13.5% of all snowboarding foot and ankle injuries.

The treatment of nondisplaced fractures of the lateral process is with a non–weight-bearing cast for 6 to 8 weeks. Displaced fractures are best treated with ORIF; however, the degree of displacement that is acceptable in a child is not clearly defined. What may be more important is the congruity of the joint surface of the talus. A step or gap in the articular surface of more than 2 to 3 mm may be useful criteria as to when to open reduce the fracture. The fracture can be held with one 3.5-mm partially threaded cancellous screw inserted from lateral to medial perpendicular to the fracture line. A below-knee cast is then worn for 6 weeks.[42,44,66]

FRACTURES OF THE OSTEOCHONDRAL SURFACE OF THE TALUS

Damage to the osteochondral surface of the talus can be caused by direct trauma or may be caused by an underlying

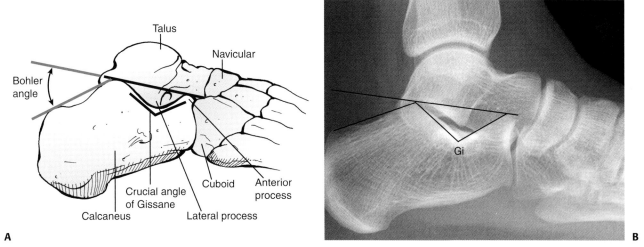

Figure 31-9. Diagrammatic (**A**) and radiographic (**B**) depictions of the crucial angle of Gissane (Gi) and the Bohler (Bo) angles. The Bohler angle is more frequently used for decision making regarding fracture management. For measuring the Bohler angle, the landmarks on the lateral radiograph of the calcaneus are the anterior and posterior facets and the superior margin of the calcaneal tuberosity.

osteochondral lesion (osteochondritis dissecans [OCD]) that may have been present for some time and has been made symptomatic by the injury. The pathogenesis and etiology of OCD are controversial; however, most authors report preceding trauma as a cause of the defects (Canale and Belding[16] 80%, Letts et al.[68] 79%, Higuera et al.[47] 63%, and Perumal et al.[95] 47%). Medial lesions are usually deeper and cup shaped compared to the thinner "wafer" type lateral lesions. Lateral lesions are more often associated with trauma and more symptomatic than medial lesions. It is postulated that medial lesions may be caused by repetitive microtrauma.[16,17] Berndt and Harty,[8] in 1959, used freshly amputated legs to biomechanically reproduce injuries to the ankle and observe the injuries inflicted. They showed that the anterolateral talus hits the medial aspect of the fibula with dorsiflexion and inversion and that plantarflexion and inversion caused posteromedial osteochondral lesions (Fig. 31-10).

The initial radiographs following an ankle injury in a child should be closely assessed for an osteochondral injury. If pain and swelling persist for over 2 months after an "ankle sprain," then further investigations should be carried out to look for an osteochondral lesion, which will initially be a further radiograph series. However, an MRI scan is often more useful at this stage to look for an osteochondral lesion as a small percentage are purely cartilaginous. Some consider an MRI arthrogram useful in further determining whether the fragment is detached as occasionally the arthrographic contrast can be seen deep in to the osteochondral lesion. The bone scan has largely been superseded by the MRI scan in the diagnosis and assessment of these lesions. The bone scan is useful, however, when it is not clear if the pain in the child's ankle is coming from the osteochondral lesion or some other pathology. A normal bone scan in the presence of a stage I or II osteochondral lesion may indicate a soft tissue lesion as being a source of the pain.

Mechanical symptoms of locking and catching are not as common as one would think but can occur with these lesions if the loose fragment becomes trapped within the joint. The pain seems to be related to the synovitis and effusion that develops secondary to the uneven articular surface. On examination, the ankle is slightly swollen and can be painful on passive movement as the loose fragment passes under the tibia. With plantarflexion of the foot, the anterolateral talus can be palpated directly, and a lesion here is painful on direct pressure.

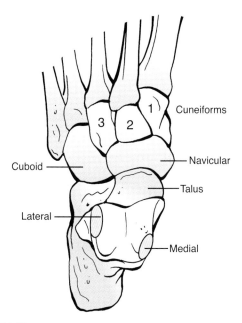

Figure 31-10. Typical positions of osteochondral lesions of the talus. Berndt and Harty[8] found that of 201 osteochondral lesions in adults 56% were on the medial side and 44% on the lateral side. Letts et al. found medial lesions in 79% of 24 children, lateral lesions in 21%, and central lesions in 1%. (Reprinted with permission from Letts M, et al. Osteochondritis dissecans of the talus in children. *J Pediatr Orthop.* 2003;23(5):617–625.)

CLASSIFICATION OF FRACTURES OF THE OSTEOCHONDRAL SURFACE OF THE TALUS

Berndt and Henry Classification of Fractures of the Osteochondral Surface of the Talus	
Stage	**Description**
I	Subchondral trabecular compression fracture (not seen radiographically)
II	Incomplete separation of an osteochondral fragment
III	The osteochondral fragment is unattached but undisplaced
IV	A displaced osteochondral fragment

Berndt and Harty[8] classified osteochondral fractures of the talar dome into four stages based on radiographic criteria (Fig. 31-11).

Anderson et al.[4] modified this classification after correlating clinical findings with radiographs and MRI scans. They described the stage I lesion as not visible on plain radiographs but visible on an MRI scan. They also introduced a stage IIa lesion, which is an undisplaced osteochondral lesion with a subchondral cyst adjacent to the floor of the lesion. Anderson et al.[4] thought a stage IIa lesion should be treated surgically whereas a stage II lesion can initially be treated nonoperatively (Fig. 31-12).

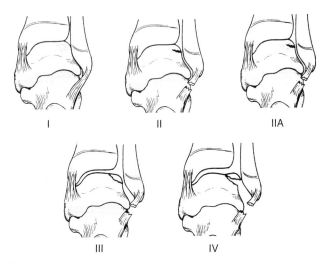

Figure 31-11. Adaptation of the Berndt and Harty[8] (1959) classification of osteochondral injuries of the talus by Anderson et al.[4] Stage I is identified only by MRI scanning, which demonstrates trabecular compression of subchondral bone. Stage II lesions have incomplete separation of the osteochondral fragment from the talus. If a subchondral cyst also is present, the lesion is designated stage IIa. Stage III lesions occur when the fragment is no longer attached to the talus but is undisplaced. Stage IV indicates both complete detachment and displacement. (Reprinted with permission from Alexander IF, et al. Osteochondral fractures of the dome of the talus. *J Bone Joint Surg Am.* 1989;71(8):1143–1152.)

Figure 31-12. This CT scan clearly shows a well-circumscribed cyst at the base of a stage II osteochondral lesion. This would be classified by Anderson et al.[4] as a stage IIa lesion.

A further classification was proposed by Pritsch et al.[100] in 1986 based on the arthroscopic appearance of the articular cartilage. The quality of the articular cartilage was placed into one of three grades:

Pritsch Classification of Fractures of the Osteochondral Surface of the Talus	
Grade	**Description**
I	Intact, firm, and shiny articular cartilage
II	Intact but soft articular cartilage
III	Frayed articular cartilage

They used this classification to determine which lesions should be treated with activity modification (grade I), which patients should have arthroscopic drilling (grade II), and finally which patients require arthroscopic curettage and microfracture (grade III).

TREATMENT OPTIONS FOR OSTEOCHONDRAL FRACTURES OF THE TALUS

The treatment of osteochondral lesions of the talus in children is challenging. Only a few papers purely address this condition in children,[47,68,95] and the rest of the literature is a combination of adult and childhood lesions. It is important to distinguish between an acute osteochondral fracture and a chronic osteochondral lesion as the two may require different treatment strategies.

To enable thorough assessment, these patients need to be followed up for a minimum of 2 years as it takes this long for the lesion to become radiographically healed despite the child often being clinically normal.[95]

Figure 31-13. A: Anterolateral stage III osteochondral lesion that was treated by arthroscopic excision and microfracture. **B:** Posteromedial stage II osteochondral lesion that was treated successfully nonoperatively.

Nonoperative Treatment

Most authors agree that the primary treatment of stage I and stage II lesions is nonoperative.[8,47,68,95] The symptomatic patient can be immobilized for 6 weeks in a below-knee walking cast or a Cam walker (Fig. 31-13). This usually relieves the acute symptoms; over the next 6 weeks, the patient has activity modification maintaining a pain-free range of movement. This allows the fracture to heal before returning to active sports. Higuera et al.[47] treated their stage III lesions nonoperatively as well and all seven patients had good outcomes.

Operative Treatment

The outcomes of surgery for osteochondral fractures of the talus are controversial. It is hard to compare results between authors as they have often used different outcome measures. Some authors use pain as their primary outcome,[68] whereas others also consider radiologic healing. The long-term outcome of an asymptomatic subchondral lucency in the talar body is unknown. In some series, the patients have had arthrotomies,[68] whereas others had arthroscopic debridement.[95] The staging of the lesions is also subject to interobserver variability.[68] With modern ankle arthroscopy equipment and newer surgical techniques, ankle arthroscopy has become the primary surgical treatment for both medial and lateral lesions of the talar dome. The anterolateral lesions are more accessible; however, with good ankle distraction and different portal placement posteromedial lesions are accessible, as well.

Perumal et al.[95] reviewed 31 patients with juvenile OCD and a minimum of 6-month follow-up. They recommended nonoperative treatment with an ankle brace and activity modification for 6 months in most cases. Only 16% of the lesions healed radiographically in that timeframe. If pain continues after this time and the lesion is still present, further immobilization and activity modification is recommended. They recommend arthroscopic surgery for patients with type II lesions who are not prepared to modify their activities longer than 6 months, and patients with type III lateral lesions, and all stage IV lesions. Thirteen of the 31 patients were treated surgically.

Arthroscopic treatment options include[62,100]:

- Drilling the lesion (antegrade or retrograde)
- Curettage and microfracture
- Internal fixation with bioabsorbable nails
- Bone grafting and internal fixation

In stage II lesions with intact articular cartilage, Kumai et al.[62] showed excellent results drilling through the lesion into the subchondral bone. The authors also found that in skeletally immature patients, there may be an increased tendency for the lesion to heal when compared to the adult patients. Retrograde drilling can be performed using specific tip directed instrumentation. This approach avoids damage to the articular cartilage and may prevent fragmentation of a small lesion. Access to a posteromedial lesion can be difficult. One approach is to use a transmalleolar portal after drilling a 3.5-mm drill through the medial malleolus or to use a posteromedial portal, taking care to avoid damaging the neurovascular bundle.

Curettage and microfracture is a very effective, relatively straightforward procedure. It is particularly useful in small stage III and stage IV lesions where the fragment is too small to internally fix or there is no subchondral bone on the lesion for healing. The articular cartilage is debrided back to stable tissue and the subchondral bone is curettaged until bleeding occurs. Either a microfracture pick or 2-mm drill is then used in the subchondral bone. Anderson et al.[4] would suggest this treatment for all stage IIa lesions in which a subchondral cyst is present.

Internal fixation with or without bone grafting is a difficult procedure for an inexperienced arthroscopist. It is preferable to use absorbable pegs or nails rather than metallic implants. In large stage III and IV acute osteochondral lesions, this is probably the treatment of choice rather than excising the fragment.

Author's Preferred Technique for Talus OCD Injuries (Algorithm 31-1)

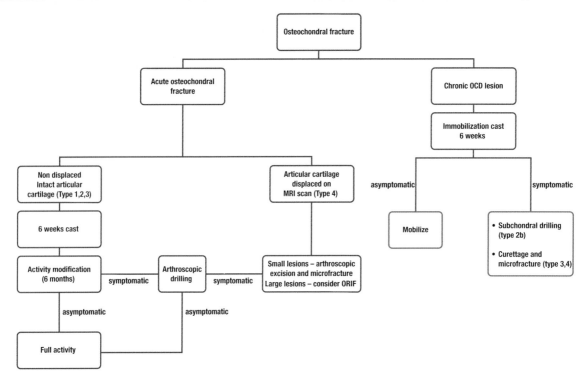

Algorithm 31-1. Authors preferred treatment for talus OCD injuries.

For simple undisplaced fractures, a below-knee nonwalking cast is applied for 6 weeks.

Displaced lateral process fractures need to be anatomically reduced especially if they are intra-articular and there is 2 to 3 mm of incongruity in the joint surface. A lateral approach is used and a single compression screw inserted across the fracture. The foot is immobilized in a below-knee cast for 6 weeks.

Displaced talar neck fractures should be operated on as soon as possible. If the fracture can be reduced closed, the authors prefer a posterolateral approach to insert the compression screws as this helps preserve the tenuous blood supply (see Fig. 31-7). These screws are best inserted through this open approach so an accurate starting point can be found and neurovascular structures protected. The authors have no hesitation to use an anteromedial approach as well to help with fracture reduction before inserting the screws. Through this approach, the neck fragment can be stabilized while the screws are being compressed and anatomic fracture reduction can be seen. Usually, two 4.5-mm partially threaded titanium screws are used depending on the size of the talus and degree of fragmentation. The titanium screws allow MRI postoperatively if osteonecrosis is suspected.

Acute osteochondral injuries need to be recognized and distinguished from osteochondritis dissecans (OCD) lesions. Acute lesions should be repaired after assessing the amount of bone present on the lesion. This can be initially assessed arthrocopically but is repaired through an arthrotomy depending on the position on the talus. The author prefers to repair the lesion with dissolvable nails.

The authors treat types I to III OCD lesions nonoperatively for 6 months. Initially, the child or adolescent wears a Cam walker for 4 to 6 weeks to help the symptoms settle and then an elastic ankle support and activity modification. If symptoms persist, the authors perform a repeat MRI scan and, if the staging has worsened, proceeds to an arthroscopic debridement and microfracture or stabilization. For patients with displaced fragments on presentation (stage IV), the authors recommend arthroscopic removal and microfracture or repair if possible.

MANAGEMENT OF EXPECTED ADVERSE OUTCOMES AND UNEXPECTED COMPLICATIONS RELATED TO TALAR FRACTURES

Osteonecrosis of the talus is the most serious complication of talus fractures. It has been reported in a number of large series of predominantly adult patients. Osteonecrosis of the body of the talus occurs when the blood supply has been disrupted by a fracture of the talar neck. The result is necrosis of the talar dome and possible collapse of the articular surface. Hawkins[42] described the presence of a subchondral lucent line, the "Hawkins sign," as prognostic of a good outcome as it indicates adequate blood flow to the talar body. The absence of the sign on a

6- to 8-week radiograph implies there is inadequate blood supply and osteonecrosis may evolve. In adults, a negative Hawkins sign has been found to be highly sensitive but not specific for future development of AVN.[127]

In adults, the incidence of osteonecrosis seems directly related to the Hawkins classification type. Hawkins[42] showed that type I fractures had a 0% to 10% AVN rate, type II fractures a 20% to 50% AVN rate, type III an 80% to 100% AVN rate, and all type IV fractures develop AVN. Canale and Kelly[17] had similar long-term results.

Osteonecrosis has also been seen in pediatric talus fractures, with multiple reports of talus AVN.[103,126] The Hawkins sign was described in adults, and Ogden[92] suggested this sign may not be as reliable in the cartilaginous talar dome of a child. The rate of AVN after pediatric talus fractures is uncertain, with series ranging from 0% to 20%.[32,55] More recently, a series of 25 pediatric talus fractures reported no cases of AVN a final follow-up in patients less than 12 years old. This finding suggests that, while case reports exist of AVN in young patients,[103,126] the outcome can be expected to be favorable in patients younger than 12 years old who have sustained a talus fracture.[32]

The dilemma for the treating surgeon is what to advise the patient regarding weight bearing when the Hawkins sign is not present by 8 weeks. AVN may occur 6 months after the injury and not resolve for many years. There does not appear to be any series comparing outcomes in patients who bear weight over this period and those who do not. If the Hawkins sign is not present, it is advisable to perform an MRI scan at 3 months to establish whether AVN is present.[45,127] If present, it may be advisable to encourage the child to avoid impact activities to prevent collapse rather than have a prolonged period of non–weight bearing.

Calcaneal Fractures

INTRODUCTION TO CALCANEAL FRACTURES

Fractures of the calcaneus are rare in children, with an incidence of only 1 in 100,000 fractures.[137] The treatment of these fractures has historically been nonoperative, relying on the largely cartilaginous bone to remodel with time. The majority of fractures in children are extra-articular,[82] whereas in older children, the fracture pattern resembles that in adults. Children appear to have more coexisting lower limb fractures than adults but fewer fractures of the axial skeleton.[116]

Calcaneal fractures in young children are often missed or are diagnosed late. At the other end of the spectrum, the adolescent patient has often had a major fall and has a displaced intra-articular fracture. This older age group should be treated like the adult population—with ORIF to restore the joint congruity and calcaneal height and width.[87] The challenge for the surgeon is at what age and what degree of displacement is this more aggressive treatment indicated in a group of patients traditionally treated nonoperatively.

ASSESSMENT OF CALCANEAL FRACTURES

MECHANISMS OF INJURY FOR CALCANEAL FRACTURES

By far the most common mechanism of injury is a fall from a height.[12,53] The axial load drives the talus into the calcaneus resulting in the fracture. The degree of comminution appears to be less in children even though they often fall from greater heights than adults.[13] Wiley and Profitt[137] found that in young children, the fall was usually less than 4 feet and in children older than 10 years the fall was greater than 14 feet. They noted that the minor falls in the younger children often resulted in undisplaced fractures that were diagnosed late.

In Schmidt and Weiner's[116] review of pediatric calcaneal fractures they found that children less than 14 years of age predominantly had extra-articular fractures, hypothesizing that the calcaneus in this age bracket absorbs the compression force rather than dissipating it through the joint. This finding is supported by Mora et al.,[82] who found 78% extra-articular fractures in their series of pediatric calcaneus fractures.

Vehicle-related injuries were the second biggest cause of calcaneal fractures in both Schmidt and Weiner[116] and Wiley and Profitt's reviews.[137] Fractures of the calcaneus can also occur in major crush injuries when compartment syndrome may coexist, and open fractures are common in lawnmower injuries.

SIGNS AND SYMPTOMS OF CALCANEAL FRACTURES

Any child who has fallen from a height and landed on their feet should be examined carefully for a calcaneal fracture. Associated injuries should also be evaluated with a thorough secondary survey, especially of the lower limbs, distal radius, and spine.

The foot will often be extremely swollen with bruising around the heel and dorsum of the foot. Symptoms and signs of compartment syndrome, including excessive pain, pallor, paresthesia, and pulselessness should be assessed. In more subtle injuries, careful palpation is necessary to elucidate areas of pain which may disclose an underlying undisplaced fracture.

Many calcaneal fractures in children are initially missed and diagnosed late. Often, the fracture line is not evident on the initial radiographs. Inokuchi et al.[53] reported that 44% of fractures in their series were initially missed, as were 55% of those reported by Schantz and Rasmussen[114] and 44% of those reported by Wiley and Profitt.[137]

A differential diagnosis must be kept in mind for other causes of heel pain in a child. These include Sever disease, osteomyelitis, a unicameral bone cyst, or a stress fracture.

INJURIES ASSOCIATED WITH CALCANEAL FRACTURES

Schmidt and Weiner[116] reviewed 56 children with calcaneal fractures and found a number of associated injuries. These included fractures of the lumbar spine, lower limb fractures, a pelvic fracture, and upper extremity fractures. These other skeletal injuries were more frequent in children over 13 years of age. Associated lower limb fractures occurred twice as frequently as in adults; however, injuries to the axial skeleton occurred half as often as in adults. Wiley and Profitt,[137] however, only had two patients with accompanying significant injuries in their series of 32 pediatric calcaneal fractures.

IMAGING AND OTHER DIAGNOSTIC STUDIES FOR CALCANEAL FRACTURES

Radiography

Calcaneal fractures in children are often not diagnosed initially as the radiographic findings are usually more subtle than in adults. Subsequent radiographs at 2 weeks often show the fracture line. Most of these fractures are extra-articular.

The standard views for a suspected calcaneal fracture are posteroanterior, lateral, and Harris (axial) views. The posteroanterior view shows the calcaneocuboid and talonavicular joints well. The lateral view is excellent at showing the congruity of the posterior articular facet and allows calculation of Bohler angle (see Fig. 31-9). The axial view demonstrates the tuberosity, the body, the sustentaculum tali, and the posterior facet of the calcaneus. Oblique views are also useful and will show a fracture of the anterior process more clearly (Fig. 31-14).[104] The oblique views also define the subtalar joint well and, thus, are very useful in identifying intra-articular fractures. Broden views can also be taken that look at the posterior facet of the calcaneus. These are taken with the leg internally rotated 40 degrees and the x-ray beam angled between 15 and 40 degrees toward the head.[11] This image is a difficult radiograph for the technicians to master, and almost the same information can be

Figure 31-14. Fracture of the anterior process of the calcaneus.

achieved by ordering a mortise view of the ankle to look at the posterior facet of the subtalar joint.

The lateral view is useful for measuring the Bohler angle, which is the angle between a line drawn from the highest point of the anterior process to the highest point of the posterior facet and a line drawn tangential to the highest point of the calcaneal tuberosity. The normal value in an adult is between 20 and 40 degrees. In a child, the angle is slightly less than in an adult, which may be caused by the incomplete ossification of the calcaneus. It is advisable to perform a lateral radiograph of the contralateral calcaneus to use as a comparison rather than accept the absolute value of Bohler angle. The child's calcaneus does not resemble that of an adult until after 10 years of age.[51,92] Another angle which is not easy to measure is "the crucial angle of Gissane," which is the angle formed by two strong cortical struts seen on the lateral radiograph. One runs along the lateral margin of the posterior facet and the other runs up to the anterior process of the calcaneus. This angle ranges from 95 to 105 degrees (see Fig. 31-9).

When reviewing radiographs of children's feet, it is always important to be cognizant of the ossification centers and accessory bones within the growing foot, which often are confused with fractures (see Figs. 31-1 and 31-2). The os calcis is the earliest tarsal bone to ossify with the primary ossification center appearing in the third intrauterine month. The secondary ossification center appears around 6 to 8 years and is the crescentic epiphysis seen posteriorly. This epiphysis fuses to the body of the calcaneus between 14 and 16 years of age.

The use of a technetium-labeled bone scan in diagnosing calcaneal fractures is uncommon with the ready availability of MRI scans. The bone scan has been used to evaluate a nonlocalized painful limp in a toddler. However, often clinical judgment and radiographic follow-up are sufficient in the diagnosis of pain following trauma, making a bone scan unnecessary.[115]

Computed Tomography

CT scanning has evolved as the best method to evaluate the fractured calcaneus. Not only does it clearly show the fracture lines and altered anatomy, but also reveals injuries to adjacent bones. Sanders et al.[110] have used CT scans to develop a classification system that is particularly useful in the preoperative planning of open reduction of these fractures. The primary and secondary fracture lines are identified, and the degree of comminution and position of the fragments are more accurately seen than in the radiographs. The primary fracture line usually runs obliquely from plantar medial to dorsolateral exiting the posterior facet. Secondary fracture lines that develop off this primary line are also seen and their pattern determines the classification of the fracture (Fig. 31-15). The CT scan also allows a three-dimensional reconstruction, which can be useful in preoperative planning.

Buckingham et al.[13] and Ogden[92] reviewed 9 patients with 10 calcaneal fractures and performed CT scans on all of them. They found the fracture patterns in these adolescents (average 13.4 years old) to be very similar to those found in adults. They did find less comminution in children than in adults, even though the children reportedly had fallen from greater heights.

Figure 31-15. Sanders CT-based classification of intra-articular fractures of the calcaneus in adults. (Reprinted with permission from Sanders R. Intraarticular fractures of the calcaneus: Present state of the art. *J Orthop Trauma.* 1992;6(2):252–265.)

MRI scans are largely unnecessary. They can be useful in young children when the calcaneus is still largely cartilaginous and a fracture is not seen on plain films or CT.

CLASSIFICATION OF CALCANEAL FRACTURES

Children's calcaneal fractures were traditionally classified according to their adult counterparts using the Essex-Lopresti[36] and Letournel[67] classifications. Schmidt and Weiner[116] reviewed 62 calcaneal fractures in children and compared them to the adult literature. They used the classification systems of Essex-Lopresti[36] and Chapman and Galway[21] and added a new fracture type (type VI) to develop a classification for pediatric calcaneal fractures that is in routine use today (Fig. 31-16).

For adolescent fractures, it is probably more appropriate to use the Sanders classification.[111] This adult classification system was developed after reviewing the CT scans on 120 cases preoperatively and at minimum 1-year follow-up. The follow-up CT scans were correlated with the clinical outcome scores to help validate the classification system used.

PATHOANATOMY AND APPLIED ANATOMY RELATING TO CALCANEAL FRACTURES

The calcaneus is the largest tarsal bone and has an unusual shape. It has three articular facets (anterior, middle, and posterior) on the superior surface where it articulates with the talus to form the subtalar joint (see Fig. 31-5). Anteriorly there is a saddle-shaped articular surface for the cuboid. The posterior

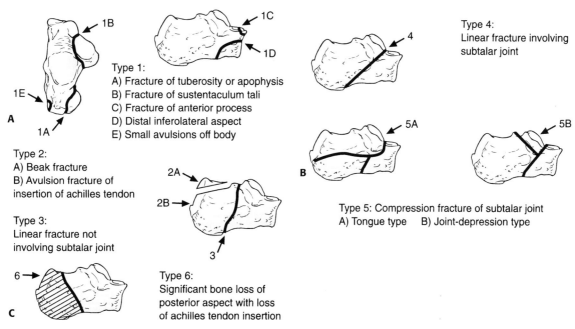

Figure 31-16. Schmidt and Weiner classification of calcaneal fracture patterns in children. **A:** Extra-articular fractures. **B:** Intra-articular fractures. **C:** Type VI fracture pattern with significant bone loss, soft tissue injury, and loss of Achilles tendon insertion. (Reprinted with permission from Schmidt TL, Weiner DS. Calcaneus fractures in children: An evaluation of the nature of injury in 56 children. *Clin Orthop Relat Res.* 1982;171:150–155.)

facet is the largest facet and is slightly convex. The middle facet is anterior and medial to the posterior facet, lying on the sustentaculum tali. It is concave like the anterior facet with which it is often contiguous. Between the middle and posterior facets lies the calcaneal groove, which forms the inferior wall of the sinus tarsi. Posteriorly, the tendo Achilles inserts into the tuberosity of the calcaneus, which is the entire area behind the posterior facet. On the lateral surface of the calcaneus are two shallow grooves with a small ridge in between (the peroneal trochlea). The peroneus longus and brevis run either side of this trochlea. The medial side is concave and is structurally stronger than the lateral side. The sustentaculum tali projects from the medial wall and supports the middle articular facet on its surface. The tendon of flexor hallucis longus runs on the undersurface of the sustentaculum. On the plantar surface are the medial and lateral processes, which represent the origin of the abductor hallucis and abductor digiti minimi muscles, respectively (Fig. 31-17).

Secondary ossification occurs in the calcaneal apophysis between the ages of 6 and 10 years. Inflammation in the apophysis around this age causes heel pain and is referred to as Sever disease.

The use of CT scans has defined the surgical anatomy of the calcaneus to help make treatment decisions. The coronal views show the important posterior facet and the sustentaculum tali and the height and width of the heel. The position of the peroneal tendons and flexor hallucis tendon can also be seen. The sagittal views provide additional information about the posterior facet and also show the anterior process well. The axial views visualize the calcaneocuboid joint well, the anteroinferior aspect of the posterior facet, and the sustentaculum tali. This information can be used in planning the reconstruction of the calcaneus.[111,112]

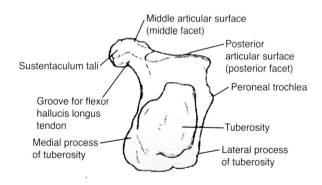

Figure 31-17. Anatomic details of various angles of the calcaneus including lateral (**A**), medial (**B**), and coronal (**C**) views through the level of the sustentaculum tali, which correlate with the CT scan view important in reconstruction of the posterior facet.

Calcaneal fractures in growing children are usually less severe than in the adult population and often do well with nonoperative treatment.[12,53] In adolescents, fracture patterns are often similar to adults and require ORIF. The challenge to the orthopaedic surgeon is to recognize the patient that requires this treatment. There is a degree of remodeling that will take place in the child and hence the amount of growth remaining, degree of ossification, and difference in morphology from the contralateral side all should be considered in making treatment decisions.

Extra-articular fractures of the calcaneus can be treated by cast immobilization for 6 weeks. The child can start weight bearing in this cast when comfortable and can be changed to a Cam walker for the final few weeks.[12,53]

Tongue-type fractures can be treated nonoperatively if the posterior gap is less than 1 cm and the Achilles tendon has not been significantly shortened by bringing the fragment up proximally. Occasionally, the technique described by Essex-Lopresti[36] for percutaneous reduction of tongue-type fractures (Fig. 31-18) is useful. A recently published survey of OTA and AOFAS members stated that 29.3% of respondents add a gastrocnemius recession at the time of definitive fixation of a tongue type calcaneus fracture in the presence of positive contralateral Silfverskiöld test.[94]

ORIF is reserved for the intra-articular fractures with displacement of the fragments and depression of the joint surfaces. These fractures occur almost exclusively in the adolescent patient, in whom the ossification process is complete. The adult literature abounds with indications for internal fixation, surgical approaches, rehabilitation, complications, and outcome measures (Fig. 31-19).[6,112] These series only have a few adolescent fractures among them, so it is difficult to draw any conclusions specifically about children's calcaneal fractures. The literature on the management of displaced intra-articular fractures in children is somewhat conflicting in the indications for

surgery. Schantz and Rasmussen[114] reported on the outcome of displaced intra-articular fractures in children less than 15 years old treated nonoperatively. Most patients had a good outcome, but four complained of pain an average of 12 years after injury. Brunet[12] asserts that the outcome does not correlate to the severity of the fracture in young patients, which is likely due to the remodeling potential of the calcaneus in this age group. Mora et al.[82] also concluded that open reduction may be suitable only for severely displaced fractures in adolescents. The difficulty is defining the age or maturity of the patient that may predict a poor outcome if the fracture is left unreduced. Using validated quality-of-life scales 2 to 8 years after surgery, O'Brien et al.[91] found that younger patients (adults under the age of 30 years) who had operative treatment had better gait satisfaction scores than those who did not have surgery. Allmacher et al.[3] questioned whether short-term or intermediate results of displaced intra-articular calcaneal fractures can predict long-term functional outcome. Using validated outcome instruments, they studied adult patients treated nonoperatively and found that nonoperative treatment often led to pain and loss of function, which increased in the second decade after injury.

Good results have been reported when ORIF has been used to treat displaced intra-articular closed calcaneus fractures in older children, mean age 11.5 to 13 years old.[97,98] In these studies, only one incisional breakdown was reported in 35 patients, which was successfully treated with wet-to-dry dressings and oral antibiotics. Ceccarelli et al.[18] found that skeletally mature children with displaced intra-articular fractures had better clinical and radiologic outcomes if treated by open reduction rather than nonoperatively. Is there any other important take-home message from this paper that would help a surgeon decide who would benefit from open reduction? Buckingham et al.[13] reviewed 10 adolescent patients and reported good or excellent outcomes in 8 patients. They had no wound complications and the motion was hardly affected in seven patients.

The surgery for these fractures is technically demanding, and, if the treating surgeon is not experienced with the approach, the child is best referred to a colleague who is.

Figure 31-18. Percutaneous reduction technique for tongue-type fractures of the calcaneus, as described by Essex-Lopresti.[36] This technique remains an alternative to conservative treatment and open reduction with internal fixation of displaced, tongue-type fractures. **A:** A pin is inserted into the tongue fragment and used as a joystick to manipulate the fragment into better position, usually with a downward force on the pin and the forefoot (plantarflexion). **B:** After reduction, the pin is driven across the fracture to maintain reduction. (Redrawn with permission from Tornetta A III. The Essex-Lopresti reduction for calcaneal fractures revisited. *J Orthop Trauma.* 1998;12(7):469–473.)

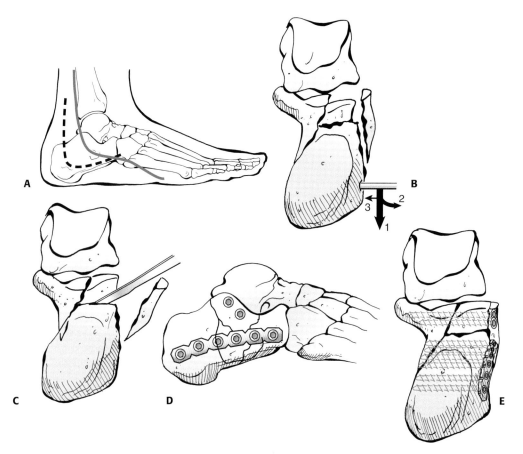

Figure 31-19. A: Lateral L-shaped approach to displaced intra-articular calcaneal fractures. The incision (*dashed line*) is laterally based, with the proximal arm approximately half the distance from the fibula to the posterior border of the foot and the distal arm halfway from the tip of the fibula to the sole of the foot. The sural nerve is illustrated. A full-thickness, subperiosteal flap exposes the entire lateral calcaneus. **B:** Reduction maneuvers 1, 2, and 3 (*densest arrow indicates greatest displacement*) with a Schanz screw are used to pull the tuberosity down and allow access to disimpact the posterior facet (**C**) after the lateral wall of the calcaneus is levered open. The posterior facet is then reduced anatomically, held provisionally with K-wires, and then fixed with two partially threaded cancellous screws (outside of plate) into the sustentaculum tali. Lateral view (**D**) of reduced calcaneus and axial view (**E**) of reduced fracture with hardware. (Redrawn with permission from Benirschke SK, Sangeorzan BJ. Extraarticular fractures of the foot: Surgical management of calcaneal fractures [Review]. *Clin Orthop Relat Res.* 1993;292:128–134.)

Author's Preferred Treatment for Calcaneal Fractures (Algorithm 31-2)

The key decision in treating children's calcaneal fractures is which require surgical intervention. Almost all closed fractures in children less than 10 years of age can be treated nonoperatively because of the remodeling potential, which includes intra-articular fractures that are displaced.

Extra-articular fractures of the calcaneus can be treated by nonoperative means with a below-knee cast for 6 weeks. Weight bearing in the cast can start after 2 to 3 weeks as the patient becomes more comfortable.

Undisplaced intra-articular fractures can also be treated in a below-knee cast. In this group of patients, it is advisable for them to be non–weight bearing for 6 weeks or until the fracture is healed to prevent further displacement.

Adolescent patients with displaced intra-articular fractures are best treated by ORIF (see Figs. 31-19 and 31-20). Prior to surgery, a thorough assessment of the skin needs to be performed. Surgery should be delayed to allow swelling to subside and fracture blisters to resolve, which will decrease some of the wound complications seen after open fixation of adult calcaneal fractures. An important point in performing this surgery is to maintain thick skin flaps, restore joint congruity, use specialized calcaneal plates, and be prepared to bone graft the defect. An outline of the surgical technique is in Table 31-2.

Algorithm 31-2. Author's preferred treatment for calcaneal fractures.

Figure 31-20. Intra-articular depressed fracture of the calcaneus in a 13-year-old boy. **A:** Preoperative sagittal CT shows the depression of the posterior facet into the body of the calcaneus. **B:** Coronal CT shows the displacement of the fracture fragments. **C:** Postoperative CT scans are useful at checking the fracture reduction and length and position of the screws. **D, E:** Postoperative radiographs confirm restoration of the Bohler angle.

TABLE 31-2. Operative Planning for Open Reduction and Internal Fixation of Intra-Articular Calcaneal Fractures in Adolescents

Equipment	Radiolucent table	Fixation	Contour 2.7-mm reconstruction plate or an Association of Osteosynthesis (AO) calcaneal plate to the lateral wall of the os calcis and fix to anterior process and the posterior tuber
	Image Intensifier	Closure	
	K-wires with driver		
	Lambotte osteotomes		Maintain posterior facet reduction with two interfragmentary screws angled well inferiorly to avoid the inferiorly curved medial surface of the calcaneal posterior facet and to engage the sustentaculum
	Periosteal elevators		
	AO modular foot set		
	Synthes calcaneal plates, 2.7-mm reconstruction plates, H cervical plates		
Positioning	Lateral decubitus on contralateral side	Irrigation	
	Upper thigh pneumatic tourniquet		Always drain
	Hip flexed 45 degrees, knee flexed 90 degrees		Two-layered closure
	Seattle cushions		2-0 Vicryl to the subcutaneous tissues (interrupted vertical. Place all sutures on clips, tie individually commencing at the apex of the incision)
	Radiolucent operating table		
Incision	L-shaped incision (Letournel, Regazzoni, Bernirschke) Curved at apex		Skin closure with interrupted 3-0 nylon Allgöwer–Donati sutures (all placed on clips and then tied individually commencing at the apex moving symmetrically to the proximal and distal extent of the wound holding multiple sutures to maintain even tension)
	Proximal extent 3-cm cephalad to tip of fibula anterior to lateral border of Achilles tendon		
	Distal extent tip of base of fifth metatarsal		
Exposure	Blunt dissection with scissors proximally to identify the short saphenous vein and sural nerve	Dressings	Gelnet dressing
	Sharp dissection with no. 15 blade direct to lateral wall of os calcaneus	Postoperative	Well-padded below-knee popliteal joint back slab supporting toes
	Subperiosteal reflection with scalpel		Elevation on two pillows
	Sharp dissection and reflection of peroneal tendons and attachment of calcaneofibular ligament dorsally		IV antibiotics
	Keep dorsal to the muscle belly of abductor digiti minimi		CT scan to check reduction and exclude screw malposition
	Protect peroneal tendons with baby Hoffmann retractors when exposing the anterior process and calcaneocuboid joint		Remove drain when drainage is less than 10 mL over an 8-hour period
	Elevate flap dorsally to expose the posterior facet of the talus and sinus tarsi		Review wound for hematoma and skin viability within 48 hours
	Maintain flap anteriorly with K-wires placed into the body and neck of the talus and the fibula		Continue splintage, elevation, and restricted mobility non–weight bearing until sutures removed 14–18 days after surgery
	Deflate tourniquet when exposure complete		
Reduction	Place Schanz pin in inferior aspect of posterior tuber		
	Reduce fracture by traction on the Schanz pin displacing posterior tuber inferiorly and thence medially		
	Reflect lateral wall laterally if necessary		
	Reduce anterior process first, then posterior facet, and finally restore alignment of the os calcis by confirming reduction and alignment of the crucial angle		
	Thus, reduce anterior to posterior, medial to lateral, and dorsal to plantar		
	Provisional reduction maintained with multiple K-wires		
	Reduction and alignment confirmed by screening with image intensifier		

Courtesy of Dr. Campbell ACL. *FRACS, Adult Foot and Ankle Surgeon.* Auckland City Hospital, New Zealand.

WOUND COMPLICATIONS

Wound dehiscence is the most common complication following open reduction of adult calcaneal fractures.[6,50]

Although reported to occur in up to 25% of adult fractures, the incidence is lower in children. Pickle et al.[98] had no wound problems in the six adolescents (age range 11–16 years) they treated with ORIF. All the patients were treated with an extensile lateral approach for an average of 10.5 days from the time of injury. The lower incidence in children reflects fewer risk factors in this group when compared to the adult population. Smoking, obesity, and diabetes can all contribute to wound problems.

Wound dehiscence can be decreased by meticulous closure of the incision. In adults, it has been shown that a two-layer closure is preferable to a single layer of sutures.[38] Wound dehiscence can occur from days to weeks after the surgery. The best initial treatment is immobilization to decrease tension on the wound edges, which is best accomplished by using a below-knee cast with a large window cut around the entire incision. This technique allows space for wound dressing changes and debridements as necessary. Oral antibiotics may be required if superficial infection is present. Once the wound is healed, gradual mobilization can be reinstated. A recent study demonstrated that using negative pressure incisional wound therapy decreased the incidence of wound dehiscence and total infections after these high-risk fractures.[124]

In serious deep wound infections, the patient will require rehospitalization, repeat surgical debridements, and intravenous (IV) antibiotics. Often, the use of a suction dressing (Vacuum Assisted Closure® [KCI Licensing, Inc., San Antonio, TX]) is advisable in recalcitrant wounds. This device has been shown to be safe and effective by Mooney et al.[81] for traumatic wounds in pediatric patients of all ages. Skin closure is usually not possible following such radical debridement. It is helpful to consult with plastic surgeons early in the course of treatment, as the patient often requires tissue transfer to cover the exposed metalware.

COMPLEX REGIONAL PAIN SYNDROME

Complex regional pain syndrome (CRPS), previously known as reflex sympathetic dystrophy (RSD), is a devastating painful disorder that can occur following operative or nonoperative management of a calcaneal fracture or other foot trauma. The condition is usually diagnosed when there is severe pain present out of proportion to the severity of the injury following the acute phase of healing. The pain is difficult to control, even with narcotics. The child will not bear weight or even allow the foot to be examined. Light touch even by water may stimulate an unusual pain response. The foot clinically demonstrates the signs of autonomic dysfunction. There is often a grayish discoloration, cold clammy skin, and decreased hair growth. Through disuse of the foot, the calf will atrophy. If radiographs are taken, the bones of the foot may show patchy disuse osteopenia.

There is a marked preponderance of lower extremity cases in children compared to adults.[133] Sarrail et al.[113] reviewed CRPS in 24 children and adolescents and found that 73% had foot or ankle injuries. Wilder et al.[134] reviewed 70 children (average age, 12.5 years) with CRPS and 87% had injuries to the lower limb. Eighty-four percent of their patients were girls, and the average time from injury to a diagnosis of CRPS was 12 months. Despite multidisciplinary treatments, 54% of patients still had persistent symptoms of CRPS at 3 years after diagnosis. They emphasized that CRPS has a different disease course in children when compared with adults and needs to be treated appropriately. CRPS occurs most commonly in girls, with the incidence peaking at or just before puberty.[133]

Most tertiary children's hospitals now have multidisciplinary pain teams that treat CRPS. These comprise a physician (anesthetist or pediatrician), a psychiatrist or clinical psychologist, a physiotherapist, and sometimes an occupational therapist. The child initially undergoes a multidisciplinary assessment that involves both schooling and social circumstances. The physiotherapist carries out a thorough functional assessment.

The treatment focuses on improving function and, therefore, extensive physiotherapy is performed initially. Analgesics need to be used to facilitate this treatment and include anti-inflammatory drugs, amitriptyline, and gabapentin. In severe cases, regional blocks can be used to control the pain. Children appear to respond to physiotherapy better than adults and they require less medication and invasive procedures. The recurrence rate of CRPS is higher in children, though they do respond well to the reinitiation of treatment.[133]

PERONEAL TENDONITIS/DISLOCATION

Peroneal tendon pain can occur in both the operated and non-operated foot. Pain in the peroneal tendons on movement or direct palpation may indicate prominent underlying implants. Simply removing the offending screw or plate may help. Buckingham et al.[13] recommended the routine removal of implants in their series of adolescent calcaneal fractures as this resulted in improved symptoms in 6 of 8 patients.

The extensile L-shaped lateral incision has largely prevented the peroneal tendon subluxation that used to occur with the Kocher incision. Care has to be taken at the proximal and distal ends of this incision as the sural nerve can be damaged and a painful neuroma can develop.

In patients with calcaneal fractures treated nonoperatively, a displaced lateral wall can sublux or even dislocate the peroneal tendons. Lateral impingement pain can also result from the fragment coming in direct contact with the fibula. Finally, residual varus angulation can result from calcaneal fractures treated nonoperatively and may lead to the need for later surgery to treat the malalignment.

Diagnostic local anesthetic injections have been useful in differentiating the cause of pain in the adult foot but its use in children is limited. However, it can be considered in adolescents.

Subtalar Dislocation

Subtalar dislocations (peritalar dislocation) occur infrequently and are particularly uncommon in children. They occur most often in young adult males. There are no series published on this condition in children.

A medial dislocation is the most common type (85%) and results from a forced inversion injury to the foot. The talonavicular and talocalcaneal ligaments rupture whereas the calcaneonavicular ligament stays intact. The result is that the bones of the foot dislocate medially whereas the talus remains in the ankle mortise (Fig. 31-21). The foot looks markedly deformed and the talar head can be palpated laterally. A lateral dislocation is caused by a forced eversion injury and results in a laterally displaced "flatfoot." Dougherty et al. presented a case report on this rare injury in a 19-month-old girl following a minor fall.[31]

Radiographs are difficult to interpret in this unusual injury (Figs. 31-22 and 31-23). The key is to look for the "empty navicular" where the talar head no longer articulates with it. A CT scan is useful to look for any associated fractures or osteochondral damage; however, it is probably more useful to perform this after a closed reduction to confirm anatomic alignment (Fig. 31-24).

The treatment for a closed subtalar dislocation is a reduction under general anesthesia. The knee should be flexed to relax the tendo Achilles and then the deformity accentuated before a reduction is carried out. Usually, the reduction is stable and anatomic reduction can be confirmed by radiographs and CT

Figure 31-22. Lateral view showing subluxation of the subtalar joint.

scan. The foot is immobilized until the child is comfortable enough to start gentle mobilizations. K-wire stabilization and 6 weeks of immobilization are necessary for unstable dislocations.

Occasionally, the subtalar dislocation is irreducible by closed means and has to be opened through an anteromedial approach. The bone or soft tissue (often the tibialis posterior tendon) is removed from the joint and the foot is reduced.

Midtarsal Injuries

Fractures and dislocations of the navicular, cuboid, and cuneiforms are rare pediatric foot injuries. The midtarsal region extends from the calcaneocuboid and talonavicular joints (Chopart joint) to the metatarsals. It includes the cuboid, navicular, and three cuneiform bones. These bones are interlinked by extremely strong ligaments especially on the plantar surface. The lateral side of the midfoot is more stable than the medial

Figure 31-21. Posterior view demonstrating cavovarus deformity of the left foot. (Courtesy of Dr. Thomas Lee, MD.)

Figure 31-23. There is incongruity of the calcaneocuboid joint on the AP x-ray associated with the subtalar subluxation.

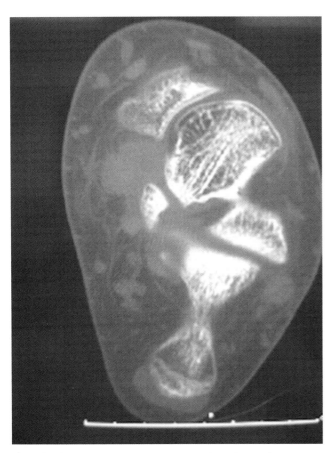

Figure 31-24. CT scan axial view shows marked talar head uncoverage ("ball is not in cup"). There is also significant incongruity of the subtalar joint. (Courtesy of Dr. Thomas Lee, MD.)

Figure 31-25. Kohler disease of the navicular that can occasionally be confused with a stress fracture.

side. The shape of these small bones and strength of their ligaments help maintain the longitudinal and transverse arch of the foot. Disruption of this rigid anatomy therefore requires a large force especially in the cartilaginous bones of a child's foot. Isolated injuries to this area are rare and one needs to look for other associated fractures and dislocations.

Hosking and Hoffman's review of four cases of midtarsal dislocations in children[49] is the only report in the literature of this injury in the pediatric age group. The children had an average age of 9.5 years, and the mechanism of injury was forced supination in three of the patients. They all had associated midtarsal injuries and presented with significant swelling. The key to making the diagnosis, which was delayed in three of the patients, was subluxation or dislocation of the calcaneocuboid joint on the lateral radiograph. The AP view only showed the dislocation in two patients and the oblique view showed it in one patient.

The dislocation can usually be reduced closed and held with percutaneous K-wires. If an anatomic reduction is not possible closed, then an open reduction must be performed.

A CT scan should be obtained to more clearly define the associated injuries to both the midtarsal bones and rest of the foot. One of the patients in Hosking and Hoffman's[49] series had an ipsilateral tibial fracture. Therefore, associated injuries may

be present due to the significant force required to cause a midfoot disruption in a child.

Isolated fractures of the midtarsal bones are rare. The navicular, cuboid, and cuneiforms are usually fractured in association with a Chopart joint (talonavicular and calcaneocuboid) dislocation or a Lisfranc injury. The navicular has a number of conditions that can mimic a fracture. Between the ages of 2 and 5 years, the navicular can become avascular (Kohler disease) and cause pain and limp while the changes seen on the radiograph can look similar to a fracture (Fig. 31-25). Likewise, an accessory navicular may mimic an avulsion fracture of the navicular tuberosity. These can be differentiated from a fracture as they have smooth, rounded edges and are usually symmetrical when a radiograph is taken of the other foot. Stress fractures of the navicular are also becoming an increasingly common problem as children and adolescents train more aggressively for competitions (see stress fractures of the foot). These stress fractures usually run in the sagittal plane in the middle third of the bone. They are often difficult to see on plain radiographs but are more easily seen on bone scans, CT, and MRI.

CUBOID FRACTURES

Cuboid fractures were considered a rare foot injury in children and were usually associated with other foot fractures. This fracture may occur more often than we thought and in isolation, however. Senaran et al.[117] reported on 28 consecutive cuboid fractures in preschool children from 1998 to 2004. They found most patients had an avoidance gait pattern and walked on the outside of their foot. They used the "nutcracker" maneuver to help diagnose the fracture. To perform this test, the heel is stabilized by the examiner and the forefoot is abducted. Pain in the lateral aspect of the foot indicates a cuboid fracture. The diagnosis was then confirmed on initial or subsequent radiographs. Initial radiographs did not demonstrate the fracture in 71% of cases. A below-knee cast or Cam walker was used for 2 to 3 weeks and all fractures healed without complications. Six patients had ipsilateral fractures in the tibia or foot. Cuboid fractures have been classified by Weber and Locher[132] into distal impaction shear-type fractures (type 1) and burst fractures (type 2).

Ceroni et al.[19] reported on four female teenagers who had equestrian injuries resulting in cuboid fractures. The mechanism of the injury was a crush to the foot when the horse fell and abduction of the forefoot while it was still in the stirrup. All four cuboid fractures were associated with other midfoot fractures and the authors recommend CT scans for patients in this age group with a cuboid fracture. Two patients underwent surgical reconstruction and had good functional outcomes with return to sports. A lateral incision was used from the tip of the fibula to the base of the fifth metatarsal. The interval was developed between the peroneal tendons and the extensor digitorum brevis. The lateral column length was restored using an allograft block.

Ruffing et al.[108] stated that extra-articular lesions are the most common type of cuboid fracture in children (69%), and a potential loss of length of the lateral column must be considered. Lower scores of the AOFAS Midfoot Scale were found with either intra-articular involvement or associated midfoot lesions.

Tarsometatarsal Injuries (Lisfranc Fracture-Dislocation)

INTRODUCTION TO TARSOMETATARSAL INJURIES

Tarsometatarsal (TMT) injuries, often referred to as a Lisfranc injury, are more common in adults than they are in children. The degree of injury varies from a subtle disruption of the Lisfranc ligament to an extensive fracture-dislocation of the forefoot. Subtle injury can be difficult to diagnose, and, if left untreated, can develop into a painful chronic problem.

Although mostly described as isolated case reports, there are a few series reported in the literature.[14,136]

ASSESSMENT OF TARSOMETATARSAL INJURIES

MECHANISMS OF INJURY FOR TARSOMETATARSAL INJURIES

TMT injuries result from either a direct blow to the foot, usually secondary to a falling object, or by indirect forces, where there is forced plantarflexion of the forefoot combined with a rotational force (Fig. 31-26).[135,136] Most are sports related.

Figure 31-26. Mechanism of Lisfranc injuries. **A:** The most common mechanism of injury: Progression from the "tiptoe" position to complete collapse of the TMT joint. **B:** Plantarflexion injury: Direct heel-to-toe compression produces acute plantar flexion of the TMT joint. **C:** Backward fall with the forefoot pinned.

Traumatic Impact in the Tiptoe Position

This mechanism is an indirect injury where a load is applied to the foot while it is in the tiptoe position, such as when jumping to the ground and landing on the toes, producing acute plantarflexion at the TMT joint. The result is a TMT joint dislocation and usually a fracture at the base of the second metatarsal. Another example would be by putting the foot down suddenly to reduce speed while riding a bike.

Heel-to-Toe Compression

In this situation, the patient is in a kneeling position when the impact load strikes the heel, which is a direct compression-type injury and usually results in lateral dislocation of the lesser metatarsals and fracture of the base of the second metatarsal.

The Fixed Forefoot

In this third mechanism, the child falls backward while the forefoot is fixed to the ground by a heavy weight. An example would be a fall backward while the foot is pinned under the wheel of a car. The patient's heel, which is resting on the ground, becomes the fulcrum for the forefoot injury.

In Wiley's[136] review of 18 patients with TMT joint injuries, 10 (56%) were a fall from a height in the "tiptoe" position, 3 (18%) suffered "heel-to-toe" compression, and 4 (22%) sustained a fall backward while their forefoot was pinned to the ground. One patient could not recall their mechanism of injury following a motorbike collision.

Atypical Lisfranc injuries have recently been reported in mini scooter injuries where the foot is planted to break speed. The resulting dorsiflexion, axial loading, and abduction cause the metatarsals to be impacted laterally. The result is a fracture of the base of the second metatarsal and a crush fracture of the cuboid.[9]

SIGNS AND SYMPTOMS OF TARSOMETATARSAL INJURIES

The diagnosis of these injuries may be difficult, and in adults as many as 20% of injuries are misdiagnosed or overlooked.[15] Some of the injuries are subtle and will present with minor pain and swelling at the base of the first and second metatarsals. This finding can be accompanied by ecchymosis on the plantar aspect of the midfoot where the TMT ligaments have been torn (Fig. 31-27).[107] Gently abducting and pronating the forefoot while the hindfoot is held fixed with the other hand would indicate the injury, though this would be quite painful acutely. Alternatively, the child can be asked to try and perform a single-limb heel lift. Pain in the midfoot often implies a TMT joint injury. With significant trauma, there is greater ligamentous injury and the resulting swelling makes it difficult to recognize any bony anatomy. It is important to assess the foot for a compartment syndrome in such circumstances, particularly when the foot has been crushed as part of the mechanism of injury. Be particularly aware of plantar bruising when assessing for these injuries.

The examiner of any child's foot following trauma needs to have a high level of suspicion for a Lisfranc injury as they are

Figure 31-27. Plantar ecchymosis sign. Ecchymosis along the plantar aspect of the midfoot is an important clinical finding in subtle Lisfranc TMT injuries. (Reprinted with permission from Ross G, et al. Plantar ecchymosis sign: A clinical aid to diagnosis of occult Lisfranc tarsometatarsal injuries. *J Orthop Trauma.* 1996;10(2):119–122.)

uncommon and difficult to diagnose but can result in a poor outcome if left untreated.

CLASSIFICATION OF TARSOMETATARSAL INJURIES

Hardcastle et al.[41] developed a classification system based on an earlier one developed by Quénu and Küss (Fig. 31-28).

Hardcastle Classification of Tarsometatarsal Injuries	
Type	**Description**
A	Total incongruity. There is total incongruity of the entire metatarsal joint in a single plane. This can be coronal, sagittal, or combined.
B	Partial incongruity. Only partial incongruity of the joint is seen involving either medial displacement of the first metatarsal or lateral displacement to the four lateral metatarsals. The medial dislocation involves displacement of the first metatarsal from the first cuneiform because of disruption of the Lisfranc ligament or fracture at the base of the metatarsal, which remains attached to the ligament.
C	Divergent pattern. The first metatarsal is displaced medially; any combination of the lateral four metatarsals may be displaced laterally. This is associated with partial or total incongruity.

This classification does not address the nondisplaced TMT joint injury, which can often be overlooked on initial assessment.

Most children's injuries are type B with minimal displacement, whereas types A and C are rare.[41,136]

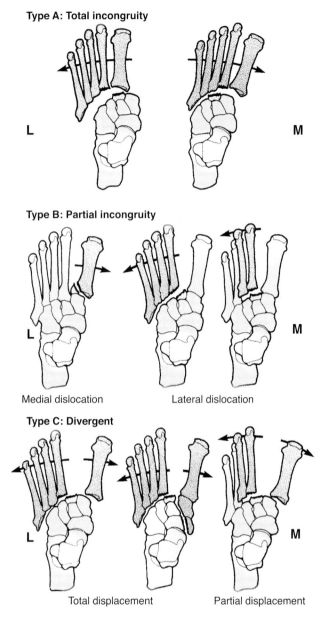

Type A: Total incongruity

L   M

Type B: Partial incongruity

L   M

Medial dislocation   Lateral dislocation

Type C: Divergent

L   M

Total displacement   Partial displacement

Figure 31-28. Classification of TMT dislocations.[28,41] L, lateral; M, medial.

Figure 31-29. Measurement of the distance between the base of first metatarsal and second metatarsal (MT1–MT2 distance, measured at 1.88 mm in this image) and between the medial cuneiform and second metatarsal (MC–MT2 distance, measured at 1.8 mm in this image).

IMAGING AND OTHER DIAGNOSTIC STUDIES FOR TARSOMETATARSAL INJURIES

The initial x-ray evaluation includes AP, lateral, and oblique views of the foot. These should be performed weight bearing if possible to stress the joint complex.

On the AP radiograph, the lateral border of the first metatarsal should be in line with the lateral border of the medial cuneiform (MC) and the medial border of the second metatarsal should line up with the medial border of the middle cuneiform. On the oblique radiograph, the medial border of the fourth metatarsal should be in line with the medial border of the cuboid. The examiner looks for a disruption in these lines. A recent radiographic review of pediatric feet non–weight-bearing AP views demonstrated normal relationships in the pediatric foot, including an MT1 to MT2 distance of less than 3 mm and an MC to MT2 distance of less than 2 mm in children older than 6 years old (Fig. 31-29).[60] It is very useful to obtain a weight-bearing radiograph of the opposite foot for comparison (Fig. 31-30). When the radiographs appear normal or minimally displaced and a Lisfranc injury is still suspected, alternative imaging with CT or MRI scans is strongly recommended. The CT scan will often show a small avulsion fracture of the first TMT ligament and will show any other associated fractures in the foot.[41,73] The MRI scan can accurately visualize a partial tear or complete rupture of the first TMT ligament.[99]

A fracture of the base of the second metatarsal should alert the examiner to the possibility of a TMT dislocation, recognizing that these injuries can spontaneously reduce. Likewise, a cuboid fracture in combination with a fracture of the base of the second metatarsal is highly suspicious for a Lisfranc injury (Fig. 31-31).

If weight-bearing radiographs are not possible, an abduction stress view can be obtained; however, in children these are difficult to obtain without general anesthesia. Bone scans may be helpful in the diagnosis of this injury when radiographs are normal, although they are not specific for the severity of the injury and are less useful than MRI or CT.

Figure 31-30. Weight-bearing radiographs show a subtle Lisfranc injury to the right foot. Weight-bearing radiographs are essential for diagnosis; using the opposite foot for comparison is also helpful.

PATHOANATOMY AND APPLIED ANATOMY RELATING TO TARSOMETATARSAL INJURIES

The TMT joint complex comprises the TMT joints, the intertarsal joints, and the intermetatarsal joints. The area represents the apex of the longitudinal and transverse arches of the foot and therefore its structural integrity is crucial in maintaining normal foot function. At the same time, there needs to be enough motion between the joints to allow the transfer of weight evenly from the hindfoot to the forefoot during the walking cycle. This intricate relationship is achieved by the anatomy of the tarsal and metatarsal bones and the arrangement of the ligaments. These midfoot bones are trapezoidal in cross-section with their base dorsal. This creates a "Roman arch" effect, which is structurally very strong and helps maintain the transverse arch in the midfoot. The TMT joint complex can be divided up into a medial column and a lateral column. The medial column is a continuation of the talus and navicular and includes the cuneiforms and the medial three metatarsals. The lateral column is a continuation of the calcaneus and comprises the cuboid and the fourth and fifth metatarsals which articulate with it. The medial column has far less mobility than the lateral column, reflecting the increased need for stability on the medial side of the foot to maintain the longitudinal arch. This stability is also provided by the second metatarsal, which is "keyed" into the step formed by the cuneiforms. This anatomy explains why the second metatarsal is usually fractured when a dislocation occurs across the TMT joint. The ligaments play a big role in maintaining stability medially and movement laterally, as well. The plantar ligaments are extremely strong compared to the weaker dorsal ligaments. The intermetatarsal ligaments help bind the lateral four metatarsals together but are absent between the first and second metatarsals. Instead, the second metatarsal is connected to the MC by the Lisfranc ligament (medial interosseous ligament) (Fig. 31-32).

The dorsalis pedis artery crosses the cuneiforms before it courses between the first and second metatarsals to form the plantar arterial branch. The deep peroneal nerve travels beside the artery but continues to supply sensation to the first web space. This neurovascular bundle can be damaged by the injury and care must be taken to protect these structures when internally fixing these fracture-dislocations. The tibialis anterior tendon inserts into the base of the first metatarsal and MC. The peroneous longus tendon inserts into the plantar surface of the base of the first metatarsal and acts as a flexor of this bone.

Figure 31-31. A: Second metatarsal is the "keystone" of the locking mechanism. **B:** Fractures of the cuboid and second metatarsal are pathognomonic signs of disruption of the TMT joints.

Figure 31-32. The ligamentous attachments at the TMT joints. There is only a flimsy connection between the bases of the first and second metatarsals (not illustrated). The second metatarsal is recessed and firmly anchored.

Together, these two muscles and their tendon insertions give added stability to the medial column of the foot.

TREATMENT OPTIONS FOR TARSOMETATARSAL INJURIES

The key to treating these injuries is to recognize the extent of the injury and the degree of instability. Appropriate treatment can then be initiated. In all these injuries, a weight-bearing radiograph at the end of treatment should confirm anatomic congruency of the TMT joint complex.

When a clinical diagnosis of a "sprain" is made, the foot should be immobilized in a below-knee cast for 6 weeks. The MRI scan may confirm a partial tear of the first TMT ligament. Regardless this painful injury takes time to heal and immobilization is the best treatment. In young adult athletes, these injuries can take a long time to heal.[79] When there is complete intraligamentous rupture or an avulsion fracture of the first TMT ligament and no displacement of the joint surfaces, a below-knee cast for 6 weeks is advised. Whether the patient should be weight bearing or not for the entire 6 weeks is debatable. Wiley[136] treated the children with undisplaced TMT joint injuries in his series with 3 to 4 weeks of immobilization with good results.

Displaced fractures of the TMT joint need to be anatomically reduced and stabilized. Myerson et al.[86] found that following a closed reduction greater than 2-mm displacement or a talometatarsal angle of greater than 15 degrees would lead to a poor outcome. A closed reduction is best carried out under a general anesthetic when the acute swelling has subsided. "Finger traps" can help with traction on the toes while the displaced metatarsals are manipulated into place. If a stable

anatomic reduction is achieved clinically and this is confirmed radiologically, a well-molded below-knee cast can be applied. Radiographs in the cast should also be taken while the patient is under anesthesia to confirm the reduction has been held. The non–weight-bearing cast is worn for 6 weeks with radiographs taken at 1 and 2 weeks to confirm the fracture-dislocation has remained reduced.

If the closed reduction results in an anatomic reduction but the fragments are unstable, K-wire fixation is used to hold the alignment of the foot. Stout 0.062-inch smooth K-wires should be used. Their placement is determined by the direction of displacement of the metatarsals and how many are involved. The most important wire is used to stabilize the second metatarsal to the MC. Additional wires can be used between the first metatarsal and the MC, and between the lesser metatarsals and their corresponding tarsal bones. A useful wire can also be passed from the first metatarsal to the second metatarsal. These K-wires are left bent over outside of the skin and are removed at 4 to 6 weeks when mobilization is initiated if the radiographs confirm healing. Again, full weight-bearing radiographs are necessary when comfort allows and after K-wire removal to confirm adequate stability. Wiley[136] used K-wire fixation in four patients. He removed these at 3 to 4 weeks, and the alignment was maintained in all the children. There were some joint incongruities from intra-articular fractures that were not surgically addressed but they did not seem to alter the clinical outcome.

ORIF is rarely required for these fractures in younger children. However, in a recent series of 56 patients with a Lisfranc injury and mean age of 14.2 years, ORIF was used in 34% of cases.[48] In this series, skeletally mature patients tended to have ORIF more than patients with open physes. ORIF is indicated if there is greater than 1 to 2 mm of joint displacement. The impediments to reduction are:

- Tibialis anterior tendon
- Interposition of fracture fragments in the second metatarsal-middle cuneiform joint
- Incongruity of the first metatarsal-MC articulation

The entire TMT joint complex can be visualized using two longitudinal incisions. One is made over the first second metatarsal space and the second is in line with the fourth metatarsal. The medial incision allows identification of the neurovascular bundle and access to the first and second metatarsal cuneiform joints. The lateral incision allows access to the lesser TMT joints. After anatomic reduction, the joints can be held reduced with K-wires or with 3.5-mm screws (Fig. 31-33). Small chondral defects can be excised and larger ones repaired. Care must be taken to avoid the proximal growth plate of the first metatarsal if screw fixation is used. The use of K-wire stabilization of the lesser metatarsals rather than screws as it is important to maintain the mobility in these joints long term. Debate exists as to when to remove the screws across these weight-bearing joints. In a child, it would seem appropriate to remove the screws once pain-free weight bearing is established as the ligaments and bone would have healed by this stage and further displacement is unlikely. Leaving the screws in for longer than 3 months risks damage to the joint and possible screw breakage.

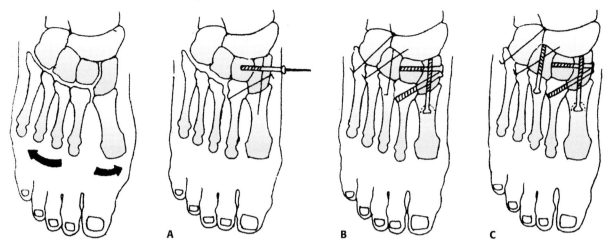

Figure 31-33. Sequence of repair for reduction and stabilization of TMT fracture-dislocations. **A:** Stabilization of the first ray by alignment of the metatarsal, medial cuneiform, and navicular. **B:** Stabilization of the Lisfranc ligament by accurate alignment of the second metatarsal to the medial cuneiform, as well as the medial and middle cuneiforms. **C:** Alignment and stabilization of the third through fifth metatarsal rays. Cannulated screws can be used instead of pins as needed for stability and compression. (Redrawn from Trevino SG, Kodros S. Controversies in tarsometatarsal injuries. *Orthop Clin North Am.* 1995;26:229–238, with permission from Elsevier.)

Author's Preferred Treatment for Tarsometatarsal Injuries (Algorithm 31-3)

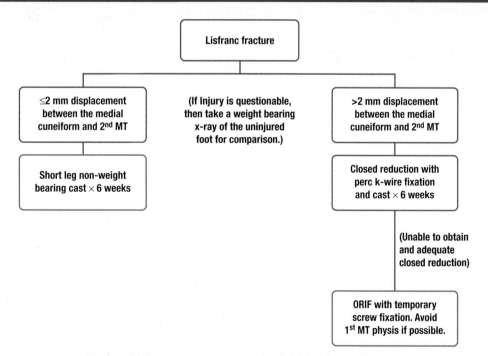

Algorithm 31-3. Author's preferred treatment for tarsometatarsal injuries.

Most children have a type B tarsometatarsal (TMT) dislocation with minimal displacement. The most important step in treatment is confirming the diagnosis and treating them until the joint is stable. If any doubt exists, the author takes a comparable radiograph of the other foot. The author routinely orders a CT scan of the midfoot to assess the extent of the injury and to look for any associated injuries.

An injury with less than 1 to 2 mm of displacement is treated in a below-knee non–weight-bearing cast for 6 weeks. Weight-bearing radiographs are taken after removal of the cast to assess stability. These radiographs are repeated 6 weeks later once pain-free weight bearing is achieved to confirm no further displacement.

If the TMT joint is displaced more than 1 to 2 mm, then the author performs a closed reduction and routinely uses percutaneous K-wire fixation with image intensifier assistance. Although these injuries can be held with cast immobilization, the author prefers the assurance of knowing the fracture-dislocation is being held internally. This fixation is especially useful when the foot is very swollen and repeated assessments are necessary to rule out compartment syndrome. In the rare circumstance of an open reduction, the

author prefers to use temporary screw fixation. These injuries are usually far more severe than a type B dislocation and the TMT joints are very unstable. After open reduction through two longitudinal incisions, 3.5-mm cortical screws are used to hold the reduction taking care to avoid the proximal growth plate of the first metatarsal. These screws are removed usually within a month of cast removal.

Regardless of the way the fracture-dislocation is treated, all these patients must be investigated at outpatient appointments with weight-bearing radiographs to confirm that the ligaments have healed and there is no residual subluxation.

MANAGEMENT OF EXPECTED ADVERSE OUTCOMES AND UNEXPECTED COMPLICATIONS RELATED TO COMPLICATIONS OF TARSOMETATARSAL INJURIES

The most common complication following TMT injuries is posttraumatic arthritis, which often occurs because the injury is "missed" and a subtle fracture-dislocation remains displaced. Another cause is a loss of reduction. Finally, the trauma itself can damage the articular cartilage and, despite an anatomic reduction, arthritis can develop.

Hardcastle et al.[41] showed that the outcomes are poor if the diagnosis is made more than 6 weeks after the injury. Curtis et al.[25] found similar results in athletes who had a delayed diagnosis. These findings reinforce the importance of making the diagnosis early and treating appropriately.

Posttraumatic arthritis is known to occur after TMT injuries in a significant percentage of adults, which is best prevented by achieving an anatomic reduction.[86] Wiss et al.[138] performed gait analysis on 11 adult patients with TMT joint fracture-dislocations and found that no patient walked normally after a displaced TMT fracture-dislocation. In Wiley's[136] series of 18 children, none of whom required open reduction, 14 patients were asymptomatic 3 to 8 months postinjury. Four patients had minor persisting TMT joint pain 1 year following injury. Two of these patients had residual angulation at the injury site. One patient had an unrecognized dislocation and had not been treated; the other had not had an anatomic reduction due to extensive intra-articular fractures. One 16-year-old patient developed asymptomatic osteonecrosis of the second metatarsal head, and this was attributed to a possible compromise of the blood supply at the time of injury. Buoncristiani et al.[14] followed eight children (3–10 years old) with indirect TMT joint injuries treated in a below-knee cast. Seven were asymptomatic at an average follow-up of 32 months; one patient developed early degenerative changes on radiographs and had midfoot pain.

The treatment for painful TMT joint arthritis is arthrodesis if conservative care fails, which is extremely unusual in children. An arthrodesis often requires extensive soft tissue release to allow anatomic reduction of the joint and rigid internal fixation

with screws. It is important not to fuse the lesser TMT joints if possible as mobility here is important for the long-term foot function.

Metatarsal Fractures

INTRODUCTION TO METATARSAL FRACTURES

Fractures of the metatarsals are the most common fractures of the foot in children, accounting for up to 60% of all pediatric foot fractures.[93,120] In a large series of metatarsal fractures, children 5 years of age or less had an isolated first metatarsal fracture in 51% of cases and children older than 5 years of age had isolated fifth metatarsal fractures in 55% of cases.[106] Owen et al. found that 7% of all metatarsal fractures and 20% of first metatarsal fractures were not diagnosed at the initial consultation.[93] Fractures of the base of the fifth metatarsal are discussed separately from the other metatarsal fractures because the anatomy, fracture patterns, and treatment indications are quite different.

ASSESSMENT OF METATARSAL FRACTURES

MECHANISMS OF INJURY FOR METATARSAL FRACTURES

Metatarsal fractures result from either a direct or indirect injury. Direct injuries are usually caused by a heavy load falling on the forefoot or a crush injury (i.e., the foot being run over by a car). The metatarsals can be fractured anywhere along the shaft but typically they are fractured middiaphyseal. Indirect injuries are caused by axial loading or torsional forces and usually produce spiral fractures of the proximal shaft or neck of the metatarsal. Singer et al.[120] found in a recent study of 125 children that if the patient was less than 5 years of age, the most common mechanism was a fall from a height occurring within the home. In children older than 5 years of age, the most common mechanism occurred playing sports and on a level playing surface.

SIGNS AND SYMPTOMS OF METATARSAL FRACTURES

Direct injuries can result in significant swelling and bruising of the foot due to soft tissue injury as well as metatarsal fractures. Careful evaluation for compartment syndrome should take place. An indirect injury usually has more subtle clinical findings and careful palpation will usually locate the site of the fracture. An infant with a metatarsal fracture due to an unwitnessed injury may present with minimal swelling but an inability to bear weight.

INJURIES ASSOCIATED WITH METATARSAL FRACTURES

Proximal fractures of the metatarsals are often associated with tarsal fractures or fracture-dislocations, which should be evaluated further with a CT scan. A fracture of the second metatarsal and a cuboid fracture are highly suggestive of a TMT joint dislocation rather than two isolated fractures. Singer et al.[120] found that the first and fifth metatarsals were more often isolated fractures, whereas if multiple metatarsals were fractured, they were always contiguous bones and involved the second, third, and fourth metatarsals.

IMAGING AND OTHER DIAGNOSTIC STUDIES FOR METATARSAL FRACTURES

Radiographic evaluation should consist of AP, lateral, and oblique views of the whole foot. The AP view often gives the impression that the fractures are minimally displaced; however, the lateral view can show significant plantar or dorsal displacement. Other associated fractures may be apparent on the plain radiographs and if any doubt exists, especially if there has been significant trauma, a CT scan of the entire foot is advised. In a young child, if a metatarsal fracture is suspected but not visible on the initial radiograph, a repeat film taken 10 to 14 days later often shows the fracture or early callus.

CLASSIFICATION OF METATARSAL FRACTURES

No classification system exists for fractures of the first through fourth metatarsals. Fractures of the fifth metatarsal are classified according to location (see section on fifth metatarsal treatment below).

TREATMENT OPTIONS FOR METATARSAL FRACTURES

Most metatarsal fractures in children can be treated nonoperatively in a below-knee cast. The child with a displaced fracture often needs to be admitted overnight for pain relief and observation for compartment syndrome. The initial treatment includes elevation for the severe swelling that coexists with the fractures. Immobilization may be performed by a well-padded cast, splint, or a Cam walker. Once the swelling subsides, a molded below-knee cast can be applied. Weight bearing can be initiated when pain allows, and the cast can usually be removed at 3 to 4 weeks at which time the patient can be transitioned to a Cam walker.

The acceptable amount of angulation or shortening in a child has not been determined. A closed reduction of the central metatarsals is indicated in an adult if there is more than 10 degrees of angulation in the dorsal plain or more than 4 mm of translation in any plane. These criteria may be appropriate for an older adolescent whose growth plates have closed but are far too stringent for a skeletally immature patient. If there is severe dorsal angulation of greater than 20 degrees or "tenting" of the skin and shortening of more than 5 mm, then a closed reduction is indicated, which is best performed under a general anesthetic when the swelling has subsided. Finger traps have been advocated by some surgeons to help with traction while the metatarsals are manipulated. A below-knee cast can be molded on both the dorsal and plantar aspects of the foot; however, the need to allow for swelling suggests implants should be used to hold fracture reduction rather than molding of a cast. To accommodate the swelling, the cast can be applied with the ankle in slight equinus. When it is changed 2 weeks later, a neutral position can be obtained.

First metatarsal fractures need careful attention, especially in an adolescent patient. The first ray is important in maintaining the longitudinal arch of the foot. The position of the first metatarsal head in relation to the lesser metatarsal heads is also important. A closed reduction should be considered if there is greater than 10 degrees of dorsal angulation or any shortening of the first metatarsal. It is unusual to have angulation in the coronal plane if the second metatarsal is intact and transverse displacement is acceptable if there is no shortening.

If a closed reduction is performed, K-wire fixation is at times required. Intramedullary placement is difficult to perform without opening the fracture and passing the wires under direct vision. Small, dorsal, longitudinal incisions are made over the fracture sites and dissection is carefully carried out down to the fracture. The wire is drilled down the distal fragment to exit the plantar skin. The wire is then withdrawn enough to allow the fracture to be reduced, then the wire is driven retrograde across the fracture site and sufficiently far enough into the proximal fragment. Another technique is to hold fracture reduction by placing K-wires across the fractured metatarsal to an adjacent nonfractured metatarsal both proximal and distal to the fracture. The K-wire is cut and bent outside the skin to facilitate removal in the outpatient clinic 3 to 4 weeks later when the patient can be placed in a walking cast for 2 more weeks to allow fracture consolidation. This technique can also be used when an open reduction is required for an irreducible fracture or the fracture is open.

FRACTURES OF THE BASE OF THE FIFTH METATARSAL

Fractures of the fifth metatarsal are the most common metatarsal fracture in children, constituting almost 50% of all metatarsal fractures in some series.[102,120] Traditionally, treatment has been based on the adult literature.

The fifth metatarsal has a number of tendinous insertions at its base. The peroneus brevis tendon inserts on the dorsal aspect of the tubercle and the peroneus tertius attaches on the dorsal aspect of the fifth metatarsal at the metaphyseal–diaphyseal

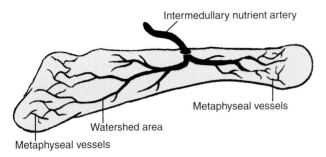

Figure 31-34. Blood supply of the proximal fifth metatarsal.

junction. The strong plantar aponeurosis inserts into the plantar aspect of the tubercle at the base.

The nutrient artery enters the shaft of the fifth metatarsal medially at the junction of the proximal and middle thirds of the diaphysis and sends intraosseous branches proximally and distally (Fig. 31-34). Proximally within the bone are the metaphyseal vessels, and the small area where these overlap with the proximal vessels from the nutrient artery is known as the watershed area. This region corresponds with zone 2 and fractures in this area have a higher rate of delayed union or nonunion in those close to maturity. The proximal apophyseal growth center of the fifth metatarsal can often be confused for a fracture. One series of diagnosed proximal fifth metatarsal fractures in children ages 7 to 16 years old found that 47% of these injuries were actually a misidentified growth center.[105] The apophyseal growth center (os vesalianum) has a longitudinal orientation roughly parallel to the metatarsal shaft, which distinguishes it from a transverse-orientated fracture (Fig. 31-35). The os vesalianum usually appears by age 9 years and unites with the metaphysis between ages 12 and 15 years (Fig. 31-36).

Classification

Fractures of the base of the fifth metatarsal are classified into one of three zones according to their location (Fig. 31-37). Zone 1 is the cancellous tuberosity, which includes the insertion of the peroneus brevis tendon, the abductor digiti minimi tendon, and the strong calcaneometatarsal ligament of the plantar fascia. Zone 2 is the distal aspect of the tuberosity where the dorsal and plantar ligamentous attachments to the fourth metatarsal attach. Zone 3 extends from distal to these ligamentous attachments to approximately the middiaphyseal area. Herrera-Soto et al.[46] classified fifth metatarsal fractures in a review of 103 children. They define a type I fracture as a "fleck" injury. A type II fracture is a tubercle fracture with an intra-articular extension. A type III fracture represents a fracture at the proximal diaphyseal region (Jones fracture).

Treatment

Traditionally, treatment has reflected the adult literature. Treatment of fractures of the base of the fifth metatarsal in children is determined primarily by the fracture zone, and, somewhat, by age.

Zone 1 Fractures

These injuries are usually traction-type injuries in which the force from the peroneus brevis tendon and the pull from the plantar aponeurosis result in an avulsion fracture of the fifth metatarsal. The fracture may be an avulsion at the origin of abductor digiti minimi. Treatment involves a weight-bearing below-knee walking cast for 3 to 6 weeks. Herrera-Soto et al.[46] found all 30 of their children with an extra-articular type 1 fracture treated in this way healed with good outcomes even

Figure 31-35. A: A normal apophysis of the base of the fifth metatarsal at the attachment of the peroneus brevis (*arrow*) in a 10-year-old girl. **B:** The *thicker arrow* points to the normal apophysis, which is roughly parallel to the metatarsal. The *thinner arrow* points toward a fracture, which is roughly perpendicular to metatarsal.

A
B

Figure 31-36. This 11-year-old girl had pain in her proximal fifth metatarsal after twisting her foot during physical education at school. No fracture was visible; however, her secondary ossification center is clearly seen running parallel to the shaft of the metatarsal.

if they were displaced. Undisplaced intra-articular tuberosity fractures also healed well in the series, but displaced (>2 mm) intra-articular fractures took significantly longer to heal. Radiographic union usually lags behind resolution of symptoms, and most patients are asymptomatic after 3 weeks.[46] This delay in radiographic union should not prevent the child returning to full activities as symptoms allow. Treatment with a Cam walker rather than a cast may be considered. Nonunion can occur but usually is asymptomatic. Although operative fixation of acute tuberosity avulsions rarely is indicated, it may be considered for significant displacement (> 3 mm) in young active patients who want to return to competitive sports sooner (Fig. 31-38).

Zone 2 Fractures

Zone 2 fractures include the Jones fracture, which is an oblique fracture in the watershed area at the proximal metaphyseal–diaphyseal junction. It typically occurs in adolescents and is thought to be caused by a combination of vertical loading and coronal shear forces at the junction of the stable proximal metaphysis and the mobile fifth metatarsal diaphysis. Frequently, these fractures are stress injuries, usually involving athletic adolescents who present with a traumatic event superimposed on prior symptoms.[24,65,109] Determining the duration of symptoms is important because chronic injuries are unlikely to respond to nonoperative treatment as well as acute fractures. Critical radiographic analysis will show cortical sclerosis in the chronic injuries.

Acute injuries should be immobilized in a short-leg non–weight-bearing cast for 6 weeks. Serial radiographs and examinations are necessary to determine adequate healing. Further non–weight-bearing immobilization may be necessary if the fracture has not healed clinically and radiographically at 6 weeks. With evidence of callus and diminished tenderness, the patient can begin protected weight bearing in a hard-soled shoe or Cam walker for an additional 4 weeks. This protected weight bearing may prevent refracture.[46] In a series of adults, successful healing in 14 of 15 patients treated with non–weight-bearing casts, whereas only 4 of 10 who were allowed to bear weight went on to union.[128] Herrera-Soto et al.[46] reported 15 fractures in this zone (type III) and found a higher rate of delayed union and refracture in patients over 13 years of age. They feel that primary internal fixation in this age group may be indicated.

For chronic zone 2 fractures with more than 3 months of symptoms, nonoperative management is unlikely to be successful. Nonetheless, it is worthwhile initially trying 6 weeks immobilization in a non–weight-bearing below-knee cast or brace. If this attempt fails, internal fixation is required. One technique is to insert an intramedullary screw from proximal to distal to stabilize the fracture site. A 4-mm cancellous screw is usually sufficient; however, in an older adolescent with a capacious intramedullary canal, a 6.5-mm cancellous screw may give better fixation and compression. It is beneficial to curette the intramedullary canal and use cancellous bone graft, which can be harvested from the distal tibia (Fig. 31-39).

Figure 31-37. The three anatomic zones of the proximal fifth metatarsal.

Figure 31-38. **A:** A 12-year-old boy who is a professional snowboarder with a displaced, intra-articular fifth metatarsal fracture. **B:** This was reduced open and internally fixed, which allowed him to compete 8 weeks after surgery.

Figure 31-39. This 15-year-old high-level basketball player sustained a proximal fifth metatarsal fracture at the metaphyseal–diaphyseal junction. The patient chose intramedullary screw fixation because of his desire to return to sports as promptly as possible, lessen his time in immobilization, and lessen the risk of delayed union or nonunion. **A:** Radiograph at time of injury. **B, C:** After intramedullary screw fixation. (Courtesy of Keith S. Hechtman, MD.)

Zone 3 Fractures

Zone 3 fractures are usually stress fractures in athletes. Acute fractures in this zone with no prodromal symptoms can be treated with a below-knee non–weight-bearing cast for 6 weeks followed by protective weight bearing for 4 weeks. In the more common scenario, involving pain with activity for several months, this period of casting is often unsuccessful but worth trying initially. The stress fracture may heal clinically with 6 to 12 weeks of immobilization and radiographs will confirm the reconstitution of the medullary canal and fracture site less sclerosis. Electrical or ultrasound stimulation may be used. If the chronic stress fracture does not heal, surgical intervention is required similar to that in a zone 2 fracture outlined above. Some authors advocate a more aggressive open debridement of the fracture site with bone grafting before introducing the intra-medullary screw.[128]

Author's Preferred Treatment of Fifth Metatarsal Fractures (Algorithm 31-4)

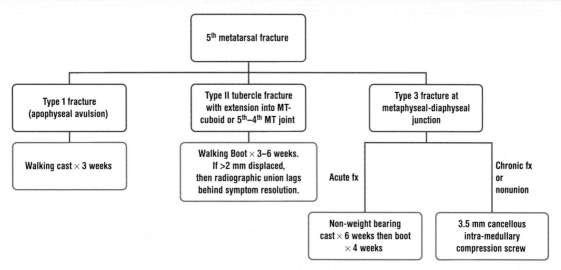

Algorithm 31-4. Author's preferred treatment of fifth metatarsal fractures.

Lesser metatarsal fractures are usually treated nonopera-tively in a below-knee walking cast for 3 to 4 weeks. Grossly displaced fractures in older children with greater than 20 degrees of dorsiflexion or more than 5 mm of shortening are treated with closed reduction under a general anesthetic and a well-molded below-knee cast. If the reduction is diffi-cult, percutaneous K-wires are used for supplementary sup-port. Except for open injuries, rarely is an open reduction through longitudinal incisions required.

A shortened or rotated distal fracture of the first or fifth metatarsal is treated by closed reduction and crossed K-wire fixation.

Proximal fifth metatarsal fractures present a more chal-lenging problem. Treatment is determined by the location of the fracture in the bone and the age and activity level of the child. If inadequately treated, they can go on to a delayed union or nonunion. For zone 1 fractures that are intra-articular and displaced greater than 3 to 4 mm, the author recommends ORIF with a 3.5-mm partially threaded screw, especially if the child is involved in competitive sports, as this will allow an earlier return to sports. This fixation is per-pendicular to the fracture line and gives maximum compres-sion. The screw is inserted through a direct lateral approach. Care must be taken to identify and protect the sural nerve,

which is usually directly under the incision. The peroneous brevis and peroneous tertius tendons are identified, and the area between them at their insertion into the proximal fifth metatarsal is a good starting point for the screw. The author prefers to insert a bicortical cannulated compression screw. This can either be a partially threaded cancellous screw or a fully threaded cortical screw. The fracture can usually be indirectly reduced and held with a K-wire. In difficult frac-ture patterns or in delayed presentations, the fracture line needs to be clearly seen and can be held reduced with a com-pression clamp.

The author treats zone 2 fractures (Jones fractures) with a non–weight-bearing cast for 6 weeks and then protected weight bearing in a moon-boot for 2 to 4 weeks as comfort allows. A study by Herrera-Soto et al.[46] showing poor results with this treatment in patients more than 13 years old indi-cates that primary internal fixation may be a better option in this age group. Acute zone 3 fractures are treated similarly, with perhaps earlier weight bearing if nondisplaced, or there are early signs of healing.

Chronic fractures or nonunions should be treated with internal fixation. The author prefers to perform this with an intramedullary screw that compresses the fracture site. If a 3.5-mm cancellous screw does not achieve adequate internal fixation in the medullary canal, increase the diameter of the screw until it does. Often, a 4-mm malleolar screw is used. Sclerotic bone can be removed with a small curette down the medullary canal. If this is not possible, the fracture site should be debrided open with small osteotomes and

rongeurs. Bone grafting is required for these chronic injuries and can be harvested from the distal tibia.

Grossly displaced shaft and distal metaphyseal fractures are treated with closed reduction and cast immobilization for 6 weeks. Occasionally, crossed K-wires are required.

MANAGEMENT OF EXPECTED ADVERSE OUTCOMES AND UNEXPECTED COMPLICATIONS RELATED TO METATARSAL FRACTURES

The most common complication of treating metatarsal fractures is nonunion, which is more common in zone 2 and zone 3 fractures of the proximal fifth metatarsal. Herrera-Soto et al.[46] concluded that pediatric fifth metatarsal fractures behaved similarly to adult fractures and can be treated the same. If a symptomatic nonunion develops and surgery is indicated, the procedure should include a thorough debridement of the sclerotic medullary canal, bone graft, and a strong appropriately sized compression screw across the fracture site.

Phalangeal Injuries

INTRODUCTION TO PHALANGEAL INJURIES

Phalangeal fractures are common in children and account for nearly one in five pediatric foot fractures. Most toe injuries are treated by primary care physicians, so orthopaedic surgeons see only the more severe fractures. Phalangeal fractures are the result of direct trauma by a falling object or indirect trauma when the unprotected toe is struck against a hard object ("stubbing"). The proximal phalanx is more commonly injured than the distal phalanges.

The toes must be closely examined for any break in the skin especially at the base of the nail as this may indicate an open Salter–Harris fracture with an associated nail bed injury. These compound injuries require a thorough debridement, repair of the nail bed, and often a single longitudinal K-wire to stabilize the fracture (Fig. 31-40). IV antibiotics should be given for 24 hours followed by 7 days of oral antibiotics. Nail bed injuries should be repaired as meticulously as in the hand with glue or sutures. A poorly repaired germinal matrix will cause abnormal nail growth and difficulty with shoe wear long after the fracture has healed.

TREATMENT OPTIONS FOR PHALANGEAL INJURIES

Closed fractures of the phalanges rarely require reduction and can be treated by simple "buddy strapping" to the adjacent toe

and immediate mobilization. A hard-soled shoe or Cam walker may help minimize pain; however, crowding in the toe box may make this more uncomfortable than bare feet. An angulated toe in both the coronal and sagittal plane usually remodels well if the growth plate is still open. In adolescents, a percutaneous K-wire can be used if the fracture is grossly unstable and unable to be held reduced by strapping alone. This wire can be passed longitudinally through the tip of the affected toe or obliquely across the fracture. It is extremely unusual to get any growth disturbance from a smooth wire crossing the growth plate in the phalanges. These pins can be removed in clinic 4 to 6 weeks later. Laterally angulated fractures of the little toe sometimes need closed reduction before strapping them to the fourth toe.

NAIL BED INJURIES

✓ Repair of Nail Bed Injuries: SURGICAL STEPS

- ❏ Use sterile tourniquet (glove)
- ❏ Remove the nail
- ❏ Thoroughly clean the nail bed gently
- ❏ Repair the nail bed with fine absorbable suture (6-0 or 7-0 rapid dissolving suture) or glue
- ❏ Protect the eponychial fold by replacing the nail or holding it open with another spacer
- ❏ Cover with sterile dressing and tape
- ❏ Leave dressing intact for 10 days then debulk dressing

Nail bed injuries to the toes should be treated similarly to those to the fingers. Failure to address the nail bed adequately can lead to abnormal nail growth and problems with shoewear (Fig. 31-41).

GREAT TOE FRACTURES

The great toe is injured by the same mechanisms as the lesser toes, with sports injury being a common etiology. Standard AP and lateral radiographs are taken. It is useful to have the patient hold the lesser toes dorsiflexed with a small towel to maximize visualization on the lateral view. Intra-articular fractures of the proximal phalanx are more common in the great toe than the other toes. They are usually Salter–Harris type III or IV fractures (Fig. 31-42).

Most of these fractures can be managed with "buddy strapping" to the second toe. If greater than 25% of the joint surface is involved and there is displacement of more than 2 to 3 mm of the joint surface, reduction should be performed. Fracture reduction may be held by strapping to the second toe or a percutaneous K-wire. In the rare occasion that this is not successful,

Figure 31-40. A: This 7-year-old boy "stubbed" his toe barefoot on his bike and sustained an open fracture of the tuft of the distal phalanx and associated laceration of the germinal matrix. **B:** Preoperative radiograph shows the small tuft fracture. **C, D:** The wound was thoroughly debrided, germinal matrix repaired, and a K-wire passed across the fracture to hold the fragment and soft tissues reduced.

Figure 31-41. Second toe distal phalangeal fracture with nail bed split. **A:** Before repair of nail bed. **B:** Nail bed repaired with absorbable suture and nail glued back.

an open reduction can be performed either through a midlateral or dorsal incision. However, caution should be advised when pursuing open reduction of these injuries as Kramer et al.[61] reported significant complications in six of nine patients treated with open reduction in their series. With diaphyseal fractures,

axial alignment, and rotation both need to be addressed with the closed reduction. Often, the clinical appearance of the toe following the reduction is more useful than the postreduction radiograph as the toe usually looks "fine" even though the radiograph shows malalignment.

Figure 31-42. A: An 11-year-old boy with an intra-articular fracture of the proximal phalanx of the great toe. Successful treatment was achieved with simple buddy strapping. **B:** A lateral radiograph of the great toe is best taken with the lesser toes held flexed with a bandage.

Other Injuries to the Foot

LAWNMOWER AND OTHER MUTILATING INJURIES

There are approximately 9,400 lawnmower injuries a year in the United States affecting children 20 years or younger, with an average age of 10.7 years.[129] These accidents occur with all types of lawnmowers, but the most common and severe injuries involve a riding mower.[58,64,129] Most children who have severe lawnmower injuries are bystanders,[129] though some fall off the mower and are run over. Seventy-eight percent of all lawnmower accidents occur in boys.[129] Loder et al.[71] reviewed 235 children who had a traumatic amputation and found that these injuries are more common in the spring and summer. Garay et al.[39] recommended annual springtime "publicity campaigns" to remind the public of the dangers involved with lawnmowers during this peak time. However, the incidence of these injuries has not decreased despite the current regulations.[58] With millions of dollars in new estimated annual burdens in prosthetic costs for children with amputations due to lawnmowers, the cost of a public relations campaign would likely be dwarfed in comparison. Children under the age of 14 years are most susceptible to injury with those under the age of 6 years having the greatest risk of death.[88] Hand injuries are the most common type (34.6%), followed by the leg (18.9%) and the foot (17.7%) (Fig. 31-43).[129]

Figure 31-43. A 4-year-old boy with a severe lawnmower accident after being run over by the driver. There was extensive soft tissue loss and compound fractures to the foot. Despite multiple debridements, the leg was amputated below the knee.

The initial treatment for these children is thorough assessment of the injuries and appropriate resuscitation. Often, a large volume of blood has been lost. Once the child is stabilized, a secondary survey can be conducted to assess the extent of the injury to each limb. With regard to the foot, these injuries are mutilating and heavily contaminated with soil and grass. After inspection, the wound should be dressed and a firm bandage applied to prevent further bleeding. Antibiotics need to be administered as soon as possible and include a cephalosporin, aminoglycoside, and penicillin. The patient's tetanus status should be ascertained and tetanus prophylaxis administered if unknown.

The child then needs to be taken urgently to the operating room for the initial debridement. Considerable time should be spent meticulously removing foreign material. A water jet lavage system can be useful but should be used with care, as it can force debris further into the soft tissue envelopes. Clearly devitalized tissue should be debrided. Questionable tissue should be left as there will be return trips to the operating room, and tissue in younger children especially may have remarkable recovery at times. It is useful to involve a plastic surgeon even at this initial surgery so they can see the extent of the damage and start planning for definitive coverage. The child will generally need at least three trips to the operating room and some cases many more.[30] These return trips should be every 24 to 48 hours depending on the state of the wound. Each debridement is important and should not be left to the most junior member of the surgical team. Every piece of viable skin is vital and may be the difference between a primary closure over an amputation stump or a skin graft or tissue transfer. There is no hurry to close the wound until the soft tissue and bone is completely free of foreign material and the tissues are well perfused. Shilt et al.[118] and many others have found the use of wound vacuum closure dressing (VAC) safe and effective in managing of lawnmower injuries. Fractures need to be stabilized and initially external fixation is useful, which allows for further debridements and does not compromise later internal fixation once the soft tissue coverage has been determined.[35]

Skin grafting or flap coverage of lawnmower injuries is required in approximately 50% of cases.[30] Unlike in adults, split-thickness skin grafting can function very well on the weight-bearing surfaces in children.[30] When the soft tissue defect is large or there is exposed bone that would be better to preserve than excise, a free tissue transfer is helpful.[70] Lin et al.[71] reviewed 93 pediatric foot soft tissue defect microsurgical reconstructions. They reported excellent results with free musculocutaneous flaps or skin-grafted muscle flaps. For plantar foot reconstructions, the musculocutaneous flaps had better results with fewer tropic ulcers and fewer resurfacing procedures. They also found that reconstruction of the tendons in the immediate setting led to fewer subsequent operations than staged tendon reconstructions.[71]

One of the problems with free flaps is their bulk and subsequent problems with shoe fitting. An alternative to a free muscle flap is a free fascial flap. A common one is the temporoparietal fascial flap.[22,27] This fascia is supplied by the superficial temporal artery which is a terminal branch of the external carotid. The graft can be as large as 12 × 14 cm. This varies with the age and size of the child. It is harvested through an incision within the hairline, which results in a cosmetic closure (Fig. 31-44A). The

Figure 31-44. A: Temporoparietal fascia is harvested through the incision marked by the *green line. Red line* is markings of superficial temporal artery. **B**, **C:** Severe crush and degloving injury to the foot in a 6-year-old boy run over by a car. **D:** The incision for harvesting the temporoparietal graft heals with an excellent cosmetic result. **E**, **F:** The temporoparietal graft has healed with skin grafting to cover the defect. (Courtesy Dr. Jonathan Wheeler, Consultant Plastic Surgeon, Middlemore Hospital, Auckland, New Zealand.)

fascial flap can then be used to cover exposed bone and tendons in the foot (Fig. 31-44B–D). Split skin can then be grafted onto the fascia and any surrounding areas of full-thickness skin loss.

One of the most difficult decisions to make while treating these severe injuries is whether to salvage the affected part of the limb or amputate the questionable part. This decision is based largely on what the likely functional outcome will be and what effect prolonged treatments and hospitalizations will have on the child. A mangled extremity severity score (MESS) has been developed in adults to help surgeons make these decisions. The MESS score was validated in children by Fagelman et al.[37] However, they did not include fractures below the ankle. It is useful to ask for a colleague's advice when contemplating an amputation so the advantages and disadvantages can be discussed. If an amputation is performed, as much length of the bone should be preserved as possible, and transdiaphyseal amputation should generally be avoided to prevent problems with stump overgrowth. The functional outcome for these patients is generally satisfactory. Vosburgh et al.[130] reviewed the functional outcome of 21 children with lawnmower accidents. They found that isolated forefoot injuries resulted in 88% of normal function compared to 72% of normal function for injuries to the posterior and plantar aspects of their foot.

CRUSH INJURIES

Severe crush injuries to the foot in children are rare but the consequences of not recognizing the degree of injury can be devastating. The most common cause is the foot being run over by a car tire resulting in both a crush and shearing force (see Fig. 31-44). An alternative injury would be a heavy weight falling on the foot.

The child presents with an extremely painful, tight foot usually with the skin intact. Shoes can be difficult to remove and they may need sedation first. Initial primary and secondary surveys need to be completed and then a thorough assessment of the foot undertaken.

It is important to continually assess the child for compartment syndrome and perform fasciotomies when indicated (see compartment syndrome below).

It is common for children to have persistent neuropathic pain following these injuries.

SESAMOID FRACTURES

There are a number of sesamoid bones in the foot. The most commonly symptomatic ones are the two within the plantar plate of the first metatarsophalangeal joint and in the flexor hallucis brevis tendons. These medial and lateral sesamoid bones functioning both shock absorption and as a fulcrum to improve the biomechanical function of the tendons to the first toe.

Acute sesamoid fractures are rare in children, and diagnosis is difficult because of the variable anatomy of the medial and

lateral sesamoid bones. They can have more than one ossification center that does not unite, resulting in a partite sesamoid. The incidence of partite sesamoids varies between 19% and 31%.[29] The incidence of a partite sesamoid is approximately 10 times higher in the medial sesamoid than in the lateral one. The incidence of bilaterality varies between 25% and 85%.[23]

An acute fracture to the sesamoids is usually caused by a fall from a height onto the forefoot which may be associated with a forced dorsiflexion of the first metatarsal. The injury results in acute pain and swelling under the first metatarsal head and pain on first toe dorsiflexion. Common causes of sesamoid pain are stress fractures or inflammation of the sesamoid (sesamoiditis), which occurs from repetitive dorsiflexion of the great toe (e.g., in runners and dancers).

Radiographs need to be taken to help differentiate whether the condition is acute or chronic. AP and lateral weight-bearing views coned on the sesamoids should be requested. A tangential view is also advisable (Fig. 31-45). An acute fracture will usually be transverse and have a "jagged" appearance with sharp corners. It is not widely displaced as the fragments are contained within the plantar plate. Wide displacement would represent a major disruption to the first metatarsophalangeal joint which would be obvious clinically. Another useful tip is that the sum of the fragment sizes should add up to the "normal sesamoid size." Two partite fragments are often much larger when combined than one would normally expect with a fracture. Radiographs of the opposite foot can be helpful for comparison. However, with the variable incidence of bilaterality, a definitive diagnosis is not always possible.

Treatment for a closed injury with an intact planter plate is nonoperative. Immobilization in a below-knee plaster cast with a toe plate for 4 to 6 weeks is advisable. Alternatively, a moot-boot with a midfoot ridge to unload the forefoot can be used. Transition from the cast into a stiff-soled shoe that continues to prevent dorsiflexion will give symptomatic relief. With stress fractures and sesamoiditis a longer period of immobilization may be necessary.

Surgical intervention is rarely required. If a symptomatic nonunion occurred this can be treated by open reduction and bone grafting which is technically difficult or by excision of the smaller of the two fragments. Either way, care needs to be taken to avoid damage to the plantar plate.

COMPARTMENT SYNDROME

Compartment syndrome of the foot can occur in children with severe soft tissue injuries in the presence or absence of associated fractures.[119] Most commonly, it occurs with severe crush injuries of the forefoot where there are multiple fractures and dislocations; however, it can occur without any fracture, such as the case of a car running over a foot causing crush and shear injury to soft tissue. The symptoms are not as obvious as they are in compartment syndrome of the forearm or leg, and increased pain with passive motion of the toes is not always present. There is significant pain from the injury itself, which often requires

Figure 31-45. A: Medial sesamoid of the right foot appears fractured following a great toe injury. A radiograph of the left foot confirms a similar partite sesamoid that is asymptomatic. **B:** Asymptomatic partite patella in the contralateral uninjured foot. **C:** Tangential sesamoid views can be useful however in this case the radiograph does not show the transverse partite sesamoid. **D:** An MRI scan of the right foot 5 months after the injury for a different problem shows the partite medial sesamoid.

considerable amounts of pain relief. Pallor, pain on passive extension, paresthesia, and a dorsalis pedis pulse that is difficult to palpate likewise can be clinical signs in a large number of foot injuries. The clinician needs to have a high index of suspicion for a compartment syndrome and if any doubt exists, the compartment pressures should be measured or the child taken urgently to the operating room for a decompression of the foot.

Compartment pressure measurements are difficult to perform with invasive catheterization in an awake child with foot trauma. Often, the compartments need to be measured under a general anesthetic, so the child and parents need to be warned that the surgeon may proceed to a decompression. There are nine compartments in the foot, and it is difficult to confirm exact compartment location. It is important to measure the pressure in the calcaneal compartment as it appears to be the most sensitive.[76] When a pressure of greater than 30 mm Hg is measured in any compartment, a fasciotomy should be performed.[76,85] It may be more accurate to use a measurement that takes into account the patient's blood pressure. In adults, the threshold is a measured pressure that is less than 30 mm Hg below the patient's diastolic blood pressure.[75]

There are nine fascial compartments in the foot that contain the intrinsic muscles and short plantar flexors. All the compartments should be released during a decompression regardless of the clinical findings or compartment measurements. The most thorough way to achieve this is by using the three-incision

Figure 31-46. Surgical approaches for fasciotomy of the foot. **A:** The dorsal approach is made through an incision over the second and fourth metatarsal shafts and is more suitable for injuries of the forefoot or midfoot. **B:** The medial approach is more suitable for injuries of the hindfoot, with the incision extending from the base of the first metatarsal to the medial malleolus. A tarsal tunnel release can be done through this incision. (Reprinted by permission from Myerson MS. Experimental decompression of the fascial compartments of the foot: The basis for fasciotomy in acute compartment syndromes. *Foot Ankle.* 1988;8(6): 308–314. Copyright © 1988 SAGE Publications.)

technique (Fig. 31-46).[85] Two dorsal longitudinal incisions are made in line with the second and fourth metatarsals. Dissection is then carried out through the interosseous compartments and fascia to enable decompression of the deep plantar compartments. Puncturing the fascia and spreading with a hemostat is effective and safe. The lateral compartment is decompressed through the incision over the fourth metatarsal by dissecting deep to the fifth metatarsal. A medial incision is made along the arch of the foot as far posterior as the medial malleolus. This incision allows decompression of the medial compartment and a more thorough decompression of the deep compartments. It also allows decompression of the tarsal tunnel. Dissection is carried out on both the dorsal and plantar surfaces of the abductor hallucis muscle, freeing it from both the plantar fascia and bony attachments. Care must be taken to avoid damaging the lateral plantar nerve and vessels which lie on the quadrates plantae muscle. The deep compartments can now be easily released under direct vision. These three incisions are usually well placed to help with fracture reduction and K-wiring to stabilize the foot at the same time as the decompression. The wounds should be left open initially and closed 5 to 7 days later. Often, one of the wounds will require split-skin grafting.

Although uncommon in children, late sequelae of missed compartment syndrome can lead to disabilities including claw toe deformity, paresthesia, cavus deformity, stiffness, and residual pain.[10] While compartment syndrome of the foot in adults is sometimes observed initially with later tendon releases if needed, there has not been a similar experience reported in the growing child.

PUNCTURE WOUNDS

Puncture wounds to the foot are extremely common in children and frequently treated by primary care physicians or in the emergency department. Most injuries can be treated by simply removing the offending foreign body, irrigating the entry site, giving tetanus prophylaxis if required, and a short course of oral antibiotics. It is important to carefully assess the foreign body that is removed to make sure a small part of it has not been retained in the foot. Often, the patient will bring the offending foreign body with them if it broke off or came out spontaneously. The depth of penetration should also be assessed by looking at the length of the foreign object as well as the point of entry. This approach may help predict if a joint or tendon sheath has been penetrated. The amount of contamination can also help determine if an open debridement is necessary and the length of administration of antibiotics.

Radiographs are useful in most cases of acute puncture wounds as a foreign body may be seen. If the foreign body has

Figure 31-47. MRI scans are useful following penetrating foot injuries as the extent of the soft tissue or joint involvement can be clearly seen. This 6-year-old boy had pain 4 days after standing on a nail barefoot. Despite oral antibiotics, he had developed a septic arthritis.

punctured a joint, air may be seen as well. When a retained foreign body is suspected but not seen on radiograph, an ultrasound scan can be useful. An MRI scan is even more useful at identifying foreign bodies and has the added advantage of showing secondary changes of septic arthritis or osteomyelitis if the puncture wound is chronic (Fig. 31-47).

If a patient with a treated puncture wound does not rapidly improve clinically, further investigation is required to rule out a retained foreign body, deep soft tissue infection, septic arthritis, or osteomyelitis. Eidelman et al.[33] recommend that patients who have an established infection 24 to 36 hours after a puncture wound should be admitted to the hospital for IV antibiotics. In their series of 80 children with puncture wounds, a delay in diagnosis or presentation was associated with deep infection.[33] The most common organism causing deep infections in their study was *Staphylococcus aureus* and group A Streptococcus. A complete blood count, erythrocyte sedimentation rate, and C-reactive protein should be performed, and an MRI scan is the most accurate radiologic investigation.[52,63] The patient can then be treated accordingly with IV antibiotics and open debridement of the entry site and deeper tissues.

Septic arthritis or osteomyelitis should be suspected if a child presents with foot pain and swelling following a nail puncture wound while wearing sneakers. *Pseudomonas* osteochondritis is thought to occur when the cartilage is damaged at the initial injury. The source of the pseudomonas is debatable, but it may be from the sneakers.[63] The patient should

be admitted to the hospital. A thorough debridement of the affected soft tissues, cartilage, and bone should be carried out. IV antibiotics are administered often for 5 to 7 days or until the infection has clearly resolved.[54] The long-term sequelae of pain, growth arrests, chronic osteomyelitis, and recurrence make this an important infection to identify early and treat aggressively.

STRESS FRACTURES

Stress fractures in children have become more common because of overtraining in youth athletics and year-round sports participation.[20] The tibia, fibula, femur, and pars interarticularis are the areas commonly affected. However, stress fractures in the foot can also occur.

The predominant symptom is "pain with weight bearing," which usually coincides with the beginning of an intense period of training. The repetitive training results in bone fatigue and eventual partial or complete fracture. The normal cortical bone remodeling is accelerated and resorption occurs at a faster rate than the reparative process resulting in bone weakening and inevitable microfracture. Therefore, treatment attempts to break this cycle by activity modification and protected weight bearing to prevent further fracture and allow the reparative process to "catch up."

Patients with stress fractures in the foot present with pain on weight bearing and often no history of any particular causative injury. A thorough history of their training regimen is essential, particularly any increases or changes in technique, playing surface, or footwear. On examination, there is point tenderness but minimal swelling. Radiographs taken early in the process are often normal but later can show periosteal layering of new bone on the cortex and osteolysis at the fracture site. Bone scans are often more sensitive initially and a three-phase technetium bone scan is helpful when the radiographs are normal in the first 2 to 3 weeks after the onset of symptoms.[34] MRI has been shown to identify stress fractures before radiographic changes are evident, and, in a prospective study of collegiate basketball players, MRI demonstrated marrow edema even before stress fractures were clinically evident.[74]

As well as concentrating on the fracture, the patient should be assessed for any conditions that could predispose to stress fractures. These conditions include metabolic bone diseases, amenorrhea, eating disorders, and incorrect training techniques. A cause may be as simple as a change in footwear that has led to increased stress in a particular bone in the foot.

The second metatarsal is the most common bone in the foot to get a stress fracture, which often occurs at the neck of the metatarsal at the junction of the mobile shaft and rigid metaphysis. Treatment involves rest and partial weight bearing in a moonboot for 4 to 6 weeks. It is best to avoid a cast as during this time the athlete can maintain physical fitness with swimming, deep water running, and cycling. A gradual return to activity can be restarted when radiographs confirm adequate healing and the symptoms have abated, which often takes 8 to 12 weeks. Stress fractures of the navicular are disabling and difficult to treat. They occur most commonly in basketball players, hurdlers, and runners.[80] Bennell and Bruckner[7] reviewed 18 large studies of stress fractures and found that the incidence of navicular stress fractures can range between 0% and 28.6% of injuries among track and field athletes. These fractures are thought to arise because of overuse and the reduced vascularity that can exist in the central third of the navicular. They are difficult to diagnose, and one needs to have a high level of suspicion as with any other stress fracture. The fracture is often diagnosed by MRI, and if this is positive in the region of the navicular, a CT scan is very helpful in delineating the stress response from an acute injury. The fracture line on CT, and if present on radiograph, is vertically orientated in the middle third of the bone. Most of these fractures heal with rest and protective weight bearing. However, some do go on to delayed union or nonunion. The treatment for a painful nonunion is ORIF with autogenous bone grafting. The average time for the return to activity following a navicular stress fracture in athletes is 5.6 months.[57] Stress fractures of the base of the fifth metatarsal usually occur in zone 2 or 3 and their treatment is discussed earlier in the chapter under the section fractures of the fifth metatarsal base.

Stress fractures can also occur in the cuboid, calcaneus, and sesamoid bones of the foot.

Annotated References

Reference	Annotation
Dougherty CP, Nebergall RW, Caskey PM. Lateral subtalar dislocation in a 19-month-old female. *Am J Orthop.* 2003;32(12):598–600.	A case report of a lateral subtalar dislocation in a 19-month-old female after a minor fall. Review of the literature reveals no prior report of this injury in a patient of this age. This case illustrates the importance of thoroughly examining the pediatric patient. When fracture is not diagnosed and a child refuses to use the affected extremity, examination to rule out occult fracture or dislocation must be included. Level of Evidence: V
Eberl R, Singer G, Schalamon J, et al. Fractures of the talus—differences between children and adolescents. *J Trauma.* 2010;68:126–130.	From 1990 to 2005, 24 patients (18 males, 6 females) presented with 25 fractures of the talus. The medical records were reviewed retrospectively. Follow-up was performed by radiographical grading, and the functional outcome was measured using the Foot-Function Index. Adolescents present with more severe fractures of the talus compared with children younger than 12 years. In addition, we did not observe persistent osteonecrosis in patients younger than 12 years old, and the outcome is favorable in most cases irrespective of the mode of treatment. Level of Evidence: IV
Hill JF, Heyworth BE, Lierhaus A, et al. Lisfranc injuries in children and adolescents. *J Pediatr Orthop B.* 2017;26(2):159–163.	Fifty-six children treated for bony or ligamentous Lisfranc injuries over a 12-year period were reviewed. Overall, 51% of fractures and 82% of sprains were sports related (P = .03). A total of 34% of the cohort underwent open reduction internal fixation, which was more common among patients with closed physes (67%). Full weight bearing was allowed in open reduction internal fixation patients at a mean of 14.5 weeks, compared to 6.5 weeks in the nonoperative group. Complications were rare (4%) and included physeal arrest in one patient and a broken, retained implant in one patient. Level of Evidence: IV
Kamphuis SJ, Meijs CM, Kleinveld CM, et al. Talar fractures in children: A possible injury after go-karting accidents. *J Foot Ankle Surg.* 2015;54(6):1206–1212.	This is a case series that describes six talar fractures in four patients that resulted from go-karting accidents. Talar fractures caused severe damage to the tibiotalar joint, talocalcaneal or subtalar joint, and the talonavicular joint. This damage leads to complications such as avascular necrosis, arthritis, nonunion, delayed union, and neurapraxia, which have the potential to cause long-term disability in a child. Level of Evidence: V.
Knijnenberg LM, Dingemans SA, Terra MP, et al. Radiographic anatomy of the pediatric Lisfranc joint. *J Pediatr Orthop.* 2016. Sep 3. [Epub ahead of print].	Foot radiographs without traumatic injury taken between August 2014 and February 2015 in patients younger than 18 years were reviewed. Using a non–weight-bearing anteroposterior view of the foot the distance between the base of metatarsal 1 and metatarsal 2 (MT1–MT2) and the distance between the medial cuneiform (MC) and the base of metatarsal 2 (MC–MT2) were measured. Median normal values were calculated per age. In the analysis were 243 patients. The distance between the base of MT1–MT2 was constant below 3 mm. Measurements for both MT1–MT2 and MC–MT2 distance approached adult values at the age of 6. Level of Evidence: III.

Annotated References

Reference	Annotation
Kramer DE, Mahan ST, Hresko MT. Displaced Intra-articular Fractures of the Great Toe in Children: Intervene With Caution! *J Pediatr Orthop.* 2014;34(2):144–149.	Seven boys and three girls with a mean age of 12.6 years (range 8.7–15.7 years) were identified. The mechanism of injury was a direct blow from a stubbed toe (eight cases) or a dropped object onto the foot (two cases). There were seven intra-articular fractures of the proximal phalanx base, four of which occurred in the setting of an open physis. Mean fracture displacement was 4.4 mm. Open reduction was necessary in nine cases, with K-wire fixation used in nine cases. Median follow-up was 50.5 months (range 11–123 months). Seven fractures healed at a mean of 7.9 weeks. Nine patients returned to full activity without limitation at the latest follow-up. Six patients had significant complications: two underwent revision open reduction internal fixation (one for postoperative redisplacement and the other for painful nonunion), one suffered a refracture, one developed posttraumatic arthritis requiring interphalangeal joint fusion, one developed an asymptomatic fibrous nonunion with avascular necrosis of the fragment, and one had K-wire migration necessitating early surgical removal. Conclusions: Intra-articular fractures of the great toe primarily occur in adolescents after direct impact injuries. The most common location was the proximal phalangeal base. There is a high complication rate after surgical intervention, although most patients were asymptomatic at latest follow-up. Level of Evidence: IV
Petit CJ, Lee BM, Kasser JR, Kocher MS. Operative treatment of intraarticular calcaneal fractures in the pediatric population. *J Pediatr Orthop.* 2007;27(8):856–862.	Children with closed displaced intra-articular calcaneal fractures treated with open reduction internal fixation at Boston Children were reviewed at an average of 67 months postoperatively. Fourteen fractures in 13 patients who met the inclusion criteria were treated with open reduction internal fixation. We found seven tongue-type and seven joint depression-type fractures based on the Essex-Lopresti classification. Based on the Sanders classification, we found nine type II (two-part) fractures and five type III (three-part) fractures. The average preoperative and postoperative Bohler angles were 11.8 and 28.4 degrees (*P* < .0001), respectively. The average subjective AOFAS hindfoot score was 64 of a possible 68 points. Of 14 fractures, 13 were fixed with a buttressing plate laterally. One patient was fixed with a single 3.5-mm cortical screw and had the lowest AOFAS hindfoot score. Four minor complications in three patients were encountered. Level of Evidence: IV
Petnehazy T, Schalamon J, Hartwig C, et al. Fractures of the hallux in children. *Foot Ankle Int.* 2015;36:60–63.	Three hundred seventeen patients (mean age = 11.7 years; range 1–18 years; 65% males) sustained a fracture of the hallux. Most accidents (28%) occurred at sports facilities, and soccer was the most common cause of a fracture of the hallux (28%). Closed injuries were diagnosed in 92% of the patients; 8% of the children presented with open fractures. In 144 children, the growth plate was affected. Fifty-nine patients presented with diaphyseal fractures, 42 patients with osseous avulsions, and 40 patients with fractures of the distal part of the phalanx. Nineteen children had incomplete and 13 patients comminuted fractures. The vast majority of the children (86%) were treated conservatively. Operative interventions were required in 14% of the patients. Good outcome was achieved in both conservatively and operatively treated patients. Level of Evidence: IV
Riccardi G, Riccardi D, Marcarelli M, et al. Extremely proximal fractures of the fifth metatarsal in the developmental age. *Foot Ankle Int.* 2011;32(5):S526–S532.	Between 2001 and 2003, the radiographs of 481 patients (558 feet) between 6 months and 16 years that were diagnosed with a proximal fifth metatarsal fracture were reviewed. The x-rays were evaluated for the presence and morphology of the growth nucleus of the base of the fifth metatarsal in the 7- to 16-year age group because this is the time interval in which the nucleus becomes visible radiographically. They identified the nucleus of the base of the fifth metatarsal in 115 patients for a total of 132 feet. A fracture of the fifth metatarsal was found in 12.8%. A misdiagnosis had been made in 47%. Misdiagnosis was strictly related to the presence of the growth nucleus of the apophysis except two cases where an accessory bone was present. Level of Evidence: IV

Annotated References

Reference	Annotation
Smith JT, Curtis TA, Spencer S, et al. Complications of Talus Fractures in Children. *J Pediatr Orthop.* 2010;30(8):749–757.	This study included 29 children with talus fractures sustained between 1999 and 2008 at an average age of 13.5 years (range 1.2–17.8 years). Avascular necrosis occurred in two patients (7%), arthrosis in five (17%), delayed union in one (3%), neurapraxia in two (7%), infection in zero, and the need for further surgery in three (10%). Both high-energy mechanism and fracture displacement corresponded to a greater number of posttraumatic complications. The number and severity of talus fractures increased in older children. Level of Evidence: IV
Talkhani S, Reidy D, Fogarty E, et al. Avascular necrosis of the talus after a minimally displaced neck of talus fracture in a 6 year old child. *Injury.* 2000;31(1):63–65.	Case report of ANV after a nondisplaced talar neck fracture in a 6-year-old child. Level of Evidence: V
Tezval M, Dumont C, Stürmer KM. Prognostic reliability of the Hawkins sign in fractures of the talus. *J Orthop Trauma.* 2007;(8):538–543.	Between January 1995 and December 2000, a total of 41 patients (13 females, 28 males) with displaced talar fractures were operated on. Thirty-four patients with a mean age of 35 years (range 12 to 60 years) were followed for more than 36 months (range 36 to 52 months). The prognostic reliability of the Hawkins sign was studied in 31 of these patients using a two-by-two table. No Hawkins sign was found in the five patients who developed avascular necrosis (AVN) of the talus. In the remaining 26 patients who did not develop AVN, a positive (full) Hawkins sign was observed 11 times, a partially positive Hawkins sign 4 times, and a negative Hawkins sign 11 times. The Hawkins sign thus showed a sensitivity of 100% and a specificity of 57.7%. The Hawkins sign (if present) appeared between the sixth and the ninth week after trauma. The Hawkins sign is a good indicator of talus vascularity following fracture. If a full or partial positive Hawkins sign is detected, it is unlikely that AVN will develop at a later stage after injury. Level of Evidence: IV
Wu Y, Jiang H, Wang B. Fracture of the lateral process of the talus in children: A kind of ankle injury with frequently missed diagnosis. *J Pediatr Orthop.* 2016;36(3):289–293.	From March 2011 to October 2013, 12 children with lateral process fractures of the talus were treated. The age at the time of injury ranged from 8 to 13 years. Concomitant injuries included undisplaced calcaneus fractures in one case and distal fibula epiphysis injury in one case. Seven of the cases were initially diagnosed in our department, and the diagnosis was missed in five cases. The missed diagnosis rate was 42%. All patients were followed up for 18 months on average. Follow-up radiographs did not show avascular necrosis of the talus, nonunion, and malunion in any patient. The mean AOFAS hindfoot score was 96 points. The clinical result was found to be excellent in 10 patients, good in 1 patient, and fair in 1 patient (the success rate was 92%). The lateral process of talus fracture is a frequently missed injury. Level of Evidence: IV

REFERENCES

1. Adelaar RS. Complex fractures of the talus. *Instr Course Lect.* 1997;46:323–338.
2. Adirim TA, Cheng TL. Overview of injuries in the young athlete. *Sports Med.* 2003;33(1):75–81.
3. Allmacher DH, Galles KS, Marsh JL. Intra-articular calcaneal fractures treated nonoperatively and followed sequentially for 2 decades. *J Orthop Trauma.* 2006;20(7):464–469.
4. Anderson IF, Crichton KJ, Grattan-Smith T, et al. Osteochondral fractures of the dome of the talus. *J Bone Joint Surg Am.* 1989;71(8):1143–1152.
5. Aquino MD, Aquino L, Aquino JM. Talar neck fractures: a review of vascular supply and classification. *J Foot Surg.* 1986;25(3):188–193.
6. Benirschke SK, Kramer PA. Wound healing complications in closed and open calcaneal fractures. *J Orthop Trauma.* 2004;18(1):1–6.
7. Bennell KL, Brukner PD. Epidemiology and site specificity of stress fractures. *Clin Sports Med.* 1997;16(2):179–196.
8. Berndt AL, Harty M. Transchondral fractures (osteochondritis dissecans) of the talus. *J Bone Joint Surg Am.* 1959;41(6):988–1028.
9. Bibbo C, Davis WH, Anderson RB. Midfoot injury in children related to mini scooters. *Pediatr Emerg Care.* 2003;19(1):6–9.
10. Bibbo C, Lin SS, Cunningham FJ. Acute traumatic compartment syndrome of the foot in children. *Pediatr Emerg Care.* 2000;16(4):244–248.
11. Broden B. Roentgen examination of the subtaloid joint in fractures of the calcaneus. *Acta Radiol.* 1949;31(1):85–91.
12. Brunet JA. Calcaneal fractures in children: Long-term results of treatment. *J Bone Joint Surg Br.* 2000;82(2):211–216.
13. Buckingham R, Jackson M, Atkins R. Calcaneal fractures in adolescents. CT classification and results of operative treatment. *Injury.* 2003;34(6):454–459.
14. Buoncristiani AM, Manos RE, Mills WJ. Plantar-flexion tarsometatarsal joint injuries in children. *J Pediatr Orthop.* 2001;21(3):324–327.
15. Burroughs KE, Reimer CD, Fields KB. Lisfranc injury of the foot: a commonly missed diagnosis. *Am Fam Physician.* 1998;58(1):118–124.

16. Canale ST, Belding RH. Osteochondral lesions of the talus. *J Bone Joint Surg Am.* 1980;62(1):97–102.

17. Canale ST, Kelly FB Jr. Fractures of the neck of the talus. Long-term evaluation of 71 cases. *J Bone Joint Surg Am.* 1978;60(2):143–156.

18. Ceccarelli F, Faldini C, Piras F, Giannini S. Surgical versus nonsurgical treatment of calcaneal fractures in children: a long-term results comparative study. *Foot Ankle Int.* 2000;21(10):825–832.

19. Ceroni D, De Rosa V, De Coulon G, Kaelin A. Cuboid nutcracker fracture due to horseback riding in children: case series and review of the literature. *J Pediatr Orthop.* 2007;27(5):557–561.

20. Chambers HG. Ankle and foot disorders in skeletally immature athletes. *Orthop Clin North Am.* 2003;34(3):445–459.

21. Chapman H, Galway H. Os calcis fractures in childhood. *J Bone Joint Surg.* 1977;59B:510.

22. Cheney ML, Varvares MA, Nadol JB Jr. The temporoparietal fascial flap in head and neck reconstruction. *Arch Otolaryngol Head Neck Surg.* 1993;119:618–623.

23. Chisis D, Peyser A, Milgram C. Bone scintigraphy in the assessment of hallucial sesamoids. *Foot Ankle Int.* 1995;16:291–294.

24. Craigen MA, Clarke NM. Bilateral "Jones" fractures of the fifth metatarsal following relapse of talipes equinovarus. *Injury.* 1996;27(8):599–601.

25. Curtis MJ, Myerson M, Szura B. Tarsometatarsal joint injuries in the athlete. *Am J Sports Med.* 1993;21(4):497–502.

26. Damore DT, Metzl JD, Ramundo M, et al. Patterns in childhood sports injury. *Pediatr Emerg Care.* 2003;19(2):65–67.

27. David SK, Cheney ML. An anatomic study of the temporoparietal fascia flap. *Arch Otolaryngol Head Neck Surg.* 1995;121(10):1153–1156.

28. DeLee J. Fracture and dislocations of the foot. In: Mann RA, ed. *Surgery of the Foot and Ankle.* Mosby; 1993.

29. Dobas DC, Silvers MD. The frequency of the partite sesamoids of the first metatarsophalangeal joint. *J Am Podiatr Assoc.* 1977;67:880–882.

30. Dormans JP, Azzoni M, Davidsion RS, Drummond DS. Major lower extremity lawn mower injuries in children. *J Pediatr Orthop.* 1995;15(1):78–02.

31. Dougherty CP, Nebergall RW, Caskey PM. Lateral subtalar dislocation in a 19-month-old female. *Am J Orthop (Belle Mead NJ).* 2003;32(12):598–600.

32. Eberl R, Singer G, Schalamon J, et al. Fractures of the talus—differences between children and adolescents. *J Trauma.* 2010;68:126–130.

33. Eidelman M, Bialik V, Miller Y, Kassis I. Plantar puncture wounds in children: analysis of 80 hospitalized patients and late sequelae. *Isr Med Assoc J.* 2003;5(4):268–271.

34. Englaro EE, Gelfand MJ, Paltiel HJ. Bone scintigraphy in preschool children with lower extremity pain of unknown origin. *J Nucl Med.* 1992;33(3):351–354.

35. Erdmann D, Lee B, Roberts CD, Levin LS. Management of lawnmower injuries to the lower extremity in children and adolescents. *Ann Plast Surg.* 2000;45(6):595–600.

36. Essex-Lopresti P. The mechanism, reduction technique, and results in fractures of the os calcis. *Br J Surg.* 1952;39:395–419.

37. Fagelman MF, Epps HR, Rang M. Mangled extremity severity score in children. *J Pediatr Orthop.* 2002;22(2):182–184.

38. Folk JW, Starr AJ, Early JS. Early wound complications of operative treatment of calcaneus fractures: analysis of 190 fractures. *J Orthop Trauma.* 1999;13(5):369–372.

39. Garay M, Hennrikus WL, Hess J, et al. Lawnmowers versus children: the devastation continues. *Clin Orthop Relat Res.* 2017;475(4):950–956.

40. Gelberman RH, Mortensen WW. The arterial anatomy of the talus. *Foot Ankle.* 1983;4(2):64–72.

41. Hardcastle PH, Reschauer R, Kutshca-Lissberg E, Schoffmann W. Injuries to the tarsometatarsal joint. Incidence, classification, and treatment. *J Bone Joint Surg Br.* 1982;64(3):349–356.

42. Hawkins LG. Fracture of the lateral process of the talus. *J Bone Joint Surg Am.* 1965;47:1170–1175.

43. Hawkins LG. Fractures of the neck of the talus. *J Bone Joint Surg Am.* 1970;52(5):991–1002.

44. Heckman JD, McLean MR. Fractures of the lateral process of the talus. *Clin Orthop Relat Res.* 1985;199:108–113.

45. Henderson RC. Posttraumatic necrosis of the talus: The Hawkins sign versus magnetic resonance imaging. *J Orthop Trauma.* 1991;5(1):96–99.

46. Herrera-Soto JA, Scherb M, Duffy MF, Albright JC. Fractures of the fifth metatarsal in children and adolescents. *J Pediatr Orthop.* 2007;27(4):427–431.

47. Higuera J, Laguna R, Peral M, et al. Osteochondritis dissecans of the talus during childhood and adolescence. *J Pediatr Orthop.* 1998;18(3):328–332.

48. Hill JF, Heyworth BE, Lierhaus A, et al. Lisfranc injuries in children and adolescents. *J Pediatr Orthop B.* 2017;26(2):159–163.

49. Hosking KV, Hoffman EB. Midtarsal dislocations in children. *J Pediatr Orthop.* 1999;19(5):592–595.

50. Howard JL, Buckley R, McCormack R, et al. Complications following management of displaced intra-articular calcaneal fractures: a prospective randomized trial comparing open reduction internal fixation with nonoperative management. *J Orthop Trauma.* 2003;17(4):241–249.

51. Hubbard AM, Meyer JS, Davidson RS, et al. Relationship between the ossification center and cartilaginous anlage in the normal hindfoot in children: Study with MR imaging. *AJR Am J Roentgenol.* 1993;161(4):849–853.

52. Imoisili MA, Bonwit AM, Bulas DI. Toothpick puncture injuries of the foot in children. *Pediatr Infect Dis J.* 2004;23(1):80–82.

53. Inokuchi S, Usami N, Hiraishi E, Hashimoto T. Calcaneal fractures in children. *J Pediatr Orthop.* 1998;18(4):469–474.

54. Jarvis JG, Skipper J. Pseudomonas osteochondritis complicating puncture wounds in children. *J Pediatr Orthop.* 1994;14(6):755–759.

55. Jensen I, Wester JU, Rasmussen F, et al. Prognosis of fracture of the talus in children. 21 (7- to 34-)-year follow-up of 14 cases. *Acta Orthop Scand.* 1994;65(4):398–400.

56. Kamphuis SJM, Meijs CMEM, Kleinveld S, et al. Talar fractures in children: a possible injury after go-karting accidents. *J Foot Ankle Surg.* 2015;54(6):1206–1212.

57. Khan KM, Fuller PJ, Brukner PD, et al. Outcome of conservative and surgical management of navicular stress fracture in athletes. Eighty-six cases proven with computerized tomography. *Am J Sports Med.* 1992;20(6):657–666.

58. Khansa I, Pearson GD, Bjorklund K, et al. Pediatric lawnmower injuries: a 25-year review. *JPRAS Open.* 2021;29:135–143.

59. Kirkpatrick DP, Hunter RE, Janes PC, et al. The snowboarder's foot and ankle. *Am J Sports Med.* 1998;26(2):271–277.

60. Knijnenberg LM, Dingemans SA, Terra MP, et al. Radiographic anatomy of the pediatric Lisfranc joint. *J Pediatr Orthop.* 2018;38(10):510–513.

61. Kramer DE, Mahan ST, Hresko MT. Displaced intra-articular fractures of the great toe in children: intervene with caution! *J Pediatr Orthop.* 2014;34(2):144–149.

62. Kumai T, Takakura Y, Higashiyama I, Tamai S. Arthroscopic drilling for the treatment of osteochondral lesions of the talus. *J Bone Joint Surg Am.* 1999;81(9):1229–1235.

63. Lau LS, Bin G, Jaovisidua S, et al. Cost effectiveness of magnetic resonance imaging in diagnosing *Pseudomonas aeruginosa* infection after puncture wound. *J Foot Ankle Surg.* 1997;36(1):36–43.

64. Lau ST, Lee YH, Hess DJ, et al. Lawnmower injuries in children: a 10-year experience. *Pediatr Surg Int.* 2006;22(3):209–214.

65. Lawrence SJ, Botte MJ. Jones' fractures and related fractures of the proximal fifth metatarsal. *Foot Ankle.* 1993;14(6):358–365.

66. Leibner ED, Simanovsky N, Abu-Sneinah K, et al. Fractures of the lateral process of the talus in children. *J Pediatr Orthop B.* 2001;10(1):68–72.

67. Letournel E. Open treatment of acute calcaneal fractures. *Clin Orthop Relat Res.* 1993;290:60–67.

68. Letts M, Davidson D, Ahmer A. Osteochondritis dissecans of the talus in children. *J Pediatr Orthop.* 2003;23(5):617–625.

69. Letts RM, Gibeault D. Fractures of the neck of the talus in children. *Foot Ankle.* 1980;1(2):74–77.

70. Lickstein LH, Bentz ML. Reconstruction of pediatric foot and ankle trauma. *J Craniofac Surg.* 2003;14(4):559–565.

71. Lin CH, Mardini S, Wei FC, et al. Free flap reconstruction of foot and ankle defects in pediatric patients: long-term outcome in 91 cases. *Plast Reconstr Surg.* 2006;117(7):2478–2487.

72. Lindvall E, Haidukewych G, DiPasquale T, et al. Open reduction and stable fixation of isolated, displaced talar neck and body fractures. *J Bone Joint Surg Am.* 2004;86(10):2229–2234.

73. Lu J, Ebraheim NA, Skie M, et al. Radiographic and computed tomographic evaluation of Lisfranc dislocation: a cadaver study. *Foot Ankle Int.* 1997;18(6):351–355.

74. Major NM. Role of MRI in prevention of metatarsal stress fractures in collegiate basketball players. *AJR Am J Roentgenol.* 2006;186(1):255–258.

75. Manoli A II. Compartment syndromes of the foot: Current concepts. *Foot Ankle.* 1990;10(6):330–334.

76. Manoli A II, Fakhouri A, Weber T. Compartmental catheterization and fasciotomy of the foot. *Operative Tech Orthop.* 1992;2:203–210.

77. Mazel C, Rigault P, Padovani JP, et al. [Fractures of the talus in children. Apropos of 23 cases]. *Rev Chir Orthop Reparatrice Appar Mot.* 1986;72(3):183–195.

78. McCrory P, Bladin C. Fractures of the lateral process of the talus: a clinical review. "snowboarder's ankle." *Clin J Sport Med.* 1996;6(2):124–128.

79. Meyer SA, Callaghan JJ, Albright JP, et al. Midfoot sprains in collegiate football players. *Am J Sports Med.* 1994;22(3):392–401.

80. Monteleone GP Jr. Stress fractures in the athlete. *Orthop Clin North Am.* 1995;26(3):423–432.

81. Mooney JF III, Argenta LC, Marks MW, et al. Treatment of soft tissue defects in pediatric patients using the V.A.C. system. *Clin Orthop Relat Res.* 2000;376:26–31.

82. Mora S, Thordorson DB, Zionts LE, Reynolds RA. Pediatric calcaneal fractures. *Foot Ankle Int.* 2001;22(6):471–477.

83. Morris C, Doll H, Davies N, et al. The Oxford Ankle Foot Questionnaire for children: responsiveness and longitudinal validity. *Qual Life Res.* 2009;18(10):1367–1376.

84. Mulfinger GL, Trueta J. The blood supply of the talus. *J Bone Joint Surg Br.* 1970;52(1):160–167.

85. Myerson MS. Experimental decompression of the fascial compartments of the foot—the basis for fasciotomy in acute compartment syndromes. *Foot Ankle.* 1988;8(6):308–314.

86. Myerson MS, Fisher RT, Burgess AR, Kenzora JE. Fracture dislocations of the tarsometatarsal joints: end results correlated with pathology and treatment. *Foot Ankle.* 1986;6(5):225–242.

87. Najefi AA, Najefy A, Vemulapalli K. Paediatric calcaneal fractures: a guide to management based on a review of the literature. *Injury.* 2020;51(7):1432–1438.

88. Newman R, Miles R. *Hazard Analysis: Injuries Associated With Riding Type Mowers.* U.S.C.P.S. Commission; 1981.

89. Nicholas R, Hadley J, Paul C, James P. "Snowboarder's fracture": fracture of the lateral process of the talus. *J Am Board Fam Pract.* 1994;7(2):130–133.

90. Noble J, Royle SG. Fracture of the lateral process of the talus: computed tomographic scan diagnosis. *Br J Sports Med.* 1992;26(4):245–246.

91. O'Brien J, Buckley R, McCormack R, et al. Personal gait satisfaction after displaced intraarticular calcaneal fractures: a 2–8 year followup. *Foot Ankle Int.* 2004;25(9):657–665.

92. Ogden J. The foot. In: Ogden J, ed. *Skeletal Injury in the Child.* Springer Verlag; 2000.

93. Owen RJ, Hickey FG, Finlay DB. A study of metatarsal fractures in children. *Injury.* 1995;26(8):537–538.

94. Patterson JT, Campbell ST, Wallace SJ, et al. Triceps surae lengthening in foot and ankle trauma: a survey of OTA and AOFAS Members. *Foot Ankle Orthop.* 2022;7(3):24730114221126719.

95. Perumal V, Wall E, Babekir N. Juvenile osteochondritis dissecans of the talus. *J Pediatr Orthop.* 2007;27(7):821–825.
96. Peterson L, Romanus B, Dahlberg E. Fracture of the collum tali—an experimental study. *J Biomech.* 1976;9(4):277–279.
97. Petit CJ, Lee BM, Kasser JR, Kocher MS. Operative treatment of intraarticular calcaneal fractures in the pediatric population. *J Pediatr Orthop.* 2007;27(8):856–862.
98. Pickle A, Benaroch TE, Guy P, Harvey EJ. Clinical outcome of pediatric calcaneal fractures treated with open reduction and internal fixation. *J Pediatr Orthop.* 2004;24(2):178–180.
99. Potter HG, Deland JT, Gusmar PB, et al. Magnetic resonance imaging of the Lisfranc ligament of the foot. *Foot Ankle Int.* 1998;19(7):438–446.
100. Pritsch M, Horoshovski H, Farine I. Arthroscopic treatment of osteochondral lesions of the talus. *J Bone Joint Surg Am.* 1986;68(6):862–865.
101. Purvis JM, Burke RG. Recreational injuries in children: Incidence and prevention. *J Am Acad Orthop Surg.* 2001;9(6):365–374.
102. Quill GE Jr. Fractures of the proximal fifth metatarsal. *Orthop Clin North Am.* 1995;26(2):353–361.
103. Rammelt S, Zwipp H, Gavlik JM. Avascular necrosis after minimally displaced talus fracture in a child. *Foot Ankle Int.* 2000;21(12):1030–1036.
104. Rasmussen F, Schantz K. Radiologic aspects of calcaneal fractures in childhood and adolescence. *Acta Radiol Diagn (Stockh).* 1986;27(5):575–580.
105. Riccardi G, Riccardi D, Marcarelli M, et al. Extremely proximal fractures of the fifth metatarsal in the developmental age. *Foot Ankle Int.* 2011;32(5):526–532.
106. Robertson NB, Roocroft JH, Edmonds EW. Childhood metatarsal shaft fractures: treatment outcomes and relative indications for surgical intervention. *J Child Orthop.* 2012;6(2):125–129.
107. Ross G, Cronin R, Hauzenblas J, Juliano P. Plantar ecchymosis sign: a clinical aid to diagnosis of occult Lisfranc tarsometatarsal injuries. *J Orthop Trauma.* 1996;10(2):119–122.
108. Ruffing T, Rückauer T, Bludau F, et al. Cuboid nutcracker fracture in children: management and results. *Injury.* 2019;50(2):607–612.
109. Sammarco GJ. The Jones fracture. *Instr Course Lect.* 1993;42:201–205.
110. Sanders R, Fortin P, DiPasquale T, et al. Operative treatment in 120 displaced intraarticular calcaneal fractures. Results using a prognostic computed tomography scan. *Clin Orthop Relat Res.* 1993;290:87–95.
111. Sanders R. Fractures and fracture-dislocations of the calcaneus. In: Coughlin M, Mann R, eds. *Surgery of the Foot and Ankle.* 7th ed. Mosby; 1999.
112. Sanders R. Intra-articular fractures of the calcaneus: present state of the art. *J Orthop Trauma.* 1992;6(2):252–265.
113. Sarrail R, Launay F, Marez M. Reflex dystrophy in children and adolescents. *J Bone Joint Surg Br.* 2004;86(suppl):23.
114. Schantz K, Rasmussen F. Good prognosis after calcaneal fracture in childhood. *Acta Orthop Scand.* 1988;59(5):560–563.
115. Schindler A, Mason DE, Allington NJ. Occult fracture of the calcaneus in toddlers. *J Pediatr Orthop* 1996;16(2):201–205.
116. Schmidt TL, Weiner DS. Calcaneal fractures in children. An evaluation of the nature of the injury in 56 children. *Clin Orthop Relat Res.* 1982;171:150–155.
117. Senaran H, Mason D, De Pellegrin M. Cuboid fractures in preschool children. *J Pediatr Orthop.* 2006;26(6):741–744.
118. Shilt JS, Yoder JS, Manuck TA, et al. Role of vacuum-assisted closure in the treatment of pediatric lawnmower injuries. *J Pediatr Orthop.* 2004;24(5):482–487.
119. Silas SI, Herzenberg JE, Myerson MS, Sponseller PD. Compartment syndrome of the foot in children. *J Bone Joint Surg Am.* 1995;77(3):356–361.
120. Singer G, Cichocki M, Schalamon J, et al. A study of metatarsal fractures in children. *J Bone Joint Surg Am.* 2008;90(4):772–776.
121. Smith JT, Curtis TA, Spencer S, et al. Complications of talus fractures in children. *J Pediatr Orthop.* 2010;30(8):779–784.
122. Sneppen O, Christensen SB, Krogsoe O, Lorentzen J. Fracture of the body of the talus. *Acta Orthop Scand.* 1977;48(3):317–324.
123. Stanitski CL. Pediatric and adolescent sports injuries. *Clin Sports Med.* 1997;16(4):613–633.
124. Stannard JP, Volgas DA, McGwin G III, et al. Incisional negative pressure wound therapy after high-risk lower extremity fractures. *J Orthop Trauma.* 2012;26(1):37–42.
125. Swanson TV, Bray TJ, Holmes GB Jr. Fractures of the talar neck: a mechanical study of fixation. *J Bone Joint Surg Am.* 1992;74(4):544–551.
126. Talkhani S, Reidy D, Fogarty E, et al. Avascular necrosis of the talus after a minimally displaced neck of talus fracture in a 6 year old child. *Injury.* 2000;31(1):63–65.
127. Tezval M, Dumont C, Stürmer KM. Prognostic reliability of the Hawkins sign in fractures of the talus. *J Orthop Trauma.* 2007;(8):538–543.
128. Torg JS, Balduini FC, Zelko RR, et al. Fractures of the base of the fifth metatarsal distal to the tuberosity. Classification and guidelines for nonsurgical and surgical management. *J Bone Joint Surg Am.* 1984;66(2):209–214.
129. Vollman D, Smith GA. Epidemiology of lawnmower-related injuries to children in the United States, 1990–2004. *Pediatrics.* 2006;118(2):e273–e278.
130. Vosburgh CL, Gruel CR, Herndon WA, Sullivan JA. Lawnmower injuries of the pediatric foot and ankle: observations on prevention and management. *J Pediatr Orthop.* 1995;15(4):504–509.
131. Waseem S, Nayar SK, Vemulapalli K. Paediatric talus fractures: a guide to management based on a review of the literature. *Injury.* 2022;53(3):1029–1037.
132. Weber M, Locher S. Reconstruction of the cuboid in compression fractures: short to midterm results in 12 patients. *Foot Ankle Int.* 2002;23(11):1008–1013.
133. Wilder RT. Management of pediatric patients with complex regional pain syndrome. *Clin J Pain.* 2006;22(5):443–448.
134. Wilder RT, Berde CB, Wolohan M, et al. Reflex sympathetic dystrophy in children. Clinical characteristics and follow-up of 70 patients. *J Bone Joint Surg Am.* 1992;74(6):910–919.
135. Wiley JJ. The mechanism of tarsometatarsal joint injuries. *J Bone Joint Surg Br.* 1971;53(3):474–482.
136. Wiley JJ. Tarsometatarsal joint injuries in children. *J Pediatr Orthop.* 1981;1(3):255–260.
137. Wiley JJ, Profitt A. Fractures of the os calcis in children. *Clin Orthop Relat Res.* 1984;188:131–138.
138. Wiss DA, Kull DM, Perry J. Lisfranc fracture-dislocations of the foot: a clinical-kinesiological study. *J Orthop Trauma.* 1987;1(4):267–274.
139. Wu Y, Jiang H, Wang B, Miao W. Fracture of the lateral process of the talus in children: a kind of ankle injury with frequently missed diagnosis. *J Pediatr Orthop.* 2016;36(3):289–293.

INDEX

Page numbers followed by an *f* indicate figure; page numbers followed by a *t* indicate table.